Resources for Instructor Success—

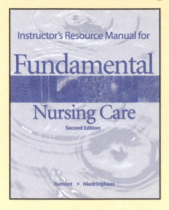

Instructor's Resource Manual
ISBN: 0-13-224979-0

This manual contains a wealth of material to help faculty plan and manage their LPN/LVN nursing courses. It includes detailed learning outcomes, lecture outlines, teaching suggestions for the classroom and clinical settings, and more for each chapter. This supplement is available to faculty upon adoption of the textbook.

Instructor's Resource CD-ROM
ISBN: 0-13-243012-6

This comprehensive resource CD-ROM provides lecture notes, animations, and illustrations integrated in PowerPoint presentations for use in the classroom. It also contains an electronic test bank and additional resources. The supplement is available to faculty upon adoption of the textbook.

Online Course Management

OneKey is an integrated online resource that brings a wide array of supplemental resources together in one convenient place for both students and faculty. OneKey features everything you and your students need for out-of-class work, conveniently organized to match your syllabus. OneKey is an online course management solution that features interactive modules, text and image PowerPoints, animations, videos, case studies, and more. OneKey also provides course management tools so faculty can customize course content, build online tests, create assignments, enter grades, post announcements, communicate with students, and much more. Testing materials, gradebooks, and other instructor resources are available in a separate section that can be accessed by instructors only. OneKey content is available in three different platforms. A nationally hosted version is available in the reliable, easy-to-use CourseCompass platform. The same content is also available for download to locally hosted versions of BlackBoard and WebCT. Please contact your Prentice Hall Sales Representative for a demonstration or go online to **http://myphlip.pearsoncmg.com/OneKey/index.html.**

OneKey is all you need.
Convenience. Simplicity. Success.

Powered by

Blackboard   WebCT   CourseCompass

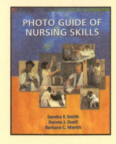

Photo Guide of Nursing Skills

Provides a full-color atlas of all basic and intermediate skills and its unique, easy-to-use format presents each procedure in logical steps—complete with appropriate illustrations, descriptions, and rationales. A critical thinking section focuses on unexpected outcomes.
ISBN: 0-8385-8174-9
Smith, Duell & Martin

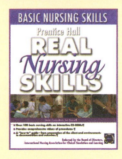

Prentice Hall Real Nursing Skills

The volumes in this series consist of CD-ROMs with comprehensive procedures and rationales demonstrated in hundreds of realistic video clips, animations, illustrations, and photographs. This is the only skills series designed to help students and practicing nurses visualize how to perform clinical nursing skills and understand the concepts and rationales for each skill.

Basic Nursing Skills
ISBN: 0-13-1915266

Brief Table of Contents

Fundamental

Nursing Care

Fundamental

Nursing Care

Second Edition

Roberta Pavy Ramont, EdD, MS, RN
North Orange County Regional Occupational Program
Anaheim, California
Educational Innovations, Owner/Consultant

Dee Maldonado Niedringhaus, BSN, RN
Instructional Administrator of Medical Programs
North County Regional Occupational Program
Anaheim, California

PEARSON
Prentice
Hall

Upper Saddle River, New Jersey 07458

Library of Congress Cataloging-in-Publication Data
Ramont, Roberta Pavy.
    Fundamental nursing care / Roberta Pavy Ramont, Dee Maldonado Niedringhaus. — 2nd ed.
        p.; cm.
    Includes bibliographical references and index.
    ISBN-13: 978-0-13-224432-9
        ISBN-10: 0-13-224432-2
    1. Nursing.   I. Niedringhaus, Dolores Maldonado.   II. Title.
    [DNLM: 1. Nursing Care.   2. Nursing Process.   3. Nursing, Practical. WY 100 R175f 2008]
    RT41. F873 2008
    610.73 — dc22   2007020661

Publisher: Julie Levin Alexander
Publisher's Assistant: Regina Bruno
Editor-in-Chief: Maura Connor
Senior Acquisitions Editor: Kelly Trakalo
Editorial Assistant: JulieAnn Oliveros
Development Editor: Rachel Bedard, Jenna Caputo
Managing Editor, Development: Marilyn Meserve
Managing Production Editor: Patrick Walsh
Production Liaison: Yagnesh Jani
Production Editor: Penny Walker, Aptara Inc.
Manufacturing Manager: Ilene Sanford
Manufacturing Buyer: Pat Brown
Design Director and Cover Designer: Mary Siener
Photographer: Patrick Watson
Director of Marketing: Karen Allman
Senior Marketing Manager: Francisco Del Castillo
Marketing Coordinator: Michael Sirinides
Associate Editor: Michael Giacobbe
Marketing Assistant: Anca David
Media Product Manager: John Jordan
Media Project Manager: Tina Rudowski
Composition: Aptara, Inc.
Printer/Binder: Courier Kendallville, Inc.
Cover Printer: Phoenix Color

Notice: Care has been taken to confirm the accuracy of information presented in this book. The authors, editors, and the publisher, however, cannot accept any responsibility for errors or omissions or for consequences from application of the information in this book and make no warranty, express or implied, with respect to its contents.

The authors and publisher have exerted every effort to ensure that drug selections and dosages set forth in this text are in accord with current recommendations and practice at time of publication. However, in view of ongoing research, changes in government regulations, and the constant flow of information relating to drug therapy and drug reactions, the reader is urged to check the package inserts of all drugs for any change in indications of dosage and for added warnings and precautions. This is particularly important when the recommended agent is a new and/or infrequently employed drug.

Water Drop Background & Image: Biren Haglwara/Jupiter Images. Lake: Getty Images Inc. Spring Waterfall: Jupiter Images. Wave: Getty Images. Pool: Martin Child/Getty Images Inc. Mountain Waterfall: Getty Images Inc. Splash: Lily Valde/Jupiter Images.

Pearson Education LTD., London
Pearson Education Singapore, Pte. Ltd
Pearson Education, Canada, Ltd
Pearson Education–Japan
Pearson Education Australia PTY, Limited

Pearson Education North Asia Ltd
Pearson Educación de Mexico, S.A. de C.V.
Pearson Education Malaysia, Pte. Ltd
Pearson Education, Upper Saddle River, New Jersey

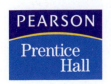

10 9 8 7 6 5 4 3 2 1
ISBN 13: 978-0-13-224432-9
ISBN 10:   0-13-224432-2

Student Success is built in from the start...

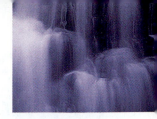

Practical and vocational nurses from around the country told us that they needed two things to succeed as students in order to achieve their LPN/LVN licenses. First, they needed books that explain what the LPN/LVN needs to know and do. Second, they needed a variety of excellent review materials to reinforce their learning. ***Fundamental Nursing Care, 2e*** contains power-packed, built-in support to ensure your success throughout your LPN/LVN education.

As you start each chapter—

Brief Outlines preview what the chapter will cover for quick access and review.

Learning Outcomes identify what you can expect to learn from each chapter and help you focus your reading.

Historical Perspectives give historical context to the chapter.

MediaLinks call your attention to the additional learning tools that are available on the Prentice Hall Nursing MediaLink CD-ROM and Companion Website that accompany your textbook, including:

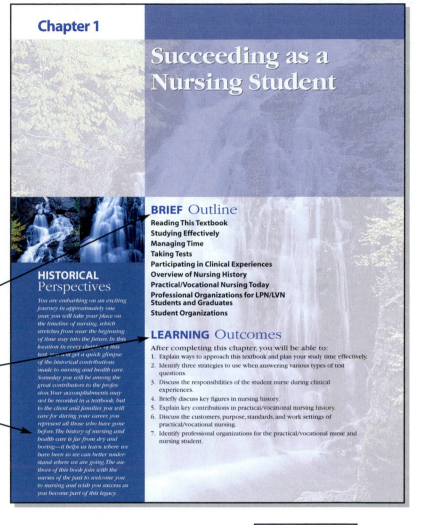

Chapter 1

Succeeding as a Nursing Student

HISTORICAL Perspectives

You are embarking on an exciting journey in approximately one year; you will take your place on the timeline of nursing, which stretches from near the beginning of time way into the future. In this location in every chapter of this text, you will get a quick glimpse of the historical contributions made to nursing and health care. Someday you will be among the great contributors to the profession. Your accomplishments may not be recorded in a textbook, but to the client and families you will care for during your career, you represent all those who have gone before. The history of nursing and health care is far from dry and boring—it helps us learn where we have been so we can better understand where we are going. The authors of this book join with the nurses of the past to welcome you to nursing and wish you success as you become part of this legacy.

BRIEF Outline

Reading This Textbook
Studying Effectively
Managing Time
Taking Tests
Participating in Clinical Experiences
Overview of Nursing History
Practical/Vocational Nursing Today
Professional Organizations for LPN/LVN Students and Graduates
Student Organizations

LEARNING Outcomes

After completing this chapter, you will be able to:
1. Explain ways to approach this textbook and plan your study time effectively.
2. Identify three strategies to use when answering various types of test questions.
3. Discuss the responsibilities of the student nurse during clinical experiences.
4. Briefly discuss key figures in nursing history.
5. Explain key contributions in practical/vocational nursing history.
6. Discuss the customers, purpose, standards, and work settings of practical/vocational nursing.
7. Identify professional organizations for the practical/vocational nurse and nursing student.

Prentice Hall Nursing MediaLink CD-ROM

- *Learning Outcomes*
- *Audio Glossary*—key terms, definitions, and pronunciations
- *NCLEX-PN® Review Questions*—unique to this CD-ROM
- *Animations & Videos*—difficult concepts brought to life

Companion Website

- *Learning Outcomes*
- *Chapter Outlines*
- *Audio Glossary*
- *NCLEX-PN® Review Questions*—unique to this website
- *Key Term Review*—matching questions and crossword puzzles to help with new terminology and definitions
- *Case Studies*—scenarios and critical-thinking questions
- *Challenge Your Knowledge*—visual critical thinking questions
- *WebLinks*—content-related hyperlinks
- *Nursing Tools*—handy reference materials

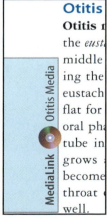

Otitis

Otitis **r**

the *eust*
middle
ing the
eustach
flat for
oral ph
tube in
grows
become
throat
well.

MediaLink Tabs prompt you to explore videos, animations, and activities on the Prentice Hall Nursing MediaLink CD-ROM and Companion Website.

Makes need-to-know information easy to find and use!

Fundamental Nursing Care, 2e contains color-coded boxes and tables with important information for you to remember.

BOX 11-4 | **POPULATION FOCUS**

Developmental Tasks of the Older Adult

- Adjusting to decreasing physical strength and health; safeguarding mental health
- Adjusting to retirement and reduced income; establishing a comfortable routine
- Adjusting to the death of a spouse
- Establishing an explicit affiliation with one's age group; keeping involved
- Meeting social and civic obligations
- Establishing satisfactory living arrangements
- Maintaining marital and family relations

Population Focus and Client Teaching boxes provide information on age-specific and other special needs of client groups, and help prepare you for client instruction.

BOX 24-6 | **CLIENT TEACHING**

Abdominal (Diaphragmatic) and Pursed-Lip Breathing Techniques

Teach client to:

- Assume a comfortable semi-sitting position in bed or on a chair or a lying position in bed with one pillow.
- Flex your knees to relax the muscles of the abdomen.
- Place one or both hands on your abdomen, just below the ribs.
- Breathe in deeply through the nose, keeping the mouth closed.
- Concentrate on feeling your abdomen rise as far as possible; stay relaxed and avoid arching your back. If you have difficulty raising your abdomen, take a quick, forceful breath through the nose.
- Then purse your lips as if about to whistle, and breathe out slowly and gently, making a slow whooshing sound without puffing out the cheeks. This pursed-lip breathing creates a resistance to air flowing out of the lungs, increases pressure within the bronchi (main air passages), and minimizes collapse of smaller airways, a common problem for people with COPD.
- Concentrate on feeling the abdomen fall or sink, and tighten (contract) the abdominal muscles while breathing out to enhance effective exhalation. Count to 7 during exhalation.
- Use this exercise whenever feeling short of breath, and increase gradually to 5 to 10 minutes four times a day. Regular practice will help you do this type of breathing without conscious effort. The exercise, once learned, can be performed when sitting upright, standing, or walking.

BOX 9-1 | **CULTURAL PULSE POINTS**

Infection

Although susceptibility to infectious/communicable diseases is frequently linked to socioeconomic factors such as overcrowding and poor nutrition, there are some ethnic factors that should be considered:

- Ethnicity appears to be a factor in the incidence of tuberculosis and hepatitis B viral infection. Native Americans living in the southwest, Vietnamese refugees, and Mexican Americans have a relatively high incidence of these diseases.
- Africans possessing sickle cell trait are known to have increased immunity to malaria.
- Childhood illnesses caused by viruses such as rubeola and varicella are considered to be benign in a majority of children. However, many countries do not have the vaccine and immunization programs in place that are standard here in the United States.
- HIV infections continue to be a major health problem, with racial/ethnic minorities suffering a disproportionate share of the disease.

Cultural Pulse Points provide insight into populations and situations nurses may meet.

BOX 9-3 | NURSING CARE CHECKLIST

Using Bactericidal and Bacteriostatic Agents

When disinfecting, remember to:

- ☑ Use the recommended concentration of the solution and keep it on the area for the required amount of time.
- ☑ Know the type and number of infectious organisms. Make certain no soap is present on the item since some disinfectants will not work when soap is present.
- ☑ Keep the room temperature within a normal range because some disinfectants will not work otherwise.
- ☑ Be certain there is no organic material (e.g., blood, pus, excretions) present because the disinfectants may be inactivated.
- ☑ Treat all exposed surface areas and crevices.

Nursing Care Checklists provide handy summaries of important nursing interventions.

Assessment boxes summarize client data, common risk factors, and manifestations you might observe.

BOX 13-1 | MANIFESTATIONS OF SENSORY DEPRIVATION

- Excessive yawning, drowsiness, sleeping
- Decreased attention span, difficulty concentrating, decreased problem solving
- Impaired memory
- Periodic disorientation, general confusion, or nocturnal confusion
- Preoccupation with somatic complaints, such as palpitations
- Hallucinations or delusions
- Crying, annoyance over small matters, depression
- Apathy, emotional lability

BOX 13-3 | MANIFESTATIONS OF SENSORY OVERLOAD

- Complaints of fatigue, sleeplessness
- Irritability, anxiety, restlessness
- Periodic or general disorientation
- Reduced problem-solving ability and task performance
- Increased muscle tension
- Scattered attention and racing thoughts

clinical ALERT

Report

LPNs/LVNs should inform the registered nurse of all concerns stated by the client that could potentially affect the client's continued progress toward wellness. Questions and concerns specifically related to discharge instructions and progress expectations should always be discussed with the registered nurse. In some instances, the registered nurse will refer questions to or obtain answers from the physician.

Clinical Alerts call your attention to clinical roles and responsibilities for heightened awareness, monitoring, and/or reporting.

Learn to prioritize nursing actions and to deliver safe, effective nursing care as a part of the healthcare team!

NURSING CARE

ASSESSING

The initial assessment should be started once the client is settled into the room. The JCAHO requires that a registered nurse perform the admission assessment. Subjective and objective data are collected throughout the interview, medical history, and physical assessment. However, the RN may delegate parts of the assessment to the LPN/LVN. This may include baseline information such as level of consciousness, vital signs, skin condition, height and weight, bowel sounds, lung sounds,

Nursing Care is presented in the five-step nursing process format, and emphasizes the scope of practice for the LPN/LVN. Rationales after each nursing action explain why the action is important and support the evidence-based nursing process.

NURSING PROCESS CARE PLAN
Client Affected by Nurse Communication Barriers

Lucy, an LPN, is assigned to care for Mr. Levowitz. He is currently in the recovery room after surgery to remove prostate cancer that had spread to his abdomen. His wife comes into the room crying. Lucy asks her what is wrong. Mrs. Levowitz continues to sob and is unable to answer. Lucy gets chairs for herself and Mrs. Levowitz and urges her to sit down. Lucy says, "Come on now. The news can't be that bad, can it?" Mrs

Nursing Process Care Plans illustrate nursing care in a "real-life" scenario.

Critical Thinking in the Nursing Process

1. What communication techniques did Lucy use?
2. What barriers to communication did Lucy use?
3. What nonverbal communication did Lucy use?

Critical Thinking questions allow you to apply your new knowledge to a specific client.

PROCEDURE 9-1 **Hand Hygiene/Washing**

Hand Washing and Gloving

Purposes
- To reduce the number of microorganisms on the hands
- To reduce the risk of transmission of microorganisms to clients
- To reduce the risk of cross-contamination among clients and equipment
- To reduce the risk of transmission of infectious organisms to oneself

Equipment
- Soap
- Warm running water
- Towels
- Alcohol-based foam or gel

MediaLink

Check order → Gather equipment → Introduce yourself → Identify client → Provide privacy → Explain procedure → Hand hygiene → Gloves as needed

Procedures give you step-by-step instructions and rationales for nursing actions. Special icons in the procedures reinforce essential preliminary steps in client care. "Live" **documentation** at the end of each procedure demonstrates samples of good recordkeeping.

Comprehensive reviews at the end of the chapter...

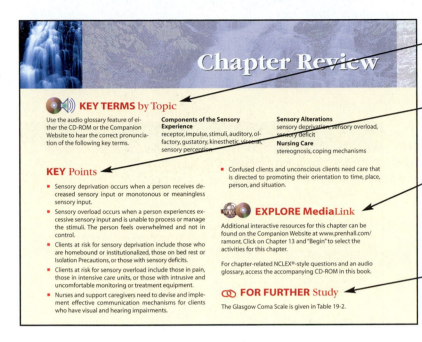

Key Terms by Topic link important new vocabulary to its content area in the chapter.

Key Points summarize need-to-know concepts from the chapter.

EXPLORE MediaLink encourages you to use the Prentice Hall Nursing MediaLink CD-ROM and Companion Website for a multi-modal review, regardless of your learning style.

For Further Study shows where related content areas are cross-referenced throughout the book.

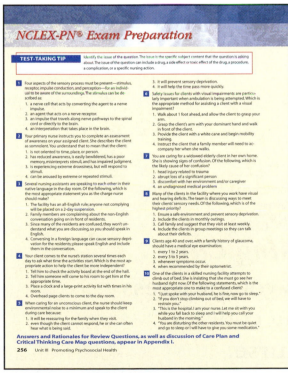

NCLEX-PN® Exam Preparation includes:

- A **Test-Taking Tip** with a focused study hint
- **NCLEX-PN®** style questions for review and test practice, with questions in both traditional and alternative formats. Answers are found in Appendix I.

Critical Thinking Care Map prepares you for success on NCLEX-PN®, in clinical, and on-the-job with a focused review of a client problem, including:

- NCLEX-PN® Focus Area
- Case Study
- Nursing Diagnosis
- Data Collection
- Reporting
- Nursing Care
- Documentation

Prepare for your career as an LPN/LVN...

After each unit in this book, use the **Thinking Strategically About . . .** pages as an opportunity to reflect on the topics you have just read in the context of important themes across the LPN/LVN curriculum. Short scenarios and project ideas spotlight the unit's content from a variety of angles. Review of concepts enables you to approach unit topics from a more integrated perspective.

Critical Thinking questions highlight specific challenges you will face as a new nurse and assist you to provide the best possible care.

Collaborative Care challenges you to think about the different healthcare settings and to envision the many healthcare workers who may participate in a client's care.

Delegating helps you determine which nursing interventions may be delegated to assistive personnel.

Management of Care highlights specific nursing interventions appropriate to the care of the client.

Communication and **Client Teaching** focus on communication methods and educational strategies necessary to teach the client and the family.

Time Management and **Priorities in Nursing Care** help you organize care and focus on the most important aspects of care first.

Documenting and Reporting helps you practice what and how to document and when to report your findings.

Cultural Care Strategies build your confidence by providing information and scenarios to familiarize you with cultural patterns and differences.

UNIT I WRAP-UP

Thinking Strategically About...

Carlos, a licensed vocational nurse with several years of experience, begins working in a long-term care facility. Within a few weeks, it becomes apparent that the night nurse is treating elderly clients unkindly, and there seems to be an increase in reported skin tears on the nights when she works. He speaks to this nurse about his concerns, but he sees no change in the situation. One morning, arriving at work early for a staff meeting, he overhears her verbally abusing a confused resident who will not take his medications. Carlos reports his observation to the director of nursing (DON). When there is still no improvement, Carlos returns to the manager and says that he is considering speaking to the administrator or making a formal complaint to the state nursing board.

The alleged abuser is a long-time employee at the facility and popular with the nursing assistants and other staff. When the supervisor finally speaks to her about the complaint, the identity of the reporter becomes clear. Carlos is ostracized by most of the staff. He is criticized in front of residents and family members, and the night nurse continuously makes racial slurs when referring to him with other staff members. After several months, Carlos feels he can no longer tolerate the working conditions and accepts a job at another facility.

COMMUNITY
Why could this nurse's action or inaction be considered a community issue?

CRITICAL THINKING
Would you consider Carlos to be a "whistle-blower?"
Was Carlos's decision to report what he observed a legal or ethical issue?
Does Carlos have any legal recourse for his treatment?

COMMUNICATION
Consider the instances of communication that occurred in this case study: between the abusive nurse and the client, between the two nurses, between Carlos and the DON, and between the staff and Carlos. In pairs or small groups, role-play these interactions as you think they probably occurred.

CONFLICT RESOLUTION
As a class or in an essay, review Carlos's decisions using the seven-step decision-making process as a guide. What other alternatives might Carlos have had? How could the DON have handled the situation differently?

Fundamental Nursing Care
will be a key resource as you progress
through your nursing courses
and become a nurse.

The nature of nursing—grow with it!

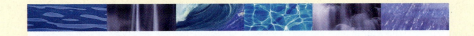

To the memory of my husband Frederick

To my three delightful grandchildren Haley and T. J. Parks and Dylan Thomas Ramont and to my great nephew Samuel and great niece Mikayla our miracle babies, you are the future.

Roberta Pavy Ramont

To my husband Lee, my children Jamie and Josh, and my mother Dora, whose love and patience have always made the difference in my life.

Dee Maldonado Niedringhaus

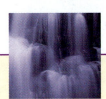

Preface

FUNDAMENTAL NURSING CARE arose from a desire to provide the best possible fundamentals book for LPNs and LVNs. For years, LPNs and LVNs in training have had to use RN-level textbooks, sifting out material and "translating" it from the RN point of view. This text, however, begins and ends with what LPNs and LVNs need to know and do. It identifies their scope of practice and affirms their importance in the larger healthcare system.

Increasingly, LPNs and LVNs are the nurses who come in direct contact with the healthcare consumer. They will be bedside nurses, team members, supervisors of unlicensed healthcare workers, and client educators. They will function in settings as diverse as acute care hospitals, long-term care facilities, and clients' homes. They must be competent, professional, articulate, and compassionate to win the confidence of their clients. We undertook this project to meet their growing needs.

To make this text "user friendly," we incorporated student feedback and our own wish lists from using other textbooks. The result is a practical book with ideas for many types of learners. By presenting solid information about studying, test taking, and time management, we help create more successful students and, in time, more successful nurses. By highlighting the role of men, we reflect the fact that nursing is becoming increasingly gender equal. By providing technology assistance with the text and support materials, we aid students in long-distance or computer-assisted programs.

FUNDAMENTAL NURSING CARE is a print and electronic product with a wealth of resources for students and instructors. It consists of a textbook (with enclosed CD-ROM), instructor's resource manual, companion website, and student workbook. Electronic media are also available, including a test bank, links to valuable LPN/LVN websites, PowerPoints, a "toolbox" of teaching adjuncts, and a variety of visuals and critical thinking exercises.

This text is in alignment with the NCLEX-PN® test plan. It does not "teach to the test," but it demonstrates how information relates to the broad categories of the test plan. It incorporates focus area information into all clinical chapters, and provides NCLEX-PN® style testing in every review section.

Organization

This book is organized to be accessible to students. Most LPN/LVN programs are designed from simple to complex, building on knowledge and skills already obtained. The chapters of FUNDAMENTAL NURSING CARE are organized in the same manner and with a consistent format.

Unit I describes the history, laws, ethics, and basic theories of nursing. It provides a sketch of the healthcare system and a full discussion of the nursing process, with specifics about the role of practical/vocational nurses. **Units II, III, and IV** cover clinical aspects of care. Only skills and competencies that are within the scope of practice are included, making this text a truly LPN/LVN-level book. The new **Unit V** discusses alternate care settings for LPNs/LVNs such as urgent care and ambulatory care. **Unit VI** discusses teamwork and leadership, the NCLEX-PN® licensure exam, and strategies for entering the workforce.

Features

- Each chapter begins with **Learning Outcomes** to help you focus your learning.
- A **Nursing Care** section demonstrates the nursing process format and includes reference to the role of the Practical/Vocational Nurse in a variety of settings. Nursing interventions are followed by rationales, to reinforce your understanding of why selected nursing actions are performed.
- **Case Studies** and **Critical Thinking** exercises are designed to bring the concepts to life and to engage you in problem-solving in situations you might encounter at work.
- **Key Terms** and **Key Points** are reviewed at the end of each chapter.
- **NCLEX-PN® Review Questions** help you practice your test-taking skills.
- **Appendices** contain invaluable reference material answers and rationales to NCLEX-PN® Review Questions, NANDA Nursing Diagnoses, and a sample Critical Pathway.

Acknowledgments

Each author owes much gratitude to a special LVN/LPN who helped her achieve her career path. With this text we hope to repay some of our debt, assisting today's LVN/LPN students to become the outstanding nurses of the 21st century.

ROBERTA RAMONT

When I was 19, nursing was the farthest thing from my mind. I was working at a job I disliked immensely, when I ended up in a hospital bed. An LPN student cared for me. She saw I was lost and looking for direction in my life, and she took time to talk. She suggested I consider a career in nursing. At first it seemed like an outrageous idea, but after a month, I signed up for a nurse's aide training class at the very same hospital. Things went well until one winter morning I bathed a client with the window open slightly. The instructor suggested I resign, saying this lack of attention would prevent me from being a good care provider. I was devastated. While I was crying in the back of the cafeteria, my LPN "guardian angel" appeared once again. She didn't coddle me or allow me to make excuses. Instead, she said that if I really wanted to be a nurse, I shouldn't let anything or anyone stand in my way. "Go to the instructor," she told me. "Tell her that you want to learn, you want to correct your mistakes, and tell her that you are not going to quit." This occurred almost 40 years ago. Since then I have learned much about caring for clients, about dealing with students, and most of all much about myself. I have learned that we as nurses must encourage people to consider health care as a life's work, and we must always try to excel, even in the midst of discouragement.

DEE NIEDRINGHAUS

In contrast to Roberta, I wanted to be a nurse ever since I could remember. I signed up to be a Candy Striper as soon as they would take me. When I started out, I was very timid; I was afraid to go into a room to make a bed! Luckily for me, I met an LVN who was kind, caring, and enjoyed being a nurse. I loved working with her. As a senior in high school, I took a nursing assistant class there, and the LVN who had had such an influence on me was still working at the hospital. When I completed my nursing assistant class, she wrote me a letter of recommendation for the Los Angeles County School of Nursing. I had no doubts; I wanted to be a nurse, and this kind of support certainly helped.

Roberta and I have worked as instructors in a vocational nursing program together and we found that most of the texts were RN, BSN level books. We had a strong desire to help our students succeed and wrote this book for all vocational nursing students. It was our way of giving back to our profession.

A project such as this could never have been accomplished without the contributions of many people. We first thank our students. In our quest to teach you nursing, we have learned much from you about persistence, motivation, culture, and life. You are our future and we are confident that you will be a credit to the profession.

We want to thank the many nursing colleagues who have provided us with their encouragement and insight and helped to shape the book. Their experience as practitioners and as instructors helped to inform the content. Our contributors provided knowledge, skill, and time to write selected chapters in the text. Reviewers provided quality assurance for the book as well as a nationwide perspective. They validated the content, and provided broader perspective as this book came into being.

This project required the support, skills, and expertise of many people. Kelly Trakalo, our editor and Jenna Caputo, our developmental editor joined the project mid-way, hit the ground running and guided us to a finished product. JulieAnn Oliveros, editorial assistant, attended to many critical details. Yagnesh Jani, production editor, tracked and recorded all the pieces of the project, problem-solved, and monitored quality.

Our special thanks are also due to many others. Marilyn Meserve, managing editor, guided important editorial aspects from behind the scenes. Patrick Walsh (managing production editor), Ilene Sanford and Pat Brown (manufacturing managers) guided scheduling, production, and manufacturing. Penny Walker and her capable staff at Aptara, Inc. copyedited and produced the book. A special thanks to our copyeditor Loretta Palagi, for her attention to details, making sure every word and punctuation mark conveyed the proper message. Mary Seiner, art director, created a visually clear and inviting format. John Jordan, Dorothy Cook and Tina Rudowski made all the media components happen and Patrick Watson oversaw the development of art and photos for the book. Our thanks to all of you!

About the Authors

Roberta Pavy Ramont

Roberta was an instructor of Vocational Nursing at The North Orange County Regional Occupational Program in Anaheim, California, for 13 years. She received her initial nursing education at The Cooper Hospital School of Nursing in Camden, New Jersey; her baccalaureate degree from the University of Redlands; a Masters in Psychology-School Counseling from the University of LaVerne; and a doctorate in Educational Leadership with an emphasis in Training and Development at Alliant International University.

Following graduation from nursing school, she began her nursing career working in intensive care. Unlike today, in 1969 very few people recovered from critical illness. She quickly learned that she wanted to focus her career on keeping people healthy. She spent several years work as a visiting nurse for an agency that provided well-child clinics, school nursing services, and home visits (e.g., crippled children's services, communicable disease care, and mental health).

When her twin daughters were two she returned to nursing. She worked part time in maternal and infant care, taught childbirth preparation classes, and worked in clinics and physicians' offices until she moved from New Jersey to California. There, in the midst of a statewide hiring freeze, she found a job working with the developmentally disabled in a state hospital and was quickly promoted to Unit Supervisor. These individuals were physically handicapped as well as having cognitive deficits, so she hired a number of LVNs to care for them. These nurses made a real difference in the residents' lives. They brought joy to their lives and concentrated on what the residents could accomplish rather than on their disabilities. Many of these LVNs were promoted to positions of increased responsibility or continued their education and achieved an RN license.

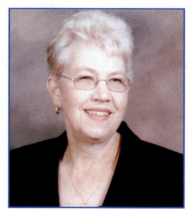

In 1981 Roberta had the opportunity to leave the state hospital system, when residents were sent to community schools to meet the "least restrictive environment and education for the handicapped" laws. She became a school nurse and continued to work with students with special needs.

The year 1985 brought a diagnosis of cancer and, over the next six years, numerous treatments and surgeries. During hospitalizations Roberta was able to observe nurses in their work. She became concerned that many of them did not seem to enjoy their work and seemed just to be doing a job. Compassionate and professional nurses were few and far between. While unemployed following an injury, she had the opportunity to teach a part time class, and this assignment presented her with a new focus. She found that she enjoyed imparting knowledge and instruction to students. She also felt she could pass on some of the "lost art" of nursing. That same summer she was hired to teach a nursing assistant class. This quickly developed in to an opportunity to teach LVNs. From 2003–2005 she oversaw Practical Nursing program in several states for Corinthian Colleges Inc. In 2006 she returned to North Orange County Regional Occupational Programs teaching part time and preparing graduates for their NCLEX®. She also started Educational Innovations—a private consultation firm, providing curriculum and program development for a number of private educational organizations, and technical assistance to new HOSA Advisors.

Over the years Roberta has been able to pass on to hundreds of students what it means to be a nurse. When teaching growth and development, she always tells her students that children only need to be given two things: Roots and Wings. She feels that this holds true for nursing students also. They need to understand the rich heritage of nursing that they will carry into the future, and they need to develop skills that will make them competent, safe nurses who can think and function with confidence.

While serving as curriculum chair for health careers education at the Regional Occupational Program, Roberta worked with the health occupations faculty to identify academic standards taught in the career technical classes. She has been involved in an extensive project to develop rubrics for alternate assessment of student work.

Roberta has served as an advisor for Health Occupation Students of America, and Cal-HOSA Inc. Board of Directors Chair in 2002. She served as President of the California Association of Health Careers Educators (CAHCE) during 2000–01. She is a member of Society of Pediatric Nurses and Pi Lambda Theta, International Honor Society in Education. She was awarded the Lillian Runge Memorial Scholarship for Continuing Education from CAHCE in 2002.

Over the years Roberta has had the privilege of serving on the NCLEX-PN® writing panel, and developing and presenting educational seminars on the adult learner and technology in the classroom. She has taught teacher credentialing classes for San Diego University and is serving on a task force with the California Department of Education of Teacher Credentialing for Health Occupation teachers.

Roberta has three children: twin daughters Amy (an RN) and Alicia (a stay-at-home mom to Haley and T. J.), and Tom a graphic-artist. When time permits she enjoys reading and traveling. She credits her entrance into nursing to an LVN student who cared for her during an illness and who recognized her potential. She also credits the continued support and encouragement of her parents, who always demonstrated that anything worth achieving is worth 100% effort.

Dee Maldonado Niedringhaus

Dee's nursing career began right after graduation from Nursing School at USC/LACMC, (Los Angeles County Medical Center), when she moved to Orange County and applied for a graduate nursing position. She was hired on the spot at what used to be Orange County Hospital. Although it was much smaller than LACMC (the rooms had only had five beds instead of eight to ten), it was a challenge. As the county hospital, it was always busy. The first year she worked pm shift on an orthopedic floor, where once there were prisoners in four rooms with guards and sometimes conditions were so crowded that clients had spaces in the halls. This was a period of growth. The doctors were interns and residents; all the staff worked together and learned how to be creative, innovative, and inventive.

After her marriage Dee transferred to a day shift position on the surgical floor, dealing with all types of surgical specialty (EENT, Plastic Surgery, Thoracic Surgery, and General Surgery). In team nursing there Dee was fortunate to have as colleagues two of the best LVNs, who did most of the dressings and wound care and helped with medications. Dee's nursing techniques developed as she learned from these nurses. After working at this hospital for twelve years in various areas, she was chosen to work a new unit as the surgical specialist. It was the first outpatient unit developed at what was now UCIMC (University of California at Irvine Medical Center).

A chance request brought her to teaching. One summer a colleague needed a substitute instructor for a Nursing Assistant program run by North Orange County Regional Occupational Program. Those two months changed her nursing career. She was hooked on and loved teaching. When she was offered a full time position teaching a day Nursing Assistant Program, she taught this for a year. She then took a position teaching Vocational Nurses, and for fifteen years taught Fundamentals I & II, Integumentary, Gastrointestinal, Endocrine and Leadership modules. She began the first HOSA (Health Occupations Students of America) chapters, which became very successful and continue today. She also instructed classes for Health Career Instructors and was the chairman for Cal-HOSA Inc. Currently Dee is an Instructional Administrator of Medical Programs at North Orange County ROP

Contributor Team

Cynthia Bartlau, RN, PHN, MSN
Faculty
Long Beach City College
Long Beach, CA

Marti Burton, RN, BS
Curriculum Design and Development
Canadian Valley Technology Center
El Reno, OK

Margaret C. Davis, PhD, MSN, RN
Assistant Professor
Georgia Southern University
Statesboro, GA

Margaret M. Gingrich, RN, MSN
Professor
Harrisburg Community College
Harrisburg, PA

Donna Halloran-Krol, RN, BSN
Faculty
Ivy Tech Community College
Valaparaiso, IN

Jeanne Hately, PhD, MSN, RN
President
Professional Nurse Consultants, LLC
Aurora, CO

Donna Walker Hubbard, MSN, RN, CNN
Assistant Professor
University of Mary Hardin-Baylor
Belton, TX

Darlene Lacy, PhD, RN, BS
Assistant Professor
Texas Tech University Health Sciences Center
Lubbock, TX

Thanh Nguyen, FF, Paramedic
North Orange Country Regional
Occupational Program
Anaheim, CA

David Oswandel, BS
Faculty
Pikes Peak Community College
Colorado Springs, CO

Kathleen O'Leary Oller, MSN, RN
Maternal & Women's Health Coordinator
Florida Community College at Jacksonville
Jacksonville, FL

Betty Richardson, PhD, RN, CNS-MHP, BS, LPC, LMFT
Professor Emeritus
Austin Community College
Private Practice Marriage and Family
    Therapy
Austin, TX

Marti Stow, MS, APRN, BC, CNOR
Assistant Professor
Lewis Clark State College
Coeur d' Alene, ID

LeeAnn Thrapp Fields, RN, BSN, MA
Founder, President
New Haven Healing Center
Bolingbrook, IL

Katherine West, BSN, MSEd, CIC
Infection Control Consultant
Infection Control/Emerging
    Concepts, Inc.
Manassas, VA

Supplement Contributors

Student CD-ROM

Diane Anderson, MS, RN, FNC-P
Professor
Texas Women's University
Denton, TX

Cathleen Kunkler, MSN, RN, ONC
Instructor
Corning Community College
Corning, NY

Student Study Guide

Traudel Cline, RN, MSN
Faculty
Milwaukee Area Technical College
Milwaukee, WI

Instructor's Resource CD-ROM

Linda Manlove Johnson, RN, MSN, MS
Faculty
City College of San Francisco
San Francisco, CA

Instructor's Resource Manual

Betty K. Rickard MSN, RN
Faculty
University of North Alabama
Florence, AL

Janelle Hernden Sorrell, RN, BS
Faculty
Northwest-Shoals Community College
Muscle Shoals, AL

Reviewer Panel

Vicki Agyekum, RN, MSN
Faculty
Savannah Technical College
Savannah, GA

Janice Ankenmann-Hill, RN, MSN, CCRN, FNP
Faculty
Napa Valley College
Napa, CA

Rebecca S. Appleton, RN, PhD
Professor
Marshall University
Huntington, WV

Marjorie L. Archer, MS, RNC, WHCNP
Dean of Health Sciences, Director of Vocational
    Nursing
North Central Texas College
Gainesville, TX

Andrea Bowden-Evans, RN, MSN, CRNP
Faculty
Shelton State Community College
Tuscaloosa, AL

Kim Cooper, RN, MSN
Assistant Professor and Department
    Chair
Ivy Tech Community College
Terre Haute, IN

Rebecca Ann Craig
Faculty
Gwinnett Technical College
Lawrenceville, GA

Francine Davis, RN, MPH
Faculty
Vance Granville Community College
Henderson, NC

Rebekah Delafield, RN
Vocational Nursing Instructor
San Jacinto College North
Houston, TX

Gail Dunham, RN, MSN
Professor of Nursing
Mid Michigan Community College
Harrison, MI

Dina Faucher, RN, PhD
Faculty
Apollo College
Phoenix, AZ

Rebecca Gesler, MSN, RN
Faculty
Spalding University
Louisville, KY

Shari Gholson, MSN, RN
Associate Professor
West Kentucky Community and
    Technical College
Paducah, KY

Helena Gunnell, RN, BSN, MEd
Practical Nursing Instructor
Jones County Junior College
Ellisville, MS

Pamela Gwin, RNC
Director, Vocational Nursing Program
Brazosport College
Lake Jackson, TX

Contents

UNIT VI *Becoming a Licensed Nurse,* 865

The Nature of Nursing

UNIT I

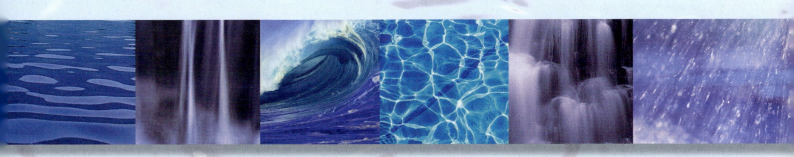

Succeeding as a Nursing Student

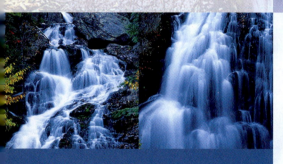

HISTORICAL Perspectives

You are embarking on an exciting journey in approximately one year, you will take your place on the timeline of nursing, which stretches from near the beginning of time way into the future. In this location in every chapter of this text, you will get a quick glimpse of the historical contributions made to nursing and health care. Someday you will be among the great contributors to the profession. Your accomplishments may not be recorded in a textbook, but to the client and families you will care for during your career, you represent all those who have gone before. The history of nursing and health care is far from dry and boring—it helps us learn where we have been so we can better understand where we are going. The authors of this book join with the nurses of the past to welcome you to nursing and wish you success as you become part of this legacy.

BRIEF Outline

Reading This Textbook
Studying Effectively
Managing Time
Taking Tests
Participating in Clinical Experiences
Overview of Nursing History
Practical/Vocational Nursing Today
Professional Organizations for LPN/LVN Students and Graduates
Student Organizations

LEARNING Outcomes

After completing this chapter, you will be able to:

1. Explain ways to approach this textbook and plan your study time effectively.
2. Identify three strategies to use when answering various types of test questions.
3. Discuss the responsibilities of the student nurse during clinical experiences.
4. Briefly discuss key figures in nursing history.
5. Explain key contributions in practical/vocational nursing history.
6. Discuss the customers, purpose, standards, and work settings of practical/vocational nursing.
7. Identify professional organizations for the practical/vocational nurse and nursing student.

Welcome to a career in nursing. You have made an excellent choice for a future helping others to regain or maintain health and function. Nursing is full of rewards and challenges while you are a student and also after you graduate. This text is designed to help you recognize and overcome those challenges as well as to appreciate the rewards.

LPN/LVN training programs can be found in many different types of schools. In some states, they are part of high schools. In others, they are in community college settings, vocational training centers, or private schools.

The length of the program is dictated by the governing nursing board in each state. Some programs can be completed in about 9 months. Others take up to 2 years. Some are full-time day programs; others are part time in the evenings and/or on weekends.

People with a variety of backgrounds enter the nursing profession. Your classmates may represent a variety of life experiences, educational backgrounds, and ethnic/cultural influences. You can learn a great deal by collaborating with fellow students during your course of study. The ages of LPN/LVN students within a class may range from young adult to near retirement. Motives may also vary. Students may be realizing a lifelong dream to become a nurse or making a career change.

It may have been a long time since you studied a subject that really mattered to you, or you may have recently been in school and studied with serious commitment. In either case, here are some academic "survival skills" to help you in your vocational/practical nursing course of study.

Reading This Textbook

Begin by reading the preface and other material in the front of the book. Become familiar with how the book is organized and any special features that will make your reading and studying easier. Review the table of contents and look over the appendices. By spending a few minutes becoming familiar with the book, you will be ready to use your book when the first reading assignment is given. The textbook is a great stand-alone reference, as well as a source for clarifying lecture material.

Read textbook assignments before the class in which the material will be covered. Reading beforehand will help you organize your thoughts, and help you spell and define words that may be used in a lecture. Although many students use highlighter pens while reading, it is much better to save the highlighter for reviewing lectures notes or marking the location of answers to the chapter's study questions (Porter, L.).

Studying Effectively

It is easy to stare at a page of text and feel that you have "spent time" studying when, in fact, you may have understood very little. When you have a block of time set aside to study, make sure you use it wisely. For hints about what is

most important in the text, look at the Learning Outcomes at the beginning of each chapter. These objectives guide you in discovering the information you need to obtain from the chapter as you read and study. When an objective states "Identify three strategies to use when . . . ," go to the text, find all three strategies, and write them down. As you study, review those three strategies and when you would use them.

Another technique to employ when studying is outlining. Some students find it helpful to outline the chapter after reading it. Under the main ideas, they organize the concepts and the information that supports those ideas. You can easily do this by using the main headings in the chapter as outline headings, then listing two or three main ideas from the paragraphs beneath those headings.

Study questions at the end of the chapter and/or in student workbooks are another way to help you pull out the most important information in a chapter. First, try to answer the questions from what you have read and understood. If you are unable to answer them correctly or at all, look up the information within the chapter to find the correct answer. This will help you remember the information better than simply looking up each answer. Some students find it helpful to make up their own study questions; they anticipate what instructors might ask by using information from class notes.

Take advantage of all available tools. Use a computer at school or at home to access the Companion Website (www.prenhall.com/ramont) or the student CD for this text. These tools provide additional questions and case studies to bring the information to life and to prepare you for future practice. The website and CD also supply links to the Internet to help you with your school projects and research.

Studying with another person or group of three or four people can be helpful in processing information and discussing ideas. To be successful, the groups must be well organized. Study groups are discussed further in the next section.

Managing Time

The "average" practical/vocational nursing student is far from average. Proposing one time management template that would work for everyone is impossible. Still, being organized and having a plan will help you work within your time limits. Learning to manage your time is a skill that will benefit you during the nursing program and also in your career and in life.

Learning how to be a good student may be the most important lesson during the first few weeks of your nursing program. Study skills will support you throughout your student days and as you prepare for exams. The time taken to perfect these skills will be hours well spent. See Figure 1-1 ■ for a sample time management schedule.

	Monday	Tuesday	Wednesday	Thursday	Friday	Saturday	Sunday
0600	Sleep	Sleep	Sleep	Shower/dress	Shower/dress	Shower/dress	Sleep
0700	Shower/dress	Shower/dress	Shower/dress	Clinical	Clinical	Work	Sleep
0800	Class	Class	Class				Shower/dress
0900							Breakfast
1000							Church
1100							
1200	Lunch	Lunch	Lunch	Lunch	Lunch	Lunch	
1300	Class	Class					
1400		Library	Group project				Dinner with family
1500							
1600							
1700	Dinner	Dinner	Dinner	Dinner	Dinner	Dinner	
1800						Movie	
1900	Study group	Study	Study	Study			Laundry
2000							Study
2100			Personal time	Personal time			
2200	Personal time	Personal time	Sleep	Sleep	Personal time		Personal time
2300	Sleep	Sleep	Sleep	Sleep	Sleep		Sleep

Figure 1-1. ■ Sample time management schedule.

The following suggestions for time management may be useful:

- Obtain a blank calendar or planner for the entire year.
- Fill in holidays, vacations, medical or dental appointments, class times, and clinical days as soon as you know them.
- Add due dates, tests, homework, and projects as they are assigned.
- Schedule study time by writing it on your calendar or planner.
- Schedule personal time for relaxation and being with other people.

Group study time can be very useful when you participate regularly. Learn to plan your group study time, just as you would plan other parts of your day. Stay focused on content, and resist the urge to talk about things that are not study material. Bring four or five questions with you to discuss with the group. This can be especially helpful if you are having difficulty understanding certain concepts.

It is a good idea to break a study session down into segments. For example, a 2-hour session might include 30 minutes of lecture note review, 20 minutes of shared questions and answers, a 10-minute break, 30 minutes of quizzing, and 30 minutes of review of class objectives. This plan gives focus to the study time. The change in activities also helps to sustain people's interest and energy levels.

Taking Tests

ANSWERING MULTIPLE-CHOICE QUESTIONS

Most tests given in nursing programs will be objective, multiple-choice tests. These are the same types of questions used on the NCLEX-PN® exam. Multiple-choice questions can evaluate your knowledge of facts, as well as your ability to apply that knowledge within a client care scenario. Each question will consist of a stem and answer choices. Read each question completely in order to understand what is being asked. Then read each of the choices. Try to eliminate one or more of the choices. Examine each choice to see if anything is incorrect within the answer itself. Watch out for choices that are correct and accurate on their own, but that do not answer the question as it is written. See Box 1-1 ■ for an example.

Multiple-choice questions can test **knowledge, comprehension, application,** and ability to **analyze.** Table 1-1 ■ provides examples and comparisons of each type.

Questions that include choices such as "all of the above" or "none of the above" have been eliminated from the NCLEX-PN® examination. However, some textbooks have them as study questions, and some instructors may test with them. A choice of this type can be confirmed or eliminated easily. If you have identified one choice as being correct, then you can eliminate "none of the above." If you can identify one choice

BOX 1-1

Example of a Multiple-Choice Question

Which of the following men was responsible for the reduction of maternal death related to infection transmitted by way of unwashed hands?

1. Joseph Lister
2. Louis Pasteur
3. Ignaz Semmelweis
4. Karl Crede

Although all four people were involved in prevention of infection and/or disease, the correct answer is 3. Ignaz Semmelweis was the person who discovered that puerperal fever was related to examination of mothers during the intra- and postpartum periods by doctors who had not washed their hands after performing autopsies.

that is incorrect, then "all of the above" can also be eliminated. If you can identify at least two answers as correct, then the question qualifies as an "all of the above" answer.

If you are able to narrow your choice to two options, don't spend too much time deciding between them. More likely than not, your first impression is correct. Once you have identified your choice, don't go back and change it unless you later figure out the correct response with absolute certainty.

Answering the study questions at the end of each chapter and in the student workbook will help you improve your ability to select correct answers in objective tests.

Most questions on the NCLEX-PN® exam are standard multiple choice, but some new types of questions are being added. The NCLEX-PN® exam is discussed in more detail in Chapter 37 ⬭.

TABLE 1-1

Test Questions and Levels of Learning

LEVEL	INFORMATION REQUIRED	EXAMPLE	RATIONALE
Knowledge question	Requires recall of information. To answer a knowledge question, you need to commit facts to memory. Knowledge questions expect you to know terminology, specific facts, trends, sequences, classifications, categories, criteria, structures, principles, generalizations, and/or theories.	What does the abbreviation BRP mean? a. bathe daily b. bedrush pt c. blood pressure reading d. bathroom privileges	To answer this question correctly, you have to know the meaning of the abbreviation BRP (bathroom priviliges answer d).
Comprehension question	Requires you to understand information. To answer a comprehension question, not only must you commit facts to memory, but it is essential that you be able to translate, interpret, and determine the implications of the information. You demonstrate understanding when you translate or paraphrase information, interpret or summarize information, or determine the implications, consequences, corollaries, or effects of information. Comprehension questions expect you not only to know but also to understand the information being tested. You do not necessarily have to relate it to other material or see its fullest implications.	To evaluate the therapeutic effect of a cathartic, the nurse should assess the client for: a. increased urinary output. b. a decrease in anxiety. c. a bowel movement. d. pain relief.	To answer this question, you not only have to know that a cathartic is a potent laxative that stimulates the bowel, but that the increase in peristalsis will result in a bowel movement (answer c).
Application question	Requires you to utilize knowledge. To answer an application question, you must take remembered and comprehended concepts and apply them to concrete situations. The abstractions may be theories, technical principles, rules of procedures, generalizations, or ideas that have to be applied in a scenario. Application questions test your ability to use information in a new situation.	An elderly client's skin looks dry, thin, and fragile. When providing back care, the nurse should: a. apply a moisturizing body lotion. b. wash back with soap and water. c. massage back using short kneading strokes. d. leave excess lubricant on the client's skin.	To answer this question, you must know that dry, thin, fragile skin is common in the elderly and that moisturizing lotion helps the skin to retain water and become more supple. When presented with this scenario, you have to apply your knowledge concerning developmental changes in the elderly and the benefits of using moisturizing lotion (answer a).

(continued)

TABLE 1-1

Test Questions and Levels of Learning (*continued*)

LEVEL	INFORMATION REQUIRED	EXAMPLE	RATIONALE
Analysis question	Requires you to interpret a variety of data and recognize the commonalities, differences, and interrelationships among present ideas. Analysis questions make assumptions that you know, understand, and can apply information. Now you must identify, examine, dissect, evaluate, or investigate the organization, systematic arrangement, or structure of the information presented in the question. This type of question tests your analytical ability.	A client who is undergoing cancer chemotherapy says to the nurse, "This is no way to live." Which of the following responses uses reflective technique? a. "Tell me more about what you are thinking." b. "You sound discouraged today." c. "Life is not worth living?" d. "What are you saying?"	To answer this question, you must understand the communication techniques of reflection, clarification, and paraphrasing. You must also analyze the statements and identify which techniques are represented. This question requires you to understand, interpret, and differentiate information to know that the correct answer is c.

Several techniques are useful in calling information to mind during a test. For example, by using visualization, you may be able to picture something the instructor wrote on the board during a lecture. You may be able to "see" in your mind a poster or handout that was used during a class presentation. With some practice, you may be able to visualize a word or a passage that you read in the textbook.

ANSWERING ESSAY, SHORT-ANSWER, AND CALCULATION QUESTIONS

Answers to essay, short-answer, and calculation questions will need to be extracted from your memory. Read the question carefully to determine what is being asked. Some students find it helpful to develop a brief outline before beginning an essay question. Check with the instructor to see if this can be written on the test paper or if you are permitted to use an additional sheet. The outline can help you organize your thoughts and can serve as a checkpoint that all important information was included. Usually, a number of key introductory words appear in essay questions (Table 1-2 ■). Look for these words, and do only what is required of you. Many low grades are caused by ignoring these key words.

Calculation questions are particularly troubling for many students who have convinced themselves that they cannot do math. Although math may be difficult, it is a necessary skill for a nurse. With extra practice, calculations are possible to learn. Several methods are used to do calculations (see Chapter 29 ⚭).

It is important to show your work on calculations. If you are unable to arrive at the correct answer, your instructor can review your work, and will be able to tell you where you went wrong. Memorizing formulas and frequently used conversions will make calculations on tests and in the clinical area much easier.

TABLE 1-2

Key Words in Essay Exams

KEY WORD	EXPLANATION
Compare	To point out similarities and differences
Contrast	To point out differences only
Define	Several connotations: (1) to give the meaning of, (2) to explain or describe essential qualities, (3) to place it in the class to which it belongs and set it off from other items in the same class
Describe	Enumerate (list) the special features of the topic Show how the topic is different from similar or related items Give an account of, tell about, and give a word picture of
Discuss	Present various sides or points, talk over, consider the different sides; a discussion is usually longer than an explanation of the same subject
Explain	Make plain or clear, interpret, tell "how" to do
Identify	Show recognition
Illustrate	Describe in narrative form using "word pictures" to provide examples
Justify	Provide supporting data for opinions or actions
List or name	Present a group of names or items in a category
Outline	Give information systematically in headings and subheadings
Summarize	Present in condensed form; give main points briefly

Participating in Clinical Experiences

A major part of your learning will occur during your clinical experiences. You will be assigned to assist with the care of one or more clients in a healthcare setting. This experience is extremely valuable in preparing you for the profession you have chosen. You will find that observing signs and symptoms of an illness firsthand is far more impressive than reading about them.

At first you will care for just one client, with assistance from other healthcare workers as needed. As you progress through your course of study, you will be assigned more responsibility and more clients. The clients you care for will have more complex illnesses and needs. When you study and learn about performing skills and signs to watch for, you are learning what you need to know to be a safe healthcare practitioner.

As a student, your responsibilities in preparing for clinical experience include:

- Ensuring that you understand what you read and how to apply it to the care of real clients
- Practicing skills repeatedly so that you know exactly what to do when called on to perform those skills quickly and efficiently in the clinical setting
- Researching information about an assigned client's medical diagnosis, nursing diagnoses, problems, and needs so that you are prepared and can anticipate what could happen as you care for that client
- Asking for help when you are not sure how to proceed, but proceeding when you are sure of what you need to do
- Reporting any and all deviations from baseline that you observe while caring for clients (You may not realize the significance of your observation, especially early in the program, but other healthcare professionals will know what actions to take.)
- Taking advantage of all learning opportunities in the clinical setting. If a procedure is being done, ask if you can observe, even though the client may not be assigned to you. Spend any "downtime" during your clinical experience observing, assisting, or listening to healthcare staff.

Overview of Nursing History

To fully appreciate your position as a contemporary practical/vocational nurse, you need to understand a bit about the history of nursing. Many women and men have been influential in developing nursing into the profession it is today.

NIGHTINGALE (1820–1910)

Florence Nightingale's contributions to nursing are well documented. Her achievements in improving the standards

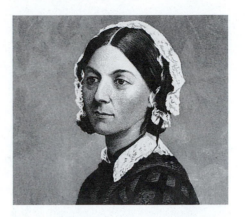

Figure 1-2. ■ Considered to be the founder of modern nursing, Florence Nightingale (1820–1910) was influential in developing nursing education, practice, and administration. Her 1859 publication *Notes on Nursing: What It Is, and What It Is Not* was intended for all women. (*Source:* © Bettmann/CORBIS. Reprinted with permission.)

for the care of war casualties in Crimea earned her the title "Lady with the Lamp" (Figure 1-2 ■). Her efforts in reforming hospitals and in producing and implementing public health policies also made her an accomplished political nurse. She was the first nurse to exert political pressure on government. She is also recognized as nursing's first scientist-theorist for her work *Notes on Nursing: What It Is, and What It Is Not.*

When she returned from Crimea, a grateful English public gave Nightingale an honorarium of £4,500. She used this money to establish the Nightingale Training School for Nurses in 1860. At St. Thomas Hospital in London, England, she taught her straightforward requirements.

Nightingale believed that nursing education should develop both the intellect and character of the nurse. She gave students a solid background in science to understand the theory behind their care. To develop character, by increasing their understanding of human ethics and morals, she assigned readings in the humanities. She believed that nurses should never stop learning. To her nurses she wrote, "[Nursing] is a field of which one may safely say: there is no end in what we may be learning everyday" (Schuyler, 1992). The school served as a model for other training schools. Its graduates traveled to other countries to manage hospitals and to institute training programs for nurses.

Nightingale's vision of nursing, which included public health and health promotion roles for nurses, was only partially addressed in the early days. The focus first was on developing the profession within hospitals. Although Miss Nightingale died in 1910, her influence continues in nursing today.

BARTON (1821–1912)

Clara Barton (Figure 1-3 ■) was a schoolteacher who volunteered as a nurse during the American Civil War. Her

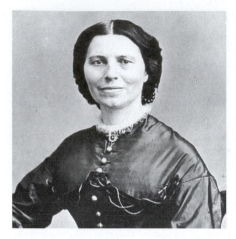

Figure 1-3. ■ Clara Barton (1821–1912) organized the American Red Cross, which linked with the International Red Cross when the U.S. Congress ratified the Geneva Convention in 1882. (*Source:* © Bettmann/CORBIS. Reprinted with permission.)

responsibility was to organize the nursing services. Barton is noted for her role in establishing the American Red Cross, which linked with the International Red Cross when the United States Congress ratified the Treaty of Geneva (Geneva Convention). In 1882, Barton persuaded Congress to ratify this treaty so that the Red Cross could perform humanitarian efforts in times of peace.

WALD (1867–1940)

Lillian Wald (Figure 1-4 ■) is considered the founder of public health nursing. Wald and Mary Brewster were the first to offer trained nursing services to the poor in the New York slums. They founded the Henry Street Settlement, and Visiting Nurse Service, which provided nursing and social services, and also organized educational and cultural activities. Soon after the founding of the Henry Street Settlement, school nursing was established as an adjunct to visiting nursing.

DOCK (1858–1956)

Lavinia L. Dock (Figure 1-5 ■) was a feminist, as well as a prolific writer, political activist, suffragist, and friend of Wald. She participated in protest movements for women's rights that resulted in the 1920 passage of the 19th Amendment to the U.S. Constitution, which granted women the right to vote. In addition, Dock campaigned for legislation to allow nurses rather than physicians to control their profession. In 1893, Dock, Mary Adelaide Nutting, and Isabel Hampton Robb founded the American Society of Superintendents of Training Schools for Nurses of the United States and Canada. This was a precursor to the current National League for Nursing (NLN).

MALE NURSES IN HISTORY

Women were not the sole providers of nursing services. The first nursing school in the world was started in India in about 250 B.C. Only men were considered to be "pure" enough to fulfill the role of nurse at that time. In Jesus's parable in the New Testament, the good Samaritan paid an innkeeper to provide care for the injured man. Paying a man to provide nursing care was fairly common. During the Crusades, several orders of knights provided nursing care to their sick and injured comrades and also built hospitals. The organization and management of their hospitals set a standard for the administration of hospitals throughout Europe at that time. St. Camillus de Lellis started out as a soldier and later turned to nursing. He started the sign of the Red Cross and developed the first ambulance service.

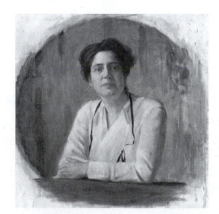

Figure 1-4. ■ Lillian Wald (1867–1940) founded the Henry Street Settlement and Visiting Nurse Service (circa 1893), which provided nursing and social services and organized educational and cultural activities. She is considered to be founder of public health nursing. (*Source:* University of Iowa, College of Nursing, Iowa City, IA.)

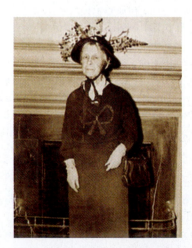

Figure 1-5. ■ Nursing leader and suffragist Lavinia L. Dock (1858–1956) was active in the protest movement for women's rights that resulted in the 1920 U.S. constitutional amendment allowing women to vote. (*Source:* Courtesy of Millbank Memorial Library, Teachers' College, Columbia University. Reprinted with permission.)

Friar Juan de Mena was shipwrecked off the south Texas coast in 1554. He is the first identified nurse in what would become the United States. James Derham, a black slave who worked as a nurse in New Orleans in the late 1700s, saved the money he earned to purchase his freedom. Later, he studied medicine and became a well-respected physician in Philadelphia. During the Civil War, both sides had military men who cared for the sick and wounded.

In 1876, only three years after the first U.S. nurse received her diploma from New England Hospital for Women and Children, the Alexian brothers opened their first hospital in the United States and a school to educate men in nursing.

During the years from the Civil War to the Korean War, men were not permitted to serve as nurses in the military. Today, men have resumed their historical place in the profession. As the history of nursing continues to be written, men and women will work side by side (Figure 1-6 ■).

HISTORY OF LPNS/LVNS

The first training for practical nurses was at the Young Women's Christian Association (YWCA) in New York City in 1892. The following year this became the Ballard School. The program of study was 3 months long, and the participants studied special techniques for caring for the sick as well as a variety of homemaking techniques. Much of the care during this time was done in the client's home, making the licensed practical nurse (LPN) a home health or visiting nurse. Eleven years later, a second school, the Thompson Practical Nursing School, was established.

In 1914, the state legislature in Mississippi passed the first laws governing the practice of practical nurses. Other states were slow to follow. By 1940, only six states had passed such laws. In 1955, the state board test pool of the NLN Education Committee established the procedures for testing graduates of approved practical/vocational education programs in all states. Graduates who passed the examination became LPNs or, in California and Texas, licensed vocational nurses (LVNs). Each state set its own passing score.

Today, a graduate of an approved LPN/LVN training program is eligible to take the National Council Licensure Examination for Practical Nursing (**NCLEX-PN**®). The examination is computerized, with a "pass" score that is standardized throughout the United States. All states have licensing laws. *Interstate endorsement* (reciprocity between states) exists. This means that an LPN/LVN from one state can apply for licensure in another state without retesting. It is the responsibility of the individual nurse to contact the board of nursing in the jurisdiction where he or she wishes to work. The nurse must apply for licensure and for information regarding the scope of practice within that state. Table 1-3 ■ lists important events in the history of practical/vocational nursing.

Practical/Vocational Nursing Today

OUR CUSTOMERS

The "customers" we serve in nursing today are sometimes called consumers, sometimes patients, and sometimes clients. A **consumer** is an individual, a group of people, or a community that uses a service or commodity. People who use healthcare products or services are consumers of health care. A **patient** is a person who is waiting for or undergoing medical treatment and care. The word *patient* comes from a Latin word meaning "to suffer" or "to bear." Traditionally, the person receiving health care has been called a patient. People become patients when they seek assistance because of illness. Some nurses believe that the word *patient* implies passive acceptance of the decisions and care of health professionals. Because nurses interact with family, friends, and healthy people as well as those who are ill, nurses increasingly refer to recipients of health care as *clients*.

A **client** is a person who engages the advice or services of someone who is qualified to provide the service. Therefore, a client is a collaborator, a person who is also responsible for his or her own health. The health status of a client is the responsibility of the individual in collaboration with health professionals. In this book, *client* is the preferred term, although *consumer* and *patient* may be used in some instances.

OUR PURPOSE

Nurses provide care for individuals, families, and communities. The scope of nursing practice involves four areas: promoting health and wellness, preventing illness, restoring health, and caring for the dying.

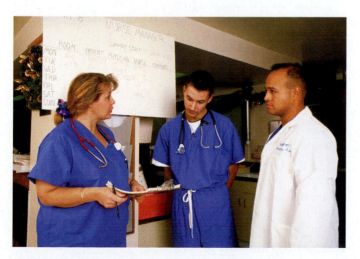

Figure 1-6. ■ Modern male nurses work side by side with their female colleagues to provide care to hospitalized clients.

TABLE 1-3

Important Historical Events for LPNs/LVNs

DATE	EVENT	IMPORTANCE
1893	Ballard School at YMCA, Brooklyn, New York	First formal training for practical nurses.
1914	Mississippi legislature passed license laws for practical nurses	First laws passed to govern the practice of practical nurses.
1917	Smith-Hughes Act	Provided federal funding for vocationally oriented schools of practical nursing.
1918	Third school established	Even with new schools and federal assistance, the need for nurses could not be met because of the demand created by the war and epidemics.
1941	The Association of Practical Nurse Schools was founded; the name was changed to National Association for Practical Nurse Education (NAPNE) in 1942	Standards for practical nurse education were established.
1944	U.S. Department of Education commissioned an intensive study differentiating tasks of the practical nurse	The outcome of the study differentiated tasks performed by the practical nurse from those performed by the registered nurse. State boards of nursing established tasks that could be performed by both groups.
1945	New York established mandatory licensure for practical nurses	The first state to require licensure; by 1955 all other states had followed suit.
1949	The National Federation of Licensed Practical Nurses (NFLPN) was founded by Lillian Kuster; the name was changed to the National Association for Licensed Practical Nurse Education and Services in 1959	The discipline now had an official organization with membership limited to LPNs/LVNs.
1955	All states passed licensing laws for practical/vocational nurses	Practice of nursing by licensed practical nursing was regulated in all states.
1961	The National League of Nursing established a Department of Practical Nursing	Through this department, schools of practical nursing could be accredited by the NLN.
1965	American Nurses Association published a position paper that influenced attitudes about practical/vocational nursing	The paper clearly defined the two levels of nursing: registered nursing and technical nursing. The exclusion of the term *practical/vocational nurse* necessitated that the LPN/LVN prove his or her worth to provide valuable nursing interventions under the direction of a registered nurse.
1994	Computerized NCLEX-PN® examination available to graduates of practical/vocational nursing programs in all states	Allowed for more availability of test dates and interstate endorsement of licensure.

Promoting Health and Wellness

Wellness is a state of well-being. It means engaging in attitudes and behavior that enhance the quality of life and maximize personal potential. Nurses promote wellness in individuals and groups who are healthy or ill. Nurses may hold blood pressure clinics, teach about healthy lifestyles, give talks about drug and alcohol abuse, and instruct about safety in the home and workplace. Nurses who work in public health, community clinics, mental health facilities, and in occupation health settings promote health and wellness.

Preventing Illness

Illness may be defined as the highly individualized response a person has to a disease. The goal of illness prevention programs is to maintain optimal health by preventing disease. Nurses in physician's offices or health clinics administer immunizations, provide prenatal and infant care, and teach about the prevention of sexually transmitted infections.

Restoring Health

Restoring health means focusing on the ill client from early detection of disease through the recovery period. Nurses in acute care and rehabilitation facilities perform all of the following:

- Provide direct care to the ill person, such as administering medications, assisting with activities of daily living, and performing specific procedures and treatments.
- Perform diagnostic and assessment procedures, such as measuring blood pressure and examining feces for occult blood.
- Consult with other healthcare professionals about client problems.
- Teach clients about recovery activities, such as exercises that will hasten recovery after a stroke.
- Rehabilitate clients to their optimal functional level following physical or mental illness, injury, or chemical addiction.

Caring for the Dying

This area of nursing practice involves comforting and caring for people of all ages who are dying. It includes helping clients live as comfortably as possible until death and helping clients' support persons cope with death. Nurses carry out these activities in homes, hospitals, and extended care facilities. Some agencies, called hospices, are specifically designed for this purpose (see Chapter 17 ⚭).

OUR STANDARDS

Nurse practice acts, or legal acts for professional nursing practice, regulate the practice of nursing in the United States and Canada. Each state in the United States and each province in Canada has its own act.

Although practice acts may differ in various jurisdictions, they all have a common purpose: to protect the public. The title of *nurse* can legally be used *only* by an individual who is licensed as a registered nurse or a licensed practical or vocational nurse. For additional information, see Chapter 37 ⚭.

During your nursing education program, you will develop, clarify, and internalize professional values. The National Federation of Licensed Practical Nurses Inc. has identified specific standards (Box 1-2 ■). LPNs/LVNs in all areas of practice should adhere to these standards.

OUR WORK SETTINGS

In the past, the acute care hospital was the major practice setting open to most nurses. Today the LPN/LVN works in hospitals, clients' homes, community agencies, ambulatory clinics, health maintenance organizations, and skilled nursing facilities (see Chapter 7 ⚭). See also Chapter 38 ⚭ for a description of opportunities available to the LPN/LVN.

LPNs/LVNs work under their own license under direct supervision of a physician or a registered nurse. LPNs/LVNs may be involved in clinical planning meetings because of their expertise, but they are required to do this less than other licensed healthcare providers. Their primary duty is to deliver care to the client.

Professional Organizations for LPN/LVN Students and Graduates

When a professional organization is in place to oversee the operation of a group, it becomes a **profession** rather than an occupation. Several organizations oversee the profession of practical/vocational nursing.

NATIONAL ASSOCIATION FOR PRACTICAL NURSE EDUCATION AND SERVICE

The National Association for Practical Nurse Education and Service (NAPNES) was established in 1941. This was the first national organization for the practical/vocational level of nursing. NAPNES was responsible for the accreditation of LPN/LVN education programs from 1945 until 1984. Students can join this organization, and NAPNES publishes a journal called *The Journal of Practical Nursing.*

NATIONAL LEAGUE FOR NURSING

The National League for Nursing, formed in 1952, is an organization of both individuals and agencies. In 1961, the NLN established the Council for Practical Nursing Programs. This arm of the organization assumed responsibility for promoting the interests of LPNs/LVNs in the NLN. All of these organizations provide continuing education opportunities and publish literature of interest to the LPN/LVN.

NATIONAL FEDERATION OF LICENSED PRACTICAL NURSES

In 1949, Lillian Custer founded the National Federation of Licensed Practical Nurses (NFLPN). This organization is considered to be the official membership organization for LPNs and LVNs. Affiliate memberships are also available for those interested in the work of NFLPN but who are not LPNs/LVNs.

NFLPN welcomes LVN/LPN students as members. NFLPN provides leadership for nearly 1 million licensed practical and vocational nurses employed in the United States. It also fosters high standards of practical/vocational nursing education and practice so that the best nursing care will be available to every client.

The NFLPN serves as the central source of information on what is new and changing in practical/vocational nursing education and practice on the local, state, and national level. The organization is a three-tiered concept of local, state, and national enrollment. By participating in local, state, and national meetings and conferences, the practical/vocational nursing student can learn firsthand how a professional organization works to maintain the professional status of the membership. NFLPN also encourages continuing education and publishes a quarterly magazine, *Practical Nursing Today.*

BOX 1-2

Nursing Practice Standards for the Licensed Practical/Vocational Nurse

Education
The licensed practical/vocational nurse:

1. Shall complete a formal education program in practical nursing approved by the appropriate nursing authority in a state.
2. Shall successfully pass the National Council Licensure Examination for Practical Nurses.
3. Shall participate in initial orientation within the employing institution.

Legal/Ethical Status
The licensed practical/vocational nurse:

1. Shall hold a current license to practice nursing as an LP/VN in accordance with the law of the state wherein employed.
2. Shall know the scope of nursing practice authorized by the Nursing Practice Act in the state wherein employed.
3. Shall have a personal commitment to fulfill the legal responsibilities inherent in good nursing practice.
4. Shall take responsible actions in situations wherein there is unprofessional conduct by a peer or other health care provider.
5. Shall recognize and commit to meet the ethical and moral obligations of the practice of nursing.
6. Shall not accept or perform professional responsibilities that the individual knows (s)he is not competent to perform.

Practice
The licensed practical/vocational nurse:

1. Shall accept assigned responsibilities as an accountable member of the health care team.
2. Shall function within the limits of educational preparation and experience, as related to the assigned duties.
3. Shall function with other members of the health care team in promoting and maintaining health, preventing disease and disability, caring for and rehabilitating individuals who are experiencing an altered health state, and contributing to the ultimate quality of life until death.
4. Shall know and utilize the nursing process in planning, implementing, and evaluating health services and nursing care for the individual patient or group.
   a. Planning: The planning of nursing includes:
      1. Assessment of health status of the individual patient, the family, and community groups
      2. Analysis of the information gained from assessment
      3. Identification of health goals
   b. Implementation: The plan for nursing care is put into practice to achieve the stated goals and includes:
      1. Observing, recording, and reporting significant changes that require intervention or different goals
      2. Applying nursing knowledge and skills to promote and maintain health, to prevent disease and disability, and to optimize functional capabilities of an individual patient

   3. Assisting the patient and family with activities of daily living and encouraging self-care as appropriate
   4. Carrying out therapeutic regimens and protocols prescribed by an RN, physician, or other persons authorized by state law
   c. Evaluation: The plan for nursing care and its implementations are evaluated to measure the progress toward the stated goals and will include appropriate persons and/or groups to determine:
      1. The relevancy of current goals in relation to the progress of the individual patient
      2. The involvement of the recipients of care in the evaluation process
      3. The quality of the nursing action in the implementation of the plan
      4. A reordering of priorities or new goal setting in the care plan
5. Shall participate in peer review and other evaluation processes.
6. Shall participate in the development of policies concerning the health and nursing needs of society and in the roles and functions of the LP/VN.

Continuing Education
The licensed practical/vocational nurse:

1. Shall be responsible for maintaining the highest possible level of professional competence at all times.
2. Shall periodically reassess career goals and select continuing education activities that will help to achieve these goals.
3. Shall take advantage of continuing education opportunities that will lead to personal growth and professional development.
4. Shall seek and participate in continuing education activities that are approved for credit by appropriate organizations, such as the NFLPN.

Specialized Nursing Practice
The licensed practical/vocational nurse:

1. Shall have had at least one year's experience in nursing at the staff level.
2. Shall present personal qualifications that are indicative of potential abilities for practice in the chosen specialized nursing area.
3. Shall present evidence of completion of a program or course that is approved by an appropriate agency to provide the knowledge and skills necessary for effective nursing services in the specialized field.
4. Shall meet all of the standards of practice as set forth in this document.

Source: National Federation of Licensed Practical Nurses, Inc. Copyright © 1991.

Through relationships with the National Council of State Boards of Nursing and the U.S. Congress, the NFLPN enables policy makers to better understand the role of practical/vocational nursing in the nation's healthcare delivery system (NFLPN, 2003).

Student Organizations

HEALTH OCCUPATIONS STUDENTS OF AMERICA (HOSA)

HOSA is a nationally recognized technical career student organization, which was founded in 1976. HOSA provides a unique program of leadership and team-building development, motivation, and recognition experience. HOSA is an instructional tool integrated into the health careers classroom by the instructor. It is *intracurricular* (occurring within the framework of the school curriculum). It reinforces technical skills and supports service to the community. HOSA helps to develop the "total person." The national organization is made up of health occupations students from 42 affiliated states and Puerto Rico. HOSA's membership is made up of secondary, postsecondary, and collegiate students. Healthcare professionals, alumni, and business and industry members are welcome. There is also an associate membership category for students who are interested in health careers but who are not enrolled in a program. Through participation, the LPN/LVN student can network with other health career students. Involvement in a student organization demonstrates to students the benefits of participating in professional organizations once they have graduated.

Note: The references and resources for this and all chapters have been compiled at the back of the book.

KEY TERMS by Topic

Use the audio glossary feature of either the CD-ROM or the Companion Website to hear the correct pronunciation of the following key terms.

Taking Tests
knowledge, comprehension, application, analyze

Overview of Nursing History
NCLEX-PN®

Practical/Vocational Nursing Today
consumer, patient, client, wellness, illness, nurse practice acts

Professional Organizations for LPN/LVN Students and Graduates
profession

KEY Points

- Learning good study skills now will serve you for the rest of your career. Knowing how to get an overview of a task, organize your time, and break large job into smaller tasks are all life skills that will help you both inside and outside of nursing.

- Nursing values have traditionally included compassion, devotion to duty, and hard work. Nurses today are regarded as a vital part of the healthcare team. All levels of staff work together to provide the best possible care for clients.

- Practical and vocational schools have existed since the late 1800s, but it was only in the 1950s that a procedure was established to test graduates of approved schools in all states. Individual states still govern many factors of LPN/LVN practice.

- The terms *consumer, patient,* and *client* all refer to the recipient of healthcare services. The term *client* indicates that the person is actively involved in all phases of decision making and planning care.

- The scope of nursing practice includes promoting wellness, preventing illness, restoring health, and caring for the dying.

- Nurse practice acts vary among states and provinces, and nurses are responsible for knowing the act that governs their practice.

- Standards of clinical nursing practice provide measurement criteria for the effectiveness of nursing care and for professional performance behaviors.

- Traditionally, the majority of nurses were employed in hospital settings. Today, more nurses are working in home health care, ambulatory care, and community health settings.

- Professional and student organizations help the nursing profession and individual nurses. Participation in nursing associations encourages individual growth and helps nurses influence policies that affect nursing practice.

EXPLORE MediaLink

Additional interactive resources for this chapter can be found on the Companion Website at www.prenhall.com/ramont. Click on Chapter 1 and "Begin" to select the activities for this chapter.

For chapter-related NCLEX®-style questions and an audio glossary, access the accompanying CD-ROM in this book.

Video
- The History of Nursing

⌘ FOR FURTHER Study

LPNs/LVNs work in hospitals, in clients' homes, community agencies, ambulatory clinics, health maintenance organizations, and skilled nursing facilities (see Chapter 7).

Some agencies, called hospices, are specifically designed for this purpose (see Chapter 17).

Several methods are used to do calculations (see Chapter 29).

The NCLEX-PN® exam is discussed in more detail in Chapter 37.

Licensure as a licensed practical or vocational nurse is discussed further in Chapter 37.

See also Chapter 38 for a description of opportunities available to the LPN/LVN.

NCLEX-PN® Exam Preparation

1 A question that requires you to use knowledge, as well as take remembered and comprehended abstractions and apply them to concrete situations, is what type of question?
1. knowledge
2. comprehension
3. application
4. analysis

2 The NCLEX-PN® examination consists of:
1. essay questions and math calculations.
2. a practical demonstration to evaluate skills.
3. multiple-choice questions that test knowledge, comprehension, application, and analysis.
4. a different test for each licensure jurisdiction.

3 Which of the following indicates that a student needs more understanding of roles and responsibilities in the clinical situation?
1. The student has read about the clinical situation and understands how to apply the information to the care of individual clients.
2. The student has practiced a skill repeatedly and can perform it quickly and efficiently in the clinical setting.
3. The student is not sure how to proceed but makes an educated guess and completes the procedure.
4. The student reports deviations from baseline to the team leader.

4 Why is the term *client* used to refer to a healthcare recipient?
1. It indicates that the person needing health care can sue if he or she is unsatisfied with treatment.
2. The person is paying for the services.
3. The person is an active participant in determining the plan for care.
4. The person accepts the decisions and judgments of healthcare professionals.

5 Florence Nightingale is considered to be nursing's first scientist-theorist because:
1. she reformed hospitals and pressured government to implement public health policies.
2. she described the basic elements of the nursing profession in her work *Notes on Nursing: What It Is, and What It Is Not.*
3. she believed that nurses should never stop learning.
4. she taught that an understanding of human ethics and morals was essential to the development of nursing students.

6 In what decade were procedures established for testing of practical/vocational nurse graduates?
1. 1950s
2. 1890s
3. 1940s
4. 1990s

7 What is the significance of the Smith-Hughes Act for LPNs/LVNs?
1. It required licensure for practical nurses.
2. It differentiated the practice of LPNs and LVNs from RNs.
3. It provided federal funds to support practical nurse education.
4. It established computerized testing centers for licensure exams.

8 What differentiates a profession from an occupation?
1. required licensure
2. educational programs
3. an overseeing organization
4. nationally recognized testing

9 In 1949, Lillian Kuster founded which of the following organizations?
1. Health Occupations Students of America (HOSA)
2. National Council of State Boards of Nursing
3. National Federation of Licensed Practical Nurses (NFLPN)
4. Henry Street Settlement House

10 The nurse practice act provides:
1. the NCLEX-PN® test plan.
2. the scope of practice for LPNs/LVNs in individual states.
3. guidelines for the ethical practice of nursing.
4. questions to prepare for the licensing exam.

Answers and Rationales for Review Questions, as well as discussion of Care Plan and Critical Thinking Care Map questions, appear in Appendix I.

Chapter 2

Promoting Culturally Proficient Care

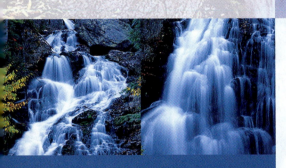

BRIEF Outline

Development of Transcultural Nursing
Theoretical Basis of Transcultural Nursing
Culturally Based Communication
Transcultural Communication and Client Concerns
Subculture of Health Care

HISTORICAL Perspectives

Transcultural nursing originated with Dr. Madeleine Leininger. She developed her theory of cultural care diversity and universality in the early 1950s, at a time when few if any professional nurses had knowledge of anthropologic concepts or cultural factors affecting health care, and at a time when articles written about transcultural nursing were rejected by editors. The concept of transcultural nursing had limited interest for nurses until the 1970s, and it was 1996 before cultural care was included in plans of study for nursing education at the University of Colorado where Leininger was professor of anthropology and nursing.

LEARNING Outcomes

After completing this chapter, you will be able to:

1. Understand the history and terminology of transcultural nursing.
2. Identify the importance of intercultural communication in today's world.
3. Describe the 12 domains of culture.
4. Identify the role of the nurse in delivering culturally proficient care to hospitalized clients and their families.
5. List the components of a cultural assessment.

For more than 30 years, nursing has been concerned with the cultural differences among clients. In the early years, culture was equated with ethnicity. Ethnicity was identified by a code on the client's chart or on the addressograph plate. As the profession became aware of the need to provide for the client holistically, the words **cultural awareness** (knowing about the similarities and differences among cultures) crept into the professional vocabulary. The goal of cultural awareness was to end prejudice and discrimination. In fact, though, awareness often resulted in a focus on differences, without providing the nurse with the tools to meet the culturally related needs of the client.

To break down the barriers among cultures, there was a movement toward **cultural sensitivity** (being aware of the needs and feelings of your own culture and of other cultures). Since the 1990s, a new term has been added. The profession has been talking about **cultural competence**—a set of practice skills, knowledge, and attitudes that must encompass the following elements:

1. Awareness and acceptance of differences
2. Awareness of one's own cultural values
3. Understanding of the dynamics of difference
4. Development of cultural knowledge
5. Ability to adapt practice skills to fit the cultural context of the client.

Now it is time to take the next step past competency to culturally proficient care. For culturally proficient nurses, the five components of cultural care will be second nature. Care for clients will include consideration of their physical, psychosocial, emotional, spiritual, and cultural components.

Development of Transcultural Nursing

The study of transcultural nursing began in the 1950s, when Dr. Madeleine Leininger noted differences in culture among clients and nurses. As she studied cultural differences, she realized that health and illness are influenced by culture. Dr. Leininger's work encouraged a broader awareness of cultural issues (Box 2-1 ■) and led to the study of culture within the nursing curriculum.

Although diversity of population can be one of a country's greatest assets, it also represents a range of health improvement challenges. Nurses need to be prepared to meet the holistic needs of their clients, including those affected by client culture.

One pitfall in communicating with a person from a different culture is ethnocentrism. **Ethnocentrism** means interpreting the beliefs and behavior of others in terms of one's own cultural values and traditions. It assumes that one's own culture is superior. It is difficult to avoid the ten-

---

BOX 2-1	

Events in the History of Cultural Care

1974	Transcultural Nursing Society was established as the official organization of transcultural nursing.
1991	Dr. Leininger published theory of cultural care diversity and universality.
2000	The U.S. Department of Health and Human Services (USDHHS) stated, "*Healthy People 2010* is firmly dedicated to the principle that—regardless of age, gender, race or ethnicity, income, education, geographical location, disability and sexual orientation—every person in every community across the nation deserves equal access to comprehensive, culturally competent, community-based health care systems that are committed to serving the needs of the individual and promoting community health" (USDHHS, 2000).

---

dency toward ethnocentrism. Nurses, though, must be extra diligent to avoid **stereotypes** (oversimplified conceptions, opinions, or beliefs about some aspect of a group of people). Individuals vary greatly within any ethnic group, just as children vary within one family. The nurse must look for ways to care for each client as a unique person, regardless of category.

Theoretical Basis of Transcultural Nursing

Nursing theories base their views on four concepts: nursing, person/client, health, and environment. (See Chapter 4 ◐ for more information on nursing models and theories.) Leininger's cultural care diversity and universality theory (see Table 4-4 ◐) is still the only theory focused specifically on transcultural nursing with a cultural care focus. It is used worldwide today. Leininger's "Sunrise" model is probably the best known of all nursing theories related to culture. Figure 2-1 ■ provides a visual representation of Dr. Leininger's theory.

Leininger's theory can be used with individuals, families, groups, communities, and institutions. Her ideas are important to nursing care today, not only because of the diversity of the healthcare clients, but also because travel and communication have made us a global society. A competent, effective nurse must be aware of his or her feelings and behaviors and must be able to view the client without **prejudice** (prejudgment or bias based on characteristics such as race, age, or gender).

Dorothea Orem's theory (see selected nursing theories in Table 4-4 ◐), which looks at self-care deficits and the client's level of performance of self-care, must be considered

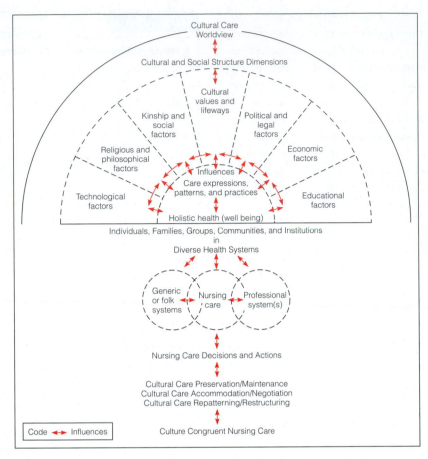

Figure 2-1. ■ Leininger's "Sunrise" model, depicting the cultural care diversity and universality theory. (*Source:* From *Cultural Care Diversity and Universality: A Theory of Nursing,* by M. M. Leininger, 1991, New York: National League for Nursing Press. Reprinted by permission.)

in light of a client's culture. Orem added several observations about cultural issues in nursing. She recognized that some ethnic or cultural groups tend not to seek Western-style health care. They may either try folk remedies or avoid care altogether. In many instances, this can result in a self-care deficit and worsening of the condition. Healthcare professionals and community health educators need to be aware of this resistance and work to provide clients with the skills they need to develop self-care. The lack of access can also be a problem. If individuals have been unable to obtain health care in the past, they may avoid seeking it in the future. This again compounds the health issues.

Larry Purnell and B. J. Paulanka (1998) developed a model for cultural competence that describes 12 domains of culture. This assessment tool identifies ethnocultural attributes of an individual, family, or group. Box 2-2 ■ provides a list of these domains.

In everyday practice as a practical or vocational nurse, you will need to be aware of these domains. You will develop knowledge of different cultures, especially those in the area where you live and work. This should include becoming familiar with the part of the world where those

cultures were established and the heritage of the people. It is also important for you to realize that individuals within a particular culture may have characteristics that don't "fit" their group. It is important not to generalize and stereotype a member of a group (Purnell & Paulanka, 1998).

BOX 2-2

Twelve Domains of Culture

1. Overview, inhabited localities, and topography
2. Communication
3. Family roles and organization
4. Workforce issues
5. Biocultural ecology
6. High-risk health behaviors
7. Nutrition
8. Pregnancy and childbearing practices
9. Death rituals
10. Spirituality
11. Healthcare practices
12. Healthcare practitioners

The American Nurses Association (ANA) has recognized the importance of understanding the concepts of transcultural nursing. Its *Position Statement on Cultural Diversity in Nursing Practice, 1991,* maintains that:

- Cultural assessment of the client is an expected nursing function.
- Sensitive nursing care and appropriate client advocacy cannot be accomplished without knowledge of cultural diversity.

SEGREGATION AND DISCRIMINATION

Segregation (physical separation of housing and services based on race) and **discrimination** (unfair and unequal treatment or access to services based on race, culture, or other bias) have permeated the global community. Although the United States has moved beyond segregation in many areas, there are still inequalities based on lack of access to equal health care. Discrimination, as it relates to health services, can involve more than just race or ethnicity. The nurse must also guard against unequal treatment related to an individual's gender, sexual orientation, or legal status. If a client feels that the nurse is being judgmental because of his or her differences, the therapeutic relationship is compromised.

Culturally Based Communication

Intercultural communication occurs when members of two or more cultures exchange messages in a manner that is influenced by their different cultural perceptions (Adler et al., 1998). Communication is interrelated with all other domains. It includes verbal communication (dialects, the context in which language is used, etc.) and nonverbal communication. Clients may communicate quite differently with family and close friends than with unfamiliar healthcare professionals.

VERBAL COMMUNICATION

One of the first questions that should be asked in any healthcare situation is "What language do you normally use to communicate?" Even though a client may understand English in a casual conversation, he or she may not be able to communicate on the technical level required during a health interview. Healthcare workers need to be aware of the dominant language of an area, as well as problems that may be caused by particular dialects. Clients from Mexico may speak 1 of more than 50 dialects. People from the Philippines may speak 1 of 87. The dialect may pose a communication barrier even if a nurse speaks the same language. Dialect differences increase the difficulty of obtaining accurate information.

NONVERBAL COMMUNICATION

Many times much more is learned from what is not said than from what is said. Nonverbal communication is vital to communicating with clients, but here cultural variations can have a big impact. For example, in Western cultures, people are expected to make eye contact during communication. In other cultures, Asian specifically, making eye contact is a demonstration of lack of respect.

Nurses can learn ways of identifying a particular client's normal behavior. For example, in any culture a client may be reluctant to make eye contact with the health professional when sensitive issues are being discussed. The nurse may wonder whether embarrassment about the topic or cultural behavior is the reason. To assess the situation, the nurse can move to a less sensitive topic and observe the client's response. If the client continues to avoid eye contact, the nurse who is culturally sensitive will be able to interpret such behavior accurately.

Touch can convey much, but again, cultures differ on what they permit and accept. It is important for the nurse to be aware of the client's reaction to touch. During the first contact with a client, the nurse should ask permission to touch the client. When performing a procedure that involves touch, the nurse should fully explain the procedure before touching the client.

Personal space must be respected, both when caring for multicultural clients and when interacting with coworkers. For example, European Americans usually keep a minimum of 18 inches between themselves and the person with whom they are communicating. Middle Easterners tend to stand very close and stare during conversation. A European American nurse who does not know about this difference may feel threatened during a conversation with a Middle Eastern physician. The nurse may feel the physician is invading his or her personal space. Information about cultural norms is important to staff education to preserve a comfortable work environment.

Facial expressions and hand gestures also have different meanings from one culture to another. For example, individuals of Jewish, Hispanic, and Italian heritage rarely smile because showing one's teeth can be viewed as a sign of aggression. A therapeutic relationship can be promoted or hampered by the nurse's understanding of transcultural communication.

Transcultural Communication and Client Concerns

PREVENTING ERRORS AND NONCOMPLIANCE

Transcultural communication is applicable in all healthcare situations. It can help to prevent errors and noncompliance during client teaching. For example, the nurse may tell a mother with limited English to give her child Tylenol (acetaminophen) elixir if the child develops a fever. Medication to lower a fever is the usual intervention in American culture. A mother from an Asian or Latin American culture, however, may view the fever as resulting from an upset of body balance. It is important for the nurse to teach the mother that a fever in a young child can spike very quickly and may even result in a seizure. For this reason, cooling measures and antipyretic medication (like acetaminophen) should be used when the fever reaches 38.3°C (101°F). Besides giving clear and specific instructions, nurses should also make sure instructions are understood before ending the communication.

ENSURING INFORMED CONSENT

Informed consent can also present enormous difficulties. Whenever possible, family members (especially children) should not be used to interpret medical information. Although they may have better English skills than the client, they may be too emotionally involved to give clear information. They may not have the language skills to ensure a clear understanding of the procedures to which the client is consenting. Also, including a family member in discussions can involve violations of confidentiality. Newly instituted Health Insurance Portability and Accountability Act (HIPAA) regulations prevent information from being given to a family member without specific permission from the client. The hospital or healthcare institution must make provisions for maintaining privacy. (See more about HIPAA in Chapter 3 ⬤⬤.)

Many healthcare facilities designate qualified employees to provide translation services. Each unit will have contact information for these individuals. Frequently these staff members are compensated for their skill. Nurses who have the ability to speak, write, or translate another language should provide that information to their facilities' human resources departments.

REDUCING CLIENT STRESS AND ANXIETY

Stress and anxiety are alleviated when there is adequate understanding and communication. Clients whose questions and concerns are addressed in a language with which they are comfortable will be more cooperative, less anxious, and more able to cope with hospitalization than clients who are having communication problems.

PROVIDING CUSTOMER SATISFACTION

Good communication is also important because customer service has become an important part of health care. Health care is a service industry, and clients are increasingly aware consumers. Clients frequently research their disease and the available treatments. When they come for a consultation, they expect to be given all the appropriate information. If information is not given to their satisfaction, they may look elsewhere for care. They may change doctors or refuse to

allow a particular healthcare professional to administer treatment to them. Taking time to communicate effectively on first contact is not wasting time. In fact, it may save time, because corrections will not have to be made. Further, a well-informed client is likely to be more willing to participate in the treatment plan than one who is not well informed.

Subculture of Health Care

No matter how proficient the nurse is in understanding his or her own culture, there is an added barrier to communication. The healthcare profession itself is a kind of subculture, and all nurses are members of it. The subculture of nursing affects the nurse's views and actions, no matter what the culture of origin. A Hispanic nurse may have been raised in an environment where folk medicine, a variety of prayers, poultices, and herbs were used to treat illness. After training, the nurse may view certain health-seeking behaviors of clients as being primitive or even foolish, even when members of the nurse's own family practice those behaviors. The client may treat the nurse as a member of the "establishment" and an oppressor rather than as someone who shares the same background and has experienced the same social treatment. Nurses cannot prevent their education and training from affecting their thinking and perhaps even their cultural values. However, if they have insight into their own changes in thinking, their interactions with clients will be more positive. They will be able to interact with clients with more acceptance and empathy.

Healthcare facilities can provide training and policies to encourage culturally proficient care, but staff attitudes are another important consideration. Facilities must regularly assess staff attitudes and take steps to correct those that hamper the mission of delivering culturally proficient care. Box 2-3 ■ offers some questions for reviewing your own attitudes.

BOX 2-3

Reviewing Your Attitudes Toward Cultural Diversity

- Do you react negatively if the client has an accent?
- Are you open to differences among cultures and different way of doing things?
- Do you respect diverse practices and requests without judgment?
- Do you recognize and actively accommodate clients' choices about their care?
- Do you assume you know the client's wants or needs?
- Do you identify the need for resources to overcome barriers, such as poor or insufficient English proficiency or lack of support networks?
- Do you identify the need for, and obtain knowledge of, sources of extra social support, such as community organizations?

CULTURAL EMPATHY

Cultural empathy involves the ability to experience "as" the client experiences rather than "how" they experience themselves. It is the ability to express genuine interest in the struggles, challenges, and conflicts surrounding the client's health-related problems (Andrews & Boyle, 1999). The nurse has a responsibility to help the client explore his or her feelings, thoughts, and behaviors. It is important to validate the client's feelings and to demonstrate genuine concern. Without these positive actions, the client is not likely to perceive that the nurse cares.

NURSING CARE

Nurses at all levels have the responsibility to deliver culturally proficient care. Because LPNs/LVNs work so closely with clients and families, they carry a large share of this responsibility.

Before nurses can provide proficient transcultural care, they must have an understanding of their own culture. For example, if a nurse discovers that immigrants of his own culture (French) once competed heavily for jobs with Irish immigrants, he might reconsider his "instant dislike" for Irish clients. He may also understand why some of his Irish clients react negatively toward him "for no reason." By recognizing this bias in his culture, the nurse will be able to identify those unhelpful reactions and learn to overcome them.

Both the nurse and the client are influenced by their cultural identity, ethnic history, values, kinship, and family. Illness and stress may cause these aspects of a person's life and cultural, religious, and spiritual beliefs to become more pronounced. Philosophic points of view and moral and ethical perspectives also influence the nurse–client relationship.

ASSESSING

To meet the holistic needs of clients, it is important for the nurse to complete a holistic assessment, not just a physical assessment. This includes information about the client's physical, psychosocial, emotional, and spiritual status, as well as cultural status. It may be necessary to work with an interpreter while completing the assessment. The team leader or RN usually obtains the full assessment, but ongoing assessment requires the same full awareness. Box 2-4 ■ provides guidelines for working with interpreters.

Conducting the Cultural Assessment

Nurses learn general concepts about transcultural nursing and specific facts about various cultures so that we can provide ethical and effective care to all our clients. We must

---

BOX 2-4

Working with Interpreters

- Obtain an interpreter from the facility's designated interpreters list (when available).*
- Avoid using family members.
- Confirm the issue of confidentiality with the interpreter and reassure the client of same.
- Allow additional time for the assessment or interview.
- Brief the interpreter and provide background information prior to the encounter with the client.
- Use simple language and pause between sentences to allow the interpreter to translate every word.
- Talk directly to the client, not the interpreter. The interpreter is just a voice.
- If the client and the interpreter begin to talk to each other, ask for a translation. Do not be left out.
- If possible, use the same interpreter for all such contacts with the client.
- Validate the client's understanding by asking for brief summaries. Important ideas can be lost during translation.
- Encourage the interpreter to inform the nurse of any cultural differences that may lead to misunderstanding or lack of compliance. (Interpreters are usually bicultural as well as bilingual; they can be a source of information about the culture, customs, and worldview of the client.)
- Respect the interpreter's suggestions but do not allow him or her to take over.

A list is usually available through the human resources or social services department.

---

understand how ideas from other cultures agree with or differ from our own. We must be sensitive to issues of race, gender, sexual orientation, social class, and economic situation in our everyday work.

A cultural assessment has four basic elements. These data can be collected by the LPN/LVN.

1. *The cultural identity of the client.* How does the client identify himself or herself culturally? Does the client feel closer to the native culture or to the host culture? What is the client's language preference?

2. *The cultural factors related to the client's psychosocial environment.* What stressors are there in the local environment? What role does religion play in the individual's life? What kind of support systems does the client have?

3. *The cultural elements of the relationship between the healthcare provider and the client.* What kind of experiences has the client had with healthcare providers, either now or in the past? (The nurse should also consider what differences exist between the provider's and the client's culture and social status. These differences are important in communicating and in negotiating an appropriate relationship.)

4. *The cultural explanation of the client's illness.* What is the client's cultural explanation of the illness? What idioms does the client use to describe it? (For example, the client may say she is suffering from *ataque de nervios*—an attack of the nerves. This is a syndrome in Hispanic cultures that closely resembles anxiety and depressive disorders.) Is there a name or category used by the client's family or community to identify the condition? In order for care to be client centered, no matter what culture the client is, the nurse has to elicit specific information from the client and use it to organize strategies for care.

When performing the cultural assessment, the nurse needs to consider many of the cultural domains that were mentioned earlier (see Box 2-2).

Heritage and residence are important. Immigrants commonly relocate to an area where there is an established population of the same background. When individuals settle and work in ethnic communities, their primary social support is enhanced. However, **acculturation** (the modification of a group's or individual's culture as a result of contact with another group) may be hindered. The nurse can increase the opportunities for clients to cooperate in health promotion, health maintenance, and disease prevention by being aware of the geographic location of a cultural group. Communities with large cultural groups may have specific services available to meet their population's healthcare needs while also considering their cultural practices.

Educational status must also be considered. Primary learning styles vary among individuals from different cultures. The nurse adjusts teaching strategies to fit the individual's educational values and modes of learning.

The client's occupation is also of importance. Being knowledgeable about a client's current *work and work history* is essential for health screening. For example, individuals who worked in the mines in their home country may need to be evaluated for respiratory conditions.

Family roles and organization may need to be considered. Dominant family roles determine who will make healthcare decisions. Some cultures (such as Italian and Filipino families) are patriarchal. (No major health decisions would be made without consulting with the male head-of-the-house.) The African American family is primarily matriarchal. European American families are more egalitarian. Family roles also describe gender-related roles of men and women in the family system.

Biocultural ecology involves the assessment of skin color and biologic variations. The skin color may pose special problems or concerns for healthcare professionals. For example, to collect data about anemia in an African American client, the nurse needs to know to assess the oral mucosa.

Nurses must also identify biologic variations in body structure. For example, many Asian children are small by American standards. This must be considered by the nurse when gathering data on a standard growth chart.

The nurse will need to identify *specific risk factors* related to topography or climate. Hereditary or genetic diseases or conditions, as well as endemic diseases specific to a cultural or ethnic group, must be identified. Some groups have an increased susceptibility to certain diseases or health conditions. This knowledge is important for health screening and prevention. Finally, variations in drug metabolism, interaction, and related side effects should be considered.

Assessment should take into consideration specific *high-risk behaviors* that are common among the client's culture of origin. The nurse should explore behaviors related to the use of tobacco, alcohol, and recreational drugs. Healthcare practices, or the client's reluctance to follow safety practices, may provide some essential information. The client should be assessed for the level of physical activity in his or her lifestyle. Clients should also be asked about the use of safety measures, such as seat belts or motorcycle or bike helmets.

Healthcare practices and the use of health practitioners are also part of the cultural assessment. Questions related to *lifespan issues,* specifically pregnancy and childbearing practices and death rituals, can provide vital information. For a complete cultural assessment, the nurse may explore the client's views and practices related to fertility control and pregnancy. Many cultures have prescriptive, restrictive, and taboo practices related to childbearing. These may interfere with instructions given by the healthcare provider. By identifying these issues, the client and the provider can address them while maintaining an open therapeutic relationship. During the cultural assessment, practices related to food, exercise, intercourse, and avoidance of weather-related conditions should also be addressed.

Many nurses may find it uncomfortable to discuss the client's views on *death and dying.* However, this too is a key part of the cultural assessment. It is important for the nurse to understand the mourning practices of cultural groups, so that respect and privacy can be provided for the family. The nurse must also be aware of the client's individual desires. Some may want to talk about the meaning of death, dying, and the afterlife. Others may feel that this is private and not something to be discussed.

Pain Expression

Pain and pain expression are an important area of consideration in nursing. Pain is a universal occurrence. Pain is the most frequent reason for seeking health care, and chronic pain is now the leading cause of disability in the country.

It is difficult to define pain, partly because of its complex nature and partly because of the many different perspectives on pain that exist. The medical definition of pain, established in the late 1800s, is a sensation associated with real or potential tissue damage involving chemical disturbances along neurologic pathways. However, we know that pain is much more. It is a very personal experience. Perception of pain is based on cultural learning, the meaning of the situation, and factors unique to each individual.

Responses to pain culturally have been divided into two categories: *stoic* and *emotive.* Stoic clients are less expressive of their pain and tend to "grin and bear it." They tend to withdraw socially. Emotive clients are more likely to verbalize their expressions of pain. They desire people around to react to their pain and assist them with their suffering. Expressive clients often come from Hispanic, Middle Eastern, and Mediterranean backgrounds. Stoic clients often come from Northern European and Asian backgrounds. However, ethnicity alone does not predict accurately how a person will respond to pain. Some individuals tolerate even the most severe pain with little more than a clenched jaw and frequently refuse pain medication.

Pain has both personal and cultural meanings. It is a subjective and universal experience of human existence that affects individuals of every age and every culture. Pain has physical, emotional, social, and spiritual components. There are vast differences in the expression of pain, and culture plays a major role in these pain experiences. Culture significantly affects the assessment and management of people in pain.

Cultural diversity affects care of the client in pain. The influx of minorities from other countries is predicted to continue, along with the growth of the proportion of minorities within the United States. This changing population means that we as healthcare providers must learn how to respond to pain in a wide range of clients. Cultural background affects pain perception. Cultural background has long been recognized as having a major influence on how one perceives and reacts to painful situations. Pain has both personal and cultural meanings. Although clients from two different cultures may experience a similar condition or surgical procedure, their pain response may differ dramatically. An understanding of pain from a cultural perspective is vital if healthcare providers are to respond to clients in a helpful manner.

Caregivers must also be aware that people within cultural groups may differ biologically from those in other groups. This is true with medications affecting the central nervous system that may be used for pain or symptoms related to pain. Clients with a genetic alteration in a drug-metabolizing enzyme cannot metabolize codeine to morphine properly, so they do not experience an analgesic response. About 5% to 10% of the population does not receive an analgesic effect from codeine.

When treating a client from a different culture, the *client's concern for symptoms* must be treated with as much concern as the actual physical symptoms that are present. People often attribute meaning to their pain. Clients attempt to order the experience of their pain (what it means to them and those close to them) through personal narratives of their illness. These stories are not fixed, but constantly told and retold. In a sense, the narratives not only reflect the pain experience but create it. Key metaphors and rhetorical devices appear to be chosen by the client as a way to make sense of the pain experience.

Nurses' Views about Pain Response

Nursing, medical, and hospital cultures influence pain assessment, decision making, and care. An understanding of the impact of culture on the pain experience is crucial to providing effective care. Because cultural or religious reasons may keep a person from requesting pain medication even when it is medically necessary, it is often best to anticipate a client's pain needs.

DIAGNOSING, PLANNING, AND IMPLEMENTING

The nurse's number one responsibility is to establish an open nurse–client relationship. Nurses must always present themselves as supportive, effective, competent, and empathetic professionals. The nurse–client relationship should be one of respect, genuineness, and warmth. These behaviors constitute the essence of transcultural nursing. If the client gets the impression that the nurse is looking down on him or her, the relationship will be damaged.

The nurse must respect the client as an individual, whether the nurse is meeting the client's physical or psychosocial needs. When the professional loses sight of the individual, stereotyping based on culture can occur. Prejudging a client's needs can place the client in jeopardy. One example of this is related to protocols for breast cancer treatment. A client who has a mixed heritage of African American and Native American will usually be African American in appearance. However, African Americans and Native Americans may have quite different responses to chemotherapeutic drugs. The physician may prescribe treatment according to protocols developed through research with an African American group. The assumption that the client is genetically identical to the research group may lead to unexpected reactions. In this instance, cultural assessment could have provided the physician with valuable information. Collaboration with the RN or the physician on cultural information can be an important function of the LPN/LVN.

Partly as a result of the nursing subculture, nurses often expect people to be objective about a really subjective experience. In clinical practice, the nurse may expect clients to give a detailed description of their pain, and to give the description without displaying an emotional response. When a client complains, cries, or screams, he or she may be labeled as overreacting or having an excessive need for additional medication.

Extensive research has been done about nurses' reactions to clients in pain. Nurses bring their own attitudes about pain to each interaction. It is important for them to identify their beliefs and opinions about pain relief. They should also examine how they express and manage their own pain. Then, they must begin to understand that there is no right or wrong way to express pain. Only when nurses have dealt with their own attitudes about pain will they be able to help their clients who are in pain.

EVALUATING

Discharge planning is also a responsibility of the nurse. Depending on the type of healthcare facility, the LPN/LVN will participate to a greater or lesser degree. Cultural care should continue throughout the nursing process. Points that are considered especially important for clients from diverse cultural backgrounds are listed in Box 2-5 ■.

It is no longer acceptable to treat a client without considering his or her culture throughout the hospital stay. As you work your way through this text, you will find cultural appli-

---

BOX 2-5

Discharge Planning

The nurse should consider the following questions when evaluating discharge planning:

- Do you use an interpreter when necessary to facilitate communication about discharge planning?
- Do you start discharge planning as early as possible in the hospitalization period?
- Do you consider the client's medical and nonmedical needs?
- Do you employ a multidisciplinary approach?
- Do you allow clients and their families to be involved in planning their care?
- Do you check that the clients, family/support people, and care providers fully understand the proposed plan?
- Do you ensure that post-hospital care involves cooperation and collaboration among the hospital, home care agencies, community services, or alternate care facilities?

---

cations in every chapter called "Cultural Pulse Points." They will be found as a box for easy reference.

Technology and travel have expanded our community such that now we are part of a global community. As we develop a fuller understanding of the cultures of the people with whom we come in contact, we as nurses can become more accepting of differences. As we become more accepting, we will be able to provide culturally proficient nursing care.

Note: The references and resources for this and all chapters have been compiled at the back of the book.

Chapter Review

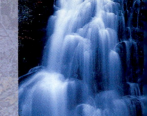

 KEY TERMS by Topic

Use the audio glossary feature of either the CD-ROM or the Companion Website to hear the correct pronunciation of the following key terms.

Introduction
cultural awareness, cultural sensitivity, cultural competence

Development of Transcultural Nursing
ethnocentrism, stereotypes

Theoretical Basis for Transcultural Nursing
prejudice, segregation, discrimination

Culturally Based Communication
intercultural communication

Subculture of Health Care
cultural empathy

Nursing Care
acculturation, biocultural ecology

KEY Points

- The goal of cultural awareness is to end prejudice and discrimination.

- Theories of transcultural nursing, begun by Dr. Madeleine Leininger in the 1950s, are a vital part of nursing care in our diverse society.

- Ethnocentrism is a common tendency. Nurses must be extra careful not to stereotype their clients, because their work depends on their ability to see each client as unique.

- The LPN/LVN will need to develop knowledge of different cultures, especially those that relate to groups where the nurse lives and works.

- Nonverbal communication is vital to communicating with clients. Cultural variations have a big impact on nonverbal communication.

- Transcultural communication is applicable in all healthcare situations. It can help to prevent error and noncompliance during client teaching.

- Whenever possible, family members (especially children) should not be used to interpret medical information.

- A trained nurse may view the health-seeking behaviors of clients as being primitive or even foolish, even when members of the nurse's own family practice those behaviors.

- Healthcare practices and the use of health practitioners are part of the cultural assessment.

 EXPLORE Media Link

Additional interactive resources for this chapter can be found on the Companion Website at www.prenhall.com/ramont. Click on Chapter 2 and "Begin" to select the activities for this chapter.

For chapter-related NCLEX®-style questions and an audio glossary, access the accompanying CD-ROM in this book.

FOR FURTHER Study

For discussion about HIPAA, see Chapter 3.

For more information on Dorothea Orem's theory and other nursing theories, see Chapter 4 (Table 4-4).

NCLEX-PN® Exam Preparation

1 During shift report, the night nurse states, "Maria Sanchez in Room 402 has been yelling all night 'delaude, delaude,' but she doesn't look like she is in pain. You know those people have a very low pain tolerance." The nurse is using:

1. stereotypes.
2. ethnocentrism.
3. acculturation.
4. cultural awareness.

2 The only theory focused specifically on transcultural nursing with a culture care focus was developed by:

1. Dorothea Orem
2. Martha Rogers
3. Madeleine Leininger
4. Betty Neuman

3 Cultural competence encompasses awareness and acceptance of differences, understanding of the dynamics of difference, awareness of one's own cultural values, development of cultural knowledge, and the ability to:

1. communicate in the client's native language.
2. adapt practice skills to fit the cultural context of the client.
3. ignore cultural differences while providing nursing care.
4. provide complementary or alternative health care to culturally diverse clients.

4 The nurse should ask what role religion plays in the client's life. Why is this important to the understanding of a client's culture?

1. When people are seriously ill, they decide it is important to follow the religious practices of their family.
2. The hospital requires that a religious preference be noted on the admission forms.
3. Religious practices vary among cultural groups, especially as they relate to death and dying.
4. The nurse needs to be able to call the appropriate clergy when a client is near death.

5 A Caucasian nurse raised in the American culture and viewing Western medicine as the only option can be said to be:

1. prejudiced.
2. culturally sensitive.
3. ethnocentric.
4. culturally competent.

6 When a nurse makes a statement based on ethnic stereotyping ("Italians have no pain tolerance"), the nurse assumes:

1. all members of an ethnic group are alike.
2. all members of a cultural group have the same health beliefs.
3. commonalities occur among cultures.
4. individuals of specific groups respond to medical treatment differently.

7 An Asian mother brings in her child for follow-up after an ear infection. The physician suggests surgery to place ear tubes. The mother becomes agitated when pushed to schedule surgery. With your knowledge of cultural responses, you determine that:

1. she doesn't understand why the procedure must be done.
2. it is important to consider who has the authority to make healthcare decisions in the family.
3. she is concerned that her health insurance may not pay for the procedure.
4. an interpreter should be provided when consent for surgery is being obtained.

8 A Hispanic mother who had expressed a desire to breast feed is giving her baby a bottle. She states, "I don't have any milk yet. I will breast feed when I get home." From her statement you would conclude the following:

1. She does not understand the importance of colostrum to provide immunity for the baby.
2. She does not understand the concept of supply and demand for milk production.
3. Some cultural groups are extremely modest and are only comfortable breast feeding in private.
4. She really doesn't plan to breast feed. She just feels pressured by the staff to agree to it.

9 A Jewish rabbi in traction refuses your help to eat roast pork, vegetables, roll, and butter and drink a carton of milk. Which statement would be appropriate to encourage him to eat?

1. "It is very important that you have a diet high in protein and calcium in order for your body to heal."
2. "If you don't like the meal they have sent, I can see what else is available."
3. "I know it is difficult to be dependent. Once you are out of traction you will be able to do it on your own."
4. "Do you follow kosher dietary laws? I will have the dietitian speak with you about your special needs."

10 Why might insufficient health information be received if the family interprets for a non-English speaking client?

1. The family members do not understand the medical questions asked.
2. The client does not wish family members to know about her problem.
3. The client is reluctant to answer personal questions.
4. The client feels the nurse will not try to understand her problem because of the language barrier.

Answers and Rationales for Review Questions, as well as discussion of Care Plan and Critical Thinking Care Map questions, appear in Appendix I.

Chapter 3

Legal and Ethical Issues of Nursing

BRIEF Outline

UNDERSTANDING LEGAL ISSUES

Kinds of Legal Actions

Regulation of Nursing Practice

Legal Roles of Nurses

Nursing Responsibilities and Protections

Selected Legal Aspects of Nursing Practice

UNDERSTANDING ETHICAL ISSUES

Ethical Concepts

Moral Concepts

Nursing Ethics

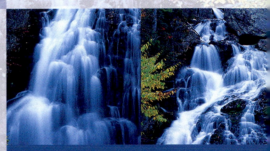

LEARNING Outcomes

After completing this chapter, you will be able to:

1. Differentiate crimes from torts, and give examples in nursing.
2. Define unprofessional conduct: negligence, assault/battery, false imprisonment, invasion of privacy, and defamation.
3. Describe standards of care, agency policies, and nurse practice acts that affect the scope of nursing practice.
4. Describe Good Samaritan acts and the Americans with Disabilities Act.
5. Identify ways nurses and nursing students can minimize their chances of liability and explain the purpose of professional liability insurance.
6. Discuss privileged communication in the nurse–client relationship.
7. Describe the purpose and essential elements of informed consent.
8. List information that needs to be included in an incident report.
9. Explain the uses and limitations of professional codes of ethics.
10. Discuss common legal and ethical issues currently facing healthcare professionals.
11. Discuss the advocacy role of the nurse.

HISTORICAL Perspectives

"That the female head in charge of any building does not think that it is necessary to visit every hole and corner of it everyday. How can she expect those who are under her to be more careful to maintain her house in a healthy condition than she who is in charge of it?" (Nightingale, 1992/1859). Although Nightingale was speaking of managing houses and servants, this quote seems appropriate to the discussion of ethics. Can we expect outside groups to do a better job than the heads of nursing, as well as each nurse individually and collectively, in examining issues of competence?

Nursing practice is governed by many legal concepts. It is important for nurses to know the basics of legal concepts because nurses are accountable for their professional judgments and actions. You must know laws that regulate and affect nursing practice for two reasons:

1. To ensure that your decisions and actions are consistent with current legal principles.
2. To protect you from liability.

UNDERSTANDING LEGAL ISSUES

Law can be defined as "those rules made by humans which regulate social conduct in a formally prescribed and legally binding manner" (Bernzweig, 1996, p. 3).

The law serves a number of functions in nursing:

- It provides a framework for establishing which nursing actions in the care of clients are legal.
- It differentiates the nurse's responsibilities from those of other healthcare professionals.
- It helps establish the boundaries of independent nursing action.
- It assists in maintaining a standard of nursing practice by making nurses accountable under the law.

The regulation of nursing is a function of state law in the United States and of provincial law in Canada. State or provincial legislatures pass statutes that define and regulate nursing, that is, nurse practice acts. These acts, however, must be consistent with constitutional and federal provisions. See Table 3-1 ■ for selected categories of law affecting nurses.

Kinds of Legal Actions

There are two kinds of legal actions: civil or private actions, and criminal actions. Civil actions deal with the relationships among individuals in society. For example, a man may file a suit against a person who he believes cheated him. Civil actions that are of concern to nurses include the contracts and torts listed in Table 3-1. Criminal actions deal with disputes between an individual and the society as a whole. For example, if a man shoots a person, society brings him to trial. The major difference between criminal and civil law is the potential outcome for the defendant. If found guilty in a civil action, such as malpractice, the defendant will have to pay a sum of money. If found guilty in a criminal action, the defendant may lose money, be jailed, or be executed. Nurses could lose their license. The action of a lawsuit is called *litigation,* and lawyers who participate in lawsuits may be referred to as *litigators.*

CIVIL LAW

A **tort** is a civil wrong committed against a person or a person's property. Torts are usually litigated in court by civil action between individuals. In other words, the person or persons claimed to be responsible for the tort are sued for damages. Tort liability almost always is based on fault, that is, something was done incorrectly (an unreasonable act of commission) or something should have been done but was not (an act of omission).

Torts may be classified as unintentional or intentional.

Unintentional Torts

Negligence and malpractice are examples of unintentional torts that may occur in the healthcare setting. **Negligence** is misconduct or practice that is below the standard expected of an ordinary, reasonable, and prudent practitioner, which places another person at risk for harm. Gross negligence

TABLE 3-1	
Selected Categories of Laws Affecting Nurses	
CATEGORY	**EXAMPLES**
Constitutional	Due process
	Equal protection
Statutory (legislative)	Nurse practice acts
	Good Samaritan acts
	Child and adult abuse laws
	Living wills
	Sexual harassment laws
	Americans with Disabilities Act
Criminal (public)	Homicide, manslaughter
	Theft
	Arson
	Active euthanasia
	Sexual assault
	Illegal possession of controlled drugs
Contracts (private/civil)	Nurse and client
	Nurse and employer
	Nurse and insurance
	Client and agency
Torts (private/civil)	Negligence
	Assault and battery
	False imprisonment
	Invasion of privacy
	Libel and slander

involves an extreme lack of knowledge, skill, or decision making. The person clearly should have known that such behavior would put clients at risk for harm. **Malpractice** is negligence that occurred while the person was performing as a professional. Malpractice applies to physicians, dentists, lawyers, and, in some cases, nurses. Four elements must be present for a case of nursing negligence or malpractice to be proven:

1. The nurse has a working relationship with the client (duty).
2. The nurse fails to uphold the appropriate standard of care (breach).
3. The client must have suffered harm, injury, or damage (harm).
4. The harm has to be a direct result of the nurse's failure to provide appropriate care (causation).

If a lawsuit is filed for a negligent act performed by a nurse, it will also name the nurse's employer. In addition, employers may be held liable for negligence if they fail to provide adequate human and material resources for nursing care, to properly educate nurses on the use of new equipment or procedures, or to orient nurses to the facility. Sometimes the harm cannot be traced to a specific healthcare provider or standard but does not normally occur unless there has been a negligent act. An example is harm that results when surgical instruments or sponges are accidentally left in a client during surgery.

To defend against a negligence suit, the nurse must prove that one or more of the required elements is not met. There is also a limit to the amount of time that can pass between recognition of harm and the bringing of a suit. This is referred to as the **statute of limitations**. In some cases, an additional defense is "contributory or comparative negligence" on the part of the injured client. In these situations, the client was at least partly responsible for his or her own injury. When clients choose not to follow healthcare advice, such as remaining in bed while recovering from a treatment, the court may reduce any verdict against the nurse by an amount considered to be the plaintiff's own contribution.

To avoid charges of malpractice, nurses need to recognize those nursing situations in which negligent actions are most likely to occur and to take measures to prevent them (Box 3-1 ■). The most common situation is the medication error. Because of the large number of medications on the market today and the variety of methods of administration, these errors may be on the increase. Nurses always need to check medications very carefully (see Chapter 29 ⬀). Even after checking, the nurse is wise to recheck the medication order and the medication before administering it if the client states, for example, "I did not have a green pill before."

A relatively frequent malpractice action attributed to nurses is causing a burn to a client. Elderly, comatose, and

---

> ## BOX 3-1
>
> ### Basic Nursing Care Errors Resulting in Negligence
>
> #### Assessment Errors
> Failing to
> - Gather and chart client information adequately.
> - Recognize the significance of certain information (e.g., laboratory values, vital signs).
>
> #### Planning Errors
> Failing to
> - Chart each identified problem.
> - Use language in the care plan that other caregivers understand.
> - Ensure continuity of care by ignoring the care plan.
> - Give discharge instructions that the client understands.
>
> #### Intervention Errors
> Failing to
> - Administer and document medications correctly.
> - Interpret and carry out a doctor's orders.
> - Perform nursing tasks correctly.
> - Pursue the physician if the doctor doesn't respond to calls or notify the nurse-manager if the physician is unavailable.

---

diabetic people are particularly vulnerable to burns because of their decreased sensitivity to pain and temperature. Hot objects can burn these people before they notice it.

Clients often fall accidentally, sometimes with resultant injury. Some falls can be prevented by elevating the side rails on the cribs, beds, and stretchers of babies and small children and, when necessary, of adults. If a nurse leaves the rails down or leaves a baby unattended on a bath table, that nurse is guilty of malpractice if the client falls and is injured as a direct result. The nurse needs to follow facility policies regarding side rails and injury prevention. Information about providing a safe environment for the client can be found in Chapter 8 ⬀.

In some instances, ignoring a client's complaints can constitute malpractice. This type of malpractice is termed *failure to observe and take appropriate action.* If a nurse does not report a client's complaint of acute abdominal pain and the client sustains a ruptured appendix, the nurse is negligent and may be found guilty of malpractice. If a nurse fails to check vital signs and the dressing of a client who has just had surgery, important assessments are omitted. If the client hemorrhages and dies, the nurse may be held responsible for the death as a result of this malpractice.

Incorrectly identifying clients is a problem, particularly in busy hospital units. Failure to check identification bands before administering medication can result in injury to the client if the medication is given to the wrong person. Checking the medication administration record (MAR) against the armband at the bedside every time can prevent cases of mistaken identity, which are costly to the client and render the nurse liable for malpractice.

Intentional Torts

In the United States, the terms *assault* and *battery* are often heard together, but each has its own meaning. **Assault** can be described as an attempt or threat to touch another person unjustifiably. Assault precedes battery; it is the act that causes the person to believe a battery is about to occur. For example, the person who threatens someone by making a menacing gesture with a club or a closed fist is guilty of assault. In nursing, a nurse who threatens a client with an injection after the client refuses to take the medication orally would be committing assault.

Battery is the willful touching of a person (or the person's clothes, or even something the person is carrying) that may or may not cause harm. To be illegal, however, the touching must be wrong in some way. For example, it must be done without permission, be embarrassing, or cause injury. In the previous example, if the nurse followed through on the threat and gave the injection without the client's consent, the nurse would be committing battery. Even though the physician ordered the medication and even if the client benefits from the administration of the medication, the nurse is still liable.

In Canada, the term *battery* is not used. Instead, there are three categories of assault: assault with intent to injure (e.g., threatening someone with a knife), assault causing bodily injury, and sexual assault.

To perform procedures without consent is considered battery. (See discussion on informed consent later in this chapter.)

False imprisonment is the "unlawful restraint or detention of another person against his or her wishes." False imprisonment does not require force; the fear of force to restrain or detain the individual is sufficient (Bernzweig, 1996). False imprisonment accompanied by forceful restraint or threat of restraint is battery.

Nurses may suggest under certain circumstances that a client remain in the hospital room or in bed, but the client must not be detained against the client's will. The client has a right to insist on leaving, even though it may be detrimental to his or her health. The client can leave by signing an absence without authority (AWA) or against medical advice (AMA) form. As with assault or battery, client competency is a factor in determining whether there is a case of false imprisonment or a situation of protecting a client from injury. Agencies usually have clear policies about the application of restraints to guide nurses in such dilemmas. See Chapter 8 ⚭ for information about restraints.

Invasion of privacy is a direct wrong of a personal nature that injures the feelings of the person and does not take into account the effect of revealed information on the standing of the person in the community. Privacy is the right of individuals to withhold themselves and their lives from public scrutiny, or the right to be left alone. Liability can result if the nurse breaches confidentiality by passing along confidential client information to others or by intruding into the client's private domain.

Necessary discussion about a client's medical condition is usually considered appropriate, but unnecessary discussions and gossip are considered a breach of confidentiality. Necessary discussion involves only those people engaged in the client's care. Four major categories of confidential client information must be reported: (1) vital statistics, such as births and deaths; (2) infections and communicable diseases, such as syphilis; (3) child or elder abuse; and (4) violent incidents, such as knife wounds. As of April 14, 2003, healthcare agencies and providers must adhere to the Health Insurance Portability and Accountability Act of 1996 (HIPAA). See Chapter 7 ⚭ for HIPAA guidelines.

False Communication

Defamation is communication that is false, or made with a careless disregard for the truth, and that results in injury to the reputation of a person. Both libel and slander are wrongful actions that come under the heading of defamation. **Libel** is defamation by means of print, writing, or pictures. Writing in the nurse's notes that a physician is incompetent because he didn't respond immediately to a call is an example of libel. **Slander** is defamation by the spoken word, stating information or false words that can cause damage to a person's reputation. An example of slander would be for the nurse to tell a client that another nurse is incompetent.

If a comment that criticizes a person's competence is made to that person in private, it is not defamation because a third party did not hear it. It is slander only if the comment is communicated to a third party.

Nurses are allowed to make statements that could be considered defamatory, but only as a part of nursing practice and only to a physician or another healthcare team member caring directly for the client, for example, "The client exhibits inappropriate sexual behavior."

Loss of Client Property

Client property, such as jewelry, money, eyeglasses, and dentures, is a constant concern to hospital personnel. Today, agencies are taking less responsibility for property and are generally requesting clients to sign a waiver on admission relieving the hospital and its employees of any responsibility for property. Situations arise, however, in which the client cannot sign a waiver and the nursing staff must follow prescribed policies for safeguarding the client's property (see Chapter 10 ⚭). Nurses are expected to take reasonable precautions to safeguard a client's property, and they can be held liable for its loss or damage if they do not exercise reasonable care.

CRIMINAL LAW

A **crime** is an act committed in violation of public (criminal) law and punishable by a fine or imprisonment. A crime does not have to be intended in order to be a crime. For example, a nurse may commit a crime by accidentally giving a client an additional and lethal dose of a narcotic to relieve discomfort.

Crimes are classified as either felonies (or in Canada, indictable offenses) or misdemeanors (or in Canada, summary conviction offenses). Crimes are punished through criminal action by the state or province against an individual. A *felony* is a crime of a serious nature, such as murder, punishable by a term in prison. In some areas, second-degree murder is called *manslaughter*. A nurse who accidentally gives an additional and lethal dose of a narcotic can be accused of manslaughter.

A *misdemeanor* is a less serious offense than a felony and is usually punishable by a fine, a short-term jail sentence, or both. A nurse who slaps a client's face could be charged with a misdemeanor.

Regulation of Nursing Practice

CREDENTIALING

Credentialing is the process of determining and maintaining competence in nursing practice. The credentialing process is one way in which the nursing profession maintains standards of practice and accountability for the educational preparation of its members. Credentialing includes licensure, registration, certification, and accreditation.

Licensure and Registration

There are two types of licensure and registration: mandatory and permissive. In the United States, nursing licensure is mandatory in all states. In Canada, permissive licensure and registration are allowed in some provinces, which means that people who are not licensed or registered can perform nursing duties. Note, however, that licensure and registration are mandatory in most Canadian provinces.

A nurse in any state or province can have his or her license revoked for just cause. These causes are defined in the nurse practice acts. They include incompetent nursing practice, professional misconduct, and conviction of a crime such as using illegal drugs or selling drugs illegally. In each situation, all of the facts are generally reviewed by a committee at a hearing. Nurses are entitled to be represented by legal counsel at such a hearing. If the nurse's license is revoked as a result of the hearing, either the nurse can appeal the decision to a court of law or, in some states, an agency is designated to review the decision before any court action is initiated.

Certification

Most certifications are awarded to advanced practice nurses. However, an LPN/LVN can be certified in long-term care and IV therapy through the National Federation of Licensed Practical Nurses (NFLPN).

Accreditation/Approval of Basic Nursing Education Programs

Accreditation is a process by which a private organization, such as the National League for Nursing, or a governmental agency, such as the state board of nursing, appraises and grants accredited status to institutions, programs, or services that meet predetermined standards. Minimum standards for basic nursing education programs are established in each state of the United States and in each province in Canada. State accreditation or provincial approval is granted to schools of nursing that meet the minimum criteria.

NURSE PRACTICE ACTS

Each state in the United States has a nurse practice act, and each province in Canada has a nurse practice act or an act for professional nursing practice. Nurse practice acts legally define and describe the scope of nursing practice, which the law seeks to regulate, thereby protecting the public as well. See the website of the National Council of State Boards of Nursing for more information. State boards of nursing also have Internet websites that provide valuable information on the nurse practice acts and scope of practice for the LPN/LVN.

STANDARDS OF PRACTICE

Another way the nursing profession attempts to ensure that its practitioners are competent and safe to practice is through the establishment of standards of practice. These standards are often used to evaluate the quality of care nurses provide. Standards of practice for the LPN/LVN are outlined in the **scope of practice**, a document developed by the board of nursing that governs practice within each state.

Legal Roles of Nurses

Nurses have three separate, interdependent legal roles, each with rights and associated responsibilities: provider of service, employee or contractor for service, and citizen. As the nurse carries out these roles, the issue of liability must be considered. **Liability** means being legally responsible for one's acts and omissions. When a nurse carries out treatments ordered by the physician, the responsibility for the nursing activity is the nurse's. When a nurse is asked to carry out an activity that the nurse believes could injure the client, the nurse's legal responsibility is to refuse to carry out the order and report this to the nurse's supervisor.

PROVIDER OF SERVICE

The nurse is expected to provide safe and competent care so that harm (physical, psychological, or material) to the recipient of the service is prevented.

EMPLOYEE OR CONTRACTOR FOR SERVICE

A nurse who is employed by an agency works as a representative of the agency. A nurse who is employed directly by a client, for example, a private nurse, may have a written contract with that client to provide professional services for a certain fee. If the nurse becomes ill or dies and cannot fulfill the contract, that is understood. But if a nurse does not fulfill the contract because his or her car broke down or because of personal problems, the nurse broke the contract.

A nurse employed by a hospital functions within an employer–employee relationship, in which the nurse represents and acts for the hospital and therefore must function within the policies of the employing agency. The employer assumes responsibility for the conduct of the employee and can also be held responsible for malpractice by the employee. The nurse's conduct, therefore, is the hospital's responsibility.

This does not mean that the nurse cannot be held liable as an individual. If the employee's actions are extraordinarily inappropriate, the employer might not be held liable. For example, if a nurse hits a client in the face, the employer would not be responsible because this behavior is inappropriate. Criminal acts, such as assisting with criminal abortions or taking drugs from a client's supply for personal use, would also be considered extraordinarily inappropriate behavior. Nurses can be held liable for failure to act as well. For example, a nurse who sees another nurse hitting a client and fails to do anything to protect the client may be considered negligent.

The nurse has obligations to the employer, the client, and other personnel. Nurses must give appropriate care and perform only those responsibilities that they are competent to perform.

The nurse is expected to respect the rights and responsibilities of other healthcare team members. For example, the nurse explains nursing activities to a client but does not have the right to comment on the client's medical care in a way that disturbs the client or criticizes the physician. The nurse also has the right to expect reasonable and prudent conduct from other healthcare professionals.

Collective Bargaining

Collective bargaining is the formalized decision-making process between representatives of management and representatives of labor to negotiate wages and conditions of employment, including work hours, working environment, and fringe benefits of employment (e.g., vacation time, sick leave, and personal leave). Through a written agreement, both employer and employees legally commit themselves to observe the terms and conditions of employment.

When collective bargaining breaks down because an agreement cannot be reached, the employees usually call a strike. A *strike* is an organized work stoppage by a group of employees to express a grievance, enforce a demand for changes in conditions of employment, or solve a dispute with management.

Because nursing practice is a service to people (often ill people), striking presents a moral dilemma to many nurses. Actions taken by nurses can affect the safety of people. When faced with a strike, each nurse must make an individual decision to cross or not to cross a picket line.

Arbitration (an agreement negotiated by a designated impartial person) may be required to prevent a strike or to settle a strike.

CITIZEN

The rights and responsibilities of the nurse in the role of citizen are the same as those of any individual under the legal system. Nurses move in and out of these roles when carrying out professional and personal responsibilities.

Nursing Responsibilities and Protections

GOOD SAMARITAN ACTS

Good Samaritan acts are laws designed to protect healthcare providers who provide assistance at the scene of an emergency against claims of malpractice unless it can be shown that there was a gross departure from the normal standard of care or willful wrongdoing on their part. Gross negligence usually involves further injury or harm to the person. For example, an injured child left on the side of the road may be struck by an automobile when the nurse leaves to obtain help.

In the United States, most state statutes do not require citizens to render aid to people in distress. Such assistance is considered more of an ethical than a legal duty. A few states and provinces, however, have enacted legislation that requires people to stop and aid persons in danger (Fletcher, 1996, p. 139). In Canada, some provinces specify that it is the responsibility of people to give aid at the scene of an emergency.

To encourage citizens to be "Good Samaritans," most states have now enacted legislation releasing a Good Samaritan from legal liability for injuries caused under such circumstances, even if the injuries resulted from negligence of the person offering emergency aid.

It is generally believed that a person who renders help in an emergency, at a level that would be provided by any reasonably prudent person under similar circumstances, cannot be held liable. The same reasoning applies to nurses, who are among the people best prepared to help at an emergency scene. If the level of care a nurse provides is of the caliber that would have been provided by any other nurse, then the nurse will not be held liable. Guidelines for nurses who choose to render emergency care are:

- Limit actions to those normally considered first aid if possible.
- Do not perform actions that you do not know how to do.
- Offer assistance, but do not insist.
- Do not leave the scene until the injured person leaves or another qualified person takes over.

PROFESSIONAL LIABILITY INSURANCE

Because of the increase in the number of malpractice lawsuits against health professionals, nurses are advised in many areas to carry their own liability insurance. Most hospitals have liability insurance that covers all employees, including all nurses. However, some smaller facilities, such as "walk-in" clinics, may not. Thus the nurse should always check with the employer at the time of hiring to see what coverage the facility provides. A physician or a hospital can be sued because of the negligent conduct of a nurse, and the nurse can also be sued and held liable for negligence or malpractice. Because hospitals have been known to countersue nurses when they have been found negligent and the hospital was required to pay, nurses are advised to provide their own insurance coverage and not rely on hospital-provided insurance.

Additionally, nurses often provide nursing services outside of employment-related activities, such as being available for first aid at children's sport or social activities or providing health screening and education at health fairs. Neighbors or friends may seek advice about illnesses or treatment for themselves or family members. In such situations, the nurse may be tempted to give advice, but it is always advisable for the nurse to refer the friend or neighbor to the family physician. The nurse may be protected from liability under Good Samaritan acts when nursing service is volunteered. However, if the nurse receives any compensation or if there is a written or verbal agreement outlining the nurse's responsibility to the group, the nurse needs liability coverage to cover legal expenses in the event that the nurse is sued.

Students and teachers of nursing are unlikely to be covered by the insurance carried by hospitals and health agencies. It is advisable for them to check with their school about the coverage that applies to them. In some states, hospitals do not allow nursing students to provide nursing care without liability insurance.

NURSES AS WITNESSES

A nurse may be called to testify in a legal action for a variety of reasons. The nurse may be a defendant in a malpractice or negligence action or may have been a member of the healthcare team that provided care to the plaintiff. If a nurse is going to testify, he or she should consult an attorney first. If the action is against the nurse's employer, the same attorney will assist the nurse. If the action is against the nurse, he or she should retain a separate attorney.

A nurse may also be asked to provide testimony as an expert witness. An *expert witness* has special training, experience, or skill and offers an opinion on some issue within the nurse's area of expertise. Nurses usually are called to help a judge or jury understand evidence pertaining to the extent of damage or the standard of care.

STUDENT NURSES

Nursing students are responsible for their own actions and liable for their own acts of negligence committed during the course of clinical experiences. When they perform duties that are within the scope of professional nursing, such as administering an injection, they are legally held to the same standard of skill and competence as a licensed nurse. Lower standards are not applied to the actions of nursing students.

Students in clinical situations must be assigned activity within their capabilities and be given reasonable guidance and supervision. Nursing instructors are responsible for assigning students to the care of clients and for providing reasonable supervision.

To fulfill responsibilities to clients and to minimize chances for liability, nursing students need to:

- Make sure they are prepared to carry out the necessary care for assigned clients.
- Ask for additional help or supervision in situations for which they feel inadequately prepared.
- Comply with the policies of the agency in which they obtain their clinical experience.
- Comply with the policies and definitions of responsibility supplied by the school of nursing.

Students who work as part-time or temporary nursing assistants or aides must also remember that legally they can perform only those tasks that appear in the job description of a nurse's aide or assistant. Even though a student may have received instruction and acquired competence in administering injections or suctioning a tracheostomy tube, the student cannot legally perform these tasks while employed as an aide or assistant. While acting as a paid worker, the student is covered for negligent acts by the employer, not the school of nursing.

Selected Legal Aspects of Nursing Practice

PRIVILEGED COMMUNICATION

A *privileged communication* is information given to a professional person who is forbidden by law from disclosing the information in a court without the consent of the person who provided it. See the earlier discussion of invasion of privacy.

Legislation regarding privileged communications is highly complicated. Many states with statutes granting privileged communications among the client and various healthcare providers do not extend the privilege to nurse–client communication.

INFORMED CONSENT

Informed consent is an agreement by a client to accept a course of treatment or a procedure after complete information has been provided by a healthcare provider. Information includes the risks of the treatment and facts relating to it. Usually, the client signs a form provided by the agency. The form is a record of the informed consent, not the informed consent itself.

Obtaining informed consent for specific medical and surgical treatments is the responsibility of a physician. This responsibility is delegated to nurses in some agencies, and no laws prohibit the nurse from being part of the information-giving process. However, it is not appropriate for the nurse to obtain informed consent.

Witnessing Informed Consent

Often, the nurse's responsibility is to witness the giving of informed consent for medical procedures. This involves the following:

- Witnessing the exchange between the client and the physician.
- Establishing that the client really did understand, that is, was really informed.
- Witnessing the client's signature.

If a nurse witnesses only the client's signature and not the exchange between the client and the physician, the nurse should write "witnessing signature only" on the form. If the nurse finds that the client really does not understand the physician's explanation, then the physician must be notified.

Obtaining informed consent for nursing procedures is the responsibility of nurses when they perform direct care such as insertion of nasogastric tubes or medication administration.

It can be a challenge to determine the amount and type of information required for the client to make an informed decision. General guidelines include:

- The purposes of the treatment
- What the client can expect to feel or experience
- The intended benefits of the treatment
- Possible risks or negative outcomes of the treatment
- Advantages and disadvantages of possible alternatives to the treatment (including no treatment).

There are three major elements of informed consent:

1. The consent must be given voluntarily.
2. The client must have the capacity and competence to understand.
3. The client must be given enough information to be the ultimate decision maker.

To give informed consent voluntarily, the client must not feel coerced. Sometimes fear of disapproval by a health professional can be the reason the client gives consent. Such consent is not voluntarily given.

Technical words and language barriers can keep clients from understanding information about the procedure. If a client cannot read, the consent form must be read to the client before it is signed. If the client does not speak the same language as the health professional who is giving the information, an interpreter must be provided.

A client who is confused, disoriented, or sedated is not considered functionally competent (able to understand and give informed consent).

Ensuring informed consent is also important when providing nursing care in the home. Because home care often occurs over an extended period of time, the nurse has many opportunities to ensure that the plan of treatment is accepted.

Exceptions

Three groups of people cannot provide consent. The first is a dependent child, under the age of 18 (minor). In most areas, a parent or guardian must give consent before minors can obtain treatment. Adults who have the mental capacity of a child and who have an appointed guardian also fall into this category. There are some exceptions. Some states allow minors to give consent for such procedures as blood donations, treatment for drug dependence and sexually transmitted infections, and procedures for obstetric care. Minors who are married, pregnant, parents, members of the military, or emancipated (living on their own) may be legally allowed to give their own consent. These statutes may vary by state or province.

The second group includes persons who are unconscious or injured so that they are unable to give consent. In these situations, consent is usually obtained from the closest adult relative if existing statutes permit. In a life-threatening emergency, if consent cannot be obtained from the client or a relative, the law generally agrees that consent is implied (agreed to).

The third group consists of people with mental illnesses who have been judged by professionals to be incompetent. State and provincial mental health acts or similar statutes generally provide definitions of mental illness and specify the rights of the mentally ill under the law as well as the rights of the staff caring for such clients.

CARRYING OUT PHYSICIANS' ORDERS

Nurses are expected to analyze procedures and medications ordered by the physician. It is the nurse's responsibility to seek clarification of ambiguous or seemingly erroneous orders from the prescribing physician. Clarification from any other source is unacceptable and regarded as a departure from competent nursing practice.

There are several categories of orders that nurses must question to protect themselves legally:

- Question any order a client questions. For example, if a client who has been receiving an intramuscular injection tells the nurse that the doctor changed the order from an injectable to an oral medication, the nurse should recheck the order before giving the medication.
- Question any order if the client's condition has changed. The nurse is considered responsible for notifying the physician of any significant changes in the client's condition, whether the physician requests notification or not. For example, if a client who is receiving an intravenous infusion suddenly develops a rapid pulse, chest pain, and a cough, the nurse must notify the physician immediately and question continuance of the ordered rate of infusion.
- Question and record verbal orders to avoid miscommunications. In addition to recording the time, the date, the physician's name, and the orders, the nurse documents the circumstances that occasioned the call to the physician, reads the orders back to the physician, and documents that the physician confirmed the orders as the nurse read them back.
- Question any order that is illegible, unclear, or incomplete. Misinterpretations in the name of a drug or in dose, for example, can easily occur with handwritten orders. The nurse is responsible for ensuring that the order is interpreted the way it was intended and that it is a safe and appropriate order.

PROVIDING COMPETENT NURSING CARE

Competent practice is a major legal safeguard for nurses. Nurses need to provide care that is within the legal boundaries of their practice and within the boundaries of agency policies and procedures. Nurses, therefore, must be familiar with their various job descriptions, which may be different from agency to agency. All nurses are responsible for ensuring that their various education and experience are adequate to meet the responsibilities delineated in their job descriptions.

Competency also involves care that protects clients from harm. Nurses need to anticipate sources of client injury, educate clients about hazards, and implement measures to prevent injury.

Application of the nursing process is another essential aspect of providing safe and effective client care. Clients need to be assessed and monitored appropriately and involved in care decisions. All assessments and care must be documented accurately. Effective communication can also protect the nurse from negligence claims. Nurses need to approach every client with sincere concern and include the client in conversations. In addition, nurses should always acknowledge when they do not know the answer to a client's questions, tell the client they will find out the answer, and then follow through.

Methods of legal protection for nurses are summarized in Box 3-2 ■.

RECORD KEEPING

The client's medical record is a legal document and can be produced in court as evidence. Often, the record is used to remind a witness of events surrounding a lawsuit, because several months or years can elapse before a suit goes to trial. The effectiveness of a witness's testimony can depend on the accuracy of such records. Nurses, therefore, need to keep accurate and complete records of nursing care provided to clients. Failure to keep proper records can constitute negligence and be the basis for tort liability. Insufficient or inaccurate assessments and documentation can hinder proper diagnosis and treatment and result in injury to the client. See Chapter 6 🔗 for types of records and facts about recording.

THE INCIDENT REPORT

An incident report is an agency record of an accident or unusual occurrence. Incident reports are used to make all the facts available to agency personnel, to contribute to statistical data about injuries or incidents, and to help healthcare personnel prevent future incidents or injuries. All injuries are usually reported on incident forms. Some agencies also report other incidents, such as the occurrence of client infection or the loss of personal effects. Box 3-3 ■ lists the information to be included in an incident report. The report should be completed as soon as possible and filed according to agency policy. Because incident reports are not part of the client's medical record, the facts of the incident should also be noted in the medical record. Do not record in the client record that an incident report has been completed.

The incident report should be completed by the person who identifies that the incident occurred. This may not be the same person actually involved with the incident. For example, the nurse who discovers that an incorrect medication has been administered completes the form even if it was another nurse who administered the medication. In addition, all witnesses to an incident, such as a client fall, are listed on the incident form even if they were not directly involved.

Incident reports are often reviewed by an agency risk management committee, which decides whether to investigate the incident further. Nurses may be required to answer questions such as what they believe precipitated the incident, how it could have been prevented, and whether any equipment should be adjusted. Incident reports are discussed further in Chapter 36 🔗.

REPORTING CRIMES, TORTS, AND UNSAFE PRACTICES

Nurses may need to report nursing colleagues or other health professionals for practices that endanger the health and safety of clients. For instance, alcohol and drug use, theft from a

---

BOX 3-2 **NURSING CARE CHECKLIST**

Legal Precautions for Nurses

☑ Function within the scope of your education, job description, and area nurse practice act. This enables you to function within the scope of the description and know what is and what is not expected.

☑ Follow the procedures and policies of the employing agency.

☑ Build and maintain good rapport with clients. Keeping clients informed about diagnostic and treatment plans, giving feedback on their progress, and showing concern for the outcome of their care prevent a sense of powerlessness and a buildup of hostility in the client.

☑ Always identify clients, particularly before initiating major interventions (e.g., surgical or other invasive procedures or when administering medications or blood transfusions).

☑ Observe and monitor the client accurately. Communicate and record significant changes in the client's condition to the physician.

☑ Promptly and accurately document all assessments and care given. Records must show that the nurse provided and supervised the client's care daily.

☑ Be alert when implementing nursing interventions and give each task your full attention and skill.

☑ Perform procedures appropriately. Negligent incidents during procedures generally relate to equipment failure, improper technique, and improper performance of the procedure. For instance, the nurse must know how to

safeguard the client in the event that a respirator or other equipment fails.

☑ Make sure the correct medications are given in the correct dose, by the right route, at the scheduled time, and to the right client. See Chapter 29 ⚭ for more detailed information about the administration of medications.

☑ When delegating nursing responsibilities, make sure that the person who is delegated a task understands what to do and that the person has the required knowledge and skill. As the delegating nurse, you can be held liable for harm caused by the person to whom the care was delegated.

☑ Protect clients from injury. Inform clients of hazards and use appropriate safety devices and measures to prevent falls, burns, or other injuries.

☑ Report all incidents involving clients. Prompt reporting enables those responsible to attend to the client's well-being, to analyze why the incident occurred, and to prevent recurrences.

☑ Always check any order that a client questions and ensure that verbal orders are accurate and documented appropriately. Question and confirm standing orders if you are inexperienced in a particular area.

☑ Know your own strengths and weaknesses. Ask for assistance and supervision in situations for which you feel inadequately prepared.

☑ Maintain your clinical competence. For students, this demands study and practice before caring for clients. For graduate nurses, it means continued study, including maintaining and updating clinical knowledge and skills.

---

client or agency, and unsafe nursing practice should be reported. Reporting a colleague is not easy. The person reporting may feel disloyal, incur the disapproval of others, or perceive that chances for promotion are endangered. When reporting an incident or series of incidents, the nurse must be careful to describe observed behavior only and not make inferences as to what might be happening. Reporting these events is referred to as *whistle-blowing*. Many states have laws that prevent wrongful termination of whistle-blowers by employers. Reporting illegal, unethical, or incompetent performance is an expectation found in the code of ethics of the NFLPN.

AMERICANS WITH DISABILITIES ACT

The Americans with Disabilities Act (ADA), passed by the U.S. Congress in 1990 and fully implemented in 1994, prohibits discrimination on the basis of disability in employment, public services, and public accommodations. The purposes of the act are:

- To provide a clear and comprehensive national mandate for eliminating discrimination against individuals with disabilities.

- To provide clear, strong, consistent, enforceable standards addressing discrimination against individuals with disabilities.

- To ensure that the federal government plays a central role in enforcing standards established under the act.

BOX 3-3

Information to Include in an Incident Report

- Identify the client by name, initials, and hospital or identification number.
- Give the date, time, and place of the incident.
- Describe the facts of the incident. Avoid any conclusions or blame. Describe the incident as you saw it even if your impressions differ from those of others.
- Identify all witnesses to the incident.
- Identify any equipment by number and any medication by name and number.
- Document any circumstance surrounding the incident, for example, that another client was experiencing cardiac arrest.

An employer may not refuse to hire a nurse with disabilities if the nurse is able to fulfill the duties of the work role. The ADA also enables individuals of normal intelligence who have a physical or learning disability to pursue a nursing curriculum through alternative learning methods.

CONTROLLED SUBSTANCES

Laws in the United States and Canada regulate the distribution and use of controlled substances such as narcotics, depressants, stimulants, and hallucinogens. Misuse of controlled substances leads to criminal penalties. See Chapter 29 🔗 for the legal aspects of drug administration.

The Impaired Nurse

The term **impaired nurse** refers to a nurse whose practice has been negatively affected because of chemical abuse, specifically the use of alcohol and drugs. Chemical dependence in healthcare workers has become a problem because of the high levels of stress involved in many healthcare settings and the easy access to addictive drugs. Substance abuse is the most common reason for actions against nurses' licenses. Between 10% and 15% of nurses are estimated to be chemically impaired. This is about the same percentage as in the general population. Employers must have sound policies and procedures for identifying situations that involve a possibly impaired nurse. Intervention in such situations is important to protect clients and to get treatment for the impaired nurse quickly.

A variety of programs have been developed to assist impaired nurses to recover. In many states, impaired nurses who enter an intervention program for treatment (diversion program) are closely supervised and restricted in practice, but do not have to surrender their nursing license.

SEXUAL HARASSMENT

Sexual harassment is a violation of the individual's rights and a form of discrimination. In 1987, the law prohibiting sexual discrimination was clarified to apply to all educational and employing institutions receiving federal funding. The Equal Employment Opportunity Commission (EEOC) defines sexual harassment as "unwelcome sexual advances, requests for sexual favors, and other verbal or physical conduct of a sexual nature" occurring in the following circumstances (EEOC, 1980, sections 3950.10–3950.11):

- When submission to such conduct is considered, either explicitly or implicitly, a condition of an individual's employment
- When submission to or rejection of such conduct is used as the basis for employment decisions affecting the individual
- When such conduct interferes with an individual's work performance or creates an "intimidating, hostile, or offensive working environment."

In health care, both clients and healthcare professionals may experience sexual harassment. Because sexual harassment is generally related to a power imbalance, female nurses are more likely than male nurses to experience sexual harassment from male physicians or administrators. Nurses may be "sexually propositioned," "suggestively touched," or "sexually insulted" during their careers. Such behavior is considered sexual harassment and can negatively affect client care. For example, to avoid uncomfortable situations, a nurse may refuse to care for the clients of a particular offensive physician or work on a unit with an offensive administrator, or a nurse may avoid calling a physician to report changes in client status or to suggest changes to improve client care.

The victim or the harasser may be male or female. The victim does not have to be of the opposite sex. Furthermore, the victim does not have to be the person harassed. Anyone who is affected by the offensive conduct may be considered a victim. Nurses must develop skills of assertiveness to deter sexual harassment in the workplace. (See also Box 15-7 🔗, Nursing Strategies for Dealing with Inappropriate Sexual Behavior.)

Nurses must be familiar with the sexual harassment policy and procedures that are in place in every institution. These will include information regarding the grievance policy, the person to whom incidents should be reported, and the resolution process.

UNDERSTANDING ETHICAL ISSUES

In the course of their daily work, nurses deal with such fundamental events as birth, suffering, and death. They must decide the morality of their own actions when they face these ethical issues. The present cost-driven environment of managed care tends to give highest priority to business values. This creates new moral problems and exaggerates old ones. It is more critical than ever for nurses to make sound moral decisions. Therefore, nurses need to develop an understanding of the ethical dimensions of nursing practice by examining their values. Early on in their practice, nurses must look ahead to the kinds of moral problems they are likely to face and begin to understand how values influence their decisions.

Ethical Concepts

Values are freely chosen, enduring beliefs or attitudes about the worth of a person, object, idea, or action. Values are important because they influence decisions and actions. Values are often taken for granted. In the same way that people are not aware of their breathing, they usually do not think about their values; they simply accept them and act on them. The word *values* usually brings to mind things such as honesty, fairness, friendship, safety, or family unity. Of course, not all values are moral values. For example, some people hold money, work, power, and politics as values in their lives.

Although values consist of freely chosen and enduring beliefs and attitudes, beliefs and attitudes are related, but not identical, to values.

Values are learned through observation and experience. They are transmitted to others through the influence of environment—that is, by family and peer groups, by cultural, ethnic, and religious groups. For example, if a parent consistently demonstrates honesty in dealing with others, the child will probably begin to value honesty. Nurses should keep in mind the influence of values on health. In some cultures, folk healers are valued over treatment by a physician.

Beliefs or opinions are interpretations or conclusions that people accept as being true; they do not necessarily involve values. For example, the statement "I believe if I study hard I will get a good grade" expresses a belief that does not involve a value. By contrast, the statement "Good grades are really important to me. I believe I must study hard to obtain good grades" involves both a belief and a value.

Attitudes are mental positions or feelings toward a person, object, or idea (e.g., acceptance, compassion, openness). Attitudes are often judged as good or bad, positive or negative, whereas beliefs are judged as correct or incorrect.

The term **ethics** has several meanings in common use. It refers to (1) a method of inquiry that helps people to understand the morality of human behavior (i.e., it is the study of morality), (2) the practices or beliefs of a certain group (e.g., medical ethics, nursing ethics), and (3) the expected standards of moral behavior of a particular group as described in the group's formal code of professional ethics. **Bioethics** is ethics as applied to life (e.g., decisions about abortion or euthanasia). Nursing ethics refers to ethical issues that occur in nursing practice. The NFLPN holds nurses accountable for their legal and ethical conduct in the *Nursing Practice Standards for the Licensed Practical/Vocational Nurse* (2003).

Moral Concepts

Morality (or morals) is similar to ethics, and many people use the terms interchangeably. *Morality* usually refers to private, personal standards of what is right and wrong in conduct, character, and attitude. Sometimes the first clue to the moral nature of a situation is an aroused conscience or an awareness of feelings such as guilt, hope, or shame. Another indicator is the tendency to respond to the situation with words such as *ought, should, right, wrong, good,* and *bad.* Moral issues are concerned with important social values and norms; they are not about trivial things.

Nurses should distinguish between morality and law. An action can be legal but not moral. For example, an order for full resuscitation of a dying client is legal, but one could still question whether the act is moral. On the other hand, an action can be moral but illegal. For example, if a child at home stops breathing, it is moral but not legal to exceed the speed limit when driving to the hospital.

Moral principles are statements about broad, general, philosophic concepts such as autonomy and justice. They provide the foundation for moral rules, which are specific prescriptions for actions. Principles are useful in ethical discussions because even if people disagree about which action is right in a situation, they may be able to agree on the principles that apply. Such an agreement can serve as the basis for a solution that is acceptable to all parties. Ethical issues are looked at differently among people of different cultures; the nurse must consider these differences when providing care. See Box 3-4 ■ for cultural pulse points related to legal and ethical considerations.

BOX 3-4	**CULTURAL PULSE POINTS**

Because of the increase in the number of immigrants now living in the United States, nurses working in a multicultural setting may encounter families who wish to have procedures such as female circumcision performed on their daughters. This presents a real ethical issue for healthcare professionals in this country. The procedure is widely performed in 27 different countries. Members of societies where these procedures are widely practiced do not consider them to be mutilation, as do many healthcare professionals in the United States. Many immediate and long-term health effects are related to the procedures. Nursing intervention strategies for ethical problems of traditional cultural practices include:

- Addressing problematic practice honestly and with respect
- Listening and valuing the perspective of the client and family
- Conducting interactions that engage the client as an equal partner.

While expressing respect for the practices of all cultures, there must be a recognition that traditional practices may need to be viewed differently. This can be done by collaborating with the client to:

- Identify the current values.
- Prioritize the values.
- Identify the goals of the values.
- Identify alternative methods to achieve the same goal.

Source: Excerpt from *Transcultural Concepts in Nursing Care* (3rd ed.) by M. M. Andrews and V. S. Boyle, 1999, Philadelphia: Lippincott.

Autonomy refers to the right to make one's own decisions. Nurses who follow this principle recognize that each client is unique, has the right to be what that person is, and has the right to choose personal goals.

Honoring the principle of autonomy means that the nurse respects a client's right to make decisions even when those choices seem not to be in the client's best interest. It also means treating others with consideration. In a healthcare setting, this principle is violated, for example, when a nurse disregards a client's report of the severity of his or her pain.

Nonmaleficence is duty to do no harm. Although this would seem to be a simple principle to follow, in reality it is complex. Harm can mean intentional harm, risk of harm, and unintentional harm. In nursing, intentional harm is never acceptable. However, the risk of harm is not always clear. A client may be at risk of harm during a nursing intervention that is intended to be helpful. For example, a client may react adversely to a medication, and caregivers may or may not always agree on the degree to which a risk is morally permissible.

Beneficence means "doing good." Nurses are obligated to do good, that is, to implement actions that benefit clients and their support persons. However, doing good can also pose a risk of doing harm. For example, a nurse may advise a client about a strenuous exercise program to improve general health, but should not do so if the client is at risk of a heart attack.

Justice is often referred to as fairness. Nurses often face decisions in which a sense of justice should prevail. For example, a nurse making home visits finds one client tearful and depressed, and knows she could help by staying for 30 more minutes to talk. However, that would take time from her next client, who is a diabetic who needs a great deal of teaching and observation. The nurse will need to weigh the facts of each situation carefully in order to divide her time justly among her clients.

Fidelity means to be faithful to agreements and promises. By virtue of their standing as professional caregivers, nurses have responsibilities to clients, employers, the government, and society, as well as to themselves. Nurses often make promises such as "I'll be right back with your pain medication," "You'll be all right," or "I'll find out for you." Clients take such promises seriously, and so should nurses.

Veracity refers to telling the truth. Although this seems straightforward, in practice, choices are not always clear. Should a nurse tell the truth when it is known that it will cause harm? Does a nurse tell a lie when it is known that the lie will relieve anxiety and fear? The loss of trust in the nurse and the anxiety caused by not knowing the truth, for example, usually outweigh any benefits derived from lying. Lying to sick or dying people is rarely justified.

Nursing Ethics

In the past, nurses looked on ethical decision making as the physician's responsibility. However, no one profession is responsible for ethical decisions, nor does expertise in one discipline such as medicine or nursing necessarily make a person an expert in ethics. As situations become more complex, input from all caregivers becomes increasingly important.

Most healthcare institutions have ethics committees. Ethical standards of the Joint Commission on Accreditation of Healthcare Organizations support nurses' involvement on these committees. Ethics committees typically review cases, write guidelines and policies, and provide education and counseling. They ensure that relevant facts of a case are brought out, provide a forum in which diverse views can be expressed, provide support for caregivers, and can reduce legal risks.

A **code of ethics** is a formal statement of a group's ideals and values. It is a set of ethical principles that (1) is shared by members of the group, (2) reflects their moral judgments over time, and (3) serves as a standard for their professional actions. Codes of ethics usually have higher requirements than legal standards, and they are never lower than the legal standards of the profession. Nurses are responsible for being familiar with the code that governs their practice.

International, national, state, and provincial nursing associations have established codes of ethics.

Nursing codes of ethics have the following purposes:

1. Inform the public about the minimum standards of the profession and help them understand professional nursing conduct.
2. Provide a sign of the profession's commitment to the public it serves.
3. Outline the major ethical considerations of the profession.
4. Provide general guidelines for professional behavior.
5. Guide the profession in self-regulation.
6. Remind nurses of the special responsibility they assume when caring for the sick.

ORIGINS OF ETHICAL PROBLEMS IN NURSING

Nurses' growing awareness of ethical problems has occurred largely because of (1) social and technologic changes and (2) nurses' conflicting loyalties and obligations.

Social and Technologic Changes

Social changes, such as the women's movement and a growing consumerism, expose ethical problems. Presently, the large number of people without health insurance, the high cost of health care, and workplace redesign under managed care are all raising issues of fairness and allocation of resources.

Technology creates new issues that did not exist in earlier, simpler times. Before monitors, ventilators, and parenteral feedings, there was no question about whether to "allow" an 800-gram premature infant to die. Today, with treatments that can prolong biologic life almost indefinitely, the questions are: Should we do what we know we can? Who should be treated—everyone, only those who can pay, only those who have a chance to improve?

Conflicting Loyalties and Obligations

Because of their unique position in the healthcare system, nurses experience conflicts among their loyalties and obligations to clients, families, physicians, employing institutions, and licensing bodies. Client needs may conflict with institutional policies, physician preferences, needs of the client's family, or even laws of the state. According to the nursing code of ethics, the nurse's first loyalty is to the client. However, it is not always easy to determine which action best serves the client's needs. For instance, a nurse may think that a client needs to be told a truth that others have been withholding. But this might damage the client–physician relationship, in the long run causing harm to the client rather than the intended good.

MAKING ETHICAL DECISIONS

Responsible ethical reasoning is rational and systematic. It should be based on ethical principles and codes rather than on emotions, intuition, fixed policies, or precedent. (A precedent is an earlier similar occurrence.)

A good decision is one that is in the client's best interest and at the same time preserves the integrity of all involved. Nurses have ethical obligations to their clients, to the agency that employs them, and to physicians. Therefore, nurses must weigh competing factors when making ethical decisions (Box 3-5 ■). See also Chapter 4 ⚭, the section on critical thinking.

Although the nurse's input is important, in reality several people are usually involved in making an ethical decision. Therefore, collaboration, communication, and compromise

---

BOX 3-5

Examples of Nurses' Obligations in Ethical Decisions

- Maximize the client's well-being.
- Balance the client's need for autonomy with family members' responsibilities for the client's well-being.
- Support each family member and enhance the family support system.
- Carry out hospital policies.
- Protect other clients' well-being.
- Protect the nurse's own standards of care.

BOX 3-6

Strategies to Enhance Ethical Nursing Practice

- Become aware of your own values and the ethical aspects of nursing.
- Be familiar with nursing codes of ethics.
- Respect the values, opinions, and responsibilities of other healthcare professionals that may be different from your own.
- Participate in or establish ethics rounds. Ethics rounds using hypothetical cases based on real situations incorporate the traditional teaching approach for clinical rounds, but focus on the ethical dimensions of client care rather than the client's clinical diagnosis and treatment.
- Serve on institutional ethics committees.
- Strive for collaborative practice in which nurses function effectively in cooperation with other healthcare professionals.

---

are important skills for health professionals. When nurses do not have the autonomy to act on their moral or ethical choices, compromise becomes essential.

Integrity-preserving compromises are most likely to be produced by collaborative decision making. See Box 3-6 ■ for strategies to enhance ethical decisions and practice.

SPECIFIC ETHICAL ISSUES

The American Nurses Association (ANA) Center for Ethics and Human Rights conducted a survey at the 1994 ANA convention that indicated the following as some of the ethical problems nurses encounter most frequently: cost-containment issues that jeopardize client welfare and access to healthcare (resource allocation), end-of-life decisions, breaches of client confidentiality (e.g., computerized information management), use of advance directives, informed consent and procedures, and issues in the care of HIV/AIDS clients (Scanlon, 2003). These and other issues are discussed in this section.

Acquired Immune Deficiency Syndrome (AIDS)

Because of its association with sexual behavior, prostitution, illicit drug use, and inevitable physical decline and death, AIDS bears a social stigma. Nurses caring for AIDS clients frequently have conflicting feelings of anger, fear, sympathy, fatigue, helplessness, and self-enhancement.

According to an ANA position statement titled *HIV Infections and Nursing Students,* "Nursing Curriculum including current HIV information should be provided by faculty with expertise in HIV disease at the onset of the academic program and as applicable throughout their course. . . . Each school of nursing should demonstrate the availability of a post-exposure management program for students who sustain exposure to blood and certain body fluids in the clinical practice setting. . . . Nursing students should be assured workplace/clinical setting protections consistent with those of employees according to OSHA Standards. . . . Nursing students and applicants to nursing programs should not be deprived of access to schools of nursing nor dismissed based solely on HIV positive status. . . . There must be confidentiality of all HIV-related information to safeguard nursing students' right to privacy" (ANA, 2001).

Other ethical issues center on testing for HIV status and for the presence of AIDS in health professionals and clients. Questions arise as to whether testing should be mandatory or voluntary and to whom test results should be given. The Centers for Disease Control and Prevention (CDC) provides recommendations as to which persons should be considered for HIV antibody counseling and testing. It also recommends that voluntary testing be made available to anyone, including all healthcare professionals. In addition, the CDC recommends that HIV-positive healthcare professionals avoid performing "exposure prone procedures" (CDC, 2001).

Abortion

Abortion is a highly publicized issue about which many people, including nurses, feel very strongly. Debate continues, pitting the principle of sanctity of life against the principle of autonomy and the woman's right to control her own body. This is an especially volatile issue because no public consensus has yet been reached.

Most state and provincial laws have provisions known as conscience clauses that permit individual physicians and nurses, as well as institutions, to refuse to assist with an abortion if doing so violates their religious or moral principles. However, nurses have no right to impose their values on a client. Abortion laws provide specific guidelines for nurses about what is legally permissible, although the U.S. Supreme Court and state legislatures continue to struggle with the issue of abortion.

Organ Transplantation

Organs for transplantation may come from living donors or from donors who have just died. Many living people choose to become donors by giving consent under the Uniform Anatomical Gift Act. Ethical issues related to organ transplantation include allocation of organs, selling of body parts, involvement of children as potential donors, consent, clear definition of death, and conflicts of interest between potential donors and recipients. In some situations, a person's religious beliefs may also present conflict. For example, certain religions forbid the mutilation of the body, even for the benefit of another person.

End-of-Life Issues

Some of the most frequent disturbing ethical problems for nurses involve issues that arise around death and dying. These include euthanasia, assisted suicide, termination of life-sustaining treatment, and the withdrawing or withholding of food and fluids.

Many moral problems surrounding the end of life can be resolved if clients complete advance directives. Presently, all 50 of the United States have enacted advance directive legislation (Scanlon, 2003, p. 94). Advance directives direct caregivers as to the client's wishes about treatments, providing an ongoing voice for clients when they have lost the capacity to make or communicate their decisions. See Chapter 17 ⬤⬤ for a full discussion of advance directives.

EUTHANASIA AND ASSISTED SUICIDE. *Euthanasia,* a Greek word meaning "good death," is popularly known as "mercy killing." Active euthanasia involves actions to directly bring about the client's death, with or without client consent. An example of this would be the administration of a lethal medication to end the client's suffering. Regardless of the caregiver's intent, active euthanasia is forbidden by law and can result in criminal charges of murder.

Active euthanasia includes assisted suicide, or giving clients the means to kill themselves if they request it (e.g., providing pills or a weapon). Nurses should recall that legality and morality are not one and the same. Determining whether an action is legal is only one aspect of deciding whether it is ethical. The questions of suicide and assisted suicide are still controversial in our society. The ANA's position statement on assisted suicide (1995) states that active euthanasia and assisted suicide are in violation of the Code for Nurses.

Passive euthanasia involves the withdrawal of extraordinary means of life support, such as removing a ventilator or making a client a "no code (do not resuscitate). The legality of passive euthanasia is dependent on the laws of a particular jurisdiction and/or facility, even though not a violation of the ANA code." (1995)

TERMINATION OF LIFE-SUSTAINING TREATMENT. Antibiotics, organ transplants, and technologic advances (e.g., ventilators) help to prolong life, but not necessarily to restore health. Clients may specify that they wish to have life-sustaining measures withdrawn, they may have advance directives on this matter, or they may appoint a surrogate decision maker. There is no ethical or legal distinction between the withholding or withdrawing of treatments. However, it is usually more troubling for healthcare professionals to withdraw a treatment than to decide initially not to begin it. Nurses must understand that a decision to withdraw treatment is not a decision to withdraw care. As the primary caregivers, nurses must ensure that sensitive care

MediaLink Understanding Legal and Ethical Issues

and comfort measures are given as the client's illness progresses.

WITHDRAWING OR WITHHOLDING FOOD AND FLUIDS. It is generally accepted that providing food and fluids is part of ordinary nursing practice and, therefore, a moral duty. However, when food and fluids are administered by tube to a dying client, or are given over a long period of time to an unconscious client who is not expected to improve, then some consider it to be an extraordinary, or heroic, measure. A nurse is morally obligated to withhold food and fluids when it is more harmful to administer them than to withhold them. In addition, "It is morally as well as legally permissible for nurses to honor the refusal of food and fluids by competent patients in their care" (ANA, 1998, p. 3). The ANA Code for Nurses supports this position through the nurse's role as a client advocate and through the moral principle of autonomy.

ALLOCATION OF HEALTH RESOURCES

Allocation of healthcare goods and services, including organ transplants, artificial joints, and the services of specialists, has become an especially urgent issue as medical costs continue to rise and more stringent cost-containment measures are implemented.

Nursing care is also a health resource. Most institutions have been implementing "workplace redesign" in order to cut costs. As a result, nursing units are staffed with fewer nurses and more unlicensed caregivers. Nurses must continue to look for ways to balance economics and caring in the allocation of health resources.

MANAGEMENT OF COMPUTERIZED INFORMATION

In keeping with the principle of autonomy, nurses are obligated to respect clients' privacy and confidentiality. Clients must be able to trust that nurses will reveal details of their situations only as appropriate and will communicate only the information necessary to provide for their healthcare. Computerized client records make sensitive data accessible to more people and accent issues of confidentiality. Nurses should help develop and follow security measures and policies to ensure appropriate use of client data. For example, nurses should not give their system security codes to unauthorized persons.

BOX 3-7

Values Basic to Client Advocacy

- The client is a holistic, autonomous being who has the right to make choices and decisions.
- Clients have the right to expect a nurse–client relationship that is based on shared respect, trust, and collaboration in solving problems related to health and healthcare needs, and consideration of their thoughts and feelings.
- Clients are responsible for their own health.
- It is the nurse's responsibility to ensure the client has access to healthcare services that meet health needs.

ADVOCACY

An **advocate** is one who expresses and defends the cause of another. A client advocate is an advocate for clients' rights. The healthcare system is complex, and many clients are too ill to deal with it. If they are to keep from "falling through the cracks," clients need an advocate to cut through the layers of bureaucracy and help them get what they require. Values basic to client advocacy are shown in Box 3-7 ■.

The overall goal of the client advocate is to protect clients' rights. Being an effective client advocate involves

- Being assertive
- Recognizing that the rights and values of clients and families must take precedence when they conflict with those of healthcare providers
- Being aware that conflicts may arise over issues that require consultation, confrontation, or negotiation between the nurse and administrative personnel or between the nurse and physician
- Working with unfamiliar community agencies and lay practitioners
- Knowing that advocacy may require political action—communicating a client's healthcare needs to government and other officials who have the authority to do something about these needs.

Note: The references and resources for this and all chapters have been compiled at the back of the book.

Chapter Review

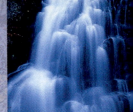

 KEY TERMS by Topic

Use the audio glossary feature of either the CD-ROM or the Companion Website to hear the correct pronunciation of the following key terms.

Understanding Legal Issues
law

Kinds of Legal Actions
tort, negligence, malpractice statute of limitations, assault, battery, false

imprisonment, invasion of privacy, defamation, libel, slander, crime

Regulation of Nursing Practice
scope of practice

Legal Roles of Nurses
liability

Selected Legal Aspects of Nursing Practice
impaired nurse, sexual harassment

Ethical Concepts
values, beliefs, attitudes, ethics, bioethics

Moral Concepts
autonomy

Nursing Ethics
code of ethics, advocate

KEY Points

- Accountability is an essential concept of professional nursing practice under the law.

- Nurses need to understand laws that regulate and affect nursing practice to ensure that the nurses' actions are consistent with current legal principles and to protect the nurse from liability.

- Nurse practice acts legally define and describe the scope of nursing practice that the law seeks to regulate.

- Nurses can be held liable for intentional torts, such as invasion of privacy, defamation, assault and battery, and false imprisonment; and for unintentional torts, such as negligence and malpractice.

- Negligence or malpractice of nurses can be established when (1) the nurse (defendant) owed a duty to the client, (2) the nurse failed to carry out that duty according to standards, (3) the client (plaintiff) was injured, and (4) the client's injury was caused by the nurse's failure to follow the standard.

- Good Samaritan acts protect health professionals from claims of malpractice when they offer assistance at the scene of an emergency, provided that there is no willful wrongdoing or gross departure from normal standards of care.

- Chemical dependence in healthcare workers has become a problem because of the high levels of stress involved in many healthcare settings and the easy access to addictive drugs. The nurse needs to know the proper procedure for reporting nursing colleagues who are chemically impaired.

- Sexual harassment is a violation of the individual's right and a form of discrimination. Sexual harassment can happen to both nurses and clients. The nurse needs to be aware of strategies to deter harassing behavior.

- Nursing students need to make certain that they are prepared to provide the necessary care to assigned clients and to ask for help or supervision in situations for which they feel inadequately prepared.

- Moral issues and ethical problems are created as a result of advances in technology and nurses' conflicting loyalties and obligations.

- Client advocacy involves concern for an action on behalf of another person or organization in order to bring about change.

 EXPLORE MediaLink

Additional interactive resources for this chapter can be found on the Companion Website at www.prenhall.com/ramont. Click on Chapter 3 and "Begin" to select the activities for this chapter.

For chapter-related NCLEX®-style questions and an audio glossary, access the accompanying CD-ROM in this book.

Videos
- Collective Bargaining
- Understanding Legal and Ethical Issues

FOR FURTHER Study

See Chapter 6 for information about types of records and how to document care.

See Chapter 7 for more information on HIPAA and on incident reports.

See Chapter 8 for more information about providing a safe client environment and the correct use of restraints.

See Chapter 10 for policies for safeguarding clients' property.

See Chapter 15 for ways to deal with sexual harassment.

See Chapter 17 for more information about advance directives.

See Chapter 29 for information about administering medications and documenting their administration.

NCLEX-PN® Exam Preparation

1 A client has signed the consent for surgery, which is scheduled for the morning. You enter the room and find the client crying. The client tells you, "I don't want to have surgery, but the doctor and my family tell me I must." You should consider which of the following dilemmas? (Select all that apply.)
   1. Has the client given informed consent?
   2. Do the client and family disagree on treatment?
   3. Has the client already signed the consent?
   4. Has the treatment team followed the principle of beneficence?

2 You are assigned a client who has been placed in restraints. You fail to follow the hospital policy on frequency of assessment and periodic release of restraints. Your behavior could be considered which of the following?
   1. negligence
   2. false imprisonment
   3. ethical misconduct
   4. defamation

3 In the course of administering medications, your client states, "I don't take that yellow pill every day and I took it at home yesterday." Without verifying the physician's orders, you say to the client, "Your doctor wants you to have this, so you must take it now!" Later, you check the order and find that it is an every-other-day order. You are guilty of which of the following?
   1. a crime
   2. assault
   3. negligence
   4. misdemeanor

4 As you are performing your morning assessment on a client, you notice there is a bruise in the area where the last injection was given. When you ask the client to turn onto that side, she complains that it is sore. You state, "The night nurse is incompetent; no one gets a bruise like that from an injection." You have used which type of false communication?
   1. libel
   2. slander
   3. breach of confidence
   4. invasion of privacy

5 If a nurse fails to report a client's complaint, resulting in client suffering, the nurse can be liable for which type of malpractice?
   1. mistaken identity
   2. failure to observe and take appropriate action
   3. intentional tort
   4. performing a procedure without consent

6 Which of the following is a responsibility of the National League for Nursing?
   1. enforcing nurse practice acts
   2. issuing nursing licenses once the exam has been passed
   3. providing approval and accreditation of basic nursing programs
   4. assessing credentials of non–U.S.-trained nurses

7 An incident report should be completed by which of the following individuals?
   1. the nurse involved in the incident
   2. the immediate supervisor of the nurse involved in the incident
   3. the nurse who discovers the incident
   4. the risk management department of the facility

8 The Americans with Disabilities Act:
   1. can be interpreted by the employer.
   2. enables a person with a learning disability, who is physically able, to pursue a nursing curriculum through alternate methods.
   3. provides retraining for nurses who have been injured on the job.
   4. prohibits setting lifting requirements for nursing jobs.

9 The right of the person to make his or her own decisions is related to which principle?
   1. respect for the person
   2. autonomy
   3. justice
   4. nonmaleficence

10 Your supervisor has asked you to serve on the committee to develop guidelines for the new computerized client record system. Coworkers are concerned about confidentiality. The best response to their concerns would be:
   1. "Medical records on the Internet are guaranteed to be secure."
   2. "The best ways we can protect the client's information is by following security policies and keeping our security codes private."
   3. "There is no way to protect confidentiality, but the benefits of the system outweigh the risks."
   4. "As long as we save after each entry, the records are secure."

Answers and Rationales for Review Questions, as well as discussion of Care Plan and Critical Thinking Care Map questions, appear in Appendix I.

Chapter 4

Critical Thinking and Nursing Theory/Models

BRIEF Outline

Critical Thinking
Theories and Models

LEARNING Outcomes

After completing this chapter, you will be able to:

1. Discuss characteristics, skills, and attitudes of critical thinking.
2. Explain the importance of critical thinking to the nursing process.
3. Define nursing theory.
4. Compare selected theories of nursing in terms of client, environment, health, and nursing.
5. Identify areas in which LPNs/LVNs can incorporate nursing theory into their nursing practice.

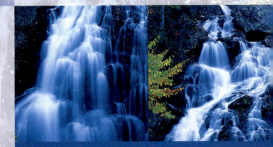

HISTORICAL Perspectives

Nursing theories and models are usually thought of as a contribution to nursing during the later part of the 20th century, but nursing historians know that the mother of modern-day nursing, Florence Nightingale, became the first nursing theorist in 1859.

Nursing instructors as well as staff nurses in the clinical setting continually challenge nursing students to become critical thinkers. You may ask a question about a client, only to be asked a question in return. Your instructor or staff nurse is trying to help you think like a nurse. For example, you may ask, "Can my client ambulate in the hall?" And your instructor may reply, "Think about your client's diagnosis and the results of the ultrasound of her leg this morning. What could happen if she ambulates?" Beginning LPN/LVN students certainly may be puzzled when confronted with such a situation. From the very beginning of the training program, the LPN/LVN student is challenged to begin to think like a nurse. Thinking like a nurse is different from thinking like a doctor or a teacher or a lawyer. Seeing the client as a whole person and dealing with problems that arise when providing care are what defines thinking for the nurse.

A nurse's thinking is not limited to problem solving or decision making. Nurses must also make reliable observations, draw sound conclusions, create new information and ideas, evaluate other people's ways of reasoning, and improve their own self-knowledge. Critical thinking goes hand in hand with the nursing process. As you work your way through this chapter and Chapter 5, you will begin to see how the pieces fit together.

You will develop many critical-thinking skills and abilities, such as information gathering, focusing, remembering, organizing, analyzing, generating, integrating, and evaluating. As you progress through your program, you will encounter increasingly more complex situations. This is the challenge of nursing: *thoughtful, thorough nursing practice based on sound reasoning and committed to safe and effective client care.* To accomplish this goal, you will be required to reason about nursing by reading, writing, listening, and speaking critically. By thinking critically about nursing, you will gain in-depth knowledge about the practice of nursing as a professional.

Critical Thinking

The thinking process that guides nursing practice must be organized, logical, purposeful, and disciplined rather than random or undirected. Paul and Elder (2001) describe **critical thinking** as "the art of thinking about thinking." *Critical,* in this context, does not mean "eager to find fault," but instead "capable of judging carefully and accurately."

METHODS OF PROBLEM SOLVING

When solving problems, the nurse makes inferences, sorts out facts from opinions, evaluates the credibility of information sources, and uses a variety of other cognitive skills. The LPN/LVN employs questioning skills when listening to an end-of-shift report, reviewing a history or progress notes, or

planning care, or discussing a client's care with colleagues. For example, during the end-of-shift report about a client who has just been diagnosed with terminal cancer, the nurse coming on shift may ask, "What has the family been told about the client's prognosis?" This helps the staff understand the family's knowledge level and their needs. Asking such questions gives the nurse additional information to use when applying inductive and deductive reasoning.

Types of Reasoning

The nurse learns to approach problems from several angles in order to apply reasoning skills. Figure 4-1 ■ highlights the different factors that go into the process of reasoning.

Two other skills used in critical thinking are inductive and deductive reasoning.

- **Inductive reasoning** forms generalizations. Inductive reasoning is like looking at the pieces of a jigsaw puzzle and attempting to describe the whole (without seeing a picture of the completed puzzle). As the person puts more and more pieces together, the whole picture becomes clearer. For example, the nurse who observes that a client has dry skin, poor turgor, sunken eyes, and dark amber urine may make the generalization that the client appears dehydrated.

- **Deductive reasoning** is reasoning from the general to the specific. In deductive reasoning, the thinker sees the whole picture (from the puzzle box cover) and puts the puzzle together by organizing the pieces into border pieces, or colors, or some other grouping. For example,

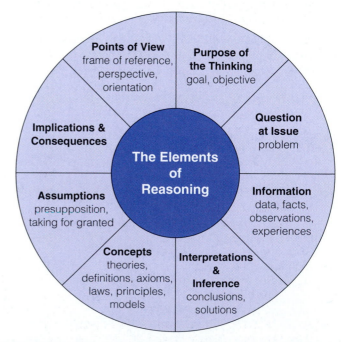

Figure 4-1. ■ The elements of reasoning. (*Source:* Adapted from "Critical Thinking" by R. Paul, 1993, Dillon Beach, CA: Foundation for Critical Thinking, www.criticalthinking.org. Reprinted with permission.)

TABLE 4-1

Differentiating Types of Statements

STATEMENT	DESCRIPTION	EXAMPLE
Facts	Can be verified through investigation	Birth control pills do not protect against sexually transmitted infections (STIs).
Inferences	Conclusions drawn from the facts; going beyond facts to make a statement about something not currently known	A person in a sexual relationship with a client with an STI should not rely on birth control pills alone but should consider using a method that provides a physical barrier.
Judgments	Evaluation of facts or information that reflect values or other criteria; a type of opinion	Having multiple sexual partners can lead to serious health consequences.
Opinions	Beliefs formed over time that include judgments and may fit facts or be in error	It is wrong not to wait until marriage to have sex.

nurses know that people who have experienced several days of vomiting and diarrhea are likely to be dehydrated. In a client who has had vomiting and diarrhea for 2 days, the nurse would confirm this generalization deductively by checking skin turgor, appearance of the client's eyes, and color and quantity of the client's urine.

By using critical thinking, the nurse will also separate facts, inferences, judgments, and opinions (Table 4-1 ■). Box 4-1 ■ lists the characteristics of a critical thinker.

APPLYING CRITICAL THINKING TO NURSING

LPNs/LVNs use their critical-thinking skills in a variety of ways. Nursing students must take knowledge from the classroom and apply it to real-life client situations. You will study life span development, nutrition, communication, and psychosocial issues in addition to nursing courses so

that you can acquire a strong foundation on which to build your nursing knowledge and skill. You will use the knowledge from all of your courses when you care for your clients. For example, you may be assigned to care for a 17-year-old with Crohn's disease, a disorder of the small intestine. Your client will have needs in a variety of areas:

- She is a normal adolescent with the same needs as any 17-year-old.
- She has nutritional needs due to poor absorption of nutrients from her small intestine.
- She has communication needs regarding her feelings and issues about hospitalization and illness.
- She has psychological needs because she is away from her friends and family and her "normal life."

These needs are in addition to the technical aspects of her nursing care, which may include managing total parenteral nutrition, IV therapy, medications, and pain. You will pull together concepts from many different courses when you care for this client.

Nurses deal with change in stressful **environments**. Treatments, medications, and technology change constantly, and a client's condition may change from minute to minute. When unexpected situations arise, critical thinking enables the nurse to recognize important cues, respond quickly, and adapt interventions to meet specific client needs. An example of this is the client about to be discharged who is stable when you arrive on shift, but over the next several hours has a drop in blood pressure, an increase in pulse, and develops an irregular heart rate. Although the plan was to discharge the client and admit another person into the room, the nurse must assess the situation and respond to changes that have occurred. In addition to responding to the changes in the client's vital signs and implementing care to stabilize him, the nurse must notify the physician, cancel the discharge, and let admitting know that a new person cannot be admitted to the room.

BOX 4-1

Characteristics of Critical Thinkers

As Critical Thinkers:

- We analyze our thinking.
- We subject the egocentric (self-centered) root of our thinking to close scrutiny.
- We expose inappropriate standards and replace them with sound ones.
- We learn how to raise our thinking to conscious examination, to free ourselves from traps of undisciplined, instinctive thought.
- We develop tools for analyzing and assessing our participation in logical systems in which we live.
- We take explicit intellectual and emotional command of who we are, what we are, and the ends to which our lives are tending.
- We learn how to govern the thoughts that govern us.

During the course of a workday, nurses make vital decisions of many kinds. These decisions may be made independently by the LPN/LVN or in collaboration with an RN or other team member. It is important that the decisions be sound. LPNs/LVNs use critical-thinking skills when collecting information. For example, consider a nurse who is caring for a client. The client states that he feels itchy on his back. The nurse must recognize that this itchy feeling could be a sign of a reaction to a medication. The nurse must decide if this problem is indeed a possible drug reaction and must notify the physician if that is the case. The nurse may decide to seek collaboration with the RN to determine whether a drug reaction is taking place. Or, the nurse may decide it is not a serious problem and take steps to make the client more comfortable, while still monitoring the situation for any changes.

Nurses do not always have to think critically and make critical decisions. Some things come naturally without too much thought, like selecting clothes or deciding what to eat for lunch. Nurses often do familiar tasks, such as taking vital signs, without thinking much about how to do the job. But the higher order skills of critical thinking are put into play as soon as a new idea is encountered or a less-than-routine decision must be made. An example of this is the nurse who uses critical thinking when deciding which clients need to be cared for first, second, or third as the shift begins.

USING CRITICAL THINKING TO MAKE NURSING DECISIONS

The Nursing Process

One model for making decisions is the nursing process, which is a systematic method of assessing, planning, implementing, and evaluating nursing care (see Chapter 5 ⬤⬤). Critical thinking is used throughout the nursing process (Table 4-2 ▪).

Nurses use critical thinking to resolve problems related to client care. The nurse obtains information that clarifies the nature of the problem and suggests possible solutions. The nurse then carefully evaluates the possible solutions and chooses the best one to implement. The nurse monitors the situation carefully over time to ensure its initial and continued effectiveness. The nurse does not discard the other solutions but keeps them in mind. They may be useful if the first solution is not effective, or if a different client with a similar problem prefers an alternative solution. For example, a nurse may be attempting to solve the problem of a client who refuses most of the food on his tray. The nurse considers possible solutions: asking for a consult with the dietician, talking with the client about his food likes and dislikes, checking to see if chewing or swallowing is difficult for him, and asking questions that might indicate if he is discouraged and therefore not eating. The

TABLE 4-2	
Questions about Critical Thinking Throughout the Nursing Process	
NURSING PROCESS	**QUESTIONS TO ASK**
COLLECTING DATA FOR THE ASSESSMENT	
	Are the data complete?
	What other data do I need?
	What are the possible sources of the data?
	What assumptions and biases do I have about the situation?
	What is the client's point of view?
PLANNING FOR AND IMPLEMENTING THE NURSING DIAGNOSIS	
Diagnosing	What do these data mean?
	What else could be happening?
	Are there any gaps in the data?
	How are these data similar and how are they different?
	What assumptions or biases do I have in this situation?
	Have my assumptions affected my interpretation of the data?
Planning	What are the goals for the client?
	What do I want to accomplish?
	How are my goals related to what the client wants to accomplish?
	What are the expected outcomes for this client?
	What interventions are to be used?
	How much involvement can the client and family have at this time?
Implementing	What is the client's current status?
	What are the most critical steps in this intervention?
	How must I alter the interventions to best meet this client's needs and maintain the principles of safety?
	What is the client's response during and after the intervention?
	Is there a need to alter the intervention in any way? If so, how?
Evaluating	Were the interventions successful in helping the client to meet the desired goals?
	How could things have been done differently?
	What data do I need to make new decisions?
	Where will I get the data?
	Were there assumptions, biases, or points of view that I missed that affected the outcomes?

nurse chooses the best solution to implement by checking to see if the client has difficulty chewing or swallowing and determines that no problem exists. The nurse next checks with the client about his food preferences and includes this information in his care plan. The nurse then evaluates how the client is eating for the next several days and, if needed, asks for a dietary consult. The next time the nurse encounters a similar client situation, this problem-solving experience will be remembered and drawn on.

Nursing Decisions

Nurses make many types of decisions throughout the day. They make value decisions, such as ways to keep client information confidential, and time management decisions, such as taking clean linen to the client's room at the same time as the medication in order to save steps. They make scheduling decisions, such as the decision to bathe the client before scheduled physical therapy, and priority decisions, such as preparing a client for surgery before giving a bath to another client.

Decision making is a critical-thinking process for choosing the best actions to meet a desired goal. Nurses must make decisions and assist clients to make decisions. When two call lights are ringing, an IV pump is beeping, and a physician is calling, the nurse must decide which situation to handle first. When a client is faced with choices about chemotherapy and radiation therapy to treat cancer, the nurse may need to provide information or resources the client can use in making a decision. See Table 4-3 ■ for a description of a seven-step decision-making process.

TABLE 4-3	
Seven-Step Decision-Making Process	
STEP	**EXPLANATION**
Identify the purpose.	Identify the why and what.
Set the criteria.	Question what needs to be achieved, preserved, avoided.
Weigh the criteria.	Set priorities in order of importance.
Seek alternatives.	Identify all possibilities for meeting the criteria.
Test alternatives.	Study alternatives for objective rationales for choosing one alternative over another.
Troubleshoot.	Determine what might go wrong and develop a plan to prevent, minimize, or overcome problems.
Evaluate the action.	Determine how effective the actions were and if they achieved the purpose.

PRACTICING CRITICAL THINKING

The day in and day out use of critical thinking and problem solving takes a great deal of practice. As a student, you may feel overwhelmed right now. That is why your instructors and other healthcare professionals will continue to challenge your thinking and decision making throughout your course of study. Every chapter in this text provides review questions to strengthen your thinking. Chapters 5 through 35 also provide care plans and care maps to encourage you to apply your critical-thinking skills to nursing situations.

Critical Thinking Care Map

As LPNs/LVNs collect assessment data about a client, they use critical-thinking skills to organize data into **subjective data** (apparent only to the person being affected) and **objective data** (detectable by an observer). These data contribute to the development of nursing diagnoses (see Chapter 5 ∞). For example, an LPN/LVN assesses a client who has not been taking his medication consistently. The blood pressure is elevated, and the nurse reports it to the physician. The physician orders an increase in the dose of blood pressure medication. The nurse knows the client is not compliant in taking the medication due to lack of understanding of its importance. The client is at risk for complications of elevated blood pressure and stroke. LPNs/LVNs also use critical thinking to determine which interventions would be appropriate for specific nursing diagnoses. They think critically when they frame their narrative notes for the client's chart.

A sample Critical Thinking Care Map is shown on page 50. The case studies supplied in Chapters 5 through 35 will focus on one of the NCLEX-PN® focus areas, to help you think in terms of the broad categories of nursing you will master. An appropriate nursing diagnosis will be supplied, and you will select and sort objective and subjective data that apply to this nursing diagnosis. You will decide which of the data you would report immediately to a supervisor or physician. You will select appropriate interventions from the list provided. You will also practice documenting the important information. When you take time to complete these Critical Thinking Care Maps, you will practice and sharpen your critical-thinking skills.

Theories and Models

Besides thinking critically about a client's condition and care, nurses must also think critically about nursing itself. Starting with Florence Nightingale, nurses have been doing just that. Several have developed theories of nursing. **Theories** are ways of looking at a discipline, such as nursing, in clear, explicit terms that can be communicated to others.

This line provides an appropriate nursing diagnosis.

This line provides the appropriate NCLEX-PN® focus area.

This information is provided to give you basic information about the client.

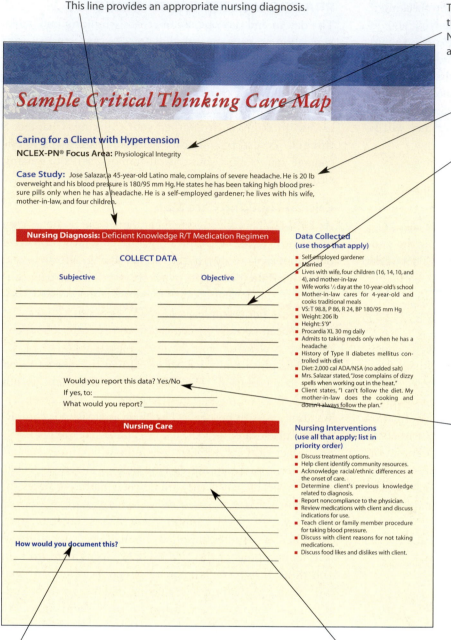

Sample Critical Thinking Care Map

Caring for a Client with Hypertension
NCLEX-PN® Focus Area: Physiological Integrity

Case Study: Jose Salazar, a 45-year-old Latino male, complains of severe headache. He is 20 lb overweight and his blood pressure is 180/95 mm Hg. He states he has been taking high blood pressure pills only when he has a headache. He is a self-employed gardener; he lives with his wife, mother-in-law, and four children.

Nursing Diagnosis: Deficient Knowledge R/T Medication Regimen

COLLECT DATA

Subjective	Objective
_____	_____
_____	_____
_____	_____
_____	_____
_____	_____
_____	_____

Would you report this data? Yes/No
If yes, to: _____
What would you report? _____

Nursing Care
_____
_____
_____
_____
_____
_____
_____
_____
_____

How would you document this? _____
_____
_____

Data Collected
(use those that apply)
- Self-employed gardener
- Married
- Lives with wife, four children (16, 14, 10, and 4), and mother-in-law
- Wife works ½ day at the 10-year-old's school
- Mother-in-law cares for 4-year-old and cooks traditional meals
- VS: T 98.8, P 86, R 24, BP 180/95 mm Hg
- Weight: 206 lb
- Height: 5'9"
- Procardia XL 30 mg daily
- Admits to taking meds only when he has a headache
- History of Type II diabetes mellitus controlled with diet
- Diet: 2,000 cal ADA/NSA (no added salt)
- Mrs. Salazar stated, "Jose complains of dizzy spells when working out in the heat."
- Client states, "I can't follow the diet. My mother-in-law does the cooking and doesn't always follow the plan."

Nursing Interventions
(use all that apply; list in priority order)
- Discuss treatment options.
- Help client identify community resources.
- Acknowledge racial/ethnic differences at the onset of care.
- Determine client's previous knowledge related to diagnosis.
- Report noncompliance to the physician.
- Review medications with client and discuss indications for use.
- Teach client or family member procedure for taking blood pressure.
- Discuss with client reasons for not taking medications.
- Discuss food likes and dislikes with client.

Carefully consider the data. What statements and data collected would support this nursing diagnosis? What data are subjective and what data are objective? What data are not relevant?

Subjective data: Only takes blood pressure medication when he has a headache, severe headache, dizzy when working outside in heat, not following diet

Objective data: VS: T 98.8, P 86, R 24, BP 180/95 mm Hg, weight 206, height 5'9", 2,000 cal ADA diet (no salt added), Procardia XL 30 mg daily

Irrelevant data: Self-employed gardener; married; lives with wife, four children (16, 14, 10, and 4), and mother-in-law; wife works ½ day at the 10-year-old's school; mother-in-law cares for 4-year-old and cooks traditional meals.

Think about the data you have collected. Are any of the data abnormal? Would they indicate deficient knowledge that could have a negative impact on the client's health? Would it be important to report this information? If so, to which person? **Yes, report dizziness and blood pressure reading to physician.**

This question allows you to practice your documentation. It is not necessary to document all the data or interventions for this exercise. For example, the assessment documentation might be:

1/5/08 Client admitted through E.R following dizzy spell at work. BP 150/95, complaining of severe headache. Hx of hypertension treated with Procardia KL 30mg qd. Client admits to taking meds only when he has a headache

Marge Smith LPN

Consider the client's deficient knowledge about the medication regimen. Make a decision about which interventions are relevant and which are not relevant.

Relevant interventions: Acknowledge racial/ethnic differences at the onset of care. Determine client's previous knowledge related to diagnosis. Review medications with client and discuss indications for use. Teach client or family member procedure for taking blood pressure. Discuss with client reasons for not taking medications. Report noncompliance to the physician.

Irrelevant interventions: Discuss treatment options. Help client identify community resources. Discuss food likes and dislikes with client.

INTRODUCTION TO NURSING THEORIES

Until 1859, when Florence Nightingale penned her *Notes on Nursing: What It Is, and What It Is Not,* nursing practice was based on borrowed theory from medicine. Nursing continues to draw on the medical communities for knowledge, but since the middle of the twentieth century, nursing has begun to develop its unique theory. Theory development gained momentum in the 1960s and has progressed since then through the work of several nurse-theorists and nurses. Each theory bears the name of the person or group that developed it and reflects the beliefs of the developer.

Essential Elements in Nursing Theory

Nursing theories address and specify relationships about four major ideas. These four concepts are central to nursing:

1. Nursing—the attributes, characteristics, and actions of the nurse providing care on behalf of, or in conjunction with, the client
2. Person or client—the recipient of nursing care (includes individuals, families, and communities)
3. Health—the degree of wellness or well-being that the client experiences
4. Environment—the internal and external surroundings that affect the client, including people in the physical environment, such as families, friends, and significant others.

Each nurse-theorist's definitions of the four major concepts vary in accordance with personal philosophy, scientific orientation, and experience in nursing. See Table 4-4 ■ for selected theorists' definitions and descriptions of nursing, person/client, health, and environment.

NON-NURSING MODELS

Models and theories of health and wellness are also used by nurses, even though they are not specifically about nursing.

Wellness Model

Nurses use wellness models to assist clients to identify health risks and to explore lifestyle habits and health behaviors, beliefs, values, and attitudes that influence levels of wellness. Such models generally include the following:

- Health history
- Physical fitness evaluation
- Nutritional assessment
- Life-stress analysis
- Lifestyle and health habits
- Health beliefs
- Sexual health
- Spiritual health
- Relationships
- Health risk appraisal.

Non-nursing models are included in LPN/LVN training programs to assist the nurse in gathering data and processing it.

Nurses usually will use more than one model at a time in order to obtain a complete history.

Body Systems Model

Closely related to the medical model, the body systems model focuses on abnormalities. The client is assessed and treated according to the body system that is affected by the primary or presenting diagnosis. The model does have one very significant downfall: It is not effective when treating a client with a disease process that has multisystem effects.

Body systems covered by this model include:

- Integumentary system
- Respiratory system
- Cardiovascular system
- Nervous system
- Musculoskeletal system
- Gastrointestinal system
- Genitourinary system
- Reproductive system.

Maslow's Hierarchy of Needs

Maslow's hierarchy of needs theory assists the nurse in identifying needs and setting priorities. It clusters data pertaining to the following:

- Physiological needs (survival needs)
- Safety and security needs
- Love and belonging needs
- Self-esteem needs
- Self-actualization needs.

See Chapter 11 ⚭ for detailed information about this theory.

Developmental Theories

Developmental theories assist the nurse in treating the client holistically. Several physical, psychosocial, cognitive, and moral developmental theories may be used by the nurse in specific situations. Examples include the following:

- Freud's five stages of development
- Erikson's eight stages of development
- Piaget's phases of cognitive development
- Kohlberg's stages of moral development.

The theories and theorists are discussed in Chapter 11 ⚭ as they relate to life span development.

SIGNIFICANCE OF MODELS AND THEORIES

Why is it important for an LPN/LVN to have an understanding of nursing theories? A theoretical understanding of nursing helps you view your clients as more than a medical diagnosis from which you will perform nursing tasks. This understanding will help you develop a personal nursing philosophy. It will help you to understand and participate in the nursing process and collaborate with registered nurses and other staff. It will also help you to discern the differences in

TABLE 4-4

Selected Nursing Theories and the Nursing Process

THEORY	NURSING	PERSON/CLIENT	HEALTH	ENVIRONMENT	COLLECTING DATA FOR ASSESSMENT	PLANNING AND IMPLEMENTING THE DIAGNOSIS	EVALUATING
Florence Nightingale's environmental theory (1859)	Provision of optimal conditions to enhance the person's reparative processes and prevent the reparative process from being interrupted.	An individual with vital reparative processes to deal with disease and desirous of health but passive in terms of influencing the environment or nurse.	Health: being well and using one's powers to the fullest extent. Health is maintained through prevention of disease via environmental health factors. Disease is a reparative process nature institutes because of some want of attention.	Environment: The major concepts for health are ventilation, warmth, light, diet, cleanliness, and absence of noise. Although the environment has social, emotional, and physical aspects, Nightingale emphasized the physical aspects.	"The most important practical lesson that can be given to nurses is to teach them what to observe, how to observe, what symptoms indicate improvement, what the reverse indicates, which are of importance, which are not, which are the evidence of neglect, and what kind of neglect." In this statement Nightingale was teaching the first step.	**Diagnosing/ Planning:** The concept of nursing diagnoses came much later, but she did identify particular needs and problems presented by the client. Through observation she was able to title problems such as lack of appetite or difficulty breathing so that they could be addressed immediately. Nurses were able to plan care, basing it on the prioritizing of patients' needs. **Implementing:** The plan of care was directly related to Nightingale's theory of environment. Nurses were responsible not only for personal care of the patient but also for washing the floors and walls and maintenance of the stove to provide warmth in the environment.	The client's progress was evaluated and reassessed by observation. She determined that the evaluation of the client's status was critical to the process of providing adequate care, and to determine if care should be continued or altered.

TABLE 4-4

Selected Nursing Theories and the Nursing Process (*continued*)

THEORY	NURSING	PERSON/CLIENT	HEALTH	ENVIRONMENT	COLLECTING DATA FOR ASSESSMENT	PLANNING AND IMPLEMENTING THE DIAGNOSIS	EVALUATING
Dorothea Orem's general theory of nursing (1980)	A helping or assisting service to persons who are wholly or partly dependent—infants, children, and adults—when they, their parents, guardians, or other adults responsible for their care are no longer able to give or supervise their care. A creative effort of one human being to help another human being. Nursing is deliberate action, a function of the practical intelligence of nurses, and action to bring about humanely desirable conditions in persons and their environments. It is distinguished from other human services and other forms of care by its focus on human beings.	A unity who can be viewed as functioning biologically, symbolically, and socially and who initiates and performs self-care activities on own behalf in maintaining life, health, and well-being; self-care activities deal with air, water, food, elimination, activity and rest, solitude and social interaction, prevention of hazards to life and well-being, and promotion of human functioning.	Health is a state that is characterized by soundness or wholeness of developed human structures and of bodily and mental functioning. It includes physical, psychological, interpersonal, and social aspects. Well-being is used in the sense of individuals' perceived condition of existence. Well-being is a state characterized by experiences of contentment, pleasure, and certain kinds of happiness; by spiritual experiences; by movement toward fulfillment of one's self-ideal; and by continuing personalization. Well-being is associated with health, with success in personal endeavors, and with sufficiency of resources.	The environment is linked to the individual, forming an integrated and interactive system.	Involves collecting data about the client's capacities (knowledge, skills, and motivation) to perform universal, developmental, and health-deviation self-care requisites. Determines self-care deficits.	**Diagnosing:** Stated in terms of the client's limitations for maintaining self-care (a deficit in self-care agency). **Planning:** Involves considering and designing, with the client's participation, an appropriate nursing system (wholly compensatory, partially compensatory, supportive-educative, or a mix) that will help the client achieve an optimal level of self-care (i.e., enhance the client's self-care agency). **Implementing:** Assisting the client by acting for or doing for, guiding, supporting, providing a developmental environment, and teaching.	Determining the client's level of achievement in resolving self-care deficits and in performing self-care.

(*continued*)

TABLE 4-4

Selected Nursing Theories and the Nursing Process (*continued*)

THEORY	NURSING	PERSON/CLIENT	HEALTH	ENVIRONMENT	COLLECTING DATA FOR ASSESSMENT	PLANNING AND IMPLEMENTING THE DIAGNOSIS	EVALUATING
Betty Neuman's system model (1982)	A unique profession in that it is concerned with all of the variables affecting an individual's response to stressors, which are intra-, inter-, and extrapersonal in nature. The concern of nursing is to prevent stress invasion, or, following stress invasion, to protect the client's basic structure and obtain or maintain a maximum level of wellness. The nurse helps the client, through primary, secondary, and tertiary prevention modes, to adjust to environmental stressors and maintain client system stability.	Open system consisting of a basic structure or central core of survival factors surrounded by concentric rings that are bounded by lines of resistance, a normal line of defense, and a flexible line of defense. The total person is a composite of physiological, psychological, sociocultural, and developmental variables.	Wellness is the condition in which all parts and subparts of an individual are in harmony with the whole system. Wholeness is based on interrelationships of variables that determine the resistance of an individual to any stressor. Illness indicates lack of harmony among the parts and subparts of the system of the individual. Health is viewed as a point along a continuum from wellness to illness; health is dynamic (i.e., constantly subject to change). Optimal wellness or stability indicates that all a person's needs are being met. A reduced state of wellness is the result of unmet systemic needs. The individual is in a dynamic state of wellness–illness, in varying degrees, at any given time.	Both internal and external environments exist, and a person maintains varying degrees of harmony and balance between them. It is all factors affecting and affected by the system.	Proper assessment requires consideration of both the client's and the caregiver's perceptions of the basic structure, the lines of resistance and defense, and the internal and external environments.	**Diagnosing:** The nursing diagnosis must be a comprehensive statement that encompasses the client's general condition and circumstances, including actual and potential variances from wellness. **Planning:** The diagnostic statements are used to formulate and prioritize the client's needs and to identify interactions. **Implementing:** Nursing interventions focus on retaining or maintaining system stability. Interventions are carried out on three preventive levels: primary, secondary, and tertiary.	The final stage of the nursing process according to Neuman occurs when the client's outcomes are evaluated to confirm their attainment or guide reformulation of the goals.

THEORY	NURSING	PERSON/CLIENT	HEALTH	ENVIRONMENT	COLLECTING DATA FOR ASSESSMENT	PLANNING AND IMPLEMENTING THE DIAGNOSIS	EVALUATING
Sister Callista Roy's adaptation model (1970)	Nursing involves the care and well-being of human persons; the value-based stance of the discipline is rooted in beliefs about the human person. As a science, nursing is a developing system of knowledge about persons used to serve, classify, and relate the processes by which persons positively affect their health status. As a practice discipline, nursing's scientific body of knowledge is used to provide an essential service to people, that is, to promote the ability to affect health positively.	A biopsychosocial being who is in constant interaction with the environment and who has four modes of adaptation, based on physiological needs, self-concept (physical self, moral-ethical self, self-consistency, self-ideal and expectancy, and self-esteem), role function, and interdependence relations. Persons are coextensive with their physical and social environments. Persons and the earth are one; they are in God and of God.	A state and a process of being and becoming an integrated and whole person. Lack of integration represents lack of health.	All the conditions, circumstances, and influences surrounding and affecting the development and behavior of persons or groups; the input into the person as an adaptive system involving both internal and external factors.	Involves two levels. First-level assessment includes collecting data about output behaviors related to the four adaptive modes (physiological, self-concept, role function, and interdependence modes). Second-level assessment includes collecting data about internal and external stimuli (focal, contextual, or residual) that are influencing the identified behaviors.	**Diagnosing:** Focuses on adaptation problems and uses one of three alternative methods: 1. Stating behaviors within one mode with their most relevant influencing stimuli. 2. Clustering behavioral information and labeling it according to indicators of positive adaptation and a typology of common adaptation problems related to each mode. Roy provides a typology of indicators of positive adaptation and a typology of commonly recurring adaptation problems according to each of the four modes. 3. Labeling a behavioral pattern when more than one mode is being affected by the same stimuli. **Planning:** Setting goals in terms of behaviors the client is to achieve and planning nursing	Determining the client's output behaviors with those identified in the goals.

(*continued*)

TABLE 4-4

Selected Nursing Theories and the Nursing Process (*continued*)

THEORY	NURSING	PERSON/CLIENT	HEALTH	ENVIRONMENT	COLLECTING DATA FOR ASSESSMENT	PLANNING AND IMPLEMENTING THE DIAGNOSIS	EVALUATING
						interventions to promote the effectiveness of the client's coping mechanisms and adaptive behaviors. **Implementing:** Altering and manipulating the focal, contextual, and residual stimuli by increasing, decreasing, or maintaining them.	
Madeleine Leininger's cultural care diversity and universality theory (1991)	A learned humanistic art and science that focuses on personalized behaviors, functions, and processes to promote and maintain health or recovery from illness. It has physical, psychosocial, and cultural significance for those being assisted. It uses a problem-solving approach, as depicted in the Sunrise model, and uses three models of action: culture care preservation, culture care accommodation, and culture care repatterning.	Human beings are caring and capable of feeling concern for others; caring about human beings is universal, but ways of caring vary across cultures.	A state of well-being that is culturally defined, valued, and practiced. It is universal across cultures but is defined differently by each culture. It includes health systems, healthcare practices, health patterns, and health maintenance and promotion.	Not specifically defined, but concepts of world view, social structure, and environmental context are closely related to the concept of culture.	Must take into account biocultural variations in health and illness (e.g., assessing cyanosis, jaundice, anemia, and related clinical manifestations of disease in darkly pigmented clients).	**Diagnosing:** Focuses on meeting healthcare needs in the context of clients' patterns. **Planning:** The nurse plans, negotiates, and accommodates the client's specific cultural wants and needs (e.g, food preferences, religious practices, and treatment practices). **Implementing:** Healthcare personnel should work toward an understanding of care and the values, health beliefs, and lifestyles of different cultures, which will form the basis for providing culture-specific care.	When the client chooses to follow only folk medicine/treatment and refuses all prescribed medical or nursing interventions, nursing goals for the client need to be adjusted.

BOX 4-2	CULTURAL PULSE POINTS

Thinking Clearly about Clients of Other Cultures

When culture is an issue in the delivery of client care, the nurse must make use of his or her critical-thinking ability. Cultural awareness does not take the process far enough. Cultural awareness can be used to categorize, rather than individualize, care. Focusing too heavily on race, culture, and ethnicity is one danger associated with transcultural nursing theories and models.

Nurses must not label people by culture and race. Do not assume that the characteristics of a certain cultural group are true for every client who belongs to that racial, ethnic, or cultural group. The information we learn about cultural groups is no more than an overview. To fill in the picture would take many books. Nurses must always be aware of what people may be thinking that may differ from our own thoughts, and that other sources outside the traditional medical community exist to help the client.

scope among levels of nursing practice. It will help you provide culturally competent care (Box 4-2 ■). Most schools of nursing and healthcare agencies have developed their own structured assessment tools. Many of these are based on selected nursing theories.

Today the LPN/LVN has a great deal of responsibility and must think critically to make sound decisions. Understanding the four concepts that are central to nursing will help the LPN/LVN process information and make appropriate judgments. As nurses progress in formal education or lifelong learning, they will develop a personal theory of nursing. Understanding the basic principles will prepare the LPN/LVN for nursing of the future.

Note: The references and resources for this and all chapters have been compiled at the back of the book.

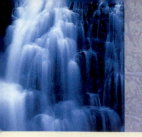
 KEY TERMS by Topic

Use the audio glossary feature of either the CD-ROM or the Companion Website to hear the correct pronunciation of the following key terms.

Critical Thinking
critical thinking, inductive reasoning, deductive reasoning, environments, subjective data, objective data

Theories and Models
theories

KEY Points

- Critical thinking is a purposeful, organized, logical, and disciplined mental activity in which ideas are produced and evaluated and judgments made.

- Critical thinking is reasonable, rational, reflective, autonomous, creative, fair, and inspires an attitude of inquiry that focuses on deciding what to believe or do.

- Critical thinkers have certain attributes: independence of thought, humility, courage, integrity, perseverance, empathy, and fair-mindedness.

- Everyone has at least some level of critical-thinking skill, and that skill can be developed with practice.

- Nursing theories help us view the client more completely or understand the goals of nursing better.

- Nursing theories explore the meaning of "client environment, health, and nursing" and add perspective to our own individual way of approaching our profession.

- Non-nursing theories help nurses as they gather and process data, particularly when completing a client history.

 EXPLORE Media Link

Additional interactive resources for this chapter can be found on the Companion Website at www.prenhall.com/ramont. Click on Chapter 4 and "Begin" to select the activities for this chapter.

For chapter-related NCLEX®-style questions and an audio glossary, access the accompanying CD-ROM in this book.
Video
- Thinking Critically, Making Decisions, Solving Problems

FOR FURTHER Study

See Chapter 5 for more information on critical thinking and the nursing process.

See Chapter 11 for details about Maslow's hierarchy of needs theory and other theories as they relate to life span development.

NCLEX-PN® Exam Preparation

TEST-TAKING TIP Identify the components of the question. The case situation gives you the information about the clinical health problem and the information you need to consider when answering the question. Always read all of the information and every word of the case situation.

1. Critical thinking can be described as:
   1. finding fault with statements of fact.
   2. the art of thinking about thinking.
   3. making decisions considering only one point of view.
   4. random and undirected.

2. Critical thinking and the nursing process go hand in hand. The nurse should consider personal assumptions or biases about the situation during what phase of the nursing process?
   1. assessment/data collection
   2. diagnosing
   3. planning
   4. evaluation

3. An application of critical thinking to the client teaching process requires that the nurse be aware of potential pitfalls and limitations in thinking. Which of the following actions take this into account?
   1. Evaluate the cognitive ability of the client.
   2. Give the client written instructions and allow time to read them.
   3. Instruct the client to call the home health nurse if problems develop.
   4. Arrange for a family member to be present during teaching.

4. In the seven-step decision-making process which of the following steps is explained as identify all possibilities for meeting the criteria?
   1. Set the criteria
   2. Weigh the criteria
   3. Seek alternatives
   4. Test alternatives

5. Your neighbor is a nurse at the community hospital. She is a member of the union. The union has called for a strike. All of the nurses at the hospital will go on strike. This sequence of thinking is called:
   1. inductive reasoning.
   2. deductive reasoning.
   3. opinion.
   4. belief.

6. Research has shown that children under 18 years who are given aspirin products during a viral infection are at risk for developing Reye's syndrome. Of the following statements, which is an example of deductive reasoning about this subject?
   1. The American Academy of Pediatrics recommends that children under the age of 18 not be given aspirin products.
   2. Children receiving aspirin are at risk for developing Reye's syndrome.
   3. Parents who give children aspirin during a viral infection are negligent.
   4. Parents should treat fever with cooling measures rather than medication.

7. Four concepts are central to nursing theory: nursing, person/client, environment, and health. Which of the following interventions is aimed at addressing the environment?
   1. teaching a community class on proper nutrition
   2. actively listening to a client who expresses concerns about upcoming surgery
   3. limiting external stimulation for a client who has increased intracranial pressure
   4. instructing a client to do range-of-motion exercises in preparation for walking following a cerebrovascular accident

8. The Neuman system model's unique focus is on:
   1. responses to a constantly changing environment.
   2. clients' reactions to stress.
   3. nurses' actions related to therapeutic self-care.
   4. culturally competent care.

9. The environment theory is attributed to which of the following nursing theorists?
   1. Florence Nightingale
   2. Sister Callista Roy
   3. Betty Neuman
   4. Madeleine Leininger

10. The dominant, distinctive, and unifying feature of nursing was identified as human caring by which of the following theorists?
    1. Dorothea Orem
    2. Sister Callista Roy
    3. Betty Neuman
    4. Madeleine Leininger

Answers and Rationales for Review Questions, as well as discussion of Care Plan and Critical Thinking Care Map questions, appear in Appendix I.

The LPN/LVN and the Nursing Process

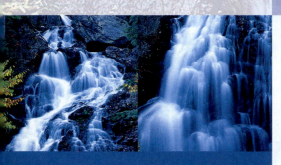

HISTORICAL Perspectives

The nursing process was based on theory developed by Ida Jean Orlando in the late 1950s. The nursing process is the most effective and practical, yet most misunderstood nursing theory. It takes time for students and new nurses to become comfortable with its use. All nursing personnel take part in the nursing process; however, the RN has the primary responsibility.

LEARNING Outcomes

After completing this chapter, you will be able to:

1. Identify essential characteristics of the nursing process.
2. Describe the components of the nursing process.
3. Identify the purpose of assessing.
4. Differentiate objective and subjective data, and primary and secondary data.
5. Identify three methods of data collection, and give examples of how each is useful.
6. Describe the importance and the elements of nursing diagnoses.
7. Discuss the planning step of the nursing process.
8. Discuss the activities of the implementing phase.
9. Explain the value of evaluating and how evaluating relates to other phases of the nursing process.

In 1961, the nursing process was defined at the Catholic University of America. It was developed as a template for thinking that was exclusively for nursing. The process was designed with the RN in mind, but use of the nursing process provides a common way of thinking for all licensed nurses. All licensed nurses collect data for assessment. They plan, implement, and evaluate. Although RNs are responsible for diagnosing, LPNs and LVNs contribute to the diagnosis through the data they collect and through their ongoing evaluation of the client.

The Nursing Process

The **nursing process** is a systematic, logical method of providing individualized nursing care. The purpose of the nursing process is to identify a client's health status and actual or potential healthcare problems or needs, to establish plans to meet the identified needs, and to deliver specific nursing interventions to meet those needs.

The components of the nursing process follow a logical sequence, but more than one component may be involved at any one time (Figure 5-1 ■). The nursing process consists of five steps: assessing, diagnosing, planning, implementing, and evaluating. Nursing theorists may use different terms to describe these steps. For example, nursing diagnosis may sometimes be called analysis. Implementation (implementing) may be called intervention or intervening. However, the activities of the nurse using the process are similar. An overview of the five-phase nursing process is shown in Table 5-1 ■.

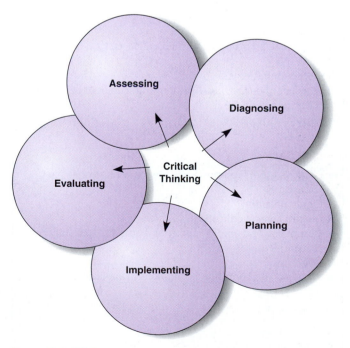

Figure 5-1. ■ The nursing process in action.

Assessing

Diagnosing

Critical Thinking

Evaluating

Planning

Implementing

TABLE 5-1	
Overview of the Nursing Process	
COMPONENT AND DESCRIPTION	**PURPOSE**
Assessing Collecting, organizing, validating, and documenting client data	To establish a database about the client's response to health concerns or illness and the ability to manage healthcare needs
Diagnosing Analyzing and synthesizing data	To identify client strengths and health problems that can be prevented or resolved by collaborative and independent nursing interventions To develop a list of nursing diagnoses and collaborative problems
Planning Determining how to prevent, reduce, or resolve the identified client problems; how to support client strengths; and how to implement nursing interventions in an organized, individualized, and goal-directed manner	To develop an individualized care plan that specifies client goals/desired outcomes and related nursing interventions
Implementing Carrying out the planned nursing interventions	To assist the client in meeting desired goals/outcomes, promote wellness, prevent illness and disease, restore health, and facilitate coping with altered functioning
Evaluating Measuring the degree to which goals/outcomes have been achieved and identifying factors that positively or negatively influence goal achievement	To determine whether to continue, modify, or terminate the plan of care

The nursing process "provides the framework in which nurses use their knowledge and skills to express human caring" and to help clients meet their actual and potential health problems (Wilkinson, 2007, p. 10). The nursing process has unique properties that enable it to respond to the changing health status of the client.

ROLE OF THE LPN/LVN IN THE NURSING PROCESS

LPNs/LVNs, as important members of the healthcare team, should be educated to use all aspects of the nursing process that fall within their scope of practice. Within each step there will be functions delegated to the LPN/LVN, functions carried out in collaboration with or under the direction of the RN, and functions implemented by the RN. It is very important for the LPN/LVN to understand the entire nursing process.

The nursing process helps students to think critically and to transfer classroom knowledge to the clinical setting. (See also Chapter 4 ⚭.) It provides both structure and guidance for LPN/LVNs as they provide client care. This chapter will define specific duties that can be carried out by the LPN/LVN. Guidelines for scope of practice do vary, however, so the nurse must always check state regulations.

Assessment

Assessment is the systematic collection, organization, *validation* (proving or supporting), and documentation of data. All phases of the nursing process depend on accurate and complete collection of data (information). Nursing assessments focus on a client's responses to a health problem. The Joint Commission on Accreditation of Healthcare Organizations (JCAHO; 2002) recommended that each client receive a documented assessment on admission to an agency. The initial assessment is done by or in collaboration with the RN.

In some situations, ongoing assessments are done only by RNs. This may be stated in the nurse practice act of the state or may be a management decision of a particular facility. The LPN/LVN is responsible for contributing by collecting data.

clinical ALERT

The LPN/LVN is responsible for reading the assessment *prior to* beginning care of assigned clients.

The assessment process involves four closely related activities: collecting data, organizing data, validating data, and documenting data.

COLLECTING DATA

Data collection is the process of gathering information about a client. It must be both systematic and continuous, and it must reflect a client's changing health status.

A client's **database** (baseline data) includes information from many sources: (1) the nursing health history (Box 5-1 ■), (2) the nurse's physical assessment, (3) the physician's history and physical examination, (4) results of laboratory and diagnostic tests, and (5) information contributed by other health personnel.

Client data should include past history as well as current problems. For example, a history of an allergic reaction to

BOX 5-1

Components of a Nursing Health History

Biographic Data
- Client's name, address, age, sex, marital status, occupation, religious preference, healthcare financing, and usual source of medical care

Chief Complaint or Reason for Visit
- The answer given to the question "Why did you come here today?"

History of Present Illness
- Provocation or palliation: what causes it, what relieves it
- Quality and quantity: type of pain and intensity
- Region or radiation: where it is, where it goes
- Scale of pain: 1 to 10
- Timing: when it began, how long it lasts, and how often it occurs

Past History
- Childhood illnesses
- Childhood immunizations
- Allergies
- Injuries
- Hospitalization for serious illnesses
- Medication: all currently used prescription and over-the-counter medication, such as aspirin, nasal spray, vitamins, or laxatives

Family History of Illness
- Heart disease, cancer, genetic abnormalities

Lifestyle
- Personal habits: tobacco, alcohol, coffee, etc.
- Diet
- Sleep/rest patterns
- Activities of daily living (ADLs): any difficulties in performing the basic activities
- Recreation/hobbies

Social Data
- Client's support system: family, friends, professional counseling
- Ethnic affiliation
- Highest level of education
- Occupation and employment: Has illness affected ability to work?
- Health insurance
- Home and neighborhood conditions (if applicable)

Psychological Data
- Major stressors
- Usual coping pattern
- Communication style

Assessing Across Cultural Differences

The assessment step of the nursing process is extremely important when clients and nurses have different ethnic backgrounds. To gather data about a client of a culture different from your own, you need to view the person in the context within which he or she exists. It is important to ask, not to assume, information. A helpful strategy is to repeat back information as a question, in order to validate what the client has said.

penicillin is a vital piece of historical data. Current data relate to present circumstances, such as pain, nausea, or sleep patterns. To collect data accurately, both the client and nurse must participate actively. The assessment should also consider the culture of each client (Box 5-2 ■).

TYPES OF DATA

Data can be subjective or objective. **Subjective data**, also referred to as **symptoms**, are apparent only to the person affected. Itching, pain, and feelings of worry are examples of subjective data. Subjective data include the client's sensations, feelings, values, beliefs, attitudes, and perception of personal health status and life situation. Information supplied by family members and significant others is also considered subjective. The following statements are examples of subjective data:

- "I feel weak all over when I exert myself."
- "I'm short of breath."
- "He doesn't seem so sad today," wife states.
- Client states he has a cramping pain in his abdomen. States, "I feel sick to my stomach."
- "I would like to see the chaplain before surgery."

Objective data, also referred to as **signs**, are detectable by an observer or can be tested against an accepted standard. They can be seen, heard, felt, or smelled. The following data are examples of objective data:

- Blood pressure 90/50
- Apical pulse 104
- Skin pale and diaphoretic
- Vomited 100 mL green-tinged fluid
- Cried during interview
- Lung sounds clear bilaterally
- Holding open Bible.

During the head-to-toe assessment, the nurse obtains the objective data needed to validate subjective data. A complete database of both subjective and objective data provides a baseline for comparing the client's responses to nursing and medical interventions. Together, subjective and objective data are called **manifestations**.

SOURCES OF DATA

The client is the *primary source* of data. All sources other than the client are considered *secondary sources*. The nurse should indicate on the nursing history when the data are obtained from a secondary source (a parent, a cousin, a friend).

The nurse must always consider the information in client records in light of the present situation. For example, if the most recent medical record is 10 years old, it is likely that the client's health practices and coping behaviors have changed.

DATA COLLECTION METHODS

The primary methods used to collect data are observing, interviewing, and examining.

Observing

Observation is gathering data by using the senses. Observation occurs whenever the nurse is in contact with the client or support persons. Although nurses observe mainly through sight, most of the senses are engaged during careful observations. Examples of client data observed through four of the five senses are shown in Table 5-2 ■.

Observation involves interpretation of data. The LPN/LVN and the RN work together (*collaborate*) to determine the meaning of the observation.

Interviewing

An **interview** is a planned communication or a conversation with a purpose. Interviewing is used mainly while taking the nursing health history. In interviews, the nurse gets or gives information, identifies problems of mutual concern, evaluates change, teaches, and provides support, counseling, or therapy. Interviewing is a process the nurse applies in most phases of the nursing process. During the assessment phase, however, the primary purpose of the interview is to gather data. (See Chapter 12 ⚭ for interviewing and communication techniques.)

TABLE 5-2
Observational Skills

SENSES	EXAMPLES OF CLIENT DATA
Vision	Overall appearance (body size, general weight, posture, grooming); signs of distress or discomfort; facial and body gestures; skin color and lesions; abnormalities of movement; nonverbal demeanor (e.g., signs of anger or anxiety); religious or cultural artifacts (e.g., books, icons, candles, beads)
Smell	Body or breath odors
Hearing	Breath and heart sounds; bowel sounds; ability to communicate; language spoken; ability to initiate conversation; ability to respond when spoken to; orientation to time, person, and place; thoughts and feelings about self, others, and health status
Touch	Skin temperature and moisture (e.g., hand grip); pulse rate, rhythm, and volume; palpatory lesions (e.g., lumps, masses, nodules)

Examining

The physical **examination** or physical assessment is a systematic data collection method. To conduct the examination, the nurse uses techniques of inspection, auscultation, palpation, and percussion. These techniques are discussed in Chapter 19 ⚭.

DOCUMENTING DATA

To complete the assessment phase, the nurse records client data. Accurate documentation is essential and should include all data collected about the client's health status. Data are recorded in a factual manner and not interpreted by the nurse. For example, the nurse records the client's breakfast intake (objective data) as "coffee 240 mL, juice 120 mL, 1 egg, and 1 slice of toast," not as "appetite good" (a judgment). A judgment or conclusion such as "appetite good" or "normal appetite" may have different meanings for different people.

To increase accuracy, the nurse records subjective data in the client's own words. Rewording what someone says increases the chance of changing the original meaning. Details of recording are discussed in Chapter 6 ⚭.

Diagnosis

Diagnosing is the second phase of the nursing process. In this phase, nurses use critical-thinking skills to interpret assessment data and identify client strengths and problems.

As mentioned earlier, this phase is the responsibility of the RN. The LPN/LVN discusses the collected data with the RN. The RN identifies appropriate nursing diagnoses for the client and initiates the nursing care plan.

A **nursing diagnosis** is a statement about an alteration in the client's health status. It refers to a condition that nurses are licensed to treat. A *medical diagnosis* is made by a physician and refers to a condition that only a physician can treat. Table 5-3 ■ compares nursing and medical diagnoses.

The identification and development of nursing diagnoses began formally in 1973, and international recognition came in 1977 with the First Canadian Conference. In 1982, the conference group accepted the name North American Nursing Diagnosis Association (NANDA, now NANDA International), recognizing the participation and contributions of nurses in the United States and Canada. NANDA updates its list of nursing diagnoses every 2 years (see Appendix II ⚭).

DEFINITIONS

In 1990, NANDA adopted an official working definition for the term *nursing diagnosis:* "Nursing diagnosis is a clinical judgment about individual, family, or community responses to actual and potential health problems/life processes. Nursing diagnoses provide the basis for selection of nursing interventions to achieve outcomes for which the nurse is accountable." They also defined the term *wellness diagnosis* as follows: "A wellness diagnosis is a clinical judgment about

---

TABLE 5-3

Comparison of Medical Diagnosis, Nursing Diagnosis, and Collaborative Problem

CATEGORY	MEDICAL DIAGNOSIS	NURSING DIAGNOSIS	COLLABORATIVE PROBLEM
Description	Describes disease and pathology; does not consider other human response; usually consists of not more than three words	Describes human responses to disease process or health problems; consists of a one-, two-, or three-part statement, usually including problem and etiology	Involves human responses, mainly physiological complications of disease, test, or treatments; consists of a two-part statement of situation/pathophysiology and the potential complication
Example	Myocardial infarction	*Activity Intolerance* related to decreased cardiac output	Potential complication of myocardial infarction: congestive heart failure
Duration	Remains the same while disease is present	Can change frequently	Present when disease or situation is present
Treatment orders	Physician orders primary interventions to prevent and treat	Nurse plans interventions to prevent and treat the nursing diagnosis	Nurse collaborates with physician and other healthcare professionals to prevent and treat
Nursing focus	Implement medical orders for treatment and monitor status of condition	Provide interventions for the nursing diagnosis	Prevent and monitor for onset or status of condition

an individual, family, or community in transition from a specific level of wellness to a higher level of wellness." *Readiness for Enhanced Spiritual Well-Being* and *Readiness for Enhanced Nutrition* are examples of possible wellness diagnoses.

Linda Carpenito (2005b) provided a definition of nursing diagnosis that is perhaps easier to understand. According to her, nursing diagnoses are "... actual or potential health problems which nurses, by virtue of their education and experience, are capable and licensed to treat."

Both of these definitions imply the following:

- Registered nurses are responsible for making nursing diagnoses, even though other nursing personnel may contribute data to the process of diagnosing and may implement specified nursing care.
- Nursing diagnoses describe a continuum of health states: deviations from health, presence of risk factors, and areas of enriched personal growth or areas of improved health.
- The domain of nursing diagnosis includes *only* those health states that nurses are educated and licensed to treat. For example, nurses are not educated to diagnose or treat diseases such as diabetes mellitus. This task is legally within the practice of medicine. Yet nurses can diagnose and treat *Deficient Knowledge, Ineffective Individual Coping,* or *Imbalanced Nutrition,* all of which may accompany diabetes mellitus.
- A nursing diagnosis is a statement made only after thorough, systematic data collection.

COMPONENTS OF A NANDA NURSING DIAGNOSIS

A nursing diagnosis has three components: the problem, defining characteristics, and etiology. Each diagnostic label approved by NANDA carries a definition that clarifies its meaning. For example, the definition of the label *Activity Intolerance* is: A state in which an individual has insufficient physiological or psychological energy to endure or complete required or desired daily activities.

Problem (Diagnostic Label)

The problem statement, or *diagnostic label,* describes the client's health problem or response for which nursing theory is given in clear, concise terms. (See Appendix II ⬭.) The purpose of the nursing diagnosis is to direct the formation of client goals and desired outcomes. It may also suggest some nursing interventions.

Defining Characteristics

Defining characteristics are the cluster of manifestations (signs and symptoms) that indicate the presence of a particular diagnostic statement. *Major and critical defining characteristics* are those that must be present for the diagnosis to be valid. For example, if the nursing diagnosis is *Activity Intolerance,* the client must have manifestations that include:

- Altered response to activity (such as dyspnea, tachypnea, shortness of breath)
- A weak, thready, or irregular pulse; tachycardia; increased pulse that does not return to resting heart rate after 3 minutes
- Blood pressure that does not increase with activity, hypotension, increased diastolic pressure of 15 mm Hg
- Weakness and fatigue.

Minor characteristics may or may not be present. The client with *Activity Intolerance* might or might not have the following manifestations:

- Pallor
- Cyanosis
- Vertigo
- Diaphoresis
- Confusion.

For *actual* nursing diagnoses, the defining characteristics are the client's signs and symptoms. For *risk* nursing diagnoses, characteristics are the factors that cause the client to be more than "normally" vulnerable to the problem.

Qualifiers

When a NANDA label is followed by the word (*specify*), the nurse states the area in which the problem occurs. For example, *Deficient Knowledge* (medications) and *Deficient Knowledge* (dietary adjustments) specify the particular area in which teaching is needed.

Qualifiers are added to some NANDA statements to give additional meaning to the diagnostic statement. For example, NANDA uses these qualifications:

- *Imbalanced* (a change from baseline)
- *Impaired* (made worse, weakened, damaged, reduced, deteriorated)
- *Decreased* (smaller in size, amount, or degree)
- *Ineffective* (not producing the desired effect)
- *Acute* (severe or of short duration)
- *Chronic* (lasting a long time, recurring, or constant).

Etiology

The **etiology** piece (related and risk factors) of the nursing diagnosis identifies probable causes of the health problem. It gives direction to the required nursing therapy, and enables nurses to individualize the client's care.

Take the example of a nursing diagnosis of *Constipation.* In one client, the etiology of constipation may be long-term laxative use. In another, it may be inactivity and insufficient fluid intake. In a third, it may be a diet that is very low in fiber and high in refined and processed foods.

TWO-PART AND THREE-PART NURSING DIAGNOSIS STATEMENTS

Most nursing diagnoses are written as two-part or three-part statements. Basic two-part statements are used for potential

Basic Three-Part Diagnostic Statement

Problem

Situatational Low Self-Esteem related to (r/t)

Etiology

Rejection by husband as manifested by (a.m.b.)

Signs and Symptoms

Hypersensitivity to criticism; states, "I don't know if I can manage by myself" and rejects positive feedback.

problems or "at risk for" statements. The basic two-part statement includes the following:

1. Problem (P): statement of the client's response (NANDA label)
2. Etiology (E): factors contributing to or probable causes of the responses.

The two parts are joined by the words *related to* to imply a relationship (such as *Ineffective Breastfeeding* related to breast engorgement).

Basic three-part statements are used for actual problems. The basic three-part nursing diagnosis statement is in the PES format and includes:

1. Problem (P): statement of the client's response (NANDA label)
2. Etiology (E): factors contributing to or probable causes of the response
3. Signs and symptoms (S): defining characteristics manifested by the client.

Box 5-3 ■ provides an example of a three-part diagnostic statement.

Planning

Planning is the third step in the nursing process. Planning is the process of designing nursing activities required to prevent, reduce, or eliminate a client's health problems. It involves decision making and problem solving. In planning, the nurse refers to the client's assessment data and diagnostic statements for direction in formulating client goals. All planning is aimed at preventing, reducing, or eliminating the client's health problems. The product of the planning phase is a client **care plan**.

The input of the LPN/LVN and support persons is essential if a plan is to be effective. Nurses do not plan for the client, but encourage the client to participate as actively as possible in making a plan together. In a home setting, the client's support people and caregivers are the ones who implement the plan of care. They should help create the care plan because its effectiveness depends largely on them.

According to the NCLEX-PN® test plan, the LPN's/LVN's role in the planning phase is to do the following:

1. Assist in the formation of the goals of care:
   - Participate in identifying nursing interventions required to achieve goals.
   - Communicate client needs that may require alteration of the goals of care.
2. Assist in developing the plan of care:
   - Involve the client and healthcare team members in the selection of nursing interventions.
   - Plan for the client's safety, comfort, and maintenance of optimum functioning.
   - Select nursing interventions for delivery of client's care (Anderson, 2005, p. 234).

TYPES OF PLANNING

Planning begins with the first client contact and continues until the nurse–client relationship ends, usually when the client is discharged from the healthcare agency.

The RN who performs the admission assessment usually develops the *initial comprehensive plan of care.* Planning should be initiated as soon as possible after the initial assessment, especially because of the trend toward shorter hospital stays. The LPN/LVN assists with data collection.

Ongoing planning is done by all nurses who work with the client. As nurses obtain new information and evaluate the client's responses to care, they can individualize the initial care plan further.

Discharge planning involves anticipating and planning for needs after discharge. It is a crucial part of comprehensive health care and should be addressed in each client's care plan. Although many clients are discharged to other agencies (e.g., nursing homes), follow-up care is increasingly being delivered in the home. Effective discharge planning begins at first client contact and involves comprehensive and ongoing assessment to obtain information about the client's ongoing needs. For details about discharge planning, see Chapter 10 ∞.

NURSING CARE PLANS

The end product of the planning phase of the nursing process is a formal or informal plan of care. An informal plan is a plan of action that exists in the nurse's mind. For example, the nurse may think, "Mrs. Phan is very tired. I will need to reinforce her teaching after she is rested." A formal nursing care plan is a written guide that organizes information about the client's care. The most obvious benefit of a formal written care plan is that it provides continuity of care. When nurses use the client's nursing diagnoses to develop goals and nursing interventions, the result is a holistic, individualized plan of care that will best meet the client's unique needs.

Standardized care plans (Figure 5-2 ■) specify the nursing care for groups of clients with common needs (e.g., all clients

Standardized Care Plan for Nursing Diagnosis of DEFICIENT FLUID VOLUME		
Etiology	**Desired Outcomes**	**Nursing Order** (Identify Frequency)
✓Decreased oral intake	✓Urinary output > 30 mL/hr	✓Monitor intake and output q _1_ h
✓Nausea		✓Weigh daily
__Depression	✓Urine specific gravity 1.005±1.025	✓Monitor serum electrolyte levels X 1 *or until normal*
✓Fatigue, weakness	✓Serum Na⁺ normal	✓Check skin turgor and mucus membranes q _8 h_
__Difficulty swallowing	✓Mucus membranes moist	✓Monitor temperature q _4 h_
__Other:_____	✓Skin turgor good	✓Administer prescribed IV therapy (Monitor according to protocol for Intravenous Therapy) *1000 mL D₅ LR*
✓Excess fluid loss	✓No weight loss	
✓Fever or increased metabolic rate	✓8-hour intake =	✓Offer oral liquids q _1_ h *at 100 mL/hr*
✓Diaphoresis	____400 mL oral____	Type _clear, cold_____
✓Vomiting	Other:	✓Instruct client regarding amount, type, and schedule of fluid intake
__Diarrhea		✓Assess understanding of type of fluid loss; teach accordingly
__Burns		✓Mouth care prn with _mouthwash_
__Other_____		✓Institute measures to reduce fever (e.g., lower room temperature, remove bed covers, offer cold liquids)
		Other Nursing Orders:_____
Defining Characteristics		_Monitor urine specific gravity_____
✓Insufficient intake		_q shift_____
✓Negative balance of intake and output		_____
✓Dry mucus membranes		_____
✓Poor skin turgor		_____
__Concentrated urine		_____
__Hypernatremia		_____
✓Rapid, weak pulse		
__Falling B/P		
__Weight loss		

Plan Initiated by: _M. Medina RN_____ Date _[date]_____

Plan/outcomes evaluated_____ Date_____

Plan/outcomes evaluated_____ Date_____

Client: _Amanda Aquilini_____

Figure 5-2. ■ A standardized care plan for the nursing diagnosis of *Deficient Fluid Volume*.

with myocardial infarction). Individualized care plans are tailored to meet the unique needs of a specific client—needs that are not addressed by the standardized plans.

Kardex Care Plans

Kardex is a trade name for a system in which client information and instructions for some of the client's care are kept on a large card in a central file, making information quickly accessible. The Kardex usually contains information about diet, activity levels, self-care/hygiene needs, treatments, and procedures (Figure 5-3 ■). Kardex information may change frequently. It is usually recorded in pencil so that the Kardex can be changed and kept up to date. For more information, see Chapter 6.

Computerized Care Plans

Computers are increasingly being used to create and store nursing care plans. The computer can also generate both standardized and individualized care plans. Nurses access the client's stored care plan from a centrally located terminal at the nurses' station or from terminals in client rooms.

Regardless of whether care plans are handwritten, computerized, or standardized, nursing care must be individualized to fit the unique needs of each client. The nurse uses standardized care plans for predictable, commonly occurring problems. Individual plans are used for unusual problems or problems that need special attention.

Student Care Plans

Because student care plans are a learning activity as well as a plan of care, they may be more lengthy and detailed than care plans used by working nurses. To help students learn to write a care plan, educators generally require that it be individualized. They may also modify the care plan by adding a column for "Rationale" after the nursing orders column (Table 5-4 ■). A **rationale** is the scientific principle given as the reason for selecting a particular nursing intervention.

The student may find it helpful to follow these guidelines when writing nursing care plans:

1. Use these category headings: "Nursing Diagnoses," "Goals/Desired Outcomes," "Evaluation Statement," "Nursing Orders/Interventions," "Rationales," and include a date for the evaluation of each goal.
2. Use standardized medical or English abbreviations and key words, not complete sentences, to communicate your ideas. Be sure to use only acceptable JCAHO

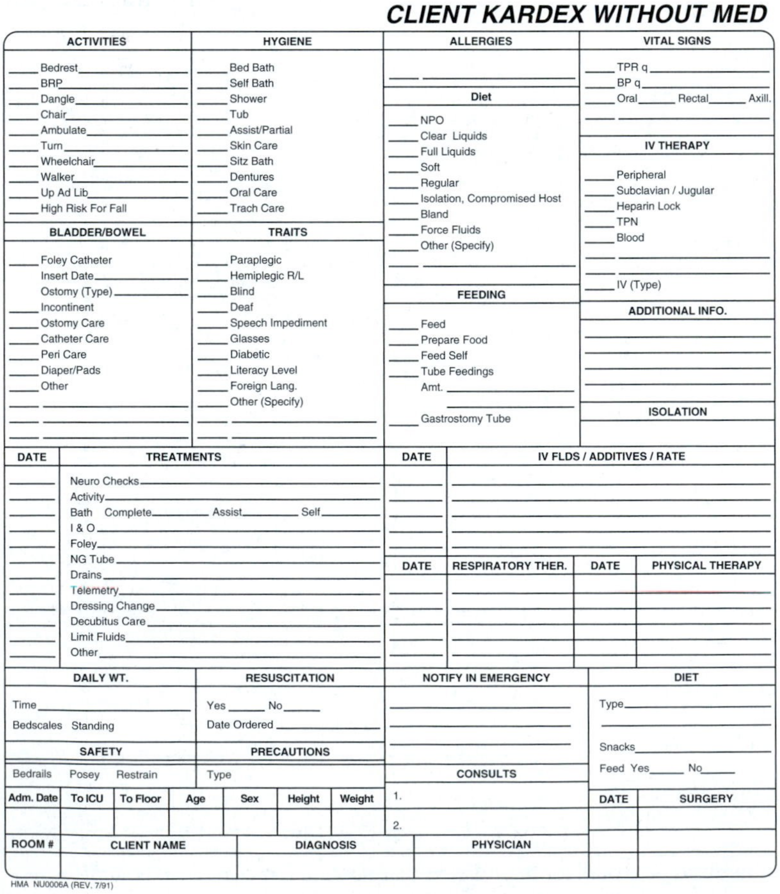
CLIENT KARDEX WITHOUT MED

ACTIVITIES: Bedrest; BRP; Dangle; Chair; Ambulate; Turn; Wheelchair; Walker; Up Ad Lib; High Risk For Fall

HYGIENE: Bed Bath; Self Bath; Shower; Tub; Assist/Partial; Skin Care; Sitz Bath; Dentures; Oral Care; Trach Care

ALLERGIES

Diet: NPO; Clear Liquids; Full Liquids; Soft; Regular; Isolation, Compromised Host; Bland; Force Fluids; Other (Specify)

VITAL SIGNS: TPR q; BP q; Oral Rectal Axill.

IV THERAPY: Peripheral; Subclavian / Jugular; Heparin Lock; TPN; Blood; IV (Type)

BLADDER/BOWEL: Foley Catheter; Insert Date; Ostomy (Type); Incontinent; Ostomy Care; Catheter Care; Peri Care; Diaper/Pads; Other

TRAITS: Paraplegic; Hemiplegic R/L; Blind; Deaf; Speech Impediment; Glasses; Diabetic; Literacy Level; Foreign Lang.; Other (Specify)

FEEDING: Feed; Prepare Food; Feed Self; Tube Feedings; Amt.; Gastrostomy Tube

ADDITIONAL INFO.

ISOLATION

DATE | TREATMENTS: Neuro Checks; Activity; Bath Complete Assist Self; I & O; Foley; NG Tube; Drains; Telemetry; Dressing Change; Decubitus Care; Limit Fluids; Other

DATE | IV FLDS / ADDITIVES / RATE

DATE | RESPIRATORY THER. | DATE | PHYSICAL THERAPY

DAILY WT.: Time; Bedscales Standing

RESUSCITATION: Yes No; Date Ordered

NOTIFY IN EMERGENCY

DIET: Type; Snacks; Feed Yes No

SAFETY: Bedrails Posey Restrain

PRECAUTIONS: Type

CONSULTS: 1. 2.

Adm. Date | To ICU | To Floor | Age | Sex | Height | Weight

DATE | SURGERY

ROOM # | CLIENT NAME | DIAGNOSIS | PHYSICIAN

HMA NU0006A (REV. 7/91)

Figure 5-3. ■ Kardex. (*Source:* Courtesy of Community Hospital of Lancaster, PA.)

TABLE 5-4

Partial Care Plan for a Client with Pneumonia

Nursing Diagnosis: *Ineffective Airway Clearance* related to viscous secretions and shallow chest expansion secondary to deficient fluid volume, pain, and fatigue.

DESIRED/EXPECTED OUTCOMES	EVALUATION STATEMENTS	NURSING ORDERS/ INTERVENTIONS	RATIONALE
Demonstrates adequate air exchange, as evidenced by 1. Absence of pallor and cyanosis (skin and mucous membranes)	1. Goal partially met. Skin and mucous membranes not cyanotic, but still pale.	a. Monitor respiratory status every 4 h; rate, depth, effort, skin color, mucous membranes, amount and color of sputum. b. Monitor results of blood gases, chest x-ray studies, and incentive spirometer volume as available. c. Monitor level of consciousness. d. Auscultate lungs every 4 h.	a, b, c, d. To identify progress toward or deviations from goal. *Ineffective Airway Clearance* leads to poor oxygenation, evidenced by pallor, cyanosis, lethargy, and drowsiness. *Retain nursing orders to continue to identify progress. Goal status indicates problem not resolved.*
2. Using correct breathing/ coughing technique after instruction	2. Goal partially met. Uses correct technique when pain well controlled by narcotic analgesics.	e. Vital signs every 4 h (TPR, BP).	e. Inadequate oxygenation causes increased pulse rate. Respiratory rate may be decreased by narcotic analgesics or increased by dyspnea and anxiety.
3. Productive cough	3. Goal met. Cough productive of moderate amounts of thick, yellow, pink-tinged sputum.	f. Instruct in breathing and coughing techniques. Remind to perform and assist every 3 h. Support and encourage. g. Administer prescribed expectorant; schedule for maximum effectiveness.	f. Does not need to be reinstructed as client demonstrates correct techniques. May still need support and encouragement because of fatigue and pain. g. Helps loosen secretions so they can be coughed up and expelled.
4. Demonstrating symmetric chest excursion of at least 4 cm	4. Goal not met. Chest excursion = 3 cm.	h. Maintain Fowler's or semi-Fowler's position.	h. Gravity allows for fuller lung expansion by decreasing pressure of abdomen on diaphragm.

abbreviations. See Table 6-1 for a list of standard medical abbreviations.

3. Refer to procedure books or other sources of information rather than including all the steps on a written plan.

4. Tailor the plan to the unique characteristics of the client by ensuring that the client's choices, such as preferences about the times of care and the methods used, are included. This reinforces the client's individuality and sense of control. For example, the written nursing order "Provide prune juice at breakfast rather than regular

juice" indicates that the client was given a choice of beverages.

5. Ensure that the nursing plan incorporates preventive and health maintenance aspects as well as restorative ones. For example, carrying out the order "Provide active-assistance ROM [range-of-motion] exercises to affected limbs every 2 h" prevents joint contractures and maintains muscle strength and joint mobility.

6. Ensure that the plan contains orders for ongoing assessment of the client (e.g., "Inspect incision every 8 h").

7. Include collaborative and coordination activities in the plan. For example, the RN may write orders to ask a nutritionist or physical therapist about specific aspects of the client's care.
8. Include plans for the client's discharge and home care needs. It is often necessary to consult and make arrangements with the community health nurse, social worker, and specific agencies that supply client information and needed equipment.
9. Date and sign the plan. The date the plan is written is essential for evaluation, review, and future planning. The nurse's signature demonstrates accountability to the client and to the nursing profession, since the effectiveness of nursing actions can be evaluated.

Chapters 6 through 35 ∞ provide Nursing Process Care Plans like the sample one given here. You will be asked to review the care plans and answer questions that call on your critical thinking skills.

NURSING PROCESS CARE PLAN
Client with Pneumonia

Amanda Aquilini is a 28-year-old female attorney who lives with her husband and 3-year-old daughter; her husband is on a business trip and will return tomorrow. The child is staying with a neighbor until her husband returns. Amanda was admitted to an acute care facility with shortness of breath (S.O.B.) on exertion, lung pain and fever, following a chest cold of two weeks' duration.

Assessment. The client states, "The doctor says I have pneumonia"; anxious, "I can't breath when lying down"; states "I feel weak"; experiencing chills; VS: T 103, P 92, R 28, BP 122/80 sitting, pulse ox 95% on room air; skin dry, cheeks are flushed; respirations shallow, productive cough—pale pink sputum, inspiratory crackles right upper and lower chest, diminished breath sounds on right side.

Nursing Diagnosis. The following important nursing diagnosis (among others) is established for this client:

- *Ineffective Airway Clearance*

Expected Outcomes. The expected outcomes specify that Ms. Aquilini will:

- Demonstrate adequate air exchange:
  - AEB absence of pallor and cyanosis
  - Use of correct breathing/coughing technique after instruction
  - Productive cough
  - Symmetric chest excursion of at least 4 cm

- Verbalizing chest pain of less than 4 on a 1–10 scale within 30 minutes after receiving PO analgesic.

Planning and Implementation. The following nursing interventions are planned and implemented:

- Monitor respiratory status every 4 h: rate, depth, effort, skin color, mucous membranes, amount and color of sputum.
- Monitor results of blood gases, chest x-ray studies, and incentive spirometer volume as available.
- Monitor level of consciousness.
- Auscultate lungs every 4 h.
- Take vital signs every 4 h (TPR, BP).
- Instruct in breathing and coughing techniques.
- Administer prescribed expectorant.
- Administer prescribed analgesic.
- Administer oxygen by nasal cannula.
- Assist with postural drainage daily.
- Administer prescribed antibiotic to maintain blood level.

Evaluation. Skin and mucous membranes not cyanotic, but still pale. Uses correct technique when pain well controlled by narcotic analgesics. Cough productive of moderate amounts of thick, yellow, pink-tinged sputum. Chest excursion = 3 cm. Stated "Easier to breath," rated pain at 3, and cough effective 30 minutes after oral analgesics. Scattered crackles throughout right anterior and posterior chest on auscultation. Respirations 26/min, pulse 96.

The physician orders:

- Chest x-ray
- Sputum culture and sensitivity
- Antibiotic therapy
- Expectorant
- Analgesics.

Critical Thinking in the Nursing Process

1. Identify and prioritize your nursing activities at this time.
2. Why does the physician order culture and sensitivity? Why must this be done prior to beginning antibiotic therapy?
3. Ms. Aquilini states, "I can't breath." What nursing activities can you perform to relieve her anxiety and ease her breathing?
4. What discharge teaching should be given to continue recovery and prevent another respiratory infection?

Note: Discussion of Critical Thinking questions appears in Appendix I.

LPN/LVN Long-Term Care Planning
The LPN/LVN working in long-term or home care may be assigned greater responsibilities related to care planning.

Once the initial assessment has been completed by the RN, the care plan will be developed as a collaborative process. The LPN/LVN will be responsible for implementing, evaluating, and reporting back to the RN on the achievement of the client's goals. Most long-term facilities and home care agencies have regularly scheduled client care conferences so that the healthcare team can interact and plan for the client's future needs.

SETTING PRIORITIES

Priority setting is the process of identifying nursing diagnoses and interventions in order from most important or critical to least important. Life-threatening problems, such as loss of respiratory or cardiac function, are given highest priority. Health-threatening problems, such as pain and decreased coping ability, are assigned medium priority because they may result in delayed development or cause destructive physical or emotional changes. A low-priority problem is one that arises from normal developmental needs or that requires only minimal nursing support.

Nurses frequently use Maslow's hierarchy of needs when setting priorities. In Maslow's hierarchy, physiologic needs that are basic to life (like air, food, and water) are listed at the base of the pyramid (Figure 5-4 ■). They receive higher priority than the need for security or activity. Growth needs, such as self-esteem, are not perceived as "basic" in this framework. So, nursing diagnoses such as *Ineffective Airway Clearance* and *Impaired Gas Exchange* would take priority over nursing diagnoses such as *Anxiety* or *Ineffective Coping*. See Table 5-5 ■ for an example of high, medium, and low priorities for a client.

Establishing Client Goals/Expected Outcomes

After establishing priorities, the nurse and client set goals for each nursing diagnosis. (*Note:* The terms *goal* and *expected outcome* are used interchangeably in this text.) On a care plan, the **goals** or **desired/expected-outcomes** describe, in terms of observable client responses, what the nurse hopes the client will achieve by implementing the nursing orders.

LONG-TERM AND SHORT-TERM GOALS. Goals may be short term or long term. A short-term goal might be "Client will raise right arm to shoulder height by Friday." In the same context, a long-term goal might be "Client will regain full use of right arm in 6 weeks." Long-term goals are often used for clients who live at home and have chronic health problems and for clients in nursing homes, extended care facilities, and rehabilitation centers.

DEVELOPING DESIRED OUTCOMES FROM NURSING DIAGNOSES. Goals are derived from and relate to the client's nursing diagnoses. For every nursing diagnosis, there will be at least one desired outcome that, when achieved, directly helps resolve the problem. When developing goals/desired outcomes, ask the following questions:

1. What is the problem statement?
2. What is the opposite, healthy response?

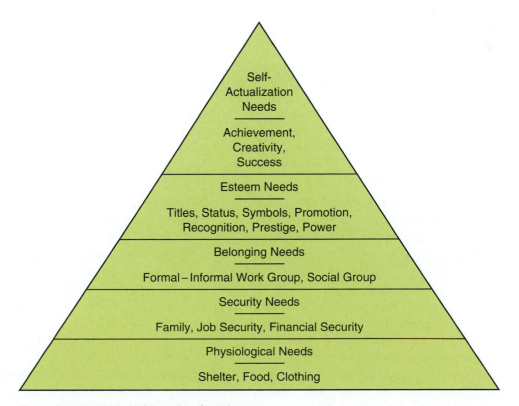

Figure 5-4. ■ Maslow's hierarchy of needs.

TABLE 5-5

Prioritizing Nursing Diagnoses for a Client with Pneumonia

NURSING DIAGNOSIS	PRIORITY	RATIONALE
Ineffective Airway Clearance related to (1) viscous secretions secondary to deficient fluid volume and (2) shallow chest expansion secondary to pain and fatigue	High priority	Loss of respiratory functioning is a life-threatening problem. The nurse's primary concern must be to promote the client's oxygenation by addressing the etiologies of this problem.
Deficient Fluid Volume: intake insufficient to replace fluid loss related to fever and diaphoresis	High priority	Severe fluid volume deficit is life threatening. Although not that severe for this client, it is a high-priority problem because it is also a contributing factor for *Ineffective Airway Clearance.* Collaborative efforts to improve hydration have already begun (intravenous fluids). The nurse must immediately and continuously assess and promote hydration.
Anxiety related to (1) difficulty breathing and (2) concerns over work and parenting roles	Medium priority	Although the client is concerned about work and parenting roles, these are not a threat to life. Also, treatment of her high-priority problem, *Ineffective Airway Clearance,* will relieve one of the etiologies of this problem (dyspnea). Meanwhile, the nurse must provide symptomatic relief of the client's anxiety during periods of dyspnea because extreme anxiety could further compromise oxygenation by causing her to breathe ineffectively and increasing the rate at which she uses oxygen.
Imbalanced Nutrition: Less than Body Requirements related to decreased appetite, nausea, and increased metabolism secondary to disease process	Low priority	This problem is not currently health threatening, but it could be if it were to persist. It will almost certainly resolve in a day or two as the medical problem is treated. If the medical problem does not resolve quickly, this will change to a medium priority.
Interrupted Family Processes related to mother's illness and temporary unavailability of father to provide child care	Low priority	Client's child is currently being cared for. If the husband returns as planned, this potential problem will not develop into an actual problem. No interventions are needed at present, except for continued assessment and reassurance.

3. How will the client look or behave if the healthy response is achieved? (What will I be able to see, hear, palpate, smell, or otherwise observe with my senses?)
4. What must the client do and how well must the client do it to demonstrate problem resolution or to demonstrate the ability to resolve the problem?

For example, if the nursing diagnosis is "*Risk for Deficient Fluid Volume* related to diarrhea and inadequate intake secondary to nausea," the related goal statement might be "Maintain fluid balance, as evidenced by urinary output in balance with fluid intake, normal skin turgor, and moist mucous membranes." In this example, a general goal (fluid balance) is stated as the opposite of the problem (deficient fluid volume) and then followed by a list of observable desired outcomes. If achieved, the outcomes would be evidence that the problem, *Deficient Fluid Volume,* has been prevented. See Table 5-6 ■ for examples of establishing goals and desired outcomes from nursing diagnoses.

WRITING DESIRED OUTCOME STATEMENTS. Goals/desired outcome statements should usually have the following four elements:

1. *Subject.* The subject is the client, any part of the client, or some attribute of the client (such as the client's pulse or urinary output). You do not need to write "the client" or "the client's pulse" in each statement, although as you begin to write care plans, stating, "the client will," will make sure you are writing a client outcome. It is assumed that the subject is the client unless otherwise stated.
2. *Action verb.* The verb specifies an action the client is to perform, for example, what the client is to do, learn, or experience. Some action verbs that express directly observable behaviors are *apply, describe, explain, inject, move, sleep, turn,* and *verbalize.*
3. *Measurable modifiers.* Conditions or modifiers may be added to the verb to explain the circumstances under which the behavior is to be performed. They explain:

TABLE 5-6

Deriving Desired Outcomes from Nursing Diagnoses

NURSING DIAGNOSIS	OPPOSITE HEALTHY RESPONSE (GOALS)	DESIRED OUTCOMES
Impaired Physical Mobility: inability to bear weight on left leg, related to inflammation of knee joint	Improved mobility: ability to bear weight on left leg	Ambulate with crutches by end of the week. Be able to stand without assistance by end of the month.
Ineffective Airway Clearance related to poor cough effort, secondary to incision pain and fear of damaging sutures	Effective airway clearance	Lungs will be clear to auscultation during entire postoperative period. No skin pallor or cyanosis by 12 hours post-operation. Within 24 hours after surgery, will demonstrate good cough effort.

- *How*—"Walks with the help of a walker."
- *When*—"After attending two group diabetes classes, lists signs and symptoms of diabetes."
- *Where*—"When at home, maintains weight at existing level."
- *What*—"Discusses food pyramid and recommended daily servings."

4. *Criteria of desired performance.* The criteria indicate the standard by which a performance is evaluated, or the level at which the client will perform the behavior. These criteria may specify time or speed, accuracy, distance, and quality. Examples follow:

- To establish a time-achievement criterion, the nurse asks *"How long?"*—"Weighs 75 kg by April."
- To establish an accuracy criterion, the nurse asks *"How well?"*—"Lists five out of six signs of diabetes in 2 weeks."
- To establish distance, the nurse asks *"How far?"*—"Walks one block per day."
- To establish quality, the nurse asks *"What is the expected standard?"*—"Administers insulin using aseptic technique in 3 days."

Students can use the guidelines listed in Box 5-4 ■ to help them develop useful outcome statements.

BOX 5-4   NURSING CARE CHECKLIST

Student Guidelines for Writing Desired Outcomes

☑ Write goals/outcomes in terms of client responses, not nurse activities. Begin each goal statement with "The client will" to focus it on client behaviors and responses. Avoid statements that start with *enable, facilitate, allow, let, permit.* These indicate what the *nurse* hopes to accomplish, not what the *client* will do.

   Correct: The client will drink 100 mL of water per hour. (*client behavior*)

   Incorrect: Maintain client hydration. (*nursing action*)

☑ Be sure that desired outcomes are realistic for the client's capabilities, limitations, and designated time span, if it is indicated. Limitations include finances, equipment, family support, social services, physical and mental condition, and time. For example, the outcome "Measures insulin accurately" may be unrealistic for a client who has poor vision due to cataracts.

☑ Ensure that the desired outcomes are compatible with the therapies of other professionals. For example, the outcome "The client will increase the time spent out of bed by 15 minutes each day" is not compatible with a physician's prescribed therapy of bed rest.

☑ Make sure that each goal is derived from only one nursing diagnosis. For example, the goal "The client will increase the amount of nutrients ingested and show progress in the ability to feed self" is derived from two nursing diagnoses: *Feeding Self-Care Deficit* and *Imbalanced Nutrition: Less than Body Requirements.*

☑ Use observable, measurable terms for outcomes. Avoid words that are vague and require interpretation or judgment by the observer. Phrases such as "increase daily exercise" and "improve knowledge of nutrition" can mean different things to different people. They are not clear and specific enough to guide the nurse when evaluating client responses.

☑ Make sure the client considers the goals important and values them. The nurse must actively listen to the client to determine personal values, goals, and desired outcomes in relation to current health concerns. Clients are usually motivated to reach goals they consider important. They may resist goals they feel they are told they "should do."

Implementation

Implementation is the fourth step of the nursing process, in which selected nursing interventions and activities occur. Nursing **interventions** are the actions that are initiated by the nurse to achieve client goals. The specific strategies should focus on eliminating or reducing the cause of the nursing diagnosis.

The process of implementing normally includes five steps: (1) reassessing the client, (2) determining the nurse's need for assistance, (3) implementing nursing orders, (4) delegating and supervising, and (5) documenting nursing actions.

REASSESSING THE CLIENT

Just before implementing an order, the nurse must reassess the client to make sure the intervention is still needed, because the client's condition may have changed. For example, Gayle Fischer has a nursing diagnosis of *Disturbed Sleep Pattern* related to anxiety and unfamiliar surroundings. During rounds, the nurse discovers that Gayle is sleeping and therefore does not perform the back rub that had been planned as a relaxation strategy.

New data may indicate a need to change the priorities of care or the nursing strategies. For example, a nurse begins to teach Ms. Eves, who has diabetes, how to give herself insulin injections. Shortly after beginning the teaching, the nurse realizes that Ms. Eves is not concentrating on the lesson. In discussion, the nurse learns that Ms. Eves is worried about her eyesight and fears she is going blind. Realizing that the client's level of stress is interfering with her learning, the nurse ends the lesson. She documents the client's response to the teaching and discusses Ms. Eves' concerns with the RN. The nurse continues to provide support to help the client cope with her stress.

DETERMINING THE NURSE'S NEED FOR ASSISTANCE

When implementing some nursing strategies, the nurse may require assistance for one of the following reasons:

- The nurse is unable to implement the nursing strategies safely alone (e.g., turning an obese client in bed).
- Assistance would reduce stress on the client (e.g., turning a person who experiences acute pain when moved).
- The nurse lacks the knowledge or skills to implement a particular nursing activity (e.g., a nurse who is not familiar with a particular model of oxygen mask needs assistance the first time it is applied).

IMPLEMENTING NURSING ORDERS (STRATEGIES)

It is important to explain to the client what will be done, what sensations to expect, and what the client is expected to do. For many nursing actions, it is also important to ensure the client's privacy, for example by closing doors, pulling curtains, or draping the client.

DELEGATING AND SUPERVISING

The LPN/LVN may have the opportunity to delegate to nursing assistants or other unlicensed staff. It is the responsibility of the delegator to assess the abilities of the staff member being assigned the task. Delegating does not relieve the nurse of the ultimate responsibility for the task. When in doubt, the nurse and the unlicensed person should work together until the unlicensed person's understanding of the assigned task and ability to perform it are confirmed.

DOCUMENTING AND REPORTING NURSING ACTIONS

After carrying out the nursing orders, the nurse completes the implementing phase by recording the interventions and client responses in the nursing progress notes. These are a part of the agency's permanent record for the client. Nursing actions must not be recorded in advance because, on reassessment, the nurse may find that the action should not or cannot be implemented. For example, a nurse is authorized to inject 10 mg of morphine sulfate subcutaneously to a client, but the nurse finds that the client's respiratory rate is 4 breaths per minute. This finding contraindicates the administration of morphine (a respiratory depressant). The nurse withholds the morphine and reports the client's respiratory rate to the nurse in charge and/or physician.

The nurse may record routine or recurring activities (e.g., mouth care) at the end of a shift. In the meantime, the nurse maintains a personal record of these interventions. Many agencies have special forms for this type of recording.

> ### clinical ALERT
>
> In some instances, it is important to record a nursing action immediately after it is implemented. Recorded data about a client must be up to date, accurate, and available to other nurses and healthcare professionals. This is particularly true of the administration of medications and treatments. For example, immediate recording helps safeguard the client from receiving a second dose of medication.

Nursing actions are communicated verbally as well as in writing. When a client's health is changing rapidly, the charge nurse and/or the physician may want to be kept up to date with verbal reports.

Interdisciplinary documentation forms require the nurse to chart in a timely manner. When others are using the same form, delayed charting may find the nurse without a place to document, making it necessary to document a late entry.

Nurses also give verbal reports at a change of shift and on a client's discharge to another unit or health agency. For information on documenting and reporting, see Chapter 6 ⬤⬤.

TYPES OF NURSING INTERVENTIONS

Nursing interventions that were identified and written during the planning step of the nursing process are performed during the implementing step. McCloskey and Bulechek (2003) define a nursing intervention as "any treatment, based upon clinical judgment and knowledge, that a nurse performs to enhance patient/client outcomes." Nursing interventions include:

- *Direct care*—An intervention performed through interaction with the client, such as giving a back massage.
- *Indirect care*—An intervention performed away from but on behalf of the client, such as obtaining a referral for physical therapy.
- **Independent interventions**—Independent or nurse-initiated interventions are those activities that nurses are licensed to do on the basis of their knowledge and skills. An example of an independent action is planning and providing special mouth care for a client based on a nursing diagnosis of *Impaired Oral Mucous Membranes.*
- **Dependent interventions**—Dependent (physician-initiated) interventions are activities carried out under the physician's orders or supervision, or according to specified routines.
- **Collaborative interventions**—These are nursing activities that reflect the overlapping responsibilities among healthcare personnel. A collaborative problem is a type of potential problem that nurses manage using both independent and physician-prescribed interventions.

Independent nursing interventions for a collaborative problem focus mainly on monitoring the client's condition and preventing development of the potential complication. For example, the physician might order physical therapy to teach the client crutch-walking. The nurse would be responsible for informing the physical therapy department and for coordinating the client's care to include the physical therapy sessions. When the client returns to the nursing unit, the nurse would assist with crutch-walking and collaborate with the physical therapist to evaluate the client's progress.

The nurse is responsible for explaining, assessing the need for, and administering the medical orders. The RN may write nursing orders to individualize the medical order based on the client's status. For example, for a medical order of "Progressive ambulation, as tolerated," the nursing orders might be:

1. Dangle for 5 min, 12 h postop.
2. Stand at bedside 24 h postop; observe for pallor, dizziness, and weakness.
3. Check pulse before and after ambulating. Do not progress if pulse 110.

The nurse should consider the consequences of each strategy and develop an understanding of the rationale for performing each intervention. Usually several possible interventions can be identified for each nursing diagnosis. The nurse's task is to choose those that are most likely to achieve the desired client outcomes. An intervention may have more than one consequence. For example, the strategy "Provide accurate information" could result in the following client behaviors:

- Increased anxiety
- Decreased anxiety
- Wish to talk with the physician
- Desire to leave the hospital
- Relaxation.

After considering the consequences of the alternative interventions, the nurse chooses one or more that are likely to be most effective. Although the nurse bases this decision on knowledge and experience, the client's input is important. The LPN/LVN must use judgment (or critical thinking) in implementing them.

The following criteria can help the nurse choose the best nursing strategy. The planned action must be:

- Safe and appropriate for the individual's age, health, and condition.
- Achievable with the resources available. For example, a home care nurse might wish to include a nursing order for an elderly client to "Check blood glucose daily," but if the client is legally blind, a daily visit by a capable support person or a home care nurse must be available and affordable.
- Compatible with the client's values, beliefs, and culture.
- Compatible with other therapies (e.g., if the client is not permitted food, the strategy of taking medication with an evening snack is not workable).
- Based on nursing knowledge and experience or on scientific knowledge (i.e., based on a rationale). For examples of rationales, refer to Table 5-5.
- Within established standards of care as determined by state laws and the policies of the institution.

IMPLEMENTATION SKILLS

Nurses employ a wide variety of skills in providing client care:

1. *Cognitive* (intellectual) skills include problem solving, decision making, critical thinking, and creative thinking. They are crucial to safe, intelligent nursing care.
2. *Interpersonal* skills are all the verbal and nonverbal activities people use when communicating directly with one another. The effectiveness of a nursing action often depends largely on the nurse's ability to communicate with others. Even when giving medication to a client, the nurse needs to understand the client and in turn be understood. A nurse who is delegating a nursing action also needs to be understood. Communication skills are discussed in detail in Chapter 12 ⦂

Interpersonal skills are necessary for all nursing activities. Caring, comforting, referring, counseling, and supporting are just a few. Interpersonal skills also include conveying knowledge, attitudes, feelings, interest, and appreciation of the client's cultural values and lifestyle.

3. *Technical skills* or **procedures** are "hands-on" skills such as manipulating equipment, giving injections, doing dressing changes, and moving, lifting, and repositioning clients. Procedures, also called psychomotor skills, always require communicating with the client. However, they also require knowledge and, frequently, manual dexterity. The number of technical skills expected of a nurse has greatly increased in recent years because of the increased use of technology, especially in acute care hospitals.

ESSENTIAL PROCEDURES IN IMPLEMENTING CARE

The procedures provided in this book give you some of the basic skills you will need to provide excellent client care. Procedures should always begin with an initial set of actions that ensure a safe, efficient, and caring environment. See Procedure 5-1 ■ for an example. These actions will become second nature to you as you continue your nursing training. Icons will be used to represent this initial set of actions at the start of each procedure. In some instances, an action may be optional. However, most are not. The icons (Figure 5-5 ■) are a reminder to do these basic, important interventions in nursing care:

1. Check the physician's order (Figure 5-5A).
2. Gather the necessary equipment (Figure 5-5B).
3. Introduce yourself to the client (Figure 5-5C).
4. Identify the client (check the client's wristband against the chart [Figure 5-5D]).
5. Provide privacy as needed (close the curtain [Figure 5-5E]).
6. Explain the procedure (Figure 5-5F).
7. Wash your hands. Hand hygiene is the single most effective way to prevent disease transmission (Figure 5-5G).
8. Don gloves as needed. (If the client is wet, wear gloves.) (Figure 5-5H)

Evaluation

Evaluation is the fifth and last phase of the nursing process, but many times the evaluation phase is overlooked. **Evaluation** is a planned, ongoing, purposeful activity in which client and healthcare professionals determine the client's progress toward goal achievement and the effectiveness of the nursing care plan. Without evaluation, an intervention

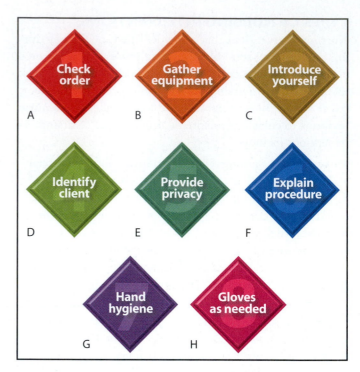

Figure 5-5. ■ Icons of initial nursing actions. **A.** Check the physician's order. **B.** Gather the necessary equipment. **C.** Introduce yourself to the client. **D.** Identify the client (check the client's wristband against the chart). **E.** Provide privacy as needed (close the curtain). **F.** Explain the procedure. **G.** Wash your hands. Hand hygiene is the single most effective way to prevent disease transmission. **H.** Don gloves as needed. (If the client is wet, wear gloves.)

may be discarded as ineffective without taking time to discover why it did not work. One thing that sets the LPN/LVN apart from a certified nursing assistant (CNA) is the knowledge and ability to evaluate.

Clients need to be evaluated all day long. The best way to evaluate an intervention is to determine if the objective from the written care plan has been met, and if not, why not. Through evaluating, nurses accept responsibility for their actions. They indicate interest in the results of the nursing actions. They also demonstrate a desire to replace ineffective actions with more effective ones. After determining whether a goal has been met, the nurse writes an evaluative statement (either on the care plan or in the nurse's notes). These notes help the RN to review and modify the nursing care plan so that individualized nursing care can continue. Once the care plan is modified, the nursing process cycle begins again.

Note: The references and resources for this and all chapters have been compiled at the back of the book.

Basic Procedure Steps and Admission Information

Purpose

- To obtain all pertinent data on hospital admission.

Equipment

- Admission kit
- Thermometer
- Blood pressure cuff and stethoscope
- Appropriate scale of client's need
- Urine container (if UA needed)
- Kardex, care plan
- Client's medical record

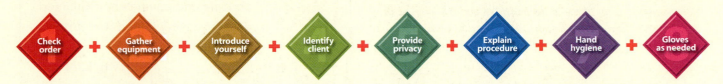

Interventions

1. Check physician's orders. *All dependent nursing interventions require a physician's order.*

2. Gather the necessary equipment. *Collecting all necessary equipment prior to beginning procedure will save steps, time, and assure that you will have what you need to complete procedure correctly.*

3. Introduce yourself. Address the client by Mr., Mrs., Ms., followed by first and last name.

4. Compare the wristband to the name and medical record number on the client's chart, in order to make sure procedure is being done on the correct client.

5. Provide privacy. *By closing the door or pulling the bed curtain, you can assure the client that confidentiality will be maintained.*

6. Explain the procedure. *This will help relieve client anxiety and help establish rapport between you and the client.*

7. Wash hands. *Hand hygiene is the most important thing that the nurse can do to stop the spread of infectious disease. This should be done prior to any client contact.*

8. Put on gloves if necessary. Some facilities say, "If it's wet and you are not, put on gloves." Other facilities may require gloves for all client contact. *(Note: Throughout the text, steps 1–8 will be identified with icons only to remind you to complete the steps before starting the procedure.) Rationales follow the procedure steps in italics.*

9. Place a hospital gown on the client and assist him or her into bed. *Wearing a hospital gown will be necessary during the physical assessment, and the client will be more comfortable in bed during the assessment.*

10. Explain equipment and hospital routine. *To assist the client to adjust to hospital environment with minimal distress.*

11. Open and place admission kit on the bedside table. Fill and place water pitcher and cup on the overbed table unless the client is NPO (nothing by mouth). *Supplies and water will be easily accessible to the client.*

12. Record personal belongings on the admission form and encourage family to take valuables home. (Valuables can be placed in the hospital safe if no family available.) *This will serve as a checklist on discharge to be sure all belongings are sent home with the client. Valuables should not be kept at the bedside to prevent loss.*

13. Obtain client's height and weight using a bed or floor scale. *Height and weight need to be available for physician and pharmacy for proper dosage of medication, and as a baseline of client's nutritional status.*

14. Take vital signs. *This is a baseline to determine the client's status.*

15. Collect data for the client's health history. *A complete history provides a total picture of client's condition and present health problems.*

16. Complete the bedside assessment (if this is within the LPN/LVN's scope in your area of practice). *To obtain as much data as possible about the client's chief complaint.*

17. Document the procedure. *"If it is not documented, it is not done." (Each procedure in the clinical chapters will provide a sample documentation.)*

18. Obtain a urine specimen, and notify laboratory, x-ray, and ECG of client's admission. *Client may need to have admission laboratory studies, ECG, and chest x-ray done as a baseline.*

19. Document all findings in the client's medial record on the admission form. *Complete, accurate, timely documentation is necessary to provide continuity of care.*

20. Collaborate with the RN to write and initiate the care plan. *Initiation of care plan will be the first step on client's road to recovery.*

21. Notify the physician that the client has been admitted and obtain orders if they are not on the floor. *It is important that the physician be notified in a timely manner so that treatment can begin as soon as possible.*

SAMPLE CHARTING (DOCUMENTATION)

[date]
[time]

Admission procedure completed on a 28-year-old female, admitted with pneumonia. See admission form for vital signs and assessment. V.A. obtained and sent to lab. Blood sample drawn by lab for CBC and blood culture. Bedside portable chest obtained. Hospital routine and equipment explained. Client resting in bed. Dr. Katz's exchange notified.

_____M. Smith, LPN

Chapter Review

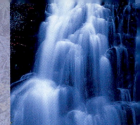

 KEY TERMS by Topic

Use the audio glossary feature of either the CD-ROM or the Companion Website to hear the correct pronunciation of the following key terms.

Nursing Process
nursing process

Assessment
assessment, database, subjective data (symptoms), objective data (signs),
manifestations, observation, interview, examination

Diagnosis
diagnosing, nursing diagnosis, etiology

Planning
planning, care plan, rationale, goals, desired/expected outcomes

Implementation
implementation, interventions, independent interventions, dependent interventions, collaborative interventions, procedures

Evaluation
evaluation

KEY Points

- The nursing process is a systematic, rational method of planning and providing individualized nursing care for individuals, families, groups, and communities.

- The nursing process can be used in all healthcare settings. It is client centered, interpersonal, and collaborative. It provides a framework for nurses' accountability and responsibility.

- The five phases of the nursing process—assessing, diagnosing, planning, implementing, and evaluating—are ongoing and interconnected. The primary functions of the LPN/LVN are gathering data for assessment, implementing, and evaluating.

- The nurse collects data for assessment (1) to help establish nursing diagnoses and care plans, (2) to ensure that the ordered intervention is appropriate, and (3) to evaluate whether nursing actions have been effective.

- Nursing diagnoses define health conditions that nurses are legally qualified to treat. A nursing diagnosis has three components: the problem, the etiology (cause), and the defining characteristics (signs and symptoms). Professional standards require that RNs establish nursing diagnoses.

- Planning involves establishing goals and designing nursing activities to prevent, reduce, or eliminate a client's health problems. The client and family should be involved in establishing desired outcomes.

- Planning is generally done by registered nurses, but LPNs/LVNs in long-term care may be called on to identify problems and initiate the plan of care.

- Implementing is carrying out or delegating the nursing interventions. It incorporates all of the activities performed to promote health, prevent complications, treat present problems, and facilitate the client's coping with chronic alterations in health status. Documenting is an important piece of this step of care.

- Evaluating is the process of comparing client responses to established goals/outcomes to determine whether goals have been met. It includes review and modification of the care plan.

- Goal statements and desired outcomes are written in terms of the client's behavior. They describe specific and measurable client responses and help the nurse evaluate the effectiveness of the nursing interventions.

- The desired outcomes determine the data that must be collected to evaluate the client's health status. The data are used to confirm or change the nursing diagnoses, maintain or alter the plan of care, and continue or change nursing interventions.

 EXPLORE Media Link

Additional interactive resources for this chapter can be found on the Companion Website at www.prenhall.com/ramont. Click on Chapter 5 and "Begin" to select the activities for this chapter.

For chapter-related NCLEX®-style questions and an audio glossary, access the accompanying CD-ROM in this book.

FOR FURTHER Study

For more about the critical-thinking process, see Chapter 4.
For information on documenting and reporting, see Chapter 6.
For more information on the Kardex system, see Chapter 6.
See Table 6-1 for a list of standard medical abbreviations.
For details about discharge planning, see Chapter 10.
See Chapter 12 for interviewing and communication techniques.
For a full discussion on examination techniques see Chapter 19.

Critical Thinking Care Map

Caring for a Client with Alzheimer's
NCLEX-PN® Focus Area: Nursing Process

Case Study: Charles Weldon, a 78-year-old male, was diagnosed with Alzheimer's disease 3 years ago. His wife Mary has been his primary caregiver. They reside in their own retirement apartment in Lakeview Manor, a full-care retirement community. Mr. Weldon has being admitted to the skilled nursing area on a trial basis while Mrs. Weldon attends her granddaughter's college graduation out of state. She comes to visit to tell him good-bye before her trip. He says he doesn't know her and that they won't give him any food. She begins to cry and says, "It was a bad idea to plan this trip. I should stay and take Charles home with me."

Nursing Diagnosis: Compromised Family Coping

COLLECT DATA

Subjective	Objective
_____	_____
_____	_____
_____	_____
_____	_____
_____	_____
_____	_____
_____	_____

Would you report this data? Yes/No

If yes, to: _____

What would you report? _____

Nursing Care

_____
_____
_____
_____
_____
_____
_____
_____
_____
_____

How would you document this? _____
_____
_____

Data Collected
(use those that apply)

- Articef
- Coreg 6.125 mg every day (hold if SBP < 110)
- Ativan 1 mg prn every 6 h for anxiety
- Regular insulin per sliding scale ac and at bedtime
- NPH Humulin 30 units every am
- Diet: mechanical soft diet
- VS: T 98.2, P 68, R 16, BP 104/60

Nursing Interventions
(use those that apply; list in priority order)

- Assist significant person with expanding repertoire of coping skills.
- Observe for any symptoms of elder abuse.
- Assess the client's awareness of deficits that may result from normal aging.
- Assess for dietary intake of essential nutrients.
- Help family members recognize the need for help and teach them how to ask for it.
- Encourage family members to verbalize feelings.
- Provide finger food and place in hands as needed to cue.
- Validate the family's feelings regarding the impact of client's illness on family lifestyle.

Compare your documentation to the sample provided in Appendix I.

NCLEX-PN® Exam Preparation

1   Assessment can be distinguished from evaluation in which of the following ways?

1. Assessment is done throughout the nursing process; evaluation is done only when the client is ready for discharge.
2. Assessment is done by the LPN/LVN, evaluation is always done by the RN.
3. Assessment identifies the client's current status, while evaluation determines the client's progress toward a desired outcome.
4. Assessment is based on subjective data, while evaluation is based on objective data.

2   The second phase of the nursing process involves analyzing data and identifying health problems, risks, and strengths. This phase is known as:

1. planning.
2. evaluating.
3. diagnosing.
4. implementing.

3   In your collaboration with the RN, it is determined that the client has a nursing diagnosis of *Impaired Mobility*. Which of the following statements is an appropriately written client goal for this problem?

1. Encourage ambulation 3×/day.
2. Client will walk the length of the hall 2×/day, with the assistance of two staff members, in 2 days.
3. Client's ability to ambulate will improve by the second day of hospitalization.
4. Assist client to sit in chair for meals.

4   Rationales can be described as:

1. scientific reasons that support the choice of a particular nursing intervention.
2. subjective data for identifying client problems.
3. methods used to evaluate client outcomes.
4. steps of nursing procedures.

5   The final nursing task of the planning phase is:

1. choosing the appropriate interventions.
2. evaluating the effectiveness of the interventions.
3. delegating interventions to unlicensed personnel.
4. writing the care plan.

6   From the following statements from a care plan, identify which one is a rationale.

1. Vital signs every 4 h (T and BP).
2. Cough productive of moderate amount of pink-tinged sputum.
3. Inadequate oxygenation causes increase in pulse rate.
4. Demonstrates adequate air exchange as evidenced by absence of cyanosis.

7   The nursing care plan is put into action during which phase of the nursing process?

1. planning
2. implementing
3. assessing
4. evaluating

8   Delegating and supervision occurs in which stage of the nursing process?

1. assessing
2. diagnosis
3. planning
4. implementing

9   Evaluation statements consist of two parts:

1. conclusion and supporting data
2. desired outcome and rationale
3. problem status and client's response
4. reassessment and data comparison

10   The nursing process can be described as a(n):

1. strategy for implementing evidence-based nursing practice.
2. holistic nursing assessment.
3. organized framework for professional nursing practice.
4. contributing factors for nursing diagnosis.

Answers and Rationales for Review Questions, as well as discussion of Care Plan and Critical Thinking Care Map questions, appear in Appendix I.

Thinking Strategically About. . .

Carlos, a licensed vocational nurse with several years of experience, begins working in a long-term care facility. Within a few weeks, it becomes apparent that the night nurse is treating elderly clients unkindly, and there seems to be an increase in reported skin tears on the nights when she works. He speaks to this nurse about his concerns, but he sees no change in the situation. One morning, arriving at work early for a staff meeting, he overhears her verbally abusing a confused resident who will not take his medications. Carlos reports his observation to the director of nursing (DON). When there is still no improvement, Carlos returns to the manager and says that he is considering speaking to the administrator or making a formal complaint to the state nursing board.

The alleged abuser is a long-time employee at the facility and popular with the nursing assistants and other staff. When the supervisor finally speaks to her about the complaint, the identity of the reporter becomes clear. Carlos is ostracized by most of the staff. He is criticized in front of residents and family members, and the night nurse continuously makes racial slurs when referring to him with other staff members. After several months, Carlos feels he can no longer tolerate the working conditions and accepts a job at another facility.

COMMUNITY

Why could this nurse's action or inaction be considered a community issue?

CRITICAL THINKING

- Would you consider Carlos to be a "whistle-blower?"
- Was Carlos's decision to report what he observed a legal or ethical issue?
- Does Carlos have any legal recourse for his treatment?

COMMUNICATION

Consider the instances of communication that occurred in this case study: between the abusive nurse and the client, between the two nurses, between Carlos and the DON, and between the staff and Carlos. In pairs or small groups, role-play these interactions as you think they probably occurred.

CONFLICT RESOLUTION

As a class or in an essay, review Carlos's decisions using the seven-step decision-making process as a guide. What other alternatives might Carlos have had? How could the DON have handled the situation differently?

Introduction to Clinical Practice

UNIT II

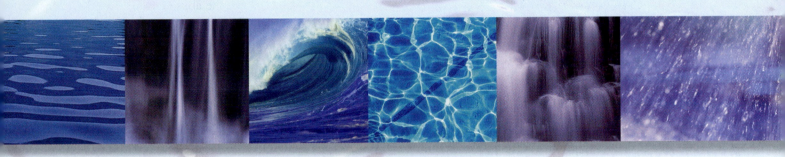

Chapter 6

Documenting and Reporting

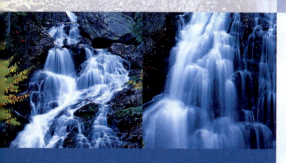

HISTORICAL Perspectives

Walt Whitman was a volunteer nurse during the Civil War. He created one of the first documentations of care in a narrative form. In his book of poetry entitled Drum Taps, *you will find poems from his years as a psychological nurse to sick and wounded soldiers. Whitman was known to constantly scribble in little notebooks filled with bits of poetry, and notes concerning the needs of the wounded soldiers. Whitman writes, "The expression of American personality through this war is not to be looked for in the great campaign, & the battle-fights. It is to be looked for ... in the hospitals, among the wounded." Louisa May Alcott published* Hospital Sketches *(1865) after a brief time as a nurse during December 1862 and January 1863. Her work was cut short when she became ill with typhoid fever.*

BRIEF Outline

Purposes of Client Records
Guidelines for Recording
Confidentiality of Client Records
Documentation Systems
Types of Documentation Methods
Reporting

LEARNING Outcomes

After completing this chapter, you will be able to:

1. Discuss reasons for keeping client records.
2. Identify and discuss guidelines for effective recording that meet legal and ethical standards.
3. List the measures used to maintain the confidentiality of records, including computer records.
4. Identify abbreviations and symbols commonly used for charting.
5. Compare and contrast different documentation systems.
6. Explain how various forms in the client record are used to document steps of the nursing process.
7. Compare and contrast the documentation needed for clients in acute care, home health care, and long-term care settings.
8. Identify essential guidelines for reporting client data.
9. Describe the nurse's role in reporting, conferring, and making referrals.

Effective communication among health professionals is vital to the quality of client care. Generally, health personnel communicate through discussion, reports, and records. A *discussion* is an informal conversation between two or more healthcare personnel to identify a problem or establish strategies to resolve a problem. A **report** is an oral, written, or computer-based communication intended to convey information to others. For example, nurses always report on clients at the end of a work shift. A **record** is a written or computer-based collection of data. The process of making an entry on a client record is called *recording,* **charting**, or **documenting**. A **clinical record**, also called a *chart* or *client record,* is the formal, legal document that provides evidence of a client's care. Although healthcare organizations use different systems and forms for documentation, all client records contain similar information.

Each healthcare organization has policies about recording and reporting client data, and each nurse is accountable for practicing in accordance with these standards. Agencies also indicate which nursing assessments and interventions must be recorded by a nurse and those items that may be delegated to unlicensed personnel. In addition, the Joint Commission on Accreditation of Healthcare Organizations (JCAHO) has policies on information management which specify that record keeping should be timely, accurate, confidential, and client specific (JCAHO, 2000).

Purposes of Client Records

COMMUNICATION
The client record serves as the vehicle by which different health professionals who interact with a client communicate with each other. This prevents fragmentation, repetition, and delays in client care. The record also provides a central location for notifying health professionals of the client's needs, progress, and current health status.

PLANNING CLIENT CARE
Each health professional uses data from the client's record to plan care for that client. A physician, for example, may determine that laboratory tests reveal the presence of a certain microorganism and then orders an antibiotic. Nurses then use baseline and ongoing assessments to determine the effectiveness of interventions and the nursing care plan. The record also provides a base from which all healthcare disciplines may coordinate the client's care.

LEGAL DOCUMENTATION
The client's record is a legal document and is admissible in court as evidence. In some jurisdictions, however, the record is considered inadmissible as evidence when the client objects, because information the client gives to the physician is confidential.

EDUCATION, RESEARCH, AND HEALTHCARE ANALYSIS
Students use client records as an essential educational tool. A record can frequently provide a comprehensive view of the client, the illness, treatment strategies, and factors that affect the outcome of the illness. The information contained in a record can be a valuable source of data for research. Review of treatment plans for clients with similar health problems can yield helpful information when treating new clients with the same problems.

Likewise, information from records may assist healthcare planners to identify agency needs. It can highlight overused and underused hospital services. It can identify services that cost the agency money and those that generate revenue.

AUDITING
An audit is a review of records. Client records are audited for quality improvement. Accrediting agencies such as the JCAHO may review client records to determine if a particular health agency is meeting its stated standards.

REIMBURSEMENT
Documentation also helps a facility receive reimbursement from the federal government. For a facility to obtain payment through Medicare, the client's clinical record must contain the correct diagnosis-related group (DRG) codes and reveal that the appropriate care has been given.

Guidelines for Recording

Because the client's record is a legal document and may be used to provide evidence in court, many factors are considered in recording. Healthcare personnel must not only maintain the confidentiality of the client's record but also meet legal standards in the process of recording.

DATE AND TIME
- Document the date and time with each entry.
- Make entries as soon as possible after performing an assessment or intervention.
- Record the time either using conventional time, denoting A.M. or P.M., or using the 24-hour clock (military time) (Figure 6-1 ■). Follow agency policy.
- Avoid block-style charting in which an entire shift is documented under one date and time.

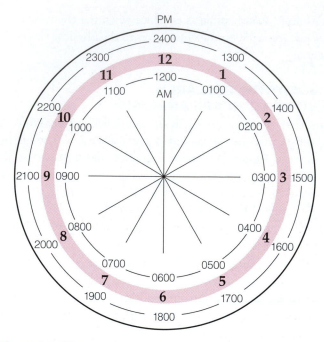

Figure 6-1. ■ The 24-hour clock.

TIMING

■ Follow agency policy regarding the frequency of documenting.
■ Adjust frequency of documentation as a client's condition indicates. An unstable client requires more frequent assessment and documentation than a stable client.
■ Never record nursing care before it is provided.

LEGIBILITY

■ Make all entries legible and easy to read to prevent interpretation errors.
■ Print your entries if your cursive writing is difficult to read.
■ Follow agency policy regarding handwritten recording of nurses' notes.

PERMANENCE

■ Make all entries on the client's record in permanent, nonerasable blue or black ink according to agency policy. This ensures that the record is permanent and that changes can be identified.

ACCEPTED TERMINOLOGY

■ Use only commonly accepted abbreviations, symbols, and terms specified by agency policy. See Table 6-1 ■ for common abbreviations and Table 6-2 ■ for common symbols. See Chapter 29 ⬭ for abbreviations related to medication administration. Access the JCAHO website for more information.

■ Write a term out in full if in doubt about whether to use an abbreviation.

CORRECT SPELLING

■ Use correct spelling to ensure accuracy in documentation.
■ Look words up in a dictionary or other resource book if unsure of the correct spelling.
■ Spell similar medication names correctly to avoid medication errors. (For example, *Celebrex* and *Cerebyx* are two decidedly different medications.)

SIGNATURE

■ Sign entries made in the nurses' notes at the time you make the entry.
■ Use your name and title in the signature. For example, the signatures "Susan J. Green, LPN" or "S. Green, LPN" would be correct, depending on facility policy.
■ Full signature should appear at least once on each page.
■ Use correct title abbreviations: RN for registered nurse, LPN for licensed practical nurse, LVN for licensed vocational nurse, SN for student nurse in an RN program, and SVN/SPN for student vocational/practical nurse. (Some schools use VNS or PNS for vocational/practical nursing student.)

ACCURACY

■ Check that you have the correct chart by verifying the client's name and identification information stamped or written on each page before making any entry or filing a report.
■ Make accurate notations—ones that consist of facts or observations rather than opinions or interpretations. Describe what you see and hear, not what you think or interpret for client actions.
■ Quote the client directly in the client's exact words when documenting client's concerns. For example, "Stated: 'I'm worried about my leg.'"
■ Chart specific data rather than using general terms such as *large, good,* or *normal* that can be misinterpreted. For example, "2 cm by 3 cm bruise" is more accurate than "large bruise."
■ Document a description of behavior you observed rather than using terms such as *anxiety* or *agitation.*
■ Document objectively—what you see, hear, feel, smell. . . .
■ Correct an error in documentation by drawing a single line through it and writing the word *error* above it, with your initials or name, depending on agency policy.
■ Do not erase, overwrite, blot out, or use correction fluid. The original entry must remain visible.
■ Write on every line but never between lines.

TABLE 6-1

Commonly Used Abbreviations

ABBREVIATION	TERM	ABBREVIATION	TERM
abd	abdomen	H_2O	water
ABO	the main blood group system	hs	at bedtime (hora somni)
ac	before meals (ante cibum)	I&O	intake and output
ad lib	as desired (ad libitum)	IV	intravenous
ADLs	activities of daily living	Lab	laboratory
adm	admitted or admission	liq	liquid
am	morning (ante meridiem)	LMP	last menstrual period
amb	ambulatory	lt (L)	left
amt	amount	meds	medications
approx	approximately (about)	mL (ml)	milliliter
bid	twice daily (bis in die)	mod	moderate
BM (bm)	bowel movement	neg	negative
BP	blood pressure	nil	none
BR	bed rest	no. (#)	number
BRP	bathroom privileges	NPO (NBM)	nothing by mouth (per os)
c̄	with	NS (N/S)	normal saline
C	Celsius (centigrade)	O_2	oxygen
CBC	complete blood count	od	daily (omni die)
CBR	complete bed rest	OD	overdose
Cl	client	OOB	out of bed
c/o	complains of	os	mouth or opening
DAT	diet as tolerated	pc	after meals (post cibum)
dc (disc)	discontinue	PE (PX)	physical examination
drsg	dressing	per	by or through
Dx	diagnosis	pm	afternoon (post meridiem)
ECG (EKG)	electrocardiogram	PO	by mouth (per os)
F	Fahrenheit	postop	postoperative (ly)
fld	fluid	preop	preoperative (ly)
GI	gastrointestinal	prep	preparation
GP	general practitioner	prn	when necessary (pro re nata)
gtt	drops (guttae)	pt	patient
h (hr)	hour (hora)	q	every (quaque)

(continued)

TABLE 6-1

Commonly Used Abbreviations (*continued*)

ABBREVIATION	TERM	ABBREVIATION	TERM
qh (q1h)	every hour (quaque hora)	tid	three times a day (ter in die)
q2h, q3h, and so on	every 2 hours, 3 hours, and so on	TL	team leader
qhs	every night at bedtime (quaque hora somni)	TLC	tender loving care
qid	four times a day (quater in die)	TPR	temperature, pulse, respirations
req	requisition	Tr	tincture
Rt (rt, R)	right	VO	verbal order
s̄	without (sine)	VS (vs)	vital signs
SI	seriously ill	WNL	within normal limits
spec	specimen	wt	weight
stat	at once, immediately (statim)		

- Draw a line through any blank space and sign the notation. In this way, no additional information can be recorded at any other time or by any other person.
- Never leave blank lines above your entry or between your entries (Figure 6-2 ■).

TABLE 6-2

Commonly Used Symbols

SYMBOL	TERM	SYMBOL	TERM
=	equal to	i	1
↑	increased	ii	2
↓	decreased	iii	3
♀	female	iv	4
♂	male	v	5
°	degree	vi	6
#	number; fracture	vii	7
		viii	8
ʒ	dram	ix	9
℥	ounce	x	10
×	times	ss	1/2

SEQUENCE

- Document events in the order in which they occur: assessments, interventions, and client responses.
- Make a late entry by clearly labeling your entry as late according to facility policy. For example, "Late entry [date] [time]" or "[date] [time] Late entry" could be correct. See Figure 6-2.
- Do not make a late entry more than 24 hours after the event. This is not usually permitted.

CONTINUED NOTES

- Continue entries to another page by indicating that the note continues and signing the entry. On the next page, enter the date/time of the note and start it by indicating that it is a continuation (see Figure 6-2).

APPROPRIATENESS AND COMPLETENESS

- Record only information that pertains to the client's health problems and care.
- Record all assessments, dependent and independent nursing interventions, client problems, client comments and responses to interventions and tests, progress toward goals, and communication with other disciplines.
- Document any care that was omitted and include why it was omitted and who was notified.
- Use descriptions that are appropriate and accurate. Avoid stereotyping (Box 6-1 ■).

Date	Time	Nursing Note
1/1/08	0015	BP 150/82, P 92 irregular/irregular EKG leads in place, Resp 22
		unlabored O$_2$ 2L/min via N/C. NG tube placement verified via
		auscultation and litmus strip testing, low intermittent suction
		continues. C/O nausea, phenergan 25mg suppository given rectally.
		Color normal for race, skin warm and dry to touch. --------S. Oradei LPN
----------	--------	--- ----
1/1/08	0200	Wakeful, watching TV, states relief of nausea. ----------------S. Oradei LPN
1/1/08	0600	~~BP 152/90~~ error S.O. -- BP 152/80, P 90 irregular/irregular EKG leads
		in place. Resp 24 unlabored O$_2$ 2L/min via NC occasional dry
		non-productive cough, lung sounds clear to auscultation. Denies
		nausea at this time. --S. Oradei LPN
1/1/08	0400	Late entry – Telemetry unit reports irregular signal. Leads checked,
		lead left low chest loose, pad replaced and lead reattached. Verified
		signal with telemetry.--S. Oradei LPN
1/1/08	0700	Vomited approximately 100cc of dark green liquid, black flecks noted
		in emesis. Denies nausea prior to emesis---(Continued) --S. Oradai LPN
Jones, Adam (male - 51y/o) / 410A / Dr. A. Amsterdamm / Partial Gastrectomy , A.Fib, HTN / NKDA		

Date	Time	Nursing Notes
1/1/08	0700	(Continued) – and denies nausea at this time. BP 168/90, P 100
		irregular/irregular, Resp 26 O$_2$ 2L/min via N/C, no cough noted at this
		time. Color pale, skin moist. .----------------------------------S. Oradai LPN
1/1/08	0715	Dr. Amsterdamm notified of client condition, no new orders noted.
		---S. Oradai LPN
01/01/08	0800	Dr. Amsterdamm to see client. New orders noted for IV Zantac bid, and
		labs to be drawn stat. Lab & Pharmacy notified.------------ *K. Hamrick LPN*

Figure 6-2. ■ Sample narrative notes with error correction, a skipped line, and a continued note.

CONCISENESS

■ Do not use the client's name when charting. Some people feel that use of the words *client, resident,* and *patient* in charting is repetitive because this *is* the client's chart, so they suggest avoiding these terms when charting in order to keep notes brief and save time. In many facilities, however, the use of these terms is common practice. Check policies and procedures for your facility.

■ End each thought or sentence with a period; it is not necessary to use complete sentences.

BOX 6-1	CULTURAL PULSE POINTS

Documentation

When documenting information in nurses' notes or on a cultural or psychosocial assessment, it is important to use terminology that is free of derogatory racial terms. Biological variations, as well as cultural beliefs and practices, do need to be recorded. They give the health care team essential information. However, take care to use exact and appropriate terms in all documentation.

■ Write notes so that data that follows a comma is associated with the data that preceded it.

LEGAL PRUDENCE

■ Document accurately and completely to protect the healthcare staff, the facility, and the client. The clinical record is a legal document that provides proof of the quality of care given to a client.

■ Follow the general principle, "If it isn't charted, it wasn't done."

■ Follow agency policy and procedures for intervention and documentation in all situations, especially high-risk situations.

ADDITIONAL TIPS FOR DOCUMENTATION

Special care is needed when caring for clients with the same last name to prevent documentation mistakes. Many agencies have a policy about flagging charts when name confusion could occur. Do not identify charts by room number only.

LEGAL AND ETHICAL ASPECTS OF DOCUMENTATION

As has already been stated, the client record is a legal document, admissible in a court of law. All information in the document is open to scrutiny by attorneys; however, a client may object to having the record admitted into court because of the confidential information it contains. It is very important that nurses remember that the chart could someday be read in court when they enter information in it.

The client's record is usually considered the property of the agency. The client generally has a right to a copy of the information, though the client will need to make a written request and may need to pay a copying fee. The client can also sign a release allowing access to the record by his or her attorney.

When you are charting, be sure to use objective, factual information rather than opinions or interpretations. It is more accurate, for example, to write that a client "refused medication" (fact) than to write that the client "was uncooperative" (opinion). To write that a client "was crying" (observation) is preferable to noting that the client "was depressed" (interpretation). Avoid using the word *seems* regarding the client. Write that the client is "resting in bed with eyes closed" rather than the client "seems to be sleeping."

Not all data about a client should be recorded. Any personal information the client shares that does not pertain to the client's health problems and care is inappropriate for the record. Recording irrelevant information may be considered an invasion of the client's privacy and could be considered libelous.

For the best legal protection, the nurse should not only adhere to professional standards of nursing care but also follow agency policy and procedures for intervention and documentation in all situations, especially high-risk situations. Below is an example of such documentation:

> 1100 hours—Complained of feeling dizzy. Raised side rails and instructed to stay in bed and ring call bell if requiring assistance. 1130 hours—found beside bed on floor. Said, "I climbed over these rails all by myself." When asked about pain, replied, "I feel fine but a little dizzy." BP 100/60 P 90 R 24. Assessed for injuries. No complaints of pain or discomfort in limbs or trunk. Assisted back to bed. Dr. RJ Naden notified. _____ R.S. Woo, LVN

Documentation is the determining factor in a great percentage of malpractice cases involving client care, so it is important that you document client care clearly, concisely, and accurately.

Confidentiality of Client Records

The client's record is protected legally as a private record of the client's care. Access to the record is restricted to health professionals directly involved in giving care to the client. Insurance companies, for example, have no legal right to de-

mand access to medical records, even though they may be determining compensation to the client. Therefore, a client who is making a claim for compensation may ask to have the medical history used as evidence. In order for an agency to provide the requested information, the client must sign an authorization for review, copying, or release of information from the record. This form must specifically indicate what information is to be released and to whom. A nurse should not allow access to a client's record by significant others or any person other than the healthcare providers who are directly involved in the care of the client.

For purposes of education and research, most agencies allow student and graduate health professionals access to client records. The records are used in client conferences, clinics, rounds, and written papers or client studies. The student is bound by a strict ethical code to hold all information in confidence. It is the responsibility of the student and health professionals to protect the client's privacy by not using a name or any statements in the notations that would identify the client. Additionally, it is very important for staff and students to maintain confidentiality with worksheets and assignment sheets. Caution must be used to ensure that papers are not left where visitors and clients may see them. For additional information see the discussion in Chapter 3 about the Health Insurance Portability and Accountability Act (HIPAA).

ENSURING CONFIDENTIALITY OF COMPUTER RECORDS

Because of the increased use of computerized client records, healthcare agencies have developed policies and procedures to ensure the privacy and confidentiality of client information stored in computers. The following are some suggestions for ensuring the confidentiality of computerized records:

1. Each healthcare worker needs a password to enter and sign off computer files. Do not share this password with anyone. Do not write down your password where others may find it.
2. After logging on, never leave a computer terminal unattended. If your agency provides handheld computers, ensure that you do not leave them unattended.
3. Do not leave client information displayed on the monitor where others may see it.
4. Follow agency procedures for documenting sensitive material. Conditions of confidentiality for computerized documents are the same as those for paper charts.

Documentation Systems

A number of documentation systems are in current use: source-oriented record, problem-oriented record, PIE, Focus Charting, charting by exception, FACT, CORE, outcome documentation, computerized documentation, and case management.

SOURCE-ORIENTED RECORD

The traditional client record is source oriented. Each person or department makes notations in a separate section or sections of the client's chart. In the **source-oriented record**, information about a particular problem is distributed throughout the record. For example, if a client had *left hemiplegia* (paralysis of the left side of the body), data about this problem might be found in the physician's history sheet, on the physician's order sheet, in the nurses' notes, in the physical therapist's record, and in the social service record. See Table 6-3 ■ for the components of a source-oriented record.

Narrative charting is a traditional part of the source-oriented record. It consists of written notes that include routine care, normal findings, and client problems. There is no right or wrong order to the information, although chronological order is most frequently used. Currently, narrative

TABLE 6-3

Components of the Source-Oriented Record

FORM	INFORMATION
Admission (face) sheet	Legal name, birth date, age Social Security number Address Marital status; closest relatives or person to notify in case of emergency Date, time, and admitting diagnosis Food or drug allergies Name of admitting (attending) physician Insurance information Any assigned DRG
Initial nursing assessment	Findings from the initial nursing history and physical health assessment
Graphic record	Body temperature, pulse rate, respiratory rate, blood pressure, daily weight, and special measurements, such as fluid intake and output
Daily care record	Activity, diet, bathing, and elimination records; may also include restraints, isolation precautions
Special flow sheets	Examples: 24-hour fluid balance record
Medication record (see Chapter 29 ⚭)	Name, dosage, route, time, date, site of regularly administered medications Name or initials of person administering the medication
Narrative nurses' notes	Pertinent assessment of client Specific nursing care including teaching and client's responses Client's complaints and how client is coping
Medical history and physical examination	Past and family medical history, present medical problems, differential or current diagnoses, findings of physical examination by the physician
Physician's order sheet	Medical orders for medications, treatments, and so on
Physician's progress notes	Medical observations, treatments, client progress, and so on
Consultation records	Reports by medical and clinical specialists
Diagnostic reports	Examples: laboratory reports, x-ray reports, CT scan reports
Consultation reports	Physical therapy, respiratory therapy
Client discharge plan and referral summary	Started on admission and completed upon discharge; includes nursing problems, general information, and referral data

recording is being replaced by other systems, such as PIE and Focus. Narrative charting is expedient in emergency situations or when the space provided on a flow sheet is insufficient for the information that needs to be documented (see Figure 6-2 for an example of a narrative note).

Source-oriented records are convenient because care providers from each discipline can easily locate the forms on which to record data, and it is easy to trace the information specific to one's discipline. The disadvantage is that information about a specific problem is scattered throughout the chart, so it can be difficult to find chronological information on a client's problems and progress.

PROBLEM-ORIENTED MEDICAL RECORD

In the **problem-oriented medical record (POMR)**, or *problem-oriented record (POR)*, established by Lawrence Weed in the 1960s, the data are arranged according to the individual problems the client has rather than the source of the information. All of the members of the healthcare team contribute to the same problem list, plan of care, and progress notes. Plans for each active or potential problem are drawn up, and progress notes are recorded for each problem.

The advantages of POMR are that it encourages collaboration, and that the problem list in the front of the chart alerts caregivers to the client's needs and makes it easier to track the status of each problem. Its disadvantages are that caregivers differ in their ability to use the required charting format, it takes constant vigilance to maintain an up-to-date problem list, and it is somewhat inefficient because assessments and interventions that apply to more than one problem must be repeated.

The POMR has four basic components: database, problem list, plan of care, and progress notes. In addition, flow sheets and discharge notes are added to the record as needed.

The **database** contains all information known about the client from the nursing assessment, physician's history, and the family. This database is updated as needed. The problem list (Figure 6-3 ■) is kept at the front of the chart and serves as an index for the numbered entries in the progress notes. As problems are resolved they are marked off. As new ones appear they are identified and numbered. As the client's needs change, problems are redefined (see problems 1B and 1C in Figure 6-3). All caregivers may contribute to

No.	Date Entered	Date Inactive	Client Problem
#1	3/9/08		CVA resulting in Rt hemiplegia and left-sided weakness
#1A	3/9/08		Self-care deficit (hygiene, toileting, grooming, feeding)
#1B	3/9/08		Impaired physical mobility (unable to turn and position self) *Redefined 2/7/07*
#1C	3/9/08		Total urinary incontinence *Redefined 1/17/07*
#1D	3/9/08		Progressive dysphasia
#2	3/9/08		Constipation r/t immobility *Redefined 6/10/06*
#3	3/9/08		History of depression
#4	3/9/08		Essential hypertension
~~#5~~	~~6/6/08~~	~~7/11/08~~	~~Pruritus~~
#2	6/10/08		*Risk for constipation r/t insufficient fiber intake*
#1C	1/17/08		Nocturnal urinary incontinence
#1B	2/7/08		Impaired physical mobility (needs major assistance to transfer and walk)

Figure 6-3. ■ Client problem list in the POMR system.

the problem list. The plan of care is based on the list of active problems and includes both physician's orders and nursing orders (generally written by RNs) aimed at resolving the problems. All healthcare professionals involved in the client's care make progress notes, numbered to correspond to the problems on the list.

Types of Documentation Methods

Several methods are available for documenting data in the progress notes: SOAP, which has evolved into SOAPIE and SOAPIER in some facilities; PIE or APIE; Focus Charting; FACT, CORE, or DAE format; charting by exception; outcome documentation; computerized documentation; and case management.

SOAP

SOAP is an acronym for subjective data, objective data, assessment, and planning.

S—Subjective data are information obtained from what the client says. They describe the client's perceptions and experience of the problem. When possible, the nurse quotes the client's words; otherwise, they are summarized. Subjective data are included only when they are important and relevant to the problem. Refer to the section on accuracy for more information regarding quoting the client.

O—Objective data consist of information that is measured or observed by use of the senses (e.g., vital signs, laboratory and x-ray results). Examples of subjective and objective data are provided in Chapter 5 🔗.

A—Assessment is the interpretation or conclusions drawn about the subjective and objective data. During the initial assessment, the problem list is created from the database, so the initial "A" entry should be a statement of the problem, such as in a nursing diagnosis. In all subsequent SOAP notes for that problem, the "A" should describe the client's condition and level of progress rather than merely restating the diagnosis or problem.

P—The plan is the plan of care designed to resolve the stated problem. The person who entered the problem into the record writes the initial plan. All subsequent plans, including revisions, are entered into the progress notes.

Over the years, the SOAP format has been modified. The acronyms SOAPIE and SOAPIER refer to formats that add interventions, evaluation, and revision.

I—Intervention refers to the specific interventions that have actually been performed by the caregiver.

E—Evaluation includes client responses to nursing interventions and medical treatments. This is primarily reassessment data.

R—Revision reflects care plan modifications suggested by the evaluation. Changes may be made in desired outcomes, interventions, or target dates.

See Figure 6-4 ■ for an example of progress notes using the SOAP, SOAPIER, and PIE formats.

PIE/APIE CHARTING

PIE charting, which is similar to SOAPIE charting, stands for problem, intervention, and evaluation and is based on the nursing process. PIE charting consists mainly of assessment flow sheets and progress notes. On admission, the nurse, generally an RN, completes a thorough assessment and identifies and documents specific problems on the progress notes using NANDA diagnoses. If there is no NANDA diagnosis for the client's particular problem, then a problem statement is formulated based on the NANDA format (see Chapter 5). Each problem is numbered P1, P2, P3, and so on. As problems are revised, the numbers are changed to P1A, P1B, and so on. Interventions and evaluations are numbered similarly.

After the initial assessment, 24-hour flow sheets are used, which include specific assessment criteria in a structured format. Some PIE systems use APIE wherein "A" stands for assessment. The assessment data are included in your problem list to support the PIE portion of the documentation.

The PIE or APIE system eliminates the traditional care plan by incorporating an ongoing care plan into the progress notes. The major disadvantage is that the nurse must review all of the progress notes before giving care, to determine which problems are current and which interventions were effective.

FOCUS CHARTING

Focus Charting is intended to make the client and client concerns and strengths the focus of care. Three columns for recording are usually used: date and time, focus, and progress notes (see the example at the end of this section). The focus may be a condition, a nursing diagnosis, a behavior, a sign or symptom, an acute change in the client's condition, or a client's strength. The progress notes are organized into data (**D**), action (**A**), and response (**R**), referred to as **DAR**. The data category consists of observations of client status and behaviors, including data from flow sheets (e.g., vital signs, pupil reactivity). The nurse records both subjective and objective data in this section.

The action category includes immediate and future nursing actions. It may also include any changes to the plan of care. The response category describes the client's response to any nursing and medical care.

SOAP Format

[date] #5 Generalized pruritus

[time] S—"My skin is itchy on my back and arms, and it's been like this for a week."

O—Skin appears clear—no rash or irritations noted. Marks where client has scratched noted on left and right forearms. Allergic to elastoplast but has not been in contact.
No previous history of pruritus.

A—Altered comfort (pruritus): cause unknown.

P—Instructed to not scratch skin.
- Applied calamine lotion to back and arms at 1430 h.
- Cut fingernails.
- Assess further to determine whether recurrence associated with specific drugs or foods.
- Refer to physician and pharmacist for assessment.

SOAPIER Format

[date] #5 Generalized pruritus

[time] S—"My skin is itchy on my back and arms, and it's been like this for a week."

O—Skin appears clear—no rash or irritation noted. Marks where client has scratched noted on left and right forearms. Allergic to elastoplast but has not been in contact.
No previous history of pruritus.

A—Altered comfort.

P—Instruct to not scratch skin.
- Apply calamine lotion as necessary.
- Cut nails to avoid scratches.
- Assess further to determine whether recurrence associated with specific drugs or foods.
- Refer to physician and pharmacist for assessment.

I —Instructed not to scratch skin. Applied calamine lotion to back and arms at 1430 h. Assisted to cut fingernails. Notified physician and pharmacist of problem.

[time] E—States, "I'm still itchy. That lotion didn't help."

R—Remove calamine lotion and apply hydrocortisone ungt. as ordered.

PIE Format

[date] #5 Generalized pruritus r/t unknown cause

[time] P—Instruct not to scratch skin.
- Apply calamine lotion as necessary.
- Cut nails to avoid scratches.
- Assess further to determine whether recurrence associated with specific drugs or foods.
- Refer to doctor and pharmacist for assessment.

I —Instructed not to scratch skin. Applied calamine lotion to back and arms at 1430 h. Assisted to cut fingernails. Notified physician and pharmacist of problem.

E—States, "I'm still itchy. That lotion didn't help."

Figure 6-4. ■ SOAPIER and PIE charting examples. Nurse's signature is required whenever charting is done.

The Focus Charting system provides a holistic perspective of the client and the client's needs. It also provides a framework for the progress notes (DAR). The three components do not need to be recorded in order, and each note does not need to have all three categories. Flow sheets are frequently used on the client's chart to augment recording data.

Date/Hour	Focus	Progress Notes
[date]	Neuro	**D:** Unresponsive to verbal
[time]	status	stimuli; responsive to painful
		stimuli.
		Pupils pinpoint and equal.
		Dr. Ward visited.
		A: Neuro assessment and VS
		every 2 h.
		R: See flow sheets.
		S. Myers, LVN

CORE

The CORE documentation system focuses on the nursing process. It consists of a database, plans of care, flow sheets, progress notes, and discharge summary. CORE documentation calls for assessing the client's functional and cognitive status within 8 hours of admission (Springhouse, 1995, p. 91).

The progress notes use a DAE format:

Data
Action
Evaluation.

This system has been found to be most useful in acute care and long-term care facilities.

CHARTING BY EXCEPTION

Charting by exception (CBE) is a documentation system in which only significant findings or exceptions to norms are recorded. CBE involves three distinct components:

1. Unique flow sheets that highlight significant findings and define assessment parameters and findings. The flow sheets include a sheet for the nursing and physician orders to perform assessments or interventions, the graphic record (see Figure 6-5 ■), the client teaching record, and the client discharge note.

2. Documentation by reference to the agency's printed standards of nursing practice. This eliminates much of the repetitive charting of routine care. An agency using CBE must develop its own specific standards or definitions of nursing practice that identify the minimum criteria for client care or status regardless of clinical area. Some units may also have unit-specific standards unique to their type of client; for example, "The nurse

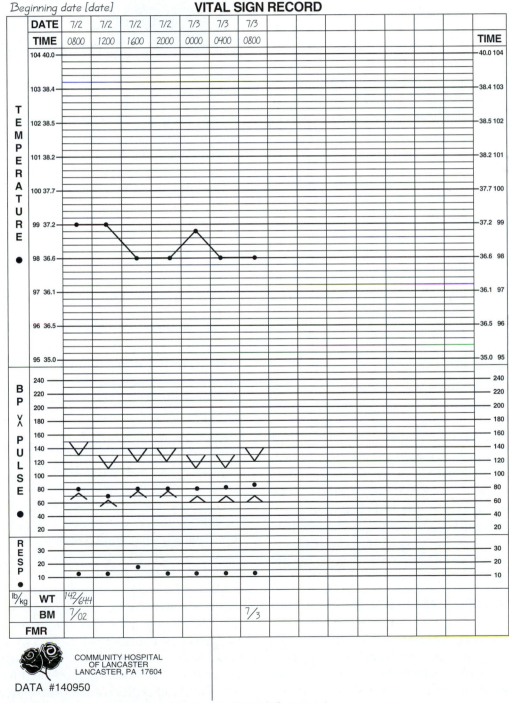

Figure 6-5. ■ Graphic flow sheet. (*Source:* Courtesy of Community Hospital of Lancaster.)

must ensure that the unconscious client has oral care at least every 4 h." Documentation of care according to these specified standards involves only a check mark in the routine standards box on the graphic record. If all of the standards are not implemented, an asterisk or other mark is made on the flow sheet with reference to the nurses' notes. All exceptions to the standards are fully described in narrative form on the nurses' notes.

3. Documentation forms at the bedside. Flow sheets are kept at the client's bedside for immediate recording. This eliminates the need to transcribe data from the nurse's worksheet to the permanent record.

FACT

The FACT system of documentation is named for its elements. It has many similarities to CBE and is designed to eliminate redundant and irrelevant data and inconsistencies in recording. The four main elements are:

Flow sheets that are individualized
Assessment sheet that is standardized with baseline parameters
Concise integrated progress notes and flowsheets that are used to document the client's condition and response
Timely entries that are recorded after care is given.

To use FACT documentation, the nurse must start with a complete database on each client. Only significant information and exceptions to the normal are recorded. The comprehensive assessment is recorded on an assessment action flow sheet. Another flow sheet is used for frequent assessments, such as blood pressure or neurologic assessments. Progress notes are written in narrative style to document a client's clinical progress and any significant changes in health status.

This system of documentation is computer ready, and it eliminates duplication and supports consistent language.

OUTCOME DOCUMENTATION

This system of documentation focuses on a client's behavior. It presents the client's condition in relation to predetermined outcomes, such as "The client's blood pressure will be 120/80 while sitting by the time of discharge."

The standards that are used to evaluate outcomes are specific client behavior, a specific standard, the conditions under which the behaviors occur, and a target date or time by which the behaviors occur.

COMPUTERIZED DOCUMENTATION

Computerized clinical record systems are rapidly being developed as a way to manage the huge volume of information required in contemporary health care. Nurses use computers to store the client's database, add new data, create and revise care plans, and document client progress (Figure 6-6 ■). Some institutions have a computer terminal at each client's

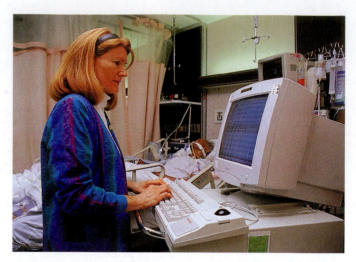

Figure 6-6. ■ The nurse using a bedside computer. (Photographer Elena Dorfman.)

bedside, or nurses carry a small handheld unit, enabling the nurse to document care immediately after it is given.

Use of the computer in documentation has drastically changed the amount of time needed for charting. Since the systems are linked to various sources of information, requests and results are sent and received quickly. Some monitoring equipment is connected directly to bedside computers, eliminating the need for the nurse to record the readings. If a nurse neglects to record important information, the program will prompt the nurse to do so. In some cases, the nurse cannot exit the page until all critical information has been entered.

Multiple flow sheets are not needed in computerized record systems. Information can be easily retrieved in a variety of formats, because the data are cross-indexed within the computer's program. For example, the computer can provide results of a client's blood test, a schedule of all clients on the unit who are to have surgery during the day, a suggested list of interventions for a nursing diagnosis, a graphic chart of a client's vital signs, or a printout of all the progress notes for a client. Many systems can generate a work list for the shift, with a list of all the treatments, procedures, and medications needed by the client. It is also possible to run a computer query to find out whether documentation was missed or medication is due. Some facilities use e-mail between departments so that questions about client care can be answered quickly.

Other advantages of computerized documentation over written documentation include the fact that the date and time of the entry is automatically recorded and all entries are legible. Reimbursement to the facility is quicker because the documentation done by a computer is complete and accurate. This eliminates the need for the third-party payer to ask for additional information or the correction of inconsistent information.

TABLE 6-4

Examples of Variance Documentation (Portion of a Critical Pathway)

An elderly client has had a below-the-knee amputation. On the third postoperative day, he has a temperature of 38.8°C (102°F). Lung sounds are clear, and he is not coughing. The nurse notices redness and skin breakdown over the client's sacrum. The critical pathway outcomes specified for Day 3 are "Oral temperature <37.7°C (100°F)" and "Skin intact over bony prominences." The nurse should chart the following variances:

DATE/TIME	VARIATION	CAUSE	ACTION TAKEN/PLANS
[date] [time]	Elevated temperature	Possible sepsis	[date]—Blood cultures ×3 per order. Monitor temp. every 1 h. Monitor I&O, hydration, and mental status.
[date] [time]	*Impaired Skin Integrity:* pressure sore on sacrum	Client does not move about in bed unless reminded	[date]—Positioned on L side. Turn side-to-side every 2 h while awake. On every client contact, remind client to move about in bed. Apply DuoDERM daily after bath.

Computers make care planning and documentation relatively easy. In most facilities, nurses record nursing actions and client responses by choosing from standardized lists of care and interventions using a touch screen. The nurse can also type narrative information into the computer for further explanation or to note exceptions. Some computer programs produce a flow sheet with expected outcomes and nursing interventions. The nurse chooses the appropriate interventions for the specific client and initials them, indicating they were implemented. Others use the problem-oriented format, producing a problem list in priority order. The nurse then selects the appropriate nursing diagnoses, expected outcomes, and nursing interventions by using a light-pen on the screen. The nurse uses the keyboard to type in additional information.

In the future, automated speech-recognition technology may allow nurses to enter data by voice and have it converted to written documentation. Handwriting-recognition technology reduces the need for typing on the handheld units.

As documentation on computers becomes more prevalent, the problems related to use of computers are being overcome. The issue that is most often cited is that system downtime makes information temporarily unavailable and documenting impossible. Client confidentiality is always of concern. Making systems secure and protecting information on computer screens both require constant vigilance.

CASE MANAGEMENT

The case management model emphasizes quality, cost-effective care delivered within an established length of stay. This model uses a multidisciplinary approach to planning and documenting client care, using critical pathways, and is most effective when there is a predictable outcome. These forms identify the outcomes that certain groups of clients

are expected to achieve on each day of care, along with the interventions necessary for each day. See Chapter 7 ∞ for more information about critical pathways and case management. See Appendix III ∞ for a sample critical pathway.

Along with critical pathways, the case management model incorporates graphics and flow sheets. Progress notes typically use some type of charting by exception. For example, if goals are met, no further charting is required. Goals that are not met are called *variances.* Deviations or variances are unexpected occurrences that affect the planned care or the client's responses to care. When a variance occurs, the nurse writes a note documenting the unexpected event, the cause, and actions taken to correct it. Or, the note may justify the actions taken. See Table 6-4 ■ for an example of how a variance might be documented.

The case management model promotes collaboration and teamwork among caregivers, helps to decrease length of stay, and makes efficient use of time. Because care is goal focused, the quality may improve. However, critical pathways work best for clients with one or two diagnoses and few individualized needs. Clients with multiple diagnoses (e.g., a client with a hip fracture, pneumonia, diabetes, and pressure sore) or those with an unpredictable course of symptoms (e.g., a neurologic client with seizures) are difficult to document on a critical path.

Reporting

Reports can be either oral or written. The purpose of reporting is to communicate specific information to a person or group of people. A report should be concise, including pertinent information but no extraneous detail.

CHANGE-OF-SHIFT REPORTS

A **change-of-shift report** is a report given to all nurses on the next shift. Its purpose is to provide continuity of

---

BOX 6-2

Key Elements of a Change-of-Shift Report

- Follow a particular order (e.g., follow room numbers in a hospital).
- Provide basic identifying information for each client (e.g., name, room number, bed designation).
- For new clients, provide the reason for admission or medical diagnosis (or diagnoses), pertinent medical history, surgery (date), diagnostic tests, and therapies in past 24 hours.
- Include significant changes in client's condition and present information in order (i.e., assessment, nursing diagnoses, interventions, outcomes, and evaluation). For example, "Mr. Ronald Oakes said he had an aching pain in his left calf at 1400 hours. Inspection revealed no other signs. Calf pain is related to altered blood circulation. Rest and elevation of his legs on a footstool for 30 minutes provided relief."
- Provide exact information, such as "Ms. Jessie Jones received Demerol 100 mg intramuscularly at 2000 hours," not "Ms. Jessie Jones received some Demerol during the evening."
- Report clients' need for special emotional support. For example, a client who has just learned that his biopsy results revealed malignancy and who is now scheduled for a laryngectomy

needs time to discuss his feelings before preoperative teaching is begun.
- Include current nurse-prescribed and physician-prescribed orders.
- Provide a summary of newly admitted clients, including diagnosis, age, general condition, plan of therapy, and significant information about the client's support people.
- Report clients who have been transferred or discharged from the unit.
- Clearly state priorities of care and care that is due after the shift begins. For example, in a 7:00 A.M. report, the nurse might say, "Mr. Li's vital signs are due at 0730, and his IV bag will need to be replaced by 0800." Give this information at the end of that client's report, because memory is best for the first and last information given.
- Be concise. Don't elaborate on background data or routine care (e.g., do not report "Vital signs at 0800 and 1200" when that is the unit standard). Do not report coming and going of visitors unless there is a problem or concern, or visitors are involved in teaching and care. Social support and visits are the norm.

---

care for clients by providing the new caregivers with a quick summary of client needs and details of care to be given.

Change-of-shift reports may be written or given orally, either in a face-to-face exchange or by audiotape recording. The face-to-face report permits the listener to ask questions during the report. Written and tape-recorded reports are often briefer and less time consuming. Reports are sometimes given at the bedside, and clients as well as nurses may participate in the exchange of information. See Box 6-2 ■ for key elements of a change-of-shift report. Also see information on reporting in Chapter 36 🔗.

TELEPHONE REPORTS

Health professionals frequently report about a client by telephone. Nurses inform physicians about a change in a client's condition; a radiologist reports the results of an x-ray study; a nurse may confer with a nurse on another unit about a transferred client.

The nurse receiving a telephone report should document the date and time, the name of the person giving the information, and what information was received, and should sign the notation. For example:

[date] [time] GL Messina, laboratory technician, reported by telephone that Mrs. Sara Ames's hematocrit was 39/100 mL. _____ Barbara Ireland, LPN

If there is any doubt about the information given over the telephone, the person receiving the information should repeat it back to the sender to ensure accuracy.

When giving a telephone report to a physician, it is important that the nurse be concise and accurate. Begin with name and relationship to the client (e.g., "This is Jana Gomez; I'm calling about your patient, Dorothy Mendes. I'm her nurse on the 7 P.M. to 7 A.M. shift.").

Telephone reports usually include the client's name and medical diagnosis, changes in nursing assessment, vital signs related to baseline vital signs, significant laboratory data, and related nursing interventions. The nurse should have the client's chart ready to give the physician any further information.

After reporting, the nurse should document the date, time, and content of the call. (See Table 36-3 🔗 for guidelines for calling a physician.) For example: [date] [time] 24-year-old Asian female admitted from ED to Room 301B with c/o burning and pain URQ. BP 120/80, P 100, R 22, T 99.8. Had received Demerol 100 mg IM in ED at 11:10. States pain "10" on a scale of 1 to 10. See Admission Sheet for admission assessment. _____K. Hamrick, LVN. [date] [time] states pain unchanged. Color pale and perspiring profusely. BP 100/60, P 105, R 24, T 100.4. Dr. Burns notified via telephone new order noted for stat MRI of abd. _____K. Hamrick, LVN

TELEPHONE ORDERS

Physicians often order a therapy (e.g., a medication) for a client by telephone. Most agencies have specific policies about telephone orders. Some agency policies require that only registered nurses take telephone orders. (See also Chapter 36 🔗.) *Note:* JCAHO requires that any information given over the phone (lab results, doctors orders, etc.) be repeated to the caller and documented as "100% read-back."

When the physician gives the order, write it down and repeat it back to the physician to ensure accuracy. Question the physician about any order that is ambiguous, unusual (e.g., an abnormally high dosage of a medication), or contraindicated by the client's condition. When preparing to receive verbal or telephone orders, you should have the client's chart with you so that you may verify allergies or review current medication orders while the physician is talking to you. These efforts will prevent you from having to contact the physician to clarify the order or provide omitted information. Then transcribe the order onto the physician's order sheet, indicating it as a verbal order or telephone order. Refer to Box 6-3 ■ for guidelines concerning telephone orders.

Once the order is transcribed on the physician's order sheet, the order must be countersigned by the physician within a time period described by agency policy. Many acute care hospitals require that this be done within 24 hours, while most long-term care facilities require physician signatures within 72 hours.

FAX AND E-MAIL COMMUNICATION

Faxing and e-mailing are convenient ways of sending large amounts of information, laboratory results, or copies of progress notes. These routes of communication should not be used in emergency situations as a primary method of communication. In the nurse's notes, document how the information was sent and the date and time of the fax or e-mail.

BOX 6-3   NURSING CARE CHECKLIST

Guidelines for Telephone Orders

- ☑ Do not accept an order from a prescriber you do not know.
- ☑ Ask the prescriber to speak slowly and clearly.
- ☑ Ask the prescriber to spell out the name of the medication.
- ☑ Question the drug, dosage, or changes if they seem inappropriate for this client.
- ☑ Read the order back to the prescriber at the end. Use words for abbreviations (i.e., three times a day for *tid*).
- ☑ When writing a dosage, always put a zero (0) before a decimal (i.e., 0.3 mL) but never after a decimal (i.e., 6 mg, not 6.0 mg).
- ☑ Write out units (i.e., 20 units of insulin, not 20 U of insulin).
- ☑ Follow agency protocol about the prescriber's protocol for signing telephone orders (e.g., within 24 hours).
- ☑ Note that 100% readback is required by JCAHO for all telephone orders.

When faxing or e-mailing information, a follow-up phone call is needed to ensure that the information was received. You should also document the follow-up call. Include the person's name who verified receipt of the fax or e-mail, as well as the date and time of your call.

NURSING CARE CONFERENCE

A **nursing care conference** is a meeting of a group of nurses to discuss possible solutions to certain problems of a client, such as inability to cope with an event or lack of progress toward reaching goals.

To **confer** is to consult another person or persons for advice, information, ideas, or instructions. Nursing conferences are most effective when there is a climate of respect—that is, nonjudgmental acceptance of others even though their values, opinions, and beliefs may seem different. Nurses will gain the most information and insight about a client's situation by listening with an open mind to what others are saying, even when there is disagreement (see Chapter 4 ⚭).

NURSING ROUNDS

Nursing rounds are procedures in which a group of nurses visit selected clients at each client's bedside to:

- Obtain information that will help plan nursing care
- Provide clients the opportunity to discuss their care
- Evaluate the nursing care the client has received.

To help clients participate in nursing rounds, nurses need to use terms that clients can understand.

INTERDISCIPLINARY CARE PLAN MEETINGS

Skilled nursing units, rehabilitation facilities, and long-term care facilities have regularly scheduled meetings where care is coordinated for a common care plan. Often nursing services or social workers are the primary coordinators for these meetings.

INCIDENT REPORTS

An **incident** can be defined as any unexpected event. A medication error and a fall are examples of incidents. Each agency defines what it considers an incident, which forms need to be completed, and which protocols are to be implemented. An incident event needs to be documented in the nurse's notes. However, the words "incident report completed" should not be included in the nurse's notes. Incident reports are for the agency's use. They are not generally part of the client's medical record. Incident reports are discussed in Chapter 36 ⚭.

NURSING CARE

The client record should describe the client's ongoing status and reflect the full range of the nursing process. Regardless of the records system used in an agency, nurses document

TABLE 6-5

Documenting the Nursing Process

STEP[a]	DOCUMENTATION FORMS
Assessment	Initial assessment form, various flow sheets
Nursing diagnosis	Nursing care plan, Kardex, critical path, progress notes, problem list
Planning	Nursing care plan, critical path
Intervention	Progress notes, flow sheets
Evaluation	Progress notes

[a]All steps are recorded on discharge/referral summaries.

the same types of evidence of the nursing process on a variety of forms throughout the clinical record (Table 6-5 ■).

ASSESSING

Admission Nursing Assessment

A comprehensive admission assessment, also referred to as an initial assessment, initial database, nursing history, or nursing assessment, is completed when the client is admitted to the nursing unit. The initial nursing assessment is a snapshot of the client's condition and needs upon admission. This comprehensive and accurate evaluation of the client guides care and interventions. See Figure 10-1 ⚭ for an example of an admission assessment document.

DIAGNOSING, PLANNING, AND IMPLEMENTING

Nursing Care Plans

The JCAHO *Accreditation Manual for Hospitals* (2000) requires that the clinical record include evidence of client assessments, nursing diagnoses and/or client needs, nursing interventions, and client outcomes, but the standards no longer require a separate nursing care plan. Depending on the records system being used, the nursing care plan may be separate from the client's chart, recorded in progress notes and other forms in the client record, or incorporated into a multidisciplinary plan of care.

There are two types of nursing care plans: traditional and standardized. The traditional care plan is written for each client. The form varies from agency to agency according to the needs of the client and the department. Most forms have three columns: one for nursing diagnoses, a second for expected outcomes, and a third for nursing interventions. See Chapter 5 ⚭ for additional information.

Standardized care plans have been developed to save documentation time. These plans are based on an institution's standards of practice; they help maintain the quality of nursing care. However, the nurse must individualize standardized plans in order to address individual client needs well. To do this, the nurse selects from a list of interventions relating to a specific nursing diagnosis, then fills in data specific to the client.

Kardexes

The **Kardex** (see Figure 5-3 ⚭) is a widely used, concise method of organizing and recording data about a client, making information quickly accessible to all health professionals. The system consists of a single card or a series of cards kept in a portable index file or on computer-generated forms. The cards for a particular client can be quickly turned up to reveal specific data. The Kardex may or may not become a part of the client's permanent record. In some organizations, it is a temporary worksheet written in pencil for ease in recording when frequent changes in details of a client's care must be made. The information on Kardexes may be organized into sections, for example:

- Pertinent information about the client, such as name, room number, age, religion, marital status, admission date, physician's name, diagnosis, type of surgery and date, occupation, and next of kin
- List of intravenous fluids, with dates of infusions; medications may also be listed
- List of daily treatments and procedures, such as dressing changes, postural drainage, or measurement of vital signs
- List of diagnostic procedures ordered
- Allergies
- Specific data on how the client's physical needs are to be met, such as type of diet, assistance needed with feeding, elimination devices, activity, hygienic needs, and safety precautions (e.g., use of side rails)
- A problem list, stated goals, and a list of nursing approaches to meet the goals and relieve the problems.

Although much of the information on the Kardex may be recorded by the nurse in charge or a delegate (e.g., the ward clerk), any nurse who cares for the client plays a key role in initiating the record and keeping the data current. Students must avoid planning care based solely on information found on the Kardex, because it is necessary to check orders with the physician's orders.

Flow Sheets

Flow sheets, also called abbreviated progress notes, enable nurses to record nursing data quickly and concisely and provide an easy-to-read record of the client's condition over time (see Figure 6-5).

The time parameters for flow sheets can vary from minutes to months. In a hospital intensive care unit, a client's blood pressure may be monitored by the minute, whereas in an ambulatory clinic, a client's blood glucose level may be recorded once a month.

Flow sheets commonly used are the graphic (clinical) record, the fluid intake and output record, the medication record, and daily nursing care records.

Graphic (Clinical) Record.
This record (see Figure 6-5) indicates body temperature, pulse, respiratory rate, blood pressure, weight, and, in some agencies, other significant clinical data such as admission or postoperative day, bowel movements, appetite, and activity.

24-Hour Fluid Balance Record.
All routes of fluid intake and all routes of fluid loss or output are measured and recorded on this form. Information about ways to measure and record specific amounts of fluid intake and output are described in Chapter 26 ⚭. This record is often called an I&O sheet.

Medication Record.
Medication flow sheets are also called medication administration records (MARs). They usually include designated areas for the date of the medication order, the expiration date, the medication name and dose, the frequency of administration and route, and the nurse's signature. Some records also include a place to document the client's allergies. A sample medication record is shown in Chapter 29 ⚭. When changes are made to the MAR, the initials of the nurse making the changes and the date and time of the changes should be included. Frequently, facilities will use a colored highlighter to cross through medications that have been discontinued (dc), for easy identification.

Daily Nursing Care Record.
Daily nursing care for activities of daily living (ADLs) are most frequently recorded on a flow sheet such as the one in Figure 6-7 ■. These records may include categories related to diet, hygiene, activity, elimination, treatments, protective precautions, diagnostic studies, and so on. Depending on the agency, licensed nurses may delegate the completion of this flow sheet to unlicensed staff.

Progress Notes
Progress notes made by nurses provide information about the progress a client is making toward achieving the desired outcomes. Therefore, in addition to assessment and reassessment data, progress notes include information about client problems and nursing interventions. The format used depends on the documentation system in place in the institution. Various kinds of nursing progress notes were discussed earlier in this chapter.

Nursing Discharge/Referral Summaries
Discharge notes are completed when the client is being discharged, although discharge planning is an ongoing process that begins at the time of admission. See Figure 10-4 ⚭ in the discharge planning section of Chapter 10 ⚭ and the assessment parameters suggested when preparing clients to go home. Many discharge forms combine the discharge plan, including instructions for care, and the final progress note. Many forms are designed with checklists to facilitate data recording.

If the client is being transferred to another institution or to a home setting where a visit by a home health nurse is required, the discharge note takes the form of a referral summary. Regardless of format, the nurse includes some or all of the elements noted in Box 6-4 ■ in discharge and referral summaries.

Long-Term Care Documentation
Requirements for documentation in long-term care settings are based on professional standards, federal and state regulations, and the policies of the healthcare agency. The kind and frequency of documentation required are determined by the Health Care Financing Administration (HCFA), a branch of the Department of Health and Human Services, and the Omnibus Budget Reconciliation Act (OBRA) of 1987. The OBRA law, for example, requires that (1) a comprehensive assessment (the Minimum Data Set [MDS] for Resident Assessment and Care Screening) be performed within 14 days of a client's admission to a long-term care facility, (2) a formulated plan of care be completed within 7 days of completion of the MDS, and (3) the comprehensive assessment and care screening process be reviewed every 90 days.

> ### clinical ALERT
>
> The ability of the nurse to be aware of his or her clients' status is essential for identifying changes in condition. In long-term care, a client's condition can change significantly in hours, and the nurse must be alert to these changes.
>
> **Report**
>
> The nurse must document and report changes in a client's condition within 24 hours to the physician and the client's family, and institute appropriate care measures.

Documentation also must comply with requirements set by Medicare and Medicaid. These requirements vary with the level of service provided and other factors. For example, Medicare provides little reimbursement for care provided in long-term care facilities except for services that require skilled care such as chemotherapy, tube feedings, and ventilators. For such clients, the nurse must provide daily documentation to verify the need for service and reimbursement.

PeaceHealth

MED/SURG/TELE/ONC
DAILY CARE RECORD

Date: _____

12	13	14	15	16	17	18	19	20	21	22	23

Pain Intervention Key:
1. Medicated   4. Repositioned
2. Cold   5. Diversion
3. Heat   6. PCA/Epidural

Sedation Scale:
0 – None; alert
1 – Mild; occasionally drowsy,
    easy to arouse
2 – Moderate; frequently drowsy,
    easy to arouse
3 – Severe; somnolent, difficult to
    arouse

Diversion Therapies Key:
A - Audio   V - Visual   T - Tactile

Hygiene Key:
S–Self   A–Assist   D–Depend
CB – Complete bath
SH – Shower   PC – Peri Care
OC – Oral Care   HS – HS Care
FC – Foley Care

Toileting Key:
BRP – Bathroom Privileges
C – Commode   U – Urinal
BP – Bed Pan   I – Incontinent
FC – Foley Catheter

Activity Key:
S–Self   A–Assist   D–Depend

BR – Bed Rest   T – Turn
C – Chair   AMB – Ambulate

Positioning Key:
R – Right   L – Left   S – Supine

12	13	14	15	16	17	18	19	20	21	22	23

Pulmonary Toilet Key:
IS – Incentive Spirometer
C&DB – Cough & Deep Breathe
RT – Respiratory Therapy

Diet Function Key:
FS – Feeds Self
A – Setup Assist
CS – Constant Supervision
F – Total Feed
FF – Force Fluids
RF – Restrict Fluids

Dysphagia Eval Key:
CH – Choke   CO – Cough
V – Change in Voice   N – None

Oversight of Care:

Initials Indicate RN Delegation and Oversight of Care:

Initials	Signature	Initials	Signature	Initials	Signature

Figure 6-7. ■ Daily record of care. (*Source:* Courtesy of PeaceHealth St. John Medical Center, Longview, WA. Used with permission.)

BOX 6-4 | **NURSING CARE CHECKLIST**

Discharge or Referral Summary

The nurse would include some or all of the following in the client summary for discharge or referral:

☑ Description of client's physical, mental, and emotional status at discharge or transfer

☑ Resolved health problems

☑ Unresolved continuing health problems and continuing care needs; may include a review-of-systems checklist (e.g., integumentary, respiratory, cardiovascular problems)

☑ Treatments that are to be continued (e.g., wound care, oxygen therapy)

☑ Current medications

☑ Restrictions that relate to

  ☑ Activity such as lifting, stair climbing, walking, driving, work

  ☑ Diet

  ☑ Bathing such as sponge bath, tub, or shower

☑ Functional/self-care abilities in terms of vision, hearing, speech, mobility with or without aids, meal preparation and eating, preparation and administration of medications, and so on

☑ Comfort level

☑ Support networks including family, significant others, religious adviser, community self-help groups, and home care and other community agencies available

☑ Client education provided in relation to disease process, activities and exercise, special diet, medications, specialized care or treatments, follow-up appointments, and so on

☑ Discharge destination (e.g., home, nursing home) and mode of discharge (e.g., walking, wheelchair, ambulance)

☑ Referral services (e.g., social worker, home health nurse)

Nurses need to familiarize themselves with regulations that influence the kind and frequency of documentation required in long-term care facilities. Usually, the nurse completes a nursing care summary at least once a week for clients requiring skilled care and every 2 to 4 weeks for those requiring intermediate care. Clients in a skilled nursing unit within a long-term care facility should be assessed daily or each shift, depending on the skilled services needed by the client. Summaries should address the following:

- Specific problems noted in the care plan
- Mental status
- ADLs
- Rehabilitative or restorative interventions, with comments about progress made
- Hydration and nutrition status
- Safety measures needed (e.g., bed rails)

- Medications and treatments
- Skin condition and wound treatments if applicable
- Preventive measures.

Nurses should also keep a record of visits and phone calls to the client from family, friends, and others.

Home Care Documentation

The HCFA mandated that home healthcare agencies standardize their documentation methods to meet requirements for Medicare and Medicaid and other third-party disbursements. Two records are required: (1) a home health certification and plan of treatment form and (2) a medical update and client information form. The nurse assigned to the home care client usually completes the forms, which must be signed by both the nurse and the attending physician. Box 6-5 ■ provides guidelines for home healthcare documentation.

Some home health agencies provide nurses with laptop or handheld computers to make records available in multiple locations. With the use of a modem, the nurse can add new

BOX 6-5 | **NURSING CARE CHECKLIST**

Home Healthcare Documentation

☑ Complete a comprehensive nursing assessment and develop a plan of care to meet Medicare and other third-party payer requirements. Some agencies use the certification and plan of treatment form as the client's official plan of care.

☑ Write a progress note at each client visit, noting any changes in the client's condition; nursing interventions performed (including education and instructional brochures and materials provided to the client and home caregiver); client responses to nursing care; and vital signs as indicated.

☑ Provide a monthly progress nursing summary to the attending physician and to the reimburser to confirm the need to continue services.

☑ Keep a copy of the care plan in the client's home and update it as the client's condition changes.

☑ Report changes in the plan of care to the physician and document that these were reported. Medicare and Medicaid will reimburse only for the skilled services provided that are reported to the physician.

☑ Encourage the client or home caregiver to record data when appropriate.

☑ Write a discharge summary for the physician to approve the discharge and to notify the reimbursers that services have been discontinued. Include all services provided, the client's health status at discharge, outcomes achieved, and recommendations for further care.

client information to records at the agency without traveling to the office.

EVALUATING

Evaluation of client status, goals, and outcomes is an ongoing part of the nursing process. Documentation of client changes is recorded on progress notes daily. Periodic evaluations are performed and documented at regular intervals, depending on client status and institutional policy.

NURSING PROCESS CARE PLAN
Client with Ineffective Protection

Amy is a 14-year-old girl who is popular in school. She has recently been diagnosed with leukemia. Amy lives with her mother, father, and two brothers who are also active in school activities. The physician has ordered Amy be started on chemotherapeutics and corticosteroids.

Assessment. VS: 99.2/72/16, BP 124/68. Height: 5 ft, 2 inches. Weight: 105 lbs.

Client states:

"I have several of my friends coming to visit me tonight."
"I don't like to eat much. I have to keep my weight down."
"I have leukemia. I'm not sure what that means."
"I get tired easily."

Nursing Diagnosis. The following important nursing diagnoses (among others) are established for this client:

- *Ineffective Protection* related to chemotherapy and cortisone therapy
- *Imbalanced Nutrition: Less than body requirements*

Expected Outcomes

- Client will not have symptoms of infection.
- Client will demonstrate knowledge and understanding of asepsis.
- Client will demonstrate understanding of need for balanced diet.
- Client will demonstrate understanding of need for energy conservation.

Planning and Implementation

- VS every 4 hours.
- Monitor WBC levels.
- Administer medications per doctor's orders.
- Post signs regarding neutropenic precautions.
- Provide age-appropriate education (to client and family) regarding the following:
  - Client teaching regarding hand hygiene and need for asepsis.

- Observe return demonstration of proper hand hygiene.
- Client will verbalize understanding of asepsis.
- Client teaching regarding neutropenic precautions.
- Client verbalizes understanding of precautions.
- Client verbalizes willingness to comply with precautions.
- Age-appropriate education for visiting friends.
- Client education regarding proper nutrition.
- Client verbalizes understanding of need for balanced diet (without raw/uncooked foods).
- Obtain dietitian consult regarding dietary needs.
- Client teaching regarding energy conservation.
- Client verbalizes understanding regarding grouping activities and resting between activities.
- Client teaching regarding signs and symptoms of infection.
- Client is able to verbalize signs and symptoms of infection and verbalizes understanding of need to immediately report signs/symptoms if noted.

Evaluation. Two days after admission, Amy has met all of her educational needs. She verbalizes that she is unhappy about not being able to have plants in her room but is willing to comply. You note that she is washing her hands regularly and wears a mask when her friends come to visit. The dietitian reports that Amy is not eating a balanced diet and has scheduled further meetings with both Amy and her parents. She must be reminded to rest during the day, especially when friends are visiting. Amy's parents are supportive and cooperative with protocols. Amy is 48 hours into her chemotherapy and corticosteroids treatments, and is free of any signs of infection at this time.

Critical Thinking in the Nursing Process

1. What is Amy's priority need at this time?
2. Amy's friends do not understand why Amy wears a mask. They say that they thought you couldn't catch cancer. How will you explain this to them?
3. Four days into her treatment, Amy reports a sore throat. Her VS are T 101.4°F, P 92, R 18, BP 136/74. What is your next action and why?
4. Ten days into her treatment, Amy is upset about her "fat face" and wants to know what is causing it. When you tell her it is a side effect of the steroids, she wants to know why she's taking them. How will you answer her?

Note: Discussion of Critical Thinking questions appears in Appendix I.

Note: The references and resources for this and all chapters have been compiled at the back of the book.

Chapter Review

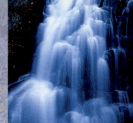

 KEY TERMS by Topic

Use the audio glossary feature of either the CD-ROM or the Companion Website to hear the correct pronunciation of the following key terms.

Introduction
report, record, charting, documenting, clinical record

Documentation Systems
source-oriented record, problem-oriented medical record (POMR), database, DAR

Reporting
change-of-shift report, nursing care conference, confer, nursing rounds, incident

Nursing Care
Kardex, flow sheets

KEY Points

- Nurses must accurately document each step of the nursing process in a timely manner, regardless of the documentation system used.

- Entries into the client's record must be legible, concise, sequential, complete, and signed by the healthcare provider making the entry.

- The client record is a legal document. All parts of the client's record are admissible into a court of law as evidence.

- The most common documentation systems are SOAP, (E) PIE, Focus Charting, CORE, CBE, FACT, outcome documentation, and case management.

- Computers have increased the ease of documenting most nursing interventions. Most documentation systems can be adapted to computer use. Terminals at bedsides and handheld units permit immediate documentation of care.

- Case management uses critical pathways that incorporate the care plan into the documentation form.

- Long-term care documentation is essentially the same as documentation made in the acute care setting but has a different focus. Acute care charting focuses on progress toward a wellness goal. Long-term care charting focuses on daily functioning and maintenance of function with the use of restorative and preventive measures. Long-term care charting is also less frequent.

- Accuracy is important in the home care setting because there are fewer caregivers. Documentation in the home care setting is used to obtain reimbursement from third-party payers and to justify continued home care.

- Confidentiality must be maintained at all times, regardless of location of care, documentation method, or whether or not computers are used.

 EXPLORE Media Link

Additional interactive resources for this chapter can be found on the Companion Website at www.prenhall.com/ramont. Click on Chapter 6 and "Begin" to select the activities for this chapter.

For chapter-related NCLEX®-style questions and an audio glossary, access the accompanying CD-ROM in this book.

FOR FURTHER Study

See Chapter 3 for a discussion of HIPAA.

For further discussion regarding critical thinking, see Chapter 4.

For additional information about subjective and objective data, planning care, and formulating NANDA diagnoses, see Chapter 5.

For additional discussion about critical pathways and case management, see Chapter 7.

For additional information about discharge planning, see Chapter 10.

See Figure 10-1 for an example of an admission assessment document, and Figure 10-4 for a discharge document.

For additional information about fluid monitoring, see Chapter 26.

For more information about abbreviations used for medication administration and a sample MAR, see Chapter 29.

For additional information on taking telephone orders and reporting, including incident reporting, see Chapter 36.

See Appendix III for a sample critical pathway.

Critical Thinking Care Map

Caring for a Client Who Is Grieving
NCLEX-PN® Focus Area: Coping and Adaptation

Case Study: Mrs. Estella Rodriguez is an 87-year-old female admitted 3 days ago for treatment of bilateral pneumonia. She has lost 1 kilogram (2.2 lbs) since admission, and her records note that she does not eat well at mealtimes. The dietitian reports that Mrs. Rodriguez does not fill out her menus and declines assistance. When her son visits later in the shift, you ask him about food preferences. Her son reports that she hasn't had much of an appetite since his father died 2 years ago, and has lost "quite a bit" of weight. He also reports that she used to be very active in church and hardly leaves the house anymore. The daughter-in-law comments that Mrs. Rodriguez cries frequently and occasionally talks as if her husband is still alive. The son tells you that they had been married 62 years.

Nursing Diagnosis: Dysfunctional Grieving Related to Loss of Spouse

COLLECT DATA

Subjective	Objective
_____	_____
_____	_____
_____	_____
_____	_____
_____	_____
_____	_____
_____	_____

Would you report this data? Yes/No

If yes, to: _____

What would you report? _____

Nursing Care

_____
_____
_____
_____
_____
_____
_____

How would you document this? _____
_____
_____
_____

Data Collected
(use those that apply)

- 87 years old
- Weight 36.63 kg (85 lbs)
- Weight loss since admission
- Height 152 cm (5'2")
- Crying
- Talks as if spouse alive
- States "I don't know how to cook for one person."
- Not wearing makeup, hair not combed
- Decreased social activity
- Belongs to the Catholic Church
- VS: T 98.2°F, P 84, R 18, BP 150/82
- Complains of hunger
- Watches TV much of day
- Decreased interest in surroundings

Nursing Interventions
(use those that apply; list in priority order)

- Obtain referral to grief counselor.
- Encourage family to choose an adult singles group for their mother.
- Obtain referral to appropriate grief support group.
- Dietitian consult for meal planning upon discharge.
- Suggest to family that the client's priest should visit regularly.
- Provide reality orientation.
- Suggest weight gain program and recommend a 6.5-kg weight gain by end of the month.
- Schedule follow-up visit in doctor's office, for 1 week from today.
- Schedule time during the shift where you can spend one-on-one time with client.
- Encourage client to talk about spouse.

Compare your documentation to the sample provided in Appendix I.

NCLEX-PN® Exam Preparation

1 Mrs. Smith has told you that she wishes she were dead. When you ask her about her feelings, she tells you that since her husband died a year ago nothing has mattered to her. You would best document this as:

1. client has suicidal tendencies.
2. client is grieving for her spouse.
3. client expressing dysfunctional grieving and states that she wishes she were dead. Physician notified.
4. referral for psychiatric evaluation made at this time.

2 Which of the following would be a breach of confidentiality?

1. Notifying the pharmacist of the blood level of an antibiotic
2. Discussing the progress of a rehabilitation client with the case manager
3. Explaining what the "contact isolation" notice on a family member's door means
4. Telling a coworker about a suicide attempt that a client made on another unit

3 You are a student nurse on a unit and request permission to make copies of the medication administration record. Which of the following is not an appropriate action for you to take?

1. Mark through the identifying information with a thick marker, to protect confidentiality.
2. Remember to initial the copy as you give medications.
3. Return the forms at the end of the day for shredding.
4. Tell the unit manager how you plan to keep the copies secure during your shift.

4 Mr. Alexander tells you that he didn't like his care and is going to sue. He is demanding a copy of his records. You would tell him that:

1. he will need to contact medical records and complete necessary paperwork before he may receive a copy.
2. because he's going to sue, he cannot have a copy of his records for legal reasons.
3. the chart belongs to the facility and he has no right to it.
4. there is a $100 copy fee and it will take 6 to 8 weeks to receive it.

5 You are making an entry into the nurses' notes and discovered that you forgot to enter something that happened half an hour ago. You would best correct this omission by:

1. crossing through the entry you are now making, writing *error,* initialing it, and then making the entry you forgot to enter earlier.
2. making the entry now with the current time since that is when you are documenting it.
3. making the entry with the time the event happened, and labeling it as a late entry.
4. doing nothing—it is too late.

6 Dr. Jones has seen two of your clients and has left new orders. After Dr. Jones has left the unit, you discover that you cannot read some of the orders. You should first:

1. do the best you can and leave a note for him to clarify the remaining orders.
2. page him immediately.
3. contact your charge nurse for assistance in reading the orders.
4. contact the pharmacy to see what Dr. Jones usually orders in these situations.

7 You are an LPN/LVN who has been working in a large county hospital. At that hospital, you were accustomed to a wide range of responsibility. You have recently accepted a job at a new hospital. You will expect your duties to include:

1. all the same duties that you had at your last job.
2. fewer duties than you had at your last job.
3. more duties than you had before.
4. client assessment, intervention, and teaching within the scope of the job description.

8 You are working the 7-to-3 shift on an oncology unit. At 7:30 this morning, you changed a client's surgical dressing and assessed the site. You are documenting it at 8:00. What time would you enter into the nurse's notes?

1. 0730
2. 0800
3. 7-to-3 shift
4. No time is needed if you use the flow sheet.

9 You are working at a long-term care facility and lab reports have just come in. You plan to fax the lab results to the individual doctors. You should:

1. not fax lab reports, because faxing is unreliable.
2. follow up with a phone call to the physician's office to ensure receipt of the fax.
3. fax the lab results and include a request for the office staff to call you if they don't get the fax.
4. call the abnormal lab values in to the office.

10 You are doing walking rounds with the on-coming nurse. You come to Room 402 and stand in the doorway to discuss the conditions and progress of the clients in bed A and bed B. You should be aware that:

1. this is normal procedure.
2. if you are not careful, you may create a breach of confidentiality.
3. walking rounds are done only on critical care units.
4. taped reports are a better form of shift-to-shift communication.

Answers and Rationales for Review Questions, as well as discussion of Care Plan and Critical Thinking Care Map questions, appear in Appendix I.

Chapter 7

Healthcare Delivery Systems

LEARNING Outcomes

After completing this chapter, you will be able to:

1. Differentiate primary, secondary, and tertiary healthcare delivery services.
2. Compare the characteristics of nursing in the outpatient setting to those of institutionalized nursing care.
3. Describe the functions and purposes of the healthcare agencies outlined in this chapter.
4. Discuss healthcare as a right and the essentials of the Patient's Bill of Rights.
5. Identify the roles of various healthcare professionals.
6. Differentiate between the various models of care.
7. Compare various systems of payment for healthcare services.

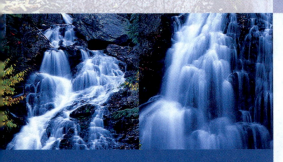

HISTORICAL Perspectives

Since 1950, the American Public Health Association (APHA) has vigorously supported and promoted the concept of universal health care throughout the U.S. A 1966 APHA Policy Statement on the Nationwide Coverage by Organized Public Health Services stated, "It is neither defensible nor acceptable that in 1966 there still are geographic regions without even the structure for public health services and many other areas with the structure largely on paper. APHA supports the position that Federal, state and local governments begin to implement policies and procedures to achieve the goal of complete geographic health coverage with official health programs. Elected officials must take the steps necessary to realize true universal coverage through legislative initiatives, administrative actions and substantial funding."

A **healthcare system** is the totality of services offered by all health disciplines. Healthcare services are commonly categorized according to type and level.

Types of Health Care

Three types of services are often described: (1) health promotion and illness prevention, (2) diagnosis and treatment, and (3) rehabilitation and health restoration.

HEALTH PROMOTION AND ILLNESS PREVENTION

Based on the notion of maintaining an optimum level of wellness, the U.S. Department of Health and Human Services (DHHS) has developed a systematic approach to health improvement. A DHHS report, *Healthy People 2010* (2000), "focuses on improving health—the health of each individual, the health of the communities, and the health of the nation." However, the *Healthy People 2010* goals and objectives cannot by themselves improve the health status of the nation; instead, they need to be recognized as a part of a larger systemic approach to health improvement.

Since the 1980s, more and more people have recognized the advantages of staying healthy and avoiding illness. Health promotion programs address areas such as adequate and proper nutrition, weight control and exercise, and stress reduction. Health promotion activities emphasize the important role clients play in maintaining their own health and encourage them to maintain the highest level of wellness they can achieve. Recent transitions in healthcare also reflect a growing support for community-based nursing and health care that capitalizes on health promotion activities.

The healthcare delivery system also offers illness prevention programs. They may be directed at the client or the community and involve such practices as providing immunizations, identifying risk factors for illnesses (e.g., cardiovascular disease), and helping people take measures to prevent these illnesses from occurring.

DIAGNOSIS AND TREATMENT

Traditionally, the largest segment of the healthcare delivery system has been dedicated to the diagnosis and treatment of illness. Hospitals and physicians' offices were the major agencies offering these services. More recently, however, community-based agencies have been instrumental in providing these services. For example, clinics in some communities provide mammograms and education regarding the early detection of cancer of the breast. Voluntary HIV testing and counseling is another example of the shift in services from traditional healthcare settings to community-based agencies. Some shopping malls and shopping centers have walk-in clinics that provide diagnostic screening tests, such as screening for cholesterol and high blood pressure.

REHABILITATION AND HEALTH RESTORATION

Rehabilitation is a process of restoring ill or injured people to optimum and functional levels of wellness. Rehabilitative care emphasizes the importance of assisting clients to function adequately in the physical, mental, social, economic, and vocational areas of their lives. The goal of rehabilitation is to help people move to their previous level of health (i.e., to their previous capabilities) or to the highest level they are capable of given their current health status. Rehabilitation may begin in the hospital but will eventually lead clients back out into the community for further treatment and follow-up once health has been restored.

Levels of Health Care

Healthcare delivery services can also be categorized according to the complexity or level of the services provided: primary, secondary, or tertiary. See Table 7-1 ■ for the levels of care and the kinds of services provided at each level. Nurses play a key role in health promotion activities and in providing primary health care, whether in the hospital or in the community.

Types of Healthcare Settings

Healthcare agencies and settings are both varied and numerous. Some agencies provide a number of services; for example, a hospital may provide acute inpatient services, outpatient or ambulatory care services, and emergency services. In addition, the same services may be found in other community-based agencies. For example, hospice

TABLE 7-1	
Types of Healthcare Services by Increasing Complexity	
LEVEL	**NURSING SERVICES**
Primary	Health promotion
	Preventive care (e.g., immunization)
	Health education
	Environmental protection
	Early detection and treatment
Secondary	Emergency care
	Diagnosis and treatment (complex)
	Acute care
Tertiary	Long-term care
	Care of the dying
	Rehabilitation

services may be provided in the hospital, in the home, or in another agency within the community.

A client may be categorized as an inpatient or an outpatient. An *inpatient* is a person who enters a setting such as a hospital and remains for at least 24 hours. An *outpatient* is a person who requires healthcare but does not need to stay in an institution such as a hospital.

Because the array of healthcare services and agencies is so great, nurses often need to help clients choose the service that best suits their needs. Clients may be seen in any number of these agencies, depending on their care and ability to pay for the services. Traditional nursing roles and responsibilities are also changing in response to the movement of client care from the hospital into the community. The LPN/LVN is currently being employed in almost every type of healthcare setting.

OUTPATIENT SETTINGS

Public Health

Health agencies at the state, county, or city level vary according to the needs of the area. Their funds, usually generated from taxes, are administered by elected or appointed officials. Local health departments (county, bicounty, or tricounty) traditionally have responsibility for developing programs to meet the health needs of the people, providing the necessary staff and facilities to carry out these programs, continually evaluating the effectiveness of the programs, and monitoring changing needs. State health organizations are responsible for assisting the local health departments. In some remote areas, state departments also provide direct services to people.

The Centers for Disease Control and Prevention (CDC) in Atlanta, Georgia, administers a broad program related to surveillance of diseases. By means of laboratory and epidemiologic investigations, data are made available to the appropriate authorities. The CDC also publishes recommendations about the prevention and control of infections and administers a national health program. The federal government also administers a number of Veterans Administration services in the United States.

Physicians' Offices

In North America, the physician's office is a traditional primary care setting. The majority of physicians either have their own offices or work with several other physicians in a group practice. Clients usually go to a physician's office for routine health screening, illness diagnosis, and treatment. People often seek consultation from physicians when they are experiencing symptoms of illness or when a significant other considers the person to be ill.

Nurses employed in physician's offices have a variety of roles and responsibilities. Some nurses carry out traditional functions including client registration, preparing the client for an examination, obtaining health information, and providing information. Other functions may include obtaining specimens, assisting with procedures, and providing some treatments.

Ambulatory Care Centers

Ambulatory care centers are being used more frequently in many communities. Most ambulatory care centers have diagnostic and treatment facilities providing medical, nursing, laboratory, and radiologic services, and they may or may not be attached to or associated with an acute care hospital. Some ambulatory care centers provide services to people who require minor surgical procedures that can be performed outside the hospital. Nurses in ambulatory care centers may have specialized knowledge and skills to enable them to assist physicians with procedures. The term *ambulatory care center* has replaced the term *clinic* in many places.

General Clinics

The term *clinic* can refer to a department inside or outside the hospital, managed by a group of physicians or by nurses. Some may provide a specialized type of health service such as infant immunizations. Nurses in clinics perform many of the same functions as nurses employed in a physician's office.

Industrial Clinics

The industrial clinics are gaining importance as a setting for employee health care. Employee health has long been recognized as important to productivity. Nursing functions in industrial health care include work safety and health education, annual employee health screening for tuberculosis, and maintaining immunization information. Other functions may include screening for such health problems as hypertension and obesity, caring for employees following injury, and counseling.

Home Healthcare Agencies

The implementation of prospective payment (discussed later in this chapter) and the resulting earlier discharge of clients from hospitals have made home care an essential aspect of the healthcare delivery system. As concerns about the cost of health care have escalated, the use of the home as a care delivery site has increased. In addition, the scope of services offered in the home has broadened. Home healthcare agencies offer education to clients and families and also provide comprehensive care to acute, chronic, and terminally ill clients. Once the RN has opened the home care case, the LPN/LVN may be assigned to provide care and to supervise the home health aide or the individual providing homemaker services.

There are several different types of home health agencies:

- Official or public agencies are operated by state or local governments and financed primarily by tax funds.
- Voluntary or private not-for-profit agencies are supported by donations, endowments, charities such as the United Way, and third-party reimbursement. Because these agencies are not for profit, they are exempt from federal income tax.
- Private, proprietary agencies are for-profit organizations and are governed by either individual owners or national corporations. Some of these agencies participate in third-party reimbursement; others rely on "private-pay" sources.
- Institution-based agencies operate under a parent organization, such as a hospital.

Regardless of the type of agency, all home health agencies must meet specific standards for licensing, certification, and accreditation. See Box 7-1 ■ for the unique aspects of home care nursing.

Day Care Centers

Day care centers serve many functions and many age groups. A relatively new concept is centers that provide care for adults who cannot be left at home alone but do not need to be in an institution. Elder care centers often provide care involving socializing, exercise programs, and stimulation.

BOX 7-1

Unique Aspects of Home Health Nursing

The nurse:

- Functions independently.
- Must establish rapport with client and family.
- Provides care while family is present.

The family:

- May feel more free to question advice than when in the hospital setting.
- Will set their own schedule and priorities.
- Has more responsibility for care of client.

Positive Aspects

- Setting is more intimate and relaxed.
- Behaviors are more natural.
- Cultural beliefs and practices are more visible.
- Multigenerational interaction can take place.

Negative Aspects

- Caregiver demands may continue for months or years.
- Living conditions and support systems may be inadequate.
- There is risk of psychological or physical problems for caregiver.

Some centers provide counseling and physical therapy. Nurses who are employed in adult day care centers may provide medications, treatments, and counseling, thereby facilitating continuity between day care and home care. Adult day care is another work opportunity for the LPN/LVN.

INPATIENT SETTINGS

Hospitals

Hospitals traditionally have provided restorative care to the ill and injured. Although hospitals are chiefly viewed as institutions that provide care, they have other functions, such as providing sources for health-related research and teaching.

Hospitals are classified by the services they provide. General hospitals admit clients requiring a variety of services, such as medical, surgical, obstetric, pediatric, and psychiatric services. Other hospitals offer only specialty services, such as psychiatric or pediatric care. Hospitals can be further described as acute care or chronic (long-term) care. An acute care hospital provides assistance to clients who are acutely ill or whose illness and need for hospitalization are relatively short term. Long-term care hospitals provide services for longer periods, sometimes for years or the remainder of the client's life.

The variety of healthcare services hospitals provide usually depends on their size and location. The large urban hospitals usually have inpatient beds, emergency services, diagnostic facilities, ambulatory surgery centers, pharmacy services, intensive and coronary care services, and multiple outpatient services provided by clinics. Some large hospitals have other specialized services such as spinal cord injury and burn units, oncology services, and infusion and dialysis units. In addition, some hospitals have substance abuse treatment units and health promotion units. Small rural hospitals often are limited to inpatient beds, radiology and laboratory services, and basic emergency services. The number of services a rural hospital provides is usually directly related to its size and its distance from an urban center.

Hospitals in the United States have undergone massive changes. Many hospitals have merged with other hospitals or have been sold to large multihospital for-profit corporations.

Another change relates to the client population. Most clients in hospitals are seriously ill and require complex nursing care. With the increasing acuity (severity) of illness among clients, general hospitals have virtually become complex care centers. Because so many of the seriously ill are elderly, some general hospitals are becoming acute care hospitals solely for the elderly.

Nurses in hospitals have multiple responsibilities including the coordination of client care, assessing and monitoring client health, and providing direct care. The LPN/LVN works closely with the RN and provides much of the direct client care. While working in the acute care hospital, LPN/LVNs have excellent opportunities to continue their education and then obtain RN positions.

Extended Care (Long-Term Care) Facilities

Traditionally, all extended care facilities were called nursing homes. Extended care facilities now include skilled nursing facilities (intermediate care) and extended care facilities (long-term care) that provide personal care for those who are chronically ill or are unable to care for themselves without assistance. Traditionally, extended care facilities provided care only for elderly clients, but now they provide care to clients of all ages who require rehabilitation or custodial care. Because clients are being discharged earlier from acute care hospitals, some clients may still require supplemental care in an extended care facility before they return home.

Because long-term illness occurs most often in the elderly, long-term care facilities have programs that are oriented to the needs of this age group. These facilities are intended for people who require not only personal services (bathing, hygiene, assistance with daily activities, etc.), but also some regular nursing care and occasional medical attention. However, the type of care provided varies considerably. Some facilities admit and retain only residents who are able to dress themselves and are ambulatory. Other extended care facilities provide bed care for clients who are more incapacitated. These facilities can, in effect, become the client's home, and consequently the people who live there are frequently referred to as residents rather than patients or clients.

In 1987, as part of the **Omnibus Budget Reconciliation Act (OBRA)**, the Congress of the United States passed legislation to bring a measure of quality improvement to the nursing home and extended care facility industry. In response to a growing concern about whether minimal essential standards were being met in many facilities, OBRA instituted requirements for nurse's aide training. Specific requirements include a 75-hour training program for nurse's aides and competence evaluations of the aides.

Specific guidelines govern the admission procedures for clients admitted to an extended care facility. Insurance criteria, treatment needs, and nursing care requirements must all be assessed beforehand. Many skilled nursing facilities exist as units within a hospital but are regulated by federal, state, and local governmental bodies to make sure they are meeting the requirements for a long-term care facility. If a client in a hospital needs to be transferred to such a unit, the client is discharged from the hospital and then admitted to the long-term care unit. Extended care and skilled nursing facilities are becoming increasingly popular means for

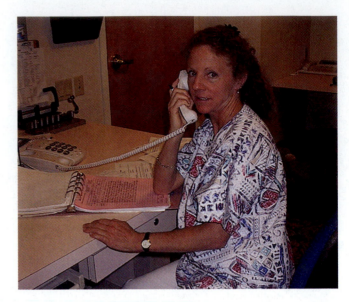

Figure 7-1. ■ The LPN/LVN charge nurse in the long-term setting serves as a liasion between resident, family, and physician.

managing the healthcare needs of clients who require additional care but do not meet the criteria for remaining in the hospital. Often, these extended care facilities have client waiting lists for admission. Nurses in extended care facilities assist clients with their daily activities, provide care when necessary, and coordinate rehabilitation activities (Figure 7-1 ■).

LPNs/LVNs have an increased level of responsibility in the long-term care setting. They may function in a charge nurse position, being responsible for coordination of client care, working with physicians, and supervision of unlicensed nursing assistants. They will administer medications and treatments and serve as a liaison between families and needed services.

Retirement and Assisted Living Centers

Retirement or assisted living centers consist of separate houses, condominiums, or apartments for residents. Residents live relatively independently. However, many of these facilities offer meals, laundry services, nursing care, transportation, and social activities. Some centers have a separate hospital to care for residents with short-term or long-term illness. Often, these centers also work collaboratively with other community services including case managers, social services, and a hospice to meet the needs of the residents who live there. The retirement or assisted living center is intended to meet the needs of people who are unable to remain at home but do not require hospital or nursing home care. Nurses in retirement and assisted living centers provide limited care to residents, usually related to the administration of medications and minor treatments. An LPN/LVN may be the only licensed nurse in an assisted living facility.

Rehabilitation Centers

Rehabilitation centers usually are independent community centers or special units. However, because rehabilitation ideally starts the moment the client enters the healthcare system, nurses who are employed on pediatric, psychiatric, or surgical units of hospitals also help to rehabilitate clients. Rehabilitation centers play an important role in assisting clients to restore their health and recuperate. Drug and alcohol rehabilitation centers, for example, help free clients of drug and alcohol dependence, and assist them to reenter the community. Physical rehabilitation centers help clients to regain purpose, function, and dignity. The focus is on assisting them to function at the maximum level possible and return to their community. Today, the concept of rehabilitation is applied to all illness (physical and mental), to injury, and to chemical addiction. Nurses in the rehabilitation setting coordinate client activities and ensure that clients are complying with their treatments. This type of nursing often requires specialized skills and knowledge.

MIXED SETTINGS

Hospice Services

The hospice movement provides a variety of services to clients who are terminally ill, their families, and support persons. In the 1970s, the movement gained momentum, through the work of such people as Elisabeth Kübler-Ross, whose books challenged prevailing attitudes, and Cicely Saunders, founder of St. Christopher's Hospice in London, England. Saunders believed that the physical and social environments of dying people are as important as medical interventions on their behalf. The central concept of the hospice movement, as distinct from the acute care model, is not saving life but improving or maintaining the quality of life until death. The LPN/LVN works under the direction of an RN case manager to provide care for clients who are terminally in their home, long-term care facilities, or in inpatient hospice centers. For additional information, see Chapter 17 .

Crisis Centers

Crisis centers provide emergency services to clients experiencing life crises. These centers may operate out of a hospital or in the community, and most provide 24-hour telephone service. Some also provide direct counseling to people at the center or in their homes. The primary purpose of a crisis center is to help people cope with an immediate crisis and then provide guidance and support for long-term therapy. The LPN/LVN with specialized training may be employed and work with RNs, counselors, and psychologists in these settings.

Mutual Support and Self-Help Groups

Mutual support or self-help groups exist for nearly every major health problem or life crisis people experience. Alcoholics Anonymous, which formed in 1935, served as the model for many of these groups. The National Self-Help Clearinghouse provides information on current support groups and guidelines about how to start a self-help group. Many of these groups are facilitated by lay volunteers, although social workers or other healthcare professionals may carry out responsibilities for self-help groups.

Rights and Health Care

The movement for clients' rights in health care arose in the late 1960s. Today, clients are also seeking more self-determination and control over their own bodies when they are ill. Informed consent, confidentiality, and the right of the client to refuse treatment are all aspects of this self-determination. Today, the goals of health include the return of autonomy and independence to the client and the acceptance of good health as a responsibility of the client, the care providers, and society. These goals cannot be met unless clients accept active responsibility for their health and health care, and unless clients and care providers have mutual respect.

When people are ill, they are frequently unable to assert their rights as they would if they were healthy. Asserting rights requires energy and an underlying awareness of one's rights in the situation.

PATIENT'S BILL OF RIGHTS

In 1973, the American Hospital Association (AHA) published *A Patient's Bill of Rights* to promote the rights of hospitalized clients. The publication was revised in 1992. Included in this bill of rights are the right of clients to considerate and respectful care; consideration of privacy for clients, including confidentiality of all records and communications regarding their care; and the right to make decisions about their care, including the right to refuse a treatment or plan of care. In addition, clients have a right to make a statement such as a living will, which should be followed by the agency as permitted by law.

The AHA bill of rights states that clients have the right to review all of their medical records and have them explained; to receive requested care and services, provided these are reasonable; and to be informed of any business arrangements among institutions or people involved in their care. In addition, clients have the right to be informed of resources that can be used to resolve a dispute or grievance and of hospital policies and practices that relate to client care, treatment, and responsibilities, and to be informed of hospital charges and available payment methods. Furthermore, the AHA bill states that clients have the right to refuse to participate in any research study, to expect reasonable continuity of care, and to have options explained when hospital care is no longer appropriate.

The Patient's Bill of Rights, by federal law, must be explained verbally and signed by the client before care can be provided. Verification of compliance is an important nursing function at the time of admission. The client should be asked about any advance directive (e.g., not to be resuscitated in the event of a cardiac arrest), and this information must be on the client's record. If the hospital's policy limits its ability to implement any advance directive, the client has a right to be informed of this before any problem arises. See details about advance directives in Chapter 17 ⬭.

If a client lacks decision-making capacity, is legally incompetent, or is a minor, these rights can be exercised on the client's behalf by a designated surrogate or proxy decision maker.

Providers of Health Care

The providers of health care, also referred to as the healthcare team or health professionals, are health personnel from different disciplines who coordinate their skills to assist clients and perhaps their support persons. Their mutual goal is to restore a client's health and promote wellness. The choice of personnel for a particular client depends on the needs of the client. In the present system of health care in North America, health teams commonly include the personnel discussed in the following subsections.

NURSE

The role of the nurse varies with the needs of the client. As nursing roles have expanded, new dimensions for nursing practice have been established. See Chapter 1 ⬭ for the roles of the nurse. Nurses can pursue a variety of practice specialties (e.g., critical care, mental health, oncology). An RN assesses a client's health status, identifies health problems, and develops and coordinates care. An LPN/LVN provides direct client care under the direction of a registered nurse.

NURSE PRACTITIONER

A nurse practitioner is a registered nurse who has advanced training and a master of science in nursing degree. These nurses are responsible for screening, diagnosis, and treatment of uncomplicated illnesses and injury. They have prescriptive authority and may order diagnostic tests. They often work directly with a physician in his or her office. In some settings, the nurse practitioner may have a solo practice, but generally will work closely with a physician for referral if necessary.

PHYSICIAN

The physician is responsible for determining medical diagnoses and for determining the therapy required by a person who has a disease or injury. The physician's traditional role is the treatment of disease and trauma (injury); however, many physicians are now including health promotion and disease prevention in their practice. Some physicians specialize in specific areas such as surgery or oncology.

PHYSICIAN'S ASSISTANT

Physician's assistants (PAs) perform certain tasks under the direction of a physician. They diagnose and treat certain diseases and injuries. In most states, physician's assistants also have limited prescriptive authority.

UNLICENSED ASSISTIVE PERSONNEL

Unlicensed assistive personnel (UAPs) are healthcare staff such as certified nurse assistants, hospital attendants, nurse technicians, and orderlies who assume aspects of client care that do not require nursing judgment. These tasks include bathing, assisting with feeding, exercise, and range of motion. Individual facilities may provide training for unlicensed personnel to perform additional tasks.

DENTIST

Dentists diagnose and treat dental problems. Dentists are also actively involved in preventive measures to maintain healthy oral structures (e.g., teeth and gums). Many hospitals, especially long-term care facilities, have dentists on staff.

PHARMACIST

A pharmacist prepares and dispenses pharmaceuticals in hospital and community settings. The role of the pharmacist in monitoring and evaluating the actions and effects of medications on clients is becoming increasingly prominent. A clinical pharmacist is a specialist who guides physicians in prescribing medications. A pharmacy technician/assistant is also recognized in some states. This person administers medications to clients or works in the pharmacy under the direction of the pharmacist.

DIETITIAN OR NUTRITIONIST

When dietary and nutritional services are required, the dietitian or nutritionist may be a member of a health team. A dietitian, often a registered dietitian (RD), has special knowledge about the diets required to maintain health and to treat disease. Dietitians in hospitals generally are concerned with therapeutic diets, may design special diets to meet the nutritional needs of individual clients, and supervise the preparation of the meals to ensure that clients receive the proper diet.

A nutritionist is a person who has special knowledge about nutrition and food. The nutritionist in a community setting recommends healthy diets and gives broad advisory services about the purchase and preparation of foods. Community nutritionists often function at the preventive level. They promote health and prevent disease, for example, by advising families about balanced diets for growing children and pregnant women.

PHYSICAL THERAPIST

The physical therapist (PT), assists clients with musculoskeletal problems. He or she provides physical therapy in response to a physician's order. The physiotherapist's functions include assessing clients' mobility and strength, providing therapeutic measures (e.g., exercises and heat applications to improve mobility and strength), and teaching new skills (e.g., how to walk with an artificial leg). Some physiotherapists provide their services in hospitals; often, however, independent practitioners establish offices in communities and serve clients either at the office or in the home.

RESPIRATORY THERAPIST

A respiratory therapist (RT) is skilled in therapeutic measures used in the care of clients with respiratory problems. These therapists are knowledgeable about oxygen therapy devices, intermittent positive-pressure breathing respirators, artificial mechanical ventilators, and accessory devices used in inhalation therapy.

OCCUPATIONAL THERAPIST

An occupational therapist (OT) assists clients with impaired function to gain the skills needed to perform activities of daily living. The therapist also teaches skills that are therapeutic and at the same time provide some satisfaction, such as crafts, puzzles, woodworking, and needlework.

PARAMEDICAL TECHNOLOGISTS

Paramedical means having some connection with medicine. Laboratory technologists examine specimens such as urine, feces, blood, and discharges from wounds to provide exact information that facilitates the medical diagnosis and the prescription of a therapeutic regimen. The radiologic technologist assists with a wide variety of x-ray film procedures, from simple chest radiography to more complex fluoroscopy. The nuclear medicine technologist uses radioactive substances to provide diagnostic information.

SOCIAL WORKER

A social worker counsels clients and support persons about social problems, such as finances, family interactions, parenting, and adoption. It is not unusual for health problems to produce problems in living and vice versa. Social workers usually make the placement arrangements for acute care hospital clients who require rehabilitation services in skilled nursing facilities or in the home. They also help families make choices when loved ones can no longer live at home.

SPIRITUAL SUPPORT PERSON

Chaplains, pastors, rabbis, priests, and so on serve as part of the healthcare team by attending to the spiritual needs of clients. In most facilities, local clergy volunteer their services

---

BOX 7-2

Alternative Care Providers

- Chiropractor—provides care by manipulating spinal vertebrae to relieve interference with nerve function.
- Herbalist—provides information and consultation regarding the use of herbal remedies for various symptoms and illnesses.
- Acupuncturist—provides relief of pain and other symptoms by gently inserting long, hollow needles at various points in the body to stimulate the flow of energy along meridians.
- Homeopathist—provides treatment for certain illnesses by giving small doses of substances that help build up the body's natural defenses against the specific disease or illness.
- Massage therapist—provides relief of muscle pain, spasm, and tension by stroking and kneading soft tissue.

---

on a regular or on-call basis. Hospitals affiliated with specific religions, as well as many large medical centers, have full-time chaplains on staff. They usually offer regularly scheduled religious services. The nurse is often instrumental in identifying the client's desire for spiritual support and notifying the appropriate person. A relatively new nursing specialty is that of parish nurse. A parish nurse helps meet the health needs in the community while including spiritual aspects of care. They are affiliated with a church or group of churches and provide health screening and information for church members and the surrounding community.

Case Managers

The case manager's role is to ensure fiscally sound, appropriate care in the best setting. This role is often filled by the member of the healthcare team who is most involved in the client's care. Depending on the nature of the client's concerns, the case manager may be a nurse, a social worker, an OT, a PT, or any member of the healthcare team.

Alternative Care Providers

Chiropractors, herbalists, acupuncturists, and other nontraditional healthcare providers are playing increasing roles in the contemporary healthcare system. These providers may practice alongside traditional healthcare providers, or clients may use their services in conjunction with, or in lieu of, traditional therapies. See Box 7-2 ■ for the types of alternative care providers.

Factors Affecting Healthcare Delivery

Today's healthcare consumers have greater knowledge about their health than in previous years, and they are increasingly influencing healthcare delivery. Formerly, people expected a physician to make decisions about their care; today, however, consumers expect to be involved in making any decisions. Consumers have also become aware of how lifestyle affects health. As a result, they desire more information and services related to health promotion and illness prevention. A number of other factors affect the healthcare delivery system.

INCREASING NUMBER OF ELDERLY

By the year 2020, it is estimated that the number of adults over the age of 65 years will be nearly 56 million in the United States (Abrams, et al., 2004). Long-term illnesses are prevalent among this group and frequently require special housing, treatment services, financial support, and social networks.

The frail elderly, considered to be people over age 85, are projected to be the fastest growing population in North America and will constitute 9.6 million by 2030 (Lee & Estes, 2003, p. 77).

Because only 5 percent of older people with health problems are institutionalized, substantial home management and nursing support services are required to assist those in their homes and communities.

ADVANCES IN TECHNOLOGY

Scientific knowledge and technology related to health care are rapidly increasing. Improved diagnostic procedures and sophisticated equipment permit early recognition of diseases that might otherwise have remained undetected. New antibiotics and medications are continually being manufactured to treat infections and multiple-drug-resistant organisms. Surgical procedures that were nonexistent 20 years ago are common today. Laser and microscopic procedures streamline the treatment of diseases that required surgery in the past. Computers, bedside charting, and the ability to store and retrieve large volumes of information in databases are commonplace in healthcare organizations. All the technologic advances and specialized treatments and procedures come, unfortunately, with a high price tag.

WOMEN'S HEALTH

The women's movement has been instrumental in changing healthcare practices. Examples are the provision of childbirth services in more relaxed settings such as birthing centers, and the provision of overnight facilities for parents in children's hospitals. Traditionally, women's health issues have focused on the reproductive aspects of health, disregarding many healthcare concerns that are unique to women. Today, research and treatment focuses on many areas of women's health care such as breast cancer, osteoporosis, abuse, treatment of sexually transmitted infections, and issues on aging. An expert panel on women's health of the American Academy of Nursing (AAN) recommends that "understanding women's health requires more than a biomedical view; it requires awareness of the context of women's lives" (AAN Panel on Women's Health, 1997, p. 7).

UNEVEN DISTRIBUTION OF SERVICES

Serious problems in the distribution of health services exist in the United States. In many remote and rural locations, insufficient healthcare professionals and services are available to meet the healthcare needs of individuals. Uneven distribution is evidenced by the relatively higher number of physicians and nurses per capita in the New England states than in the South, which has the lowest number per capita.

Because of the highly specialized techniques and new knowledge that have emerged during the past 30 years, an increasing number of healthcare personnel provide specialized services. This specialization leads to fragmentation of care and, often, increased cost of care. To clients, it may mean receiving care from 5 to 30 people during their hospital experience. This seemingly endless stream of personnel is often confusing and frightening.

ACCESS TO HEALTH CARE

Another problem plaguing individuals is access to health care. Low income has been associated with relatively higher rates of infectious diseases, problems with substance abuse, rape, violence, and chronic diseases. The use of healthcare services is also affected by unemployment and poverty. Even though some government assistance is available, eligibility for such assistance and type of benefits vary considerably from state to state.

HOMELESS POPULATIONS

The growing number of homeless individuals in towns and cities is a major health problem. The homeless differ from those who are poor. They are alone, lack some type of permanent residence, and are disaffiliated from family and friends. Limited access to healthcare services and compliance from the client contributes to the general poor health of the homeless in the United States. See Box 7-3 ■ for factors contributing to health problems among the homeless.

BOX 7-3	POPULATION FOCUS

Risk Factors for Health Problems among the Homeless

- Poor physical environment resulting in increased susceptibility to infections
- Inadequate rest and privacy
- Improper nutrition
- Poor access to facilities for personal hygiene
- Exposure to the elements
- Lack of social support
- Few personal resources
- Questionable personal safety (physical assault is a constant threat)
- Inadequate health care
- Poor compliance with treatment plans

BOX 7-4   CULTURAL PULSE POINTS

Healthcare Delivery Systems

A number of elements can enhance a healthcare agency's ability to provide culturally proficient care. These include but are not limited to:

- Service delivery that reflects an understanding of cultural diversity (as evidenced by signs such as "Se habla espanol")
- Institutionalized knowledge of culture (a statistical database that can aid in diagnosis and care)
- Consciousness of dynamics that are inherent when cultures interact (as in workshops or seminars on areas of conflict)
- Valuing diversity (hiring people of varied cultural, racial, or ethnic backgrounds)
- Capacity for cultural self-assessment (awareness and review from the administrative level down to assess the facility's own functioning)

DEMOGRAPHIC CHANGES

The characteristics of the North American family have changed considerably in the last few decades. The number of single-parent families and alternative family structures has increased markedly. Most of the single-parent families are headed by women, many of whom work and require assistance with child care or when a child is sick at home.

Recognition of cultural and ethnic diversity is also increasing. Healthcare professionals and agencies are aware of this diversity and are employing means to meet the challenges it presents (Box 7-4 ■).

Contemporary Frameworks for Care

Approaches to client care which support continuity of care and cost effectiveness include managed care and case management.

MANAGED CARE

Managed care describes a healthcare system whose goals are to provide cost-effective, quality care that focuses on improved outcomes for groups of clients. The care of a client is carefully planned from initial contact to the conclusion of the specific health problem. In managed care, healthcare providers and agencies collaborate so as to render the most appropriate, fiscally responsible care possible. Managed care emphasizes cost controls, customer satisfaction, health promotion, and preventive services. Health maintenance organizations and preferred provider organizations are examples of provider systems committed to managed care.

CASE MANAGEMENT

Case management describes a range of models for integrating healthcare services for individuals or groups. Various case management models strive to provide cost-effective care and ensure quality outcomes. Generally, case management involves nurse–physician teams that assume collaborative responsibility for planning, assessing needs, and coordinating, implementing, and evaluating care for groups of clients from preadmission to discharge or transfer and recuperation. A case manager, however, may be a social worker or other appropriate professional.

Case management may be used as a cost-containment strategy in managed care. Case management is usually the responsibility of the RN. Occasionally in a long-term care setting, an LPN/LVN may be specially trained to carry out these duties. Both case management and managed care systems often use clinical pathways to track the client's progress (Figure 7-2 ■). **Clinical pathways** provide an expected path of client needs, care, teaching, and progress for specific diagnoses. Case managers use them for planning care and anticipating potential problems in the progression of a client's recovery.

CRITICAL PATHWAY: TOTAL HIP REPLACEMENT

	DOS/Day 1	Days 2–3
Pain Management	Outcome: • Verbalizes comfort or tolerance of pain Circle: V NV Variance:	Outcome: • Verbalizes comfort with pain control measures Circle: V NV Variance:
Respiratory	Outcomes: • Breath sounds clear to auscultation • Achieves 50% of volume goal on incentive spirometer Circle: V NV Variance:	Outcomes: • Breath sounds clear to auscultation • Achieves 100% of volume goal on incentive spirometer Circle: V NV Variance:
Key: V = Variance NV = No Variance		
Signature:	Initials:	
Signature:	Initials:	

Figure 7-2. ■ Excerpt from a critical pathway documentation form.

Models of Care

Contemporary configurations for the delivery of nursing include collaborative arrangements such as managed care, case management, and client-focused care. Other models specifically designed for the provision of nursing are the case method, the functional method, team nursing, and primary nursing.

CLIENT-FOCUSED CARE

Client-focused care is a delivery model that brings all services and care providers to the clients. The supposition is that if activities normally provided by auxiliary personnel (e.g., physical therapy, respiratory therapy, electrocardiographic [ECG] testing, and phlebotomy) are moved closer to the client, the number of personnel involved and the number of steps involved to get the work done are decreased. Proponents of this type of system believe that clients will perceive improved care and service and the agency will achieve cost savings.

Cross-training, development of multiskilled workers who can perform tasks or functions in more than one discipline, is an essential element of client-focused care. For example, a healthcare worker may be taught to obtain a 12-lead ECG and perform phlebotomy. Individuals who are already certified in one profession can take on a second certification such as medical laboratory and x-ray technology, nursing and respiratory therapy, physical therapy and occupational therapy. Cross-training will be integral to the managed care system in the future.

CASE METHOD

The **case method**, also referred to as total care, is one of the earliest nursing models developed. In this client-centered method, one nurse is assigned to and is responsible for the comprehensive care of a group of clients during an 8- or 12-hour shift. Facilities that function under the case method employ RNs only for bedside care. With the shortage of nursing personnel during World War II, the case method could no longer be the chief mode of care for clients. Many hospitals reinstituted a form of total care, called primary care, beginning in the mid-1970s and continuing for many years.

FUNCTIONAL METHOD

The **functional method** focuses on the jobs to be completed (e.g., bed making, temperature measurement). In this task-oriented approach, personnel with less preparation than the professional nurse perform less complex care requirements. It is based on a production and efficiency model that gives authority and responsibility to the person assigning the work, for example, the head nurse. Clearly defined job descriptions, procedures, policies, and lines of communication are required. The functional approach to nursing is economical and efficient and permits centralized direction and control. Its disadvantages are fragmentation of care and the possibility that nonquantifiable aspects of care, such as meeting the client's emotional needs, may be overlooked.

TEAM NURSING

In the early 1950s, Eleanor Lambertson and her colleagues proposed a system of team nursing to overcome the fragmentation of care resulting from the task-oriented functional approach and to meet increasing demands for professional nurses created by advances in technologic aspects of care. **Team nursing** is the delivery of individualized nursing care to clients by a nursing team led by a professional nurse. A nursing team consists of RNs, LPNs/LVNs, and often nurse's aides. This team is responsible for providing coordinated nursing care to a group of clients during an 8- or 12-hour shift.

With the advent of managed care, team nursing is experiencing a resurgence. In this revisited form of team nursing, licensed nursing personnel (RNs and LPNs) are frequently paired with a UAPs. The licensed nurse retains responsibility and authority for client care but delegates appropriate tasks to the UAP. Contemporary proponents of this model believe the team approach increases the efficiency of the licensed nurse. Opponents state that inpatients' high acuity of illness leaves little to be delegated.

PRIMARY NURSING

Primary nursing, a system in which one nurse is responsible for total care of a number of clients 24 hours a day, 7 days a week, was introduced at the Loeb Center for Nursing and Rehabilitation, the Bronx, New York, in the early 1960s. It is a method of providing comprehensive, individualized, and consistent care.

Primary nursing uses the nurse's technical knowledge and management skills. The primary nurse assesses and prioritizes each client's needs, identifies nursing diagnoses, develops a plan of care with the client, and evaluates the effectiveness of care. Associates provide some care, but the primary nurse coordinates it and communicates information about the client's health to other nurses and other health professionals. Primary nursing encompasses all aspects of the professional role (RN), including teaching, advocacy, decision making, and continuity of care. The primary nurse is the first-line manager of the client's care with all of its inherent accountabilities and responsibilities. With today's nursing shortage and high cost of health care, this model of nursing care is being replaced.

Healthcare Economics

Although efforts have been made to control the costs of health care, these costs continue to increase. Employers, legislators, insurers, and healthcare providers continue to collaborate in efforts to resolve the issues surrounding how to best finance healthcare costs.

PAYMENT SOURCES

Medicare and Medicaid

In the United States, the 1965 Medicare amendments (Title 18) to the Social Security Act provided a national and state health insurance program for older adults. **Medicare** is divided into two parts: Part A is available to people with disabilities and people age 65 years and over. It provides insurance toward hospitalization, home care, and hospice care. Part B is voluntary and provides partial coverage of physician services to people eligible for Part A. Clients pay a monthly premium for this coverage. Medicare does not cover dental care, dentures, eyeglasses, hearing aids, or examinations to prescribe and fit hearing aids. Most preventive care, including routine physical examinations and associated diagnostic tests, is also not included.

In 2006, Medicare prescription drug coverage was instituted. Everyone with Medicare is eligible for the coverage regardless of income and resources, health status, or current prescription expense.

Participants must select a plan during the open enrollment period, normally November 15–December 31. Choosing an appropriate plan may be a daunting task for an older individual. Family members and healthcare providers should become familiar with available plans in order to assist the client.

Medicaid was also established in 1965 under Title 19 of the Social Security Act. **Medicaid** is a federal public assistance program paid out of general taxes to people who require financial assistance. Medicaid is paid by federal and state governments. Each state program is distinct. Some states provide very limited coverage, whereas others pay for dental care, eyeglasses, and prescription drugs.

Supplemental Security Income

In addition, people who are blind or have a disability may be eligible for special payments called **Supplemental Security Income (SSI)** benefits. These benefits are also available to people not eligible for Social Security, and payments are not restricted to healthcare costs. Clients often use this money to purchase medicines or to cover costs of extended health care.

PROSPECTIVE PAYMENT SYSTEM

In 1983 the United States Congress passed legislation putting the **prospective payment system (PPS)** into effect. This legislation limits the amount paid to hospitals that are reimbursed by Medicare. Reimbursement is made according to a classification system known as **diagnostic-related groups (DRGs)**. Prospective payment or billing is formulated before the client is even admitted to the hospital; thus, the record of admission, rather than the record of treatment, now governs payment. DRG rates are set in advance of the prospective year during which they apply and are considered fixed except for major, uncontrollable occurrences.

INSURANCE PLANS

A variety of plans have come into existence to finance health care in the United States. These include private insurance and group insurance. Each individual and group plan offers different options for consumers to consider when choosing a prepaid healthcare program.

Private Insurance

Commercial health insurance carriers offer a wide range of coverage plans. There are two types of private insurance: not-for-profit (e.g., Blue Shield) and for-profit companies (e.g., commercial companies such as Metropolitan Life, Travelers, and Aetna). Private health insurance is known as third-party reimbursement because the insurance company pays either the entire bill or, more often, 80 percent of the costs of healthcare services. With private health insurance plans, the insurance company reimburses the healthcare provider a fee for each service provided (fee-for-service).

These insurance plans may be purchased either as an individual plan or as part of a group plan through a person's employer, union, student association, or similar organization.

Group Plans

Healthcare group plans provide blanket medical service in exchange for a predetermined monthly payment. Each group plan offers different options for consumers to consider when choosing a prepaid healthcare program.

HEALTH MAINTENANCE ORGANIZATIONS. A **health maintenance organization (HMO)** is a group healthcare agency that provides basic and supplemental health maintenance and treatment services to voluntary enrollees. A fee is set without regard to the amount or kind of services provided.

The HMO plan emphasizes client wellness; the better the health of the person, the fewer HMO services are needed and the greater the agency's profit. Members of HMOs choose a primary care provider (PCP), who evaluates their health status and coordinates their care. The PCP has two options: Treat the condition or refer the client to a specialist. To reduce costs, HMOs will pay for a specialty physician's services only if the PCP has made the referral. It is an expectation between the HMO and physicians being reimbursed under their plans that PCPs will treat clients and reduce costs whenever possible. Thus, under HMO plans, clients are limited in their ability to select healthcare providers and services. Because health promotion and illness prevention are highly emphasized in HMOs, nurses in HMOs focus on these aspects of care.

PREFERRED PROVIDER ORGANIZATIONS. The **preferred provider organization (PPO)** has emerged as another alternative in the healthcare delivery system. PPOs consist of a group of physicians and perhaps a healthcare agency (often a hospital) that provide an insurance company or employer with health services at a discounted rate. One advantage of the PPO is that it provides clients with a choice of healthcare providers and services. Physicians can belong to one or several PPOs, and the client can choose among the physicians belonging to the PPO. A disadvantage of PPOs is that they tend to be slightly more expensive than HMO plans, and if individuals wish to join a PPO, they might have to pay more for the additional choices. PPOs were first established in 1980 in the United States.

PREFERRED PROVIDER ARRANGEMENTS. **Preferred provider arrangements (PPAs)** are similar to PPOs. The main difference is that the PPAs can be contracted with individual healthcare providers, whereas PPOs involve an organization of healthcare providers.

INDEPENDENT PRACTICE ASSOCIATIONS. **Independent practice associations (IPAs)** are somewhat like HMOs and PPOs. The difference is that clients pay a fixed prospective payment to the IPA, and the IPA pays the provider. The provider receives a fixed fee for services given. At the end of the fiscal year, any surplus money is divided among the providers; any loss is assumed by the IPA.

PHYSICIAN/HOSPITAL ORGANIZATIONS. Physician/hospital organizations (PHOs) are joint ventures between a group of private practice physicians and a hospital. PHOs combine both resources and personnel to provide managed care alternatives and medical services. PHOs work with a variety of insurers to provide services. A typical PHO will include primary care providers and specialists.

A PHO may be part of an **integrated delivery system (IDS)**. Such a system incorporates acute care services, home healthcare, extended and skilled care facilities, and outpatient services. Most integrated delivery systems provide care throughout the life span. An IDS enhances continuity of care and communication among professionals and various agencies providing managed care.

Note: The references and resources for this and all chapters have been compiled at the back of the book.

Chapter Review

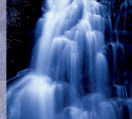

 KEY TERMS by Topic

Use the audio glossary feature of either the CD-ROM or the Companion Website to hear the correct pronunciation of the following key terms.

Introduction
healthcare system

Types of Healthcare Settings
Omnibus Budget Reconciliation Act (OBRA)

Contemporary Frameworks for Care
managed care, case management, clinical pathways

Models of Care
client-focused care, case method, functional method, team nursing, primary nursing

Healthcare Economics
Medicare, Medicaid, Supplemental

Security Income (SSI), prospective payment system (PPS), diagnostic-related groups (DRGs), health maintenance organization (HMO), preferred provider organization (PPO), preferred provider arrangements (PPAs), independent practice associations (IPAs), integrated delivery system (IDS)

KEY Points

- Healthcare delivery services can be categorized as primary, secondary, or tertiary, and generally, they can also be grouped by the type of service: (1) health promotion and illness prevention, (2) diagnosis and treatment, and (3) rehabilitation.

- Health care can be considered a right of all people.

- Hospitals provide a wide variety of services on an inpatient and outpatient basis. Hospitals can be categorized as for-profit or not-for-profit, public or private, acute care or long-term care facilities. Many other settings, such as clinics, offices, and day care centers, also provide care.

- Various providers of health care coordinate their skills to assist a client. Their mutual goal is to restore a client's health and promote wellness.

- The many factors affecting healthcare delivery include increased participation in their own care by healthcare consumers, economic factors, increased costs, the increasing number of elderly people, advances in knowledge and technology, women's health, uneven distribution of health services, access to health care, health care of the homeless, and demographic changes.

- There are a number of frameworks for client health care, including managed care, case management, and client-focused care.

- In the United States, health care is financed largely through government agencies and private organizations that provide healthcare insurance, prepaid plans, and federally funded programs.

 EXPLORE Media Link

Additional interactive resources for this chapter can be found on the Companion Website at www.prenhall.com/ramont. Click on Chapter 7 and "Begin" to select the activities for this chapter.

For chapter-related NCLEX®-style questions and an audio glossary, access the accompanying CD-ROM in this book.

Video
- Long-term Care Facilities

FOR FURTHER Study

To find out more about the roles of nurses, see Chapter 1.

For more information about hospice services, see Chapter 17.

For additional information about advance directives, see Chapter 17.

NCLEX-PN® Exam Preparation

1 Which is NOT a right of hospitalized clients according to the Patient's Bill of Rights?
1. the right to considerate and respectful care
2. the right to determine the schedule of care
3. the right to make decisions about care
4. the right to refuse treatment or care

2 The Omnibus Budget Reconciliation Act is important in health care because it:
1. instituted specific training requirements for nurse's aides working long-term care.
2. outlined guidelines for death with dignity.
3. governs Medicare payments for individuals receiving Social Security.
4. set the nurse–client ratio in acute care hospitals.

3 A homeless client is brought by a police officer to the emergency department for treatment. Which of the following would you recognize as a major contributing factor for his or her health problems?
1. mistrust of the system and healthcare providers
2. transportation for follow-up visits
3. poor physical environment exacerbating chronic health problems
4. lack of motivation to work and provide for self

4 Which model of nursing care is more favorable under managed care?
1. primary care
2. case method
3. client-focused care
4. team nursing

5 A person who is over age 65 may have national health insurance called:
1. Medicaid.
2. Medi-cal.
3. Medi-soft.
4. Medicare.

6 Diagnostic-related groups were developed to:
1. create physician groups that specialize in diagnostic procedures.
2. provide special insurance for persons with disabilities.
3. limit amounts paid to hospitals by Medicare.
4. provide medical care for groups of people with the same diagnoses.

7 Which of the following is not considered to be a paramedical technologist?
1. occupational therapist
2. physiotherapist
3. laboratory technician
4. spiritual support person

8 One of the benefits of managed care can be to:
1. emphasize wellness through access to a primary care physician.
2. offer insurance companies health services for a discounted rate.
3. increase the amount of time nurses spend with each patient.
4. provide payment to physicians for each service provided.

9 The physician's office where you work is paid monthly by the insurance company by the number of enrollees, not the service provided. You understand that the office is part of a(n):
1. IPA—independent practice association.
2. HMO—health maintenance organization.
3. PPO—preferred provider organization.
4. PHO—physician/hospital organization.

10 Preventive care such as immunizations are classified as what type of healthcare service?
1. primary
2. secondary
3. tertiary
4. prospective

Answers and Rationales for Review Questions, as well as discussion of Care Plan and Critical Thinking Care Map questions, appear in Appendix I.

Chapter 8

Safety

BRIEF Outline

Factors That Affect Safety
Preventing Specific Hazards
Preventing Procedure- and Equipment-Related Injury
Hospital and Institutional Safety
Restraining Clients
Personal Safety for Nurses

LEARNING Outcomes

After completing this chapter, you will be able to:

1. Discuss factors that affect people's ability to protect themselves from injury.
2. Provide safety teaching for clients of various ages.
3. Identify common potential hazards in the home and in healthcare settings.
4. Plan strategies to maintain safety in the healthcare setting, home, and community.
5. Describe the use and legal implications of restraints.
6. List desired outcomes to use in evaluating the selected strategies for injury prevention.
7. Describe proper techniques for lifting and transferring patients.
8. Describe ways to prevent back injuries while delivering client care.

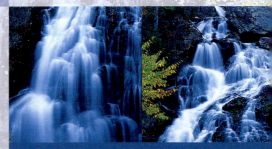

HISTORICAL Perspectives

The Centers for Disease Control and Prevention (CDC) published the Recommendations for Prevention of HIV Transmission in Health-Care Settings *in 1987. These recommendations were developed because at the time no reliable method was available for distinguishing HIV-positive clients from other clients. The CDC was also concerned about the number of healthcare workers who tested positive for HIV or hepatitis B after an occupational exposure. After the publication of the CDC recommendations, the Occupational Safety and Health Administration (OSHA) published its* Proposed Rulemaking for Bloodborne Pathogens *in the Federal Register in 1987. On March 5, 1992, OSHA's* Occupational Exposure to Bloodborne Pathogens Rule *went into effect.*

A fundamental concern of nurses, which extends from the bedside to the home and to the community, is prevention of injury, as well as assisting the injured. Motor vehicle crashes, falls, drowning, fire and burns, poisoning, inhalation and ingestion of foreign objects, and firearm use are major causes of injury and death.

Nurses need to be aware of what constitutes a safe environment for a particular person, or for a group of people, in a variety of healthcare settings. Injuries are often caused by human conduct and can be prevented.

Factors That Affect Safety

The ability of people to protect themselves from injury is affected by such factors as age and development, lifestyle, mobility and health status, sensory–perceptual alterations, cognitive awareness, emotional state, ability to communicate, safety awareness, and the environment. Nurses need to assess each of these factors when they plan care or teach clients to protect themselves.

AGE AND DEVELOPMENT

Through knowledge and accurate assessment of the environment, people learn to protect themselves from many injuries. Young children's curiosity often exceeds their judgment. However, through knowledge and experience, children do learn what is safe and what is potentially harmful. Elderly people can have difficulty with movement and diminished senses, which contribute to the likelihood of injury.

Measures to ensure the safety of people of all ages focus on two things:

1. Observation or prediction of potentially harmful situations so that harm can be avoided.
2. Client education that empowers clients to safeguard themselves and their families from injury.

Specific age-related potential hazards and preventive measures are discussed later in this chapter. See Box 8-1 ■ for safety measures for each age group. See Box 8-2 ■ for cultural issues related to safety.

BOX 8-1	**Population Focus**

Safety Measures Throughout the Life Span

Newborns and Infants

- Use a federally approved car seat at all times (including coming home from the hospital). Place children in the back seat when traveling in a car. If the child must ride in the front seat, ensure that the car seat is facing toward the rear of the car. The air bag on the passenger side of the front seat should also be disengaged in this situation.
- Never leave the infant unattended on a raised surface.
- Check the temperature of the infant's bath water and formula by using the inside of your wrist.
- Hold the infant upright during feeding. Do not prop the bottle. Cut food in small pieces, and do not feed the infant peanuts or popcorn.
- Investigate the infant's crib for compliance with federal safety regulations: slats no more than 2⅜ inches apart, lead-free paint, height of crib sides, tight fit of mattress to crib.
- Use a playpen with sides made of small-sized netting. Never leave playpen sides down.
- Provide large, soft toys with no small detachable or sharp-edged parts.
- Use guard gates on stairs and screens on windows. Supervise the infant in the walker, swing, and highchair.
- Cover electric outlets. Coil cords out of reach.
- Place plants, household cleaners, and wastebaskets out of reach. Lock away potential poisons, such as medicines, paint, and gasoline.

Toddlers

- Continue to use federally approved car seat or seat belts at all times.

- Teach children not to put objects in the mouth, including pills (unless given by parent).
- Keep objects with sharp edges (such as furniture and knives) out of children's reach.
- Place hot pots on back burners with handles turned inward.
- Keep cleaning solutions, insecticides, and medicines in locked cupboards.
- Keep windows and balconies screened.
- Teach children to swim. Fence in pools, and supervise at all times. Do not overfill bathtub. Do not let toddlers play near ditches or wells.
- Teach children not to run or ride a tricycle into the street.
- Obtain a low bed when the child begins to climb.
- Cover outlets with safety covers or plugs.

Preschoolers

- Do not allow children to run with candy or other objects in the mouth.
- Teach children not to put small objects in the mouth, nose, and ears.
- Remove doors from unused equipment, such as refrigerators.
- Teach preschoolers to cross streets safely and obey traffic signals.
- Check Halloween treats before allowing children to eat them. Discard loose or open candy.
- Teach children to play in safe areas, not on streets and railroad tracks.
- Teach preschoolers the dangers of playing with matches and playing near barbeque grills, fire, and heating appliances.

- Teach children to keep parents informed of their whereabouts and to avoid strangers.
- Teach preschoolers not to walk in front of swings and not to push others off playground equipment.

School-Age Children

- Teach children safety rules for recreational and sports activities: Never swim alone; always wear a life jacket when in a boat; and wear a protective helmet and knee and elbow pads when needed.
- Supervise contact sports and activities in which children aim at a target (e.g., archery or darts).
- Teach children to obey all traffic and safety rules for bicycling, skateboarding, and roller skating.
- Teach children to use light or reflective clothing when walking or cycling at night.
- Teach children safe ways to use the stove, garden tools, and other equipment.
- Supervise children when they use saws, electric appliances, tools, and other potentially dangerous equipment.
- Teach children not to play with fireworks, gunpowder, or firearms. Keep firearms unloaded, locked up, and out of reach.
- Teach children to avoid excavations, quarries, vacant buildings, and playing around heavy machinery.
- Teach children the effects of drugs and alcohol on judgment and coordination.

Adolescents

- Have adolescents complete a driver's education course, and take practice drives with them in various kinds of weather.
- Set firm limits on automobile use, namely, never to drive after drinking or using drugs, and never to ride with a driver who has done so. Encourage adolescents to call home for a ride if they have been drinking, assuring them they can do so without a reprimand.
- Teach adolescents to wear a safety helmet when riding motorcycles, scooters, and other sports vehicles. Teach safety rules for water sports.
- Encourage adolescents to use proper equipment when participating in sports. Schedule a physical examination before participation, and be certain there is medical supervision for all athletic activities.

- Encourage adolescents to swim, jog, and go boating in groups so they can obtain help in case of an emergency.
- Teach rules for hunting and the proper care and use of firearms.
- Inform the adolescent of the dangers of drugs, alcohol, and unprotected sex. Be alert to changes in the adolescent's mood and behavior. Listen to and maintain open communication with the adolescent. Open communication is a powerful preventive measure.
- Set a good example of behavior that the adolescent can follow.

Young Adults

- Reinforce motor vehicle safety: Drive defensively, use "designated drivers" if alcohol is consumed, routinely check brakes and tires, and use seat and shoulder belts or car seats for all passengers.
- Remind the young adult to repair potential fire hazards, such as electric wiring.
- Reinforce water safety: Know the depth of a pool before diving; supervise backyard pools and other water activities.
- Discuss evaluating the potential for workplace injuries or death when making decisions about a career or occupation. Encourage the young adult to participate actively in programs that reduce occupational hazards.
- Discuss avoiding excessive sun radiation by limiting exposure, using sun-blocking agents, and wearing protective clothing. Explain the skin changes that may indicate a cancerous condition.
- Encourage young adults who are unable to cope with the pressures, responsibilities, and expectations of adulthood to seek counseling.

Middle-Aged Adults

- Reinforce motor vehicle safety: Use seat belts and drive within the speed limit. Test visual acuity periodically.
- Make certain stairways are well lighted and uncluttered.
- Equip bathrooms with grab bars and nonskid bath mats.
- Test smoke detectors and fire alarms regularly.
- Keep all machines and tools in good working condition at work and at home. Follow safety precautions when using machinery.

Older Adults

- Encourage the client to have regular vision and hearing tests.
- Assist the client with setting up a home hazard appraisal.
- Encourage the client to keep as active as possible.

LIFESTYLE

Lifestyle factors that place people at risk include unsafe work environments; residence in neighborhoods with high crime rates; access to guns and ammunition; insufficient income to buy safety equipment or make necessary repairs; and access to illicit drugs, which may also be contaminated by harmful additives. Risk-taking behavior is a factor in some accidents.

MOBILITY AND HEALTH STATUS

People who have impaired mobility due to paralysis, muscle weakness, and poor balance or coordination are obviously prone to injury. Clients with spinal cord injury and

paralysis of both legs may be unable to move even when they perceive discomfort. Hemiplegic clients or clients with leg casts often have poor balance and fall easily. Clients weakened by illness or surgery are not always fully aware of their condition.

SENSORY–PERCEPTUAL ALTERATIONS

Accurate sensory perception of environmental stimuli is vital to safety. People with impaired touch perception, hearing, taste, smell, and vision are highly susceptible to injury. A person who does not see well may trip over a toy or not see an electric cord. People with impaired hearing may not

Safety

Cultural Issues Related to Safety

Injuries are the number one leading cause of death in the 0- to 40-year age group. Some ethnic groups have higher incidents of certain types of injuries:

- The majority of deaths among Native Americans under the age of 45 are unintentional injuries. In the 15- to 24-year age group, the death rate is more than two times higher than in the rest of the population.

- Homicide is the leading cause of death in African American males. The incidence is 18% higher than in the rest of the population.

- Automobile-related deaths are highest in the Caucasian populations from infants to middle adulthood. (There has been a recent slight decrease, probably due to increased state laws for the use of child safety seats and seat belts.)

hear a siren in traffic, and people with impaired olfactory sense may not smell burning food or escaping gas.

COGNITIVE AWARENESS

Awareness is the ability to perceive environmental stimuli and body reactions and to respond appropriately through thought and action. Clients with impaired awareness include people lacking in sleep, unconscious or semiconscious persons, disoriented people (i.e., those who may not understand where they are or what to do to help themselves), people who perceive stimuli that do not exist, and people whose judgment is altered by disease or medications (such as narcotics, tranquilizers, hypnotics, and sedatives). Mildly confused clients may momentarily forget where they are, wander from their rooms, or misplace personal belongings.

EMOTIONAL STATE

Extreme emotional states can alter the ability to perceive environmental hazards. Stressful situations can reduce a person's level of concentration, cause errors of judgment, and decrease awareness of external stimuli. Depressed people may think and react to environmental stimuli more slowly than usual.

ABILITY TO COMMUNICATE

People with diminished ability to receive and convey information are also at risk for injury. Aphasic clients, people with language barriers, and those unable to read are among them. For example, a person who cannot interpret the sign "No smoking—Oxygen in use" may cause a fire.

SAFETY AWARENESS

Information is crucial to safety. Clients in unfamiliar environments frequently need specific safety information. Lack of knowledge about unfamiliar equipment, such as oxygen tanks, intravenous tubing, and hot packs, is a potential hazard. Healthy clients need knowledge about water safety, car safety, fire prevention, ways to prevent the ingestion of

harmful substances, and preventive measures for age-related hazards.

ENVIRONMENT

The environment in which people live and work can increase their risk for injury. Nurses should assess the home environment for potential hazards such as living in an area where there are environmental contaminants from chemicals and other industrial wastes. Nurses should encourage parents to remove all mercury thermometers from the home and replace these thermometers with a digital thermometer. In addition, parents should be instructed to avoid smoking due to the risks of secondhand smoke. In the employment setting, nurses should assess the environment for exposure to hazardous chemicals through inhalation or contact, dangerous equipment, and excessive noise.

Preventing Specific Hazards

Measures to prevent specific hazards or injuries (such as burns, fire, poisoning, falls, suffocation, excessive noise, electrocution, and radiation injury) are critical aspects of nursing care. Teaching clients about safety is another important aspect. Nurses usually have opportunities to teach while providing care.

SCALDS AND BURNS

A *scald* is a burn from a hot liquid or vapor, such as steam. A burn results from excessive exposure to thermal, chemical, electric, or radioactive agents.

In healthcare agencies, the risk of scalds and burns is greater for clients whose skin sensitivity to temperature is impaired. Scalds can occur from overly hot bath water, and burns can occur from therapeutic applications of heat (see Chapter 23 ⦻). Nurses should assess their clients' skin at regular intervals to ensure therapeutic appliances have not malfunctioned and resulted in injury. It is important for the nurse to assess how well clients can protect themselves and what special precautions, if any, need to be taken.

FIRES

Fires continue to be a constant risk in both healthcare settings and homes. Agency fires usually result from malfunctioning electric equipment or combustion of anesthetic gas. In the home, fires can result from cooking, heating appliances such as kerosene or natural gas heaters, and smoking. Children may also start fires in the home if they have access to matches or lighters.

Agency Fires

In healthcare agencies, fire is particularly hazardous when people are incapacitated and unable to leave the building without assistance. This makes it extremely important for nurses to be aware of the fire safety regulations and fire prevention practices of the agency in which they work. When a fire occurs, the

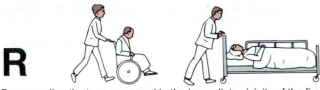

R

Remove all patients or personnel in the immediate vicinity of the fire.

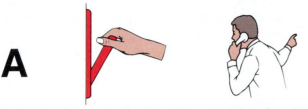

A

Activate the alarm and notify other staff members that a fire exists.

C

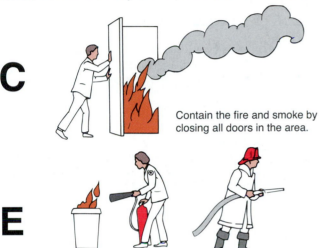

Contain the fire and smoke by closing all doors in the area.

E

Extinguish the fire, if it is a very small fire, or allow the fire department to extinguish it.

Figure 8-1. ■ The RACE system for protecting clients in case of fire.

nurse follows four sequential priorities. Using the acronym RACE can help you remember the procedure (Figure 8-1 ■):

Rescue clients in immediate danger.
Alarm (Pull alarm or call to report.)
Contain the fire.
Extinguish the fire.

Extinguishing the fire requires knowledge of three categories of fire, classified according to the type of material that is burning:

Class A: Paper, wood, upholstery, rags, ordinary rubbish
Class B: Flammable liquids and gases
Class C: Electrical.

The right type of extinguisher must be used to fight the fire. Each extinguisher has picture symbols showing the type of fire for which it is to be used. Directions for use are also attached. When using an extinguisher, remember PASS:

Point
Aim
Squeeze
Sweep.

Home Fires

In the home, adults should be educated about measures to reduce their risk of fires. If they use a kerosene or natural gas heater, they need to be certain to keep all combustible materials including paper and cloth products away from the heater. The risks of fires from cooking can be reduced by educating adults to be vigilant when cooking with oils and to avoid cooking when they are very tired and likely to fall asleep. A fire extinguisher should also be kept close to cooking areas with all family members familiar with its operation. The nurse should encourage the family to maintain working smoke detectors near sleeping and cooking areas. The smoke detectors should be checked at least every 3 months and batteries changed every 6 months. Many community fire departments offer the homeowner a free fire risk assessment and will install smoke detectors in the home for free or a minimal fee. Children should also be educated to avoid playing with matches and how to respond in case of fire. A fire escape plan should be developed by all families. In homes with bars or other protective coverings over the windows to prevent burglary, the family needs to have an escape route or a way to remove the covering to escape through a window. In an upstairs room, an escape plan is particularly important since people can become trapped if the fire starts in the downstairs living area. An outside stairwell or ladder that can be attached to the window and lowered to the ground can be effective measures to prevent trapping. Families should be encouraged to practice their fire escape plan so that all family members are familiar with it.

POISONING

Accidental poisoning can occur through swallowing or inhaling toxic substances, from bites and stings, or through contact with poisonous items such as poison ivy. Infants and children are prone to swallowing substances they may find as they explore. Adolescent and adult poisonings are usually related to the ingestion of recreational drugs or suicide attempts. Older adults are at risk for poisoning through overdoses of prescribed medications.

Prevent accidental poisonings by keeping toxic substances locked up and out of reach. Both young children and elders with dementia should have a "safe" environment with plants, flowers, medications, and small objects kept out of reach. Food poisoning can be prevented by properly washing and cooking foods. The Poison Control Center (800-222-1222) can provide current information about potential hazards and recommended treatments.

Clients and staff in healthcare facilities can be at risk for poisonings because of potential toxic substances in the environment, such as cleaning solutions. Healthcare facilities will generally have posted instructions and alerts for accidental ingestion of poisonous substances. Medication errors can lead to drug interactions and overdoses, and medication administration procedures should always be followed to prevent errors from occurring (see Chapter 29 ⬤).

FALLS

People of any age can fall, but infants and older adults are particularly prone to falling and serious injury. Falls are the leading cause of injury among older adults. They are also a major cause of hospital and nursing home admissions. Most falls occur in the home and are a major threat to the independence of older adults. Fear of falling is common in older adults, even in those who have not experienced a fall. This fear is of particular concern for those who live alone and who anticipate being helpless and unable to summon help after a fall. For these individuals the nurse can make the following recommendations:

- Encourage daily or more frequent contact with a friend or family member.
- Install a personal emergency response system.
- Maintain a physical environment that prevents falls.

Risk factors and associated preventive measures are shown in Table 8-1 ■.

Prevention of falls in healthcare agencies is an ongoing concern. Healthcare environments are designed with many safety features. These include railings along corridors; call bells at each bedside; safety bars and emergency pull cords

---

TABLE 8-1

Risk Factors for Falls and Preventive Measures

RISK FACTOR	PREVENTIVE MEASURES
Poor vision	Ensure eyeglasses are functional. Ensure appropriate lighting. Mark doorways and edges of steps as needed. Keep the environment tidy.
Cognitive dysfunction (confusion, disorientation, impaired memory or judgment)	Set safe limits to activities. Remove unsafe objects.
Impaired gait or balance and difficulty walking because of lower extremity dysfunction (e.g., arthritis)	Wear shoes or well-fitted slippers with nonskid soles. Use ambulatory devices as necessary (cane, crutches, walker, braces, and wheelchair). Provide assistance with ambulation as needed. Monitor gait and balance. Adapt living arrangements to one floor if necessary. Encourage exercise and activity as tolerated to maintain muscle strength, joint flexibility, and balance. Ensure uncluttered environment with securely fastened rugs. Adjust activity to time period when client has increased mobility.
Difficulty getting in and out of chair or in and out of bed	Encourage client to request assistance. Keep the bed in the low position. Install grab bars in bathroom. Provide raised toilet seat.
Orthostatic hypotension	Instruct client to rise slowly from a lying to sitting to standing position, and to stand in place for several seconds before walking.
Urinary frequency or receiving diuretics	Provide a bedside commode. Assist with voiding on a frequent and scheduled basis.
Weakness from disease process or therapy	Encourage client to summon help. Monitor activity tolerance.
Current medication regimen that includes sedatives, hypnotics, tranquilizers, narcotic analgesics, diuretics	Attach side rails to the bed. Keep side rails in place when the bed is in the lowest position. Monitor orientation and alertness status. Encourage annual or more frequent review of all medications prescribed.

Preventing Falls in Healthcare Agencies

☑ Orient clients on admission to their surroundings, and explain the call system.

☑ Carefully assess each client's risk for falling.

☑ Alert all personnel to the client's risk for falling.

☑ Assign clients at risk for falls to rooms near the nursing station where they can be more closely supervised.

☑ Encourage the client and family to use the call bell to request assistance; ensure that the bell is within easy reach.

☑ Answer call bells promptly.

☑ Place bedside tables and overbed tables near the bed or chair so that clients do not overreach and consequently lose their balance.

☑ Always keep hospital beds in the low position when not providing care so that clients can move in or out of bed easily.

☑ Keep side rails up and the bed in the low position for sedated and unconscious clients when they are unattended.

☑ Lock wheels on beds, wheelchairs, and stretchers.

☑ Ensure that the client wears nonskid footwear.

☑ Use bed or chair safety monitoring devices as needed.

in toilet areas; locks on beds, wheelchairs, and stretchers; side rails on beds; and night-lights. In addition, nurses can implement measures to decrease the incidence of falls, as described in Box 8-3 ■.

Safety monitoring devices are also available to prevent falls. Some monitoring systems use a chair or bed sensor (Figure 8-2 ■); others use a leg band. These devices trigger an alarm when the client attempts to get out of bed or a chair

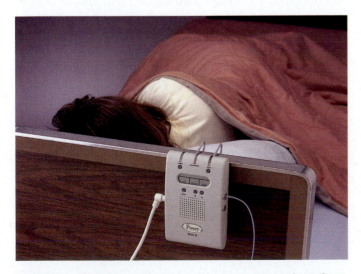

Figure 8-2. ■ Bed exit monitoring device; sounds an alarm if client exists bed. (*Source:* Courtesy of J. T. Posey Company. Reprinted with permission.)

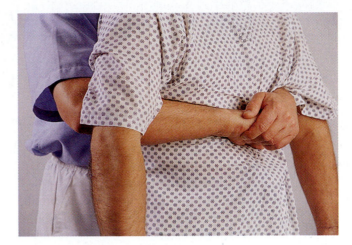

Figure 8-3. ■ Performing the Heimlich maneuver. (Photographer Elena Dorfman.)

unassisted. Procedure 8-1 ■ on page 144 describes how to use these devices.

SUFFOCATION OR CHOKING

Suffocation, or *asphyxiation,* is lack of oxygen due to interrupted breathing. Suffocation occurs when the air source is cut off for any reason. One common reason for choking is that food or a foreign object becomes lodged in the throat. The universal sign of distress in this case is observation of the victim's grasping and pointing to the neck and throat area without speaking. The emergency response is the Heimlich maneuver, or abdominal thrust, which can dislodge the foreign object and reestablish an airway (Figure 8-3 ■).

EXCESSIVE NOISE

Excessive noise is a health hazard that can cause hearing loss, depending on the overall level of noise, the frequency range of the noise, the duration of exposure, and individual susceptibility. When ill or injured, people are frequently sensitive to noises that normally would not disturb them. Loud voices, the clatter of dishes, and even a nearby television can disturb clients, some of whom react angrily. Physiological effects of noise include (1) increased heart and respiratory rates, (2) increased muscular activity, (3) nausea, and (4) hearing loss, if the noise is sufficiently loud.

Noise can be minimized in several ways. Acoustic tile on ceilings, walls, and floors as well as drapes and carpeting absorb sound. Background music can mask noise and have a calming effect on some people. During the change-of-shift reports, nurses should be careful to keep their voices low or to give reports in areas away from clients' rooms. It is important for nurses to minimize noise in the hospital setting and to encourage clients to protect their hearing as much as possible.

ELECTRICAL HAZARDS

All electric equipment must be properly grounded. The electric plug of grounded equipment has three prongs. The

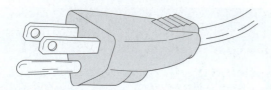

Figure 8-4. ■ Three-pronged grounded plug. (*Source: Ambularm Co.*)

two short prongs transmit the power to the equipment. The third, longer prong is the grounding device, which carries short circuits or stray electric current to the ground (Figure 8-4 ■). Grounding prongs offer a path of least resistance to stray electric currents.

Faulty equipment (e.g., equipment with a frayed cord) presents a danger of electric shock or may start a fire. For example, an electric spark near certain anesthetic gases or a high concentration of oxygen can cause a serious fire. Electric shock occurs when a current travels through the body to the ground rather than through electric wiring, or from static electricity that builds up on the body. Using machines in good repair, wearing shoes with rubber soles, standing on a nonconductive floor, and using nonconductive gloves are all ways to prevent shock. If the nurse identifies faulty equipment, the nurse is responsible for removing this equipment from service and making a report to the appropriate person at the healthcare facility.

RADIATION

Radiation injury can occur from overexposure to radioactive materials used in diagnostic and therapeutic procedures. Clients being examined using radiography or fluoroscopy generally receive minimal exposure, and few precautions are necessary. Nurses need to protect themselves, however, from radiation when some clients are receiving radiation therapy. Exposure to radiation can be minimized by (1) limiting the time near the source, (2) providing as much distance as possible from the source, and (3) using shielding devices such as lead aprons when near the source. Nurses need to become familiar with agency protocols related to radiation therapy.

Preventing Procedure- and Equipment-Related Injury

Risk assessment in the healthcare setting must include risks related to procedures and equipment. Whether giving a medication or assisting a client out of bed, nurses need to follow safeguards to prevent errors or injuries. Most healthcare agencies establish protocols that are designed to prevent injuries. When in doubt about a course of action, the nurse should consult the appropriate written guidelines before proceeding.

When an injury or error does occur, most agencies require that the incident be reported. The nurse completes the report immediately after taking whatever action is required to safeguard the client, and notifying the charge nurse. For additional information about incident reports, see Chapters 3 ⚭ and 36 ⚭.

Hospital and Institutional Safety

The Occupational Safety and Health Administration is under the Department of Labor of the federal government. Its purpose is to make sure that every worker in the United States is employed in a safe environment. Employees are required to follow OSHA regulations. Fines are imposed for violations. Student nurses are not specifically addressed in the regulations; however, they are expected to comply with healthcare facility policies and procedures.

SAFETY DEVICES

To protect healthcare workers' safety, OSHA has implemented several requirements for the use of safety devices in the healthcare setting. One example of these safety devices is the use of needleless systems to prevent needle-stick injury to healthcare workers. OSHA has also encouraged the use of assistive equipment to prevent musculoskeletal injuries. Musculoskeletal injuries are one of the most common injuries of healthcare workers today. These injuries can be so severe that the employee can no longer provide direct client care.

INFECTIOUS WASTE

OSHA has developed two standards dealing with infection control activities in the healthcare setting: the *Bloodborne Pathogens Standards* and the *Occupational Exposure to Tuberculosis Standard*. Healthcare facilities are required to develop exposure control plans. In addition, healthcare facilities must provide training to employees. When an employee is exposed to infectious agents, the facility must have a plan in place to provide appropriate intervention and follow-up. It is important that students and nurses be familiar with the requirements for controlling exposure.

Disposal of Used or Soiled Equipment from an Isolation Room

Most facilities have policies and procedures in place that state specifically how to dispose of equipment and supplies that have been contaminated. Be familiar with these policies! Materials may be disposed of, cleaned, disinfected, or sterilized. Some equipment and supplies are for single use only. Other materials are meant to be used many times.

Bagging is a technique recommended by the CDC for removal of materials from a client's room. The purpose is to prevent exposure from items contaminated with body secretions. The bag must be impervious to microorganisms. The bags may come in specific colors (e.g., red) and have labels that indicate they contain infectious materials.

The CDC recommends placing contaminated disposable items in the plastic bags that line the waste containers. Nondisposable or reusable items should be put into a labeled bag before being removed from the client's room and sent to a central processing area for decontamination. Rubber, plastic, metal, and glass items should be bagged separately. (Metal and glass can be autoclaved, but rubber and plastic need to be exposed to gas sterilization.)

Special procedure trays should be disassembled and bagged as indicated above. Soiled linens or clothing should be bagged and sent to the facility laundry or home. Linens should be handled as little as possible. They should be rolled into a bundle before being placed in the bag (do not shake the linens). Laboratory specimens should be put into a leakproof container. If the container is contaminated on the outside, it should be put in a plastic bag before sending it to the laboratory. Dishes are often made of paper and are disposed of in the refuse container. Blood pressure equipment, if kept in the room, needs no special precautions. If it becomes contaminated, follow the agency's cleaning procedures. Nondisposable thermometers should be disinfected after use according to agency protocols. Needles, syringes, and other "sharps" should be placed in a puncture-resistant container kept in the room. Clients' personal objects (such as toys) that are contaminated should be bagged and sent home for cleaning. For additional information on infection control, see Chapter 9 🔗.

HAZARDOUS WASTE

Every work area is responsible for having Material Safety Data Sheets (MSDS) available for all chemicals used in that work area. Common substances considered to be hazardous include bleach and other disinfectants. Chemotherapeutic or antineoplastic agents are among the most hazardous substances for nurses. As an LPN/LVN, you will not be administering these drugs without special training.

Each person is responsible for knowing the chemical used and any potential risks to themselves and their clients. The containers must be labeled with the chemical name as well as the function. The labels must also tell any danger or hazard that may exist with that chemical or ingredients and the name, address, and phone number of the manufacturer. Always read the label before using. If labels become illegible, do not use the bottle and report it so the bottle or label can be replaced. Know where the MSDS are kept and how to access them. Extensive information about the chemical can be found on the sheets. See Box 8-4 ■ for required information.

BOX 8-4

MSDS Required Information

- The name of the substance, the manufacturer, and the date the MSDS was prepared.
- Other names the chemical(s) may be called by or listed as, and exposure limits.
- Physical characteristics are described. This may include how a chemical looks and smells, melting and boiling points, how easily it dissolves or if it does not dissolve, and whether it floats or sinks in water.
- Fire and explosion data tell you if a substance is flammable or combustible and the lowest temperature at which it could catch fire. It also tells you the safest way to put out a fire with this chemical.
- The reactivity section tells you what happens when the chemical comes in contact with air, water, or other chemicals. This part tells you when it might burn, explode, or release dangerous vapors.
- The health hazards section lists how a chemical might enter your body (e.g., inhalation, ingestion, absorption through skin, or injection).
- The information on use, handling, and storage describes how to clear up a spill or leak in addition to handling, storage, and disposal of the chemical.
- Special protective precautions explain any need for personal protective equipment (such as goggles or a respirator) or signs or other equipment (such as a ventilation hood over a lab or pharmacy area) when using the chemical.

DISASTER PLAN

Disasters can be external or internal or a combination of both for a healthcare facility. **External disasters** include events outside the hospital that produce a large number of victims (e.g., fires, plane or train crashes, earthquakes, or violent civil disturbances). **Internal disasters** are events within the hospital that interrupt services and produce victims (e.g., utility interruption or chemical spill). Disasters such as earthquakes with building damage, tornadoes, and floods can be both internal and external.

Teamwork and cooperation are essential to any disaster plan. Many communities hold annual disaster drills in cooperation with hospitals, police and fire departments, and public works offices. Mock disasters can provide much valuable information for all involved agencies.

Triage is an important consideration during a disaster. Clients in the hospital will be assessed for possible discharge if necessary. Victims are prioritized according to their care needs, from most severe to least. Victims are identified by universal emergency medical services (EMS) disaster triage codes:

- *Red:* The most severely injured—likely to need surgery or hospitalization in the intensive care unit (ICU)

- *Yellow:* Significant injuries—require quick attention to prevent worsening of condition; may require hospitalization after treatment
- *Green:* Persons who are "walking wounded" and have non–life-threatening injuries that must eventually be treated to restore client to normal functioning; may not require hospitalization
- *Black:* Deceased, DOA, code blue; transport to morgue.

Not all victims arrive at the hospital with an EMS triage tag. The "walking wounded" may arrive by private car and will need to be assessed in the emergency department.

During a disaster, healthcare workers must be willing to perform tasks as assigned by the supervisor. During this time, personal communication should be put on hold in order not to tie up communication systems. It is important to observe client confidentiality and not perpetuate rumors. Each person should stay in his or her assigned area until directed to do otherwise. The facility will usually have a public information officer who will make statements to the media; it is imperative that all questions be referred to that person or office. Do not fall into the trap of giving unauthorized information.

EMERGENCY CODES

All healthcare facilities have emergency codes. Eleven codes have been identified. There is a real push to have all hospitals use a universal code system. Code Red and Code Blue are widely accepted, but much work is needed to bring other codes into line in all facilities. See Box 8-5 ■ for commonly used emergency codes. It is important that both students and nurses know the specific codes used in each facility where they work or are affiliated.

BOX 8-5

Emergency Codes

- *Code Red:* Fire
- *Code Blue:* Medical emergency adult
- *Code White:* Medical emergency pediatric
- *Code Pink:* Infant abduction
- *Code Purple:* Child abduction
- *Code Yellow:* Bomb threat
- *Code Gray:* Combative person
- *Code Silver:* Person with a weapon and/or hostage situation
- *Code Orange:* Hazardous material spill/release
- *Code Triage Internal:* An internal disaster
- *Code Triage External:* An external disaster

Note: Codes may vary by facility. Be sure to know the color coding of the facility in which you work!

EMERGENCY NURSING AND FIRST AID

You may be called on to deal with healthcare emergencies inside and outside of the healthcare facility. Nurses who give emergency care in the community should seek first aid training. Such training provides the individual with specific skills that can be used to serve and protect the community. It is important to administer first aid treatment and/or cardiopulmonary resuscitation (CPR) in the manner in which you have been trained (Figure 8-5 ■).

Any nurse who volunteers his or her time at community activities to provide first aid should contact a local certifying agency (such as the Red Cross) to obtain a first aid certification. As long as you provide appropriate and safe care within the guidelines of your state practice act, most states offer you protection under Good Samaritan laws.

CARDIOPULMONARY RESUSCITATION

CPR certification is required for healthcare professionals by most healthcare facilities (Box 8-6 ■). Several different agencies including the American Heart Association (AHA) and the Red Cross provide certification programs that meet these requirements. Many facilities and schools provide the classes for employees and students. It is important to maintain current certification as a nurse as well as a responsible citizen. In 2005, the AHA issued new guidelines for CPR. Those holding a CPR card should refer to the guidelines frequently and practice the skills on a regular basis. For more information, contact a local provider of CPR certification classes.

Restraining Clients

Restraints are protective devices used to limit the physical activity of the client or a part of the body. They can be classified as physical or chemical. Physical restraints are any manual method or physical or mechanical device, material, or equipment attached to the client's body. They cannot be removed easily, and they restrict the client's movement. Chemical restraints are psychotropic agents used to control disruptive behavior.

The purpose of restraints is to ensure the physical safety of the person who is being restrained, or of other persons whom the restrained person may otherwise harm. Nurses are encouraged to reduce the use of restraints and use safe alternatives whenever possible. Alternatives to restraints are listed in Box 8-7 ■.

To safeguard clients in long-term care facilities, the U.S. government regulated the use of mechanical restraints. The Omnibus Budget Reconciliation Act clearly states that restraints should be applied only as a last resort. Regulations also require that (1) restraints be applied only under a physician's written order, one that specifies why the restraint is

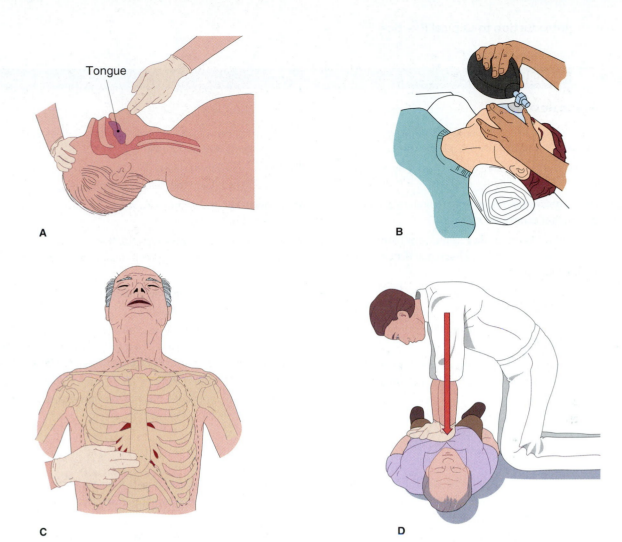

Figure 8-5. ■ CPR. **A.** Use the head tilt/chin lift method to open the airway. **B.** If not breathing, give two full breaths using a pocket mask, mouth shield, or bag-valve-mask. Observe the chest rise and fall during ventilation. **C.** Locate the compression site by following the edge of the rib cage to the notch where the ribs join the sternum. **D.** Position your hands and begin chest compressions with your arms vertical over the victim.

BOX 8-6

CPR Overview

CPR for Adults by Healthcare Provider

If you find an unresponsive adult, place flat on back on a firm surface. Move an injured adult only if necessary, and turn head, neck, and body as a unit. If the rescuer suspects the collapse is the result of asphyxiation due to an obstructed airway, the rescuer should perform approximately 2 minutes of CPR and then call for help and retrieve the automated external defibrillator (AED).

1. Shout for help. If alone, phone the emergency response number or 911 and retrieve the AED and emergency equipment.
2. **A** Open the airway:
   Perform a head tilt/chin lift maneuver.
   If neck injury is suspected, use jaw thrust.
3. **B** Check for breathing (look, listen, and feel).
   If breathing is not adequate, provide 2 breaths.
   Use bag–valve–mask device with oxygen or barrier device.
   Be sure chest rises with each breath.
   If chest does not rise, reopen the airway and try again.
4. **C** Check for signs of circulation (pulse, breathing, coughing, or movement).

Signs of circulation but no breathing:
- Provide rescue breathing (one breath every 5 to 6 seconds).

No pulse, no signs of circulation present:
- *If AED is available:* Power on, attach electrodes, follow prompts.

One shock should be delivered followed immediately by CPR.
- *If no AED available:* Perform chest compressions:
  —Compress lower half of sternum.
  —Rate approximately 100 times per minute.
  —30 compressions, then two breaths (repeat).

5. CPR: Provide 30 compressions and two breaths (repeat) until client is intubated. If client is intubated, compressions are given continually, without pauses for breaths (8 to 10 breaths per minute are provided while compressions are being given).

If the nurse is working with infants or children, they should be familiar with the current emergency care guidelines.

Source: Adapted from guidelines of American Heart Association (2005).

133

BOX 8-7	NURSING CARE CHECKLIST

Alternatives to Restraints

☑ Assign nurses in pairs to act as "buddies" so that one nurse can observe the client when the other leaves the unit.

☑ Place unstable clients in an area that is constantly or closely supervised.

☑ Prepare clients before a move, in order to limit relocation shock and resultant confusion.

☑ Stay with a client using a bedside commode or bathroom if the client is confused or sedated or has a gait disturbance or a high-risk score for falling.

☑ Monitor all of the client's medications and, if possible, attempt to lower or eliminate dosages of sedatives or psychotropic drugs.

☑ Position beds at their lowest level from the floor to facilitate getting in and out of bed.

☑ Replace full-length side rails with half- or three-quarter-length rails to prevent confused clients from climbing over rails or falling from the end of the bed.

☑ Use rocking chairs to help confused clients expend some of their energy so that they will be less inclined to wander.

☑ Wedge pillows or pads against the sides of wheelchairs to keep clients well positioned.

☑ Place a removable lap tray on a wheelchair to provide support and help keep the client in place.

☑ To quiet agitated clients, try a warm beverage, soft lights, a back rub, or a walk.

☑ Use "environmental restraints," such as pieces of furniture or large plants as barriers, to keep clients from wandering beyond appropriate areas.

☑ Place a picture or other personal item on the door to clients' rooms to help them identify their room.

☑ Try to determine the causes of the client's *sundown syndrome* (nocturnal wandering and disorientation as darkness falls, associated with dementia). Possible causes include poor hearing, poor eyesight, or pain.

☑ Establish ongoing assessment to monitor changes in physical and cognitive functional abilities and risk factors.

being used and for how long it will be used; (2) the client agrees to be restrained; and (3) the client be free of physical restraints not required to treat the client's medical symptoms.

LEGAL IMPLICATIONS OF RESTRAINTS

Because restraints restrict a person's ability to move freely, their use has legal implications. See Box 8-8 ■ for the legal implications of using restraints.

SELECTING A RESTRAINT

Before selecting a restraint, nurses need to understand clearly its purpose and measure it against the following five criteria:

1. It restricts the client's movement as little as possible. If a client needs to have one arm restrained, do not restrain the entire body.

2. It does not interfere with the client's treatment or health problem. If a client has poor blood circulation to the hands, apply a restraint that will not aggravate that circulatory problem.

3. It is readily changeable. Restraints need to be changed frequently, especially if they become soiled. Keeping other guidelines in mind, choose a restraint that can be changed with minimal disturbance to the client.

4. It is safe for the particular client. Choose a restraint with which the client cannot self-inflict injury. For example, a physically active child could incur injury

trying to climb out of a crib if one wrist is tied to the side of the crib. A jacket restraint would restrain the child more safely.

5. It is the least obvious to others. Both clients and visitors are often embarrassed by a restraint, even though they understand why it is being used. The less obvious the restraint, the more comfortable people feel.

KINDS OF RESTRAINTS

There are several kinds of restraints (Figures 8-6 ■ through 8-8 ■). Among the most common are the jacket restraint, the belt restraint, the mitt or hand restraint, limb restraints, elbow restraints, mummy restraints, and crib nets. Geri chairs and wheelchairs used to confine client activity can also be considered restraints. There are several types of vest restraints, but all are essentially sleeveless jackets (vests) with straps (tails) that can be tied to the bed frame under the mattress (see Figure 8-7) or to the legs of a chair. These body restraints are used to ensure the safety of confused or sedated clients in beds or wheelchairs. The Food and Drug Administration (FDA) advises that manufacturers place "front" and "back" labels on vest restraints.

Belt or safety strap body restraints (see Figure 8-6B) are used to ensure the safety of all clients who are being moved on stretchers or in wheelchairs. Some wheelchairs have a soft padded safety bar that attaches to side brackets that are

BOX 8-8

Legal Implications for Use of Restraints

To protect clients and to avoid legal problems, the nurse should follow these guidelines:

- Know the agency's restraint policies. Policies should cover all types of physical and chemical restraints and specify how and when to apply them and what procedures to follow.
- When determining the need for a restraint, always assess the underlying reason for a client's restlessness, agitation, or confusion.
- Apply restraints only when necessary for the client's health and safety, not for convenience or to cope with understaffing.
- Avoid being influenced by a family member's advice not to restrain the client, even when the person offers to sit with the client. Nurses cannot legally delegate responsibility to a family member.
- Try to obtain a physician's order before applying a restraint. If the client needs to be restrained immediately, apply the restraint and then notify the physician as soon as possible. In many agencies, standing orders allow the use of restraints under certain circumstances, provided that a written order is obtained from the physician within 24 hours.
- Recognize the competent adult's right to make decisions regarding personal care and treatment, and obtain appropriate consent. Check agency policies if necessary restraint is refused.

An agency may require the client to sign a release of liability should injury result; otherwise, the agency has the option of refusing to continue care. For clients who are declared legally incompetent, obtain consent from an appointed guardian or surrogate as permitted by law.

- Keep in mind the principle of least restriction; that is, restrain the client only to the extent necessary to accomplish the restraint's purpose.
- Make sure that a physical restraint fits properly.
- When a restraint is applied, document:
  a. The specific behavior that made it necessary
  b. The type of restraint used
  c. The substance of explanations given to the client and support persons
  d. The client's consent
  e. The exact times the restraint was applied and removed
  f. The client's behavior while the restraint was applied
  g. The frequency of care given while the restraint was applied and removed (e.g., assessment of circulation and range-of-motion exercises)
  h. Notification of the physician.
- Periodically reevaluate the need for the restraint.

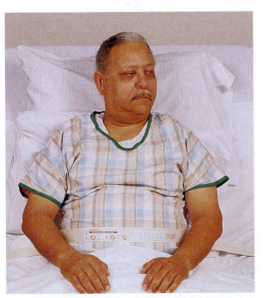

A

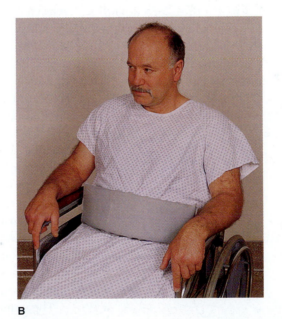

B

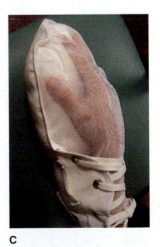

C

Figure 8-6. ■ **A.** Poncho-type vest restraint. Put vest on client, with front/back opening placed according to manufacturer's recommendations. Pull the tie on the end of the vest flap across the chest, and place it through the slit on the opposite side of the chest. Repeat for the other tie. Use a half-bow knot to secure each tie. Do not tie the vest to the head of the bed. Fasten the ties together behind the chair using a square knot. Ensure that the client is positioned appropriately to enable maximum chest expansion for breathing. **B.** Belt restraint (safety belt). Attach the belt around the client's waist and fasten it at the back of the chair. If the client is bedridden or on a stretcher, one portion of the belt (the longer portion) is placed beneath the client, and the shorter portion is placed over the client's gown, with a finger width between the belt and the client. Belt restraints need to be applied to all clients on stretchers even when the side rails are up. **C.** Mitt restraint. Make sure the fingers can be slightly flexed and are not caught under the hand. Follow the manufacturer's directions for securing the mitt. Remove the mitt at least every 2 to 4 hours for washing and exercising the client's hand. Assess the client's hand circulation shortly after the mitt is applied and at regular intervals. Monitor for feelings of numbness or discomfort or inability to move the fingers. (*Source:* Jenny Thomas Photography, photos A and B.)

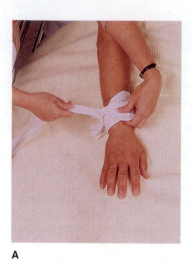
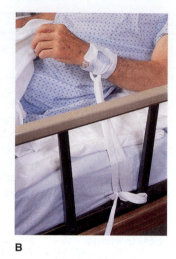
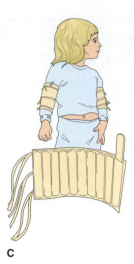

A   **B**   **C**

Figure 8-7. ■ **A, B.** Wrist or ankle restraint. Pad bony prominences to prevent skin breakdown. Pull the tie of the commercially made restraint through the slit or through the buckle, and secure the tie to the bed frame. **C.** Elbow restraint. Place the child's elbow in the center of the restraint. Make sure that the ends of the tongue depressors are covered by padded material to prevent irritation. Wrap the restraint smoothly around the arm and secure it with safety pins, ties, or tape. Pinning it to the child's shirt prevents it from sliding down the arm. Monitor for tightness and obstructed blood circulation. (*Source:* Jenny Thomas Photography, photo A.)

installed under the arm rests. To prevent the person from slumping forward, the nurse then attaches a shoulder "Y" strap to the bar and over the client's shoulders to the rear handles. Other safety belt models have a three-loop design. One loop surrounds the person's waist and attaches to the rear handles. If such restraints are unavailable, the nurse can place a folded towel or small sheet around the client's waist and fasten it at the back of the wheelchair. Belt restraints

may also be used for certain clients confined to bed or to chairs.

A mitt or hand restraint (see Figure 8-6C) is used to prevent confused clients from using their hands or fingers to scratch and injure themselves. For example, a confused client may need to be prevented from pulling at intravenous tubing or a bandage following surgery. Hand or mitt restraints allow the client to be ambulatory and/or to move the arm freely rather than be confined to a bed or a chair. (See legend for Figure 8-6C.)

Limb restraints (see Figures 8-7A and B) are generally made of cloth. They may be used to immobilize a limb, primarily for therapeutic reasons (e.g., to maintain an intravenous infusion).

Elbow restraints (see Figure 8-7C) are used to prevent infants or small children from flexing their elbows to touch or scratch a skin lesion or to reach the head when a scalp vein infusion is in place. This restraint consists of a piece of material with pockets into which plastic or wooden tongue depressors are inserted to provide rigidity.

The mummy restraint is a special folding of a blanket or sheet around a child to prevent movement during a procedure such as gastric washing, eye irrigation, or collection of a blood specimen. See Figure 8-8 for folding instructions.

General guidelines for applying and monitoring restraints are presented in Box 8-9 ■.

Attaching restraints to a bed or chair requires the use of knots, which must be secure but easily untied by staff in an emergency situation. See Figure 8-9 ■ for instructions on tying a half-bow knot and Figure 8-10 ■ for a square knot.

A   **B**

Figure 8-8. ■ Making a mummy restraint. **A.** Use a blanket about twice the length of the infant's body. Fold down one corner, and place the baby's shoulders on it in the supine position. Fold the right side of the blanket over the infant's body, leaving the left arm free (1). The right arm is in a natural position at the side. **B.** Fold the excess blanket at the bottom up under the infant (2). With the infant's left arm in a natural position beside the body, fold the left side of the blanket over the infant, including the arm, and tuck the blanket under the body (3).

BOX 8-9	**NURSING CARE CHECKLIST**

Applying and Monitoring Restraints

☑ Apply the selected restraint. Obtain consent from the client or guardian.

☑ Ensure that a physician's order has been provided, or in an emergency, obtain one within 24 hours after applying the restraint.

☑ Assure the client and the client's support people that the restraint is temporary and protective. A restraint must never be applied as punishment for any behavior or merely for the nurse's convenience.

☑ Apply the restraint in such a way that the client can move as freely as possible without defeating the purpose of the restraint.

☑ Ensure that limb restraints are applied securely but not so tightly that they impede blood circulation to any body area or extremity.

☑ Assess the restraint every 30 minutes. Some facilities have specific forms to be used to record ongoing assessment.

☑ Release all restraints at least every 2 to 4 hours, and provide range-of-motion (ROM) exercises (see Chapter 32 ⬤⬤) and skin care (see Chapter 23 ⬤⬤).

☑ If more than one limb is restrained, remove one restraint at a time. When a restraint is temporarily removed, do not leave the client unattended.

☑ Reassess the continued need for the restraint at least every 8 hours. Include an assessment of the underlying cause of the behavior necessitating use of the restraints.

☑ Immediately report to the nurse in charge and record on the client's chart any persistent reddened or broken skin areas under the restraint.

☑ At the first indication of cyanosis or pallor, coldness of a skin area, or a client's complaint of a tingling sensation, pain, or numbness, loosen the restraint and exercise the limb.

☑ Apply a restraint so that it can be released quickly in case of an emergency and with the body part in a normal anatomic position.

☑ Provide emotional support verbally and through touch.

☑ Determine that restraint is in good condition and is the appropriate size for the client.

☑ Explain to client and support people the purpose and procedure for using the restraint.

☑ Document relevant information for all types of restraints.

☑ Record on the client's chart the time the physician was notified, the type of restraint applied, the time it was applied, the reason for its application, the client's response to the restraint, and the times that the restraints are removed and skin care given.

☑ Record any other interventions, assessments, and explanations to client and significant others.

☑ Adjust the nursing care plan as required, for example, to include releasing the restraint every 2 h, assessing circulation, sensation, and motion of restrained extremities; and providing skin care and ROM exercises.

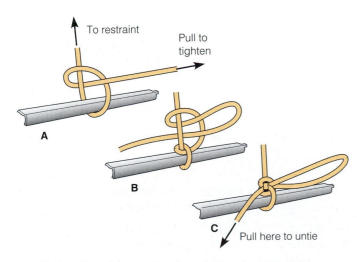

Figure 8-9. ■ To make a half-bow (quick-release) knot, first place the restraint tie under the side frame of the bed (or around a chair leg). **A.** Bring the free end up, around, under, and over the attached end of the tie and pull it tight. **B.** Again take the free end over and under the attached end of the tie, but this time make a half-bow loop. **C.** Tighten the free end of the tie and the bow until the knot is secure. To untie the knot, pull the end of the tie and then loosen the first cross over the tie.

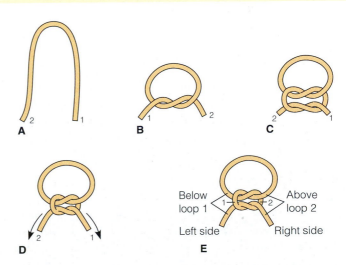

Figure 8-10. ■ To make a square (reef) knot: **A.** Form a "U" loop. **B.** Pass one end (1) over and under the other. **C.** Take the same end (1), and pass it over, under, and over the other. **D.** Pull knot tight. **E.** When the knot is tied correctly, the ties on each side are both either above or below the loop. Attach the other end of the commercial restraint to the movable portion of the bed frame, never to the side rails or to the nonmoving bed frame. If the ties are attached to the movable portion, the wrist or ankle will not be pulled when the bed position is changed.

NURSING CARE

ASSESSING

Assessing clients at risk for injury involves (1) noting risk indicators in the nursing history and physical examination, (2) using specifically developed risk assessment tools, and (3) evaluating the client's home environment.

The nursing history and physical examination can reveal considerable data about the client's safety practices and risks for injury. Data include age and developmental level; general health status; mobility status; presence or absence of physiologic or perceptual deficits such as olfactory, visual, tactile, taste, or other sensory impairments; altered thought processes or other impaired cognitive or emotional capabilities; substance abuse; any indications of abuse or neglect; and an injury history. A safety history also needs to include the client's awareness of hazards, knowledge of safety precautions both at home and work, and any perceived threats to safety.

Risk Assessment Tools

Risk assessment tools are available to determine clients at risk both for specific kinds of injury, such as falls, or skin impairment. In general, these tools direct the nurse to appraise the factors affecting safety as they have been outlined earlier. See Figure 23-14 ⚭ for one skin impairment assessment tool.

DIAGNOSING, PLANNING, AND IMPLEMENTING

A primary NANDA diagnostic label related to safety issues is *Risk for Injury,* a state in which the individual is at risk for injury as a result of environmental conditions interacting with the individual's adaptive and defense resources. One of the subcategories of this diagnosis may be preferred when the nurse wants to isolate suitable interventions. These subcategories are:

- *Risk for Poisoning*
- *Risk for Suffocation*
- *Risk for Trauma*
- *Impaired Home Maintenance*
- *Ineffective Protection.*

(Refer to Appendix II ⚭ for a complete list of nursing diagnoses related to safety.)

When planning care to prevent injury, the nurse considers all factors affecting the client's safety, specifies desired outcomes, and selects nursing activities to meet these outcomes. The major goal for clients with safety risks is to prevent injury. To meet this goal, clients often need to change their health behavior and may need to modify the environment.

Desired outcomes associated with preventing injury depend on the individual client. Examples of desired outcomes follow. The nurse needs to individualize these for clients. The client:

- Describes methods to prevent specific hazards (e.g., falls, suffocation, choking, fires, drowning, electric shock).
- Reports use of home safety measures (e.g., fire safety measures, smoke detector maintenance, fall prevention strategies, burn prevention measures, poison prevention measures, safe storage of hazardous materials, firearm safety precautions, electrocution prevention, water safety precautions, bicycle safety, motor vehicle safety).
- Alters home physical environment to reduce the risk of injury.
- Describes emergency procedures for poisoning and fire.
- Describes age-specific risks, work safety risks, or community safety risks.
- Demonstrates correct use of child safety seats.
- Demonstrates correct administration of cardiopulmonary resuscitation.

Nursing interventions to meet desired outcomes are largely directed toward helping the client and family to:

- Identify environmental hazards in home and community.
- Demonstrate safety practices appropriate to the home healthcare agency, community, and workplace.
- Demonstrate safe childrearing practices or lifestyle practices.

EVALUATING

In preventing client injury, the nurse's role is largely one of education. The nurse evaluates whether the client has learned about safety hazards, incorporated safety practice into behavior, and acquired skills to perform in the event of certain emergencies.

CONTINUING CARE

If clients require an alarm system when they return home, caregivers would need instruction in its setup and use. Instruct them to test the monitoring device every 12 to 24 hours to ensure that it is working. Also, have them check the volume of the alarm to be sure they can hear it.

If a client is in danger of falling, remind caregivers to:

- Clear the floor of wires or loose rugs.
- Provide lighting at night between bedroom and bathroom.
- Encourage clients to rise in stages from lying to sitting to standing, and to get their balance before starting to walk.
- Provide assistive devices (e.g., cane, walker) as needed.

If the client has a visual impairment, instruct the family members that the client needs to be informed of any changes to the environment. Otherwise, the change in the client's environment may pose a risk because many clients with visual impairments will memorize the layout of their home.

NURSING PROCESS CARE PLAN
Client with Fractured Hip

Mr. Moore is a 72-year-old widower who is recovering from a fall in which he fractured his hip and underwent surgical repair 1 week ago. He is returning home after staying with his son for 2 weeks. Once he is home, his son will visit nightly after work. He will receive Meals-on-Wheels once a day, and a home healthcare attendant will visit weekly to assist him with hygienic care until he is more independent. Mr. Moore's wife died 3 years ago, but he has remained independent and continued his social functions. He lives in a small three-bedroom house with his dog and cat, and he enjoys gardening. Prior to fracturing his hip, he walked his dog daily. After the initial visit from the RN, you will be his home healthcare nurse.

Assessment. Home care nurse (LPN/LVN) visited on the second day in client's own home. The home health attendant assisted with shower and dressing. The client is doing well physically with no complaints of pain. VS stable: 98.2/74/18, BP 132/84. Surgical incision well healed with no redness or drainage, open to air. AAO ×3. Throw rugs and furniture in pathway from bed to bathroom. Safety devices installed in bathroom: grab bar and raised toilet seat. Family members' phone numbers are programmed on speed dial on phone. Client states, "It is so good to be home, I had the best night's sleep last night." Walked 20 feet from front door to car using a walker. Client reports he is looking forward to being able to walk his dog.

Nursing Diagnosis. The following important nursing diagnoses (among others) are established for this client:

- *Impaired Health Maintenance*
- *Impaired Physical Mobility*
- *Risk for Injury*

Expected Outcomes. Mr. Moore will:

- Follow mutually agreed-on healthcare maintenance plan.
- Participate in activities of daily living at the maximum of functional ability.
- Demonstrate use of adaptive equipment (e.g., walker) to increase mobility.

Planning and Implementation

- Assess client's awareness of deficits that may result from normal aging.

- Give client information about community resources for the elderly (home visitors, emergency call systems, and transportation to appointments).
- Evaluate the client's knowledge of and compliance with hip precautions.
- Monitor client for physiological complaints, including pain and medication effects.
- Monitor the use of any assistive devices needed for activity in coordination with the physical therapist (PT).
- Initiate a walking program in coordination with the PT in which the client walks with or without help every day as part of his daily routine.
- Ensure the removal of the throw rugs and other obstacles in the client's path from the bed to the bathroom.

Evaluation. Two weeks after discharge, Mr. Moore is in his own home. You make your first home visit.

- Client and family have established regular schedule of caretakers' and family members' visits to allow independence.
- Meals-on-Wheels scheduled 6 days per week.
- Client spending one weekend day with family.
- Mr. Moore is able to shower and dress with assistance of home health attendant. Home safety evaluation reveals that night-lights have been installed and furniture has been rearranged for easy access from bedroom to bath.
- PT home visits 2× per week. Able to get in and out of bed. Using walker in house and outside when accompanied.
- Client demonstrates compliance with hip precautions.
- No complaints of pain or medication side effects.

Critical Thinking in the Nursing Process

1. While hospitalized, Mr. Moore tried to get out of bed without assistance and almost fell, but his nurses decided not to restrain him. What are the best reasons for avoiding the use of restraints for clients such as Mr. Moore? What are some alternatives to restraints that could be used in this situation?
2. What strengths do you note about Mr. Moore's case that may protect him from injury when he returns home?
3. What other safety issues are important to consider in this situation?

Note: Discussion of Critical Thinking questions appears in Appendix I.

Personal Safety for Nurses

Nurses routinely protect the safety of the client for whom they care. However, little thought is given to the nurse's personal safety until the nurse sustains an injury. A nurse cannot provide for clients effectively unless he or she is free from injury.

BODY MECHANICS

Body mechanics is the term used to describe safe, efficient use of the body to move objects and carry out activities of daily living. The purpose of body mechanics is to ensure safe and efficient use of appropriate muscle groups to maintain balance, reduce fatigue and energy expended, and prevent injury.

Body mechanics involves the concepts of alignment and posture. When a person moves, the center of gravity shifts continuously in the direction of moving body parts. The closer the line of gravity is to the center of the base of support, the greater the person's stability (Figure 8-11A ■). Conversely, the closer the line of gravity is to the edge of the base of support, the more precarious the balance (Figure 8-11B). If the line of gravity falls outside the base of support, the person falls (Figure 8-11C).

Body balance can be greatly enhanced by (1) widening the base of support and (2) lowering the center of gravity, bringing it closer to the base of support. The base of support may be easily widened by spreading the feet farther apart. The center of gravity is readily lowered by flexing the hips and knees until a squatting position is achieved. Use of these two techniques is vital to nurses to prevent work-related back injuries.

Preventing Back Injuries

Many factors increase the potential for lower back injury. Low back pain can be caused by a number of factors, from

injuries to the effects of aging. The American Nurses Association has initiated a campaign called Handle with Care. This campaign is designed to reduce the risks for injury to nurses and other healthcare workers who provide direct client care. The focus of the campaign is to encourage facilities to purchase equipment to assist employees in moving clients and to implement safety committees to review policy and evaluate risks for injury as a result of lifting.

Undesirable **twisting** can be prevented by facing the direction of movement squarely, whether pushing, pulling, or sliding, and by moving the object directly toward or away from one's center of gravity (Figure 8-12 ■).

clinical ALERT

Twisting (rotation) of the thoracolumbar spine and stooping (acute flexion of the back with hips and knees straight) must always be avoided because of their potential for causing back injury.

LOW BACK SPRAIN AND STRAIN. The muscles of the low back provide power and strength for activities such as standing, walking, and lifting. A strain of the muscle can occur when the muscle is poorly conditioned or overworked. The ligaments of the low back interconnect the five vertebral bones and provide support or stability for the low back. A sprain of the low back can occur when a sudden, forceful movement injures a ligament that has become stiff or weak through poor conditioning or overuse. These injuries, or sprain and strain, are the most common causes

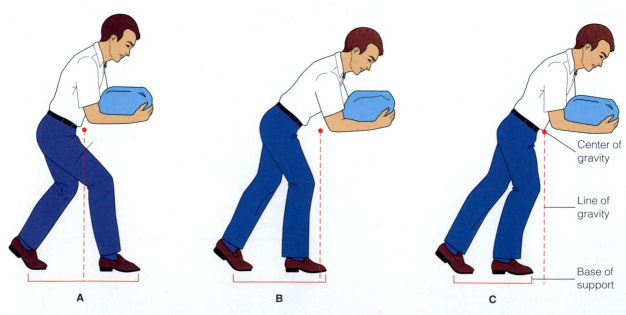

Center of gravity

Line of gravity

Base of support

A   **B**   **C**

Figure 8-11. ■ **A.** Balance is maintained when the line of gravity falls close to the base of support. **B.** Balance is precarious when the line of gravity falls at the edge of the base of support. **C.** Balance cannot be maintained when the line of gravity falls outside the base of support.

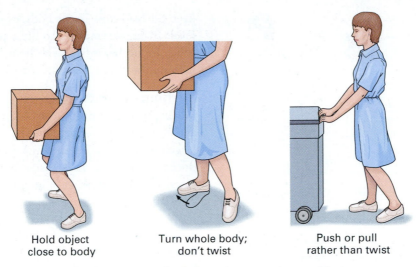

Hold object
close to body

Turn whole body;
don't twist

Push or pull
rather than twist

Figure 8-12. ■ Correct body mechanics for the proper method of carrying or moving an object.

of low back pain. Although you cannot totally halt the progress of these effects, they can be slowed by regular exercise, knowing the proper way to lift and move objects, proper nutrition, and good posture. See Box 8-10 ■ for guidelines for preventing back injury in nurses or in clients.

Lifting

When a person lifts or carries an object, the object's weight becomes part of body weight. This weight change affects the center of gravity, which becomes displaced in the direction

of the added weight. To counteract this potential imbalance, body parts (e.g., arm, trunk) move away from the weight, so the center of gravity is maintained at the same point in the base of support. By holding an object as close to the body as possible, the lifter avoids displacing the center of gravity and achieves greater stability.

People can lift more weight when using a lever. Human bones function as levers—the joint is the **fulcrum** (fixed point about which a lever moves) and the muscles exert the force (Figure 8-13 ■). Lifting involves movement against gravity, so the nurse must use major muscle groups of the thighs, knees, upper and lower arms, abdomen, and pelvis to prevent back strain.

Another technique based on the principle of leverage may be used when lifting objects from floor to waist level. In this technique, the back and knees are flexed until the load is at thigh level. Then the back straightens slowly while the knees remain flexed to provide thrust (Figure 8-14 ■). This maneuver provides for better balance and leverage. The muscles work together (in *synchronization*), which helps prevent

BOX 8-10	CLIENT TEACHING

How to Prevent Back Injuries

- Become consciously aware of your posture and body mechanics.
- When standing for a period of time, periodically flex one hip and knee and rest your foot on an object if possible.
- When sitting, keep your knees slightly higher than your hips.
- Use a firm mattress that provides good body support at natural body curvatures.
- Exercise regularly to maintain overall physical condition; include exercises that strengthen the pelvic, abdominal, and lumbar muscles.
- Avoid exercises that cause pain or require spinal flexion with straight legs (e.g., toe-touching and sit-ups) or spinal rotation (twisting).
- When moving an object, spread your feet apart to provide a wide base of support.
- When lifting an object, distribute the weight between large muscles of the legs and arms.
- Wear clothing that allows you to use good body mechanics and comfortable low-heeled shoes that provide good foot support and will not cause you to slip, stumble, or turn your ankle.

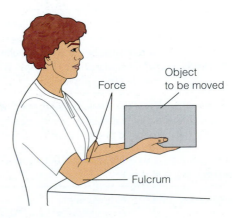

Force

Object
to be moved

Fulcrum

Figure 8-13. ■ Using the arm as a lever.

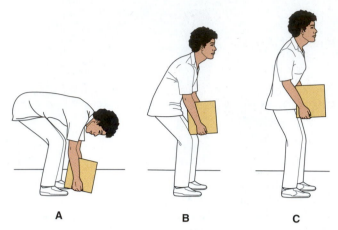

A   **B**   **C**

Figure 8-14. ■ Stages in lifting an object from the floor to the waist: **A.** Move close to the object, and begin with the back and knees flexed to grasp the object. **B.** Start the lift by keeping the back flexed while the knees begin to straighten so that the leg muscles can exert an upward thrust. **C.** Keep the back and knees in a less flexed, but not straight, position.

injury. When an object is lifted to knee level, the abdominal and lumbar muscles contract for leverage and pull. The thigh and leg muscles exert the upward thrust to bring the object off the floor. When an object is lifted from mid-thigh to waist level, force is primarily exerted by leg and thigh muscles, while back and lumbar muscles remain contracted.

For all lifting positions, it is necessary to maintain a distance of 30 cm (12 inches) or more between the feet and to keep the load close to the body, especially when it is at knee level. Before attempting to lift, the nurse must ensure that there are no hazards on the floor, there is a clear path for moving the object, and the nurse's base of support is secure.

Pushing and Pulling

When pushing or pulling an object, a person maintains balance with the least effort when the base of the support is enlarged in the direction in which the movement is to be produced or opposed. It is easier and safer to pull an object toward one's own center of gravity than to push it away, because the person can exert more control of the object's movement when pulling it.

Pivoting

Pivoting is a technique in which the body is turned in such a way to avoid twisting of the spine. To pivot, place one foot ahead of the other, raise the heels very slightly, and put the weight on the balls of the feet. When the weight is off the heels, the frictional surface is decreased and the knees are not twisted when turning. Keeping the body aligned, turn (pivot) about 90 degrees in the desired direction. The foot that was forward will now be behind. A summary of principles and guidelines related to body mechanics is shown in Table 8-2 ■.

Note: The references and resources for this and all chapters have been compiled at the back of the book.

TABLE 8-2

Summary of Guidelines and Principles Related to Body Mechanics

GUIDELINES	PRINCIPLES
Plan the move or transfer carefully. Free the surrounding area of obstacles and move required equipment near the head or foot of the bed.	Appropriate preparation prevents potential falls and injury and safeguards the client and equipment.
Obtain the assistance of other people or use mechanical devices to move objects that are too heavy. Encourage clients to assist as much as possible by pushing or pulling themselves to reduce your muscular effort. Use arms as levers whenever possible to increase lifting power.	The heavier an object, the greater the force needed to move the object.
Adjust the working area to waist level, and keep the body close to the area. Elevate adjustable beds and overbed tables or lower the side rails of beds to prevent stretching and reaching.	Objects that are close to the center of gravity are moved with the least effort.
Provide a firm, smooth, dry bed foundation before moving a client in bed or use a pull sheet.	Less energy is required when you reduce the friction between the object moved and the surface on which it is moved.
Always face the direction of the movement.	Ineffective use of major muscle groups occurs when the spine is rotated or twisted.

TABLE 8-2

Summary of Guidelines and Principles Related to Body Mechanics (*continued*)

GUIDELINES	PRINCIPLES
Start any body movement with proper alignment. Stand as close as possible to the object to be moved. Avoid stretching, reaching, and twisting, which may place the line of gravity outside the base of support.	Balance is maintained and muscle strain is avoided as long as the line of gravity passes through the base of support.
Before moving an object, increase your stability by widening your stance and flexing your knees, hips, and ankles.	The wider the base of support and the lower the center of gravity, the greater the stability.
Before moving an object, contract your gluteal, abdominal, leg, and arm muscles to prepare them for action.	The greater the preparatory isometric tensing, or contraction of muscles, before moving an object, the less energy required to move it, and the less likelihood of musculoskeletal strain and injury.
Avoid working against gravity. Pull, push, roll, or turn objects instead of lifting them. Lower the head of the client's bed before moving the client up in bed.	Moving an object along a level surface requires less energy than moving an object up an inclined surface or lifting it against the force of gravity. Pulling creates less friction than pushing.
Use your gluteal and leg muscles rather than the sacrospinal muscles of your back to exert an upward thrust when lifting. Distribute the workload between both arms and legs to prevent back strain. Balance is maintained with minimal effort when the base of support is enlarged in the direction in which the movement will occur.	The synchronized use of as many large muscle groups as possible during an activity increases overall strength and prevents muscle fatigue and injury.
When *pushing* an object, enlarge the base of support by moving the front foot forward. When *pulling* an object, enlarge the base of support by either moving the rear leg back if facing the object or moving the front foot forward if facing away from the object.	Balance is maintained with minimal effort when the base of support is enlarged in the direction in which the movement will occur.
When moving or carrying objects, hold them as close as possible to your center of gravity.	The closer the line of gravity to the center of the base of support, the greater the stability.
Use the weight of the body as a force for pulling or pushing, by rocking on the feet or leaning forward or backward.	Body weight adds force to counteract the weight of the object and reduces the amount of strain on the arms and back.
Alternate rest periods with periods of muscle use to help prevent fatigue.	Continuous muscle exertion can result in muscle strain and injury.

Using a Bed or Chair Exit Safety Monitoring Device

A bed or chair safety monitor (Figure 8-15 ■) is an electronic device with a position-sensitive switch that triggers an audio alarm when the client attempts to get out of the bed or chair unassisted. When activated, the alarm alerts the nurse and provides an opportunity for the nurse to intervene.

Purposes
- To alert the nurse that the client is attempting to get out of bed
- To help decrease the risk of client falls

Equipment
- Alarm and control device
- Connection to nurse call system (optional)
- Sensor device

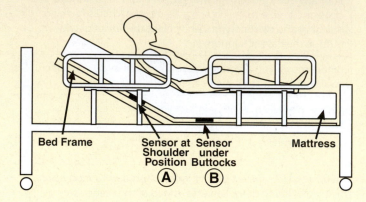

Figure 8-15. ■ Bed exit monitoring device; the sensor is usually placed under the client's buttocks. (*Source:* Courtesy of J.T. Posey Company. Reprinted with permission.)

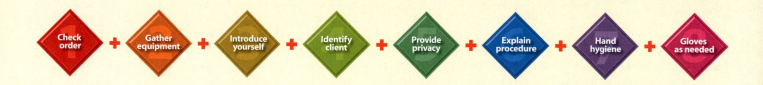

Check order + Gather equipment + Introduce yourself + Identify client + Provide privacy + Explain procedure + Hand hygiene + Gloves as needed

Interventions

1. Explain to the client and support people the purpose and procedure for using safety monitoring.
   - Explain that the device does not limit mobility in any manner; rather, it alerts the staff when the client is about to get out of bed or a chair.
   - Explain that the nurse must be called when the client needs to get out of bed. *These measures reduce anxiety and protect the client from injury.*
2. Obtain the appropriate sensor device and control unit.
3. Test the battery device and alarm sound. *This ensures that the device is functioning properly prior to use.*
4. Apply the sensor pad or leg band.
   - Place the leg band according to the manufacturer's recommendations. The usual position for a bed or chair sensor is under the mattress (see Figure 8-15) or chair cushion directly beneath the client's buttocks. For clients at high risk of falling, the sensor may be placed under the shoulders. *Placement must be individualized to the client's needs.*
   - For a bed or chair device, set the time delay for determining the client's movement patterns from 1 to 12 seconds.

- Connect the sensor pad to the control unit and the nurse call system. *The alarm device is position sensitive. For example, when a leg band approaches a near-vertical position (such as in walking, crawling, or kneeling as the client attempts to get out of bed), the audio alarm is triggered, causing a sharp, shrill sound.*
5. Instruct the client to call the nurse when the client wants or needs to get up, and assist as required. *This reassures the client that he or she will not be confined indefinitely.*
   - Before assisting the client to rise, deactivate the alarm by unsnapping the alarm device from the elastic band. *This prevents the alarm from being triggered.*
   - Assist the client back to bed, and reattach the alarm device to the sensor. *The alarm provides a safeguard against client injury.*
6. Ensure client safety with additional safety precautions.
   - Place call light within client reach, lift all side rails, and lower the bed to its lowest position. *The alarm device is not a substitute for other precautionary measures.*
   - Place monitoring device stickers on the client's door, chart, and Kardex. *This communicates use of the alarm to other personnel.*

7. Document relevant data. *An action that is not documented is not legally considered to be done.*
   ■ Record that monitoring device is intact when applied.
   ■ Record all assessments.

■ Record all safety precautions and interventions discussed and employed. *Documentation is crucial for client safety and to ensure quality of care.*

SAMPLE DOCUMENTATION

[date]	Focus		
0930	Safety	D	Attempting to climb out of bed over side rail. Confused. Stated "I need to go home and feed my dogs."
		A	Reoriented, placed call light within reach. Instructed to call before attempting to get out of bed. Wander-guard® attached to left ankle. Relocated to room close to nurses' station. Explained that the alarm will sound if he leaves the bed. Contacted family members to reassure client that the dogs are being cared for. Instruct nursing assistant to check every 15 min and respond immediately to alarm.
1030		R	Alarm activated 3 times within one hour. Asked that alarm be removed. Offered reassurance, explained purpose of alarm. Alarm remains in place. Resting quietly after reorientation. K. Adams, LPN

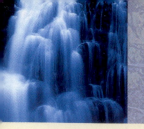

Chapter Review

 KEY TERMS by Topic

Use the audio glossary feature of either the CD-ROM or the Companion Website to hear the correct pronunciation of the following key terms.

Preventing Specific Hazards
suffocation

Hospital and Institutional Safety
bagging, external disasters, internal disasters, triage

Personal Safety for Nurses
body mechanics, twisting, fulcrum

KEY Points

- Education is a major health protection strategy in preventing injuries.

- When planning to meet safety needs of clients, nurses need to consider physical factors in the environment and the psychological and physiological state of the individual.

- Injuries are a major cause of death among individuals of all ages in the United States and Canada.

- Hazards to safety occur at all ages and vary according to the age and development of the individual.

- To ensure safety, focus on (1) observing or predicting situations that are potentially harmful and (2) educating clients to safeguard themselves and their families. It is often necessary to modify the environment to make it safe.

- Nurses must be familiar with the fire procedures in the healthcare agency where they practice. In the event of a fire, the nurse must (1) protect clients from injury, (2) report, (3) contain, and (4) put out the fire.

- To prevent falls, the nurse must provide constant surveillance for infants and young children and assess older clients' safety needs carefully.

- Prolonged exposure to excessive noise can produce hearing loss. Ill or injured people may be especially sensitive to noises.

- Electrical injuries can be prevented by using grounded outlets and plugs, putting protective covers over outlets, and making sure that electric wiring and circuits meet safety standards.

- In hospitals, radioactive substances are used for both diagnostic and treatment purposes. Follow agency policy to safeguard clients and staff from exposure.

- Side rails and handrails protect hospitalized clients from falls. Restraints keep clients from inflicting injuries on themselves and others.

- Because restraints restrict a client's basic freedom to move, they should be used as a last resort. Careful assessment and accurate, complete documentation are important when restraints are used.

- A nurse cannot provide for clients effectively unless he or she is free from injury.

- Planning moves or transfers will help prevent falls and injuries and safeguard the client and equipment.

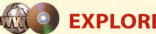 **EXPLORE MediaLink**

Additional interactive resources for this chapter can be found on the Companion Website at www.prenhall.com/ramont. Click on Chapter 8 and "Begin" to select the activities for this chapter.

For chapter-related NCLEX®-style questions and an audio glossary, access the accompanying CD-ROM in this book.

Videos
- Applying a Mummy Wrap
- Lead Poisoning

FOR FURTHER Study

For additional information about incident reports, see Chapter 3 and Chapter 36.

For additional information on infection control, see Chapter 9.

See Chapter 23 for skin care and Figure 23-14 in particular for an example of a skin assessment tool.

For therapeutic applications of heat and cold, see Chapter 23.

Chapter 29 provides information about avoiding medication errors.

For directions on passive ROM exercises, see Chapter 32.

Appendix II lists nursing diagnoses related to safety.

Caring for a Client with Risk for Injury

NCLEX-PN® Focus Area: Safety

Case Study: George Whitman is a 75-year-old man with a history of Parkinson's disease. He was admitted to the hospital following a fall, which resulted in an intertrochanteric fracture of his right hip. The fracture was treated with an open reduction internal fixation (ORIF). For the past 7 days he has been in the transitional care unit receiving physical therapy and mobility training. He is currently able to ambulate with a walker.

Nursing Diagnosis: Ineffective Protection

COLLECT DATA

Subjective	Objective
_____	_____
_____	_____
_____	_____
_____	_____
_____	_____
_____	_____
_____	_____

Would you report this data? Yes/No

If yes, to: _____

What would you report? _____

Nursing Care

_____
_____
_____
_____
_____
_____
_____
_____
_____
_____
_____

How would you document this?_____
_____
_____
_____

Compare your documentation to the sample provided in Appendix I.

Data Collected
(use those that apply)

- Client's wife expressed concerns about his upcoming discharge
- Lives with wife in a two-story house
- Does yard work
- Socializes with the neighbors
- Daughter and three grandchildren live 75 miles away
- Mrs. Whitman and the daughter feel the couple should move to a retirement apartment
- Mr. Whitman expressed, "Selling the house would be a sign that I am just giving up."
- Rigidity due to the Parkinson's
- Soft diet—difficulty in swallowing
- Large bruise on his left leg and right forearm
- Routine medications: Sinemet 25/100 tid, Tasmar 100 tid, DSS capsule 100 mg daily, ferrous sulfate 325 mg daily, heparin 5,000 units SQ bid
- VS: T 98.2, P 76, R 20, BP 140/88
- Lab results: H&H 13.2 40.4, PT 13.5 sec, PTT 90 sec

Nursing Interventions
(use those that apply; list in priority order)

- Monitor risk for bleeding.
- Assess pain severity on 1–10 scale.
- Help client perform prescribed exercises every 8 h.
- Refer family to appropriate community resources.
- Observe client for cause of impaired mobility.
- Evaluate client for signs of depression.
- Observe for causes of inability to feed self independently.
- Take temperature, pulse, and blood pressure every 4 h.
- Observe nutritional status.
- Teach client and family signs of bleeding, precautions to take to prevent bleeding.
- Work with dietitian to improve nutritional status.
- Teach caregiver feeding techniques that prevent choking.

NCLEX-PN® Exam Preparation

1 You are asked to teach a parenting class on safety at a community center. One of the parents asks why young children are so prone to injury. Of the following, which is the best answer?

1. Young children are uncoordinated, so they are more likely to fall.
2. Misbehavior results in many injuries to children.
3. Young children's curiosity exceeds their judgment.
4. Children are unable to remember safety instructions.

2 The nurse is preparing to restrain a client who has been pulling at the intravenous lines and surgical incision. The most appropriate restraint device in this situation would be:

1. a vest restraint.
2. mitt restraints.
3. bed alarm.
4. arm restraints.

3 A nurse is working in a facility where she uses a variety of chemicals. Which is the most important safety consideration for this nurse?

1. the name of the chemical
2. the nurse's access to MSDS
3. the nurse's years of experience using these chemicals
4. the nurse's previous exposure to the chemicals

4 Your client is being discharged following a total hip replacement. You provide discharge instructions involving home safety in the presence of the son. Which of the following statements would demonstrate the need for more teaching?

1. "Dad will be staying with us until he is completely recovered."
2. "We have removed the throw rugs from the bedroom and bathroom."
3. "Dad will need to use the walker only when leaving the house."
4. "When Dad gets out of bed, we will have him get up slowly and gain his balance before walking."

5 The safe and efficient use of the body to move objects and carry out activities of daily living is:

1. physical therapy.
2. body mechanics.
3. a nursing intervention.
4. occupational therapy.

6 The government agency responsible for a safe work environment is the:

1. CDC.
2. OSHA.
3. JCAHO.
4. Department of Labor.

7 You are assigned to care for a client in isolation. After you have changed the bed, you need to remove the soiled linen from the room. What is the procedure for dealing with soiled linen?

1. Linen remains in the room until the client is discharged.
2. Carry the rolled-up linen without touching your uniform.
3. Place the soiled linen in a bag, which is held by another person outside the isolation room.
4. Dispose of the linen in the refuse container.

8 The nurse is providing education regarding home fire prevention to a group of families. The nurse should include which instruction?

1. Avoid the use of electric heaters.
2. Keep paper and cloth away from heating appliances.
3. Use of bars over windows can increase fire safety.
4. Fire extinguishers should be stored close to sleeping areas.

9 The nurse is preparing to assist a client to transfer from the bed to a wheelchair. To safely transfer this client, the nurse would:

1. keep the client at arm's length.
2. have both feet close together.
3. encourage the client to perform the transfer while the nurse is standing close to the client's side.
4. hold the client close to the nurse's center of gravity with feet about hip-width apart.

10 When discovering a fire in a client's room, the nurse would take which of the following actions? (Select all that apply.)

1. Remove the client from the area.
2. Contact the client's physician.
3. Activate the alarm system.
4. Contain the fire by closing doors.

Answers and Rationales for Review Questions, as well as discussion of Care Plan and Critical Thinking Care Map questions, appear in Appendix I.

Chapter 9

Infection Control and Asepsis

BRIEF Outline

Microorganisms
Infection
Controlling Microorganisms in the Environment

LEARNING Outcomes

After completing this chapter, you will be able to:

1. Discuss helpful and harmful actions of microorganisms.
2. Name six links in the chain of infection.
3. Define nosocomial infection.
4. Explain the difference between nonspecific and specific defense systems of the body.
5. Describe client risk factors for developing an infection.
6. List relevant nursing diagnoses for clients with an infection or at risk of developing an infection.
7. Explain the meaning of medical and surgical asepsis.
8. Describe Standard Precautions and Transmission-based Precautions.
9. Demonstrate aseptic techniques including hand hygiene, donning and removing sterile gloves, donning personal protective equipment, and establishing and maintaining a sterile field.

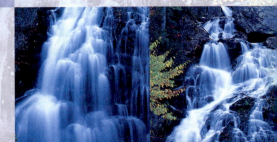

HISTORICAL Perspective

Dr. Ignaz Semmelweis, the "father of infection control," observed in 1847 that women who delivered by physicians had a much higher rate of post-delivery mortality than women who delivered by midwives. He concluded that the higher rates were associated with physicians performing autopsies before attending the pregnant women, something midwives did not do. He conducted a study in which the intervention was hand washing. Dr. Semmelweis initiated a mandatory hand washing policy for medical students and physicians. Believe it or not, his superior did not accept his conclusions. Dr. Semmelweis was the first healthcare professional to demonstrate experimentally that hand washing could prevent infections.

Infection control is a primary concern in nursing care. Nurses play an important role in establishing a biologically safe environment for their patients.

Microorganisms

Microorganisms are tiny living bodies that are visible only with a microscope. The most common are classified as bacteria, viruses, fungi, and parasites. Microorganisms are present in the environment and on body surfaces (such as the skin), in the intestinal tract, mouth, upper respiratory tract, lower urinary tract, and vaginal tract. These are referred to as *normal flora*. Although we frequently refer to microorganisms as "germs," most are harmless and some are even helpful because they perform essential functions for the body. For example, normal flora is the body's first line of protection against infection for patients and care providers.

TYPES OF MICROORGANISMS

Bacteria are the most common type of disease-causing microorganisms. They can live in and be transported through the air, water, food, soil, inanimate objects, and body tissues or fluids. **Viruses** are the smallest known disease-causing agent. They must enter living cells in order to reproduce. Viruses cannot survive or maintain their infectiousness outside a living host. Viral infections are generally self-limiting (e.g., rhinovirus, which causes the common cold). Others can cause serious illness or death (hepatitis, herpes, and human immunodeficiency virus [HIV]). **Fungi** are either yeasts or molds. Examples are the fungi that cause athlete's foot and yeast infections. **Parasites** live on other living organisms. Examples are protozoa (which cause malaria), helminths (worms), and arthropods (mites, ticks, and fleas).

HELPFUL ACTIONS OF MICROORGANISMS

Resident flora (normal flora) are harmless microorganisms. They can be found in and on the body. Many of them perform useful protective functions. For example, intestinal flora help to synthesize vitamin K, which is important to the body's blood-clotting mechanism. Various other microorganisms make antibiotic-like substances and toxic substances that slow or stop the growth of other organisms.

The process of *colonization* occurs when strains of microorganisms become resident flora. Resident flora can grow in or on the body and not cause disease. However, if a person's defenses are weak, flora may invade a part of the body they normally would not, and cause illness or infection. *Escherichia coli (E. coli),* a normal resident flora of the intestinal tract, causes illness if transmitted elsewhere. For example, if proper hygiene is not used after a bowel movement, *E. coli* may be moved to the urethra and cause a urinary tract infection. (See Table 9-1 ■ for some common resident organisms.)

TABLE 9-1

Examples of Normal Flora

BODY AREA	ORGANISMS
Skin	*Staphylococcus epidermidis*
	Propionibacterium acnes
	Staphylococcus aureus
	Coagulase negative staphylococci
	Bacillus species
	Pityrosporum ovale (yeast)
Nasal passages	Coagulase negative staphylococci
	Staphylococcus epidermidis
	Neisseria species
	Haemophilus species
Oropharynx	*Streptococcus pneumoniae*
Bronchi, lungs	None
Mouth	Coagulase negative staphylococci
	Lactobacillus
	Bacteroides
	Actinomyces
Stomach	None
Esophagus	None
Intestine	*Bacteroides*
	Fusobacterium
	Eubacterium
	Lactobacillus
	Streptococcus
	Enterobacteriaceae
	Escherichia coli
	Klebsiella species
Urethral orifice	*Staphylococcus epidermidis*
Urethra (lower)	*Proteus*
Bladder, ureters, kidneys	None
Vagina	*Lactobacillus*
	Bacteroides
	Clostridium
	Candida albicans
Blood, lymph system	None

HARMFUL ACTIONS OF MICROORGANISMS

An **infection** is defined as an invasion of the body by a disease-causing organism called the *infectious agent*. Microorganisms that cause disease are called **pathogens**. A "true" pathogen causes disease or infection in a healthy person. An *opportunistic pathogen* causes a disease only in a susceptible person, that is, someone whose immune system is not functioning as a defense system.

When an infection occurs, the signs and symptoms of the infection are distinctive, and the person's health is recognized as being different from the normal. **Disease** causes a detectable change in the way the body functions. In some cases, the microorganism will not cause any signs or symptoms of disease, and the infection is called *asymptomatic* or *subclinical*. For example, many cases of mumps are asymptomatic.

Various microorganisms are stronger than others and are called more *virulent*. **Virulence** refers to the organism's ability to produce disease and survive both inside and outside the body. Microorganisms also differ in their strength and their communicability (how easily they can be spread). The cold or the annual strain of influenza can be easily spread by hands and coughing or sneezing, whereas bloodborne pathogens such as hepatitis C and AIDS are not easily transmitted. They require blood-to-blood contact to pose a risk for transmission. A **communicable disease** is one that is spread or transmitted by direct or indirect contact. The transmission of an organism can be caused by a **vector** or vehicle (an insect, or a used drinking glass, for instance). West Nile virus is the newest vector-borne disease. It has been in the United States only a short period of time but has been spread across the United States by migrating birds. Birds contract the disease and die. Mosquitoes then pick up the virus from dead birds and pass the disease on to humans. Microorganisms can also be airborne and carried by air currents. For example, an airborne disease such as tuberculosis (TB) can be transmitted from one person to another in a close living situation. Although not a highly communicable disease, the disease has been the cause of epidemics for centuries.

Microorganisms that develop resistance to various antibiotics can lead to outbreaks of infections in both the medical facility and community. One example is methicillin-resistant *Staphylococcus aureus* (MRSA); this strain of staph has been responsible for deaths in hospitals and in the community setting. This infection has become an issue in gyms, prisons, and school locker rooms.

CONTROLLING COMMUNICABLE DISEASES

Infectious/communicable diseases are the major cause of death throughout the world. They account for a significant threat to public health and for many deaths annually in the United States. The World Health Organization works on the international level to protect people from communicable forms of disease. An infectious disease is primarily one that affects the patient. It is not necessarily one that can be transmitted to another person. For example, most pneumonias are infectious. If caused by staphylococcus bacteria, they may be communicable. A communicable disease can be transmitted from one person to another under certain conditions.

In the United States, the U.S. Public Health Service/Centers for Disease Control and Prevention (CDC) is the main agency concerned with protecting the public from disease and controlling its spread on a national level. The CDC also surveys for trends in all aspects of health and safety. Health departments in states, counties, and cities follow epidemics and illnesses when hospitals, physicians, and other healthcare providers make reports. These reports are required by law and are reported to the CDC each month and tabulated each year to assist with trend/need identification. The U.S. Public Health Service and the CDC are part of the Department of Health and Human Services. They are not part of the Department of Homeland Security.

Infection

TYPES OF INFECTION

Disease may be referred to as being infectious or communicable. Infectious disease presents as illness in the patient but may not be transmissible to others. Communicable diseases are transmissible to others. Infection in a patient may be either local or systemic. A **local infection** occurs when the microorganisms are in only a specific part of the body. A **systemic infection** exists when the microorganisms spread to other body areas. The person has *bacteremia* if the microorganisms enter the bloodstream. When bacteremia spreads through all of the body's systems, the condition is called **septicemia**.

Acute infections occur suddenly or last a short time. *Chronic infections* happen slowly over a long period of time and may last months or years. For example, an ear infection may be described as an acute infection. Hepatitis C viral infection may be described as a chronic infection in some patients.

Infections that occur after hospital admission, and for which the patient had no symptoms at the time of admission, are called **nosocomial infections** (hospital-acquired infections). Many factors contribute to nosocomial infections. An example of this would be bacteremia caused by an infected or contaminated intravenous (IV) site. An infection directly caused by any diagnostic or therapeutic source is called an **iatrogenic infection**. An example would be a negative result from a patient being given the wrong medication.

A microorganism that comes from the patient's own body and causes a nosocomial infection is referred to as being from an *endogenous* source. If the organism causing the infection comes from the healthcare environment or personnel, it is from an *exogenous* source. The three most common microorganisms causing exogenous infections are *E. coli*, *S. aureus*, and *Enterococcus* species (Table 9-2 ■).

TABLE 9-2

Nosocomial Infections

MOST COMMON ORGANISMS	CAUSES
Urinary Tract	
Escherichia coli	Catheterization technique
Enterococcus species	Contamination of closed drainage system
Pseudomonas aeruginosa	Inadequate hand hygiene
Surgical Sites	
Staphylococcus aureus	Inadequate hand hygiene
Enterococcus species	Improper dressing change technique
Pseudomonas aeruginosa	Environmental contamination
Bloodstream	
Coagulase-negative staphylococci	Inadequate hand hygiene
Staphylococcus aureus	Improper intravenous fluid, tubing, and site care technique, site prep prior to insertion
Enterococcus species	
Pneumonia	
Staphylococcus aureus	Inadequate hand hygiene
Pseudomonas aeruginosa	Improper suctioning technique, improper positioning, lack of respiratory care after anesthesia
Enterobacter species	

FACTORS IN THE CHAIN OF INFECTION

The chain of infection is made up of six factors (Figure 9-1 ■): agent, reservoir, portal of exit, method or mode of transmission, portal of entry, and susceptibility of the host.

Agent/Microorganism

The first link in the chain of infection is the infectious *(etiologic) agent.* Several factors affect whether or not a microorganism invades the body and causes an infection. These factors include the number of organisms present (dose), how virulent or potent they are, and whether the organisms can live in the host's body. Some organisms, bacteria, survive well outside the body in the presence of nutrients and the proper temperature. Others, like the viruses, do not. For example, HIV virus does not survive outside the body. Some organisms can be present in a person and not present with signs and symptoms. This person may be called a *carrier.* A **carrier** is a potential source of infection for others. For example, a person infected with hepatitis B may be a carrier and be able to transmit the disease to others through his or her blood or through sexual contact.

Reservoir

The second link in the chain of infection is the place where the microorganism naturally lives, its reservoir. The source, or **reservoir**, of the microorganism can be many different places:

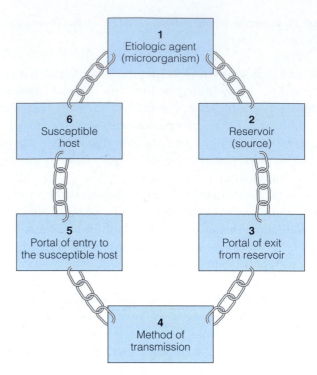

Figure 9-1. ■ The chain of infection.

the individual, other humans, animals, plants, insects, birds, or the environment. Food, water, milk, or anything that can be ingested could also be considered a reservoir (Table 9-3 ■). The more a person's resistance is lowered, the more susceptible the person becomes and the more easily he or she will be infected from the reservoir of microorganisms.

Portal of Exit from the Reservoir

The third link in the chain is the *portal of exit,* a way of leaving the reservoir. The microorganism must leave the reservoir in order to spread the infection. Any body fluid can provide an exit from the source. Wound drainage, blood, urine, feces, mucus, or any break in the skin or mucous membrane can all provide a portal of exit.

Methods or Modes of Transmission

The fourth link in the chain of infection is a method, or mode, of **transmission**. It is the manner in which the microorganism gets to the host. There are three modes of transmission. The first is direct contact. This occurs differently for different diseases. For bloodborne diseases, blood-to-blood contact must occur.

The second method is indirect contact. An example would be that of a nurse who has an open cut on her hand and picks up a piece of equipment that has blood on it. Another example is *vector-borne transmission* which could occur when an animal or insect bites or injects the microorganism through saliva into the host, or leaves feces or other material on the host's traumatized skin. An example is West Nile virus infection. Water, food, blood products, or contact with a *fomite* (an

TABLE 9-3

Human Reservoirs, Common Infectious Microorganisms, and Portals of Exit

BODY AREA (SOURCE)	COMMON INFECTIOUS ORGANISMS	PORTALS OF EXIT
Respiratory tract	Parainfluenza virus *Mycobacterium tuberculosis* *Staphylococcus aureus*	Nose or mouth through sneezing, coughing, talking; endotracheal tubes or tracheostomies
Gastrointestinal tract	Hepatitis A virus *Salmonella* species	Mouth: saliva, vomitus; anus: feces; ostomies: drainage tubes (e.g., nasogastric or T-tubes)
Urinary tract	*Escherichia coli* enterococci *Pseudomonas aeruginosa*	Urethral meatus and urinary diversion ostomies
Reproductive tract (including genitals)	*Neisseria gonorrhoeae* *Treponema pallidum* Herpes simplex virus type 2 Hepatitis B virus	Vagina: vaginal discharge; urinary meatus: urine semen (hepatitis B virus, hepatitis C virus, HIV virus via sexual contact)
Blood	Hepatitis B virus (HBV) Hepatitis C (HCV) HIV *Staphylococcus aureus* *Staphylococcus epidermidis*	Open wound, needle puncture site, any disruption of intact skin or mucous membrane surfaces
Tissue	*Staphylococcus aureus* *Escherichia coli* *Proteus* species *Streptococcus* betahemolytic A or B	Drainage from cut or wound

inanimate object such as a toy, cooking or eating utensil, or contaminated instrument) are all examples of *vehicle-borne transmission.* When a person eats poorly cooked chicken contaminated with the *Salmonella* species and becomes ill, the microorganism was transmitted by a vehicle.

The third method of transmission is droplet or airborne transmission. These modes usually involve droplet nuclei, the remains of droplets coming from an infected person, which are suspended in the air. An example of airborne transmission is when someone infected with untreated pulmonary tuberculosis coughs. The bacteria are expelled into the air, and another individual then inhales it into his or her lungs. An example of droplet transmission is influenza (flu). Dust particles can also carry infectious spores, viruses, and bacteria. Microorganisms can be inhaled into the lungs when dust is disturbed and becomes airborne. An example of this might be anthrax.

Portal of Entry

The fifth link in the chain of infection is a *portal of entry* into the host. Intact skin is a barrier to pathogenic microorganisms. However, broken skin provides a portal of entry for a pathogen. Most microorganisms enter the body through

the same routes they use to leave it. For example, an organism that was inhaled into the lungs can be then coughed out to infect someone else.

Susceptible Host

The sixth link in the chain of infection is the *susceptibility of the host.* The body provides natural defenses to fight off infection. Immune response serves to protect from infection even if an exposure were to occur. An individual who has impaired immune response and is at risk for developing an infection is called a **susceptible host**. A *compromised host* is someone who has a higher risk for getting an infection, for one or more reasons. An example would be a geriatric patient with emphysema; this person is at a higher risk for developing pneumonia than someone of the same age without emphysema.

It is important to recognize that these six factors must all come together for transmission to possibly result in infection. They cannot function independently and cause infection. And, even if they all come together, that does not mean infection will occur because the immune system may respond and protect the person. In the provision of health care, it is important to remember that exposure does not always mean infection.

FACTORS THAT REDUCE HOST RESISTANCE

Some factors will impact and reduce the body's immune response. Age is a factor influencing the risk of infection. Both the very young and the elderly have reduced defenses. Newborns have immature immune systems and are protected for only the first 2 or 3 months by immunities they received from their mother. Immunizations against communicable diseases are started at about 2 months of age, when the infant's immune system can respond.

The immune system becomes weak in the elderly, and as they age they develop infections more easily or suffer from chronic disease. The CDC recommends annual immunizations for them against influenza and pneumonia, particularly if they have histories of cardiac, renal, respiratory, or metabolic diseases. Heredity may also influence the development of infections. People may have a genetic susceptibility to them.

Stressors in life can influence susceptibility to infection. Stressors can be physical, emotional, or both. The nature, number, and duration of the stressors may all influence whether or not the individual develops an infection. Stressors elevate blood cortisol. Cortisol is a hormone in the body that is secreted by the adrenal glands. This hormone is responsible for regulating blood pressure, immune function, and proper glucose metabolism. Small increases in cortisol can result in some very positive effects: (1) increased energy, (2) increased immunity, (3) lower sensitivity to pain, and (4) heightened memory. Prolonged elevation of cortisol decreases anti-inflammatory responses; drains energy stores, causing exhaustion; decreases resistance to infection; impairs cognitive performance; suppresses thyroid function; decreases bone density; and creates sugar imbalances.

Nutrition plays a role in resistance to infection. Good nutrition provides ample proteins, which allow the body to manufacture antibodies. Medical therapies may contribute to the development of infection. Radiation treatments for cancer and diagnostic procedures that penetrate the skin or sterile body cavities are examples of procedures that increase infection risk.

Some medications can increase the chance of infection by depressing bone marrow production of white blood cells (leukocytes). Also, corticosteroids (steroids) slow down the inflammatory response needed to fight infection. Antibiotics, however, may kill not only infectious organisms but also the resident flora. This would allow other strains, which would not normally grow, to multiply. Some microorganisms may become resistant to certain medications, making them more difficult to treat. Smoking has been clearly recognized as a factor that impacts or lowers immune response.

Chronic diseases (*pathologies*) that lessen the body's defense system increase the risk for infection. Some examples are pulmonary diseases (emphysema, asthma), burns, peripheral vascular diseases, diseases of the blood, and diabetes mellitus.

NONSPECIFIC DEFENSES

The body has normal defenses to protect it against infection. **Nonspecific defenses** include anatomic and physiological barriers and the inflammatory response:

- Intact skin protects against pathogens. Organisms can live on the skin but cannot penetrate it. Resident flora (bacteria) on the skin stop other bacteria from growing. The skin's slight acidity also inhibits bacterial growth.
- Moist mucous membranes and cilia in the nose trap microorganisms, dust, and foreign materials.
- Special cells in the lungs (called macrophages or phagocytes) ingest microorganisms and foreign particles.
- Saliva in the mouth helps to prevent infection by its washing action. The presence of enzymes also serves as a protective measure.
- Tears (which have an enzyme in them) wash away organisms and protect the eyes. Tears also reduce the number load (dose) of organisms present.
- Stomach acids protect the stomach from infection. Resident flora in the large intestine stop the growth of other microorganisms.
- Vaginal secretions have a pH that stops the growth of many disease-producing bacteria.
- The flow of urine flushes the urethra and keeps bacteria from entering the bladder. Urine is a sterile body fluid.
- Gastric acids and bile serve to kill some organisms.
- Chemical agents in the immune system, such as interferon, kill viruses.

SPECIFIC OR IMMUNE DEFENSES

Specific defenses are also known as *immune defenses*. They work against identified foreign proteins such as bacteria, fungi, viruses, and other infectious agents, which are considered to be invading agents and are called **antigens**.

The resistance of the body to infection is known as **immunity** (see Table 9-4 ■). In *active immunity*, the body produces its own antibodies to natural antigens (e.g., infection) or artificial antigens (e.g., vaccines). For example, if you acquire chickenpox, you will develop acquired immunity. The same is true if you receive the chickenpox vaccine. *Passive immunity* deals with receipt of natural antibodies (e.g., from a nursing mother). Two systems are working and overlapping during the immune response. See Box 9-1 ■ for specific cultural immunity issues.

Antibody-Mediated Defense

Immune response is made up of two separate but interrelated systems. These systems are medicated by B and T lymphocytes. B cells originated in the bone marrow from stem cells. T cells also originate in the bone marrow but in more primitive stem cells.

TABLE 9-4

Types of Acquired Immunity

TYPE	ANTIGEN OR ANTIBODY SOURCE	DURATION
Active	Antibodies are produced by the body in response to an antigen.	Long
Natural	Antibodies are formed in the presence of active infection in the body.	Lifelong
Artificial	Antigens (vaccines or toxoids) are administered to stimulate antibody production.	Many years: the immunity must be reinforced by booster inoculations
Passive	Antibodies are produced by another source, animal or human.	Short
Natural	Antibodies are transferred naturally from an immune mother to her baby through the placenta or in colostrum.	6 months to 1 year
Artificial	Immune serum (antibody) from an animal or another human is injected.	2 to 3 weeks

The *antibody-mediated defense* (also called circulating or *humoral immunity*) depends primarily on the B lymphocytes. They are mediated by antibodies produced from B cells, which flow through the bloodstream. These antibodies are also called *immunoglobulins (Ig)* and are part of the body's plasma proteins. The B cells are activated and attack when they recognize a foreign invader (antigens). B cells secrete antibodies to assist in the destruction of antigens. B cells bind to the antigens, which makes it easier for phagocytes to get to the antigens. Their response makes five different classes of antibody molecules:

IgM—refers to a current infection.

IgG—refers to a past infection with the development of immunity.

IgA—Binds to organisms trying to bind to mucous membranes; highly effective in preventing virus infections (secretory antibody).

IgD—functions late in immune response (before IgG appears).

IgE—the principal allergy-inducing immunoglobulin.

Cell-Mediated Defense

The *cell-mediated defense* acts through the T-cell system. When a person is exposed to an antigen, the lymphoid tissue produces and releases large numbers of T cells into the lymphatic fluid and system. If T-cell immunity is lost, people cannot defend themselves against most viral, bacterial, and fungal infections. An example of depressed T-cell function is HIV infection. This system serves as the first line of protection from illness and disease.

Inflammatory Response

The **inflammatory response** is a local nonspecific defense reaction of tissues when they are exposed to infection or injury. The inflammatory response destroys or dilutes microorganisms and prevents their spread. There are five primary signs of inflammation: pain, swelling, redness, heat, and (if there is severe injury) weakened function of a body part. Inflammation of a part is indicated by the suffix *-itis*. For example, appendicitis is inflammation of the appendix.

There are three stages to the inflammatory response:

- *First stage: vascular and cellular response.* During the cellular and vascular response, blood vessels first constrict at the site of injury. This is quickly followed by dilation of small vessels in the area, which causes increased blood flow and redness (*hyperemia*) with increased warmth. Fluid enters the interstitial space, causing edema and irritation to the nerve endings and producing pain. Blood flow eventually slows down in the capillaries, and *leukocytes* (white blood cells) move out of them into the tissues to work against the microorganisms.
- *Second stage: exudate production.* The exudate consists of dead phagocytic cells (cells that attacked the microorganism). During this stage the microorganisms are killed. The exudate is removed when it drains into the lymphatic system channels or leaves the body as drainage.

BOX 9-1   **CULTURAL PULSE POINTS**

Infection

Although susceptibility to infectious/communicable diseases is frequently linked to socioeconomic factors such as overcrowding and poor nutrition, there are some ethnic factors that should be considered:

- Ethnicity appears to be a factor in the incidence of tuberculosis and hepatitis B viral infection. Native Americans living in the southwest, Vietnamese refugees, and Mexican Americans have a relatively high incidence of these diseases.
- Africans possessing sickle cell trait are known to have increased immunity to malaria.
- Childhood illnesses caused by viruses such as rubeola and varicella are considered to be benign in a majority of children. However, many countries do not have the vaccine and immunization programs in place that are standard here in the United States.
- HIV infections continue to be a major health problem, with racial/ethnic minorities suffering a disproportionate share of the disease.

The major types of exudates are serous, purulent, and hemorrhagic (sanguineous). (See types of cultures in Chapters 23, 24, 27, and 28 ⊂⊃.)

- *Third stage: reparative phase.* In the reparative phase, the tissues regenerate cells that are similar or identical in structure and function to the dead cells. Some tissues (like skin) regenerate well; others (like nerve tissue) regenerate little if at all. The sequence of repair of damaged tissue is discussed in detail in Chapter 23 ⊂⊃.

CLINICAL GUIDELINES

Recommendations by the CDC for hand hygiene and hand antisepsis follow:

- When hands are visibly dirty or contaminated with proteinaceous material or are visibly soiled with blood or body fluids, wash hands with either a non-antimicrobial soap and water or an antimicrobial soap and water.
- If hands are not visibly soiled, use alcohol-based hand rub for routinely decontaminating hands in all other clinical situations.
- When decontaminating hands with an alcohol-based hand rub, apply product to palm of one hand and rub together, covering all surfaces of hands and fingers, until hands are dry.
- Hands should also be washed after glove removal (CDC, 2002).

See Procedure 9-1 ■ on page 164 for hand hygiene instructions.

DRUG-RESISTANT ORGANISMS

During the past two decades, there has been rising concern regarding the increased incidence of nosocomial (hospital-acquired) infections involving drug-resistant organisms. The overuse and misuse of antibiotics, as well as the tendency of clients not to complete a prescribed course of treatment, have impacted the development of resistant organisms. In the 1980s, drug companies were not developing new antibiotics. There seemed to be a feeling that bacterial infections were a thing of the past. Bacteria can become resistant to antibiotics "naturally." This happens because when antibiotics are taken and bacteria are killed, the antibiotic will leave behind some bacteria that caused resistance to occur. Added to this is the fact that when new antibiotics are developed, physicians tend to prescribe them in mass, overlooking common and less expensive antibiotics. Resistance develops, and the number of antibiotics available to treat an infection are fewer. Clients often demand that their physicians give them antibiotics even when they are not needed. For example, clients may ask for antibiotics when they have the flu, but an antibiotic is not effective against the flu virus.

Another factor that may lead to the development of resistance is failure to complete a full course of prescribed medication. For example, when clients with tuberculosis do not complete their full course of treatment, they may develop drug-resistant tuberculosis. Currently, the three most prominent types of drug-resistant organisms are MRSA, vancomycin-resistant enterococci (VRE), and multi-drug-resistant TB. Hospitalized clients whose immune systems are already compromised are at the greatest risk. MRSA can cause illness in persons outside the hospital and healthcare facilities. Community acquired or CA-MRSA has become more apparent. Cases of CA-MRSA have been associated with transmission in contact sports, the sharing of towels in gyms, and living in crowded areas such as correctional facilities.

Failure to perform appropriate hand hygiene is considered to be the leading cause of healthcare-associated infections and spread of multi-drug-resistant organisms and has been recognized as a substantial contributor to outbreaks (CDC, 2002). See Box 9-2 ■ for teaching clients about taking their medications.

Controlling Microorganisms in the Environment

Maintaining a clean environment helps to inhibit the growth and multiplication of organisms. The very process of cleaning slows down the growth of microorganisms. **Antiseptics** (agents that inhibit the growth of some microorganisms) and **disinfectants** (agents that destroy pathogens other than spores) help to keep control of organisms in the environment.

Disinfection requires the use of a disinfectant solution that contains a chemical preparation, such as phenol, bleach, or other chemical compounds. These substances should not

---

BOX 9-2	CLIENT TEACHING

Taking Antibiotics

Client Teaching	Rational
Complete the full course of medication prescribed.	Failure to complete the full course of treatment may result in prolonged illness and the development of drug resistance.
Do not take antibiotics for viral illnesses.	Antibiotics are for the treatment of bacterial infections only.
Older, more common antibiotics work well.	Overuse of new, more powerful antibiotics may lead to resistance.

BOX 9-3   NURSING CARE CHECKLIST

Using Bactericidal and Bacteriostatic Agents

When disinfecting, remember to:

- ☑ Use the recommended concentration of the solution and keep it on the area for the required amount of time.
- ☑ Know the type and number of infectious organisms. Make certain no soap is present on the item since some disinfectants will not work when soap is present.
- ☑ Keep the room temperature within a normal range because some disinfectants will not work otherwise.
- ☑ Be certain there is no organic material (e.g., blood, pus, excretions) present because the disinfectants may be inactivated.
- ☑ Treat all exposed surface areas and crevices.

be used on tissue because they are often caustic or toxic. Both antiseptics (which can be used on tissue) and disinfectants have bactericidal and/or bacteriostatic properties. A **bactericidal agent** destroys bacteria, whereas a **bacteriostatic agent** prevents growth and reproduction of only some bacteria. Important points to remember when disinfecting are listed in Box 9-3 ■. Using boiling water for a minimum of 15 minutes is a good method for the home setting.

Sterilization destroys all microorganisms, viruses, and spores. Moist heat (steam) can be used under pressure or as a free agent to sterilize. Autoclaves provide steam under pressure, with temperatures ranging from 121 to 123°C (250 to 254°F) and 15 to 17 lbs of pressure. Free steam at 100°C (212°F) must be used for at least 30 minutes for 3 consecutive days. Gas sterilization is effective for heat-sensitive items. An example is ethylene oxide gas. However, it is toxic, and staff working with this form of sterilization must wear badges to monitor exposure. Radiation can also be employed in sterilization. Ionizing radiation is often used for foods and drugs that are sensitive to heat, although it is a very costly process. This is not routinely used in the healthcare setting.

USING ASEPTIC TECHNIQUE

Asepsis is the absence of disease-causing microorganisms. **Sepsis** is the opposite, the presence of infection. It can take many forms in the human body. **Aseptic technique** is used to prevent the possibility of transferring microorganisms from one place or person to another.

Medical Asepsis

Medical asepsis includes all practices that are used to confine a specific microorganism to a specific area, or to limit the number of microorganisms, their growth, and their transmission. Objects are referred to as clean or dirty in medical asepsis. *Clean* means the absence of almost all microorganisms. *Dirty* (soiled or contaminated) means there are microorganisms present that may cause an infection.

Surgical Asepsis

Surgical asepsis is also called *sterile technique,* and it means every practice that keeps an object or an area completely free of microorganisms and spores. When dealing with sterile areas of the body, only surgical asepsis should be used.

PROTECTIVE PRECAUTIONS AND INFECTION CONTROL

Infection control measures are used in institutions to prevent the spread of microorganisms. **Standard Precautions** (Figure 9-2 ■) are practiced in all healthcare facilities. These precautions refer to all body fluids, especially those associated with bloodborne pathogens (e.g., hepatitis B and C, and HIV infections). In 1996, the CDC presented new guidelines for isolation precautions that included two levels: Tier 1 or Standard Precautions, and Tier 2 or Transmission-based Precautions.

Standard Precautions

Standard Precautions are used in the care of all clients. They are applied to all body fluids, blood, secretions, excretions (except sweat), mucous membranes, and nonintact skin.

Transmission-based Precautions

Transmission-based Precautions are used in addition to Standard Precautions for any client with known or suspected infections that are spread by airborne or droplet transmission or by physical contact. Airborne nuclei are those agents smaller than 3 microns (e.g., tuberculosis, measles, varicella). Droplets are particles larger than 3 microns (e.g., diphtheria, streptococcal pharyngitis, mumps, pneumonia, influenza). Contact transmission occurs by touching items in the client's environment that are contaminated. Contact precautions would be appropriate for MRSA- and VRE-infected client's.

ISOLATION PRACTICES. Isolation practices are initiated after assessing the client's condition. CDC guidelines, institutional policies, nursing assessment, and laboratory study results are used to make the decision to place an individual in an isolated environment. Other factors that must be considered are the status of the client's defense mechanisms, the source of the infection, and its mode of transmission.

TRANSPORTING PATIENTS WITH INFECTIONS. Clients with infections are not transported outside of their own rooms unless it is necessary for testing or treatment. If they need to be moved to another area, the environment must be protected to avoid contamination. The client should wear a

STANDARD PRECAUTIONS

FOR INFECTION CONTROL

Hand Hygiene
Wash after touching **body fluids**, after **removing gloves**, and between **patient contacts**. If hands are not visibly soiled, use an alcohol-based hand rub for routinely decontaminating hands.

Gloves
Wear **Gloves** before touching **body fluids**, **mucous membranes**, and **nonintact skin**.

Mask & Eye Protection or Face Shield
Protect eyes, nose, mouth during procedures that cause **splashes** or **sprays** of **body fluids**.

Gown
Wear **Gown** during procedures that may cause **splashes** or **sprays** of **body fluids**.

Patient-Care Equipment
Handle soiled equipment so as to prevent personal contamination and transfer to other patients.

Environmental Control
Follow hospital procedures for cleaning beds, equipment, and frequently touched surfaces.

Linen
Handle linen soiled with **body fluids** so as to prevent personal contamination and transfer to other patients.

Occupational Health & Bloodborne Pathogens
Prevent injuries from needles, scalpels, and other sharp devices.
Never recap needles using both hands.
Place sharps in puncture-proof sharps containers.
Use **Resuscitation Devices** as an alternative to mouth-to-mouth resuscitation.

Patient Placement
Use a Private Room for a patient who contaminates the environment.

"**Body Fluids**" include **blood**, **secretions**, and **excretions**.

Condensed Version

Form No. **SPR-C**   BREVIS CORP., 225 West 2855 South, SLC, Utah 84115   www.brevis.com   © 2004 Brevis Corp.

Figure 9-2. ■ Standard Precautions for infection control. (*Source:* Courtesy of BREVIS Corporation.)

surgical mask if the infection is airborne, and all draining wounds should be covered with dressings that will not leak. The area the client is going to should be advised of the isolation precautions ordered so that they can take precautions to maintain the environment. The client should wear clean clothing, so as not to contaminate wheelchairs or transportation carts.

COLLABORATIVE CARE

Laboratory Tests

Some laboratory work with abnormal values indicates infection. Elevated white blood cell counts with changes in specific types of cells are seen on the differential count. Neutrophils increase with bacterial infections. Lymphocytes are elevated with viral infections. The erythrocyte sedimentation rate (ESR) increases with the inflammatory response. Cultures of body fluids and any drainage can identify specific organisms.

Equipment

PERSONAL PROTECTIVE EQUIPMENT. Particular items are used to protect the personnel and the client when administering care. They include gloves, gowns, protective eyewear, and masks.

Gloves are used to protect the nurse's hands from coming in contact with body fluids and contaminated items. They also protect the patient from the nurse's microorganisms. Gloves reduce the transmission of microorganisms from one client to another, or to any object (*fomite*) where microorganisms might grow. Hands are washed before and after wearing gloves. Gloves are not a primary protection measure.

For many activities, only clean gloves are worn, and no special technique is used to put them on. Sterile gloves are worn if the nurse works with a wound or when the nurse's hands enter a body orifice. A specific technique is used to apply and remove sterile gloves (Procedure 9-2 ■ on page 166). If a gown is worn, the cuff of the glove is pulled over the gown's sleeve (Figure 9-3 ■).

Gowns are used only once before being either discarded or laundered. Gowns should be water resistant and clean. Sterile gowns are used in surgery and in cases of reverse isolation (wherein the client is protected from organisms carried by the staff) or when the nurse is changing dressings on extensive wounds (e.g., burns). No special technique is used to put on a clean gown or to take it off if it is not visibly soiled. If there is a large amount of contamination, the nurse should avoid touching the contaminated area and roll the gown up with the soiled area inside. The gown is then disposed of in the proper container. Sterile gowns are grasped at the crease near the neck and held away from the

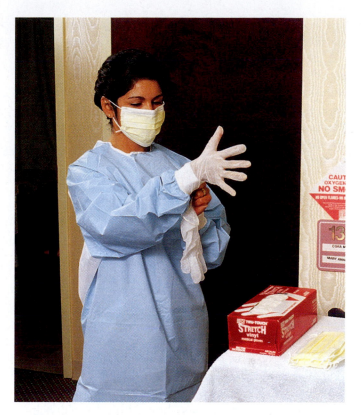

Figure 9-3. ■ Pull gloves up over the cuffs of the gown.

body. They are allowed to unfold without touching anything. If the gown's outer surface does touch something, it is contaminated. The nurse's hands are put into the shoulders and sleeves without touching the outside of the gown. The hands can be put through the cuff using the open method of sterile gloving. A coworker will tie the gown at the neck and at the back without touching the outside surface (Procedure 9-3 ■ on page 168).

Face masks are worn to stop the spread of microorganism and airborne droplets from either the nurse to the client, or the client to the nurse. They also protect against splatters from body fluids. Many face masks now have transparent protective eye coverings. Otherwise, protective glasses or goggles should be worn if there is a possibility of body fluid splatters. The CDC recommends that people within 3 feet of the client should wear masks if the infection is transmitted by large particle droplets. If the infection is transmitted by small particle or droplet nuclei, all persons entering the room should wear masks. Masks should be disposable and worn only once. They should be replaced if they become wet or soiled. They are to be disposed of in the appropriate waste container.

Particulate respirators are also used to protect against droplet transmission. Many different types are available, and some are disposable. The CDC recommends those with a rating of N95, which means a category N respirator that has 95% efficiency and meets the tuberculosis control criteria. The use of this mask by the nurse requires a medical evaluation and fit testing to ensure a proper fit and the absence of health problems that would interfere with the nurse's ability to wear a respirator. The Occupational Safety and Health Administration (OSHA) has published a specific regulation, *Respiratory Standard 1910.134,* that addresses the use of respirators.

When removing soiled protective equipment;

1. Remove the gloves first (if the gown is tied in the front, undo the ties before removing the gloves).
2. After removing the gloves, remove the mask, holding it by the strings.
3. Remove the gown next.
4. Finally, remove any eyewear.
5. Wash the hands and wrists thoroughly.

CLEANING REUSABLE EQUIPMENT. Washing items to remove any organic material is important. Cold water rinses should be done first, because hot water coagulates the protein of organic material and causes it to stick to items. Then wash items in hot water with soap to emulsify and dislodge dirt. Abrasive action with stiff-bristled brushes will help to remove material from crevices in equipment. Rinse articles with warm to hot water and dry thoroughly. Items are now considered clean. However, the process is not complete until the basin or sink and any brushes or tools used for cleaning the items are also cleaned with a disinfectant. This task is generally assigned to housekeeping or central service staff.

DISPOSAL OF USED OR SOILED EQUIPMENT FROM AN ISOLATION ROOM. Most facilities have policies and procedures in place that state specifically how to dispose of equipment and supplies that have been contaminated. Be familiar with these policies—they are based on state law! Materials may be disposed of, cleaned, disinfected, or sterilized. Some equipment and supplies are for single use only. Other materials are meant to be used multiple times.

Bagging is a technique recommended by the CDC for removal of materials from a client's room. The purpose is to prevent exposure to items contaminated with body secretions. The bag must be impervious to microorganisms. The bags may come in colors (e.g., red) and have labels that indicate they contain infectious materials.

The CDC recommends placing noncontaminated disposable items in the plastic bags that line the waste containers. Nondisposable or reusable items should be put into a labeled bag before being removed from the client's room and sent to a central processing area for decontamination. Rubber, plastic, metal, and glass items may be bagged separately. (Metal and glass can be autoclaved, but rubber and plastic need to be exposed to gas sterilization.)

Special procedure trays should be disassembled and bagged as already indicated. Soiled linens or clothing should be bagged and sent to the facility laundry or home. Linens should be handled as little as possible. They should be rolled into a bundle before being placed in the bag. (Do not shake the linens.) Laboratory specimens should be put into a leakproof container. If the container is contaminated on the outside, it should be put in a plastic bag before it is sent to the laboratory. Specimen containers must have a biohazard label on the outer surface of the container. Dishes are often made of paper and are disposed of in the refuse container. Blood pressure equipment, if kept in the room, needs no special precautions but needs to be cleaned before use on another client. If it becomes contaminated, follow the agency's cleaning procedures. Nondisposable thermometers should be disinfected after use according to agency protocols. "Sharps," including glass items, are to be placed in a puncture-resistant container kept in the room (see Chapter 29 ⌗). Clients' personal objects (such as toys) that are contaminated should be bagged and sent home for cleaning.

NURSING CARE

ASSESSING

The client history is one of the most important parts of the assessment. It gives you specific information on the client's signs/symptoms and information on what the client has tried for treatment or relief of the problem. The nursing history allows the nurse to assess the client's degree of risk for developing an infection and symptoms that suggest the presence of an infection. Along with reviewing the chart, the nurse will interview the client in order to collect objective data that are significant. Such data would include anything that might influence the development of an infection, history of recurring infections, immunization history, nutritional status, emotional stressors, and current medications and/or therapeutic measures. In light of a potential for a pandemic, travel history is also an important part of assessment especially for a client with respiratory symptoms.

Subjective data can be obtained from clients when they are asked about any symptoms they have experienced that may indicate infection. These include headache, lethargy, nausea or vomiting, rash, and pain.

Along with data already collected, the nurse looks for signs and symptoms of infection associated with specific body systems. Sneezing or watery, discolored discharge from the nose suggests sinus infection. Cloudy urine may indicate bladder infection. Vital signs also show changes, such as increased temperature, pulse, and respirations. Other observations may include anorexia and lymph node enlargement or rash.

DIAGNOSING, PLANNING, AND IMPLEMENTATING

The primary nursing diagnosis for the transmission of pathologic microorganisms is *Risk for Infection*. Some of the specific risk factors include traumatized or broken skin, stasis of body fluids, altered peristalsis, change in pH of secretions, decreased ciliary action, rash and wound contamination. Contributing factors to the nursing diagnosis include immunosuppression, anemia, and suppressed inflammatory response.

Other contributing nursing diagnoses that may result from the infection are *Impaired Physical Mobility, Imbalanced Nutrition, Pain* related to tissue damage, *Hyperthermia* related to infection, *Imbalanced Fluid Volume, Anxiety, Low Self-Esteem,* and *Impaired Social Interaction*.

Nursing goals in the planning stage of the nursing process include:

- Restoring and maintaining body defenses against infection
- Preventing the spread of infection and its complications
- Maintaining hydration to prevent fluid and electrolyte imbalances.

To achieve these goals, nursing care must include thorough aseptic technique, supporting the host's defenses, client teaching that emphasizes protective measures to prevent infections and their spread, and appropriate hydration measures. Some common nursing interventions for the patient at risk for infection include:

- Help the client as necessary with routine hygiene (including oral hygiene) and skin care. *Practicing consistent and good hygiene reduces the number of microorganisms. Maintaining intact skin prevents the possibility of infection.*
- Appropriately dispose of, or change, any clothing or linens, bandages, or dressing whenever they become soiled or wet. *Microorganisms grow easily and live in soiled or wet cloth.*
- Dispose of feces and urine appropriately. *Human waste contains many microorganisms that can cause infection or transfer bacteria and viruses to others.*
- Cover all containers of fluid (e.g., water bottles) at the client's bedside. *Uncapped containers holding liquids increase the risk of contamination and microbial growth.*
- Empty all drainage containers (e.g., suction bottles, catheter bags) before they become full, and at the end of each nursing shift, or according to agency policy. Hold containers steady and level to prevent spillage. *Body fluids and drainage contain microorganisms that grow*

and increase in numbers and can potentially be transmitted to others.

- When giving care, avoid reaching over, talking, sneezing, or coughing across open wounds. Also, cover the mouth and nose when coughing or sneezing. *This limits the number of microorganisms falling from the caregiver's skin or escaping from the respiratory tract and prevents contamination of the wound.*
- Start all client care using Standard Precautions. *Anyone may have infectious microorganisms that can potentially be transmitted to others.*
- Wash hands before and after any client contact. *Correct hand hygiene controls and prevents the spread and transmission of microorganisms.*
- Wear masks and eye protection when caring for clients who have infections transmitted by droplets from the respiratory tract, or when sprays of body fluid may occur (e.g., during wound irrigations). *Masks and eye protection reduce the spread of microorganisms from droplet secretion contamination.*
- Wear gloves (and gowns if there is a possibility of soiling clothing) when handling any secretions or excretions from the client. *Gloves and gowns prevent contamination with microorganisms by contact.*
- Provide every client with his or her own individual hygiene and personal care items. *This prevents cross-contamination of microorganisms from others.*
- Use sterile technique for all invasive procedures (e.g., injections, catheterizations, suctioning) and for open wounds. *When the body's natural defense mechanisms (e.g., skin, body cavities) are penetrated, the barriers to microorganisms are broken.*
- Use only appropriate puncture-proof containers for all disposal of used needles, knife blades, and syringes. The use of needle safe or needleless systems are now required. *Infectious diseases can be transmitted to healthcare workers and others by puncture injuries from contaminated needles, blades, and syringes. The U.S. Congress passed the Needlestick Safety and Prevention Act in 2000, which requires all sharps be needle safe or needleless. OSHA is also enforcing this mandate.*
- Provide a balanced diet for the client. *A well-balanced diet provides all the nutrients needed to maintain and build body tissues* (see Chapter 25 🔗).

Practicing Sterile Technique

Many client care procedures require the use of sterile technique. Objects are only sterile when free of all microorganisms. When practicing sterile technique, the basic principles of surgical asepsis are used.

A **sterile field** is a microorganism-free area. Nurses use sterile drapes and the inside of sterile wrappers to create the sterile field (Procedure 9-4 ▪ on page 170). Some general concepts to keep in mind when creating and working with a sterile field are listed in Box 9-4 ▪.

BOX 9-4	NURSING CARE CHECKLIST

Creating and Maintaining a Sterile Field

☑ Wear sterile gloves to work with the equipment on the field, or use sterile forceps to move items around on it.

☑ Never reach across a sterile field once it is established. (Microorganisms can be dropped on it and cause contamination.)

☑ If the field becomes wet, it is considered contaminated.

☑ If an unsterile object touches a sterile object, it is then contaminated.

☑ The edges of the sterile field are considered unsterile.

☑ If an object is below the nurse's waist level or is out of sight, it is considered unsterile.

☑ If objects must be left open to the air for a prolonged period of time, cover the sterile field with sterile drapes to prevent contamination by airborne microorganisms.

☑ Nursing qualities that are essential in maintaining a sterile field are alertness, honesty, and conscientiousness.

☑ Follow the old adage: "If there is any doubt about sterility, the object or field is unsterile."

EVALUATING

During the evaluation process, the nurse reviews both positive and negative outcomes of the care and instructions given to the client. Revisions in care are made as needed until the desired result is achieved. Examples of positive outcomes and obtaining stated goals in client care are:

- All dressings are kept dry and are changed when they are soiled or become wet.
- The client eats a well-balanced diet and has adequate fluid intake in order to maintain nutrition and hydration.
- Clients participate in self-care to the degree possible, and good hygiene is maintained.
- All contaminated equipment and linens are disposed of appropriately and according to agency standards.
- All containers holding human waste or drainage are disposed of appropriately.
- All materials used for invasive procedures (e.g., needles, syringes, catheters) are disposed of in a sharps container located at the site of use.

CONTINUING CARE

Education is an important aspect of the nurse's role in treating a client with an infection or potential for infection. Some appropriate points follow:

- Teach clients and their significant others why articles must be clean, disinfected, or sterilized. Teach how this is to be done.

- Teach clients and significant others to wash their hands before eating or handling food, after toileting, or after handling any infectious materials.
- Educate or remind clients and significant others about the importance of immunizations and booster shots.

Clients and support people must often provide home care of a person with an infectious disease or partially healed wound. The following instructions can be useful:

- Wash hands carefully before and after any hands-on care.
- Keep fingernails clean, short, and well trimmed.
- If there is no running water, use commercially available hand hygiene agents that require no water.
- Use soap and paper towels when washing hands.
- Teach young children hand hygiene as soon as they can participate.
- Keep pets out of the area when setting up for and performing sterile procedures.
- Clean and wipe dry a flat surface for the sterile field.
- Dispose of all soiled materials in a waterproof bag. Check with the home care nurse as to how to dispose of medical waste.

NURSING PROCESS CARE PLAN
Client with Respiratory Infection

Mrs. Chase is a 76-year-old woman who has a 10-year history of emphysema. She has a history of smoking a pack a day for 25 years, and continues to do so. Recently, she began coughing much more frequently and expectorating larger volumes of yellow/green-colored mucus. She was admitted to the hospital with complaints of fatigue, coughing, a poor appetite, and a fever with chills. She is sitting on the edge of the bed, coughing, with her hand pressing against her chest. There are used tissues scattered all over the bed.

Assessment. VS: T 101.4, P 90, R 22 and shallow, BP 146/88. Pain 4/10 in the chest while coughing and less between episodes. Weight is 108 lbs, height 5′ 9″. The client's skin is hot, flushed, and dry. Skin turgor is fair. She is alert and oriented, but restless and anxious. She coughs frequently and expectorates moderate amounts of thick, yellow/green-tinged mucus. She has a barrel chest, and on auscultation slight wheezes are heard in both lungs. Nail beds show slight cyanosis. Specimens of blood and sputum have already been collected. The WBC count is elevated. The sputum specimen shows a streptococcal upper respiratory tract infection. The chest x-ray shows bilateral pneumonia. Mrs. Chase states she had been caring for her young grandchild who had a "strep throat."

Nursing Diagnosis. The following important nursing diagnoses (among others) are established for this client:

- *Risk for Infection* due to decreased ciliary action in lungs
- *Deficient Fluid Volume* related to high fever and poor appetite
- *Impaired Gas Exchange* related to rapid respirations, copious secretions, alveolar destruction, and air trapping
- *Ineffective Airway Clearance* related to increased secretions and a weak cough
- *Deficient Knowledge* related to infectious process and status of compromised host.

Expected Outcomes. The expected outcomes for the plan of care are that Mrs. Chase will:

- Regain prior lung function.
- Maintain adequate hydration and circulating blood volume.
- Improve gas exchange as demonstrated by respirations within normal limits, normal pulse, and blood gases.
- Maintain a patent airway with decreased volume of secretions.
- Understand and be able to verbalize the process of contamination, susceptibility to infection, and how to prevent spread of organisms.

Planning and Implementation. The following nursing interventions are implemented for Mrs. Chase. Ongoing assessments are done to monitor her condition.

- Monitor character of respirations including rate and rhythm, blood gases, and skin color every 2 to 4 hours.
- Auscultate breath sounds. Encourage deep breathing and coughing.
- Monitor vital signs every 4 h and intake and output every shift.
- Encourage fluids. Find out what liquids she likes and offer her 8 ounces of preferred fluid every hour.
- Have client deep breathe and cough every 2 h while awake. Position in semi-Fowler's or Fowler's position. Change client's position from back to sides often.

- Document volume of secretions as well as color and character. Request order for chest physiotherapy. Suction as necessary. See also Chapter 24 🔗.
- Administer medications (antibiotics, analgesics, expectorants, antitussives) on time.
- Follow orders from respiratory therapy.
- Teach Mrs. Chase to limit her exposure to others who are ill, because her history of emphysema and advanced age make her more susceptible to infection.
- Discuss hand hygiene techniques, and emphasize that she should wash her hands after coughing or sneezing into them and after handling objects used by other ill persons.
- Remind her to throw contaminated tissues into a waste container to maintain a clean environment.

Evaluation. At the end of the shift, Mrs. Chase's lung sounds were improved with less wheezing. Mucus was clear in color, thin, and "easier to cough out." The rate, rhythm, and character of her respirations were adequate. Her blood gases were within normal limits, and she showed no signs of cyanosis. Her temperature was 99.9°F and her pulse was 82. She was resting easily with her oxygen on. She was eating and taking fluids well with good urinary output.

Critical Thinking in the Nursing Process

1. Why was caring for her ill grandchild endangering Mrs. Chase's health?
2. What is the connection between the used tissues and the spread of infection?
3. Which of Mrs. Chase's assessment findings are consistent with a bacterial infection?

Note: Discussion of Critical Thinking questions appears in Appendix I.

Note: The references and resources for this and all chapters have been compiled at the back of the book.

PROCEDURE 9-1 **Hand Hygiene/Washing**

Purposes

- To reduce the number of microorganisms on the hands
- To reduce the risk of transmission of microorganisms to clients
- To reduce the risk of cross-contamination among clients and equipment
- To reduce the risk of transmission of infectious organisms to oneself

Equipment

- Soap
- Warm running water
- Towels
- Alcohol-based foam or gel

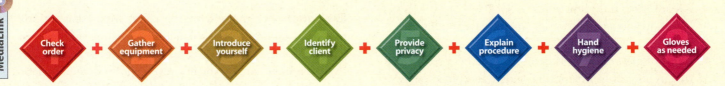

Check order + Gather equipment + Introduce yourself + Identify client + Provide privacy + Explain procedure + Hand hygiene + Gloves as needed

Interventions

1. Prepare and assess the hands.
   - File the nails short. *Short nails are less likely to harbor microorganisms, scratch a client, or puncture gloves.* Do not wear artificial nails or extensions. *These can pass organisms on to clients. Note: The CDC recommends that nail enhancements not be worn by nurses working in areas such as the OR, L&D, or NICU. Many facilities have made this recommendation a policy for all employees who have contact with clients.*
   - Remove all jewelry. Some nurses prefer to slide their watches up above their elbows. Others pin the watch to the uniform. *Microorganisms can lodge in the settings of jewelry and under rings. Removal facilitates proper cleaning.*
   - Check hands for breaks in the skin, such as hangnails or cuts. Use lotions to prevent hangnails and cracked, dry skin. *A nurse who has broken skin areas may have to wear a dressing. If the area is too large to cover, then work reassignment is required.*

2. Turn on the water and adjust the flow.
   - There are five common types of faucet controls:
     a. Hand-operated handles.
     b. Knee levers. Move these with the knee to regulate flow and temperature (Figure 9-4 ■).
     c. Foot pedals. Press these with the foot to regulate flow and temperature (Figure 9-5 ■).
     d. Elbow controls. Move these with the elbows instead of the hands.
     e. Infrared controls. The water runs when motion is detected at a preset distance.

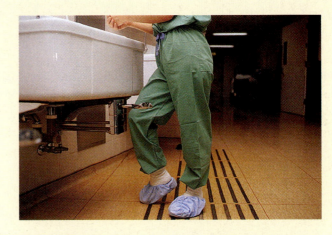

Figure 9-4. ■ A knee-lever faucet control. (Photographer: Elena Dorfman.)

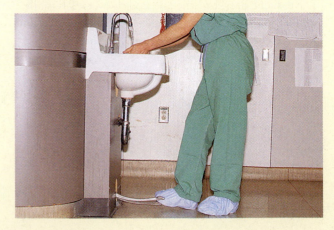

Figure 9-5. ■ A foot-pedal faucet control. (Photographer: Elena Dorfman.)

- Adjust the flow so that the water is warm. Warm water removes less of the protective oil of the skin than hot water and is more effective than cold water for producing lather.

3. Wet the hands thoroughly by holding them under the running water, and apply soap to the hands.
   - Hold the hands lower than the elbows so that the water flows from the arms to the fingertips. *The water should flow from the least contaminated to the most contaminated area; the hands are generally considered more contaminated than the lower arms.*
   - Apply 2 to 4 mL (1 tsp) of liquid soap; rub it firmly between the hands.

4. Thoroughly wash and rinse the hands.
   - Wash hands for a minimum of 10 to 15 seconds. For a more thorough washing, extend the time for wetting, washing, and rinsing.
   - Use firm rubbing and circular movements to wash the palm, back, and wrist of each hand. Interlace the fingers and thumbs and move the hands back and forth (Figure 9-6 ■), continuing the motion for 10 seconds. *The circular action helps remove microorganisms mechanically. Interlacing the fingers and thumbs cleans between the fingers.*
   - Rinse the hands.

5. Thoroughly dry the hands and arms.
   - Dry hands and arms thoroughly with a paper towel. *Moist skin becomes chapped readily; chapping produces lesions.*
   - Discard the paper towel in the appropriate container.

6. Turn off the water.
   - Use a dry paper towel to grasp a hand-operated control (Figure 9-7 ■). *This prevents the nurse from picking up microorganisms from the faucet handles.*

Hand hygiene as described is to be done when hands are visibly soiled. When not visibly soiled, alcohol-based foams and gels are to be used. They are located outside the entrance to each client room.

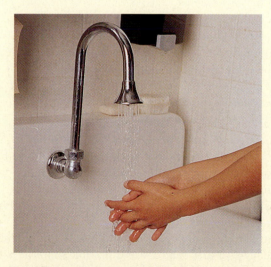

Figure 9-6. ■ Interlacing the fingers during hand hygiene. (Photographer: Elena Dorfman.)

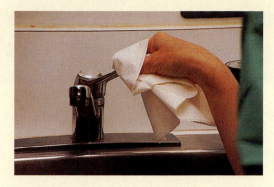

Figure 9-7. ■ Using a paper towel to grasp the hand-operated faucet. (Photographer: Elena Dorfman.)

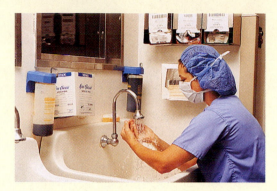

Figure 9-8. ■ The hands are held higher than the elbows during hand hygiene before a sterile technique.

VARIATION: HAND HYGIENE BEFORE STERILE TECHNIQUES

- Apply the soap and wash as described in step 3, but hold the hands higher than the elbows during this hand hygiene procedure. Wet the hands and forearms under the running water, letting it run from the fingertips to the elbows so that the hands become cleaner than the elbows (Figure 9-8 ■). *In this way, the water runs from the area with the fewest microorganisms to areas with a relatively greater number.*
- Apply the soap and wash as described earlier in step 3, maintaining the hands uppermost.
- After washing and rinsing, use a towel to dry one hand thoroughly in a rotating motion from the fingers to the elbow. Use a clean towel to dry the other hand and arm. *A clean towel prevents the transfer of microorganisms from one elbow (least clean area) to the other hand (cleanest area).*

SAMPLE DOCUMENTATION

[date]   Hand hygiene done for 3 minutes
[time]   per hospital protocol prior to
         clean dressing change.
                        _____ A. Parsons, LVN

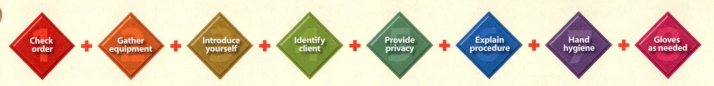

PROCEDURE 9-2

Donning and Removing Sterile Gloves (Open Method)

Purposes

■ To enable the nurse to handle sterile objects freely
■ To prevent clients at risk (e.g., those with open wounds) from becoming infected by microorganisms on the nurse's hands

Equipment

■ Package of sterile gloves

Check order + Gather equipment + Introduce yourself + Identify client + Provide privacy + Explain procedure + Hand hygiene + Gloves as needed

Interventions

1. Open the package of sterile gloves.
   ■ Place the package of gloves on a clean dry surface. *Any moisture on the surface could contaminate the gloves.*
   ■ Some gloves are packed in an inner as well as an outer package. Open the outer package without contaminating the gloves or the inner package.
   ■ Remove the inner package from the outer package.
   ■ Open the inner package as in step 2 of Procedure 9-3 or according to the manufacturer's directions. *Some manufacturers provide a numbered sequence for opening the flaps and folded tabs to grasp for opening the flaps.* If no tabs are provided, pluck the flap so that the fingers do not touch the inner surfaces. *The inner surfaces, which are next to the sterile gloves, will remain sterile.*

2. Put the first glove on the dominant hand.
   ■ If the gloves are packaged so that they lie side by side, grasp the glove for the dominant hand by its cuff (on the palmar side) with the thumb and first finger of the nondominant hand. Touch only the inside of the cuff (Figure 9-9 ■). *The hands are not sterile. By touching only the inside of the glove, the nurse avoids contaminating the outside.*

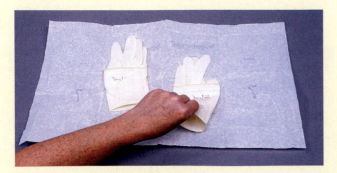

Figure 9-9. ■ Picking up the first sterile glove. (Al Dodge, Pearson Education/PH.)

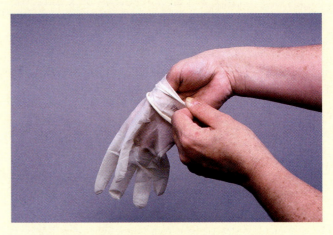

Figure 9-10. ■ Putting on the first sterile glove. (Al Dodge, Pearson Education/PH.)

or
   If the gloves are packaged one on top of the other, grasp the cuff of the top glove as above, using the opposite hand.
   ■ Insert the dominant hand into the glove and pull the glove on. Keep the thumb of the inserted hand against the palm of the hand during insertion (Figure 9-10 ■). *If the thumb is kept against the palm, it is less likely to contaminate the outside of the glove.*
   ■ Leave the cuff turned down.

3. Put the second glove on the nondominant hand.
   ■ Pick up the other glove with the sterile gloved hand, inserting the gloved fingers under the cuff and holding the gloved thumb close to the gloved palm (Figure 9-11 ■). *This helps prevent accidental contamination of the glove by the bare hand.*
   ■ Pull on the second glove carefully. Hold the thumb of the gloved first hand as far as possible from the palm (Figure 9-12 ■). *In this position, the thumb is less likely to touch the arm and become contaminated.*

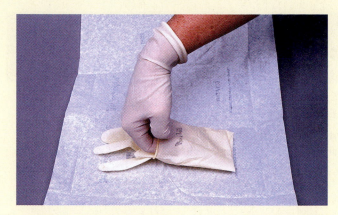

Figure 9-11. ■ Picking up the second sterile glove. (Al Dodge, Pearson Education/PH.)

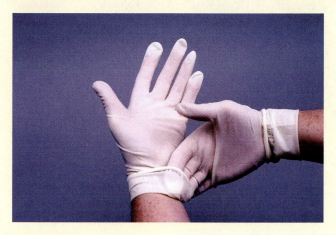

Figure 9-12. ■ Putting on the second sterile glove. (Al Dodge, Pearson Education/PH.)

- Adjust each glove so that it fits smoothly, and carefully pull the cuffs up by sliding the fingers under the cuffs.

4. Remove and dispose of used gloves.
   - To remove sterile gloves that are soiled with secretions, hold the palmar surface below the cuff and turn it inside out. Insert fingers into the second glove, and turn it inside out while removing it (Figure 9-13 ■).

SAMPLE DOCUMENTATION

[date]   Donned sterile gloves according to
[time]   institutional protocol. Changed
            dressing. Wound pink, granulation
            tissue visible.

            _____ P. Morgan, LVN

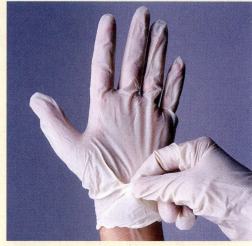

A

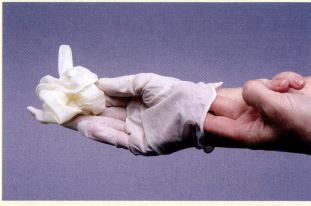

B

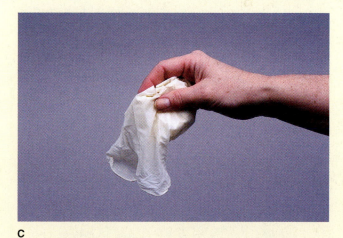

C

Figure 9-13. ■ **A.** Plucking the palmar surface below the cuff of a contaminated glove. **B.** Inserting fingers to remove the second contaminated glove. **C.** Holding contaminated gloves, which are inside out. (Al Dodge, Pearson Education/PH.)

<table>
<tr><td>PROCEDURE 9-3</td><td># Donning Personal Protective Equipment</td></tr>
</table>

Purposes

■ To enable the nurse to work close to a sterile field and handle sterile objects freely
■ To protect clients from becoming contaminated with microorganisms on the nurse's hands, arms, and clothing

Equipment

■ A sterile pack containing a sterile gown
■ A package of sterile gloves

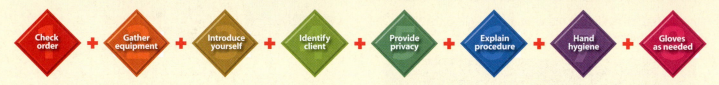

Check order + Gather equipment + Introduce yourself + Identify client + Provide privacy + Explain procedure + Hand hygiene + Gloves as needed

Interventions

DONNING A STERILE GOWN

1. Open the package of sterile gloves.
   ■ Remove the outer wrap from the sterile gloves and leave the gloves in their inner sterile wrap on the sterile field. *If the inner wrapper is not touched, it will remain sterile.*
2. Unwrap the sterile gown pack.
3. Wash and dry hands carefully. See "Variation" at the end of Procedure 9-1 and review agency practice.
4. Put on the sterile gown.
   ■ Grasp the sterile gown at the crease near the neck, hold it away from you, and permit it to unfold freely without touching anything, including the uniform. *The gown will be unsterile if its outer surface touches any unsterile objects.*
   ■ Put the hands inside the shoulders of the gown, and work the arms partway into the sleeves without touching the outside of the gown (Figure 9-14 ■).

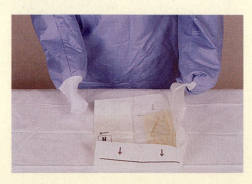

Figure 9-14. ■ Putting on a sterile gown. (Photographer: Jenny Thomas.)

■ If donning sterile gloves by using the closed method (*see below*), work the hands down the sleeves only to the proximal edge of the cuffs.

or

If donning sterile gloves by using the open method, work the hands down the sleeves and through the cuffs.

■ Have a coworker wearing a hair cover and mask grasp the neck ties without touching the outside of the gown and pull the gown upward to cover the neckline of your uniform in front and back. The coworker ties the neck ties. Gowning continues at step 5.

DONNING STERILE GLOVES (CLOSED METHOD)

1. Open the sterile wrapper containing the sterile gloves.
   ■ Open the sterile glove wrapper while the hands are still covered by the sleeves (Figure 9-15 ■).

Figure 9-15. ■ Opening the sterile glove wrapper. (Photographer: Jenny Thomas.)

2. Put the glove on the nondominant hand. Figures 9-16 through 9-18 ■ show the steps for a right-handed person.
   - With the dominant hand, pick up the opposite glove with the thumb and index finger, handling it through the sleeve.
   - Lay the glove on the opposite gown cuff, thumb side down, with the glove opening pointed toward the fingers (see Figure 9-16). Position the dominant hand palm upward inside the sleeve.
   - Use the nondominant hand to grasp the cuff of the glove through the gown cuff, and firmly anchor it.
   - With the dominant hand working through its sleeve, grasp the upper side of the glove's cuff, and stretch it

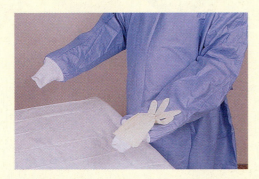

Figure 9-16. ■ Positioning the first sterile glove for the nondominant hand. (Photographer: Jenny Thomas.)

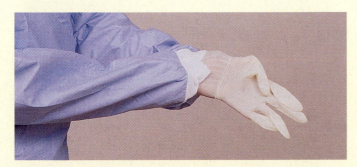

Figure 9-17. ■ Pulling on the first sterile glove. (Photographer: Jenny Thomas.)

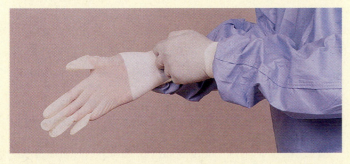

Figure 9-18. ■ Extending the fingers into the second glove of the dominant hand. (Photographer: Jenny Thomas.)

over the cuff of the gown. *This covers the nonsterile skin of the wrist and creates a solid sterile area from gloves to gown.*
   - Pull the sleeve up to draw the cuff over the wrist as you extend the fingers of the nondominant hand into the glove's fingers (see Figure 9-17).

3. Put the glove on the dominant hand.
   - Place the fingers of the gloved hand under the cuff of the remaining glove.
   - Place the glove over the cuff of the second sleeve.
   - Extend the fingers into the glove as you pull the glove up over the cuff (see Figure 9-18).

COMPLETION OF GOWNING

5. Complete gowning as follows:
   - Have a coworker wearing a hair cover and mask hold the waist tie of your gown, using sterile gloves or sterile forceps or a drape. *This approach keeps the ties sterile.*
   - Make a three-quarter turn, then take the tie and secure it in front of the gown.
   or
   - Have a coworker wearing sterile gloves take the two ties at each side of the gown and tie them at the back of the gown, making sure that your uniform is completely covered. *Both methods ensure that the back of the gown remains sterile.*
   - When worn, sterile gowns should be considered sterile in front from the waist to the shoulder. The sleeves should be considered sterile from 2 inches above the elbow to the cuff, since the arms of a scrubbed person must move across a sterile field. Moisture collection and friction areas such as the neckline, shoulders, underarms, back, and sleeve cuffs should be considered unsterile.

SAMPLE DOCUMENTATION

[date] [time]	Prior to entering reverse isolation, sterile gown, gloves, and mask applied utilizing proper procedure, and according to institutional protocol.
	_____ P. Morgan, LVN

Special note: *This type of documentation will become more important as hospitals are required by law to report hospital-acquired (nosocomial) infection rates. These rates will be available to the public at large.*

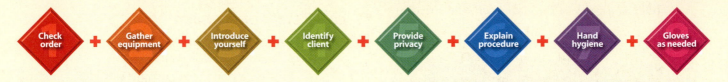

Establishing and Maintaining a Sterile Field

Purpose
■ To maintain the sterility of supplies and equipment

Equipment
■ Package containing a sterile drape
■ Sterile equipment as needed (e.g., wrapped sterile gauze, wrapped sterile bowl, antiseptic solution, sterile forceps)

Check order + Gather equipment + Introduce yourself + Identify client + Provide privacy + Explain procedure + Hand hygiene + Gloves as needed

Interventions

1. Confirm the sterility of the package.
   ■ Ensure that the package is clean and dry. *If moist, it is considered contaminated and must be discarded.*
   ■ Check the sterilization expiration dates on the package, and look for any indications that it has been previously opened.

2. Open the package.

To Open a Wrapped Package on a Surface
■ Place the package in the center of the work area so that the top flap of the wrapper opens away from you. *This position prevents the nurse from subsequently reaching directly over the exposed sterile contents, which could contaminate them.*
■ Reaching around the package (not over it), pinch the first flap on the outside of the wrapper between the thumb and index finger (Figure 9-19 ■). *Touching only the outside of the wrapper maintains the sterility of the inside of the wrapper.* Pull the flap open, laying it flat on the far surface.

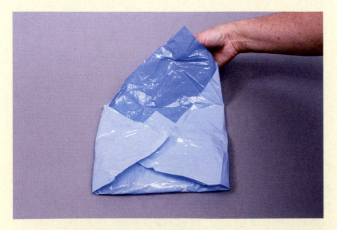

Figure 9-19. ■ Opening the first flap of a sterile, wrapped package. (Al Dodge, Pearson Education/PH.)

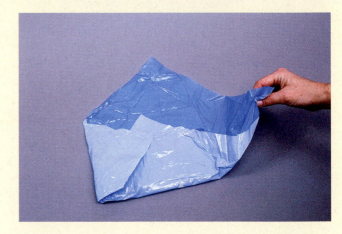

Figure 9-20. ■ Opening the second flap to the side. (Al Dodge, Pearson Education/PH.)

■ Repeat for the side flaps, opening the top one first. Use the right hand for the right flap, and the left hand for the left flap (Figure 9-20 ■). *By using both hands, the nurse avoids reaching over the sterile contents.*
■ Pull the fourth flap toward you by grasping the corner that is turned down (Figure 9-21 ■). Make sure that the flap does not touch any object. *If the inner surface touches any unsterile article, it is contaminated.* Note: One inch along the edges of a sterile package is not considered to be sterile.

To Open a Wrapped Package While Holding It
■ Hold the package in one hand with the top flap opening away from you.
■ Using the other hand, open the package as described above, pulling the corners of the flaps well back and not reaching across the contents of the package

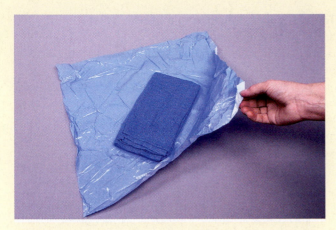

Figure 9-21. ■ Pulling the last flap toward oneself by grasping the corner. (Al Dodge, Pearson Education/PH.)

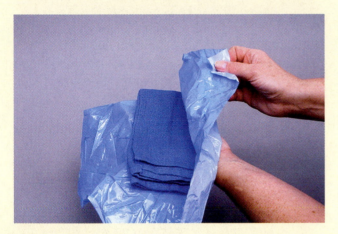

Figure 9-22. ■ Opening a wrapped package while holding it. (Al Dodge, Pearson Education/PH.)

(Figure 9-22 ■). *The hands are considered contaminated, and at no time should they touch the contents of the package.*

To Open Commercially Prepared Packages

Commercially prepared sterile packages and containers usually have manufacturer's directions for opening.

- If the flap of the package has an unsealed corner, hold the package in one hand and pull back on the flap with the other hand (Figure 9-23 ■).

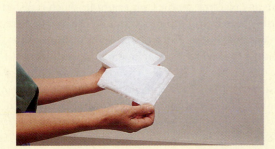

Figure 9-23. ■ Opening a sterile package that has an unsealed corner. (Photographer: Elena Dorfman.)

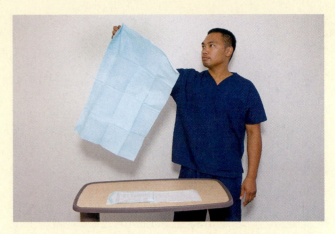

Figure 9-24. ■ Allowing a drape to open freely without touching any objects. (Patrick Watson.)

- If the package has a partially sealed edge, grasp both sides of the edge, one with each hand, and pull apart gently.

3. Establish a sterile field by using a drape.
   - Open the package containing the drape as described in step 2.
   - With one hand, pluck the corner of the drape that is folded back on the top.
   - Lift the drape out of the cover and allow it to open freely without touching any objects (Figure 9-24 ■). *If the drape touches the outside of the package or any unsterile surface or object, it is considered contaminated.*
   - Discard the cover.
   - With the other hand, carefully pick up another corner of the drape, holding it well away from yourself.
   - Lay the drape on a clean and dry surface, placing the bottom (i.e., the freely hanging side) farthest from you (Figure 9-25 ■). *By placing the lowermost side farthest away, the nurse avoids leaning over the sterile field and contaminating it.*

4. Add necessary sterile supplies.

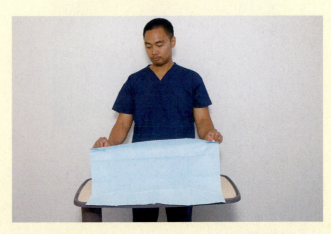

Figure 9-25. ■ Placing a drape on a surface. (Patrick Watson.)

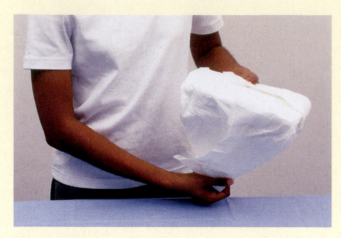

Figure 9-26. ■ Adding wrapped sterile supplies to a sterile field. (Patrick Watson.)

To Add Wrapped Supplies to a Sterile Field

- Open each wrapped package as described in the preceding steps.
- With the free hand, grasp the corners of the wrapper and hold them against the wrist of the other hand (Figure 9-26 ■). *The unsterile hand is now covered by the sterile wrapper.*
- Place the sterile bowl, drape, or other supply on the sterile field by approaching from an angle rather than holding the arm over the field.
- Discard the wrapper.

To Add Commercially Packaged Supplies to a Sterile Field

- Open each package as previously described.
- Hold the package 15 cm (6 in.) above the field and allow the contents to drop on the field (Figure 9-27 ■). *Keep in mind that 2.5 cm (1 in.) around the edge of the field is considered contaminated. At a height of 15 cm (6 in.), the outside of the package is not likely to touch and contaminate the sterile field.*

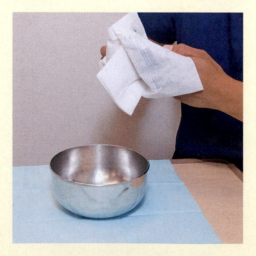

Figure 9-27. ■ Adding commercially packaged gauze to a sterile field. (Patrick Watson.)

To Add Sterile Solution to a Sterile Bowl

Sterile liquids (e.g., normal saline) frequently need to be poured into metal or nonabsorbent containers within a sterile field. *Unwrapped bottles or flasks that contain sterile solution are considered sterile on the inside and contaminated on the outside because the bottle may have been handled. Bottles used in an operating room may be sterilized on the outside as well as the inside, however, and these are handled with sterile gloves.*

- Before pouring any liquid, read the label three times to make sure you have the correct solution and concentration (strength).
- Obtain the exact amount of solution, if possible. *Once a sterile container has been opened, its sterility cannot be ensured for future use unless it is used again immediately.*
- Remove the lid or cap from the bottle and turn the lid upside down before placing it on a surface that is not sterile. *Inverting the lid keeps the inside surface sterile, because it is not allowed to touch an unsterile surface.*
- Hold the bottle at a slight angle so that the label is uppermost. *Any solution that flows down the outside of the bottle during pouring will not damage the label or make it unreadable.*
- Hold the bottle of fluid at a height of 10 to 15 cm (4 to 6 in.) over the bowl and to the side of the sterile field so that as little of the bottle as possible is over the field. *At this height, there is less likelihood of contaminating the sterile field by touching the field or by reaching an arm over it.*
- Pour the solution gently to avoid splashing the liquid. *If the sterile drape is on an unsterile surface, moisture will contaminate the field by allowing the movement of microorganisms through the sterile drape.*
- Replace the lid securely on the bottle if you plan to use it again, and provide the date and time of opening according to agency policy. *Replacing the lid immediately maintains the sterility of the inner aspect of the lid and the solution. In many agencies, a sterile container of solution that is opened is used only once and then discarded.*

5. Use sterile forceps to handle certain sterile supplies. Forceps are commonly used for such techniques as changing a sterile dressing and shortening a drain. Transfer forceps are usually used to move a sterile article from one place to another, for example, when transferring sterile gauze from its package to a sterile dressing tray. Forceps may be discarded or resterilized after use. Commonly used forceps include hemostats or artery forceps (Figure 9-28 ■) and tissue forceps (Figure 9-29 ■).

- Keep the tips of wet forceps lower than the wrist at all times, unless you are wearing sterile gloves (Figure 9-30 ■). *Gravity prevents liquids on the tips of the forceps from flowing to the handles and later back to the tips, thus making the forceps unsterile. The handles are unsterile once they are held by the bare hand.*

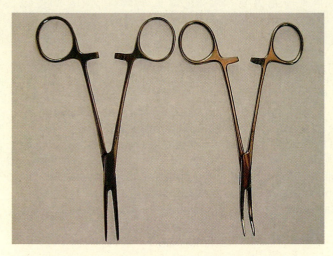

Figure 9-28. ■ Hemostats. (Alexandra Truitt & Terry Marshall.)

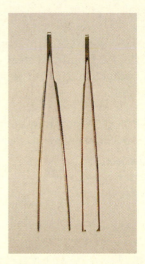

Figure 9-29. ■ Tissue forceps. (Alexandra Truitt & Terry Marshall.)

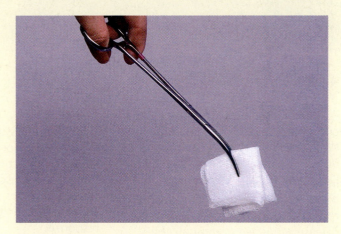

Figure 9-30. ■ Holding forceps with an ungloved hand, keeping the tips lower than the wrist. (Al Dodge, Pearson Education/PH.)

■ Hold sterile forceps above waist level. *Items held below waist level are considered contaminated.*

■ Hold sterile forceps within sight. *While out of sight, forceps may, unknown to the user, become unsterile. Any forceps that go out of sight should be considered unsterile.*

■ When using forceps to lift sterile supplies out of a commercially prepared package, be sure that the forceps do not touch the edges or outside of the wrapper. *The edges and outside of the package are exposed to the air and handled and are thus unsterile.*

■ When placing forceps whose handles were in contact with the bare hand, position the handles outside the sterile area. *The handles of these forceps harbor microorganisms from the bare hand.*

■ Deposit a sterile item on a sterile field without permitting moist forceps to touch the sterile field when the surface under the absorbent sterile field is unsterile and a barrier drape is not used. *A barrier drape is resistant to moisture (e.g., blood and antiseptics) and should be used whenever a procedure involves the use of liquids. Made of chemically treated cotton or synthetic materials, barrier drapes prevent a sterile field from becoming unsterile when the drape becomes wet. If the underlying surface is sterile (e.g., a plastic container), the field will not become unsterile when moist.*

SAMPLE DOCUMENTATION

[date]
[time]
A sterile field was set up according to hospital protocol using aseptic technique for abdominal wound irrigation and dressing change.

_____ M. Stuart, LVN

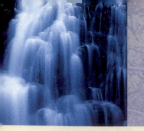

Chapter Review

KEY TERMS by Topic

Use the audio glossary feature of either the CD-ROM or the Companion Website to hear the correct pronunciation of the following key terms.

Microorganisms
bacteria, viruses, fungi, parasites, resident flora, infection, pathogens, disease, virulence, communicable disease, vector

Infection
local infection, systemic infection, septicemia, nosocomial infections, iatrogenic infection, carrier, reservoir, transmission, susceptible host, non-specific defenses, specific defenses, antigens, immunity, inflammatory response

Controlling Microorganisms in the Environment
antiseptics, disinfectants, bactericidal agent, bacteriostatic agent, asepsis, sepsis, aseptic technique, medical asepsis, surgical asepsis, Standard Precautions, Transmission-based Precautions

Nursing Care
sterile field

KEY Points

- Microorganisms are everywhere in our environment and in or on our body. Most of them are harmless and perform essential functions.

- Infections are invasions and growth of microorganisms in a body tissue or organ.

- Microorganisms are different in their strength and communicability.

- The medical and nursing communities use aseptic technique to prevent the transfer of microorganisms from one place or person to another.

- Nosocomial infections occur as a result of healthcare delivery in a healthcare setting.

- The chain of infection is composed of six links, all of which must be present to cause the infectious process.

- Specific defenses are immune defenses and work against identified foreign proteins and other infectious agents.

- Age is a factor that affects the risk of infection. Both the very young and the elderly have reduced defenses.

- Cleaning, disinfecting, and sterilizing are proven ways of inhibiting the growth and multiplication of microorganisms and of maintaining the environment.

- Isolation practices that protect the patient, the healthcare provider, and others are initiated after assessing the patient's condition. They are practiced according to institutional policies and the recommendations of the CDC.

- If there is any doubt about sterility, the object or field is unsterile.

EXPLORE MediaLink

Additional interactive resources for this chapter can be found on the Companion Website at www.prenhall.com/ramont. Click on Chapter 9 and "Begin" to select the activities for this chapter.

For chapter-related NCLEX®-style questions and an audio glossary, access the accompanying CD-ROM in this book.

Animations/Videos
- Gloving Techniques
- Handwashing & Gloving

FOR FURTHER Study

For more information on wound healing, see Chapter 23.

For more information on obtaining different types of cultures, see Chapters 23, 24, 27, and 28.

Chapter 24 provides information about oxygenation.

For further information about nutrition in healing, see Chapter 25.

For more about disposal of sharps, see Chapter 29.

Critical Thinking Care Map

Caring for a Client with a Stasis Ulcer

NCLEX-PN® Focus Area: Physiological Integrity

Case Study: George Gower has been admitted to the hospital with an open wound from an arterial stasis ulcer on his inner right lower leg. The wound has increased in size and is now draining small amounts of yellow/green secretions. There is a foul odor. The WBC count is elevated and he has an oral temperature of 101°F.

Nursing Diagnosis: Risk for Infection

COLLECT DATA

Subjective	Objective
_____	_____
_____	_____
_____	_____
_____	_____
_____	_____
_____	_____

Would you report this data? Yes/No

If yes, to: _____

What would you report? _____

Nursing Care

_____

_____

_____

_____

_____

_____

_____

_____

_____

_____

_____

How would you document this? _____

_____

_____

Data Collected
(use those that apply)

- Complains of burning pain in area of wound
- Yellow/green secretions
- Foul odor from wound and secretions
- Poor pedal pulses
- Says his foot is cold
- States elevating his foot hurts his hip
- Edema around wound, and feet are swollen
- Feet appear slightly cyanotic
- Says he has not washed right leg in several days
- States he left wound open because "air is good for it"

Nursing Interventions
(use those that apply; list in priority order)

- Administer analgesics as ordered by physician.
- Report poor pedal pulses and edema.
- Look for hazards in the environment.
- Consult with physical therapist about positioning.
- Cleanse wound and apply wound dressings as ordered.
- Keep feet warm.
- Elevate feet.
- Keep the leg uncovered.
- Put feet in a dependent position.
- Teach patient about airborne contamination.
- Consult with dietitian regarding diet.
- Keep the leg immobilized.

Compare your documentation to the sample provided in Appendix I.

NCLEX-PN® Exam Preparation

1 A man has a history of a draining wound infection in his lower right leg. He was admitted with a wet, soiled dressing and the following vital signs: T 100.6, P 90, R 20, BP 136/70. A nursing priority would be:

1. elevation of the right leg.
2. placing the person in isolation.
3. medicating the patient for an elevated temperature.
4. changing the wound dressing.

2 A client was admitted with active tuberculosis with moderate amounts of pink-tinged sputum. She was placed in isolation. The nurse knows that the type of isolation initiated would:

1. be Tier 1 or Standard Precautions.
2. be Tier 2 or Transmission-based Precautions.
3. include only the use of clean gowns.
4. require the use of masks by the client while in the room.

3 The nurse is assisting the physician by preparing the sterile tray. She knew sterility of the tray must be maintained at all times. During the process the nurse:

1. used sterile forceps while reaching across the tray to move the contents around.
2. wore clean gloves to handle the contents of the tray.
3. allowed the open tray to stand unattended for a period of 20 minutes and then covered it with a towel.
4. put on sterile gloves to handle the contents of the tray.

4 A child was admitted with pneumonia and placed in isolation. The exact organism had not yet been identified. The family was instructed to take all clothing and extra toys home. Client education for the parents would include:

1. instructing them to wash all the clothing and toys in very hot water before putting them away.
2. throwing all the clothes and toys away.
3. telling them nothing special needed to be done to the clothing and toys.
4. "airing" the clothes and toys to destroy the organisms.

5 A client with infectious tuberculosis needed to go to the radiology department for a chest x-ray. The nurse was aware that appropriate nursing care included:

1. calling the radiology department and telling them the client was still in isolation.
2. covering the client with a blanket and providing tissues.
3. telling the transport person to wear a mask for protection.
4. putting a mask and gloves on the client to prevent the spread of organisms.

6 After administering care to a client, the nurse removes a tray of soiled instruments from the room, and "bags" the materials. Some of the items were metal, while others were made of plastic. The nurse knew that:

1. everything could be placed into one bag as long as it was labeled properly.
2. the metal items must be bagged and sent for autoclaving, and the plastic items could be disposed.
3. the items must be separated into plastic in one bag for gas sterilization, and metal into another to be autoclaved.
4. The type of bag did not matter as long as it was labeled "isolation."

7 A client who was admitted with pneumonia and placed in isolation has a history of HIV+ (AIDS). Before leaving the room, the nurse will remove all soiled personal protective equipment. The nurse knew the order of removal was:

1. remove the gown, then mask, then gloves.
2. take off the mask, the gloves, and then the gown.
3. remove the gloves, then the mask, and finally the gown.
4. take off the gown first, then either the mask or gloves.

8 An 82-year-old client with a history of emphysema was being seen for a possible upper respiratory tract infection (URI). Several family members had been ill with colds during the previous week. The nurse is aware that the client may be considered:

1. a susceptible host.
2. a compromised host.
3. to be in no special danger of the infection since the family was ill last week.
4. to have a chronic URI.

9 You have been assigned to the infectious control committee. The committee is discussing hand hygiene recommendations. Of the following guidelines suggested for implementation, which one demonstrates an understanding of the CDC's recommendations?

1. Healthcare providers will wear gloves (nonlatex) when practicing Standard Precautions. Studies have shown that the overuse and misuse of latex gloves has lead to healthcare workers developing latex allergy or sensitivity.
2. Disinfecting hands following glove removal is not necessary.
3. Waterless hand cleaner is effective on hands that are not visibly soiled with blood and body fluids.
4. Waterless alcohol-based hand cleaner must be removed with paper towels in order to remove pathogens from hands. No artificial finger nails or extensions are permitted to be worn by healthcare workers.

10 A clinic client had already developed an inflammatory response in the area of a wound on the left hand. The nurse knew this was an appropriate observation when he noted:

1. the client complaining of itching around the area of the wound.
2. a moderate amount of drainage weeping from the wound.
3. swelling, redness, and heat around the wound.
4. bruising around the wound.

Answers and Rationales for Review Questions, as well as discussion of Care Plan and Critical Thinking Care Map questions, appear in Appendix I.

Chapter 10

Admission, Transfer, and Discharge

BRIEF Outline

Admitting a Client
Transferring a Client
Discharging a Client

LEARNING Outcomes

After completing this chapter, you will be able to:

1. Discuss the common reactions that a client might have to the admission, transfer, and discharge processes.
2. Describe the environment in which the client may experience dehumanization.
3. Describe the procedural steps for admission, transfer, and discharge.
4. Discuss how the nursing process applies to admission, transfer, and discharge.
5. Discuss the importance of discharge planning.
6. Explain the nurse's responsibility related to discharge instructions.

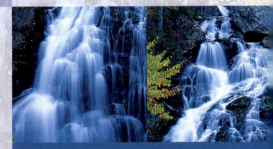

HISTORICAL Perspectives

Since April 14, 2003, regulations related to client privacy and ranging from admission to discharge have been governed by federal law. The Health Insurance Portability and Accountability Act (HIPAA) of 1996 not only provided for health insurance to follow an employee from one employer to the next, it also sent down strict guidelines for maintaining client privacy and confidentiality. Nurses ethically have always striven to protect clients' privacy, but with the institution of the HIPAA, all healthcare providers are required to follow the regulations.

Everyone, during the course of a lifetime, experiences changes in health status. At times, these changes will require medical treatment in a hospital or other healthcare facility. The person in need of such medical care, the client, will be admitted, possibly transferred, and eventually discharged from the hospital or other healthcare setting.

This chapter addresses the processes of admission, transfer, and discharge of clients in these settings. It also includes the responsibilities of the nurse in helping clients through these processes successfully, with caring attention to all clients' needs and concerns. Many research studies conducted in healthcare settings demonstrate that nursing care, and specifically the quality of the client–nurse interaction, is a part of medical treatment that affects clients' health status.

The goal of nursing care is to ensure the continuity of individualized client care during admission, transfer, and discharge. The nursing process (see Chapter 5 🔗) is used as a framework for achieving these objectives. In this chapter, the nursing process is applied in the discussion of each section: admission, transfer, and discharge.

Admitting a Client

COMMON RESPONSES TO HOSPITAL ADMISSION

Hospital admission is entry into the hospital. It is usually a very stressful time for a client and his or her family or significant others. The nurses who initially provide assistance with admission and orientation will influence the client's reaction to hospitalization and treatment. Therefore, it is important to make a positive first impression. Each individual client deserves to be greeted in a caring manner that demonstrates concern and respect.

The **admission** process elicits many different responses from clients. Clients' responses, although unique, are influenced by their particular gender, age, culture, religion, and **coping behaviors** (behaviors such as crying, acting angry, sexual "acting out," overeating, or smoking, which people perform in times of crisis or stress in an attempt to deal with their feelings). The client's responses are also related to needs identified by Maslow (see Figure 5-4 🔗 and discussion in Chapter 11 🔗).

Two of the most common responses to hospital admission are anxiety and fear of the unknown. Clients already are vulnerable to these responses because of the medical need for which they are entering the hospital. Anxiety causes emotional discomfort. It may have physical effects as well, such as an increase in vital signs. Fear of the unknown causes a sense of insecurity. Clients can be helped to feel more secure by reassuring them that their needs will be met promptly and their questions answered thoroughly.

Unfortunately, the healthcare environment promotes **dehumanization** (removal of unique human qualities) by asking clients to surrender their belongings, privacy, and independence. A loss of self-identity occurs when individuals are referred to as a number, a diagnosis, or a nickname or when they are called by their first name without having given permission. Children have other anxieties and fears that may be expressed during the admission process. For example, they are likely to experience separation anxiety if their parents are not allowed to stay with them throughout the admission procedures.

It is the nurse's responsibility to help protect the client from feeling dehumanized by anticipating and avoiding situations that are likely to provoke these feelings. In addition, the nurse must strive to help reduce the specific fears and anxieties of each client. The client's integrity and personal dignity must always be maintained (see Chapter 33 🔗).

CULTURAL CONSIDERATIONS

Culture is a set of learned attitudes and behaviors associated with particular values, ethnic traditions, and religious beliefs. Clients come from many different cultures, and so have a variety of attitudes and beliefs related to illness and medical treatment. Clients' views about health care and their behavior during hospitalization may be expressions of their cultural beliefs. Often, the client's views are different from the nurse's view. Regardless of the cultural differences between the nurse and the client, it is the nurse's obligation to provide culturally sensitive care (see Chapter 2 🔗).

Suggestions for communicating with culturally diverse clients during admission, transfer, and discharge procedures include the following:

1. Address clients by their last name. In some cultures, the informal use of first names is offensive. It is best to ask clients how they wish to be addressed.
2. Respect the clients' values and beliefs about health care and illness.
3. Use culturally sensitive language (this may include the term *African American* instead of *black, gay* or *lesbian* instead of *homosexual,* etc.). Take your cues from the client.
4. Use clear, common English. The use of slang is usually not appropriate.
5. If a language barrier exists, find an interpreter. According to Joint Commission on Accreditation of Healthcare Organizations (JCAHO) standards, the interpreter should be a medical professional to avoid miscommunication. Family members should not be relied on to interpret medical information.

Further steps to improve cultural sensitivity are discussed in detail in Chapter 2 🔗.

ADMISSION PROCEDURE GUIDELINES

Each healthcare facility has its own policies concerning admission procedures. Immediately upon entering the hospital, the client usually goes to the admitting office, where clerical personnel start the admission process. However, clients may also be admitted directly from the emergency department or physician's office.

The client's medical record is initiated in the admitting department (Figure 10-1 ■). It usually includes demographic data, such as age, gender, birthday, Social Security number, next of kin, and insurance information. At this time, clients are usually informed about their legal rights. Forms for durable power of attorney and do-not-resuscitate (DNR) orders are presented. The client may sign or waive them, but most facilities require that these forms be in the client's file. If the person does not sign the forms, a notation is made to document that the client waived the signature (see more about legal issues in Chapter 3 ⚭).

The admitting clerk places an identification bracelet on the client's arm. The bracelet is worn throughout the client's stay in the facility. Clients who have allergies will also need to have an additional armband. Some facilities have specific armbands, for example, to denote DNR status. Check with the facility to be sure that all necessary identification requirements have been met. When all appropriate information has been collected and the client is ready to be transferred to a room, the admitting personnel notify the nurse or unit clerk. The client is usually transported to the nursing unit by wheelchair.

The nurse should prepare the room before the client arrives on the unit. A room that is neat and clean, with good lighting, appropriate temperature, and equipped with basic supplies makes a client feel welcome and safe. When the client arrives on the unit, he or she should be greeted warmly and with a smile. The greeting is a way to begin the client–nurse relationship on a positive note.

Client Privacy

Hospitals and health systems are responsible for protecting the privacy and confidentiality of their clients and client information. The Health Insurance Portability and Accountability Act (HIPAA) of 1996 mandated regulations that govern privacy standards for healthcare information. HIPAA regulations specify the purposes for which information may and may not be released without authorization from the client. These regulations have been in effect since April 2003. Failure to comply with these regulations can result in fines being levied against the facility and in some cases against individuals. It is important that all hospital personnel, including nursing students, understand and adhere to these federal regulations. Refer to Table 10-1 ■ for a summary of client information that can be released.

Hospitals and other healthcare facilities usually have a staff member or department that handles the disbursement of information. All inquiries from nonfamily members for client information should be referred to that individual or department. The individual may have a title such as public information officer. Note that information also cannot be given to family or friends without the client's permission. This permission may be a formal document such as a durable power of attorney for health care or informally when a client gives permission for the individual during discussion of treatment or prognosis.

Exercise good judgment in situations where clients cannot express a preference for release of information. In some cases, clients will not have had the opportunity to state a preference related to the release of their information. For example, a client's medical condition may prevent hospital staff from asking about information preferences upon admission. In those circumstances, condition and location information should be released only if, *in the hospital's professional judgment,* releasing such information would be in the client's best interest. As soon as the client recovers sufficiently, the hospital must ask about information preferences. Each hospital should develop policies and procedures to guide staff in making these judgments.

When a client has opted out of the hospital directory (the information as to client's name and room number available through the hospital operator) by requesting information not be included, the hospital should not say that it has no information on the client or that it is unable to confirm the client's presence in the facility, since the media may then infer that the client is at the hospital. Under the HIPAA medical privacy rule, a hospital is permitted to release only directory information (i.e., the client's one-word condition {see Table 10-1} and location) to individuals who inquire about the client by name unless the client has requested that information be withheld. In response to a media inquiry about a client who has opted out of the directory, therefore, the hospital should respond by stating that the federal medical privacy regulations allow the hospital to release to the media only the information in the hospital's directory and that the hospital does not have any information about the person in its directory.

Client privacy can be protected (1) by making sure discussions between healthcare professionals are not conducted in public areas, (2) by keeping medical records and forms such as flow sheets in the nurses' station, and (3) by not posting clients' names where they can be viewed by visitors (e.g., scheduling on assignment board). Facilities who use computerized medical records are required to have safeguards in place. Computer screens should be obscured from view. Passwords must be secure, and users should always log out before leaving the computer.

ADMISSION DATA

Date _4-16-07_ Time _3:15p.m._ Primary Language _English_

Arrived Via: ☐ Wheelchair ☐ Stretcher ☑ Ambulatory

From: ☐ Admitting ☐ ER ☑ Home ☐ Nursing Home ☐ Other

Admitting M.D. _R. Katz_   Time Notified _5 p.m._

ORIENTATION TO UNIT

	YES	NO		YES	NO
Arm Band Correct	☑	☐	Visiting Hours	☑	☐
Alllergy Band	☑	☐	Smoking Policy	☑	☐
Telephone	☑	☐	TV, Lights, Bed Controls,		
Electrical Policy	☑	☐	Call Lights, Side Rails	☑	☐
Educational Mat©	☑	☐	Nurses Station	☑	☐
(TV Brochure)	☑	☐			

Family M.D. _R. Katz_

Weight _125 lb._ Height _5ft. 2in._   BP:R __ L _122 / 80_

Temp. _103F_ Pulse _92, weak_ Resp. _28, shallow_

Source Providing Information ☑ Patient ☐ Other____

Unable to Obtain History ☐

Reason for Admission (Onset, Duration, Pt. Ⓢ Perception) _"Chest cold" X2 weeks S.O.B. on exertion. "Lung pain, fever." "Dr. says I have pneumonia."_

ALLERGIES & REACTIONS

Drugs _Penicillin_

Food/Other ____

Signs & symptoms _Rash, nausea_

Blood Reaction ☐ Yes ☑ No   Dyes/Shellfish ☐ Yes ☑ No

MEDICATIONS

Current Meds	Dose/Freq.	Last Dose
Synthroid	0.1 mg. daily	4-16, 8 a.m.

Disposition of Meds: ☑ Home ☐ Pharmacy ☐ Safe *At Bedside

MEDICAL HISTORY

☑ No Major Problems   ☐ Gastro____
☐ Cardiac____   ☐ Arthritis____
☐ Hyper/Hypotension____   ☐ Stroke____
☐ Diabetes____   ☐ Seizures____
☐ Cancer____   ☐ Glaucoma____
☐ Respiratory____   ☑ Other _Childbirth - 1998_

Surgery/Procedures	Date
Appendectomy	1988
Partial thyroidectomy	2001

SPECIAL ASSISTIVE DEVICES

☐ Wheelchair ☐ Contacts ☐ Venous   ☐ Dentures
☐ Braces   ☐ Hearing Aid Access   ☐ Partial
☐ Cane/Crutches ☐ Prosthesis Device   ☐ Upper
☐ Walker   ☐ Glasses ☐ Epidural Catheter ☐ Lower
☐ Other _None_

VALUABLES

Client informed Hospital not responsible for personal belongings.

Valuables Disposition: ☐ Client ☐ Safe ☐ Given to____

Client/SO Signature _None_

PSYCHOSOCIAL HISTORY

Recent Stress _None_

Coping Mechanism _Not assessed because of fatigue_

Support System _Husband, coworkers, friends_

Calm: ☑ Yes ☐ No____

Anxious: _Facial muscles tense; trembling_

Religion _Catholic, would want Last Rites_

Tobacco Use: ☐ Yes ☑ No____

Alcohol Use: ☐ Yes ☑ No____

Drug Use: ☐ Yes ☑ No____

NEUROLOGICAL

Oriented: ☑ Person ☑ Place ☑ Time ☐ Confused ☐ Sedated
☐ Alert ☐ Restless ☑ Lethargic ☐ Comatose

Pupils: ☑ Equal ☐ Unequal ☑ Reactive ☐ Sluggish
☐ Other _3mm._

Extremity Strength: ☑ Equal ☐ Unequal

Speech: ☑ Clear ☐ Slurred ☐ Other____

MUSCULO-SKELETAL

Normal ROM of Extremities ☑ Yes ☐ No
☑ Weakness ☐ Paralysis ☐ Contractures ☐ Joint swelling ☑ Pain
☐ Other ↓ _related to fatigue_   _when coughing_

RESPIRATORY

Pattern: ☐ Even ☐ Uneven ☑ Shallow ☑ Dyspnea
☑ Other _diminished breath sounds_

Breathing Sounds: ☐ Clear ☑ Other _inspiratory crackles_

Secretions: ☐ None ☑ Other _pink, thick sputum_

Cough: ☐ None ☑ Productive ☐ Nonproductive

CARDIOVASCULAR

Pulses: Apical Rate _92-W_ ☑ Reg. ☐ Irregular ☐ Pacemaker
S = Strong W = Weak A = Absent D = Doppler

Radial R _92_ L __ Pedal R __ L __

Edema: ☑ Absent ☐ Present Site____

Perfusion: ☐ Warm ☐ Dry ☑ Diaphoretic ☐ Cool (Hot)

GASTROINTESTINAL

Oral Mucosa ☐ Normal ☑ Other _pale and dry_

Bowel Sounds: ☑ Normal ☐ Other _Abd. soft_

Wt. Change ☐ ☑ N/V Stool Frequency/Character _1/day soft_

Last B/M _4-15-07_ ☐ Ostomy (type)____

Equip.____

GENITOURINARY

Urine: Last Voided _This morning_

☐ Normal ☐ Anuria ☐ Hematuria ☐ Dysuri ☐ Incontinent
☑ Other ↓ _amount & frequency since ill_
☐ Catheter (type)____ Other____

LMP _4-1-07_ ☐ Vaginal/Penile Discharge

Other____

SELF CARE

Need Assist with: ☐ Ambulating ☐ Elimination
☐ Meals ☑ Hygiene ☐ Dressing
while fatigued

Amanda Aquilini [F. age 28]
_#4637651_

☆ NORTH BROWARD HOSPITAL DISTRICT
NURSING ADMINISTRATION ASSESSMENT

Figure 10-1. ■ Adult admission assessment. (*Source:* Courtesy of North Broward Hospital District.)

NUTRITION

General Appearance: ☑ Well Nourished ☐ Emaciated
☐ Other _____

Appetite: ☐ Good ☐ Fair ☑ Poor - *X2 days*

Diet _Liquid_ Meal Pattern _3/day_
☐ Feeds Self ☐ Assist ☐ Total Feed

SKIN ASSESSMENT

Color: ☐ Normal ☐ Flushed ☑ Pale ☐ Dusky ☐ Cyanotic
☐ Jaundiced ☑ Other _Cheeks flushed, hot_

General Description _Surgical scars;_
RLQ abdomen; anterior neck

_____
_____
_____
_____

Note Cultures Obtained _____
_____
_____

PRESSURE SORE "AT RISK" SCREENING CRITERIA

OVERALL SKIN CONDITION
Grade
- 0 Turgor (elasticity adequate, skin warm and moist)
- ☑1 Poor turgor, skin cold & dry
- 2 Areas mottled, red or denuded
- 3 Existing skin ulcer/lesions

BOWEL AND BLADDER CONTROL
Grade
- ☑0 Always able to ask for bedpan
- 1 Incontinence of urine
- 2 Incontinence of feces
- 3 Totally incontinent Confined to bed

REHABILITATIVE STATE
Grade
- 0 Fully ambulatory
- ☑1 Ambulated with assistance
- 2 Chair to bed ambulation only
- 3 Confined to bed
- 4 Immobile in bed

NUTRITIONAL STATE
Grade
- 0 Eats all
- ☑1 Eats very little
- 2 Refuses food often
- 2 Tube feeding
- 4 Intravenous feeding

MENTAL STATE
Grade
- ☑0 Alert and clear
- 1 Confused
- 2 Disoriented/senile
- 3 Stuporous
- 4 Unconscious

CHRONIC DISEASE STATUS (i.e. COPD, ASCVD. Peripheral Vascular Disease, Diabetes, or Renal Disease, Cancer, Motor or Sensory Deficits, Elderly, Other)
Grade
- ☑0 Absent
- 1 One Present
- 2 Two Present
- 3 Three or more Present

TOTAL _____ Refer to Skin Care Protocol

FALLS SCREENING

If one or more of the following are checked institute fall precautions/plan of care
☐ History of Falls ☐ Unsteady Gait ☐ Confusion/Disorientation ☐ Dizziness

If two or more of the following are checked institute fall precautions/plan of care
☐ Age over 80 ☐ Utilizes cane, walker, w/c ☐ Sleeplessness
☐ Impaired vision ☐ Urgency/frequency in elimination
☐ Multiple Diagnoses ☐ Impaired hearing
☐ Inability to understand or follow directions ☐ Medication/Sedative /Diuretic etc.

NURSE SIGNATURE/TITLE	DATE	TIME
Mary Medina, RN	[date]	[time]
NURSE SIGNATURE/TITLE	**DATE**	**TIME**

EDUCATION/DISCHARGE PLANNING

1. What do you know about your present illness? _"Dr. says I have pneumonia." "I will have an I.V."_
2. What information do you want or need about your illness?
3. Would you like family/SO involved in your care? _Husband, Michael_
4. How long do you expect to be in the hospital? _"1-2 days_
5. What concerns do you have about leaving the hospital?—

CHECK APPROPRIATE BOX

Will client need post discharge assistance with ADLs/physical functioning? ☐ Yes ☑ No ☐ Unknown

Does client have family capable of and willing to provide assistance post dishcarge?
☑ Yes ☐ No ☐ Unknown ☐ No family

Is assistance needed beyond that which family can provide?
☐ Yes ☑ No ☐ Unknown

Previous admission in the last six months?
☐ Yes ☑ No ☐ Unknown

Client lives with _Husband and child_
Planned discharge to _Home_
Comments _Fatigue and anxiety may have interfered with learning. Re-teach anything covered at admission later._

Social Services Notified ☐ Yes ☑ No

ADVANCE DIRECTIVES:

Does client have a Living Will? ☑ Yes ☐ No If Yes, please obtain a copy for the medical record. If unable to obtain a copy, document intent of Advace Directive in the medical record. Please refer to Interdisciplinary Patient/Family Education Record for documentation of Education regarding Advance Directives/Living Will.

Is the client an Organ Donor? ☑ Yes ☐ No If no, explain in progress notes.

If "No", provided information on organ donation ☐ Yes ☐ No

NARRATIVE NOTES

S--c/O sharp chest pain when coughing and dyspnea on exertion. States unable to carry out regular daily exercise for past week. Coughing relieved "if I sit up and sit still." Nausea associated with coughing. Having occasional "chills." Occasionally becomes frightened stating, "I can't breathe." Well groomed but "too tired to put on make-up."

O--Chest expansion < 3cm, no nasal flaring or use of accessory muscles. Breath sounds and insp. crackles in ® upper and lower chest.

Assesses own supports as "good" (e.g., relationship c husband). Is "worried" about daughter. States husband will be out of town until tomorrow. Left 3-year-old daughter with neighbor. Concerned too about her work (is attorney). "I'll never get caught up." Had water at noon—no food today. Informed of need to save urine for 24 hr. specimen. IV D5W LR 1000 mL started in ® arm, 100 mL/hr. Slow capillary refill. Keeping head of bed ↑ to facilitate breathing.

⁂ NORTH BROWARD HOSPITAL DISTRICT
NURSING ADMINISTRATION ASSESSMENT

Figure 10-1. ■ (continued)

TABLE 10-1

HIPAA Information Distribution Rules

INFORMATION CATEGORY	INFORMATION THAT CAN BE RELEASED WITHOUT PERMISSION	TO WHOM INFORMATION CAN BE RELEASED	CONDITIONS FOR INFORMATION RELEASE	NO INFORMATION CAN BE GIVEN
Condition and location of clients	General condition; location such as inpatient, outpatient, or emergency department	Any inquirer including the press	Released only if inquirer identifies client *specifically* by name	If the client requests that the information not be released
Inquiry from clergy	Client's name and location; religion (names of all clients of a particular religious affiliation can be given to an affiliated clergy member)	HIPAA gives specific permission to clergy	Clergy do not have to identify client by name	Hospitals are not required to ask about clients' religious affiliations, and clients do not have to supply that information
One-word condition and location	One-word condition; use the terms *undetermined, good, fair, serious,* or *critical*	To an individual who identifies client by name or to clergy	N/A	Without obtaining prior client authorization
Death of a client	Information about the cause of death must come from the client's physician, and a legal representative of the deceased must approve its release	To the authorities by the hospital, as required by law	Public information about a death will be disclosed after efforts have been made to notify the next-of-kin	Hospitals cannot share information with the media on the specifics about sudden, violent, or accidental deaths, or deaths from natural causes without the permission of the decedent's next-of-kin or other legal representative
Obstetric client	Confirm that the client is in labor and delivery or has been released from labor and delivery	Information can be released to individual who identifies client by name.	This is more information than general condition. So information cannot be released.	Without individual authorization, unless the disclosure is to family members or friends involved in the client's care or payment for the client's care
Client treated and released	A hospital may disclose, to individuals who ask for the client by name, that a client was treated and released because this only provides the client's general condition (that they were treated at the hospital) and the client's location (that the client is no longer at the hospital)	No specific health information is provided	Information, however, can be released to the client's family members or friends involved in the client's care, as long as the client has not opted out of such disclosures and such information is relevant to the person's involvement in the client's care	Although a hospital may disclose that a client was treated and released (with regard to the client's location—or lack thereof—in the hospital), it may not release information regarding the date of release or where the client went upon release without client authorization
Media access to client	Drafting a detailed statement (i.e., anything beyond the one-word condition) for approval by the client or the client's legal representative ■ Taking photographs of clients	Press or broadcast media	Require written authorization from the client	If the client is a minor, permission for any of these activities must be obtained from a parent or legal guardian. Under certain circumstances, minors can authorize disclosure of information

TABLE 10-1				
HIPAA Information Distribution Rules (*continued*)				
INFORMATION CATEGORY	INFORMATION THAT CAN BE RELEASED WITHOUT PERMISSION	TO WHOM INFORMATION CAN BE RELEASED	CONDITIONS FOR INFORMATION RELEASE	NO INFORMATION CAN BE GIVEN
	■ Interviewing clients			without parental approval or notification. State laws may vary
Information that could embarrass or endanger clients	Situations where room location information could embarrass clients include (but are not limited to) admission to a psychiatric or substance abuse unit; admission to an obstetrics unit following a miscarriage, ectopic pregnancy, or other adverse outcome; or admission to an isolation room for treatment of an infectious disease	Any inquirer	Be aware that federal laws prohibit hospitals from releasing any information regarding a client undergoing treatment for alcohol or substance abuse	Knowledge of a client's location could potentially endanger that individual (i.e., the hospital has knowledge of a stalker or abusive partner). No information of any kind should be given, including confirmation of the client's presence at the facility.

Orientation

All new clients are oriented to the hospital unit. **Orientation** is the introduction of clients to the people and the facility into which they have been admitted. It starts with the nurse introducing himself or herself and explaining the roles of the staff who will care for the client. If the client is in a semiprivate room, the roommate is also introduced. Important elements to include in the orientation are listed in Box 10-1 ■.

Client's Valuables and Clothing

Clients might bring jewelry, money, credit cards, prescription medications, and other valuables with them to the hospital. During the admission process they should be instructed to give those items to a family member to take home. If this is not possible, the valuables can usually be stored in the hospital safe. The hospital's policy for storing personal items should be explained carefully to the client and family. An inventory with a general description of each item (such as a "gold-colored ring with a clear stone," instead of "gold diamond ring") should be documented on the proper forms required by the hospital (Figure 10-2 ■). The client and a designated member of the hospital staff must sign these forms.

The client may keep personal items such as clothing, glasses, contact lenses, dentures, and hearing aids in the room. These items must also be listed on the inventory sheet. When forms are completed and signed, a copy is given to the client and a copy is placed in the client's medical record.

BOX 10-1	NURSING CARE CHECKLIST

Orienting a Client on Admission

When admitting a person to a facility, the nurse should provide the following information and instructions:

☑ The location of the room in relation to the nurse's desk

☑ How to use the intercom system

☑ How to call the nurse's station from the bed and bathroom

☑ How to use the phone

☑ How to adjust the bed (The bed should always be in the low position when the client enters.)

☑ How to operate the television

☑ Location of the bathroom

☑ How to adjust the lights

☑ Times at which meals are served

☑ Location of personal care items

☑ Hospital policies that apply to the clients, such as visiting times

☑ A gown and instructions on how to wear it (if the client doesn't have a gown or pajamas); assist client to change if necessary

☑ Explanation of why an identification band is necessary

☑ Information about when laboratory or other diagnostic tests will be performed

☑ Information about when the physician usually visits

Valuables		
Cash		
Currency		Coins
Watch and Jewelry		
Wallet		
Keys		
Driver's License		
Insurance Cards		
Credit Cards		
Documents		
Admitting Dept Use	Date Time	Received by
Disposition of Valuables	Client/Designate Signature Date	
	Witness Signature Date	

Envelope No.
This facility assumes **NO RESPONSIBILITY** for the loss or damage of personal property not enclosed within the envelope
Client Identification

Client Valuables Record

Adapted from form courtesy of Community Hospital of Lancaster, PA

Figure 10-2. ■ Excerpt from client's valuables record. (*Source:* Courtesy of Community Hospital of Lancaster.)

NURSING CARE

ASSESSING

The initial assessment should be started once the client is settled into the room. The JCAHO requires that a registered nurse perform the admission assessment. Subjective and objective data are collected throughout the interview, medical history, and physical assessment. However, the RN may delegate parts of the assessment to the LPN/LVN. This may include baseline information such as level of consciousness, vital signs, skin condition, height and weight, bowel sounds, lung sounds, specimen collection, and clarification of the client's questions and concerns. The collected data are then organized, prioritized, and reviewed. They are used to construct nursing diagnoses and to identify areas in which the client may need teaching before discharge. (See Chapter 19 ⚭ for more on focused head-to-toe assessment, Chapter 20 ⚭ for vital signs assessment, and Chapter 27 ⚭ for obtaining urine specimens.)

When the client is admitted, the physician is notified, and orders are requested if they were not sent with the client from the admitting office.

DIAGNOSING, PLANNING, AND IMPLEMENTING

As mentioned, some common nursing diagnoses of clients at admission are *Anxiety, Fear, Powerlessness, Social Isolation,* and *Disturbed Personal Identity.* For example, the RN might write *"Anxiety* related to unfamiliar hospital environment" as an admission nursing diagnosis.

As part of the planning process, the client's short- and long-term goals are set by the nurse and client. The client's choices and decisions about his or her health care are discussed and noted at this time. Nursing interventions are then planned to help the client reach these goals. Common interventions follow:

■ Orient the client to the hospital staff and environment (see Box 10-1). It is important for the client to know who should receive what information and to become acquainted with various caregiver roles. For example: "You will be visited by a laboratory technician who will draw some blood for examination." It is equally important for the client to know where the nurse's station and lounge are in relation to the room. Familiarity increases comfort.
■ Monitor client's level of understanding. Becoming familiar with the client's educational, cultural, and familial background makes communication easier. It also will make your choice of words more appropriate.
■ Provide the opportunity for clients to place belongings in the room as they wish, and assist as needed. This simple courtesy helps the client avoid feeling a loss of control and encourages a sense of ownership of the environment.
■ Provide the opportunity for the client to ask questions. Answer only what you know and obtain answers quickly to questions you do not have answers for. Do not appear hurried during the admission process. Appearing hurried will prevent the client from asking questions and will increase stress.

EVALUATING

The evaluation step is measured by assessing whether or not the goals have been met. For example, for a client with anxiety, an evaluation statement might be "Client states 'less anxious' after orientation." The plan of care is consistently reevaluated to determine if the client's changing needs are being met as treatment progresses.

NURSING PROCESS CARE PLAN
Admission of a Client from the Emergency Department

David Reynolds is a 42-year-old accounting executive with chest pain admitted from the emergency department. Janet, the admitting nurse, introduces herself and welcomes him to the cardiovascular unit. As Janet begins to obtain Mr. Reynolds's vital signs, he says: "I got this really sharp pain at work. Someone called the ambulance and also called my wife. She should have been here by now." He adds: "My father died of a heart attack at 47." While Mr. Reynolds was in the ED, he was examined by the cardiologist, who admitted him for observation and diagnostic tests. Mr. Reynolds is not receiving intravenous fluids. His right hand is on the left side of his neck. He says he is feeling his pulse.

Assessment. Mr. Reynolds's temperature is 100°F. Radial pulse is 120 and regular. Apical pulse is 118 and regular. Respirations are 28, audible and shallow. BP is 160/94.

Mr. Reynolds rates his pain as a 4 on a scale of 1 to 10. He says he is just a "little nauseated." His color is pink, and his skin is cool and dry. He is frowning, his face appears taut, and his hands are shaking. Janet is asking Mr. Reynolds about his pain—when it started, its character, and the location. She also asks him if this pain has ever been present before. He says he has never had pain this sharp or in his chest before but has had some pain in his stomach on occasion after eating a lot late at night. Mr. Reynolds interrupts Janet's questioning: "Where the heck is my wife? I could be biting the big one here! I wonder if she went to the wrong hospital."

Nursing Diagnosis. The following important nursing diagnoses (among others) are established for this client:

- *Acute Pain* (midline chest)
- *Nausea*
- *Fear*
- *Anxiety*

Expected Outcomes. The current expected outcomes specify that Mr. Reynolds will:

- Obtain relief from pain.
- Obtain relief from nausea.
- State his fears.
- Become less anxious.
- Regain and maintain vital signs within normal limits.

Planning and Implementation. The interventions indicated for Mr. Reynolds are:

- Orient to the unit.
- Explain the purpose of admission (observation and diagnosis).
- Position for greater comfort in breathing.
- Respond to need for information regarding wife.
- Encourage to talk about fears.
- Listen attentively to concerns.
- Welcome questions.
- Arrange room (client belongings) according to preferences.
- Monitor vital signs frequently as specified by physician's orders.

- Assess rate, rhythm, and character of pulse and respiration.
- Assess pain occurrence, including intensity, duration, and location.
- Assess skin color.
- Assess presence of nausea.
- Explain diagnostic procedures ordered (procedure and purpose).

Evaluation. By the third day of hospitalization, Mr. Reynolds has learned that he did not have a heart attack (myocardial infarction) but instead has a peptic ulcer. Treatment for the ulcer is continuing. Discharge planning has begun. Stress management will be one of the teaching initiatives.

Critical Thinking in the Nursing Process

1. What nursing care problems did Mr. Reynolds present at the time of admission that would be reported to the nurse team leader?
2. What aspects of Mr. Reynolds's verbal and nonverbal communication were significant indicators of fear and anxiety?
3. What effect would arranging Mr. Reynolds's room according to his preferences have in reducing his anxiety?

Note: Discussion of Critical Thinking questions appears in Appendix I.

Transferring a Client

COMMON RESPONSES TO TRANSFER

The client may require **transfer** (a move) to another unit in the hospital or to a different healthcare facility as a result of a client or physician request. The usual reasons for transfer are:

- The client may request another room (e.g., the client may need a quieter environment).
- The client's health condition may change and require more specialized nursing care (e.g., a severely elevated heart rate may require that the client be moved into intensive care).
- The client's condition may improve, permitting transfer from ICU to a medical/surgical or a transitional care unit.
- The client's condition may require a transfer to another facility (e.g., from an acute care setting to a rehab unit).
- The client may be disturbing others.

Transferring from one room, department, or facility to another is always somewhat stressful for the client and significant others. Clients may be concerned about people not being informed or about staff losing their belongings during the transfer. Anxieties tend to be lessened when the client is being transferred to a step-down or rehabilitation unit. However, when the physician orders the transfer for the purpose of having the client receive more specialized care (such as intensive care), the client's initial response is fear. Concerned that

SKILLED NURSING FACILITY (SNF)
Transfer Record

Client's Name _____ DOB _____ Insurance No. _____

SNF Name _____

Hosp. Admission Date _____ Discharge Date _____ SNF Admission Date _____

Principal Diagnosis (es):

Surgical Procedures and Dates:

Client Allergies:

Diet:

Physician Transfer Orders: (Medicines, Therapy, Lab Work, etc.)

Physician's Signature _____

Nursing Evaluation:

Date of Foley Insertion _____ Date of Last BM _____

Decubitus size / condition _____

Nursing Assessment:

Nurse's Signature _____

**Community Hospital
of Lancaster**
LANCASTER, PENNSYLVANIA

Figure 10-3. ■ Skilled nursing facility transfer record. (*Source:* Courtesy of Community Hospital of Lancaster.)

his or her condition has worsened, the client's fears may escalate into fear of death. Obviously, whatever the client's response, individualized nursing care is required.

TRANSFER GUIDELINES

Each hospital has written policies for transferring a client. The procedure usually requires the following:

1. A physician's order
2. Informing the client and family about the reason for the transfer
3. Assisting the client to gather all belongings
4. Completion of the required documentation.

Figure 10-3 ■ illustrates one type of transfer form.

NURSING CARE

ASSESSING

While it is not the practical/vocational nurse's responsibility to determine if, where, or when a client is transferred, he or she may participate in the process. The nurse may be involved in assessing and reporting client prob-

lems related to transfer. The LPN/LVN may also assist in implementing transfer procedures as directed by the registered nurse.

The following are common assessment issues related to transfer:

1. Client's health status. Physical and emotional support may be necessary throughout the process of transfer.
2. The client's and significant others' level of understanding about the reason for the transfer.
3. Safety precautions. Special equipment (such as wheelchair, stretcher, and portable IV apparatus) may be required to ensure client safety.

DIAGNOSING, PLANNING, AND IMPLEMENTING

Nursing diagnoses for clients who are being transferred are identified upon reviewing assessment issues. The following are examples:

- *Deficient Knowledge* related to need for transfer
- *Risk for Injury* related to the transfer procedure
- *Anxiety* related to a new environment.

Implementation of the care plan or nursing actions addresses client issues directly related to the nursing diagnoses. All nursing actions related to transfer should be directed toward managing the transfer process in an efficient and calm manner. These nursing actions include:

- *Explaining the transfer process.* Sharing information with the client and significant others decreases anxiety. It also generally increases compliance.
- *Taking safety precautions.* There is risk for injury in transfer situations. Also, if the transfer is delayed, there is potential for client discomfort. (For example, the client may have to wait a long time on a transfer bed or in a wheelchair. Clients in hospital gowns may become chilled.)
- *Checking and recording vital signs.* It is important to document client status before transfer. This documentation can be used as a reference point should the client's condition change.

clinical ALERT

Report

It is important to report all aspects of the transfer process immediately upon completion. Reporting completion of a transfer will allow several steps to occur:

1. Details about room number and client status at the time of transfer will be communicated.
2. The physician will be notified, usually by the unit clerk, that the client has been transferred.
3. The empty room will be cleaned and prepared for the next client.

The nurse may be directed to accompany the client to the new environment. If so, it is the nurse's responsibility to ensure that the client is greeted by the staff member of the new unit or facility who will be caring for the client. When accompanying a client to a new environment, it is also necessary to inform the registered nurse manager that transfer has occurred. Any change in the client's health status during transfer, or any problem encountered during the process, is also reported to the registered nurse who will oversee the client's care.

EVALUATING

After transfer, the nurse evaluates whether the client's vital signs and general health status have remained stable, and determines whether the transfer was completed safely. The time of transfer and the client's reaction to transfer are also noted.

Discharging a Client

Discharge is the official procedure by which the client leaves the healthcare facility and returns home or to another setting. Written permission from the physician is required for discharge. The situation of a client's leaving the hospital or healthcare facility without the written permission of a physician and **against medical advice (AMA)** is reported to the registered nurse manager immediately. If the client is rational and a court order does not exist to detain the client, he or she cannot be forcibly detained. The nurse or designated supervisor is responsible for notifying the physician. The client and supervisor sign and complete the proper forms. If the client refuses to sign the forms, this is documented in the client's medical record.

Clients are generally discharged from the hospital and return home because their condition has improved or has become stable. Client discharge to another healthcare facility, however, may occur for various reasons. For example, the discharged client may be a resident of a nursing home or may require the type of care received in a rehabilitation center. Clients may be discharged by wheelchair to their personal vehicle or by wheelchair or stretcher to some other form of transport such as an ambulance. Depending on the condition of the client at the time of discharge and the type of facility receiving the client, a nurse may accompany the client. In many healthcare facilities, there is a particular time for discharge of clients (for example, 11 A.M.), which precedes a designated admission time. Regardless of the policies and procedures in a healthcare setting, it is the nurse's responsibility to manage discharge efficiently and in a manner that ensures the client's physical and emotional comfort.

DISCHARGE GUIDELINES

Each hospital has written guidelines about the discharge procedure. They generally consist of the following:

- Written physician's order for discharge
- Completion of discharge teaching documentation (Figure 10-4 ■)
- Notification of discharge sent to the business office
- Assisting the client to prepare for discharge
- Ensuring that all client belongings are assembled for discharge
- Explanation of referral agencies and information about people or groups to contact (if this is not required prior to discharge)
- Completion of the teaching process; this includes all discharge instructions related to medication, nutrition and diet, self-care, allowable activity, and future appointments (Figure 10-5 ■ provides a sample of discharge instructions)
- Transporting the client to the discharge location.

Appointments such as those to physical therapy and referral to agencies such as home health are usually arranged by the social worker assigned to the client. Appointments and referrals are also sometimes scheduled by the nurse manager, discharge planner, or the unit clerk. The client or

Discharge Charting

Content Items marked with (✓) required on all Clients	Identified Client/Family Educational Needs		Date	Instruction Educator's Initials	Learner's Resonse	Date	Instruction Educator's Initials	Learner's Response
	Pre-op	Other						
Teaching/Miscellaneous:								
OR / PACU Routine								
Report Time to Hospital								
Waiting Area/visitors								
SCD's								
IV Therapy								
Incision / Wound Care								
NPO status								
Drain Tubes								
Other:								
Rehabilitation Needs:								
Cane/Crutch/Walker Training/Transfer Training								
Hip/Knees/Back/Ankle/Upper Extremity Exercise								
Sling/Splint/Corset/Braces								
TENS								
CPM								
Total Hip Precautions								
ADL Adaptive Equipment								
Energy Conservation / Joint Protection								
Body Mechanics								
Safety								
Other:								
Lifestyle Changes / Interventions								
Activity Level								
Other:								
Community Resources								
Specify								
Grief Counseling / Training								

 COMMUNITY HOSPITAL OF LANCASTER
LANCASTER, PENNSYLVANIA

Figure 10-4. ■ Discharge teaching from interdisciplinary client/family education record. (*Source:* Courtesy of Community Hospital of Lancaster.)

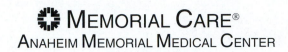

MEMORIAL CARE®
ANAHEIM MEMORIAL MEDICAL CENTER

DISCHARGE INSTRUCTIONS

For medical questions, call your physician.
For medical emergencies, dial 9-1-1 immediately.

CLIENT NAME: _____

REASON FOR YOUR HOSPITAL STAY: _____

DATE ADMITTED: _____ DATE DISCHARGED: _____

DIET: REGULAR   SPECIAL (see "special instructions" below)

BATHING: AS DESIRED LIMITS (see "special instructions" below)

PAIN MANAGEMENT: MEDICATION TREATMENT OUTPATIENT FOLLOW-UP

ACTIVITY: NORMAL LIMITS (see "special instructions" below)

YOU CAN RESUME NORMAL ACTIVITIES WHEN: _____

_____

_____

PRE-PRINTED INSTRUCTIONS PROVIDED & REVIEWED INCLUDING FOOD/DRUG AND

OTHER INTERACTIONS (LIST TITLE): _____

Home Health Services Ordered: _____

_____

_____

Co. _____ # _____
Medical Equipment Ordered: _____

_____

_____

Co. _____ # _____
Assisted Daily Living Needs: _____

_____

List of Homemaker Agencies Given? _____
Other Services Ordered/Resources Contacted?

_____

_____

Co. _____ # _____

SPECIAL INSTRUCTIONS: _____

_____

_____

THINGS TO LET YOUR DOCTOR KNOW ABOUT: _____

_____

PHYSICIAN APPOINTMENTS / REFERRALS:

1. _____
   DATE   PHYSICIAN/SPECIALTY   PHONE

2. _____
   DATE   PHYSICIAN/SPECIALTY   PHONE

3. _____
   DATE   PHYSICIAN/SPECIALTY   PHONE

4. _____
   DATE   PHYSICIAN/SPECIALTY   PHONE

MEDICATION INSTRUCTIONS

NO.	DRUG / DOSE	ROUTE	TIME(S)	PURPOSE	DATE/TIME LAST GIVEN
1					/
2					/
3					/
4					/
5					/
6					/
7					/
8					/
9					/
10					/

11 Pain Medication: _____ CALL YOUR DOCTOR WITH QUESTIONS REGARDING PAIN.

Prescription Given? ____ Yes ____ No   Medication Information Discussed? ____ Yes ____ No   Medication Side Effects Discussed? ____ Yes ____ No

Client requests additional information about medication ____ Yes ____ No   Pharmacy contacted ____ Yes ____ No   By whom: _____

Client verbalizes an understanding of above discharge instructions and states where to obtain medications.

Figure 10-5. ■ Discharge instruction sheet for client. (*Source:* Courtesy of Anaheim Memorial Medical Center.)

significant others may be instructed by the nurse or social worker in making the referral.

Referrals and appointments are ordered by the physician. An exception to a physician-ordered referral may occur when the client requests information regarding a particular problem or disease. The nurse may then refer the client to an organization by providing the name and number and perhaps some printed material. For example, a newly diagnosed diabetic client may ask where he or she can learn more about the disease and perhaps join a support group. In instances such as this, referral to community services is part of the nursing responsibility of promoting health education.

COMMON RESPONSES TO DISCHARGE

Most clients are excited and happy to be returning home. Others may be anxious about the support they will receive at home or about the consequences and nature of continued convalescence. Those who are going to an unfamiliar destination may feel uncomfortable. Clients generally feel concerned about how to care for themselves and how to follow the discharge instructions precisely.

NURSING CARE

ASSESSING

The LPN/LVN may collect data about the following issues prior to discharge:

- *Client's physical and emotional readiness for discharge.* The nurse should provide the opportunity to listen to the client's feelings related to discharge. These concerns could be related to wondering how well the client will continue to progress at home or whether medical supplies or equipment will be accessible in the home.
- *Support system for client.* Significant others must become part of the discharge process. The nurse listens to their concerns about the client's return home or to a designated facility.
- *Understanding discharge instructions.* Assessing how the client interprets the instructions is essential. Confusion about diet, medication, special procedures, or exercise and activity may be present.
- *Progress expectations.* The client may not understand what to expect regarding convalescence. Clients may wonder how long they will need certain types of treatment or how long they will have certain symptoms.
- *Home environment and safety.* Clients may feel insecure about home safety. They may feel that their living space will not accommodate the medical supplies and equipment they need.

DIAGNOSING, PLANNING, AND IMPLEMENTING

Two of the most common nursing diagnoses that are identified when discharging clients are *Self-Care Deficit* and *Deficient Knowledge.* The planning and implementation of the nursing process related to discharge occur in response to these diagnoses.

Discharge planning actually begins with hospital admission. Teaching that was identified at admission and introduced during a client's stay is reinforced on the day of discharge. Written guidelines often are provided (see Figure 10-4). Underlying all care and treatment the client receives is the goal to restore the client, if possible, to the level of wellness that preceded hospitalization.

In collaboration with the RN, the LPN/LVN helps the client to clarify goals for discharge by assisting the client in anticipating and solving problems. For example, the client who lives alone may realize that he or she will need help to carry out activities of daily living (ADLs) and to follow discharge instructions. A goal would be set to obtain help and support from significant others, home health care, or other available agencies. The social worker may be notified and may provide special assistance in obtaining help and support.

Client outcomes and timelines are also developed to help the client and family during the transition. For example, for a very weak client, an initial goal might be to work gradually toward full participation in ADLs over a period of 2 weeks (if this is in keeping with physician's orders). The plan may include slowly increasing the time spent on each activity, or selecting one or two activities to complete and gradually increasing the number as strength permits.

The example of problem solving given above relates to planning (goal setting), but it is also an example of the implementation process associated with discharge. Perhaps the most important nursing actions at discharge are those directed toward giving the client the appropriate oral presentation and written resources related to discharge instructions. For example, if a particular diet is recommended, then the nutritionist can be contacted to discuss the diet with the client and provide helpful materials and menu ideas. Printed instructions are available on many topics and in almost every language (examples: insulin self-administration, dressing changes, and mobility devices). Large-print materials are also available.

However, the nurse must not simply give the client a pack of printed brochures or information sheets and consider the discharge process complete. Printed materials are intended as an information supplement and as a reference. Every discharge instruction should be explained verbally to the client. During oral instruction, the client should be encouraged to ask questions. The client should paraphrase the instructions, and the nurse should listen carefully to determine whether the client interprets the instructions accurately. Whenever possible, the nurse should ask the client to demonstrate procedures listed in the discharge instructions.

In addition to discharge instructions related to medical care, the client should also be informed about what to expect during convalescence, what symptoms to report and to whom, and what to regard as an emergency. Often, a number of physicians in different specialties have attended the client. The client may be confused about which one to call. Review physician names and phone numbers and scheduled appointments, or give directions for scheduling appointments.

The most important fact about discharge is not a set of discharge instructions but the client's departure. Saying good-bye and wishing the client well are aspects of nursing care that, in themselves, promote client well-being. An acknowledged departure provides closure for the client and for the nursing staff and can be personally satisfying to both.

EVALUATING

Evaluation of the discharge process involves reporting to the nurse manager that discharge is completed. A release form (obtained from the business office at the time of discharge) is usually returned to the nurse manager. Details about the discharge (time, who accompanied client, type of transportation) and the client's reaction are recorded on the client's medical record.

Either at the time of discharge or shortly after (through the mail), the client is given the opportunity to evaluate the nursing care and other aspects of hospitalization. Each facility has its own procedure for reviewing and disseminating the information. Generally, though, evaluations are shared with the nursing staff in the form of reports.

Note: The references and resources for this and all chapters have been compiled at the back of the book.

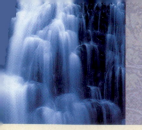

Chapter Review

 KEY TERMS by Topic

Use the audio glossary feature of either the CD-ROM or the Companion Website to hear the correct pronunciation of the following key terms.

Admitting a Client
admission, coping behaviors, dehumanization, orientation

Transferring a Client
transfer

Discharging a Client
discharge, against medical advice (AMA)

KEY Points

- Nurses can significantly affect how the client views and experiences the admission, transfer, and discharge processes.

- The client's feelings about admission help to determine the success of the hospital stay.

- The LPN/LVN participates in the baseline assessment of the new client.

- Common reactions of newly admitted clients include anxiety, feelings of loss of independence or loss of identity, and, in children, separation anxiety.

- Nurses are responsible for giving culturally sensitive care.

- The Health Insurance Portability & Accountability Act (HIPAA) provides strict guidelines for maintaining client privacy and confidentiality as well as providing for continuation of health insurance from one employer to another.

- The client's belongings and valuables must be properly identified and safely stored.

- Client transfer requires adherence to certain procedures designed to keep the client safe and comfortable during the process.

- Discharge planning and teaching actually begin during the admission process.

- The emphasis of nursing care during the discharge process is to assist the client in understanding the discharge instructions accurately and planning for any problems that may arise.

 EXPLORE Media Link

Additional interactive resources for this chapter can be found on the Companion Website at www.prenhall.com/ramont. Click on Chapter 10 and "Begin" to select the activities for this chapter.

For chapter-related NCLEX®-style questions and an audio glossary, access the accompanying CD-ROM in this book.
Animations/Videos
- Admission, Transfers, and Discharge

FOR FURTHER Study

Steps to improve cultural sensitivity are discussed in detail in Chapter 2.

For additional information about legal issues, see Chapter 3.

For more details on the nursing process, see Chapter 5.

For further information about needs as identified by Maslow, see Figure 5-4 and discussion in Chapter 11.

For further study on head-to-toe assessment, see Chapter 19; for vital signs assessment, Chapter 20; and for obtaining urine specimens, Chapter 27.

For more about maintaining the client's integrity and personal dignity, see Chapter 33.

Critical Thinking Care Map

Caring for a Client Prior to Discharge
NCLEX-PN® Focus Area: Coping and Adaptation

Case Study: Amanda Carr is an 86-year-old client being discharged from the rehabilitation unit to an assisted living center. Two months ago, after a fall, she had a hip replacement. She has been in the medical center's rehab unit since that time. Before surgery, she lived with her two cats in a second-floor apartment with an outdoor metal staircase. Mrs. Carr is scheduled to leave the hospital in 1 week. She is resisting discharge planning and insists she is returning home. "My cats need me, and I can make do."

Nursing Diagnosis: Ineffective Coping

COLLECT DATA

Subjective	Objective
_____	_____
_____	_____
_____	_____
_____	_____
_____	_____
_____	_____
_____	_____

Would you report this data? Yes/No

If yes, to: _____

What would you report? _____

Nursing Care

_____
_____
_____
_____
_____
_____
_____
_____
_____
_____

How would you document this?_____
_____
_____
_____

Data Collected
(use those that apply)

- "My cats need me, and I can make do."
- Daughter says client very independent
- Unsafe environment at home (outdoor entry and metal stairs)
- Chart indicates noncompliance with discharge plan to assisted living facility
- Height 5'9"
- Weight 100 lbs
- Reports "Nurses all mumble."

Nursing Interventions
(use those that apply; list in priority order)

- Maintain a calm, quiet manner.
- Demonstrate firmness in seeking cooperation.
- Assess level of understanding regarding discharge and transfer.
- Explain purpose of transfer to assisted living.
- Encourage statement of concerns.
- Isolate from other clients.
- Allow time to answer questions about the assisted living facility.
- Inquire about family members who live in the area.

Compare your documentation to the sample provided in Appendix I.

NCLEX-PN® Exam Preparation

1 Which statement is least dehumanizing to a client?
1. "The new total abdominal hysterectomy client has been oriented to room."
2. "Billy, the 24-year-old with the femur fracture, will need crutches ordered."
3. "The client in 256 needs a pair of slippers."
4. "Miss Smith, who just came back from surgery, is requesting a private room."

2 The nurse's understanding of culturally sensitive communication is best illustrated by:
1. referring to a Native American as Indian.
2. addressing clients by first name to reduce anxiety.
3. speaking in a loud but clear voice using simple words.
4. arranging an interpreter for the Hispanic client who speaks no English.

3 All the following tasks need to be completed prior to transfer of a client in respiratory distress. Which is the priority task?
1. Answer the client's and significant others' questions related to visiting hours in the ICU.
2. Call the RN to answer the significant others' questions related to the transfer process.
3. Give report to the RN.
4. Arrange for and place the adult client on portable oxygen prior to transfer.

4 The RN delegates the admission of a new client. In what aspects of the admission process should the LPN/LVN participate?
1. formulation of the nursing diagnosis related to anxiety caused by the admission process
2. collection of data regarding the confused client's mental status and placing him or her in restraints
3. collection of baseline subjective and objective data delegated by the RN
4. development of the treatment plan to ensure the client progresses to the optimal level of independence

5 A newly admitted adult client in an acute care facility says to the nurse, "Please put my wallet, watch, and rings in the for me." Which of the following best expresses facility policy about valuables?
1. "Don't worry, I'll leave your things in the drawer here next to your bed."
2. "Is there a family member here who could take these things home for you?"
3. "Valuables all need to be stored in the safe."
4. "I need to inventory and document your personal belongings."

6 What is the priority goal for a client during admission, transfer, and discharge?
1. ensuring the continuity of individualized care
2. beginning discharge planning after the physician writes discharge orders
3. assisting the adult client with using the proper coping skills throughout his or her stay
4. assessing the adult client's knowledge regarding the disease process

7 In caring for all of the following persons, which one is most in need of discharge planning?
1. a 70-year-old male, who is being discharged to the skilled unit for rehabilitation
2. a 24-year-old female, who broke her left tibia while skiing and who lives with her husband
3. a 38-year-old female, who is a newly diagnosed diabetic beginning insulin therapy
4. a 64-year-old African American male with a 20-year history of hypertension, controlled by medication

8 A female client is new to the unit, and diagnostic tests are ordered. The client does not have a readable identification band in place. What should the LPN/LVN do?
1. Call registration to replace the identification band before sending her for the test.
2. Report this to the charge RN, then send her for the test.
3. Replace the identification band after sending the client for the test.
4. Ask the client for her name, send her for the test so there is no delay in treatment, and replace the identification band when she returns.

9 A client is admitted to the pediatric unit. When caring for pediatric clients, which principle is most important to remember?
1. Encourage the parents to stay with the child throughout the admission process.
2. Hold the pediatric client to build trust during the admission process.
3. Speak in a normal tone and clearly.
4. Reassure the child that the shot will not hurt.

10 The LPN/LVN is preparing to transfer an adult client to the intensive care unit from the surgical unit. The nurse can improve the client's comfort by which intervention?
1. Prior to transfer, position the client on his side to allow visualization of the hall as he is transferred.
2. Call the client by his first name when you introduce him to the intensive care staff.
3. Reinforce the need for transfer to intensive care and answer any questions the client or significant others may have.
4. Give a bedside report to the ICU nurse so the client can hear that his condition is stable so he will be less anxious.

Answers and Rationales for Review Questions, as well as discussion of Care Plan and Critical Thinking Care Map questions, appear in Appendix I.

Thinking Strategically About ...

Deborah Mason, LPN, has been assigned to work with Laurene Carter, a triage nurse, in the emergency department of a large metropolitan hospital in the Southwest. Ms. Mason is responsible for conducting an "intake inquiry." This inquiry includes a brief history ("the chief complaint") and taking client vital signs. The information is charted and verbally communicated to Ms. Carter, who determines in which area of the ED the clients are to be treated and escorts them there.

Jose Suarez, age 58, arrives at the ED, accompanied by his wife Mariela. Mr. Suarez is diaphoretic and visibly short of breath. Mr. Suarez reports that he feels like he has influenza, like he had a few years ago, except he doesn't have a sore throat. Petechiae are visible on his forearms. In broken English, he explains that he picks tomatoes at a small ranch and sells them to families living on the nearby military testing base, as well as to tourists. Mrs. Suarez interrupts him repeatedly in Spanish during the intake inquiry. He gestures impatiently and says, "She wants me to tell you I had to bury four dead sheep last week at the ranch." In recent weeks, there have been three reported cases of anthrax in the state.

CRITICAL THINKING

- What is the priority nursing concern for Mr. Suarez?
- Does Mr. Suarez's condition suggest any special safety concerns?

COLLABORATIVE CARE

- Based on information gained from this scenario, what members of the healthcare team might need to be involved in assessment of Mr. Suarez?

CULTURAL COMPETENCY

- What must be done to ensure that Mr. and Mrs. Suarez have the best possible communication with hospital staff?
- What cultural influences are apparent in this case?

COMPASSIONATE CARE

- What interventions might the nurse use to assist Mr. Suarez while he is in the ED?

Promoting Psychosocial Health

UNIT III

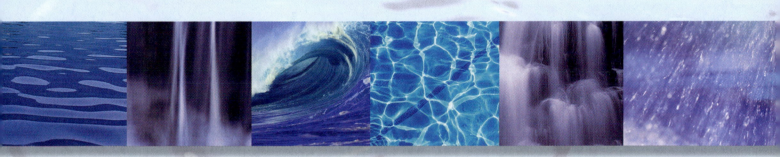

Chapter 11

Life Span Development

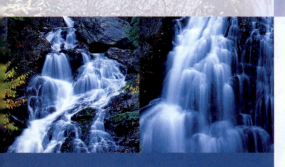

HISTORICAL Perspectives

Dr. Benjamin Spock's Baby and Child Care, *first published in 1946, was the bible of parents in the baby boom that followed World War II. The book also served as a supplemental text in many nursing programs throughout the United States. "Trust yourself," Spock told parents. "You know more than you think you do." Human development is not a strange mystery, but rather a logical journey that all must travel through.*

LEARNING Outcomes

After completing this chapter, you will be able to:

1. Differentiate growth from development.
2. List factors that influence growth and development.
3. Describe the significant characteristics and nursing implications of the stages of growth and development from infancy through old age.
4. Trace stages of psychosocial development according to Erikson.
5. Explain Piaget's phases of cognitive development.
6. Describe moral development according to Kohlberg.
7. Describe spiritual development according to Fowler.
8. Describe usual physical development through the life span.
9. Identify characteristic tasks of different stages of development.
10. Identify selected health problems associated with young, middle-aged, and older adults.
11. Identify health assessment and health promotion activities from birth through older adulthood.
12. List examples of health promotion topics for client teaching from young adulthood through old adulthood.

BOX 11-1

Principles of Growth and Development

- Growth and development are continuous, orderly, sequential processes influenced by maturational, environmental, and genetic factors.
- All humans follow the same pattern of growth and development.
- The sequence of each stage is predictable, although the time of onset, the length of the stage, and the effects of each stage vary with the person.
- Learning can either help or hinder the maturational process, depending on what is learned.
- Each developmental stage has its own characteristics.
- Growth and development occur in a cephalocaudal direction. They start at the head and move to the trunk, legs, and feet. This pattern is particularly obvious at birth, when the head of the infant is disproportionately large.
- Growth and development occur from the center of the body outward. For example, infants can roll over before they can grasp an object with the thumb and second finger.

- Development proceeds from simple to complex, or from single acts to integrated acts. To drink and swallow from a cup, for example, the child must first learn eye–hand coordination, grasping, hand–mouth coordination, controlled tipping of the cup, and then mouth, lip, and tongue movements to drink and swallow.
- Development becomes increasingly differentiated. Differentiated development begins with a generalized response and progresses to a skilled specific response. For example, an infant's initial response to a stimulus involves the total body; a 5-year-old child can respond more specifically with laughter or fear.
- Certain stages of growth and development are more critical than others. It is known that the first 10 to 12 weeks after conception are critical. The incidence of congenital anomalies as a result of exposure to certain viruses, chemicals, or drugs is greater during this stage than others.
- The pace of growth and development is uneven. Asynchronous development is demonstrated by rapid growth of the head during infancy and of the extremities at puberty.

Often used interchangeably, the terms *growth* and *development* have different meanings. **Growth** refers to physical change and increase in size. Indicators of growth include height, weight, bone size, and dentition. Although the pattern of physiological growth is similar for all people, growth rates vary during different stages of growth and development. For example, the growth rate is rapid during the prenatal, neonatal, infancy, and adolescent stages, but slows during childhood, and is minimal during adulthood.

Development is an increase in the complexity of function and skill progression. It refers to the person's capacity and skill to adapt to the environment. Development is the behavioral aspect of growth and includes the abilities to walk, to talk, and to run.

Processes of Growth and Development

Growth and development take place in an organized way, although they do not progress at the same rate with all individuals.

- *Cephalocaudally*—from the head down or literally from head (cephalo) to tail (caudal) (e.g., the infant gains head control before control of extremities)
- *Proximal to distal*—from the midline of the body to the extremities (e.g., the infant rolls over before grasp is perfected)
- *General to specific* (e.g., walking is learned before running or skipping).

Growth and development are independent, interrelated processes. For example, an infant's muscles, bones, and nervous system must grow to a certain point before the infant can sit up or walk. Growth generally takes place during the first 20 years of life; development continues after that. Principles of growth and development are described in Box 11-1 ■, and a cultural look at the stages of childhood is given in Box 11-2 ■.

BOX 11-2   CULTURAL PULSE POINTS

The Stages of Childhood

Five stages of human growth and development are common to *Homosapiens:* infancy, childhood, juvenility, adolescence, and adulthood. Margaret Mead described lap children (infants, ages 0–1), knee children (toddlers, 2–3), yard children (preschool, 4–5), and community children (juveniles in middle childhood, 6–12). Anthropologists analyze the cultural meaning of the very idea of "stages," because stages are used to account for children's behavior ("He's crying but it's okay, because he's still a toddler") and to assure and define normal and appropriate development ("She is eight and old enough to start helping run our household").

Human cultures weave wonderful variations, meanings, and stories around pan-human maturational stages of childhood. The Beng of the Ivory Coast, for example, believe that young children are still partly in yet another stage, a cultural world called *wrugbe*, where ancestors share life with prebirth children who are ambivalent about leaving that world. This helps explain for Beng why infants cry or are sickly: They want to return to *wrugbe*.

Source: Bogin, B. 1999. *Patterns of Human Growth,* 2nd ed., Cambridge University Press, New York.

The factors that influence growth and development are genetic and environmental. The genetic inheritance of an individual is established at conception. It remains unchanged throughout life and determines such characteristics as sex, physical stature, and race. Environmental factors include family, religion, climate, culture, school, community, and nutrition. For example, poorly nourished children are more likely to have infections than are well-fed children, and they may not attain their full height potential.

RELATIONSHIP BETWEEN GROWTH AND DEVELOPMENT

The rate of a person's growth and development is highly individual. However, the sequence of growth and development is predictable. Stages of growth usually correspond to certain developmental changes, as shown in Table 11-1 ■.

Growth and development are commonly thought of as having five major components:

■ **Physiological**—relating to physical processes in the human body

---

TABLE 11-1

Stages of Growth and Development

STAGE	AGE	SIGNIFICANT CHARACTERISTICS	NURSING IMPLICATIONS
Neonatal	Birth–28 days	Behavior is largely reflexive and develops to more purposeful behavior.	Assist parents to identify and meet unmet needs.
Infancy	1 month–1 year	Physical growth is rapid.	Control the infant's environment so that physical and psychological needs are met.
Toddlerhood	1–3 years	Motor development permits increased physical autonomy. Psychosocial skills increase.	Safety and risk-taking strategies must be balanced to permit growth.
Preschool	3–6 years	The preschooler's world is expanding. New experiences and the preschooler's social role are tried during play. Physical growth is slower.	Provide opportunities for play and social activity.
School age	6–12 years	Stage includes the preadolescent period (10 to 12 years). Peer group increasingly influences behavior. Physical, cognitive, and social development increases, and communication skills improve.	Allow time and energy for the school-age child to pursue hobbies and school activities. Recognize and support child's achievement.
Adolescence	12–20 years	Self-concept changes with biologic development. Values are tested. Physical growth accelerates. Stress increases, especially in the face of conflicts.	Assist adolescents to develop coping behaviors. Help adolescents develop strategies for resolving conflicts.
Young adulthood	20–40 years	A personal lifestyle develops. Person establishes a relationship with a significant other and a commitment to something.	Accept adult's chosen lifestyle and assist with necessary adjustments relating to health. Recognize the person's commitments. Support change as necessary for health.
Middle adulthood	40–65 years	Lifestyle changes due to other changes; for example, children leave home, occupational goals change.	Assist clients to plan for anticipated changes in life, to recognize the risk factors related to health, and to focus on strengths rather than weaknesses.
Older adulthood Young-old	65–74 years	Adaptation to retirement and changing physical abilities is often necessary. Chronic illness may develop.	Assist clients to keep physically and socially active and to maintain peer group interactions.
Middle-old	75–84 years	Adaptation to decline in speed of movement, reaction time, and sensory abilities and increasing dependence on others may be necessary.	Assist clients to cope with loss (e.g., hearing, eyesight, death of loved one). Provide necessary safety measures.
Old-old	85 years and older	Increasing physical problems may develop.	Assist clients with self-care as required, and with maintaining as much independence as possible.

- **Psychosocial**—pertaining to the relationship between oneself and others
- **Cognitive**—having to do with awareness of and interaction between oneself and the environment
- **Moral**—relating to judgments of right or wrong
- **Spiritual**—pertaining to relationship with God or a higher power.

A knowledge of growth and development is essential for nurses if they are to identify developmental needs and problems and participate in health assessment and promotion. Growth and development encompass the prenatal period and the life span: from the neonate to older adult including the physiological, psychosocial, cognitive, moral, and spiritual aspects of each life stage.

Conception and Prenatal Development

Prenatal or intrauterine development lasts approximately 38 to 40 weeks. Traditionally, pregnancy has been divided into three periods, called *trimesters,* each of which lasts about 3 months. Each trimester includes certain landmarks for developmental changes in the mother and the fetus. There are two phases of intrauterine life: embryonic and fetal.

The *embryonic phase* is the period during which the fertilized ovum develops into an organism with most of the features of the human. This period takes place during the first trimester of pregnancy. During the first 3 weeks:

1. The embryo is implanted.
2. Tissues differentiate into three layers. From these layers all of the body's complex organs and systems are formed.
3. Placental function starts. Its functions are to exchange nutrients and gases between the embryo or fetus and the mother.
4. The fetal membranes differentiate.

The *fetal phase* of development is characterized by a period of rapid growth in the size of the fetus. Both genetic and environmental factors affect its growth.

At the end of the second trimester, the fetus resembles a small baby. The skin appears wrinkled, red, and transparent. A protective covering (called *vernix caseosa*) begins to develop over the skin. This is a white cheeselike substance that adheres to the skin. *Lanugo,* a fine downy hair, also covers the body. At about 5 months, the mother first perceives movement by the fetus, and the first fetal heartbeat may be heard.

At the end of the third trimester, the fetus has developed to approximately 20 inches and 7.0 to 7.5 pounds. The lanugo has disappeared, and the skin is a more normal color and appears less wrinkled. The last 2 months *in utero* are largely devoted to accumulating weight.

Neonates and Infants (Birth to 1 Year)

Babies are considered neonates from birth to the end of 1 month. Infants are babies from 1 month of age to 1 year.

PHYSICAL DEVELOPMENT

An infant's basic task is survival, which requires breathing, sleeping, sucking, eating, swallowing, digesting, and eliminating. Infants undergo significant physiological change in these areas: weight, length, head growth, vision, and motor development.

Weight

Just after birth, most infants lose 5% to 10% of their birth weight because of fluid loss. This weight loss is normal, and infants usually regain that weight in about 1 week. Usual weight gain is 5 to 7 ounces weekly for 6 months. By 5 months of age infants usually reach twice their birth weight, and by age 12 months, three times their birth weight.

Length

The average length of a newborn is about 20 inches. Two recumbent lengths are measured (Figure 11-1 ■): the crown-to-rump length (the sitting length), which is approximately the same as the head circumference, and the head-to-heel length (from the top of the head to the base of the heels). By 12 months, the infant's length increases by approximately one-half of the birth length.

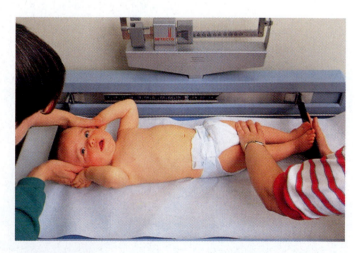

Figure 11-1. ■ Measuring an infant head to heel, from the top of the head to the base of the heels.

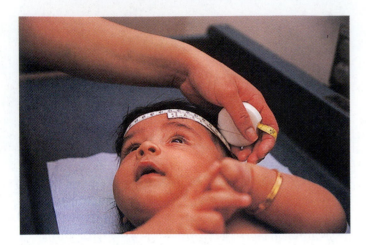

Figure 11-2. ■ An infant's head circumference is measured around the skull, above the eyebrows. (Photographer: Elena Dorfman.)

Head and Chest Circumference

Assessment of head circumference is of particular importance in infants and children to determine the growth rate of the skull and the brain. An infant's head should be measured at every visit to the physician or nurse until the child is 2 years old (Figure 11-2 ■).

Normal head circumference (*normocephaly*) is often related to chest circumference. The chest circumference of the newborn is usually less than the head circumference. As the infant grows, the chest circumference becomes larger than the head circumference.

Head Molding

The heads of most newborn babies are misshapen because of the molding of the head that occurs during vaginal deliveries. Molding of the head is made possible by **fontanelles** (unossified membranous gaps) in the bone structure of the skull and by overriding of the *sutures* (junction lines of the skull bones). Within a week of birth, a newborn's head usually regains its symmetry. The posterior fontanelle closes from 4 to 8 weeks after birth. The larger anterior fontanelle, which is diamond shaped, closes between 9 and 18 months (Figure 11-3 ■).

Sensory Abilities

VISION. The newborn can follow large moving objects and blinks in response to bright light.

- The newborn eyes cannot focus on close objects.
- At 4 months, the infant can recognize familiar objects and follow moving ones.
- At 6 months, the infant can perceive colors.
- At 9 months, most can recognize facial characteristics and often smile in response to a familiar face.
- At 12 months, depth perception has developed.

HEARING

- Newborns with intact hearing will react with a startle to a loud noise. In many locales, newborn hearing screenings are now mandated prior to hospital discharge. Computerized equipment makes this possible. Within a

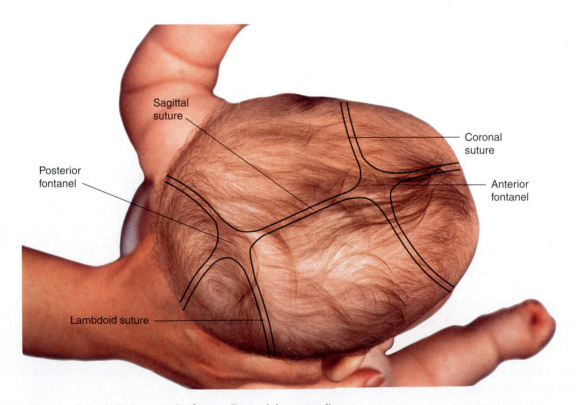

Figure 11-3. ■ The bones of the skull, showing the fontanelles and the suture lines.

BOX 11-3

Infant Reflexes

- *Sucking reflex:* A feeding reflex that occurs when the infant's lips are touched. The reflex persists throughout infancy.
- *Rooting reflex:* A feeding reflex elicited by touching the baby's cheek, causing the baby's head to turn to the side that was touched. This reflex usually disappears after 4 months.
- *Moro reflex:* Often assessed to estimate the maturity of the central nervous system. A loud noise, a sudden change in position, or an abrupt jarring of the crib elicits this reflex. The infant reacts by extending both arms and legs outward with the fingers spread, then suddenly retracting the limbs. Often, the infant cries at the same time. This reflex disappears after 4 months.
- *Palmar grasp reflex:* Occurs when a small object is placed against the palm of the hand, causing the fingers to curl around it. This reflex disappears after 3 months.
- *Plantar reflex:* Similar to the palmar grasp reflex; an object placed just beneath the toes causes them to curl around it. This reflex disappears after 8 months.
- *Tonic neck reflex or fencing reflex:* A postural reflex. When a baby who is lying on its back turns its head to the right side, for example, the left side of the body shows a flexing of the left arm and the left leg. This reflex disappears after 4 months.
- *Stepping reflex (walking or dancing reflex):* Can be elicited by holding the baby upright so that the feet touch a flat surface. The legs then move up and down as if the baby were walking. This reflex usually disappears at about 2 months.
- *Babinski reflex:* When the sole of the foot is stroked, the big toe rises and the other toes fan out. A newborn baby has a positive Babinski. After age 1, the infant exhibits a negative Babinski; that is, the toes curl downward. A positive Babinski after age 1 indicates brain damage.

few days infants can tell the difference between their mother's voice and that of another woman.

- At 5 months of age, the infant will pause while sucking in order to listen to the mother's voice.
- A 9-month-old infant is able to locate the source of sounds and recognizes familiar ones.
- At 1 year, the infant listens to sounds, begins to distinguish words, and responds to simple commands.

SMELL AND TASTE. The senses of smell and taste are functional shortly after birth. Newborns prefer sweet tastes and tend to decrease their sucking in response to liquids with a salty content. They are able to recognize the smell of their mother's milk and respond to this smell by turning toward the mother.

TOUCH. The sense of touch is well developed at birth. Skin-to-skin touching is important for an infant's development. The infant responds positively to the warmth, love, and security it perceives when touched, held, and cuddled. The newborn is also sensitive to temperature extremes and pain; however, babies react diffusely and cannot isolate the discomfort.

REFLEXES. The **reflexes** of the newborn are unconscious, involuntary responses. They are neither learned nor consciously carried out; rather, they are nervous system responses to a number of stimuli. Box 11-3 ■ describes infant reflexes.

Motor Abilities

Motor development is the development of the baby's abilities to move and to control the body (Figure 11-4 ■). See Table 11-2 ■ for examples of motor and social development in infants.

PSYCHOSOCIAL DEVELOPMENT

Erikson described eight stages of development in humans (Table 11-3 ■). According to Erikson, the central crisis at this stage is trust versus mistrust. Infants depend on the primary caregivers for all their physiological and psychological needs. The newborn reacts socially to caregivers by paying attention to the face or voice and by cuddling when held. It is able to interact with the environment by responding to various stimuli such as touch and sound.

COGNITIVE DEVELOPMENT

According to Piaget, **cognitive development** is a result of interaction between an individual and the environment. Piaget identified stages and significant behaviors for different age groups (Table 11-4 ■). Infants' initial period of cognitive development was named the sensorimotor phase.

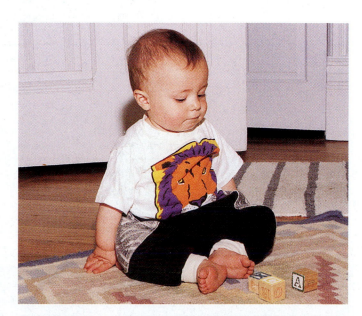

Figure 11-4. ■ An infant sits without support at 6 months of age.

TABLE 11-2

Examples of Motor and Social Development in Infancy

AGE	MOTOR DEVELOPMENT	SOCIAL DEVELOPMENT
Newborn	Turns head from side to side when in a prone position. Grasps by reflex when object is placed in palm of hand.	Displays displeasure by crying and satisfaction by soft vocalizations. Attends to adult face and voice by eye contact and quieting.
6 months	Lifts chest and shoulders off table when prone, bearing weight on hands. Manipulates small objects.	Starts to imitate sounds. Vocalizes one-syllable sounds: "ma ma," "da da."
9 months	Creeps and crawls. Beginner pincer grasp with thumb and forefinger.	Complies with simple verbal commands. Displays fear of being left alone (e.g., going to bed). Waves "bye-bye."
12 months	Walks alone with help. Uses spoon to feed self.	Clings to mother in unfamiliar situations. Demonstrates emotions such as anger and affection.

TABLE 11-3

Erikson's Eight Stages of Development

STAGE	AGE	CENTRAL TASK	INDICATORS OF POSITIVE RESOLUTION	INDICATORS OF NEGATIVE RESOLUTION
Infancy	Birth–18 months	Trust versus mistrust	Learning to trust others	Mistrust, withdrawal, estrangement
Early childhood	18 months–3 years	Autonomy versus shame and doubt	Self-control without loss of self-esteem Ability to cooperate and to express oneself	Compulsive self-restraint or compliance Willfulness and defiance
Late childhood	3–5 years	Initiative versus guilt	Learning the degree to which assertiveness and purpose influence the environment Beginning ability to evaluate one's own behavior	Lack of self-confidence Pessimism, fear of wrongdoing Overcontrol and overrestriction of own activity
School age	6–12 years	Industry versus inferiority	Beginning to create, develop, and manipulate Developing sense of competence and perseverance	Loss of hope, sense of being mediocre Withdrawal from school and peers
Adolescence	12–20 years	Identity versus role confusion	Coherent sense of self Plans to actualize one's abilities	Feelings of confusion, indecisiveness, and possible antisocial behavior
Young adulthood	18–25 years	Intimacy versus isolation	Intimate relationship with another person Commitment to work and relationships	Impersonal relationships Avoidance of relationship, career, or lifestyle commitments
Adulthood	25–65 years	Generativity versus stagnation	Creativity, productivity, concern for others	Self-indulgence, self-concern, lack of interests and commitments
Maturity	65 years to death	Integrity versus despair	Acceptance of worth and uniqueness of one's own life Acceptance of death	Sense of loss, contempt for others

Source: From *Childhood and Society,* 2nd ed. (pp. 247–274), by E. Erikson, 1963, New York: W. W. Norton. Copyright 1950, © 1963 by W. W. Norton & Company, Inc., renewed © 1978, 1991 by Erik H. Erikson. Reprinted by permission.

TABLE 11-4		
Piaget's Phases of Cognitive Development		
PHASES AND STAGES	**AGE**	**SIGNIFICANT BEHAVIOR**
Sensorimotor phase	Birth–2 years	
Stage 1: use of reflexes	Birth–1 month	Most action is reflexive.
Stage 2: primary circular reaction	1–4 months	Perception of events is centered on the body. Objects are extension of self.
Stage 3: secondary circular reaction	4–8 months	Acknowledges the external environment. Actively makes changes in the environment.
Stage 4: coordination of secondary schemata	8–12 months	Can distinguish a goal from a means of attaining it.
Stage 5: tertiary circular reaction	12–18 months	Tries and discovers new goals and ways to attain goals. Rituals are important.
Stage 6: inventions of new means	18–24 months	Interprets the environment by mental image. Uses make-believe and pretend play.
Preconceptual phase	2–4 years	Uses an egocentric approach to accommodate the demands of an environment. Everything is significant and relates to "me." Explores the environment. Language development is rapid. Associates words with objects.
Intuitive thought phase	4–7 years	Egocentric thinking diminishes. Thinks of one idea at a time. Includes others in the environment. Words express thoughts.
Concrete operations phase	7–11 years	Solves concrete problems. Begins to understand relationships such as size. Understands right and left. Cognizant of viewpoints.
Formal operations phase	11–15 years	Uses rational thinking. Reasoning is deductive and futuristic.

Source: From The Origin of Intelligence in Children, by J. Piaget, 1966, International Universities Press, Inc., Copyright © 1966. Adapted with permission.

MORAL DEVELOPMENT

Infants associate right and wrong with pleasure and pain. What gives them pleasure is right, since they are too young to reason otherwise. In later months and years, children can tell easily and quickly by changes in parental facial expressions and voice tones that their behavior is either approved or disapproved.

HEALTH ASSESSMENT AND PROMOTION

Nursing care of infants involves some specific tests. General care of infants and children is discussed in the Nursing Care section later in this chapter.

Apgar Scoring

Newborn babies can be assessed immediately by the Apgar scoring system. This provides a numeric indicator of the baby's physiological capacities to adapt to extrauterine life. Apgar scoring is usually carried out 60 seconds after birth and is repeated in 5 minutes. Those with very low scores require special resuscitative measures and care. Apgar scoring is listed in Table 11-5 ■.

During ongoing assessments, the nurse examines and observes the infant, taking into account variations that occur with developmental age and activity. Health promotion

TABLE 11-5

Apgar Scoring System to Assess the Newborn

SIGN	SCORE		
	0	1	2
1. Heart rate	Absent	Slow (below 100 per minute)	Above 100 per minute
2. Respirations	Absent	Slow, irregular	Regular rate, crying
3. Muscle tone	Flaccid	Some flexion of extremities	Active movements
4. Reflex irritability	None	Grimace	Cries
5. Color	Body pale or cyanotic	Body pink (for African American babies, pink mucous membranes), extremities blue	Body completely pink, pink mucous membranes in African American babies

guidelines for infants, toddlers, and preschoolers are shown in Table 11-6 ∎.

Developmental Screening Tests

Development can be assessed by observing the infant's behavior and by using standardized tests such as the Denver Developmental Screening Test (DDST). The DDST is used to screen children from birth to 6 years of age. The test is intended to estimate the abilities of a child compared to those of an average group of children of the same age and ethnic group.

Toddlers (1 to 3 Years)

Toddlers develop from having no voluntary control to being able to walk and speak. They also learn to control their bladder and bowels, and they acquire all kinds of information about their environment.

PHYSICAL DEVELOPMENT

Toddlers are usually chubby, with relatively short legs and a large head (Figure 11-5 ∎). The face appears small when compared to the skull. Toddlers have a pronounced lumbar lordosis and a protruding abdomen. The abdominal muscles develop gradually with growth, and the abdomen flattens.

Weight

Two-year-olds can be expected to weigh approximately four times their birth weight. The weight gain is about 5 lbs between 1 and 2 years and about 2 to 5 lbs between 2 and 3 years.

Height

A toddler's height can be measured as height or length. Height is measured while the toddler stands, and length is measured while the toddler is in a recumbent position. Be-

tween ages 1 and 2 years, the average growth in height is 4 to 5 inches, and between 2 and 3 years it slows to 2.5 to 3.5 inches.

Head Circumference

The head circumference of the toddler increases about 1 inch on average. By 24 months, the head is 80% of the average adult size and the brain is 70% of its adult size.

Sensory Abilities

Visual acuity is fairly well established at 1 year; average estimates of acuity for the toddler are 20/70 at 18 months and 20/40 at 2 years of age. Accommodation to near and far objects is fairly well developed by 18 months and continues to mature with age. Hearing in the 3-year-old is at adult levels. The taste buds of the toddler are sensitive to the natural flavors of food, and the 3-year-old prefers familiar odors and

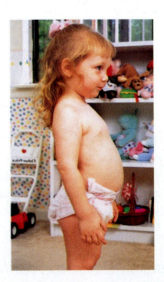

Figure 11-5. ∎ The toddler appears chubby with relatively short legs and a large head. (Photographer: Michael Newman.)

TABLE 11-6

Health Promotion Guidelines for Infants, Toddlers, and Preschoolers

GUIDELINES	INFANTS	TODDLERS	PRESCHOOLERS
Health examinations	At 2 weeks and at 2, 4, 6, and 12 months	At 15 and 18 months and then as recommended by the physician Dental visits starting at age 3 Hearing tests by 18 months or earlier	Every 1 to 2 years
Protective measures	Immunizations: diphtheria-pertussis-tetanus (DPT), oral poliovirus vaccine (OPV), measles-mumps-rubella (MMR), *Haemophilus influenzae* type B, and hepatitis B and varicella vaccines as recommended Fluoride supplements if there is inadequate water fluoridation (less than 0.7 parts per million [ppm]) Screening for tuberculosis Screening for phenylketonuria (PKU) Prompt attention for illnesses Appropriate skin hygiene and clothing	Immunizations: continuing DPT, OPV series, MMR, *Haemophilus influenzae* type B, and hepatitis B vaccines as recommended Screenings for tuberculosis and lead poisoning Fluoride supplements if there is inadequate water fluoridation (less than 0.7 ppm)	Immunizations: continuing DPT, OPV series, MMR vaccine; other immunizations as recommended Screening for tuberculosis Vision and hearing screening Regular dental screenings and fluoride treatment
Safety	Importance of supervision Car seat, crib, playpen, bath, and home environment safety measures Feeding measures (e.g., avoid propping bottle) Providing toys with no small parts or sharp edges	Importance of supervision and teaching child to obey commands Home environment safety measures (e.g., lock medicine cabinet) Outdoor safety measures (e.g., close supervision near water) Appropriate toys	Educating child about simple safety rules (e.g., crossing the street) Teaching child to play safely (e.g., bicycle and playground safety) Educating to prevent poisoning
Nutrition	Breastfeeding and bottle-feeding techniques Formula preparation Feeding schedule Introduction of solid foods Need for iron supplements at 4–6 months	Importance of nutritious meals and snacks Teaching simple mealtime manners Dental care	Importance of nutritious meals and snacks
Elimination	Characteristics and frequency of stool and urine elimination Diarrhea and its effects	Toilet training techniques	Teaching proper hygiene (e.g., washing hands after using bathroom)
Rest/sleep	Usual sleep and rest patterns	Dealing with sleep disturbances	Dealing with sleep disturbances (e.g., nightmares)
Sensory stimulation/play	Touch: holding, cuddling, rocking Vision: colorful, moving toys Hearing: soothing voice tones, music, singing Play: toys appropriate for development	Providing adequate space and a variety of activities Toys that allow "acting on" behaviors and provide motor and sensory stimulation	Providing times for group play activities Teaching child simple games that require cooperation and interaction Providing toys and dress-ups for role-playing

tastes. Touch is a very important sense, and a distressed toddler is often soothed by tactile sensations.

Motor Abilities

Fine muscle coordination and gross motor skills improve during toddlerhood. At 18 months, the child can:

- Pick up small beads and place them in a receptacle.
- Hold a spoon and a cup.
- Walk upstairs with assistance.
- Crawl down the stairs.

At 2 years, toddlers can:

- Hold a spoon and put it into the mouth correctly.
- Run (with steady gait).
- Balance on one foot.
- Ride a tricycle.

By 3 years most children are toilet trained, with occasional nighttime accidents or when playing.

PSYCHOSOCIAL DEVELOPMENT

Toddlers begin to develop their sense of autonomy by asserting themselves with the frequent use of the word *no*. Parents need to have a great deal of patience coupled with an understanding of the importance of this developmental milestone. See Table 11-3 for Erikson's stage for toddlers.

Although toddlers like to explore the environment, they always need to have a significant person nearby. During the toddler stage, receptive and expressive language skills are developing quickly. Children can understand words and follow directions long before they can actually form them into sentences. By 1 year of age, toddlers can recognize their own names.

COGNITIVE DEVELOPMENT

According to Piaget, the toddler completes the fifth and sixth stages of the sensorimotor phase and starts the preconceptual phase at about 2 years of age (see Table 11-4).

MORAL DEVELOPMENT

Kohlberg established six stages of **moral development** (Table 11-7 ■). According to Kohlberg, the first level of moral development is the preconventional when children respond to punishment and reward. During the second year of life, children begin to know that some activities elicit affection and approval.

SPIRITUAL DEVELOPMENT

Fowler theorized six stages of **spiritual development** (Table 11-8 ■). According to Fowler, the toddler's stage of spiritual development is undifferentiated. Toddlers may be

---

TABLE 11-7

Kohlberg's Stages of Moral Development

LEVEL AND STAGE	DEFINITION	EXAMPLE
Level I Preconventional		
Stage 1: Punishment and obedience orientation	The activity is wrong if one is punished, and the activity is right if one is not punished.	A nurse follows a physician's order so as not to be fired.
Stage 2: Instrumental-relativist orientation	Action is taken to satisfy one's needs.	A client in hospital agrees to stay in bed if the nurse will buy the client a newspaper.
Level II Conventional		
Stage 3: Interpersonal concordance (good boy, nice girl)	Action is taken to please another and gain approval.	A nurse gives elderly clients in hospital sedatives at bedtime because the night nurse wants all clients to sleep at night.
Stage 4: Law and order orientation	Right behavior is obeying the law and following the rules.	A nurse does not permit a worried client to phone home because hospital rules stipulate no phone calls after 9:00 P.M.
Level III Postconventional		
Stage 5: Social contract, legalistic orientation	Standard of behavior is based on adhering to laws that protect the welfare and rights of others.	A nurse arranges for an East Indian client to have privacy for prayer each evening.
Stage 6: Universal-ethical principals	Personal values and opinions are recognized, and violating the rights of others is avoided. Universal moral principles are internalized. Person respects other humans and believes that relationships are based on mutual trust.	A nurse becomes an advocate for a hospitalized client by reporting to the nursing supervisor a conversation in which a physician threatened to withhold assistance unless the client agreed to surgery.

Source: Adapted from R. Duska and M. Whelan, *Moral Development: A Guide to Piaget and Kohlberg.* Copyright 1975 by The Missionary Society of St. Paul the Apostle in the State of New York. Used by permission of Paulist Press.

TABLE 11-8

Fowler's Stages of Spiritual Development

STAGE	AGE	DESCRIPTION
0. Undifferentiated	0–3 years	Infant unable to formulate concepts about self or the environment.
1. Intuitive–projective	4–6 years	A combination of images and beliefs given by trusted others, mixed with the child's own experience and imagination.
2. Mythic–literal	7–12 years	Private world of fantasy and wonder; symbols refer to something specific; dramatic stories and myths used to communicate spiritual meanings.
3. Synthetic–conventional	Adolescent or adult	World and ultimate environment structured by the expectations and judgments of others; interpersonal focus.
4. Individuating–reflexive	After 18 years	Constructing one's own explicit system; high degree of self-consciousness.
5. Paradoxical–consolidative	After 30 years	Awareness of truth from a variety of viewpoints.
6. Universalizing	Maybe never	Becoming an incarnation of the principles of love and justice.

Source: Data from J. Fowler and S. Keen, *Life Maps: Conversations in the Journey of Faith* (Waco, TX: Word Books, 1985); and A. Hollander, *How to Help Your Child Have a Spiritual Life: A Parents' Guide to Inner Development* (New York: A & W Publishers, 1980).

aware of some religious practices, but they are primarily involved in learning knowledge and emotional reactions rather than establishing spiritual beliefs. A toddler may repeat short prayers at bedtime, conforming to a ritual, because praise and affection result.

HEALTH ASSESSMENT AND PROMOTION

Assessment activities for the toddler are similar to those for the infant in terms of measuring weight, length (height), and vital signs. Promoting health and wellness includes such areas as injury prevention, toilet training, and good dental hygiene. See Table 11-6 for health promotion guidelines. See also the Nursing Care section later in the chapter.

Preschoolers (4 and 5 Years)

During the preschool period, physical growth slows, but control of the body and coordination increase greatly.

PHYSICAL DEVELOPMENT

By the time children are 4 or 5 years old, they appear taller and thinner than toddlers. The preschooler's brain reaches almost its adult size by 5 years. The extremities of the body grow more quickly than the body trunk, making the child's body appear somewhat out of proportion.

Weight, Height, and Sensory Abilities

Weight gain in preschool children is generally slow. By 5 years, they have added only another 7 to 12 lbs to their 3-year-old weight. Preschool children grow about 2.0 to 2.5 inches each year.

VISION.   Preschool children are generally *hyperopic* (farsighted), that is, unable to focus on near objects. By the end of the preschool years, visual ability has improved to approximately 20/30.

HEARING AND TASTE.   The hearing of the preschool child has reached optimal levels, and the ability to listen (attending to and comprehending what is said) has matured since the toddler age. As for the sense of taste, preschoolers show their preferences by asking for something "yummy," and may refuse something they consider "yucky."

Motor Abilities

By 5 years of age, children are able to wash their hands and face and brush their teeth. They are self-conscious about exposing their bodies and go to the bathroom without telling others. Typically, preschool children run with increasing skill each year. By 5 years of age, they run skillfully and can jump three steps. Preschoolers can balance on their toes and dress themselves without assistance.

PSYCHOSOCIAL DEVELOPMENT

Erikson writes that the major developmental crisis of the preschooler is initiative versus guilt (see Table 11-3). Parents can enhance the self-concept of the preschooler by providing opportunities for new achievements where the child can learn, repeat, and master.

The self-concept of the preschooler is also based on gender identification. Preschoolers are aware of the two sexes and identify with the correct one. They may mimic the parent's behavior, attitudes, and appearance (Figure 11-6 ■).

Preschool children gradually emerge as social beings. At the age of 3 or 4, they learn to play with a small number of their peers. They gradually learn to play with more people as they grow older. Preschoolers also learn about

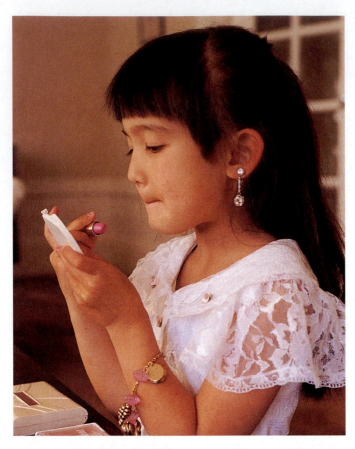

Figure 11-6. ■ Preschoolers often identify with the parent of the same sex and like to mimic behavior. (Photographer: Elena Dorfman.)

their feelings; they know the words *cry, sad,* and *laugh,* and the feelings related to them. They also begin to learn how to control their feelings and behavior. The preschooler uses the same types of coping mechanisms in response to stress as the toddler does, although protest behavior (kicking, screaming) is less likely to occur in the older preschooler.

COGNITIVE, MORAL, AND SPIRITUAL DEVELOPMENT

The preschooler's cognitive development, according to Piaget, is the phase of intuitive thought (see Table 11-4). Reading skills also start to develop at this age.

Preschoolers are capable of prosocial behavior, that is, any action that a person takes to benefit someone else. The term *prosocial* is synonymous with *kind* and connotes sharing, helping, protecting, giving aid, befriending, showing affection, and giving encouragement. Moral behavior to a preschooler may mean taking turns at play or sharing. It is important for parents to answer preschoolers' "why" questions and discuss values with them (see Table 11-7).

Many preschoolers enroll in Sunday school or faith-oriented classes. The preschooler usually enjoys the social interaction of these classes (see Table 11-8). Faith at this stage is primarily a result of the teaching of significant others, such as parents and teachers.

HEALTH ASSESSMENT AND PROMOTION

During assessment, the preschooler can often participate in answering questions with assistance from parents or caregivers. Health promotion guidelines for the preschooler are shown in Table 11-6. Further information on nursing care follows later in the chapter.

School-Age Children (6 to 12 Years)

The school-age period starts when children are about 6 years of age, when the deciduous teeth are shed. This period includes the preadolescent (*prepuberty*) period. It ends at about 12 years, with the onset of puberty. **Puberty** is the age when the reproductive organs become functional and secondary sex characteristics develop. See Chapter 15 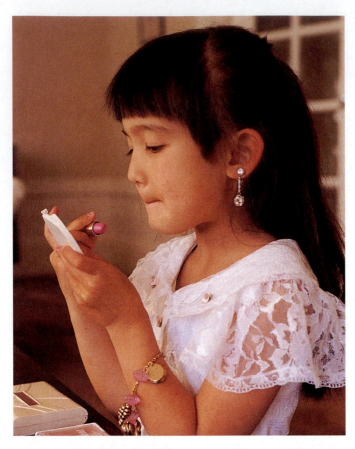 for further discussion of sexuality and sexual development. In general, the period from 6 to 12 years is one of rapid and dramatic change.

PHYSICAL DEVELOPMENT

Weight, Height, and Sensory Abilities

The school-age child gains weight rapidly and thus appears less thin than previously. At 6 years boys tend to weigh about 2 lbs more than girls. The weight gain of school children from 6 to 12 years of age averages 7 lbs per year, but the major weight gains occur from ages 10 to 12 for boys and from 9 to 12 for girls.

At 6 years both boys and girls are about the same height. Before puberty, children of both sexes have a growth spurt, girls between 10 and 12 years and boys between 12 and 14 years. Thus, girls may well be taller than boys at 12 years, but boys are usually stronger.

VISION.   The depth and distance perception of children 6 to 8 years of age is accurate. By age 6, children have full binocular vision. The eye muscles are well developed and coordinated, and both eyes can focus on one object at the same time. A child's 20/20 vision is usually well established between 9 and 11 years of age.

HEARING AND TOUCH.   Auditory perception is fully developed in school-age children, who are able to identify fine differences in voices, both in sound and in pitch. At this stage, children also have a well-developed sense of touch and are able to locate points of heat and cold on all body surfaces. They are also able to identify an unseen object, such as a pencil or a book, simply by touch. This ability is called *stereognosis.*

Prepubertal Changes

Little change takes place in the reproductive and endocrine systems until the prepuberty period. During prepuberty, at about ages 9 to 13, endocrine functions slowly increase.

This change in endocrine function can result in increased perspiration and more active sebaceous glands.

Motor Abilities

During the middle years (6 to 10), children perfect their muscular skills and coordination. By 9 years most children are becoming skilled in games of interest, such as football or baseball. These skills are often associated with school, and many of them are learned there. By 9 years most children have sufficient fine motor control for such activities as building models or sewing.

PSYCHOSOCIAL DEVELOPMENT

At this time children begin to create and develop a sense of competence and perseverance. School-age children are motivated by activities that provide a sense of worth. They concentrate on mastering skills that will help them function in the adult world (Figure 11-7 ■; see also Table 11-3).

As they grow older, schoolchildren learn to play with more children at one time. Usually, the 6- or 7-year-old is a member of a peer group. This group can have a greater influence than the family in teaching attitudes.

The schoolchild's self-concept continues to mature. Children recognize similarities and differences between themselves and others. School-age children compare themselves with others and obtain feedback from teachers and peers.

COGNITIVE, MORAL, AND SPIRITUAL DEVELOPMENT

According to Piaget, the ages 7 to 11 years mark the phase of concrete operations (see Table 11-4). During this stage, the child changes from egocentric interactions to cooperative interactions.

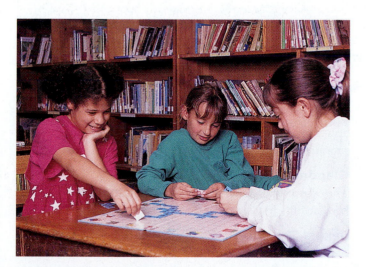

Figure 11-7. ■ Expanding cognitive skills enable school-age children to interact cooperatively in activities of an increasingly complex nature, as shown by the children playing this board game. (Photographer: Jane Wattenburg.)

Some school-age children are at Kohlberg's stage 1 of the preconventional level (punishment and obedience); that is, they act to avoid being punished. Some school-age children, however, are at stage 2 (instrumental-relativist orientation). These children do things to benefit themselves. Fairness (everyone getting a fair share or chance) becomes important (see Table 11-7).

According to Fowler, the school-age child is at stage 2 in spiritual development, the mythic–literal stage (see Table 11-8). Children learn to distinguish fantasy from fact. Spiritual facts are those beliefs that are accepted by a religious group. Parents and the minister, rabbi, or priest help the child distinguish fact from fantasy. These people still influence the child more than peers in spiritual matters.

School-age children may ask many questions about God and religion in these years and will generally believe that God is good and always present to help. Just before puberty, children become aware that their prayers are not always answered and become disappointed.

HEALTH ASSESSMENT AND PROMOTION

During the assessment interview, the nurse responds to questions from the parent or other caregiver, gives appropriate feedback, and lends encouragement and support. Promoting health and wellness includes dental hygiene and regular dental examinations, safety measures to prevent accidents, promoting physical fitness, supporting autonomy and self-esteem, and hygiene measures to prevent infections. See Table 11-9 ■ for health promotion guidelines for school-age children and adolescents.

Adolescents (12 to 18 Years)

Adolescence is the period during which the person becomes physically and psychologically mature and acquires a personal identity. At the end of this critical period in development, the person is ready to enter adulthood and assume its responsibilities. Puberty is the first stage of adolescence in which sexual organs begin to grow and mature.

PHYSICAL DEVELOPMENT

Height, Weight, and Structure

During puberty, growth is markedly accelerated compared to the slow, steady growth of the child. This period, marked by sudden and dramatic physical changes, is referred to as the adolescent growth spurt. In boys, the growth spurt usually begins between ages 12 and 16; in girls, it begins earlier, usually between ages 10 and 14. Because the growth spurt begins earlier in girls, many girls surpass boys in height at this time.

Physical growth continues throughout adolescence. Growth is fastest for boys at about 14 years, and the maximum height is often reached at about 18 or 19 years. Some

---

TABLE 11-9

Health Promotion Guidelines for School-Age Children and Adolescents

GUIDELINES	SCHOOL-AGE CHILDREN	ADOLESCENTS
Health examinations	Annual physical examination or as recommended	As recommended by the physician
Protective measures	Immunizations as recommended Screening for tuberculosis Periodic vision, speech, and hearing screenings Regular dental screenings and fluoride treatment Providing accurate information about sexual issues (e.g., reproduction, AIDS)	Immunizations as recommended, such as adult tetanus-diphtheria (Td) vaccine and hepatitis B vaccine Screening for tuberculosis Periodic vision and hearing screenings Regular dental assessments Obtaining and providing accurate information about sexual issues
Safety	Using proper equipment when participating in sports and other physical activities (e.g., helmets, pads) Encouraging child to take responsibility for own safety (e.g., participating in bicycle and water safety courses)	Adolescent's taking responsibility for using motor vehicles safely (e.g., completing a driver's education course, wearing seat belt and helmet) Making certain that proper precautions are taken during all athletic activities (e.g., medical supervision, proper equipment) Parents' keeping lines of communication open and being alert to signs of substance abuse and emotional disturbances in the adolescent
Nutrition, elimination, exercise	Importance of child not skipping meals and eating a balanced diet Experiences with food that may lead to obesity Utilizing positive approaches for elimination problems (e.g., enuresis)	Importance of healthy snacks and appropriate patterns of food intake and exercise Factors that may lead to nutritional problems (e.g., obesity, anorexia nervosa, bulimia) Balancing sedentary activities with regular exercise
Play and social interactions	Providing opportunities for a variety of organized group activities Accepting realistic expectations of child's abilities Acting as role models in acceptance of other persons who may be different Providing a home environment that limits TV viewing and video games and encourages completion of homework	Encouraging adolescent to establish relationships that promote discussion of feelings, concerns, and fears Parents' encouraging adolescent peer group activities that promote appropriate moral and spiritual values Parents' acting as role models for appropriate social interactions Parents' providing a comfortable home environment for appropriate adolescent peer group activities

men add another 1 or 2 cm to their height during their 20s as the vertebral column gradually continues to grow. During the period of 10 to 18 years of age, the average American male doubles his weight and grows about 16 inches.

Growth is noted first in the musculoskeletal system. This growth follows a sequential pattern: The head, hands, and feet are the first to grow to adult status. Next, the extremities reach their adult size. Because the extremities grow before the trunk, the adolescent looks leggy, awkward, and uncoordinated. After the trunk grows to full size, the shoulders, chest, and hips grow. Skull and facial bones

also change proportions: The forehead becomes more prominent, and the jawbones develop.

Glandular Changes

The eccrine and apocrine glands increase their secretions and become fully functional during puberty.

Sexual Characteristics

During puberty, both primary and secondary sex characteristics develop. Primary sexual characteristics relate to the organs necessary for reproduction, such as the testes, penis, vagina, and uterus. Secondary sexual characteristics differentiate the male from the female but do not relate directly to reproduction. See discussion in Chapter 15 ⚭.

The first noticeable sign that puberty has begun in males is the appearance of pubic hair. Sexual maturity is achieved by age 18.

Often, the first noticeable sign of puberty in females is the appearance of the breast bud, although the appearance of hair along the labia may precede this. The milestone of female puberty is the *menarche* (beginning of menstrual cycles), which occurs about 2 years after the breast bud appears. At first, menstrual periods are scanty and irregular and may occur without ovulation. Ovulation is usually established 1 to 2 years after menarche. Female internal reproductive organs reach adult size at about age 18 to 20.

PSYCHOSOCIAL DEVELOPMENT

The psychosocial task of the adolescent is the establishment of identity. The danger of this stage is role confusion (see Table 11-3). Because of the adolescent's dramatic body changes, the development of a stable identity is difficult. Adolescents who are accepted, loved, and valued by family and peers generally tend to gain confidence and feel good about themselves. Adolescents who have difficulty forming relationships or who are perceived by peers as too different and not included in adolescent cliques may develop less favorable self-images and have low self-esteem.

Adolescents still need guidance from their parents, although they appear to neither want it nor need it. However, adolescents need to know that their parents care about them and that their parents still want to help them. Restrictions and guidance need to be presented in a manner that makes adolescents feel loved. They need consistency in guidance and fewer restrictions than previously. They should have the independence they can handle yet know that their parents will assist them when they need help.

During adolescence, peer groups assume great importance (Figure 11-8 ■).

COGNITIVE DEVELOPMENT

Cognitive abilities mature during adolescence. Between the ages of 11 and 15, the adolescent begins the formal operations stage of cognitive development (see Table 11-4). The adolescent becomes more informed about the world and environment. Adolescents use new information to solve everyday problems and can communicate with adults on most subjects.

MORAL DEVELOPMENT

According to Kohlberg, the young adolescent is usually at the conventional level of moral development. Most still accept the Golden Rule and want to abide by social order

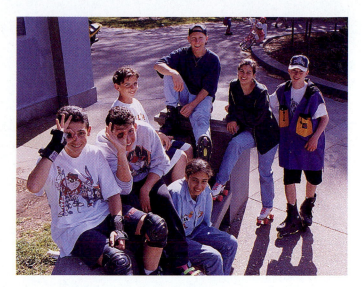

Figure 11-8. ■ Adolescent peer group relationships enhance a sense of belonging, self-esteem, and self-identity. (Photographer: Elena Dorfman.)

and existing laws. Adolescents examine their values, standards, and morals. They may discard the values they have adopted from parents in favor of values they consider more suitable. See Kohlberg's stages of moral development in Table 11-7.

SPIRITUAL DEVELOPMENT

According to Fowler, the adolescent or young adult reaches the synthetic–conventional stage of spiritual development (see Table 11-8). The adolescent may reconcile the differences in one of the following ways:

- Deciding any differences are wrong
- Compartmentalizing the differences (For example, a friend may not be able to go to dances on Friday evenings because of religious observances, but the friend can share activities on other days.)
- Obtaining advice from a significant other, such as a parent or a minister.

Often, the adolescent believes that various religious beliefs and practices have more similarities than differences.

HEALTH ASSESSMENT AND PROMOTION

Adolescents are usually self-directed in meeting their health needs. Because of maturation changes, however, they need teaching and guidance in a number of health-care areas.

Promoting health and wellness includes screening for tobacco, alcohol, and drug use and for sexual practices, and checking blood pressure, height, and weight. See Table 11-9 for health promotion guidelines for adolescents.

Young Adults (20 to 40 Years)

Legally, a person in the United States can vote at 18 years of age. Another criterion of adulthood is financial independence, which is also highly variable. Some adults are financially dependent on their families for many years during prolonged educational courses.

Adulthood may also be indicated by moving away from home and establishing one's own living arrangements. Many adults under age 30 continue to live with parents due to high housing costs and unemployment rates, as well as social issues such as high divorce rates, single parenting, and the problems resulting from substance abuse. Some young people who are employed full time receive only minimum wage and are unable to earn enough money to be totally self-supporting.

Young adults are typically busy people who face many challenges. They are expected to assume new roles at work, in the home, and in the community, and to develop interests, values, and attitudes related to these roles.

PHYSICAL DEVELOPMENT

People in their early 20s are in their prime years physically. The musculoskeletal system is well developed and coordinated. This is the period when athletic endeavors reach their peak.

Although physical changes are minimal during this stage, weight and muscle mass may change as a result of diet and exercise. In addition, extensive physical and psychosocial changes occur in pregnant and lactating women. These changes are discussed in maternal/child textbooks.

PSYCHOSOCIAL DEVELOPMENT

In contrast to the minimal physical changes, psychosocial development and stresses of the young adult are great (see Chapter 16 ⬳). Young adults face a number of new experiences and changes in lifestyle as they progress toward maturity.

Remaining single is becoming the lifestyle choice of more and more young adults. Many people choose to remain single, perhaps to pursue an education and then to have the freedom to pursue their chosen vocation. Some unmarried individuals choose to live with another person of the opposite or same sex and share living arrangements and certain expenses. Some unmarried people are gay or lesbian and live with or are involved with a partner to whom they are committed.

The multiple roles of adulthood (citizen, worker, taxpayer, homeowner, wife/husband, daughter/son, brother/sister, parent, friend, etc.) may also create stress as a result of role conflict (Figure 11-9 ■). See Table 11-3 for Erikson's stage for young adults.

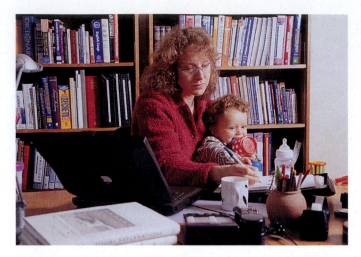

Figure 11-9. ■ Many young women combine active careers with motherhood. (Photographer: Elena Dorfman.)

COGNITIVE, MORAL, AND SPIRITUAL DEVELOPMENT

Cognitive structures were completed during the formal operations period, from roughly 11 to 15 years (see Table 11-4).

Young adults who have mastered the previous stages of Kohlberg's theory of moral development now enter the postconventional level (see Table 11-7). At this time, the person is able to separate self from the expectations and rules of others and to define morality in terms of personal principles.

According to Fowler, the individual enters the individuating–reflective period sometime after 18 years of age (see Table 11-8).

HEALTH ASSESSMENT AND PROMOTION

Young adults are usually interested in meeting their health needs. However, because of the many stresses and changes that occur throughout this 20-year period, the nurse needs to offer teaching and guidance in several healthcare areas. The nurse may wish to discuss some or all of the health promotion topics outlined for adults in Table 11-10 ■.

Middle-Aged Adults (40 to 65 Years)

The middle years, from 40 to 65, have been called the years of stability and consolidation. For most people, it is a time when children have grown and moved away or are moving away from home. Thus, partners generally have more time for and with each other and time to pursue interests they may have deferred for years.

PHYSICAL DEVELOPMENT

A number of changes take place during the middle years. At age 40, most adults can function as effectively as they did in

TABLE 11-10

Health Promotion Guidelines for Young Adults, Middle-Aged Adults, and Older Adults

GUIDELINES	YOUNG ADULTS	MIDDLE-AGED ADULTS	OLDER ADULTS
Health tests and screenings	Routine physical examination (every 1–3 years for females; every 5 years for males) Immunizations as recommended, such as Td boosters Regular dental assessments (e.g., annually) Periodic vision and hearing screenings Breast self-examination monthly, 1 week after onset of period Professional breast examination every 1–3 years Papanicolaou smear annually or at onset of sexual activity Testicular self-examination every month Screening for cardiovascular disease (e.g., cholesterol test every 5 years if results are normal; blood pressure to detect hypertension; baseline electrocardiogram at age 35 for males) Tuberculosis skin test every 2 years	Routine physical examination (annually for females; every 2–3 years or as directed by physician for males) Immunizations as recommended, such as a tetanus booster every 10–15 years and influenza and pneumococcal vaccinations Regular dental assessments (e.g., yearly) Tonometry for signs of glaucoma and other eye disease every 2–3 years or annually if indicated Breast self-examination as for young adults and first day of every month after menopause Testicular self-examination monthly Screenings for cardiovascular disease (e.g., blood pressure measurement; electrocardiogram and cholesterol test as directed by the physician) Screenings for colorectal, breast, cervical, uterine, and prostate cancer Screening for tuberculosis every 2 years	As for middle-aged adults
Safety	Motor safety reinforcement (e.g., using designated drivers when drinking, maintaining brakes and tires) Sun protection measures Workplace safety measures Water safety reinforcement (e.g., no diving in shallow water)	Motor vehicle safety reinforcement, especially when driving at night Workplace safety measures Home safety measures: keeping hallways and stairways lighted and uncluttered, using smoke detectors, using nonskid mats and handrails in the bathrooms	Home safety measures to prevent falls, fire, burns, scalds, and electrocution Motor vehicle safety reinforcement, especially when driving at night Precautions to prevent pedestrian accidents
Nutrition, exercise, and elimination	Importance of adequate iron intake in diet Nutritional and exercise factors that may lead to cardiovascular disease (e.g., obesity, cholesterol and fat intake, lack of vigorous exercise)	Importance of adequate protein, calcium, and vitamin D in diet Nutritional and exercise factors that may lead to cardiovascular disease (e.g., obesity, cholesterol and fat intake, lack of vigorous exercise) An exercise program that emphasizes skill and coordination	Importance of a well-balanced diet with fewer calories to accommodate lower metabolic rate and decreased physical activity Importance of sufficient amounts of vitamin D and calcium to prevent osteoporosis Nutritional and exercise factors that may lead to cardiovascular disease (e.g., obesity, cholesterol and fat intake, lack of exercise)

(continued)

TABLE 11-10

Health Promotion Guidelines for Young Adults, Middle-Aged Adults, and Older Adults (*continued*)

GUIDELINES	YOUNG ADULTS	MIDDLE-AGED ADULTS	OLDER ADULTS
			A regular program of moderate exercise to maintain joint mobility, muscle tone, and bone calcification Importance of adequate roughage in the diet, adequate exercise, and at least six 8-ounce glasses of fluid daily to prevent constipation
Social interactions	Encouraging personal relationships that promote discussion of feelings, concerns, and fears Setting short- and long-term goals for work and career choices	The possibility of a midlife crisis: encourage discussion of feelings, concerns, and fears Providing time to expand and review previous interests Retirement planning (financial and possible diversional activities), with partner if appropriate	Encouraging intellectual and recreational pursuits Encouraging personal relationship that promote discussion of feelings, concerns, and fears Availability of social community centers and programs for seniors.

their 20s. However, during ages 40 to 65, many physical changes take place. Normal changes of aging, which become more pronounced among older adults, are described in Table 11-11 ■.

PSYCHOSOCIAL DEVELOPMENT

Before the mid-1900s, the developmental tasks of middle-aged adults received little attention. Havighurst outlined seven tasks for this age group (Table 11-12 ■). Erikson views the developmental choice of the middle-aged adult as generativity versus stagnation (see Table 11-3). *Generativity* is defined as the concern for establishing and guiding the next generation. In other words, the concern about providing for the welfare of humankind is equal to the concern of providing for self.

The middle-aged person looks older and feels older. Although people of these ages are reaching their prime, they begin to recognize that time is at a premium and that life is finite. Youthfulness and physical strength can no longer be taken for granted.

Some researchers suggest that it is not the events themselves that make midlife a crisis, but an individual's response to these life events. Internal and external resources include physical health, family income, the social support system, intelligence, and personality. Thus, the crisis or transitions of midlife are not just within the individual but rather between the individual and the individual's world.

COGNITIVE, MORAL, AND SPIRITUAL DEVELOPMENT

The middle-aged adult's cognitive and intellectual abilities change very little. Cognitive processes include reaction time, memory, perception, learning, problem solving, and creativity. Learning continues and can be enhanced by increased motivation at this time in life.

Middle-aged adults are able to carry out all the strategies described in Piaget's phase of formal operations (see Table 11-4).

According to Kohlberg, the adult can move beyond the conventional level to the postconventional level (see Table 11-7).

Not all adults progress through Fowler's stages to the fifth, called the paradoxical–consolidative stage (see Table 11-8). At this stage, the individual can view "truth" from a number of viewpoints. In middle age, people tend to be less dogmatic about religious beliefs. People in this age group often rely on spiritual beliefs to help them deal with illness, death, and tragedy.

HEALTH ASSESSMENT AND PROMOTION

Guidelines for health promotion for the middle-aged adult are shown in Table 11-11. Further discussion of nursing care is provided in the Nursing Care section on page 222.

Older Adults (Over 65 Years)

In 2000, the number of Americans age 65 and older was about 14% of the population. By the year 2030, that percentage is projected to increase to more than 18% of the population. The group of older individuals who are 85 years and older is rapidly increasing. Census projections estimate that the population over age 85 will almost triple by the year 2020 (U.S. Bureau of the Census, 2000).

Various systems are used to categorize the aging population. *Frail elderly,* a term used to described the extremely

TABLE 11-11

Normal Physical Changes Associated with Aging

PHYSICAL CHANGES	RATIONALE
Integumentary	
Increased skin dryness	Decrease in sebaceous gland activity and tissue fluid
Increased skin pallor	Decreased vascularity
Increased skin fragility	Reduced thickness and vascularity of the dermis; loss of subcutaneous fat
Progressive wrinkling and sagging of the skin	Loss of skin elasticity, increased dryness, and decreased subcutaneous fat
Brown "age spots" (*lentigo senilis*) on exposed body parts (e.g., face, hands, arms)	Clustering of melanocytes (pigment-producing cells)
Decreased perspiration	Reduced number and function of sweat glands
Thinning and graying of scalp, pubic, and axillary hair	Progressive loss of pigment cells from the hair bulbs
Slower nail growth and increased thickening with ridges	Increased calcium deposition
Neuromuscular	
Decreased speed and power of skeletal muscle contractions	Decrease in muscle fibers
Slowed reaction time	Diminished conduction speed of nerve fibers and decreased muscle tone
Loss of height (stature)	Atrophy of intervertebral disks
Osteoporosis	Bone demineralization
Joint stiffness	Deterioration of joint cartilage
Impaired balance	Decreased muscle reaction time and coordination
Sensory/perceptual	
Loss of visual acuity	Degeneration leading to lens opacity (cataracts), thickening, and inelasticity (presbyopia)
Increased sensitivity to glare and decreased ability to adjust to darkness	Changes in the ciliary muscles; rigid pupil sphincter; decrease in pupil size
Partial or complete glossy white circle around the periphery of the cornea (*arcus senilis*)	Fatty deposits
Progressive loss of hearing (presbycusis)	Changes in the structures and nerve tissues in the inner ear; thickening of the eardrum
Decreased sense of taste, especially the sweet sensations at the tip of the tongue	Decreased number of taste buds in the tongue because of tongue atrophy
Decreased sense of smell	Atrophy of the olfactory bulb at the base of the brain (responsible for smell perception)
Increased threshold for sensations of pain, touch, and temperature	Possible nerve conduction and neuron changes
Pulmonary	
Decreased ability to expel foreign or accumulated matter	Decreased elasticity and ciliary activity
Decreased lung expansion; less effective exhalation; reduced vital capacity; and increased residual volume	Weakened thoracic muscles; calcification of costal cartilage, making the rib cage more rigid; dilation from inelasticity of alveoli
Difficult, short, heavy, rapid breathing (dyspnea) following exertion or intense exercise	Diminished delivery and diffusion of oxygen to the tissues to repay the normal oxygen debt because of changes in both respiratory and vascular tissues
Cardiovascular	
Reduced cardiac output and stroke volume, particularly during increased activity or unusual demands; may result in shortness of breath on exertion and pooling of blood in the extremities	Increased rigidity and thickness of heart valves (hence decreased filling/emptying abilities); decreased contractile strength
Reduced elasticity and increased rigidity of arteries	Increased calcium deposits in the muscular layer
Increase in diastolic and systolic blood pressure	Inelasticity of systemic arteries and increased peripheral resistance
Orthostatic hypotension	Reduced sensitivity of the blood pressure–regulating baroreceptors

(continued)

TABLE 11-11

Normal Physical Changes Associated with Aging (*continued*)

PHYSICAL CHANGES	RATIONALE
Gastrointestinal	
Delayed swallowing time	Alterations in the swallowing mechanism
Increased tendency for indigestion	Gradual decrease in digestive enzymes, reduction in gastric pH, and slower absorption rate
Increased tendency for constipation	Decreased muscle tone of the intestines; decreased peristalsis
Urinary	
Reduced filtering ability of the kidney and impaired renal function	Decreased number of functioning nephrons (basic functional units of the kidney) and arteriosclerotic changes in blood flow
Less effective concentration of urine	Decreased tubular function
Urinary urgency and urinary frequency	Enlarged prostate gland in men; weakened muscles supporting the bladder or weakness of the urinary sphincter in women
Tendency for a nocturnal frequency and retention of residual urine	Decreased bladder capacity and tone
Genitals	
Prostate enlargement (benign) in men	Exact mechanism is unclear; possible endocrine changes
Multiple changes in women (shrinkage and atrophy of the vulva, cervix, uterus, fallopian tubes, and ovaries; reduction in secretions; and changes in vaginal flora)	Diminished secretion of female hormones and more alkaline vaginal pH

TABLE 11-12

Havighurst's Age Periods and Developmental Tasks

Infancy and Early Childhood

1. Learning to walk
2. Learning to take solid foods
3. Learning to talk
4. Learning to control the elimination of body wastes
5. Learning sex differences and sexual modesty
6. Achieving psychological stability
7. Forming simple concepts of social and physical reality
8. Learning to relate emotionally to parents, siblings, and other people
9. Learning to distinguish right from wrong and developing a conscience

Middle Childhood

1. Learning physical skills necessary for ordinary games
2. Building wholesome attitudes toward oneself as a growing organism
3. Learning to get along with age-mates
4. Learning an appropriate masculine or feminine social role
5. Developing fundamental skills in reading, writing, and calculating
6. Developing concepts necessary for everyday living
7. Developing conscience, morality, and a scale of values
8. Achieving personal independence
9. Developing attitudes toward social groups and institutions

Adolescence

1. Achieving new and more mature relations with age-mates of both sexes
2. Achieving a masculine or feminine social role
3. Accepting one's physique and using the body effectively
4. Achieving emotional independence from parents and other adults
5. Achieving assurance of economic independence
6. Selecting and preparing for an occupation
7. Preparing for marriage and family life
8. Developing intellectual skills and concepts necessary for civic competence
9. Desiring and achieving socially responsible behavior
10. Acquiring a set of values and an ethical system as a guide to behavior

Early Adulthood

1. Selecting a mate
2. Learning to live with a partner
3. Starting a family
4. Rearing children
5. Managing a home
6. Getting started in an occupation
7. Taking on civic responsibility
8. Finding a congenial social group

TABLE 11-12

Havighurst's Age Periods and Developmental Tasks (*continued*)

Middle Age	Later Maturity
1. Achieving adult civic and social responsibility	1. Adjusting to decreasing physical strength and health
2. Establishing and maintaining an economic standard of living	2. Adjusting to retirement and reduced income
3. Assisting teenage children to become responsible and happy adults	3. Adjusting to death of a spouse
4. Developing adult leisure-time activities	4. Establishing an explicit affiliation with one's age group
5. Relating oneself to one's spouse as a person	5. Meeting social and civil obligations
6. Accepting and adjusting to the physiological changes of middle age	6. Establishing satisfactory physical living arrangements
7. Adjusting to aging parents	

Source: From Robert J. Havighurst, *Developmental Tasks and Education,* 3rd ed. Published by Allyn and Bacon, Boston, MA. Copyright © 1972 by Pearson Education.

---

aged, is more likely to be used to describe the elderly individual who has significant physiological and functional impairment, whatever the age.

PHYSICAL CHANGES

As the person ages, a number of physical changes occur; some are visible, some are not. Table 11-11 summarizes normal physical changes associated with aging.

PSYCHOSOCIAL DEVELOPMENT

According to Erikson, the developmental task at this time is ego integrity versus despair (see Table 11-3). People who attain ego integrity view life with a sense of wholeness and derive satisfaction from past accomplishments. They view death as an acceptable completion of life. By contrast, people who despair often believe they have made poor choices during life and wish they could live life over. For other viewpoints on developmental tasks of the older adult, see Box 11-4 ▪.

BOX 11-4   **POPULATION FOCUS**

Developmental Tasks of the Older Adult

- Adjusting to decreasing physical strength and health; safeguarding mental health
- Adjusting to retirement and reduced income; establishing a comfortable routine
- Adjusting to the death of a spouse
- Establishing an explicit affiliation with one's age group; keeping involved
- Meeting social and civic obligations
- Establishing satisfactory living arrangements
- Maintaining marital and family relations

Retirement

Today, a majority of the people over age 65 are unemployed. However, many who are healthy continue to work on a full- or part-time basis. Work offers these people a better income, a sense of self-worth, and the chance to continue long-established routines. Some need to work for economic reasons.

Retirement can be a time when projects or recreational activities deferred for a long time can be pursued (Figure 11-10 ▪). The lifestyle of later years is to a large degree

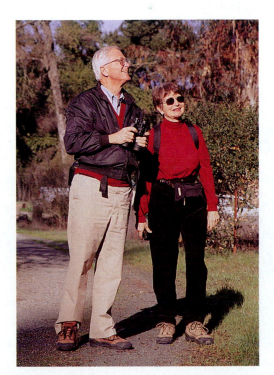

Figure 11-10. ▪ Middle-aged adults have time to pursue interests that may have been put aside for child care. (Photographer: Elena Dorfman.)

formulated in youth. People who attempt suddenly to refocus and enrich their lives at retirement usually have difficulty. The later years can foster a sense of integrity and continuity, or they can be years of despair.

Economic Changes

The financial needs of elderly people vary considerably. Food and medical costs alone are often a financial burden. Adequate financial resources enable the older person to remain independent.

Problems with income are often related to low retirement benefits, lack of pension plans for many workers, and the increased length of the retirement years. Nurses should be aware of the costs of health care. For example, the nurse or the client can request the physician to order lower priced medications.

Relocation

During late adulthood, many people experience relocation. A variety of factors may lead to this decision. The home may be too large or too expensive; maintenance may become burdensome or impossible. Decreased mobility may require living on one floor with more accessible bathroom facilities.

Leaving the family home and the neighbors and friends of several decades may be a difficult decision. Relocation for some is voluntary. The person may be seeking a more moderate climate with better recreational facilities geared to a more leisurely lifestyle. Adjustment will be much easier for the elderly person making a voluntary move.

Some elderly people must relocate to assisted living or long-term care facilities. The decision to enter a nursing home is frequently made when elderly people can no longer care for themselves, often because of problems of mobility and memory impairment. An increasing number of nursing home residents are in the very old age group (85 years and over), and most are women.

Maintaining Independence and Self-Esteem

Most elderly people thrive on independence (Figure 11-11 ■). It is important to them to be able to look after themselves even if they have to struggle to do so. Although it may be difficult for younger family members to watch an older person completing tasks in a slow, determined way, aging people need this sense of accomplishment. To maintain the elderly adult's sense of self-respect, nurses and family members need to encourage them to do as much as possible for themselves, provided that safety is maintained. Nurses need to acknowledge the elderly client's ability to think, reason, and make decisions. Most elderly people are willing to listen to suggestions and advice, but they do not want to be ordered around. The nurse can support a decision by an elderly client even if eventually the decision is reversed because of failing health.

Facing Death

Well-adjusted aging couples usually thrive on companionship. Many couples rely increasingly on their mates for this company. When a mate dies, the remaining partner

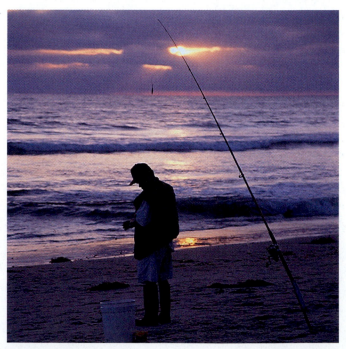

A   B

Figure 11-11. ■ **A.** Many elderly people find creative outlets during retirement. **B.** Retirement provides time for enjoying hobbies.
(**A:** Photographer: Elena Dorfman/AWL.)

MediaLink

Nursing Issues and the Elderly

inevitably experiences feelings of loss, emptiness, and loneliness. These emotions are associated with **grieving**, the process of reacting to loss. Many are capable and manage to live alone. However, reliance on younger family members increases as age advances and ill health occurs. More women than men face bereavement and solitude because women usually live longer. Older people are often reminded of the brevity of life by the death of friends. Independence established prior to loss of a mate makes this adjustment period easier. A person who has some meaningful friendships, economic security, ongoing interests in the community, or private hobbies and a peaceful philosophy of life copes more easily with bereavement. Successful relationships with children and grandchildren are also of inestimable value. See Chapter 17 ⬭ for a discussion about facing death.

COGNITIVE DEVELOPMENT

Piaget's phases of cognitive development end with the formal operations phase. Intellectual capacity includes perception, cognitive agility, memory, and learning.

Perception, or the ability to interpret the environment, depends on the acuteness of the senses. If the aging person's senses are impaired, the ability to perceive the environment and react appropriately is diminished. Changes in the nervous system may also affect perceptual capacity.

Changes in the cognitive structures occur as a person ages. It is believed that there is progressive loss of neurons. In addition, blood flow to the brain decreases, the meninges appear to thicken, and brain metabolism slows. In older adults, changes in cognitive abilities are more often a difference in speed than in ability. Overall, the older adult maintains intelligence, problem solving, judgment, creativity, and other well-practiced cognitive skills. Intellectual loss generally reflects a disease process. Most older adults do not experience cognitive impairments.

Memory is also a component of intellectual capacity. In older adults, retrieval of information from long-term memory can be slower, especially if the information is not frequently used. Most age-related differences occur in short-term memory. Older adults tend to forget the recent past. This forgetfulness can be improved by the use of memory aids, making notes or lists, and placing objects in consistent locations.

The older person should remain mentally active to maintain cognitive ability at the highest possible level. Lifelong mental activity, particularly verbal activity, helps the older person retain a high level of cognitive function and may help maintain long-term memory. Cognitive impairment that interferes with normal life is not considered part of normal aging. A decline in intellectual abilities that interferes with social or occupational functions should always be regarded as abnormal. Family members should be advised to seek prompt medical evaluation.

MORAL DEVELOPMENT

According to Kohlberg, moral development is completed in the early adult years. Most older people stay at Kohlberg's conventional level of moral development (see Table 11-7). The value and belief patterns that are important to older adults are cultural background, life experiences, gender, religion, and socioeconomic status. The nurse must identify and consider the specific values of the older client when nursing care is planned.

SPIRITUAL DEVELOPMENT

Often, the older person's knowledge becomes wisdom, an inner resource for dealing with both positive and negative life experiences. Many older people have strong religious convictions and continue to attend religious meetings or services. Involvement in religion often helps the older adult to resolve issues related to the meaning of life, to adversity, or to good fortune. The "old-old" person who cannot attend formal services often continues religious participation in a more private manner. According to Fowler, some people enter the sixth stage of spiritual development, universalizing (see Table 11-8).

HEALTH ASSESSMENT AND PROMOTION

Assessment activities may include questions about the following:

- Usual dietary pattern
- Any problems with bowel or urinary elimination
- Activity/exercise and sleep/rest patterns
- Family and social activities and interests
- Any problems with reading, writing, or problem solving
- Adjustment to retirement or loss of partner.

Healthcare professionals must also be alert for:

- Symptoms of depression
- Risk factors for suicide
- Signs of abnormal bereavement
- Changes in cognitive function
- Medications that increase risk of falls
- Signs of physical abuse or neglect
- Skin lesions (malignant and peripheral)
- Tooth decay, gingivitis, loose teeth.

Older persons are usually concerned about their health and are interested in information and behavioral strategies directed toward improving it. The nurse may wish to discuss some or all of the health promotion topics outlined in Table 11-10.

NURSING CARE

ASSESSING

Data for assessment should always take into consideration the normal growth and developmental level of the client. For example, normal assessment information for an infant would include head circumference as well as height and weight. Normal assessment data for a 14-year-old girl would include presence and frequency of menstrual cycles.

DIAGNOSING, PLANNING, AND IMPLEMENTING

Nursing diagnoses for clients with developmentally related concerns might include *Risk for Impaired Parenting, Relocation Stress Syndrome,* and *Situational Low Self-Esteem.*

Planning at all levels of nursing care should incorporate an understanding of the client's age, developmental level, and any particular issues that might affect the client's progress toward wellness.

Awareness of a client's developmental level is especially important in implementing nursing care. A young child will usually respond better if a parent or safe adult is present for nursing care. An adolescent may prefer to have the parent leave the room during physical examination (especially a parent of the opposite sex). An older adult with an age-related hearing impairment would benefit from having a family member or caregiver present to listen to discharge instructions. Sensitivity to developmental issues is a great aid to nurses both in listening and in providing teaching. (See also Chapter 33 ⚭.)

EVALUATING

The nurse collects data to determine whether outcomes have been met. If goals have not been achieved, the nurse can consider the need to adapt interventions to address developmental needs more closely.

NURSING PROCESS CARE PLAN
Client with Involutional Depression

Sandra Peterson is a 48-year-old woman experiencing perimenopause. She feels that she is "losing her mind." She constantly forgets things, and her mood is unpredictable. She often becomes irritable for no apparent reason and shortly thereafter is depressed and feels guilty for being hypercritical of her family and also herself. She has a tendency to over-

dramatize events. According to her family, she "always has to be right." In addition, Sandra accidentally burns herself every time she uses the oven, because she refuses to recognize the limitations of her aging body. Her arms have burn scars that are obviously months old. However, this time, she has sustained a severe burn. Sandra lives with her husband, but the close family frequently interacts, although she reports, "My kids continually make excuses not to attend family gatherings."

Assessment

- C/o persistent physical symptoms that do not respond to treatment: headaches, digestive disorders, chronic pain.
- Weight 135 lbs, height 62", increase of 7 lbs over the last month
- VS: T 97.2, P 76, R 18, BP 110/78; c/o palpitations
- Lab test
- H&H 12.8, 33
- T_3, T_4 within normal
- Serum calcium low

Nursing Diagnosis. The following important nursing diagnoses (among others) are established for this client:

- *Chronic Low Self-Esteem* related to repeated unmet expectations
- *Energy Field Disturbance* related to disharmony
- *Self-Mutilation* related to inability to express tension verbally

Expected Outcomes The expected outcomes for the plan of care are:

- Verbalizes increased self-acceptance through use of positive self statements.
- States feeling of relaxation.
- States appropriate ways to cope with increased psychological or physiological tension.

Planning and Implementation The following nursing interventions are implemented:

- Demonstrate and promote effective communication techniques.
- Encourage realistic and achievable goal setting; recognize the value of attempts and accomplishment.
- Assist client with evaluating the impact of family on feelings of self-worth.
- Administer therapeutic touch to induce relaxation.
- Validate the client's feelings and concerns related to sense of disharmony or energy disturbance.
- Provide medical treatment for injuries. Use careful aseptic technique when caring for burns.
- Assess for signs of depression, anxiety, and impulsivity.
- Establish trust.

Evaluation. On recheck, the client reports participating in yoga class 3× per week for relaxation. Reports that she has had no injuries this week. No digestive problems or headaches this week. Family reports she seems less stressed.

Critical Thinking in the Nursing Process

1. What might be some of the reasons for Mrs. Peterson's burns?
2. According to Erikson's developmental stages, Mrs. Peterson is in the generativity vs. stagnation stage. Her behavior demonstrates negative resolution (self-indulgence, self-concern, and lack of interest and commitments). What recommendations could you make as a nurse that would help produce positive resolution?
3. Mrs. Peterson's family is very concerned about her injuries and behavior. What can they do to help her through this difficult time?

Note: Discussion of Critical Thinking questions appears in Appendix I.

Note: The references and resources for this and all chapters have been compiled at the back of the book.

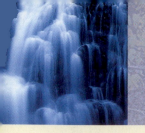

 KEY TERMS by Topic

Use the audio glossary feature of either the CD-ROM or the Companion Website to hear the correct pronunciation of the following key terms.

Introduction
growth, development

Processes of Growth and Development
physiological, psychosocial, cognitive, moral, spiritual

Neonates and Infants
fontanelles, reflexes, motor development, cognitive development

Toddlers
moral development, spiritual development

School-Age Children
puberty

Older Adults
grieving

KEY Points

- Growth and development are influenced by both genetics and environment. Development begins at conception and continues into old age.

- Growth and development have five major components: physiological, psychosocial, cognitive, moral, and spiritual.

- Developmental theories provide information to help the healthcare professional understand what is taking place within a client.

- Health assessment and promotion activities by the nurse assist the client to meet developmental milestones.

- As the population grows older, growth and development needs of the elderly will impact health care to a greater extent.

 EXPLORE MediaLink

Additional interactive resources for this chapter can be found on the Companion Website at www.prenhall.com/ramont. Click on Chapter 11 and "Begin" to select the activities for this chapter.

For chapter-related NCLEX®-style questions and an audio glossary, access the accompanying CD-ROM in this book.

Animations/Videos
- Conception
- Drowning
- Nursing Issues and the Elderly
- SIDS
- Stepping (Infant Reflex)
- Sucking (Infant Reflex)

FOR FURTHER Study

For more about sexual development and function, see Chapter 15.

For discussion about the effects of stress, See Chapter 16

For information about grief and dying, see Chapter 17.

For more about teaching clients, see Chapter 33.

Critical Thinking Care Map

Caring for a Client with Risk for Injury

NCLEX-PN® Focus Area: Safety

Case Study: Todd Underwood, a 2-year-old, is brought into the clinic by his mother, Kelly. He has been brought in for a recheck following an ear infection. When you enter the exam room to take his vital signs, you observe Kelly frantically chasing Todd around the room. He is climbing on the furniture, opening all the cupboards, and pulling the paper off the exam table. Kelly states, "I'm worn out from chasing him and worried about his safety. Over the weekend he got into the medicine cabinet and was able to open several bottles. He also has learned how to unlock the patio door, which leads to the backyard Jacuzzi." Todd lives with his parents. A 12-year-old half-sister visits on alternate weekends.

Nursing Diagnosis: Risk for Injury/Trauma

COLLECT DATA

Subjective	Objective
_____	_____
_____	_____
_____	_____
_____	_____
_____	_____
_____	_____

Would you report this data? Yes/No

If yes, to: _____

What would you report? _____

Nursing Care

_____
_____
_____
_____
_____
_____
_____
_____
_____

How would you document this? _____

_____
_____

Compare your documentation to the sample provided in Appendix I.

Data Collected
(use those that apply)

- 2-year-old male child
- Lives with parents
- Half-sister, child of father's previous marriage, visits alternate weekends
- Both parents work outside the home
- Is cared for by maternal grandmother during the week
- VS: T 98.8 (tympanic), P 80, R 18
- Weight 29 lbs
- Height 34"
- Amoxicillin 500 mg (10-day course completed 2 days ago)
- Diet: appetite fair. Grandmother has trouble getting him to sit down for meals, usually resorts to finger food. Takes a bottle at night
- Mother states opened medicine bottles from home medicine cabinet
- Able to open patio door near backyard Jacuzzi
- Mother states she is worn out from chasing Todd.

Nursing Interventions
(use those that apply; list in priority order)

- Explain individual differences in child temperaments and compare and contrast with the reality of parent expectations.
- Inform parents of available CPR and first aid training in the community.
- Assist parents in devising a plan to child-proof home.
- Advise parent to eliminate all sweets from the child's diet.
- Teach caregiver the need for close supervision of young children.
- Provide poison control number to mother.
- Initiate referrals to parent education opportunities and stress management training.
- Observe for cause of family problem.
- Help caregiver find personal time to meet own needs and learn stress management.
- Discuss sound disciplinary techniques (e.g., time out).

NCLEX-PN® Exam Preparation

1 You are assessing a 2-month-old infant. The mother tells you that he has been lifting his head and looking around but cannot roll over. She is expressing concerns about the baby's development. Your best response would be:

1. "Don't worry, he will roll over at about four months."
2. "Development is very individualized, but it does progress in an orderly manner. Once he develops head and chest control, you should expect rolling over to follow."
3. "Babies who sleep on their backs don't try to roll over as soon."
4. "Heavier babies are slower to roll over."

2 You are caring for a client who has undergone total hip replacement surgery. The physician is now recommending that the client be transferred to a long-term care facility for rehabilitation. The client states, "I would rather die than go there. My life is over. I will never be able to care for myself again." You understand that the client is in which stage of development according to Erikson's theory?

1. autonomy vs. shame and doubt
2. generativity vs. stagnation
3. integrity vs. despair
4. intimacy vs. isolation

3 A 10-year-old boy wishes to build a stand to sell lemonade on the front lawn. His mother, by encouraging his effort and desire to work, helps him achieve the development of Erikson's task of:

1. autonomy.
2. industry.
3. identity.
4. ego integrity.

4 You are assigned to measure and weigh a 5-month-old infant who has been brought into the clinic. The infant's birth weight was 7 lbs 2 oz. Using your knowledge of normal growth patterns, you would expect the weight today to be approximately:

1. 10 lbs 11 oz
2. 12 lbs
3. 14 lbs 4 oz
4. 21 lbs 6 oz

5 The extremities of the body grow more quickly than the body trunk, making the child's body appear somewhat out of proportion. This statement describes which period of development?

1. infant
2. toddler
3. preschooler
4. school age

6 You have been assigned to care for an elderly client who is scheduled for surgery in the morning. The client is anxious, cannot sleep, and wishes to phone a family member. Because the hospital rules stipulate no phone calls after 9 P.M., you do not allow the call. Your actions demonstrate which stage of moral development according to Kohlberg?

1. Stage 1: punishment and obedience orientation
2. Stage 3: interpersonal concordance
3. Stage 4: law and order orientation
4. Stage 6: universal-ethical principles

7 An adult who relies on spiritual beliefs to help him or her deal with illness, death, or tragedy is progressing to which stage of spiritual development according to Fowler?

1. intuitive–projective
2. mythical–literal
3. synthetic–conventional
4. paradoxical–consolidative

8 Establishing satisfactory physical living arrangements is a developmental task according to:

1. Erikson.
2. Fowler.
3. Kohlberg.
4. Havighurst.

9 According to Erikson, if an individual expresses a sense of loss and contempt for others, it is an indication of unmet developmental needs during which of the following stages?

1. trust vs. mistrust
2. initiative vs. guilt
3. identity vs. role confusion
4. integrity vs. despair

10 You have been studying life span development. Another member of your study groups asks which stages of psychosocial development relate to adult clients. Identify the stages from those listed below. (Choose all that apply.)

1. intimacy vs. isolation
2. identity vs. role confusion
3. generativity vs. stagnation
4. integrity vs. despair

Answers and Rationales for Review Questions, as well as discussion of Care Plan and Critical Thinking Care Map questions, appear in Appendix I.

Client Communication

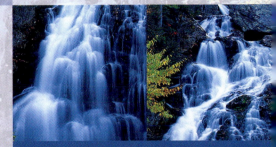

LEARNING Outcomes

After completing this chapter, you will be able to:

1. Describe essential aspects of communication and the communication process.
2. Describe factors influencing the communication process.
3. Differentiate between verbal and nonverbal communication.
4. Explain techniques the nurse can use to help the client express thoughts, feelings, and concerns.
5. Describe barriers to the development of therapeutic relationships.
6. Discuss questions and approaches to use when interviewing clients.
7. Identify factors that influence interviews with clients.

HISTORICAL Perspectives

In the more than 5,000 years since communication has become more than face-to-face use of words to convey information, the human race has come a long way. Today, more than ever before, therapeutic communication has become a benchmark of nursing care. The LPN/LVN must be able to communicate effectively with the client as well as other members of the healthcare team, verbally and nonverbally.

Communication is a critical skill for nurses. It is the primary means by which the nurse–client relationship occurs. It is the process by which humans meet their survival needs, build relationships, and experience joy. In nursing, communication is used to gather information, to teach and persuade, and to express caring and comfort.

The term **communication** has various meanings, depending on the context in which it is used. To some, communication is the exchange of information or thoughts between two or more people. This kind of communication uses talking and listening, or writing and reading. Painting, dancing, and storytelling are other methods of communication. In addition, gestures and body actions convey thoughts to others, sometimes "speaking louder than words."

The intent of any communication is to obtain a response. Communication has two main purposes: to influence others and to obtain information. **Helpful communication** encourages a sharing of information, thoughts, or feelings between two or more people. **Unhelpful communication** hinders or blocks the transfer of information and feelings. Communication techniques that help or hinder effective communication are discussed later in this chapter.

Factors Influencing Communication

Many factors influence the communication process in a therapeutic setting.

DEVELOPMENT

Language, psychosocial, and intellectual development move through stages across the life span. Knowledge of a client's developmental stage allows the nurse to modify the message to reach the listener. This is particularly true in a client teaching situation.

From an early age, females and males communicate differently. Girls tend to use language to seek confirmation, minimize differences, and establish intimacy. Boys use language to establish independence and negotiate status within a group. These differences can continue into adulthood so that the same communication may be interpreted differently by a man and a woman. Many studies have found that men and women communicate differently in both content and process of communication. There is evidence to suggest that more effective communication occurs when the care provider and the client are of the same gender.

Because each person has unique personality traits, values, and life experiences, each will perceive and interpret messages and experiences differently. It is important for the nurse to be aware of a client's values and to validate or correct perceptions to avoid creating barriers in the nurse–client relationship. (**Validation** is a form of feedback that provides confirmation that both parties have the same basic understanding of the message and the feedback.)

PERSONAL SPACE

Personal space is the distance people prefer in interactions with others. It is a natural protective instinct for people to maintain a certain amount of space immediately around them. The amount of personal space varies with individuals and cultures. When someone who wants to communicate steps too close, the receiver automatically steps back a pace or two. When providing nursing care, the nurse may need to invade a client's personal space. It is important to be aware of this and to warn the client when this will occur.

Territoriality is a concept of the space and things that an individual considers as belonging to the self. For example, clients in a hospital often consider their territory as bounded by the curtains around the bed unit. If a visitor or nurse removes a chair to use at another bed, the client may feel upset or somewhat threatened. Nurses should obtain permission from clients to remove, rearrange, or borrow objects in their hospital area.

ROLES AND RELATIONSHIPS

Roles and relationships affect the communication process. Roles vary when communication occurs. Choices of words and tone of voice are different depending on the roles of the communicators. Nursing student and instructor, client and physician, or parent and child are examples of such roles. The specific relationship between communicators is also significant. The nurse who meets with a client for the first time needs to establish a relationship with that client.

ENVIRONMENT

Communication occurs best in a comfortable, private environment. Nurses should be careful to provide for both. Environmental distractions, such as loud noises or lack of privacy, can impair and distort communication.

GROUP COMMUNICATION

A **group** is two or more people who have shared needs and goals, who take each other into account in their actions, and who thus are held together and set apart from others because of their interactions. Examples of groups are families, peer groups, work groups, and religious groups. Communication within a group depends on each member of the group and his or her motivations (the reasons for participating in the group.)

Self-help groups are composed of individuals who share a similar health, social, or daily living problem. The belief of self-help groups is that people who have experienced a similar problem understand better than those who have not experienced the problem. Examples of self-help groups include Alcoholics Anonymous (the first of this type) and groups for those who have experienced stillbirth, divorce, drug abuse, cancer, mental illness, and diabetes.

Nurses may spend time together outside of work to help relieve work-related stress. Nurses who understand work stress can help encourage and support others. They can share the joys of success and the frustration of failure.

Modes of Communication

Communication is generally carried out in two different modes: verbal and nonverbal. Verbal communication uses the spoken or written word. **Nonverbal communication** uses other forms, such as gestures or facial expressions, and touch. Although both kinds of communication occur at the same time, as much as 80% to 90% of what is actually communicated is nonverbal. Learning about nonverbal communication is very important for nurses, so they can develop effective communication patterns and relationships with clients.

VERBAL COMMUNICATION

Verbal communication is largely conscious. People choose the words they use. Their choices are often guided by their culture, socioeconomic background, age, and education. As a result, countless possibilities exist for the way ideas are exchanged.

NONVERBAL COMMUNICATION

Nonverbal communication is sometimes called body language. It includes **gestures**, body movements, touch, and physical appearance (Figure 12-1 ■). Nonverbal behavior is controlled less consciously than verbal behavior. So, nonverbal communication often tells others more about what a person is feeling than what is actually said. Nonverbal communication either reinforces or contradicts what is said verbally. If a nurse says to a client, "I'd be happy to sit here and talk to you for a while," yet glances nervously at a watch every few seconds, the actions contradict the verbal message. The client is more likely to believe the nonverbal behavior, which implies "I am very busy and need to leave."

Observing and interpreting the client's nonverbal behavior is an essential skill for nurses to develop. To observe nonverbal behavior efficiently, the nurse must make a systematic assessment of the person's overall physical appearance, posture, gait, facial expressions, and gestures. The nurse should always exercise caution in interpreting, and always confirm any observation with the client.

Nonverbal communication varies widely among cultures. Even behaviors such as smiling and handshaking can mean different things in different cultures.

Personal appearance, clothing, and adornments can say a lot about a person. Clothing may convey social and financial status, culture, religion, group association, and self-concept.

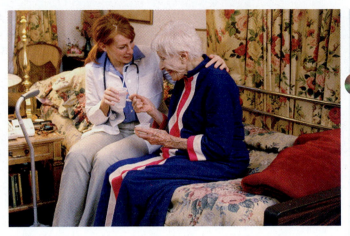

Figure 12-1. ■ Appropriate forms of touch can communicate caring.

Jewelry may be worn as a decoration or as a protection against harm. When the symbolic meaning of an object is unfamiliar, the nurse should ask about its significance. How a person dresses is often an indicator of how the person feels. When a person known for immaculate grooming becomes sloppy in appearance, the nurse may suspect a physical illness or a loss of self-esteem.

The ways people walk and carry themselves are often reliable indicators of self-concept, current mood, and health. The posture of people when they are sitting or lying can also indicate feelings or mood. The nurse can validate the interpretation of the behavior by asking, for example, "You look like it really hurts you to move. I'm wondering how your pain is and if you might need something to make you more comfortable?"

No part of the body is as expressive as the face. Facial expressions can convey surprise, fear, anger, disgust, happiness, and sadness. When the message is not clear, it is important to get feedback to be sure what the person intends.

Nurses need to be aware of their own facial expressions and what they are communicating to others (Figure 12-2 ■).

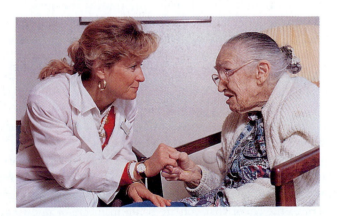

Figure 12-2. ■ The nurse's facial expression communicates warmth and caring.

Clients are quick to notice the nurse's expression, particularly when they feel unsure or uncomfortable. It is impossible to control all facial expression. However, the nurse should learn to control expressions such as fear or disgust.

Eye contact is another essential element of facial communication. In many cultures, mutual eye contact means you recognize the other person and are willing to maintain communication.

Gestures

Hand and body gestures may emphasize and clarify the spoken word. They may occur without words to indicate a particular feeling or to give a sign. Some gestures, however, may have different meanings depending on one's culture. For example, the American gesture meaning "shoo" or "go away" means "come here" or "come back" in some Asian cultures.

For people with special communication problems, such as the deaf, the hands are invaluable in communication. Many deaf people learn sign language. Ill persons who are unable to reply verbally can similarly devise a communication system using the hands. (See also Chapter 13 ☍.)

Therapeutic Communication

Therapeutic communication is client-centered, goal-directed, and time-limited communication. Nurses use therapeutic communication to determine client concerns, problems, and feelings. It is important for the nurse to know how to help clients explore their own feelings and how to avoid shutting down communication by saying the wrong thing.

THERAPEUTIC TECHNIQUES

Nurses can use a variety of responses to client's comments to help them explore or expand on the client's thoughts and feelings. This is important if the nurse is to help the client achieve goals and overcome obstacles. Table 12-1 ▪ lists therapeutic communication techniques with examples.

As you talk with clients, you will find you are most comfortable using certain techniques such as offering self, using touch, and providing general leads. However, it is good to try new techniques periodically, especially if the techniques you usually use do not seem to be working.

Communication techniques should be comfortable for you, so that the conversation flows and is not stilted. Be careful not to overuse any one technique, because it may seem to the client that you are being insincere or uncaring. Overuse of silence or reflecting, for example, may slow down communication.

BARRIERS TO COMMUNICATION

Have you ever had a conversation with someone who responded in a way that made you feel it was useless to keep talking to them? Chances are good that you experienced a barrier to communication. Everyone uses communication barriers from time to time, but nurses need to be especially careful to avoid them when speaking with clients. Communication barriers are described in Table 12-2 ▪ on page 233.

It is very important to recognize when a barrier to communication has been used. You may respond to a client and then realize that you have used a barrier. When this happens, it is perfectly acceptable to say, "Let me say that differently." Or, "I'm sorry, that did not come out the way I meant it." If you realize later that you have used a barrier and shut down communication with a client, you can speak with the client again. You can tell the client that you would like to talk about the subject again and that you did not mean to be abrupt earlier.

Effective communication in the clinical setting can be accomplished using the following communication principles:

- Use therapeutic communication techniques to communicate with clients.
- Think before you speak. Communicating with a client is different than speaking with a friend or another student. Share only what is appropriate, and always remember ethical principles and confidentiality.
- Be quiet and gentle in your communication. Do not communicate in any way that could increase the stress or discomfort of clients, families, or staff.
- Ask appropriate questions. Questions are asked to obtain information needed to care for clients, not to satisfy your curiosity. You should not make it a habit to read charts or look up information on the computer about clients to whom you are not assigned. When information is needed for educational purposes, the client's name and personal information must be removed. Client records should not be copied and removed from the hospital by a student.
- Keep information confidential. Do not talk about clients or their families in inappropriate places. Avoid discussing clients in the elevator, cafeteria, or anywhere visitors can overhear.
- Be respectful in your communication. Speak to physicians, nursing assistants, instructors, and visitors with equal respect.
- Find out what you don't know. Don't pretend that you know something if you don't. This could inadvertently harm a client. Do not expect your instructor to give you all the answers. Instead, take responsibility for your own learning.
- Give a clear concise report. Shift report is an important form of communication (see Chapter 6 ☍).

TABLE 12-1

Therapeutic Communication Techniques

TECHNIQUE	DESCRIPTION	EXAMPLES
Using silence	Accepting pauses or silences that may extend for several seconds or minutes without interjecting any verbal response.	Sitting quietly (or walking with the client) and waiting attentively until the client is able to put thoughts and feelings into words.
Providing general leads	Using statements or questions that (1) encourage the client to verbalize; (2) choose a topic of conversation; and (3) facilitate continued verbalization.	"Perhaps you would like to talk about …." "Would it help to discuss your feelings?" "Where would you like to begin?" "And then what?" "I follow what you are saying."
Being specific and tentative	Making statements that are specific rather than general, and tentative rather than absolute.	"You scratched my arm." (specific statement) "You are as clumsy as an ox." (general statement) "You seem unconcerned about Mary." (tentative statement) "You don't give a damn about Mary and you never will." (absolute statement)
Using open-ended questions	Asking broad questions that lead or invite the client to explore (elaborate, clarify, describe, compare, or illustrate) thoughts or feelings. Open-ended questions specify only the topic to be discussed and invite answers that are longer than one or two words.	"I'd like to hear more about that." "Tell me about …." "How have you been feeling lately?" "What brought you to the hospital?" "What is your opinion?" "You said you were frightened yesterday. How do you feel now?"
Using touch	Providing appropriate forms of touch to reinforce caring feelings. Because tactile contacts vary considerably among individuals, families, and cultures, the nurse must be sensitive to the differences in attitudes and practices of clients and self.	Putting an arm over the client's shoulder. Placing your hand over the client's hand.
Restating or paraphrasing	Actively listening for the client's basic message and then repeating those thoughts and/or feelings in similar words. This conveys that the nurse has listened and understood the client's basic message and also offers clients a clearer idea of what they have said.	*Client:* "I couldn't manage to eat any dinner last night—not even the dessert." *Nurse:* "You had difficulty eating yesterday." *Client:* "Yes, I was very upset after my family left." *Client:* "I have trouble talking to strangers." *Nurse:* "You find it difficult talking to people you do not know?"
Seeking clarification	A method of making the client's broad overall meaning of the message more understandable. It is used when paraphrasing is difficult or when the communication is rambling or garbled. To clarify the message, the nurse can restate the basic message or confess confusion and ask the client to repeat or restate the message. Nurses can also clarify their own message with statements.	"I'm puzzled." "I'm not sure I understand that." "Would you please say that again?" "Would you tell me more?" "I meant this rather than that." "I guess I didn't make that clear—I'll go over it again."
Perception checking or seeking consensual validation	A method similar to clarifying that verifies the meaning of specific words rather than the overall meaning of a message.	*Client:* "My husband never gives me any presents." *Nurse:* "You mean he has never given you a present for your birthday or Christmas?" *Client:* "Well—not never. He does get me something for my birthday and Christmas, but he never thinks of giving me anything at any other time."

(continued)

TABLE 12-1

Therapeutic Communication Techniques (*continued*)

TECHNIQUE	DESCRIPTION	EXAMPLES
Offering self	Suggesting one's presence, interest, or wish to understand the client without making any demands or attaching conditions that the client must comply with to receive the nurse's attention.	"I'll stay with you until your daughter arrives." "We can sit here quietly for a while; we don't need to talk unless you would like to." "I'll help you to dress to go home."
Giving information	Providing, in a simple and direct manner, specific factual information the client may or may not request. When information is not known, the nurse states this and indicates who has it or when the nurse will obtain it.	"Your surgery is scheduled for 11 A.M. tomorrow." "You will feel a pulling sensation when the tube is removed from your abdomen." "I do not know the answer to that, but I will find out from Mrs. King, the nurse in charge."
Acknowledging	Giving recognition, in a nonjudgmental way, of a change in behavior, an effort the client has made, or a contribution to a communication. Acknowledgment may be with or without understanding, verbal or nonverbal.	"You trimmed your beard and mustache and washed your hair." "I notice you keep squinting your eyes. Are you having difficulty seeing?" "You walked twice as far today with your walker."
Clarifying time or sequence	Helping the client clarify an event, situation, or happening in relationship to time.	*Client:* "I vomited this morning." *Nurse:* "Was that after breakfast?" *Client:* "I feel that I have been asleep for weeks." *Nurse:* "You had your operation Monday, and today is Tuesday."
Presenting reality	Helping the client to differentiate the real from the unreal.	"That telephone ring came from the program on television." "That's not a dead mouse in the corner; it is a discarded washcloth." "Your magazine is here in the drawer. It has not been stolen."
Focusing	Helping the client expand on and develop a topic of importance. It is important for the nurse to wait until the client finishes stating the main concerns before attempting to focus. The focus may be an idea or a feeling; however, the nurse often emphasizes a feeling to help the client recognize an emotion disguised behind words.	*Client:* "My wife says she will look after me, but I don't think she can, what with the children to take care of, and they're always after her about something— clothes, homework, what's for dinner that night." *Nurse:* "You are worried about how well she can manage."
Reflecting	Directing ideas, feelings, questions, or content back to clients to enable them to explore their own ideas and feelings about a situation.	*Client:* "What can I do?" *Nurse:* "What do you think would be helpful?" *Client:* "Do you think I should tell my husband?" *Nurse:* "You seem unsure about telling your husband."
Summarizing and planning	Stating the main points of a discussion to clarify the relevant points discussed. This technique is useful at the end of an interview or to review a health teaching session. It often acts as an introduction to future care planning.	"During the past half hour we have talked about ...." "Tomorrow afternoon we may explore this further." "In a few days I'll review what you have learned about the actions and effects of your insulin."

ATTENTIVE LISTENING

Attentive listening or active listening involves listening for key themes in communication with clients. The nurse should not interrupt the speaker, should take time to think about the message, and should ask questions to clarify or obtain additional information if needed. Attentive behaviors are a type of nonverbal communication. The nurse should lean slightly toward the client and have direct eye contact with the client. (Clients may have personal or cultural reasons for not returning eye contact. In these cases, the nurse would still make sure to make eye

TABLE 12-2

Barriers to Communication

TECHNIQUE	DESCRIPTION	EXAMPLES
Stereotyping	Offering generalized and oversimplified beliefs about groups of people that are based on experiences too limited to be valid. These responses categorize clients and negate their uniqueness as individuals.	"Two-year-olds are brats." "Women are complainers." "Men don't cry." "Most people don't have any pain after this type of surgery."
Agreeing and disagreeing	Akin to judgmental responses, agreeing and disagreeing imply that the client is either right or wrong and that the nurse is in a position to judge this. These responses deter clients from thinking through their position and may cause a client to become defensive.	*Client:* "I don't think Dr. Broad is a very good doctor. He doesn't seem interested in his patients." *Nurse:* "Dr. Broad is head of the Department of Surgery and is an excellent surgeon."
Being defensive	Attempting to protect a person or healthcare services from negative comments. These responses prevent the client from expressing true concerns. The nurse is saying "You have no right to complain." Defensive responses protect the nurse from admitting weaknesses in the healthcare services, including personal weaknesses.	*Client:* "Those night nurses must just sit around and talk all night. They didn't answer my light for over an hour." *Nurse:* "I'll have you know we literally run around on nights. You're not the only client, you know."
Challenging	Giving a response that makes clients prove their statement or point of view. These responses indicate that the nurse is failing to consider the client's feelings, making the client feel it necessary to defend a position.	*Client:* "I felt nauseated after that red pill." *Nurse:* "Surely you don't think I gave you the wrong pill?" *Client:* "I feel as if I am dying." *Nurse:* "How can you feel that way when your pulse is 60?" *Client:* "I believe my husband doesn't love me." *Nurse:* "You can't say that; why, he visits you every day."
Probing	Asking for information chiefly out of curiosity rather than with the intent to assist the client. These responses are considered prying and violate the client's privacy. Asking "why" is often probing and places the client in a defensive position.	*Client:* "I was speeding along the street and didn't see the stop sign." *Nurse:* "Why were you speeding?" *Client:* "I didn't ask the doctor when he was here." *Nurse:* "Why didn't you?"
Testing	Asking questions that make the client admit to something. These responses permit the client only limited answers and often meet the nurse's need rather than the client's.	"Who do you think you are?" (forces people to admit their status is only that of client) "Do you think I am not busy?" (forces the client to admit that the nurse really is busy)
Rejecting	Refusing to discuss certain topics with the client. These responses often make clients feel that the nurse is rejecting not only their communication but also the clients themselves.	"I don't want to discuss that. Let's talk about . . . ." "Let's discuss other areas of interest to you rather than the two problems you keep mentioning." "I can't talk now. It's time for my coffee break."
Changing topics and subjects	Directing the communication into areas of self-interest rather than considering the client's concerns is often a self-protective response to a topic that causes anxiety. These responses imply that what the nurse considers important will be discussed and that clients should not discuss certain topics.	*Client:* "I'm separated from my wife. Do you think I should have sexual relations with another woman?" *Nurse:* "I see that you're 36 and that you like gardening. This sunshine is good for my roses. I have a beautiful rose garden."
Unwarranted reassurance	Using clichés or comforting statements of advice as a means to reassure the client. These responses block the fears, feelings, and other thoughts of the client.	"You'll feel better soon." "I'm sure everything will turn out all right." "Don't worry."

(continued)

TABLE 12-2		
Barriers to Communication (*continued*)		
TECHNIQUE	**DESCRIPTION**	**EXAMPLES**
Passing judgment	Giving opinions and approving or disapproving responses, moralizing, or implying one's own values. These responses imply that the client must think as the nurse thinks, fostering client dependence.	"That's good (bad)." "You shouldn't do that." "That's not good enough." "What you did was wrong (right)."
Giving common advice	Telling the client what to do. These responses deny the client's right to be an equal partner. Note that giving expert rather than common advice is therapeutic.	*Client:* "Should I move from my home to a nursing home?" *Nurse:* "If I were you, I'd go to a nursing home, where you'll get your meals cooked for you."

contact often.) The nurse should use open and expansive gestures as well as nonverbal cues such as nodding and smiling.

Attentive listening is a highly developed skill, but it can be learned with practice. A nurse can convey attentiveness in listening to clients in various ways (Figure 12-3 ■). Common responses are nodding the head, uttering "uh huh" or "mmm," repeating the words that the client has used, or saying "I see what you mean." Each nurse has characteristic ways of responding, and the nurse must take care not to sound insincere or phony.

Interviewing

An **interview** is a planned communication or a conversation with a purpose, for example, to get or give information. Interviewing is used in most phases of the nursing process, and is especially important when obtaining the nursing health history.

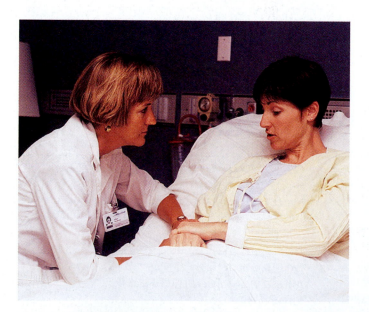

Figure 12-3. ■ The nurse conveys attentive listening through a posture of involvement.

There are two approaches to interviewing: directive and nondirective. The *directive interview* is structured and is used to discover specific information. The nurse explains the purpose of the interview and asks closed-ended questions (see the next section) that call for specific data. The client gives responses without discussion. Directive interviews are used to gather and to give information when time is limited, such as in an emergency situation.

A *nondirective interview* allows the client to control the situation. *Rapport,* an understanding between two or more people, is built in this type of interview. The nurse encourages communication by asking open-ended questions (see the next section) and by providing empathetic responses.

A combination of directive and nondirective approaches is usually appropriate during the information-gathering interview. The nurse begins by asking open-ended questions to determine areas of concern for the client. If, for example, a client expresses worry about surgery, the nurse pauses to explore the client's worry and to provide support. Simply to note the worry, without dealing with it, can leave the impression that the nurse does not care about the client's concerns or dismisses them as unimportant. As the interview evolves, the nurse may use closed-ended questions to obtain more specific data and to complete the nursing health history. See the nursing care checklist in Box 12-1 ■ for guidelines for wording verbal communication.

KINDS OF INTERVIEW QUESTIONS

Questions are classified as closed or open ended, and as neutral or leading. **Closed-ended questions**, used in the directive interview, generally require only "yes" or "no" or short factual answers giving specific information. Thus the amount of information gained is generally limited. Closed questions often begin with "when," "where," "who," "what," "do (did, does)," "is (are, was)," and sometimes "how." Examples of closed questions are "What medication did you take?" "Are you having pain now? Show me where it is." "How old are you?" "When did you fall?" The highly stressed person and the person who

BOX 12-1   NURSING CARE CHECKLIST

Guidelines for Wording Verbal Communication

☑ Pay attention to your tone of voice, manner, and pace of speech. They can change the feeling and impact of the message. Your intonation can express enthusiasm, sadness, anger, or amusement. Your pace of speech may indicate interest, anxiety, boredom, or fear.

☑ Use simple terms and give complete information. Complex technical terms become natural to nurses, but laypeople often misunderstand them. Instead of saying to a client, "The nurses will be catheterizing you tomorrow for a urine analysis," it may be more understandable to say, "Tomorrow we need to get a sample of your urine, so we will collect it by putting a small tube into your bladder." Speak clearly and briefly. A message that is direct and simple is effective. *Clarity* is saying precisely what you mean, and *brevity* is using the fewest words necessary. The result is a message that is simple and clear.

☑ Use consistency in verbal and nonverbal communication. The nurse's behavior must match the words spoken. When the nurse tells the client, "I am interested in hearing what you have to say," the nonverbal behavior would include the nurse facing the client, making eye contact, and leaning forward.

☑ Keep communication relevant and well timed. The timing of any message needs to be appropriate to ensure that words are heard. Messages should address the person's interests and concerns, and be given when the client can hear and understand them.

    Nurses need to be aware of both relevance and timing when communicating with clients. Avoid asking several questions at once or asking questions without waiting for an

answer. For example, a nurse might enter a client's room and say in one breath, "Good morning. How are you this morning? Did you sleep well last night? Your husband is coming to see you before your surgery, isn't he?" The client no doubt would wonder which question to answer first.

☑ Be adaptable when communicating. Spoken messages should be adapted to behavioral cues from the client. What the nurse says and how it is said must show sensitivity. For example, a nurse who is usually friendly and jovial may notice that a client seems very withdrawn and distressed. The nurse should modify his or her tone of speech with this client, and share observations about the client's expression and mood.

☑ Be credible (believable). Credibility may be the most important requirement for effective communication. Nurses foster credibility by being consistent, dependable, and honest. They should be knowledgeable about what is being discussed and have accurate information. Nurses should convey confidence and certainty in what they are saying. If they don't know the answer, they should say so: "I don't know the answer to that, but I will find someone who does."

☑ Use humor, but use it with care. Humor can be a positive and powerful tool in the nurse–client relationship. Humor can help clients adjust to difficult and painful situations by providing a different perspective and promoting a sense of well-being. The physical act of laughter can be both an emotional and physical release that reduces tension. Healthful humor must be distinguished from harmful humor. Healthful humor elicits laughter, it is appropriate to the situation, and it protects a person's dignity. Harmful humor ridicules other people by laughing at them. Humor is also harmful if used to avoid resolving problems.

---

has difficulty communicating will find closed-ended questions easier to answer than open-ended questions.

Open-ended questions, used in the nondirective interview, invite clients to discover and explore their thoughts or feelings. They allow clients the freedom to talk about what they wish. An open-ended question specifies only the broad topic to be discussed, and invites answers longer than one or two words. The open-ended question is useful at the beginning of an interview or to change topics and to elicit attitudes.

The type of question a nurse chooses depends on the situation. For example, the nurse asks closed-ended questions in an emergency when information must be obtained quickly. Nurses often find it necessary to use a combination of open- and closed-ended questions throughout an interview to obtain needed information. A comparisons of open- and closed-ended questions appears in Box 12-2 ■.

A *neutral question* is a question the client can answer without direction or pressure from the nurse. Examples are

BOX 12-2

Comparison of Open- and Closed-ended Questions

Open-ended questions are questions or statements that require more than a "yes" or "no" or other short response (usually begin with "what" or "how"):

    "How have you been feeling lately?"
    "What brought you to the hospital?"
    "How did you feel in that situation?"
    "Would you describe more about how you relate to your child?"
    "What would you like to talk about today?"

Closed-ended questions are questions that can be answered by "yes" or "no" or other single-word answers:

    "Are you feeling okay?"
    "Do you know why you have been admitted?"
    "Did that situation cause you to feel depressed or upset?"
    "Do you have a good relationship with your children?"
    "Would you like to talk about what is bothering you today?"

"How do you feel about that?" and "Why do you think you had the operation?" A *leading question,* by contrast, directs the client's answer. The phrasing of the question suggests what answer is expected. Examples are "You're stressed about surgery tomorrow, aren't you?" and "You will take your medicine, won't you?" The leading question gives the client less opportunity to decide whether the answer is true or not. Leading questions create problems if the client gives inaccurate responses in order to please the nurse. This can result in inaccurate data.

PLANNING THE INTERVIEW AND SETTING

Before beginning an interview, the nurse reviews available information.

Time

Nurses need to schedule interviews with hospitalized clients for a time when the client is comfortable and when interruptions are unlikely. Nurses should schedule interviews with home care clients at a time selected by the client. In all instances, the client should be comfortable and unhurried.

Place

The place for an interview should be comfortable, well lit, private, and quiet. Most people are uncomfortable about answering personal questions or expressing strong feelings in the sight or hearing of others.

Seating Arrangement

When a client is in bed, the nurse can sit at a 45-degree angle to the bed. This position is less formal than sitting behind a table or standing at the foot of the bed. During an initial admission interview, a client may feel less confronted if there is an overbed table between the client and the nurse. Sitting on a client's bed may make the client uncomfortable.

Distance

People feel uncomfortable when talking to someone who is too close or too far away. Most people feel comfortable at a distance of 3 to 4 feet during an interview. Some clients require more or less personal space, depending on their cultural and personal needs (Box 12-3 ■).

Height also affects communication. When a nurse is standing and looking down at a client, the client may feel intimidated.

STAGES OF AN INTERVIEW

An interview has three major stages: the opening or introduction, the body or development, and the closing.

The Opening

The opening can be the most important part of the interview because what is said and done at that time sets the tone for the remainder of the interview. The purposes of the opening are to establish rapport and orient the interviewee.

BOX 12-3   **CULTURAL PULSE POINTS**

Personal Space Variables

- *African:* Close personal space—touching acceptable within families and extended families.
- *Chinese:* Distant personal space—direct eye contact avoided and touch by strangers not acceptable.
- *Eastern Indian:* Direct eye contact shows lack of respect; handshake permissible only between males.
- *European-American, Canadian, and British:* Personal space at least 18 inches between individuals during conversation.
- *Filipino:* Touching permissible; if eye contact is established, must be maintained.
- *Germans:* View space as sacred; even furniture placement maintains distance.
- *Iraqi:* Touch and embracing are acceptable greetings.
- *Israeli:* Demonstrative touch.
- *Japanese:* Touch not encouraged; handshake acceptable; distant personal space; eye contact is disrespectful.
- *Mexican:* Close personal space—touch is acceptable even with those of same sex.
- *Native American:* Periods of silence during communication shows respect; close personal space—no boundaries; limited eye contact.
- *Saudi:* Handholding between men is acceptable; men may only touch females within the family.

Establishing rapport is a process of creating goodwill and trust. It can begin with a greeting ("Good morning, Mr. Johnson") or a self-introduction ("Good morning. I'm Becky James, a nursing student") accompanied by nonverbal gestures such as a smile, a handshake, and a friendly manner. A brief amount of small talk about the person, the weather, sports, and families is appropriate to develop rapport, but too much superficial talk can cause anxiety. The nurse then orients the client by explaining the purpose and nature of the interview, what information is needed, how long it will take, and what is expected of the client. The nurse usually states that the client has the right not to provide data and tells the client how the information will be used.

The following is an example of an interview introduction:

STEP 1: ESTABLISH RAPPORT

Nurse: Hello, Ms. Goodwin. I'm Sharon Fellows, and I will be assisting with your care today. I am a nursing student at the technical center.

Client: It's nice to meet you. My sister-in-law teaches at the technical center. Do you know Dorothy Goodwin?

Nurse: No, I don't believe I have met her. What does she teach?

Client: Something in computers. I don't actually understand it! Will you be bringing me my medicine today?

STEP 2: ORIENTATION

Nurse: Yes, that will be part of my responsibilities. I also need to ask you a few questions about your health and illness. Do you need any pain medicine or other medicines before we talk for about 10 minutes?

Client: No, I am fine. Just wondered if you would be doing the medicines today.

Nurse: I will. Don't hesitate to ask for anything you need.

Client: What do you need to know?

Nurse: I need to ask you about what you might need after you leave the hospital. If you don't want to discuss something I bring up, just let me know. I will be making notes so we can arrange for you to have follow-up doctor visits and nursing care if you need it.

Client: I probably will. My husband cannot do much because he is nearly blind and has a heart condition. My daughter will be coming to stay for a few days, though.

The Body

In the body of the interview, the client communicates what he or she thinks, feels, knows, and perceives in response to questions from the nurse. The nurse can make the transition from the opening stage to this stage by asking an open-ended question that is related to the stated purpose, such as "What brought you to the hospital today?"

The nurse must use communication techniques that make both parties feel comfortable and serve the purpose of the interview. Communication techniques are covered in Table 12-1. Brief guidelines for communicating during an interview are outlined in Box 12-4 ■.

The Closing

The nurse usually terminates the interview when the needed information has been obtained. In some cases, however, a client terminates it, for example, when deciding not to give any more information or when unable to offer more information for some other reason—fatigue, for example. The closing is important in maintaining rapport. The following techniques are commonly used to close an interview (Stewart & Cash, 2006, pp. 84–90):

1. Signal that the interview is coming to an end by offering to answer questions: "Do you have any questions?" "I would be glad to answer any questions you have." Be sure to allow time for the person to answer, or the offer will be regarded as insincere.

2. Declare completion of the purpose or task by saying "Well, that's about all I need to know for now" or "Well, those are all the questions I have for now." Preceding a remark with the word *well* generally signals that the end of the interaction is near.

BOX 12-4	NURSING CARE CHECKLIST

Communication during an Interview

☑ Listen attentively, using all your senses, and speak slowly and clearly.

☑ Use language the client understands, and clarify points that are not understood.

☑ Plan questions to follow a logical sequence.

☑ Ask only one question at a time. Double questions limit the client to one choice and may confuse both the nurse and the client.

☑ Allow the client the opportunity to look at things the way they appear to him or her and not the way they appear to the nurse or someone else.

☑ Do not impose your own values on the client.

☑ Avoid using personal examples, such as saying "If I were you …."

☑ Nonverbally convey respect, concern, interest, and acceptance.

☑ Use and accept silence to help the client search for more thoughts or to organize them.

☑ Use eye contact and be calm, unhurried, and sympathetic.

3. State appreciation or satisfaction about what was accomplished: "I really enjoyed meeting you, and I think we accomplished a great deal." "Those are all the questions I have. Thank you for your time and help." "The questions you have answered will be helpful in planning your nursing care."

NURSING CARE

ASSESSING

Good nursing requires an understanding of the many factors involved in communicating. A client may state that she is "all set" for the next day's gallbladder surgery. However, the nurse may observe that the client has a fearful expression and is trembling. If the nurse focuses on only the client's verbal communication, he or she is unlikely to provide good care or accurate documentation.

The nurse collects assessment data through closed- or open-ended questions, depending on the task at hand and the time available. When collecting data for a shift change, the nurse might focus on vital signs, status of IVs, and so on. When giving a client a sponge bath before sleep, the nurse might ask open-ended questions that would give the client the opportunity to reminisce and think of pleasant events.

DIAGNOSING, PLANNING, AND IMPLEMENTING

Certain nursing diagnoses that may affect communication with a client are *Anxiety, Ineffective Coping, Ineffective Denial, Hopelessness,* and *Disturbed Sensory Perception.* Be prepared to address the client's feelings, and to adapt the pace and style of your communication.

The following interventions are useful in interviewing clients:

- Before beginning an interview, know what information to collect. *Rationale: This will ensure that the exchange with the client is smooth and efficient. It will also free you to observe the client more during the interaction.*

- Schedule interviews at a time that is as convenient as possible for the client, and when interruptions are not likely to occur. Allow home care clients to select a time. *Rationale: This will allow the interview to be relaxed and unhurried. Most people are uncomfortable about answering personal questions or expressing strong feelings in the sight or hearing of others.*

- If possible, sit at a 45-degree angle to the bed or chair where the client is, and about 3 to 4 feet from the client. *Rationale: Sitting too close to, or standing over, the client can make the client feel threatened. Sitting far away may suggest lack of interest.*

- Open the interview with a friendly greeting and introduce yourself. If appropriate, start with some general conversation. Then explain why you are there. *Rationale: This approach expresses respect for the client and builds rapport. The client can be more relaxed about the interview once its purpose is stated.*

- Ask an open-ended question that is related to the stated purpose, is easy to answer, and does not embarrass or place stress on the person. *Rationale: This helps make the transition into the main part of the interview.*

- Throughout the interview, use good communication techniques. If you feel you have put up a block to communication, apologize and restate the question in a better way. If a client appears suddenly embarrassed or concerned, look for the underlying reason (Box 12-5 ■). Pay attention to both verbal and nonverbal messages from the client. *Rationale: When the nurse recognizes a communication block and attempts to correct it, communication can continue.*

- When the necessary information has been obtained, ask if the client has any questions. If the client decides to stop the interview, state what you have accomplished and, if needed, say what follow-up will be required. Suggest a follow-up time. *Rationale: If all questions have been answered, the open-ended question signals that the interview is ending. If a client is too tired or refuses to give any more information, the*

BOX 12-5	CULTURAL PULSE POINTS

Handling Miscommunications

Miscommunication is a frequent problem in hospitals. The most obvious miscommunication occurs when the client and hospital staff do not speak the same language. Language problems, however, can also occur among English-speaking people. In England, Australia, and South Africa, the word *fanny* is a derogatory term referring to a woman's vagina. Imagine the reaction of a British woman when asked to prepare for a shot in the fanny. But the more subtle problems are those that result from cultural differences in meaning of nonverbal behavior. Many Asians consider it disrespectful to look someone directly in the eye, especially if that person is a nurse. An Asian client may avoid eye contact out of respect for the superior status of the nurse. Many Middle Easterners see direct eye contact between a man and a woman as a sexual invitation. Knowing what the norm within the culture is will facilitate understanding and lessen miscommunication.

The nursing diagnosis *"Impaired Verbal Communication* related to cultural difference" is defined by NANDA as being relevant when "an individual experiences a decreased or absent ability to use or understand language in human interaction." This diagnosis implies that the client's verbal communication and ability to understand and utilize language is impaired in some way regardless of the cause. An individual who speaks a different language than that used by the healthcare provider may be capable of both use and comprehension of a familiar language when interacting with a person fluent in the language. In this situation if the client is verbally impaired, the nurse is equally impaired. It is clear that this NANDA diagnosis does not adequately address the issue of nonverbal communication, an essential assessment factor in transcultural nursing.

restatement will help them to know what has been accomplished and what more they will be asked to do at another time.

- Thank clients for their time and express hope for a positive outcome. *Rationale: This again expresses your respect and concern for them.*

EVALUATING

In evaluating professional communications with clients, the nurse first looks at the client's verbal and nonverbal expressions of comfort. Does the client seem relaxed, or does he appear flushed and tense? Does the client express satisfaction at understanding better, or does he appear anxious and confused?

The nurse also mentally reviews the interaction to determine the success of the communication process. What communication techniques were effective in the situation? Which were not effective? Did any blocks to communication arise? Was a way found to move past them? If not, can the nurse think of a possible way past the block now that the interaction is over? Has the nurse experienced any similar communications that might provide insights?

NURSING PROCESS CARE PLAN
Client Affected by Nurse Communication Barriers

Lucy, an LPN, is assigned to care for Mr. Levowitz. He is currently in the recovery room after surgery to remove prostate cancer that had spread to his abdomen. His wife comes into the room crying. Lucy asks her what is wrong. Mrs. Levowitz continues to sob and is unable to answer. Lucy gets chairs for herself and Mrs. Levowitz and urges her to sit down. Lucy says, "Come on now. The news can't be that bad, can it?" Mrs Levowitz responds by telling Lucy that the doctor has said the cancer is so bad that there is nothing they can do. Lucy then says, "I am so very sorry. That must be difficult news to hear." Mrs. Levowitz cries a bit longer, then says she doesn't know how she can live without him. Lucy tells her, "You should wait and see how the chemotherapy and radiation treatments go before you think about living without him. Things may still turn out all right." Mrs. Levowitz grasps at that hope and says, "Oh, do you really think those treatments could help him? That he doesn't really have cancer that bad?" Lucy says, "It's been known to happen. I really have to go see some other patients now. Everything will be okay for you. It will turn out just fine."

Assessment. The client and his wife live alone in a small cottage several miles outside the city. Mrs. Levowitz does not drive and has always been a stay-at-home wife. She also expresses concerns about caring for him at home and getting him to his treatment appointments. Mr. Levowitz is very controlled and sits quietly not joining in the conversation with the LPN and his wife.

Nursing Diagnosis. The following important nursing diagnoses (among others) are established for these clients:

- *Caregiver Role Strain* related to need for significant home care
- *Compromised Family Coping* related to inadequate resources available
- *Anticipatory Grieving* related to potential loss of significant others
- *Ineffective Role Performance* related to change in physical capacity to resume prior role

Expected Outcomes. The expected outcomes for the plan of care are:

- Caregiver identifies resources available to help in giving care.
- Identifies need for and seeks outside support.

- Plans for future one day at a time.
- Accepts physical limitation regarding role responsibility and considers ways to change lifestyle to accomplish goals associated with role performance.

Planning and Implementation. The following nursing interventions are implemented:

- Monitor caregiver for psychological distress and signs of depression.
- Assess health of the caregiver at intervals, especially if she has a chronic illness in addition to caregiver role.
- Help caregiver identify ways to equitably distribute workload among family.
- Assist in finding transportation for treatment and family visit.
- Refer family to appropriate resources for assistance as indicated.
- Involve client and family in planning care as much as possible.
- Use therapeutic communication with open-ended questions such as "What are your fears and thoughts?"
- Actively listen to client's/family's expression of grief; do not interrupt, do not tell own story, and do not offer meaningless platitudes such as "It will be better this way."
- Refer to family counseling if needed for adjustment of role change.
- Identify way to compensate for physical disabilities.

Evaluation. Mrs. Levowitz spoke with a social worker, and arrangements were made for her and her husband to move temporarily to an assisted living arrangement during treatment: Mrs. Levowitz expressed that "I will keep an open mind, maybe we will consider moving permanently to the assisted living apartment." Both client and wife expressed a desire to discuss the future once a therapeutic communication dialogue was started. Mr. Levowitz expressed an understanding of his physical limitation, but stated, "They can't get rid of me that easy. I am going to fight this as long as my wife is by my side."

Critical Thinking in the Nursing Process

1. What communication techniques did Lucy use?
2. What barriers to communication did Lucy use?
3. What nonverbal communication did Lucy use?

Note: Discussion of Critical Thinking questions appears in Appendix I.

Note: The references and resources for this and all chapters have been compiled at the back of the book.

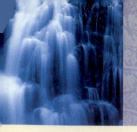

Chapter Review

 KEY TERMS by Topic

Use the audio glossary feature of either the CD-ROM or the Companion Website to hear the correct pronunciation of the following key terms.

Introduction
communication, helpful communication, unhelpful communication

Factors Influencing Communication
validation, personal space, group

Modes of Communication
nonverbal communication, gestures

Therapeutic Communication
therapeutic communication

Interviewing
interview, closed-ended questions, open-ended questions

KEY Points

- Communication is a critical nursing skill used to gather information, to teach and persuade, and to express caring and comfort.

- Communication is the exchange of information or thoughts between two or more people. Messages are both verbal and nonverbal.

- The effectiveness of verbal communication depends on many factors, including pace and intonation, simplicity, clarity and brevity, timing, relevance, adaptability, and credibility.

- Nonverbal communication includes personal appearance, posture and gait, facial expressions, and gestures. It often reveals more about a person's thoughts and feelings than words do. The "receiver" is more likely to believe a nonverbal message than a verbal one.

- When communication is effective, verbal and nonverbal expressions are consistent.

- When assessing verbal and nonverbal behaviors, nurses need to consider cultural influences. A single nonverbal expression can indicate a variety of feelings, and one word can have several meanings.

- Many techniques facilitate therapeutic communication: attentive listening; paraphrasing; clarifying; using open-ended questions and statements; focusing; being specific; using touch and silence; clarifying reality, time, or sequence; providing general leads; and summarizing.

- To communicate well, the nurse must be seen as trustworthy.

- Offering unvalidated reassurance, stating approval or disapproval, giving common (not expert) advice, stereotyping, and being defensive are barriers to communication that destroy trust.

 EXPLORE MediaLink

Additional interactive resources for this chapter can be found on the Companion Website at www.prenhall.com/ramont. Click on Chapter 12 and "Begin" to select the activities for this chapter.

For chapter-related NCLEX®-style questions and an audio glossary, access the accompanying CD-ROM in this book.

Animations/Videos
- Communicating Effectively
- Nonverbal Communication

FOR FURTHER Study

For more information on shift change reporting, see Chapter 6

See Chapter 13 for more on alternative communication techniques.

Caring for a Client with Anorexia

NCLEX-PN® Focus Area: Coping and Adaptation

Case Study: Erlene Barnes, age 18, has been diagnosed with anorexia. She expresses that she feels she is fat although she admits to losing 15 pounds in the last 2 months. She is planning to leave home to go to college in about 3 months. She has come for her college physical. Her mother accompanied her and insists on being in the room during the exam, and attempts to answer all questions directed to Ms. Barnes.

Nursing Diagnosis: Ineffective Family Therapeutic Regimen Management r/t family conflict

---

COLLECT DATA

Subjective	Objective
_____	_____
_____	_____
_____	_____
_____	_____
_____	_____
_____	_____
_____	_____

Would you report this data? Yes/No

If yes, to: _____

What would you report? _____

Nursing Care

_____
_____
_____
_____
_____
_____
_____
_____
_____
_____
_____

How would you document this? _____
_____
_____

Compare your documentation to the sample provided in Appendix I.

Data Collected
(use those that apply)

- Height 5'9"
- Weight 98 lbs, down from 117 lbs 2 months ago
- LMP 3 months ago
- VS: T 96.8, P 100, R 18, BP 90/66
- Exercises 2 hours per day in addition to cheerleading practice
- Mother states she is a straight A student and very popular; "We are so proud of Erlene. She has a full scholarship to my college; she is going to be an attorney just like her father."
- Erlene was asked what she eats on a normal day. Mother replied, "She is so busy she just grabs breakfast on the run. I am sure she eats lunch at school, 'cause she says she isn't hungry at dinner time."
- When Erlene is sent to restroom to collect a urine sample, her mother states, "She hasn't had a period in three months. Do you think she could be pregnant?"
- Takes no prescription medications; does admit to taking laxatives for "constipation"

Nursing Interventions
(use those that apply; list in priority order)

- Review with family members the congruence and incongruence of family behaviors.
- Help family to mobilize social support.
- Encourage client to use "I" statements and to accept responsibility for and consequences of actions.
- Review client's current medication.
- Facilitate modeling and role-playing for family regarding healthy ways to communicate and interact.
- Establish open and trusting relationship within the family.
- Provide knowledge to support decisions regarding therapeutic regimens.
- Assess client's level of anxiety and physical reaction to anxiety.
- Model age and cognitively appropriate caregiver skills by communicating with the client at an appropriate cognitive level.

NCLEX-PN® Exam Preparation

1 When a nursing student sits on a client's bed while conducting an admission interview, he or she is disregarding the client's need for:

1. confidentiality.
2. personal space.
3. eye contact.
4. acceptance.

2 Questions that begin with "when," "where," "who," "what," "do (did, does)," "is (are, was)," and sometimes "how" can be described as:

1. leading questions.
2. open-ended questions.
3. closed-ended questions.
4. attentive questions.

3 The opening can be the most important part of the interview because:

1. it sets the tone for the remainder of the interview, establishes rapport, and orients the interviewee.
2. it states appreciation or satisfaction about accomplishments.
3. the client communicates what he or she thinks, feels, knows, and perceives in response to questions from the nurse.
4. the nurse can make the transition by asking an open-ended question that is related to the stated purpose.

4 When the nurse makes a systematic assessment of the person's overall physical appearance, posture, gait, facial expressions, and gestures, he or she is:

1. communicating nonverbally.
2. observing or interpreting nonverbal behavior.
3. contradicting what the client is saying verbally.
4. making unfounded judgments about the client.

5 You are attempting to establish a therapeutic relationship with a client. Which of the following statements would support this attempt?

1. "I have at least 30 minutes I can spend with you, until it is time for your family session."
2. "I understand how frustrated you must be that you will have to remain in the hospital over the holidays. I had surgery one year at Thanksgiving. It was really depressing."
3. "I am sure your surgery will be fine. You have a very good doctor."
4. "If I were you I would get another opinion before I agreed to surgery."

6 The communication between you and your client has been going quite well, when you inadvertently used a communication barrier. Your best reaction would be to:

1. change the subject and continue talking with the client.
2. stop and make a statement such as "I'm sorry; that didn't come out they way I meant it."
3. ignore your mistake; the client probably didn't notice.
4. end the session, and leave the room as quickly as possible.

7 Active or attentive listening can best be described as:

1. interrupting the client to clarify information being given.
2. leaning forward slightly, making eye contact, and giving nonverbal clues while listening.
3. making notes so that you do not miss what the client is saying.
4. frequently looking at your watch or out the window, so that the client will realize that he or she has a time limit.

8 "You are stressed about your surgery tomorrow, aren't you?" is an example of a(n):

1. neutral question.
2. open-ended question.
3. leading question.
4. directed interview question.

9 The portion of the interview where the client communicates what he or she thinks, feels, knows, and perceives is known as:

1. establishing rapport.
2. the orientation.
3. the opening.
4. the body.

10 You have completed an interview with your client. Which of the following statements or actions would best signal the client that the interview is coming to an end?

1. Glance at your watch, close the chart, and stand.
2. "I really enjoyed meeting with you. I think we have accomplished a great deal."
3. "I have other clients I need to see. I will stop back later on."
4. "Time really flew. I have all the information I need."

Answers and Rationales for Review Questions, as well as discussion of Care Plan and Critical Thinking Care Map questions, appear in Appendix I.

Chapter 13

Sensory Perception

BRIEF Outline

Components of the Sensory Experience
Sensory Alterations
Factors Affecting Sensory Function
The Confused Client

LEARNING Outcomes

After completing this chapter, you will be able to:

1. Describe factors influencing the sensory experience.
2. Discuss factors that place a client at risk for sensory disturbances.
3. Describe essential components in assessing a client's sensory-perceptual function.
4. Identify clinical signs and symptoms of sensory overload and deprivation.
5. List and describe methods of preventing sensory overload and deprivation.
6. Discuss nursing interventions for managing acute sensory deficits.
7. Describe factors that affect the amount and quality of sensory stimulation.
8. Explain the key points related to diagnosis, planning, and implementing care for clients with sensory-perception problems.
9. Identify strategies to promote and maintain orientation to person, place, time, and situation for confused and unconscious clients.
10. Discuss the process of evaluation to determine if goals and outcomes have been achieved.

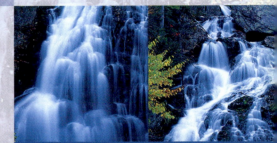

HISTORICAL Perspectives

Since the earliest days in Alexandria (circa 300 B.C.), when Euclid described the laws of reflection in Optica, the science of optics has fascinated and challenged society's most brilliant minds. Today, millions of people with optical challenges need be thankful to these pioneers for the eyeglasses, contact lenses, and other advances that have evolved from innovations dating back to as early as 1303, when Bernard of Gordon, a French physician, wrote about the use of spectacles as a way of correcting long-sightedness (hypermetropia).

An individual's senses are essential for growth, development, and survival. Sensory stimuli give meaning to events in the environment. Any alteration in people's sensory functions can affect their ability to function within the environment. For example, many clients have impaired sensory functions that put them at risk in the healthcare setting; nurses can help them find ways to function safely in this often confusing environment.

Components of the Sensory Experience

For an individual to be aware of the surroundings, four aspects of the sensory process must be present: stimulus, receptor, impulse conduction, and perception.

- *Stimulus*—An agent or act that stimulates a nerve receptor.
- *Receptor*—A nerve cell acts as a **receptor** by converting the stimulus to a nerve impulse. Most receptors are specific, that is, sensitive to only one type of stimulus, such as visual, auditory, or touch.
- *Impulse conduction*—The **impulse** travels along nerve pathways to the spinal cord or directly to the brain. For example, auditory impulses travel to the organ of Corti in the inner ear. From there the impulses travel along the eighth cranial nerve to the temporal lobe of the brain.
- *Perception*—Perception, or awareness and interpretation of stimuli, takes place in the brain, where specialized brain cells interpret the nature and the quality of the sensory stimuli. The level of consciousness affects the perception of the stimuli.

RECEPTION AND PERCEPTION

The sensory process involves two major components: reception and perception. Sensory reception is the process of receiving **stimuli** or data. These stimuli are either external or internal. External stimuli are visual (sight), **auditory** (hearing), **olfactory** (smell), tactile (touch), and **gustatory** (taste). Gustatory stimuli can be internal as well. Other types of internal stimuli are kinesthetic or visceral. **Kinesthetic** refers to awareness of the position and movement of body parts. For example, a person walking is aware of which leg is forward. **Visceral** refers to organs that may produce stimuli that make a person aware of them (e.g., a full stomach). Regardless of the type of stimuli received, **sensory perception** involves the conscious organization and translation of the data or stimuli into meaningful information.

Arousal Mechanism

For the person to receive and interpret stimuli, the brain must be alert. The brain has the capacity to adapt to sensory stimuli. For example, a person living in a city may not notice traffic noise that someone from a rural area finds loud

TABLE 13-1	
States of Awareness	
STATE	**DESCRIPTION**
Full consciousness	Alert; oriented to time, place, person; understands verbal and written words
Confused	Reduced awareness, easily bewildered; poor memory, misinterprets stimuli; impaired judgment
Disoriented	Not oriented to time, place, or person
Somnolent	Extreme drowsiness but will respond to stimuli
Semicomatose	Can be aroused by extreme or repeated stimuli
Coma[a]	Will not respond to verbal stimuli

[a]See the Glasgow Coma Scale, Table 19-2.

and disturbing. Not all sensory stimuli are acted on; some are stored by the memory to be used at a later date. *Cognition* is cerebral functioning. It involves such processes as conscious thought, reality orientation, problem solving, judgment, and comprehension.

Awareness is the ability to perceive environmental stimuli and body reactions and to respond appropriately through thought and action. The normal, alert person can assimilate many kinds of information at one time. There are several states of awareness, as listed in Table 13-1 ■.

Sensory Alterations

People become accustomed to certain sensory stimuli, and when these change markedly, the individual may experience discomfort. For example, when clients enter a hospital, they usually experience stimuli that differ in quantity and quality from those they are used to. These changes may cause clients to become confused and disoriented (see Table 13-1).

Nurses are aware of the behaviors that often result from different stimuli. More attention is now paid to color, sound, privacy, and social interaction for clients so that the stimuli more resemble those in the home environment. Factors that contribute to alterations in behavior include sensory deprivation, sensory overload, and sensory deficits.

SENSORY DEPRIVATION

Sensory deprivation is generally thought of as a decrease in or lack of meaningful stimuli. Because of this reduced stimulation, a person becomes more acutely aware of the remaining stimuli and often perceives these in a distorted manner. Thus the person often experiences alterations in perception, cognition, and emotion. See Box 13-1 ■ for the clinical signs of sensory deprivation.

BOX 13-1	MANIFESTATIONS OF SENSORY DEPRIVATION

- Excessive yawning, drowsiness, sleeping
- Decreased attention span, difficulty concentrating, decreased problem solving
- Impaired memory
- Periodic disorientation, general confusion, or nocturnal confusion
- Preoccupation with somatic complaints, such as palpitations
- Hallucinations or delusions
- Crying, annoyance over small matters, depression
- Apathy, emotional lability

Preventing Sensory Deprivation

For clients who are at risk for sensory deprivation, nurses can increase environmental stimuli in a number of ways. For example, newspapers, books, and television can stimulate the visual and auditory senses. Providing objects that are pleasant to touch, such as a pet to stroke, can provide tactile and interactive stimulation. Clocks that differentiate night from day by color can help orient a client to time. The olfactory sense can be stimulated by the presence of fresh flowers or plants.

Arrangements should also be made for people to visit and talk with the client regularly. Many church and community groups provide visitors to "shut-ins," that is, people who are confined to their homes or who reside in nursing homes. See Box 13-2 ■ for measures to prevent sensory deprivation.

SENSORY OVERLOAD

Sensory overload generally occurs when a person is unable to process or manage the amount or intensity of sensory stimuli. Three factors contribute to sensory overload:

- Increased quantity or quality of internal stimuli, such as pain, dyspnea, or anxiety
- Increased quantity or quality of external stimuli, such as a noisy healthcare setting, intrusive diagnostic studies, or contacts with many strangers
- Inability to disregard stimuli selectively, perhaps as a result of nervous system disturbances or medications that stimulate the arousal mechanism.

Sensory overload can prevent the brain from ignoring or responding to specific stimuli. The person usually feels overwhelmed and does not feel in control. It is important for nurses to remember that the sights and sounds that are familiar to them often represent overload to clients. People who have sensory overload may appear fatigued. They often cannot internalize new information and experience cognitive overload as a result of everything that is happening to them. Such factors as

BOX 13-2	NURSING CARE CHECKLIST

Preventing Sensory Deprivation

- ☑ Encourage the client to use eyeglasses and hearing aids.
- ☑ Address the client by name and touch the client while speaking if this is not culturally offensive.
- ☑ Communicate frequently with the client, and maintain meaningful interactions (e.g., discuss current events).
- ☑ Provide a telephone, radio and/or TV, clock, and calendar.
- ☑ Provide murals, pictures, sculptures, and wall hangings. Many libraries and museums will lend artwork free of charge, or a local school may provide art projects developed by their students.
- ☑ Have family and friends bring freshly cut flowers and plants.
- ☑ Consider having a resident pet such as fish, a cat, or a bird or make arrangements for pets to visit on a regular basis.
- ☑ Include different textured objects to feel such as a sheepskin pillow, silk scarf, soft blanket, or other inanimate object.
- ☑ Increase tactile stimulation through physical care measures such as back massages, hair care, and foot soaks.
- ☑ Encourage social interaction through activity groups or visits by family and friends.
- ☑ Encourage the use of crossword puzzles or games to stimulate mental function.
- ☑ Encourage environment changes such as a walk through a mall, or for an immobilized client, sitting near a window or at a place on the nursing unit where the client can watch local traffic.
- ☑ Encourage the use of self-stimulation techniques such as singing, humming, whistling, or reciting.

pain, lack of sleep, and worry can also contribute to sensory overload. See Box 13-3 ■ for common signs of sensory overload.

Preventing Sensory Overload

For clients who are at risk of overstimulation, nurses should reduce the number and type of environmental stimuli. The nurse can counteract sensory overload by blocking stimuli and by helping the client organize the stimuli and alter responses to the stimuli.

BOX 13-3	MANIFESTATIONS OF SENSORY OVERLOAD

- Complaints of fatigue, sleeplessness
- Irritability, anxiety, restlessness
- Periodic or general disorientation
- Reduced problem-solving ability and task performance
- Increased muscle tension
- Scattered attention and racing thoughts

Dark glasses can partially block light rays, and a window shade or drape can reduce visual stimulation. Earplugs reduce auditory stimuli, as do soft background music and earphones. The odor from a draining wound can be minimized by keeping the dressing dry and clean and applying a liquid deodorant on a gauze near the wound.

Another method of blocking stimuli is to provide rest intervals free of interruptions. Sometimes the number of visitors and the length of visits must be restricted. Also, if the nurse carries out several nursing measures together, the client can have a scheduled quiet period before the next activity.

By explaining sounds in the environment to help clients understand their meaning, stimuli are frequently less confusing and more easily ignored. People can also learn to alter their responses to the stimuli. Clients can employ relaxation techniques to reduce anxiety and stress despite continual sensory stimulation. See Box 13-4 ■ for nursing measures to prevent sensory overload.

SENSORY DEFICITS

A **sensory deficit** is impaired reception, perception, or both, of one or more of the senses. Blindness and deafness are sensory deficits. When only one sense is affected, other senses may become more acute to compensate for the loss. However, sudden loss of eyesight can result in disorientation.

When loss of sensory function is gradual, individuals often develop behaviors to compensate for the loss; sometimes these behaviors are unconscious. For example, a person with

gradual hearing loss in the right ear may unconsciously turn the left ear toward a speaker. When the loss is sudden, however, compensatory behavior often takes days or weeks to develop.

Some neurologic diseases cause changes in the kinesthetic sense and tactile perceptions. Diseases of the inner ear, for example, can cause loss of kinesthetic sense.

Clients with sensory deficits are at risk of both sensory deprivation and sensory overload. Persons with visual problems may be unable to read, watch television, or recognize nurses by sight. An unfamiliar environment can add to their confusion. Blind people often have highly structured home environments, and the diversity and unfamiliarity of the hospital environment can create sensory overload. At the same time, impaired vision often results in an inability to move around readily or socialize with others.

Managing Acute Sensory Deficits

When assisting clients who have a sensory deficit, the nurse needs to (1) encourage the use of sensory aids to support residual sensory function, (2) promote the use of other senses, (3) communicate effectively, and (4) ensure client safety.

Sensory Aids

Many sensory aids are available for clients who have visual and hearing deficits. Examples are shown in Box 13-5 ■.

BOX 13-4

Preventing Sensory Overload

- Minimize unnecessary light, noise, and distraction. Provide dark glasses and earplugs as needed.
- Control pain as indicated.
- Introduce yourself by name and address the client by name.
- Provide orienting cues, such as clocks, calendars, equipment, and furniture in the room.
- Provide a private room.
- Limit visitors.
- Plan care to allow for uninterrupted periods for rest or sleep.
- Schedule a routine of care so the client knows when and what to expect (post the schedule for the client wherever possible).
- Speak in a low tone of voice and in an unhurried manner.
- Provide new information gradually to enable the client to process the meaning. When providing information, ask the client to repeat it so that there are no misunderstandings.
- Describe any tests and procedures to the client beforehand.
- Reduce noxious odors. Empty a commode or bedpan immediately after use; keep wounds clean and covered; use a room deodorizer when indicated; and provide good ventilation.
- Take time to discuss the client's problems and to correct misinterpretations.
- Assist the client with stress-reducing techniques.

BOX 13-5

Sensory Aids for Visual and Hearing Deficits

Visual
- Eyeglasses of the correct prescription, clean and in good repair
- Adequate room lighting, including night-lights
- Sunglasses or shades on windows to reduce glare
- Bright contrasting colors in the environment
- Magnifying glass
- Phone dialer with large numbers
- Clock and wristwatch with large numbers
- Color code or texture code on stoves, washer, medicine containers, and so on
- Colored or raised rims on dishes
- Reading material with large print
- Braille or recorded books
- Seeing-eye dog

Hearing
- Hearing aid in good order
- Lip reading
- Sign language
- Amplified telephones
- Telecommunication device for the deaf (TDD)
- Amplified telephone ringers and doorbells
- Flashing alarm clocks
- Flashing smoke detectors

Sensory aids can be used in the healthcare setting as well as in the home. In all situations, the assistance of support people needs to be enlisted whenever possible to help the client deal with the deficit.

Factors Affecting Sensory Function

A number of factors affect the amount and quality of sensory stimulation, including a person's developmental stage, culture, level of stress, medications and illness, and lifestyle.

DEVELOPMENTAL STAGE

As children grow, they learn that certain sensations provide cues for behavior already learned, for example, parents modeling stopping and looking both ways before crossing a street. Children learn that stopping and looking at a cues is associated with safety behavior. Adults have many learned responses to sensory cues. The sudden loss or impairment of any sense, therefore, has a profound effect on both the child and adult.

CULTURE

An individual's culture often determines the amount of stimulation that a person considers usual or "normal." For example, a child raised in a large, active Latino family may be accustomed to more stimulation than an only child raised in a European American family. A sudden change in cultural surroundings experienced by immigrants or visitors to a new country, especially where there are differences in language, dress, and cultural behaviors, may also result in sensory overload or cultural shock.

It is important that nurses be sensitive to what stimulation is culturally acceptable to a client. For example, in some cultures touching is comforting; in others it is offensive.

STRESS

During times of increased stress, people may find their senses already overloaded and thus seek to decrease sensory stimulation. For example, a client dealing with physical illness, pain, hospitalization, and diagnostic tests may wish to have only close support people visit. In addition, the client may need the nurse's help to decrease unnecessary stimuli (e.g., noise) as much as possible.

MEDICATIONS AND ILLNESS

Certain medications can alter an individual's awareness of environmental stimuli. Narcotics and sedatives, for example, can decrease awareness of stimuli. Some antidepressants can alter perceptions of stimuli.

Certain diseases, such as atherosclerosis, restrict blood flow to the receptor organs and the brain, thereby decreasing awareness and slowing responses. Uncontrolled diabetes mellitus can impair vision. Some central nervous system diseases cause varying degrees of paralysis and sensory loss.

LIFESTYLE AND PERSONALITY

Lifestyle influences the quality and quantity of stimulation to which an individual is accustomed. A client who is employed in a large company may be accustomed to many diverse stimuli; a client who is self-employed and works in the home is exposed to fewer, less diverse stimuli. Personality differences also affect an individual's comfort regarding the quantity and quality of stimuli. Whereas some people delight in constantly changing stimuli and excitement, others prefer a more structured life with few changes.

The Confused Client

Confusion can occur in clients of all ages, but it is most commonly seen in older people. The causes of confusion can be physiological or situational. The most common causes of confusion are:

- Drug effects, such as potentiating effects of multiple drug use and drug intoxication
- Physiological disturbances, such as hypoxia, dehydration, metabolic or fluid imbalances, neurologic disorders, infectious processes, and nutritional deficiencies
- Abrupt loss of a significant person or persons
- Multiple losses in a short time span
- A move to a radically different environment.

Clients who are confused often know something is wrong and want help. See Box 13-6 ■ for nursing interventions to help orient the confused person to time, place, person, and situation.

NURSING CARE

ASSESSING

During the course of a head-to-toe assessment, the LPN/LVN will have the opportunity to gather information on the client's level of sensory-perceptual functioning. The examination should reveal whether the senses are impaired. Information about the client's specific visual and hearing abilities; perception of heat, cold, light touch, and pain in the limbs; and awareness of the position of the body parts will be helpful as the LPN/LVN collaborates with the RN on planning and implementation.

BOX 13-6	NURSING CARE CHECKLIST

Promoting Orientation to Time, Place, Person, and Situation

☑ Wear a readable name tag.

☑ Address the person by name and introduce yourself frequently: "Good morning, Mr. Richards. I am Alicia Gonzales. I will be your nurse today."

☑ Identify time and place as indicated: "Today is December 5th, and it is eight o'clock in the morning."

☑ Ask the client, "Where are you?" and orient the client to place (e.g., nursing home) if indicated.

☑ Place a calendar and clock in the client's room. Mark holidays with ribbons, pins, or other means.

☑ Speak clearly and calmly to the client, allowing time for your words to be processed and for the client to give a response.

☑ Provide frequent face-to-face contact.

☑ Provide clear, concise explanations of each treatment procedure or task.

☑ Reinforce reality by interpreting unfamiliar sounds, sights, and smells; correct any misconceptions of events or situations.

☑ Schedule activities (e.g., meals, bath, activity and rest periods, treatments) at the same time each day to provide a sense of security. If possible, assign the same caregivers.

☑ Keep familiar items in the client's environment (e.g., photographs), and keep the environment uncluttered. A disorganized, cluttered environment increases confusion.

☑ Encourage the client to wear familiar or personal clothing and to arrange personal hygiene articles in order of use as needed.

☑ Encourage participation in familiar activities or hobbies to emphasize the client's strengths rather than problems.

☑ Tell the client when you are leaving and when you will return.

It may be necessary to perform additional sensory tests. These tests may be performed by the LPN/LVN, the RN, or a specialist (e.g., audiologist or speech therapist). Specific sensory tests include:

- Visual acuity, using a Snellen chart or other reading material such as a newspaper, and visual fields
- Hearing acuity, by observing the client's conversation with others and by performing the whisper test and the Weber and Rinne tuning fork tests
- Olfactory sense, by identifying specific aromas
- Gustatory sense, by identifying three tastes such as lemon, salt, and sugar
- Tactile sense, by testing light touch, sharp and dull sensation, two-point discrimination, hot and cold sensation, vibration sense, position sense, and **stereognosis**, the ability to recognize objects by touching or manipulating them.

The LPN/LVN should also determine whether sensory adaptive devices that the client uses, such as eyeglasses or hearing aids, function properly. Special care should be taken to protect eyeglasses and hearing aids from breakage or loss in the hospital. A client whose glasses or hearing aids are lost or damaged will be unable to participate fully in his or her care and recovery.

Clients at Risk for Sensory Deprivation or Overload

Clients at risk for sensory-perceptual alterations need to be identified to ensure that preventive measures can be initiated. Box 13-7 ■ describes such clients.

Client Environment

The LVN/LPN must continuously be aware of quantity, quality, and type of stimuli produced in the environment. The client's environment may produce insufficient stimuli, placing the client at risk for sensory deprivation, or excessive stimuli, placing the client at risk for sensory overload. Nonstimulating environments include those that (1) severely restrict physical activity and (2) limit social contact with family and friends. Because appropriate or meaningful stimuli decrease the incidence of sensory deprivation, the nurse must consider the client's healthcare environment for the presence of the following stimuli:

- Radio or other auditory device (e.g., cassette player), television
- Clock or calendar
- Reading material (or toys for children)
- Number and compatibility of roommates
- Number of visitors.

Social Support Network

The degree of isolation a person feels is significantly influenced by the quality and quantity of support from family members and friends. It is important for the nurse to ask (1) whether the client lives alone, (2) who visits and when, and (3) about any signs indicating social deprivation, such as withdrawal from contact with others to avoid embarrassment or dependence on others, negative self-image, reports of lack of meaningful communication with others, and absence of opportunities to discuss fears or concerns that facilitate **coping mechanisms**.

DIAGNOSING, PLANNING, AND IMPLEMENTING

Following the assessment, the RN will identify diagnostic labels for sensory-perceptual problems. The LPN/LVN should become familiar with these labels in order to be

BOX 13-7

Clients at Risk for Sensory Deprivation and Overload

Sensory Deprivation

- Clients confined in a nonstimulating or monotonous environment in the home or healthcare agency
- Clients who have impaired vision or hearing
- Clients with mobility restrictions such as quadriplegia with bed rest, traction apparatus, or paraplegia
- Clients who are unable to process stimuli (e.g., clients who have brain damage or who are taking medications that affect the central nervous system)
- Clients with a communicable disease (e.g., AIDS)
- Clients who have emotional disorders (e.g., depression) and withdraw within themselves
- Clients who have limited social contact with family and friends (e.g., clients visiting from another country)

Sensory Overload

- Clients who have pain or discomfort
- Clients who are acutely ill and have been admitted to an acute care facility
- Clients who are being closely monitored in an ICU (Figure 13-1 ■) and have intrusive tubes such as IVs, catheters, or nasogastric or endotracheal tubes
- Clients who have decreased cognitive ability (e.g., head injury)

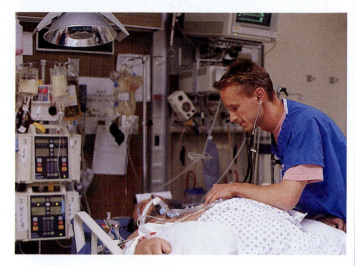

Figure 13-1. ■ A client in an intensive care unit may experience sensory overload.

prepared to collaborate with the RN. Examples of nursing diagnoses for which sensory-perceptual alterations are the etiology include:

- *Risk for Injury* related to sensory-perceptual alterations (specify). For example:
  a. Visual impairment (e.g., decreased depth perception)
  b. Reduced tactile sensation secondary to neurologic or circulatory alterations
  c. Decreased sense of smell
  d. Hearing impairment
  e. Decreased kinesthetic sense
- *Impaired Home Maintenance* related to sensory-perceptual alterations (declining visual abilities)
- *Risk for Impaired Skin Integrity* related to sensory-perceptual alterations (reduced tactile sensation)
- *Impaired Verbal Communication* related to sensory-perceptual alterations (specify). For example:
  a. Altered level of consciousness
  b. Hearing impairment
  c. Sensory overload
  d. Sensory deprivation
- *Self-Care Deficit: Bathing/Hygiene* related to sensory-perceptual alterations (specify). For example:
  a. Visual impairment
  b. Diminished kinesthetic sense

- *Social Isolation* related to sensory-perceptual alterations (specify). For example:
  a. Impaired vision
  b. Impaired hearing

Clients outcomes for sensory-perceptual alterations are to:

- Maintain the function of existing senses.
- Develop an effective communication mechanism.
- Prevent injury.
- Prevent sensory overload or deprivation.
- Reduce social isolation.
- Perform activities of daily living independently and safely.

Examples of nursing interventions for clients with sensory-perceptual alterations are:

- Increase, reduce, or eliminate environmental stimuli to achieve appropriate sensory input.
- Identify and implement appropriate safety precautions.
- Ensure access to and use of assistive devices such as eyeglasses and hearing aids.
- Promote the use of existing senses.
- Provide methods for meaningful communication through touch, writing implements, or other methods as indicated.

- Encourage social interaction with family, friends, and other components of the client's social support network.
- Provide information about social services, community resources, occupational therapy, and other appropriate resources as indicated.

Nurses can assist clients with sensory alterations by promoting healthy sensory function, by adjusting environmental stimuli, and by helping clients to manage acute sensory deficits.

Promoting Healthy Sensory Function

Early screening to detect problems in the visual and hearing functions is essential. For example, children with chronic ear infections and people who live or work in an environment where there is a high noise level should receive routine auditory testing. Women who are considering pregnancy should be advised of the importance of testing for syphilis and rubella, which can cause hearing impairments in newborns. Periodic vision screening of all newborns and children is recommended to detect congenital blindness, strabismus, and refractive errors. Newborn hearing screenings are now possible. Many states are mandating the testing, which can be completed in hospital nurseries and can be performed with relative ease and in a timely manner. The screening provides valuable information and guidelines for further testing.

Healthy sensory function can be promoted with environmental stimuli that provide appropriate sensory input. This input should vary and be neither excessive nor too limited. As many senses as possible should be stimulated. Various colors, sounds, textures, smells, and body positions can provide various sensations. Nurses can teach parents to stimulate infants and children, and family members to stimulate an elderly person. Social activities often help stimulate the mind and the senses.

Nurses should also teach clients at risk of sensory loss how to prevent the loss and should teach general health measures, such as getting regular eye examinations and controlling chronic diseases such as diabetes. Box 13-8 ■ suggests client teaching for preventing sensory impairments, and Box 13-9 ■ discusses cultural variations in the senses.

Promoting the Use of Other Senses

When one sense is lost, the nurse can teach the client to use other senses to supplement the loss. The type of stimulation needs to be adapted to the client's specific deficit. For example, for the client with a visual impairment, stimulation of hearing, taste, smell, and touch can be encouraged. A radio, audiotapes of music or books, or a clock that chimes can be used for auditory stimulation. Diets that

| BOX 13-8 | CLIENT TEACHING |

Preventing Sensory Impairments

- Have regular health examinations.
- Have regular eye examinations as recommended by the physician or pediatrician to screen for eye problems. For clients ages 40 and over, a medical eye examination is generally recommended every 3 to 5 years, or every 1 to 2 years if there is a family history of glaucoma.
- Seek early medical attention (1) if signs suggesting visual impairment arise (e.g., failure to react to light, or reduced eye contact from an infant), (2) if the child complains of an earache or has an ear infection, and (3) for persistent eye redness, discharge or increased tearing, growths on or near the eye, pupil asymmetry or other irregularity, or any pain or discomfort.
- Obtain regular immunizations of children against diseases capable of causing hearing loss (e.g., rubella, mumps, and measles).
- Avoid giving infants and toddlers toys with long pointed handles and keep pointed instruments (e.g., scissors and screwdrivers) out of reach. Supervise preschoolers when they use scissors.
- Make sure that toddlers do not walk or run with a pointed object in hand; teach preschoolers to walk carefully when carrying such objects as sticks or toy weapons.
- Teach school-age children and adolescents the proper use of sports equipment (e.g., hockey sticks) and power tools.
- Wear protective eye goggles when using power tools, riding motorcycles, spraying chemicals, and so on.
- Wear ear protectors when working in an environment with high noise levels or brief loud impulse noises (e.g., blasting).
- Wear dark glasses to avoid damage from ultraviolet rays and never look directly into the sun.

include a variety of flavors, temperatures, and textures can be planned to stimulate the taste buds. Fresh flowers, fragrances, brewing coffee, and baking can stimulate the sense of smell. Measures such as providing a massage, hair brushing, different textures in clothing and upholstery fabrics, and pets can be used to stimulate touch receptors.

| BOX 13-9 | CULTURAL PULSE POINTS |

Variations in Hearing and Vision

There are ethnic variations with both hearing and vison. Hearing gradually declines after age 40, especially at the higher frequencies. African Americans have better hearing at high and low frequencies and are less susceptible than Caucasians to noise-induced hearing loss. Visual acuity differs among cultural groups and this can be clinically significant. African Americans and Native Americans have visual acuity that is comparable to that of Caucasians. Asian Americans (especially Japanese and Chinese) have the poorest corrected vision acuity due to the high incidence of myopia in these populations.

Communicating Effectively

Communication with clients who have sensory deficits should convey respect, enhance the person's self-esteem, and ensure the exchange of correct information. A person with a hearing impairment has to concentrate more than other people and therefore tires more readily. Fatigue compounded by an illness can further reduce the person's ability to hear. A person with a visual impairment is unable to observe most nonverbal cues during communication and relies largely on the spoken word and tone of voice. Guidelines for communicating with people who have visual or hearing impairments are listed in Box 13-10 ■.

Ensuring Client Safety

Nurses must implement safety precautions in healthcare settings for clients with sensory deficits and teach them special precautions to ensure their safety at home.

Impaired Vision

For clients with visual impairments, nurses need to do the following in a healthcare setting:

- Orient the client to the arrangement of room furnishings and maintain an uncluttered environment.

- Keep pathways clear and do not rearrange furniture without orienting the client. Ensure that housekeeping personnel are informed about this.
- Organize self-care articles within the client's reach and orient the client to their location.
- Keep the call light within easy reach and place the bed in the lowest position.
- Assist with ambulation by standing to the client's side, walking about 1 foot ahead, and allowing the person to grasp your arm. Confirm whether the client prefers grasping your arm with the dominant or nondominant hand.

Impaired Hearing

Clients will need to have call lights answered in person, since they may be unable to respond to a voice on the intercom.

Caring for the Unconscious Client

The person who is unconscious and unable to respond to the spoken word nevertheless can often hear what is spoken. It is therefore important that nurses talk to the client as though he or she can understand, using a normal tone of voice and speaking before touching the client. Nurses should

---

BOX 13-10	NURSING CARE CHECKLIST

Communicating with Clients Who Have a Visual or Hearing Deficit

Visual Deficit

☑ Always announce your presence when entering the client's room and identify yourself by name.

☑ Stay in the client's field of vision if the client has a partial vision loss.

☑ Speak in a warm and pleasant tone of voice. Some people tend to speak louder than necessary when talking to a blind person.

☑ Always explain what you are about to do before touching the person.

☑ Explain the sounds in the environment.

☑ Indicate when the conversation has ended and when you are leaving the room.

Hearing Deficit

☑ Before initiating conversation, convey your presence by moving to a position where you can be seen or by gently touching the person.

☑ Decrease background noises (e.g., radio) before speaking.

☑ Talk at a moderate rate and in a normal tone of voice. Shouting does not make your voice more distinct and in some instances makes understanding more difficult.

☑ Address the person directly. Do not turn away in the middle of a remark or story. Make sure the person can see your face easily and that it is well lighted.

☑ Avoid talking when you have something in your mouth, such as chewing gum. Avoid covering your mouth with your hand.

☑ Keep your voice at about the same volume throughout each sentence, without dropping the voice at the end of each sentence.

☑ Always speak as clearly and accurately as possible. Articulate consonants with particular care.

☑ Do not "overarticulate"; mouthing or overdoing articulation is just as troublesome as mumbling. Pantomime or write ideas, or use sign language or finger spelling as appropriate.

☑ Use longer phrases, which tend to be easier to understand than short ones. For example, "Will you get me a drink of water?" presents much less difficulty than "Will you get me a drink?" Word choice is important: "Fifteen cents" and "fifty cents" may be confused, but "half a dollar" is clear.

☑ Pronounce every name with care. Make a reference to the name for easier understanding, for example, "Joan, the girl from the office" or "Sears, the big downtown store."

☑ Change to a new subject at a slower rate, making sure that the person follows the change to the new subject. A key word or two at the beginning of a new topic is a good indicator that the topic is changing.

also try to keep the environmental noises at a minimum so that the client can focus on words. The following are some additional measures nurses can take in caring for the unconscious client:

- Orient the unconscious client to self, time, and place.
- Listen carefully to the support person's concerns. Often they simply want to express them.
- Maintain the same schedule each day. Routine gives the client a sense of security.
- Touch and stroke the unconscious client.
- To the support persons, explain what is happening, and encourage them to talk to and touch the client as though the client were conscious. This auditory and tactile stimulation supports the client and may restore some degree of consciousness.
- Always address the client by name, and explain beforehand the care to be provided. Unconscious clients require bathing, skin care, turning, feeding, and assistance with elimination needs.

EVALUATING

Using the measurable desired outcomes developed during the planning stage as a guide, the nurse collects data needed to judge whether client goals and outcomes have been achieved. Examples of client goals and related outcomes are:

- Maintain or promote sensory functioning: Use protective devices (e.g., protective eyewear) appropriately.
- Maintain or improve communication: Use assistive devices for communication (e.g., hearing aid, writing implements, large print).
- Reduce social isolation: Formulate a plan to become more involved with others.

If outcomes are not achieved, the nurse and client, and support caregivers if appropriate, need to explore the reasons before modifying the care plan.

CONTINUING CARE

To provide for continuity of care, the nurse must consider the client's needs for assistance with care in the home or residential treatment setting. Some clients with severe alterations in sensory-perceptual functioning may be discharged to an assisted living facility that provides the specific support the client requires. Discharge planning incorporates a reassessment of the client's abilities for self-care, the availability and skills of support people, financial resources, and the need for referrals and home health services. Box 13-11 ■ outlines home care assessment with regard to sensory-perceptual alterations. A major aspect of discharge planning involves the instructional needs of the client and family.

BOX 13-11

Sensory-Perceptual Alterations

Client and Environment

- *Self-care abilities:* Ability to care for self while adapting to sensory impairment
- *Safety:* Physical safety of client's environment including lighting, noise, access, lack of clutter or obstructions, use of stairs, assistive devices with respect to sensory impairment, such as flashing fire alarms or telephones for hearing impaired
- *Level of knowledge:* Assistive devices available; ways to maximize use of other senses; local, regional, or national organizations that may provide education, training, support, or other assisstance, such as the National Braille Association, Guide Dogs for the Blind, the National Association of the Deaf

---

NURSING PROCESS CARE PLAN
Client in the ICU

Mrs. Dodd is a 51-year-old client who is being cared for in the critical care unit following a motor vehicle crash in which she sustained extensive traumatic injuries. Mrs. Dodd is connected to several monitoring devices, is intubated and a ventilator is assisting her with respirations. She is receiving various pain and other medications.

Assessment. VS: T 99.2, P 60, R 14 (on mechanical ventilator), BP 150/90. PCO_2 40 mm Hg. ET tube in place. Responds to verbal commands and tactile stimuli. Burr holes to evacuate epidural hematoma. Stable pelvic fracture. No evidence of internal bleeding or shock. Around-the-clock IV pain control.

Nursing Diagnosis. The following important nursing diagnosis (among others) is established for this client:

- *Disturbed Sensory Perception* related to excessive environmental stimuli

Expected Outcomes. The expected outcomes for the plan of care are:

- Demonstrates relaxed body movements and facial expression.
- Will respond to caregiver with eye blinks.

Planning and Implementation. The following nursing interventions are implemented:

- Identify name and purpose when approaching client bedside.
- Orient to time, place, person, and surroundings.
- Pay attention to client's emotional needs.
- Minimize unnecessary light, noise, and distraction.
- Monitor pain control.

- Plan care to allow for uninterrupted periods of rest.
- Describe any test and procedure or activity prior to initiating.
- Provide client with alternate form of communication.

Evaluation. Mrs. Dodd appears less anxious today as evidenced by relaxed facial expression, provided with 2 hours of uninterrupted rest every shift. Responding to yes and no questions with eye blinks. Beginning to make needs known.

Critical Thinking in the Nursing Process

1. Identify factors that place Mrs. Dodd at risk for the development of sensory deprivation or overload.

2. How can you intervene to help Mrs. Dodd during this stress event?

3. How might the care of a client in the home setting differ from the care of a client such as Mrs. Dodd who is receiving care in the critical care unit?

Note: Discussion of Critical Thinking questions appears in Appendix I.

Note: The references and resources for this and all chapters have been compiled at the back of the book.

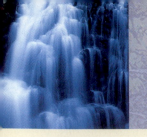

Chapter Review

 KEY TERMS by Topic

Use the audio glossary feature of either the CD-ROM or the Companion Website to hear the correct pronunciation of the following key terms.

Components of the Sensory Experience
receptor, impulse, stimuli, auditory, olfactory, gustatory, kinesthetic, visceral, sensory perception

Sensory Alterations
sensory deprivation, sensory overload, sensory deficit

Nursing Care
stereognosis, coping mechanisms

KEY Points

- Sensory deprivation occurs when a person receives decreased sensory input or monotonous or meaningless sensory input.

- Sensory overload occurs when a person experiences excessive sensory input and is unable to process or manage the stimuli. The person feels overwhelmed and not in control.

- Clients at risk for sensory deprivation include those who are homebound or institutionalized, those on bed rest or Isolation Precautions, or those with sensory deficits.

- Clients at risk for sensory overload include those in pain, those in intensive care units, or those with intrusive and uncomfortable monitoring or treatment equipment.

- Nurses and support caregivers need to devise and implement effective communication mechanisms for clients who have visual and hearing impairments.

- Confused clients and unconscious clients need care that is directed to promoting their orientation to time, place, person, and situation.

 EXPLORE MediaLink

Additional interactive resources for this chapter can be found on the Companion Website at www.prenhall.com/ramont. Click on Chapter 13 and "Begin" to select the activities for this chapter.

For chapter-related NCLEX®-style questions and an audio glossary, access the accompanying CD-ROM in this book.

FOR FURTHER Study

The Glasgow Coma Scale is given in Table 19-2.

Critical Thinking Care Map

Caring for a Client with Sensory-Perceptual Alteration
NCLEX-PN® Focus Area: Physiological Adaptation

Case Study: Julia Hagstrom is an 80-year-old widow who has recently become a resident of an extended care facility. Just prior to her admission, she underwent surgery for the removal of cataracts and also experienced more difficulty with hearing. Her children were concerned about her physical safety and lack of socialization and urged her to enter a nursing home. Mrs. Hagstrom had cared for herself independently for 15 years in her own home. Three days after admission, the nurse finds the client somewhat confused and disoriented to person, place, and time. She appears restless, withdrawn, and her syntax is sometimes inappropriate. She states, "I'm afraid of all of these strange creatures in this orphanage."

Nursing Diagnosis: Limited Vision & Hearing

COLLECT DATA

Subjective   **Objective**

Would you report this data? Yes/No

If yes, to: _____

What would you report? _____

Nursing Care

How would you document this?_____

Compare your documentation to the sample provided in Appendix I.

Data Collected
(use those that apply)

- Height 63"
- Weight 122 lbs
- VS: T 98.6, P 72, R 18, BP 128/74
- Rinne test: negative
- Diagnostic data: chest x-ray, CBC, and urinalysis all negative

Nursing Interventions
(use those that apply; list in priority order)

- Provide a consistent physical environment and a daily routine.
- Consider environmental and human factors that may limit dressing/grooming ability.
- Observe for cause of inability to feed self independently.
- Provide caregiver who is familiar to Mrs. Hagstrom.
- Provide low-stimulation environment for Mrs. Hagstrom because disorientation may be increased by overstimulation.
- Encourage independent decision making by reviewing options and their possible consequences with client.
- Provide for adequate rest, sleep, and daytime naps.
- Assess family and living environment for social dynamics.
- Facilitate use of hearing aids, as appropriate.
- Obtain Mrs. Hagstrom's attention through touch.

NCLEX-PN® Exam Preparation

1 Four aspects of the sensory process must be present—stimulus, receptor, impulse conduction, and perception—for an individual to be aware of the surroundings. The stimulus can be described as:

1. a nerve cell that acts by converting the agent to a nerve impulse.
2. an agent that acts on a nerve receptor.
3. an impulse that travels along nerve pathways to the spinal cord or directly to the brain.
4. an interpretation that takes place in the brain.

2 Your primary nurse instructs you to complete an assessment of awareness on your assigned client. She describes the client as somnolent. You understand that to mean that the client:

1. is not oriented to time, place, or person.
2. has reduced awareness, is easily bewildered, has a poor memory, misinterprets stimuli, and has impaired judgment.
3. is experiencing extreme drowsiness, but will respond to stimuli.
4. can be aroused by extreme or repeated stimuli.

3 Several nursing assistants are speaking to each other in their native language in the day room. Of the following, which is the most appropriate statement you as the charge nurse should make?

1. The facility has an all-English rule; anyone not complying will be placed on a 2-day suspension.
2. Family members are complaining about the non-English conversation going on in front of residents.
3. Since many of the residents are confused, they won't understand what you are discussing, so you should speak in English.
4. Conversing in a foreign language can cause sensory deprivation for the residents; please speak English and include them in the conversation.

4 Your client comes to the nurse's station several times each day to ask what time the activities start. Which is the most appropriate action to help the client be more independent?

1. Tell him to check the activity board at the end of the hall.
2. Tell him someone will come to his room to get him at the appropriate time.
3. Place a clock and a large-print activity list with times in his room.
4. Overhead page clients to come to the day room.

5 When caring for an unconscious client, the nurse should keep environmental noise to a minimum and speak to the client during care because:

1. it will be reassuring for the family when they visit.
2. even though the client cannot respond, he or she can often hear what is being said.

3. it will prevent sensory deprivation.
4. it will help the time pass more quickly.

6 Safety issues for clients with visual impairments are particularly important when ambulation is being attempted. Which is the appropriate method for assisting a client with a visual impairment?

1. Walk about 1 foot ahead, and allow the client to grasp your arm.
2. Grasp the client's arm with your dominant hand and walk in front of the client.
3. Provide the client with a white cane and begin mobility training.
4. Instruct the client that a family member will need to accompany her when she walks.

7 You are caring for a widowed elderly client in her own home. She is showing signs of confusion. Of the following, which is the likely cause of her confusion?

1. head injury related to trauma
2. abrupt loss of a significant person
3. discomfort with her environment and/or caregiver
4. an undiagnosed medical problem

8 Many of the clients in the facility where you work have visual and hearing deficits. The team is discussing ways to meet their clients' sensory needs. Of the following, which is of the highest priority?

1. Ensure a safe environment and prevent sensory deprivation.
2. Include the clients in monthly outings.
3. Call family and suggest that they visit at least weekly.
4. Include the clients in group meetings so they can talk about their deficits.

9 Clients age 40 and over, with a family history of glaucoma, should have a medical eye examination:

1. every 1 to 2 years.
2. every 3 to 5 years.
3. whenever symptoms occur.
4. when recommended by their optometrist.

10 One of the clients in a skilled nursing facility attempts to climb out of bed. She is insisting that she must go see her husband right now. Of the following statements, which is the most appropriate one to make to a confused client?

1. "I just spoke with your husband, he is fine, now go to sleep."
2. "If you don't stop climbing out of bed, we will have to restrain you."
3. "This is the hospital. I am your nurse. Let me sit with you while you fall back to sleep and I will help you call your husband in the morning."
4. "You are disturbing the other residents. You must be quiet and go to sleep or I will have to give you some medication."

Answers and Rationales for Review Questions, as well as discussion of Care Plan and Critical Thinking Care Map questions, appear in Appendix I.

Chapter 14

Self-Concept

BRIEF Outline

Formation of Self-Concept
Components of Self-Concept
Factors Affecting Self-Concept

LEARNING Outcomes

After completing this chapter, you will be able to:

1. Define the four personal and social dimensions of self-concept.
2. Summarize Erikson's theory of the effects of psychosocial crises on self-concept and self-esteem.
3. Describe the four components of self-concept.
4. Identify common stressors affecting self-concept and coping strategies.
5. Demonstrate nursing actions designed to achieve identified goals for clients with altered self-concept.
6. Apply ways to enhance the self-esteem of children and adults.

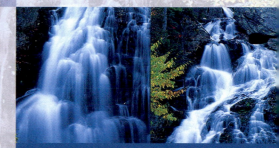

HISTORICAL Perspectives

Although the insurgence of self-concept seemed like a new and novel idea in the 1980s, it has been discussed in psychology circles since the 17th century. A milestone in human reflection about the non-physical inner self came in 1644, when René Descartes wrote Principles of Philosophy. *The idea reappeared in the 1890s in the writings of Sigmund Freud. While Freud and many of his followers hesitated to make self-concept a primary psychological unit in their theories, in 1946, Freud's daughter, Anna, gave central importance to ego development and self-interpretation. By far the most influential and eloquent voice in self-concept theory was that of Carl Rogers (1947), who introduced an entire system of helping built around the importance of the self. In Rogers' view, the self is the central ingredient in human personality and personal adjustment.*

A positive **self-concept** is essential to a person's mental and physical health. Individuals with a positive self-concept are better able to develop and maintain interpersonal relationships and resist psychological and physical illness. Nurses have a responsibility not only to identify people with a negative self-concept, but also to identify the possible causes in order to help people develop a more positive view of themselves.

A nurse's own self-concept is also important. Nurses who feel positive about themselves are better able to help clients meet their needs.

Self-concept is a complex idea that influences:

- How one thinks, talks, and acts
- How one sees and treats another person
- Choices one makes
- Ability to give and receive love
- Ability to take action and to change things.

Self-concept is a view of oneself from several angles. These include:

- *Self-knowledge:* The knowledge that one has about oneself, including insights into one's abilities, nature, and limitations.
- *Self-expectation:* What one expects of oneself; may be a realistic or unrealistic expectation.
- *Social self:* How a person is perceived by others and society.
- *Social evaluation:* The appraisal of oneself in relationship to others, events, or situations.

Formation of Self-Concept

A person is not born with a self-concept; rather, it develops as a result of social interactions with others. According to Erik Erikson, a social theorist, people face certain developmental tasks associated with eight psychosocial stages of life. The success with which a person copes with these developmental crises largely determines the development of self-concept. Inability to cope results in self-concept problems at the time, and often, later in life. See Table 14-1 ■ for

TABLE 14-1		
Examples of Behaviors Associated with Erikson's Stages of Psychosocial Development		
STAGE: DEVELOPMENTAL CRISIS	**BEHAVIORS INDICATING POSITIVE RESOLUTION**	**BEHAVIORS INDICATING NEGATIVE RESOLUTION**
Infancy: trust vs. mistrust	Requesting assistance and expecting to receive it Expressing belief of another person Sharing time, opinions, and experiences	Restricting conversation to superficialities Refusing to provide a person with information Being unable to accept assistance
Toddlerhood: autonomy vs. shame and doubt	Accepting the rules of a group but also expressing disagreement when it is felt Expressing one's own opinion Easily accepting deferment of a wish fulfillment	Failing to express needs Not expressing one's own opinion when opposed Overconcerned about being clean
Early childhood: initiative vs. guilt	Starting projects eagerly Expressing curiosity about many things Demonstrating original thought	Imitating others rather than developing independent ideas Apologizing and being very embarrassed over small mistakes Verbalizing fear about starting a new project
Early school years: industry vs. inferiority	Completing a task once it has been started Working well with others Using time effectively	Not completing tasks started Not assisting with the work of others Not organizing work
Adolescence: identity vs. role confusion	Asserting independence Planning realistically for future roles Establishing close interpersonal relationships	Failing to assume responsibility for directing one's own behavior Accepting the values of others without question Failing to set goals in life
Early adulthood: intimacy vs. isolation	Establishing a close, intense relationship with another person Accepting sexual behavior as desirable Making a commitment to that relationship, even in times of stress and sacrifice	Remaining alone Avoiding close interpersonal relationships

TABLE 14-1

Examples of Behaviors Associated with Erikson's Stages of Psychosocial Development (*continued*)

STAGE: DEVELOPMENTAL CRISIS	BEHAVIORS INDICATING POSITIVE RESOLUTION	BEHAVIORS INDICATING NEGATIVE RESOLUTION
Middle-aged adults: generativity vs. stagnation	Being willing to share with another person Guiding others Establishing a priority of needs, recognizing both self and others	Talking about oneself instead of listening to others Showing concern for oneself in spite of needs of others Being unable to accept interdependence
Older adults: integrity vs. despair	Using past experience to assist others Maintaining productivity in some areas Accepting limitations	Crying and being apathetic Not accepting changes Demanding unnecessary assistance and attention from others

behaviors indicating successful and unsuccessful resolution of these developmental crises.

There are three broad steps in the development of one's self-concept:

1. The infant learns that the physical self is separate and different from the environment.
2. The child internalizes others' attitudes toward self.
3. The child and adult internalize the standards of society.

Each person's self-concept is like a collage. At the center of the collage are the beliefs and images that are most vital to the person's identity. They constitute core self-concept. For example: "I am competent/incompetent"; "I am male/female." Images and beliefs that are less important to the person are on the periphery. For example: "I am left-/right-handed"; "I am athletic/unathletic."

People are thought to base their self-concept on how they perceive and evaluate themselves in these areas:

■ Vocational performance
■ Intellectual functioning
■ Personal appearance and physical attractiveness
■ Sexual attractiveness and performance
■ Being liked by others
■ Ability to cope with and resolve problems
■ Independence.

Components of Self-Concept

There are four components of self-concept: body image, role performance, personal identity, and self-esteem.

BODY IMAGE

The image of physical self, or **body image**, is how a person perceives the size, appearance, and functioning of the body and its parts. A person's body image develops partly from others' attitudes and responses to that person's body and partly from the individual's own exploration of the body. As the parents or caregivers respond to the child with smiles, holding, and touching, and also as the child explores its own body sensations during breastfeeding, thumb sucking, and the bath, body image develops (Figure 14-1 ■). Cultural and societal values also influence a person's body image.

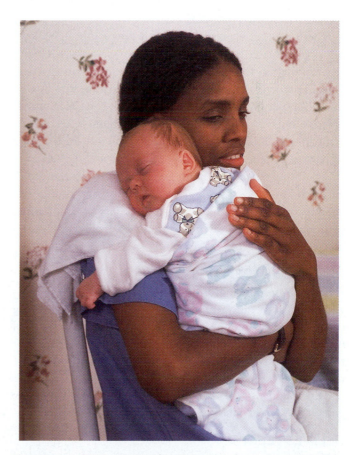

Figure 14-1. ■ Children's attitude toward themselves is learned in part by the ways they are held and touched as infants.

Body image encompasses the functioning of the body and its parts. It also includes body prostheses, such as artificial limbs, dentures, and hairpieces, as well as devices required for functioning, such as wheelchairs, canes, and eyeglasses. Past as well as present perceptions are part of one's body image.

The various information and entertainment media have played a part over the years in how individuals view themselves and others. If a person's body image closely resembles one's body ideal, the individual is more likely to think positively about the physical and nonphysical components of the self.

A person with a healthy body image will normally show concern for both health and appearance. This person will seek help if ill and will include health-promoting practices in daily activities. A person who has an unhealthy body image is likely to be overly concerned about minor illness and to neglect activities, such as sleep and a healthy diet, that are important to health.

The person with body image disturbance may ignore a body part that is significantly changed by illness or trauma (see also Chapter 31 ⬭). Some individuals may also express feelings of helplessness, hopelessness, powerlessness, and vulnerability, and may exhibit self-destructive behavior such as over- or undereating or suicide attempts.

ROLE PERFORMANCE

A **role** is a set of expectations about how a person occupying one position behaves toward a person occupying another position. Role **performance** relates what a person does in a particular role to the behaviors expected of that role. Each person usually has several roles, such as husband, parent, brother, son, employee, friend. Some roles are assumed for only limited periods, such as client, student, and ill person. People need to know who they are in relation to others and what society expects for the positions they hold. To relate or interact appropriately with others, people also need to know the role positions that others occupy. Failure to master a role creates frustration and feelings of inadequacy, often lowering self-esteem.

PERSONAL IDENTITY

A person's **personal identity** is the conscious sense of individuality and uniqueness that is continually evolving throughout life. People often view their identity in terms of name, sex, age, race, ethnic origin or culture, occupation or roles, talents, and other situational characteristics (e.g., marital status and education).

Personal identity also includes a person's beliefs and values, personality, and character.

SELF-ESTEEM

Self-esteem is one's judgment of one's own worth, that is, how that person's standards and performances compare

to those of others and also to one's ideal self. If a person's self-concept does not match with the ideal self, then low self-esteem results. Parents can encourage self-esteem.

Factors Affecting Self-Concept

Major factors that affect a person's self-concept are:

- *Development.* As an individual develops, the factors that affect the self-concept change. For example, whereas an infant requires a supportive, caring environment, a child requires freedom to explore and learn.
- *Family and culture.* A young child's values are largely influenced by the family and culture. Later on, peers influence the child and thereby affect the sense of self. When the child is confronted by differing expectations from family, culture, and peers, the child's sense of self is often confused. See Box 14-1 ■ for more about culture and self-concept.
- *Stressors.* Stressors can strengthen the self-concept as an individual copes successfully with problems. On the other hand, stressors can cause maladaptive responses including substance abuse, withdrawal, and anxiety.
- *Resources.* Internal resources such as confidence and values can affect the self-concept. External resources such as a support network, sufficient finances, and organizations can also influence self-concept. Generally, the greater the number of resources a person has and uses, the more positive the effect on the self-concept.
- *History of success and failure.* People who have a history of failures come to see themselves as a failure, whereas people with a history of successes will have a more positive self-concept, making more successes likely.
- *Illness.* Illness and trauma can also affect the self-concept. People respond to illness and aging in a variety of ways; acceptance, denial, withdrawal, and depression are common reactions.

BOX 14-1	CULTURAL PULSE POINTS

Culture and Self-Concept

Traits related to self-concept must be questioned for cultural bias. Attitudes of the dominate culture should not be used to draw stereotypical conclusions about minority cultures. Conclusions should not be drawn that the individual has a negative self-image because of a cultural difference. For example, children from some cultures do not know their precise birth date because they have never celebrated it—it is not culturally important. Other dates may be emphasized instead. Vietnamese children traditionally add a year to their age at Tet, and many children with Latin American heritage traditionally celebrate their saint's day instead.

BOX 14-2

Stressors Affecting Self-Concept

Identity Stressors

- Change in physical appearance (e.g., facial wrinkles)
- Declining physical, mental, or sensory abilities
- Inability to achieve goals
- Relationship concerns
- Sexuality concerns
- Unrealistic ideal self
- Membership in a minority group
- Cultural dissonance

Body Image Stressors

- Loss of body parts (e.g., amputation, mastectomy, hysterectomy)
- Loss of body functions (e.g., from heart disease, renal disease, spinal cord injury, cerebrovascular accident, neuromuscular disease, arthritis, declining mental or sensory abilities)
- Disfigurement (e.g., through pregnancy, severe burns, facial blemishes, colostomy, ileostomy, tracheostomy, laryngectomy)

Self-Esteem Stressors

- Lack of positive feedback from significant others
- Repeated failures
- Unrealistic expectations
- Inability to cope with life stressors
- Abusive relationship
- Loss of financial security

Role Stressors

- Loss of parent, spouse, child, or close friend
- Change or loss of job
- Retirement
- Divorce or separation
- Illness
- Hospitalization
- Ambiguous role expectations
- Conflicting role expectations
- Inability to meet role expectations

NURSING CARE

ASSESSING

Before conducting a psychosocial assessment, the nurse must establish trust and a working relationship with the client. The following guidelines are suggested for nurse–client interviewing (Neeb, 2001):

- *Be honest.* Tell the client the purpose of the interview.
- *Be assertive.* If the interview is mandatory (intake, preoperative), the client must understand that it is required. Arrange a mutually acceptable time to conduct the interview so the client will be prepared.
- *Be sensitive.* Sometimes the questions are very difficult or embarrassing for the client to answer. Assure the client that you understand his or her feelings and that information shared by the client is part of his or her medical record.
- *Use empathy.* Let the client know that you are interested in what is being said and that you are there to be helpful.
- *Use open-ended questions.* Personalize the questions as much as possible. Use this time to discuss and clarify as much information as you can to avoid having to repeat parts of the interview later.

This assessment can be used in either the acute care or home care environment. It is the nurse's responsibility to use therapeutic communication and to remain sensitive to the effect that cultural influences will have on the client's behaviors

and needs. It is also important that the nurse identify any stressors that may affect aspects of the self-concept. See Box 14-2 ■ for examples of stressors that may place a client at risk for problems with self-concept.

When stressors are identified, the nurse should also identify the client's coping style and determine whether this style is effective by asking the client such questions as:

- When you have a problem or face a stressful situation, how do you usually deal with it?
- Do these methods work?

Personal Identity

When assessing self-concept, the information the nurse first needs is about the client's personal identity. This involves who the client believes he or she is. See Box 14-3 ■ for examples of assessment questions to ask.

Body Image

If there are indications of a body image disturbance, the nurse should assess the client carefully for possible functional or physical problems. See Box 14-3 for examples of questions to ask about body image.

Self-Esteem

A nurse can ask the following questions to determine a client's self-esteem:

- Are you satisfied with your life?
- How do you feel about yourself?
- Are you accomplishing what you want?
- What goals in life are important to you?

| BOX 14-3 | ASSESSING CLIENTS: PERSONAL IDENTITY, BODY IMAGE, AND ROLE RELATIONSHIPS |

Personal Identity

- How would you describe yourself as a person?
- What do you like about yourself?
- How do others describe you as a person?
- What are your personal strengths, talents, and abilities?
- What would you change about yourself if you could?
- Does it bother you a lot if someone doesn't like you?
- Is it hard for you to say no when you want to say no?

Body Image

- Is there any part of your body you would like to change?
- Are you comfortable discussing your surgery?
- How do you feel about your appearance?
- What changes in your body do you expect after surgery?
- How have significant others in your life reacted to changes in your body?

Family Relationships

- Tell me about your family.
- What is your home like?
- Is there anyone you are especially close to or distant from in your family?

- What are your relationships like with your other relatives?
- What are your responsibilities in the family, and is there anything you would like to change?
- How well do you feel you accomplish what is expected of you?
- Do you see yourself as being treated equally in your family?
- Are you proud of your family members?
- Do you feel your family members are proud of you?
- Tell me how you spend your time each day.

Work Roles and Social Roles

- Do you like your work?
- How do you get along at work?
- What aspect of your work would you like to change if you could?
- How do you spend your free time?
- Are you involved in any community groups?
- Are you most comfortable alone, with one other person, or in a group?
- Who is most important to you?
- Whom do you seek out for help?

Some behaviors that might reflect low self-esteem are listed in Box 14-4 ■. Be sure to determine the client's cultural background first so as not to misinterpret specific cultural behaviors as indications of low self-esteem (see Chapter 2 ⚭).

Role Relationships

The nurse assesses the client's satisfactions and dissatisfactions associated with role responsibilities and relationships. Family roles are especially important to people. Relationships can be supportive and promote growth. At the opposite extreme, however, relationships can be highly stressful, especially when violence and abuse are present. To obtain information related to the client's family relationships and satisfaction or dissatisfaction with work roles and social roles, the nurse might ask some of the questions shown in Box 14-3. Questions need to be individualized according to each client's age and situation.

DIAGNOSING, PLANNING, AND IMPLEMENTING

The NANDA nursing diagnostic labels will be used by the RN. Common nursing diagnoses for this area are *Disturbed Body Image*, *Ineffective Role Performance*, and *Chronic*

Low Self-Esteem. The LPN's/LVN's role may be to collaborate with the client, the RN, or other caregivers. A list of NANDA diagnoses can be found in Appendix II ⚭.

The LPN/LVN who has little experience in intervening with clients with altered self-concept may wish to consult

| BOX 14-4 | MANIFESTATIONS OF LOW SELF-ESTEEM |

- Avoids eye contact.
- Stoops in posture and moves slowly.
- Is poorly groomed and has an unkempt appearance.
- Is hesitant or halting in speech.
- Is overly critical of self (e.g., "I'm no good," "I'm ugly," or "People don't like me.").
- May be overly critical of others.
- Is unable to accept positive remarks about self.
- Encourages reprimands from others, to punish self.
- Apologizes frequently.
- Verbalizes feelings of hopelessness, helplessness, and powerlessness, such as "I really don't care what happens," "I'll do whatever anyone wants," or "Whatever is destined will happen."

with a clinical specialist or a more experienced nurse to develop effective plans. The nurse and client set goals to enhance the client's self-concept.

The goals established vary according to the diagnoses and defining characteristics related to each individual. Examples of overall goals are:

- Develop a realistic and positive perception of body appearance and function.
- Increase feelings of self-worth.
- Perform new roles responsibly and capably.

Nurses must always establish a therapeutic relationship, in order to assist clients to evaluate themselves and make behavioral changes.

Identifying Areas of Strength

Healthy people often perceive their problems and weaknesses more clearly than they perceive their assets and strengths. When a client has difficulty identifying personality strengths and assets, the nurse needs to provide the client with a set of guidelines or a framework. Box 14-5 ■ provides a framework for identifying personality strengths.

BOX 14-5

Framework for Identifying Personality Strengths

Note past, present, and anticipated future participation in any of the following:

- Hobbies and crafts
- Expressive arts such as writing, painting, sketching, or music appreciation
- Sports and outdoor activities, including spectator sports
- Education, training, and related areas (including self-education)
- Work, vocation, job, or position.

In addition, determine which of these might apply:

- Sense of humor and the ability to laugh at oneself and take kidding
- Health status including healthy aspects of body function and good health maintenance practices
- Special aptitudes such as sales or mechanical ability; a "green thumb"; ability to recognize and enjoy beauty; ability to solve problems; a liking for adventure or pioneering; having stick-to-itiveness, perseverance, and the drive or will needed to get things done
- Relationship strengths, including the ability to make people feel comfortable, the capacity to enjoy being with people, being aware of people's needs and feelings, being able to listen
- Emotional strengths including the capacity to give and receive warmth, affection, and love; the ability to "take" anger and to feel and express a wide range of emotions; the capacity for empathy
- Spiritual strengths such as religious faith or love of God, membership and participation in church and related activities

---

Nurses can employ the following specific strategies to help clients identify personal strengths:

- Stress positive thinking rather than self-negation.
- Notice and verbally reinforce client strengths.
- Encourage the setting of attainable goals.
- Acknowledge goals that have been attained.
- Provide honest, positive feedback.

Maintaining a Sense of Self

Sometimes people who are ill not only are unaware of their strengths but also are separated from a sense of self. Nurses can use these techniques to help clients maintain a sense of self:

- Communicate worth by looks and touch (e.g., eye contact, a smile, a touch on the hand or shoulder).
- Respect the client's privacy and sensitivities.
- Provide a simple explanation before starting a procedure.
- Listen attentively to the client's concerns.
- Recognize the client's individuality by addressing the client by name.
- Accept the client's responses.

Assisting Clients with Altered Self-Concept

Nurses assisting clients who have an altered self-concept must establish a therapeutic relationship. To do this, the nurse must possess self-awareness and effective communication skills (see Chapters 12 and 33 ⚭). The following nursing interventions may help clients analyze the problem and change self-concept:

- Encourage clients to appraise the situation and express their feelings.
- Encourage clients to ask questions.
- Provide accurate information.
- Become aware of distortions, inappropriate or unrealistic standards, and faulty labels in clients' speech.
- Explore clients' positive qualities and strengths.
- Encourage clients to express positive self-evaluation more than negative self-evaluation.
- Avoid criticism.
- Teach clients to substitute negative self-talk ("I can't walk to the store anymore") with positive self-talk ("I can walk half a block each morning"). Negative self-talk reinforces a negative self-concept.

Assisting Clients with Disturbed Body Image

Surgery (ostomies, amputations, mastectomies) can have a profound effect on people's body image and self-concept. Treatments for illness, such as chemotherapy, can also radically alter a person's physical appearance (Figure 14-2 ■). Clients with conditions such as anorexia nervosa or bulimia carry a distorted self-image. To assist these clients, the nurse

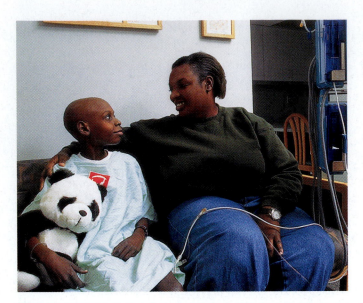

Figure 14-2. ■ One of the most common threats to body image at any age is hair loss induced by chemotherapy. Use of hats or wigs can sometimes improve self-concept.

establishes a therapeutic nursing relationship, practices good communication skills, and provides nursing care as previously described.

Many facilities use critical pathways for clients following surgery. These pathways outline expected outcomes on a day-to-day basis. For an example of a critical pathway for a client following a total mastectomy, see Appendix III ⚭.

Enhancing Self-Esteem

People who have relatively high self-esteem appear to be adjusted, happy, and competent. Box 14-6 ■ describes age-related considerations for enhancing self-esteem in children.

EVALUATING

The nurse, client, and significant others need to understand that to change beliefs, feelings, and behaviors affecting self-esteem requires time and ongoing effort. Unlike many physical problems (e.g., wounds), where healing can be observed quickly, improving one's self-concept can be a continuing concern and is not so easily evaluated. New crises can cause clients to doubt themselves and revert to former feelings of inadequacy. People learn slowly from each new situation and gradually gain new strategies for feeling satisfied with themselves.

CONTINUING CARE

Assessing the client's self concept prior to discharge is essential since negative self-concept may prevent the client from performing a health behavior. A client with a family

---

| BOX 14-6 | POPULATION FOCUS |

Ways to Enhance Self-Esteem in Children

Basic Attitudes
- Security and trust
- Identity
- Belonging
- Purpose
- Personal competence

Key Ingredients
- Love and acceptance
- Firmness
- Consistency
- Establishment of expectations

Ways to Meet Child's Needs
- Take time to be with child.
- Physical contact conveys caring better than words.
- Provide reasonable rules that can serve as guidelines for new situations.
- Give positive feedback.
- Convey faith and confidence in the child's ability to achieve goals.

---

history of diabetes mellitus and a negative self-concept may have difficulty adhering to necessary dietary restrictions. The client may feel incapable of carrying out needed self-care.

NURSING PROCESS CARE PLAN
Client with Self-Concept Issues

You are working in a community clinic. You have been assigned to do an admission workup on walk-in clients. You enter the exam room and encounter a 21-year-old young man with long hair, wearing foundation and mascara, and who is dressed somewhat effeminately. The name on his chart is Brian Breshear, yet when you address him by that name, he flinches and hardly looks up. In response to your question of what brings him in today, he softly replies, "I don't think I am supposed to be in this body. I want to learn about a sex change operation."

Assessment. Male client, height 5′6″, weight 134 lbs; speaks with almost inaudible voice; responds only to direct questions. Vital signs are within normal limits: T 98.6, P 78, R 20, BP 122/76. Client appears anxious; wringing hands and avoiding eye contact.

Nursing Diagnosis. The following important nursing diagnoses (among others) are established for this client:

- *Anxiety* related to *Disturbed Body Image*
- *Ineffective Role Performance* related to disturbed personal identity
- *Risk for Compromised Family Coping*

Expected Outcomes. The expected outcomes for the plan of care are:

- Relate an increase in psychological and physiological comfort.
- Verbalize and demonstrate increased feelings of self-concept.
- Verbalize the need for assistance with situation.
- Relate community resources available.

Planning and Implementation. The following nursing interventions are implemented:

- Be direct and nonjudgmental.
- Encourage him to express his feelings, especially about the way he feels, thinks, or views himself.
- Provide reliable information, and reinforce information already given.
- Provide for opportunity to share with others going through the same experience.
- Establish a trusting nurse–client relationship.
- Provide information on psychological and physiological counseling and referrals.
- Assess level of anxiety.
- Provide reassurance and comfort.
- Encourage realistic appraisal of the situation; dispel guilt and myths.
- If indicated, ask family members to consider the situation from Brian's perspective.

Evaluation. Brian related at his next medical visit that he had attended a counseling appointment with family members. They were able to share their feelings and concerns. His parents indicated that they will be supportive of any decision he makes. He will continue to participate in individual counseling sessions as well as attending a group. He has decided not to seek a surgical consult until a complete medical workup has been done and he has had the opportunity to work through some issues with the counselor and his family.

Critical Thinking in the Nursing Process

1. It is extremely important that the nurse establish a nonjudgmental, supportive therapeutic relationship with Brian. What are some of the communication techniques that you could use to establish this relationship?
2. Brian's father calls the clinic very upset, because the counselor wishes to see the family along with Brian. You have answered the phone. What is the most appropriate response to give to the father?
3. Brian has decided to place any plans for surgery on hold for now. How can you support him in this decision and later if he decides to go ahead with a sex change operation?

Note: Discussion of Critical Thinking questions appears in Appendix I.

Note: The references and resources for this and all chapters have been compiled at the back of the book.

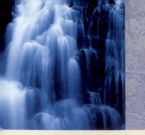

Chapter Review

 KEY TERMS by Topic

Use the audio glossary feature of either the CD-ROM or the Companion Website to hear the correct pronunciation of the following key terms.

Introduction
self-concept

Components of Self-Concept
body image, role, performance, personal identity, self-esteem

KEY Points

- A positive self-concept is essential to a person's physical and psychological well-being.
- A person's self-perception can differ from the person's perception of how others see the person and from the ideal self (how the person would like to be).
- Components of self-concept include body image, role performance, personal identity, and self-esteem.
- Because a positive self-concept is basic to health, one of the nurse's major responsibilities is to assist clients with a disturbed self-concept to develop a more positive and realistic image of themselves.
- A trusting client–nurse relationship is essential for the effective assessment of a client's self-concept, for providing help and support, and for motivating client behavior change.

 EXPLORE Media Link

Additional interactive resources for this chapter can be found on the Companion Website at www.prenhall.com/ramont. Click on Chapter 14 and "Begin" to select the activities for this chapter.

For chapter-related NCLEX®-style questions and an audio glossary, access the accompanying CD-ROM in this book.

FOR FURTHER Study

For further study of cultural awareness and culturally competent nursing, see Chapter 2.

For more information about client communication, see Chapter 12.

For more about surgery and client self-concept, see Chapter 31.

For in-depth discussion of client teaching, see Chapter 33.

A list of NANDA diagnoses can be found in Appendix II.

A critical pathway for a client following a total mastectomy is given in Appendix III.

Caring for a Client with an Amputation

NCLEX-PN® Focus Area: Safety

Case Study: Craig is a 20-year-old male college student who was involved in an automobile crash 3 days ago, resulting in a traumatic amputation of his left lower leg. Craig's mother has remained with him since the injury and is very supportive. His father is grief stricken and having difficulty dealing with Craig's condition, because Craig was captain of his college basketball team and had hopes of becoming a professional basketball player. Craig's condition is stable, and he is being placed into a rehabilitation program immediately. Soon, he will be fitted for a leg prosthesis. Usually an outgoing individual, Craig is somber and untalkative. He does not look at his leg when dressings are being changed, and he refuses to discuss his rehabilitation program.

Nursing Diagnosis: Situational Low Self-Esteem

COLLECT DATA

Subjective

_____
_____
_____
_____
_____
_____

Objective

_____
_____
_____
_____
_____
_____

Would you report this data? Yes/No

If yes, to: _____

What would you report? _____

Nursing Care

_____
_____
_____
_____
_____
_____
_____
_____
_____
_____
_____

How would you document this?_____
_____
_____

Compare your documentation to the sample provided in Appendix I.

Data Collected
(use those that apply)

- Somber and untalkative
- 20-year-old male student
- Refuses to discuss rehabilitation
- Automobile crash 3 days ago
- Father is grief stricken and having difficulty dealing with Craig's condition because of traumatic amputation of his left lower leg
- Condition is stable
- Mother at bedside
- Captain of his college basketball team; shared aspirations of becoming a professional basketball player
- To be fitted for a leg prosthesis
- Usually an outgoing individual
- Does not look at his leg when dressings are being changed
- Rehabilitation program to begin immediately
- Mother very supportive

Nursing Interventions
(use those that apply; list in priority order)

- Actively listen to, demonstrate respect for, and accept the client.
- Encourage client to get up and use crutches within 2 days.
- Assess for intergenerational family problems that can overwhelm coping abilities.
- Assess client for anger and identify previous outlets for anger.
- Have client list strengths.
- Encourage client to reminisce about basketball.
- Accept client's own pace in working through grief and crisis situation.
- Assess the strengths and deficiencies of the family system.
- Talk to family about the importance of sharing feelings and ways to do so.
- Note other stressors in the family.
- Assess for unhealthy coping mechanisms such as substance abuse.
- Provide information about support groups.
- Assess client's support system.

NCLEX-PN® Exam Preparation

1 The knowledge that one has about oneself, including insight into one's abilities and limitations, is known as:
1. self-expectation.
2. self-knowledge.
3. social self.
4. social evaluation.

2 Individuals face certain developmental tasks associated with eight psychosocial stages of development. The success with which a person copes with these developmental crises largely determines the development of self-concept. Psychosocial development was outlined by:
1. Sigmund Freud.
2. Lawrence Kohlberg.
3. Erik Erikson.
4. Aaron Beck.

3 There are three broad steps in the development of one's self-concept: learning that the physical self is separate from the environment, internalizing others' attitudes toward self, and:
1. overcoming the pressures of society.
2. overcoming separation anxiety.
3. internalizing personality development.
4. internalizing the standards of society.

4 An adolescent female with anorexia nervosa has lost more than 25% of her normal weight. When she looks in the mirror, she expresses the feeling that she is "fat." Of the following nursing diagnoses, which is appropriate for dealing with self-concept issues?
1. *Risk for Powerlessness*
2. *Disturbed Body Image*
3. *Imbalanced Nutrition: Less than Body Requirements*
4. *Ineffective Family Therapeutic Regimen Management*

5 People who are ill may be unaware of their strengths and also are separated from a sense of self. Nurses can use many techniques to help clients maintain a sense of self. Which of the following is the best way to communicate worth by looks and touch?
1. Refrain from making eye contact so as not to embarrass the client.
2. Make no physical contact with client unless necessary for care.
3. Encourage client to look at surgical site to promote self-acceptance.
4. Make eye contact and touch client lightly on hand or shoulder when providing comfort.

6 Negative self-talk reinforces a negative self-concept. Of the following statements, which would represent negative-self talk by a client?
1. "I am worried that I may have limitations when I am discharged."
2. "I can't mow my lawn anymore."
3. "Even though I may not be able to mow the lawn, I can still enjoy my flower garden."
4. "I will be glad to be in my own home even though I will need to have someone stay with me."

7 The nurse can best demonstrate empathy by which of the following statements?
1. "I know exactly how you feel."
2. "I am sure you are very devastated by your diagnosis. I know I would be."
3. "Dealing with serious illness can be very difficult. We can talk if you like, or I would be happy to just sit here with you quietly."
4. "Although things look pretty bad today, they will get better as time goes on."

8 During the course of a psychosocial interview, a nurse asks the client, "What goals in life are important to you?" The question is asked to determine:
1. the client's self-esteem.
2. the client's understanding of the care plan.
3. if the client has a disturbed body image.
4. the client's ability to cope with family roles.

9 Nurses should establish a therapeutic relationship. The purpose of this is to:
1. provide client health teaching.
2. assist clients to evaluate themselves and make behavioral changes.
3. be able to carry out the needed assessments and care.
4. provide a safe environment for the hospitalized client.

10 You are assigned to care for a client who is being discharged following a total abdominal hysterectomy. She has been given a nursing diagnosis of *Readiness for Enhanced Self-Concept.* You have learned that there are a number of stressors that affect self-concept. Of the following, which stressors can be classified as body image stressors? (Select all that apply.)
1. loss of body part
2. lack of positive feedback from significant others
3. loss of body functions
4. relationship concerns
5. disfigurement
6. sexuality concerns

Answers and Rationales for Review Questions, as well as discussion of Care Plan and Critical Thinking Care Map questions, appear in Appendix I.

Chapter 15

Sexuality

BRIEF Outline

Sex versus Sexuality
Pediatric and Adolescent Considerations
Maternal and Infant Considerations
Adult Health Considerations
Geriatric Health Considerations

LEARNING Outcomes

After completing this chapter, you will be able to:

1. Define key terms related to sexuality.
2. Describe sexual development and concerns across the life span.
3. Identify factors influencing sexuality throughout the life span.
4. Discuss essential aspects of the sexual response cycle.
5. Describe physiological changes in sexuality in males and females throughout the life span.
6. Identify the forms of male and female sexual dysfunction.
7. List the elements of a focused interview about sexual concerns.
8. Recognize health promotion teaching related to reproductive issues.

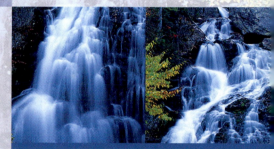

HISTORICAL Perspectives

Masters and Johnson were a pioneering team in the field of human sexuality. William Howell Masters, a gynecologist, was born in Cleveland, Ohio, in 1915. Virginia Eshelman Johnson, a psychologist, was born in Springfield, Montana, in 1925. They began a revolution in social awareness of and public attention given to human sexuality. At the time, public morality severely restricted open discussion of sexuality as a human characteristic. While some of their work generated considerable skepticism or outright criticism, they helped to revamp contemporary thinking about sex, including assisting in moving society toward a more open discussion of sexual practices and experiences.

Sexuality is important to each person's identity throughout the life span. Each person has the capacity to function as a sexual being. Clients' sexuality needs to be considered when they enter the healthcare system. The nurse must understand the normal sexual response and focus on the holistic nature of care to effectively support the sexual health of their clients during the life cycle.

Sex versus Sexuality

Sexuality is influenced by the biologic, psychological, sociologic, cultural, and spiritual aspects of being. The words *sex* and *sexuality* are used interchangeably, and often incorrectly, to define different aspects of sexual being. **Sex** is the term most commonly used to denote biologic male or female status, but it is also used to describe specific sexual behavior, such as sexual intercourse. According to Masters, Johnson, and Kolodny (1995, p. 3), "The word **sexuality** generally has a broader meaning since it refers to all aspects of being

sexual. Sexuality means a dimension of personality instead of referring to a person's capacity for erotic response alone."

Sexuality is subject to lifelong dynamic change. Normal developmental alterations and health status may necessitate adaptations in sexual expressions, but individuals continue to express sexuality in a variety of ways. To recognize if the client is sexually healthy, the nurse must explore the biologic, psychological, and sociocultural dimensions of sexuality.

Pediatric and Adolescent Considerations

From birth, infants are assigned the gender of male or female, and by 3 years of age they begin to develop a gender identity. Preschoolers become increasingly aware of their own and others' body parts. During the school-age years, gender-role behavior is learned. See Table 15-1 ■ for sexual development throughout the life span.

TABLE 15-1

Sexual Development through the Life Span

STAGE	CHARACTERISTICS	NURSING INTERVENTIONS AND TEACHING GUIDELINES
Infancy Birth to 18 months	Given gender assignment of male or female. Differentiates self from others gradually. External genitals are sensitive to touch. Male infants have penile erections; females, vaginal lubrication. Dress and toys are gender oriented.	Self-manipulation of the genitals is normal. Caregivers need to recognize these behaviors as common in children.
Toddler 1–3 years	Continues to develop gender identity. Able to identify own gender.	Body exploration and genital fondling is normal. Use correct names for body parts. Children from single-parent homes should have contact with adults of both sexes.
Preschooler 4–5 years	Becomes increasingly aware of self. Explores own and playmates' body parts. Learns correct names for body parts. Learns to control feelings and behavior. Focuses love on parent of the opposite sex.	Answer questions about "where babies come from" honestly and simply. Parental overreaction to exploration of genitals and masturbation can lead to feelings that sex is "bad."
School Age 6–12 years	Has strong identification with parent of same sex. Tends to have friends of the same sex. Has increasing awareness of self. Continues self-stimulating behavior. Learns the role and concepts of own gender as part of the total self-concept. At about 8 or 9 years becomes concerned about specific sex roles and often approaches parents with explicit concerns about sexuality and reproduction.	Provide parents and children with opportunities to express their concerns and ask questions regarding sex. Answer all questions with factual data and perhaps follow up with appropriate books and other material. Advise parents to discuss basic information about sexual intercourse, menstruation, and reproduction with children at about 10 years of age. If helpful, give children reading material and then discuss it with them.

TABLE 15-1

Sexual Development through the Life Span (*continued*)

STAGE	CHARACTERISTICS	NURSING INTERVENTIONS AND TEACHING GUIDELINES
Adolescence 12–18 or 20 years	Primary and secondary sex characteristics develop. Menarche takes place. Develops relationships with the opposite sex. Masturbation is common. May participate in sexual activity.	Adolescents require information about body changes. Peer groups have great importance at this time and assist in forming sexual roles. Dating helps adolescents prepare for adult roles. Parents influence values and beliefs regarding behavior. Teenagers require information about contraceptive measures and precautions to take with regard to sexually transmitted infections (STIs).
Young Adulthood 20–40 years	Sexual activity is common. Many prefer cohabitation instead of marriage; however, many marry and start families by age 30. Establishes own lifestyle and values. Many couples share financial obligations and household tasks.	Young adults often require information about measures to prevent unwanted pregnancies (i.e., abstinence or contraceptive devices). Require information to prevent STIs. Regular communication is required to understand partner's sexual needs and to work through problems and stresses.
Middle Adulthood 40–65 years	Men and women experience decreased hormone production. Menopause occurs in women, usually anywhere between 40 and 55 years. The climacteric occurs gradually in men. Quality rather than the number of sexual experiences becomes important. Divorce is common. Individuals establish independent moral and ethical standards.	Women and men may need help adjusting to new roles. People may require counseling to help them reevaluate and direct their energies. Encourage couples to look at the positive aspects of this time of life.
Late Adulthood 65 years and older	Interest in sexual activity may continue. Sexual activity becomes less frequent. Women's vaginal secretions diminish, and breasts atrophy. Men produce fewer sperm and need more time to achieve an erection and to ejaculate.	Elderly people can continue sexual activity. Couples may require counseling about adapting their affection and sexual needs to physical limitations.

Parents need to be the primary educators of children at an early age. However, peers, teachers, media, and toys also teach about sexual issues. Parents need to learn how to answer questions and what information to provide for their children, starting in the preschool years. Formal structured comprehensive sex education programs are available through the Sex Information and Education Council of the United States in New York. The programs are for children in kindergarten through grade 12 (Towle, 2008).

Although there is an increasing awareness today of sexuality and sexual functioning, some people still hold firmly to myths and misconceptions about sexuality. Many of these are handed down in families and cultures. Table 15-2 ■ lists some common sexual myths and misconceptions.

PUBERTY

During **puberty** in early adolescence (12 to 13 years), primary and secondary sex characteristics develop, and children need information about body changes. For boys, the testes and scrotum increase in size, the skin over the scrotum becomes darker, pubic hair grows, and axillary sweating begins. Development of the genitals to adult size takes about 5 to 6 years. For girls, the pelvis and hips broaden, the breast tissues develop, pubic hair grows, axillary

TABLE 15-2

Common Sexual Misconceptions

MISCONCEPTION	FACT
Nearly all men over 70 years old are impotent.	Sexual desire and ability decrease very little after middle age.
Masturbation causes mental instability.	Masturbation is not the cause of any mental imbalance or abnormality.
Sexual activity weakens a person.	There is no evidence that sexual activity weakens a person.
Women who have experienced orgasm are more likely to become pregnant.	Conceiving is not related to orgasm.
A large penis provides greater sexual satisfaction to women than a small penis.	Sexual satisfaction results from the entire experience of sex; size of penis is not the determining factor.
Alcohol is a sexual stimulant.	Alcohol is a relaxant and central nervous system depressant. Chronic alcoholism is associated with impotence.
Intercourse during menstruation is dangerous.	There is no physiological basis for abstinence during menses.
The face-to-face coital position is the only moral and proper one.	Various positions offer pleasure and can be acceptable.

sweating begins, vaginal secretions become milky, and menstruation begins.

Girls need to be taught about **menstruation** (monthly uterine bleeding) and related self-care. Teenagers have irregular menstruation initially, which may lead to embarrassment because of stained clothing. They can be taught to watch for signs of approaching menstruation, such as tender breasts, water retention, or the appearance of skin eruptions or pimples. Parents and nurses should advise teenage girls to wash their hands thoroughly before inserting a tampon, to change tampons frequently (at least every 4 hours), to alternate them with sanitary pads, and to use pads at night. These measures help to decrease risk of infection. Thorough cleaning of the genital area and wiping from front to back will also help to prevent *E. coli* infections and odors.

Dysmenorrhea (painful menstruation) is common among adolescent females and causes much short-term absenteeism. Cramping, lower abdominal pain radiating to the back and upper thighs, nausea, vomiting, diarrhea, and headaches result from powerful uterine contractions that cause pain. Ibuprofen (such as Motrin) is often the drug of choice for menstrual cramping.

SEXUAL ABUSE

All children need to be taught information about sexual abuse, including what it is and what to report to a responsible adult. **Sexual abuse** is any involvement of a child in an act designed to provide sexual gratification to

an adult (Clark, 2003). Of the estimated 1 million children abused each year, approximately 11% involve sexual abuse (Clark, 2003). This abuse cannot always be seen (Ball & Bindler, 2005). The child may have feelings of guilt, shame, anger, hostility, and low self-esteem that can lead to a self-destructive life and possibly suicide. Factors that increase the risk of sexual abuse are listed in Box 15-1 ■.

Children who have been victims of sexual abuse may display some or all of these symptoms: pain, itching, bruising, bleeding in the genital area, stains or blood in underwear; withdrawn or aggressive behavior; or unusual sexual behavior. Whenever a child exhibits any of these manifestations, it is important to rule out other causes, such as infection, improper genital hygiene practices, or pinworm infestation. The nurse must identify how she feels regarding this subject to be able to deal with the parents and victims of child abuse. Nursing management

BOX 15-1   **POPULATION FOCUS**

Children at Risk for Sexual Abuse

- Natural father is absent.
- Child is female.
- Mother is employed outside the home.
- Relationship with the parent is poor; conflict exists.
- Parent is substance abuser or socially isolated.

includes further prevention of injury, providing supportive care, reinforcing the importance of follow-up, and reporting suspected abuse.

clinical ALERT

All states have child abuse laws that require professionals, including nurses, to report suspected child abuse (Ball & Bindler, 2005).

Adolescents want to know about sex, but are often uneasy about discussing these concerns with their parents. Nurses, the schools, and the family need to provide accurate information. During the nursing assessment, teenagers should be asked directly what they know about sex, contraception, and reproduction. Sometimes a teenager's information is based on popular myths, not on fact. The nurse should discuss factual information about sex, sexual actions and their consequences, the individual's right to decide how to express oneself sexually, and the responsibilities that go with sexual activity.

Adolescents should be taught about **rape** (intercourse in which one person is an unwilling or unconsenting party). They should also be taught about date rape. **Date rape** occurs when a person manipulates a social interaction in order to have nonconsensual intercourse. Date rape often involves substances such as alcohol or other central nervous system (CNS) depressants, which cause the victim to fall asleep before the rape takes place. It is important to teach that rape is a violent act that should be reported, and that the victim is not to blame for being raped. Date rape drugs also often cause memory loss.

CULTURE AND SEXUALITY

Sexuality is structured and regulated by the individual's culture (see Chapter 2 ⚭). Culture influences the sexual nature of dress, rules about marriage, expectations of role behavior and social responsibilities, and specific sex practices. Societal attitudes vary widely. Attitudes about childhood sexual play, premarital sex, and homosexuality may be restrictive or permissive. Some cultures have specific sex practices. For example, puberty rites of adolescent males in native African and Australian cultures include **circumcision** (removal of the foreskin of the penis). Circumcision is also practiced on many American male infants, especially among Jewish clients as a religious ceremony.

Female circumcision or female genital mutilation (FGM) is still practiced in some parts of Africa today. It involves either excision of the clitoris, the labia minora, and the labia majora, or closure of the vagina (**infibulation**). The reasons for sexual mutilation vary. Infibulation may be done to guar-

antee the bride's virginity. Excision of the clitoris is intended to reduce sexual desire and vulnerability to temptation. In 1980, the World Health Organization and the United Nations Children's Fund unanimously recommended that all forms of female circumcision be abolished. In 1996, the U.S. Congress passed legislation making the practice of FGM on girls under age 18 a federal criminal offense in this country (Brady, 1998).

SEXUALLY TRANSMITTED INFECTION PREVENTION

Both males and females experience increased sexual motivation (*libido*) during puberty and adolescence as a result of hormonal and body changes. Responsible sexual behavior involves the prevention of sexually transmitted infections and the prevention of unwanted pregnancy. **Sexually transmitted infections (STIs)**, also sometimes called sexually transmitted diseases, are diseases transmitted by sexual activity. STIs are the most common bacterial infections among adolescents. They need education about these diseases, preventive measures, and early treatment. Table 15-3 ■ lists the common types and symptoms of STIs for which teenagers should seek medical care. The nurse should also inform the teenager about the various methods of birth control: pills, diaphragms, spermicides, intrauterine devices (IUDs), the rhythm method, and condoms to prevent an unplanned pregnancy. These are discussed later in this chapter.

The prevention of STIs is an essential part of sexual health teaching. Increases in these diseases are due to two factors: changing sexual mores that permit increased sexual activity, and an increase in the number of sexual partners. Because the term *sexually transmitted infection* raises feelings of guilt, shame, and fear, people frequently do not seek medical help as early as they should. In fact, many STIs can be treated quickly and effectively. Others may have serious consequences if they are not treated early. For example, a woman who develops pelvic inflammatory disease may have damage to the reproductive structures and become sterile.

Some infections (*Trichomonas* and *Candida*) can also be acquired nonsexually. *Trichomonas* can survive on bed linen, clothing, and towels, so it can be transmitted without direct sexual contact. *Candida* is a yeast, which usually lives harmlessly in the body, but can multiply to cause an infection. Candida infections often follow antibiotic therapy or steroids, and are often found in diabetics.

Cervical cancer, though not a sexually transmitted infection, is more of a risk for women with multiple sexual partners. Some types of human papillomavirus have an increased risk for cervical cancer, and women need to be reminded of the importance of annual Pap exams.

MediaLink HIV

TABLE 15-3

Types and Manifestations of STIs

DISEASE	MALE	FEMALE
Gonorrhea	Painful urination; urethritis with watery white discharge, which may become purulent.	May be asymptomatic; or vaginal discharge, pain, and urinary frequency may be present.
Syphilis	Chancre, usually on glans penis, which is painless and heals in 4–6 weeks; secondary symptoms—skin eruptions, low-grade fever, inflammation of lymph glands—in 6 weeks to 6 months after chancre heals.	Chancre on cervix or other genital areas, which heals in 4–6 weeks; symptoms same as for male.
Genital warts (condyloma acuminatum)	Single lesions or clusters of lesions growing beneath or on the foreskin, at the external meatus, or on the glans penis. On dry skin areas, lesions are hard and yellow-gray. On moist areas, lesions are pink or red and soft with a cauliflower-like appearance.	Lesions appear at the bottom part of the vaginal opening, on the perineum, the vaginal lips, inner walls of the vagina, and the cervix.
Herpes genitalis (herpes simplex of the genitals)	Primary herpes involves the presence of painful sores or large, discrete vesicles that last for weeks; vesicles rupture. Recurrent herpes is itchy rather than painful; it lasts for a few hours to 10 days.	Same as for males.
Chlamydia urethritis	Urinary frequency; watery, mucoid urethral discharge.	Commonly a carrier; vaginal discharge, dysuria, urinary frequency.
Trichomoniasis	Slight itching; moisture on top of penis; slight, early morning urethral discharge. Many males are asymptomatic.	Itching and redness of vulva and skin inside thighs; copious watery, frothy vaginal discharge.
Candidiasis	Itching, irritation, discharge, plaque of cheesy material under foreskin.	Itching and redness of vulva and skin inside thighs; copious watery, frothy vaginal discharge.
Acquired immune deficiency syndrome (AIDS)	Symptoms can appear anytime from several months to several years after acquiring the virus. The person has reduced immunity to other diseases. Symptoms include any of the following for which there is no other explanation: persistent heavy night sweats; extreme fatigue; severe weight loss; enlarged lymph glands in neck, axillae, or groin; persistent diarrhea; skin rashes; blurred vision or chronic headache; harsh, dry cough; thick gray-white coating on tongue or throat.	

There is still no cure for human immunodeficiency virus (HIV), which leads to AIDS, although, there are many multiple-drug treatment regimens in the United States that delay and prevent a progression to AIDS in many individuals. No cures are claimed, but more effective treatments do exist today, at least in this country, allowing some patients to live normal lives for a very long time. Access to drugs and health care is not as available in many underdeveloped countries as it is in this country. HIV-infected clients in these countries do not have a positive prognosis. Anxiety about AIDS transmission has caused many individuals to alter their sexual behavior. Lubricated condoms made of latex or polyurethane can help reduce the likelihood of STIs, but even these sometimes allow transmission of disease and pregnancy. Up to 6% of condoms break or fall off during intercourse. Although the use of condoms has been described as "safe sex," the only truly safe sex is abstinence. Even sex within a monogamous relationship (only one partner) is problematic when a partner has not been monogamous in the past. This has led to an increase in cases of HIV/AIDS among heterosexual women who thought they were in a monogamous relationship. Methods for preventing the transmission of STIs are described in Box 15-2 ■.

PREVENTION OF UNWANTED PREGNANCIES

Prevention of unwanted pregnancies should be addressed with adolescents and adults. Couples who are planning children, who want to space children, or who want to limit family size may need information about birth control. Nurses need to be familiar with various contraceptive methods and their advantages, disadvantages, contraindications, effective-

BOX 15-2   CLIENT TEACHING

Preventing Transmission of STIs

- Have one sexual partner.
- Use condoms in nonmonogamous and homosexual relationships or other relationships that have the potential for STI transmission.
- Talk openly with sexual partners about how to have "safer sex" and be honest about any history of an STI.
- Abstain from sexual activity with a partner known to have or suspected of having an STI.
- Report to a healthcare facility for examination whenever in doubt about possible exposure or when signs of an STI are evident.
- When an STI is diagnosed, notify all partners and encourage them to seek treatment.
- Avoid unnecessary transfusions of blood or blood products. Use *autologous transfusions* (donation of own blood before surgery) for elective surgery whenever possible.

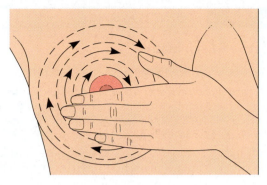

Figure 15-1. ■ Using a circular pattern to palpate the right breast.

ness, safety, and cost. Contraceptive methods are outlined in Box 15-3 ■. It is important to teach that some methods (such as coitus interruptus) are far less effective than others, and that sometimes a combination of methods can be used.

SCREENING FOR CANCER

Monthly breast self-examination (BSE) for females (Figure 15-1 ■) and monthly testicular self-examination (TSE) for males (Figure 15-2 ■) should be started in adolescence. Early detection of cancer results in a greater chance of cure and less complex treatment. Clients need to be assured that most breast lumps discovered are not cancerous. However, it is essential that all lumps or abnormalities be checked by a healthcare provider for accurate diagnosis. All nursing history assessments of clients need to include the client's

understanding and practice of BSE or TSE. Self-examination involves both inspection and palpation procedures and should be conducted once a month.

For BSE, a regular time is best, such as 1 week following menstruation, when breast tenderness and fullness caused by fluid retention have subsided. Women who examine themselves regularly become familiar with the shape and texture of their breasts. Women who no longer have their periods (i.e., after menopause or hysterectomy) should examine their breasts on the same date each month (like on the day they pay their car payment, house payment, water bill, or something else that is associated with a monthly responsibility so they don't forget to do the BSE).

The best time for TSE is after a warm bath or shower when the scrotal sac is relaxed. Men should also be taught to inspect and palpate their breasts, because they have some glandular tissue beneath each nipple, a potential site for malignancy. For specific techniques of self-examination, see Boxes 15-4 ■ and 15-5 ■. Clients should also be informed about the American Cancer Society's (ACS) cancer screening guidelines for asymptomatic people. ACS recommendations include a breast examination by a healthcare provider every 3 years from ages 20 to 39 and yearly thereafter, screening mammogram every year from age 40, annual Pap test

BOX 15-3

Methods of Contraception

- Abstinence
- Coitus interruptus (withdrawal of the penis before ejaculation)
- Fertility awareness (identification of the days of the month when conception could take place and abstaining during that time)
- Mechanical barriers: vaginal diaphragm, cervical cap, condom
- Chemical barriers: insertion of spermicidal foams, creams, jellies, or suppositories into the vagina before intercourse
- IUDs
- Hormonal barriers: oral contraceptives (birth control pills), subdermal implants of synthetic progestin
- Surgical sterilization: tubal ligation and vasectomy

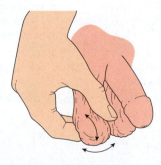

Figure 15-2. ■ Rolling the testicle between the thumb and fingers.

BOX 15-4	CLIENT TEACHING

Breast Self-Examination

Inspection in Front of a Mirror

Look for any change in size or shape; lumps or thickenings; any rashes or other skin irritations; dimpled or puckered skin; any discharge or change in the nipples (e.g., position or asymmetry). Inspect the breasts in all of the following positions:

- Stand and face the mirror with your arm relaxed at your sides or hands resting on the hips; then turn to the right and the left for a side view (look for any flattening in the side view).
- Bend forward from the waist with arms raised over the head.
- Stand straight with the arms raised over the head and move the arms slowly up and down at the sides. (Look for free movement of the breasts over the chest wall.)
- Press your hands firmly together at chin level while the elbows are raised to shoulder level.

Palpation: Lying Position

- Place a pillow under your right shoulder and place the right hand behind your head. This position distributes breast tissue more evenly on the chest.
- Use the finger pads (tips) of the three middle fingers (held together) on your left hand to feel for lumps.

- Press the breast tissue against the chest wall firmly enough to know how your breast feels. A ridge of firm tissue in the lower curve of each breast is normal.
- Use small circular motions all the way around the rim of your breast (see Figure 15-1) starting and ending at the same place (e.g., the 12 o'clock position). Then move your fingers in toward the nipple about 2 cm and feel all the way around again. Repeat this action as many times as necessary until the entire breast is covered.
- Bring your arm down to your side and feel under your armpit, where breast tissue is also located.
- Repeat the exam on your left breast, using the finger pads of your right hand.

Palpation: Standing or Sitting

- Repeat the examination of both breasts while upright with one arm behind your head. This position makes it easier to check the area where a large percentage of breast cancers are found, the upper outer part of the breast and toward the armpit.
- Report any changes to your healthcare provider promptly.
- *Optional:* Do the upright BSE in the shower. Soapy hands glide more easily over wet skin.

---

beginning at age 18 (or when sexually active), yearly rectal exam with blood test for prostate-specific antigen (PSA) for men over age 50, yearly stool exam for colon cancer, and yearly testicular exam beginning at age 15 (Nettina, 2001). (See also Chapter 19. ∞)

BOX 15-5	CLIENT TEACHING

Testicular Self-Examination

- Choose one day of each month (e.g., the first or last day of each month) to examine yourself.
- Examine yourself when you are taking a warm shower or bath.
- Place the index and middle fingers under the testicles and the thumbs on top.
- Roll each testicle between the thumb and fingers of each hand, feeling for lumps, thickening, or a hardening in consistency (see Figure 15-2). The testes should feel smooth.
- Palpate the *epididymis,* a cordlike structure on the top and back of the testicle. The epididymis feels soft and not as smooth as a testicle.
- Locate the spermatic cord, or *vas deferens,* which extends upward from the scrotum toward the base of the penis. It should feel firm and smooth.
- Using a mirror, inspect your testicles for swelling, any enlargement, or lumps in the skin of the testicle. Report any lumps or other changes to your healthcare provider promptly.

Maternal and Infant Considerations

Sexual development of the infant was outlined in Table 15-1. Sexuality begins before birth. Sex determination can be made by the 11th to the 14th week of gestation (Nettina, 2001). When an infant is born, gender is assigned. In rare cases of **hermaphroditism**, the infant has both testicular and ovarian tissue, so it may be difficult to determine gender (Anderson, 2002). This can be very upsetting and may have a profound impact on both parents and child. Chromosomal studies and other diagnostic tests may need to be completed to determine the proper gender (Novak & Broom, 1999).

PREGNANCY AND POSTPARTUM

Pregnancy may enhance sexuality for a woman and her partner, or it may decrease desire, depending on the individual. Body image, a central part of the sense of self, changes constantly during pregnancy and can affect one's sexuality. Pregnancy can affect sexual desire if it is associated with physical discomfort, fear of injury to the fetus, or perceived loss of attractiveness. Monthly BSE should continue throughout pregnancy.

Most women with normal, uncomplicated pregnancies are allowed to have intercourse until her amniotic sac (bag of water) breaks or she goes into labor. Some doctors encourage intercourse to cause labor to start. The prostaglandin in sperm often stimulates labor to begin. Alternate positions for intercourse may need to be used. Intercourse is usually prohibited in high-risk pregnancies. High-risk pregnancies have a history of repeated miscarriages, uterine abnormalities, premature labor, premature rupture of membranes, vaginal bleeding, or abdominal pain (Sherwen, et al., 1999).

Libido (sex drive) is often reduced for about 4 weeks after delivery due to decreased vaginal lubrication, thinner vaginal walls, pain or fear of pain after an episiotomy and stitches, and a slower response to stimulation. Postpartum clients should be cautioned about safe sexual activities. Sexual activity should be avoided until the episiotomy is healed and *lochia* (vaginal discharge after birth) has stopped. This helps prevent infection and trauma (Towle, 2008). Clients should be taught that as long as they are experiencing lochia, nothing should enter the vagina. This means no tampons, douching, or intercourse since traumatized tissue may become infected.

Contraception should also be addressed before the client leaves the hospital. The nurse should reinforce the fact that ovulation and pregnancy can occur before the 6-week checkup, even if the client is breastfeeding. IUDs and diaphragms are not used until the 6-week check-up. Diaphragms will need to be resized after giving birth and after weight gains or losses of over 15 pounds.

Sexuality often becomes secondary to the needs of the family. There is less time and energy for intimacy and privacy after the birth of a new baby. This often creates stress on a couple's relationship.

INFERTILITY

Infertility (inability to conceive a child) is a growing problem in the United States. About 15% of couples are unable to achieve pregnancy (Towle, 2008). Couples sometimes pursue their careers and wait until later in adulthood to have children. These individuals can have psychological reactions to infertility, including guilt, isolation, depression, and stress on the relationship. Much time, patience, and money may be invested in dealing with infertility. Culture and religion affect childbearing values and may determine infertility options. They may determine if adoption and *in vitro* fertilization treatments are an option.

Sterilization resulting from tubal ligation or vasectomy may enhance or interfere with sexual performance and pleasure. Some clients report better sex since they no longer fear an unplanned pregnancy. Other clients may need to mourn the loss of a part of their sexual identity. Each client will interpret the sterilization differently. Tubal ligation and vasectomy should be considered permanent sterilization.

Adult Health Considerations

Sexuality and sexual identity are important to clients. Sexual identity consists of biological sex, gender identity, and sexual orientation. Traditional family and cultural values influence gender identity. Traditional adult male roles included being the breadwinner, heterosexual lover and father, and expressing feelings in a controlled fashion. Women were traditionally expected to express their emotions more freely, to be more gentle and sensitive, and to be more concerned than men with clothing and appearance. Many people now challenge these stereotypes. Men are freer to be sensitive, and women are capably functioning as competitive and assertive executives and world leaders. Gender identity also includes one's comfort with his or her biological sex. Occasionally, a person has the genitalia, secondary sex characteristics, and hormonal influence of one gender, but truly identifies with the opposite gender.

SEXUAL ORIENTATION

Sexual orientation is the preference of a person for one sex or the other. Types of sexual orientation are listed in Box 15-6 ■. The determiners of sexual orientation are unknown. It is believed that homosexual identity often begins in childhood and may have a genetic basis. Estimates of the population with a homosexual orientation vary from 2% or 3% to at least 10%. Accurate figures have not been established since most individuals grow up acutely aware of the discrimination they face in many countries and cultures. See also Chapter 14 ⚭.

It is important for the nurse to understand characteristics of sexual development throughout the life span in order to determine variations. Young adults usually develop a value system and learn to respect the values of others. Cohabitation may be chosen instead of marriage. Sexual activity is common and may include experimentation with various sexual devices and expressions.

BOX 15-6

Types of Sexual Orientation

- *Heterosexual:* A person who is sexually attracted to persons of the opposite gender
- *Bisexual:* A person who is sexually attracted to persons of both sexes
- *Homosexual:* A person who is sexually attracted to persons of the same gender
- *Transsexual:* A person who is of a certain biologic gender but who has feelings of the opposite sex
- *Transvestite:* A person who desires to wear clothes or take on the role of the opposite sex

MediaLink

Gender Identity: Sexual Preference

NORMAL SEXUAL RESPONSE

Young men and women are often concerned about normal sexual response, both for themselves and their partners. Many problems arise in relationships because of basic differences in the male and female sexual response patterns. Couples need to communicate their needs to one another early in their courtship so that a successful intimate relationship can develop and grow. Young adults should also be aware that because sexual needs and responses may change, each partner should listen and respond to the needs of the other.

There are many methods of sexual stimulation. Manual or oral stimulation of the genital area can be used as a prelude to genital **intercourse** (the sexual union of two persons, most commonly by penetration of the penis into the vagina).

The most common form of sexual activity is heterosexual genital intercourse, called **coitus** or *copulation.* A variety of positions are used in sexual intercourse. The choice of intercourse positions and activities depends on physical comfort, beliefs, values, and attitudes about different practices.

During sexual arousal, two primary physiological changes occur: *vasocongestion* (congestion of the blood vessels in the genital area) and *myotonia* (increased muscle tension). One model of physiological response identifies four phases of physiological changes: excitement, plateau, orgasm, and resolution (Masters & Johnson, 1966, p. 4). Table 15-4 ■ summarizes the physiological changes associated with each of the phases of the sexual response cycle in both males and females. It is important for the nurse to understand the normal sexual response, and to remember that many variations in this cycle also are considered normal.

Anal intercourse is a key risk factor in the spread of HIV due to rectal trauma, which gives the virus immediate access to the bloodstream. Although diverse sexual activity is more widely accepted today, it is necessary to note that in many jurisdictions, anal intercourse has been legally defined as sodomy, an offense punishable by law.

Condoms help reduce STIs such as HIV/AIDS and prevent pregnancy when used correctly. Contraception was discussed in the Maternal and Infant Considerations section.

---

clinical ALERT

The use of condoms during anal sex is particularly important. Because anorectal tissue is not self-lubricating, a lubricant must be used on the condom. Also, since normal bacterial flora from the bowel can produce infections in other parts of the body, the used condom should be removed and another applied before inserting the penis into other body orifices.

Some alternative forms of sexual expression for the adult may be illegal or harmful to others. These include *voyeurism* (seeking sexual arousal by observing the body of another); *sadomasochistic bondage* (heterosexual or homosexual activities that involve inflicting pain or experiencing pain during sexual stimulation); and *pedophilia* (sexual acts with children).

Some clients may act out sexually or be sexually aggressive toward other clients or the nurse. Their behaviors may infringe on the rights of others or be harmful to others. Nurses need to respond to this behavior as unacceptable. However, they also need to recognize it as a possible expression of a sexual concern or problem that the client may be experiencing (Box 15-7 ■ on page 280).

Some clients experience **sexual dysfunction** (undesired, altered sexual function). The ability to engage in genital intercourse is very important to most people. Many people experience transient problems with their ability to respond to sexual stimulation or to maintain the response. A smaller percentage of people experience long-standing problems. Many factors may interfere with sexual response including physical dysfunction, stress, illness, overwork, and conflicts with religious beliefs. Sexual dysfunction can be further divided into male and female dysfunction.

Three types of male dysfunction are erectile dysfunction, premature ejaculation, and retarded ejaculation. **Erectile dysfunction**, more commonly referred to as **impotence**, is the inability to achieve or maintain an erection sufficient for sexual satisfaction for oneself or one's partner and can occur at any age. Erectile dysfunction can be caused by physiological or psychological factors. Physiological factors include (1) neurologic disorders created by spinal cord injuries, injury to the genitals or perineal nerves, extensive surgery such as abdominal–perineal bowel resections, radical perineal prostatectomy, diabetes mellitus, multiple sclerosis, and Parkinson's disease; (2) prolonged use of drugs, such as alcohol, sedatives, heroin, antidepressants, antipsychotics (phenothiazines), and antihypertensives; (3) traumatic early sexual experiences such as abuse or rejection; and (4) boredom associated with the specific partner.

Females have four dysfunctions. These are orgasmic dysfunction, vaginismus, dyspareunia, and vulvodynia. **Orgasmic dysfunction** is the inability of a woman to achieve orgasm. Orgasmic dysfunction can be caused by drugs, alcohol, aging, and anatomic abnormalities of the genitals. Most cases have psychological causes, including hostility between partners, fear or guilt about enjoying the sexual act, and concern about performance. Therapy usually involves helping both partners to establish new attitudes about sex. Pelvic muscle exercises (Kegel exercises) can also increase the woman's capacity to achieve orgasm by increasing the strength of the pubococcygeal muscles.

TABLE 15-4			
Physiological Changes in the Sexual Response Cycle			
PHASE OF THE SEXUAL RESPONSE CYCLE	**SIGNS PRESENT IN BOTH SEXES**	**SIGNS PRESENT IN MALES ONLY**	**SIGNS PRESENT IN FEMALES ONLY**
Excitement	Increased muscle tension Moderate increase in heart rate, respirations, and blood pressure Sex flush (less prevalent in men than in women; present in 75% of women) Nipple erection (60% of men and most women)	Penile erection Tensing, thickening, and elevation of the scrotum Partial elevation and increase in size of testicles	Enlargement of the clitoral glans Vaginal lubrication Widening and lengthening of vaginal barrels Separation and flattening of the labia majora Reddening of the labia minora and vaginal wall Breast tumescence (enlargement) and enlarged areolae
Plateau	Increased voluntary and involuntary myotonia Abdominal, intercostal, anal, and facial muscle contraction Accelerated heart rate and respiratory rate, and increased blood pressure Sex flush (appearance in some men late in the phase; spread over the entire body in women)	Increase in penile circumference at the coronal ridge (base of the prepuce), and deepening of color 50% increase in testicular size, and elevation close to the perineum Appearance of a few drops of mucoid secretions from the bulbourethral glands at tip of penis; may contain sperm	Retraction of the clitoris under the hood Appearance of the orgasmic platform (increase in the size of the outer one-third of the vagina and the labia minora) Slight increase in the width and depth of the inner two-thirds of the vagina Further reddening of the labia minora Appearance of a few drops of mucoid secretion from the Bartholin's glands to lubricate inner labia Further increase in breast size and areolar enlargement
Orgasm	Involuntary spasms of muscle groups throughout the body Diminished sensory awareness Involuntary contractions of the anal sphincter Peak heart rate (110–180 bpm), respiratory rate (40/min or greater), and blood pressure (systolic 30–80 mm Hg and diastolic 20–50 mm Hg above normal)	Rhythmic, expulsive contractions of the penis at 0.8-sec intervals Emission of seminal fluid into the prostatic urethra from contraction of the vas deferens and accessory organs (stage 1 of the expulsive process) Closing of the internal bladder sphincter just before ejaculation to prevent retrograde ejaculation into bladder Orgasm may occur without ejaculation Ejaculation of semen through the penile urethra and expulsion from the urethral meatus; the force of ejaculation varies from man to man and at different times but diminishes after the first two to three contractions (stage 2 of the expulsive process)	Approximately 5–12 contractions in the orgasmic platform at 0.8-sec intervals Contraction of the muscles of the pelvic floor and the uterine muscles Varied pattern of orgasms, including minor surges and contractions, multiple orgasms, or a single intense orgasm similar to that of the male

(*continued*)

TABLE 15-4

Physiological Changes in the Sexual Response Cycle (*continued*)

PHASE OF THE SEXUAL RESPONSE CYCLE	SIGNS PRESENT IN BOTH SEXES	SIGNS PRESENT IN MALES ONLY	SIGNS PRESENT IN FEMALES ONLY
Resolution	Reversal of vasocongestion in 10–30 min; disappearance of all signs of myotonia within 5 min Genitals and breasts return to their preexcitement states Sex flush disappears in reverse order of appearance Heart rate, respiratory rate, and blood pressure return to normal Other reactions include sleepiness, relaxation, and emotional outbursts such as crying or laughing	A refractory period during which the body will not respond to sexual stimulation; varies, depending on age and other factors, from a few moments to hours or days	

BOX 15-7

Nursing Strategies for Dealing with Inappropriate Sexual Behavior

- Identify the behavior you expect: "Please call me by my name, not 'honey'" or "I expect you to keep yourself covered when I am in the room. If you are feeling hot or something is uncomfortable, let me know, and I will try to make you more comfortable."
- Set firm limits: Take the client's hand and move it away, use direct eye contact, and say, "Don't do that!"
- Communicate that the behavior is not acceptable by saying, for example, "I really do not like the things you are saying" or "I see you are not dressed. I will be back in 10 minutes and will help you with breakfast when you have your clothes on."
- Tell the client how the behavior makes you feel: "When you act like that toward me, I don't want to come into your room. It embarrasses me and makes it hard for me to give you the kind of nursing care you need."
- Try to refocus clients from the inappropriate behavior to their real concerns and fears. Sometimes people talk inappropriately when they are concerned about the sexual part of their life and how their illness will affect them. Offer to discuss sexuality concerns: "All morning you have been making very personal sexual comments about yourself. Are there things that you have questions about or would like to talk about?"
- Clarify the consequences of continued inappropriate behavior (avoidance, withdrawal of services, no chance to help resolve underlying concerns of client).
- Report the incident to your nursing instructor, charge nurse, or clinical nurse specialist. Discuss the incident, your feelings, and possible interventions.
- If you feel you are not being successful in getting the client to change behavior, ask your supervisor to assign another nurse to the client.

Many medications have effects on sexuality. These include prescription medications and social drugs that can affect sexual desire and response. Table 15-5 ■ lists various medications that affect sexual function (Clayton & Stock, 2001). Early traumatic sexual experiences or

TABLE 15-5

Drugs Affecting Sexual Function

Antihypertensive
Thiazide diuretics
Beta blockers
Alpha-adrenergic blockers
Sympatholytics
Spironolactone

Central Nervous System Depressants
Phenothiazines
Monoamine oxidase inhibitors
Serotonin reuptake inhibitors

Cardiovascular
Digoxin
Clofibrate
Gemfibrozil

Miscellaneous Agents
Substances of abuse (alcohol, cocaine, marijuana, nicotine)
Alkylating agents
Anabolic steroids
Estrogens
Corticosteroids
Cimetidine
5-alpha-reductase inhibitors

boredom with a sexual partner can also depress sexual responsiveness.

The nurse can assist the client in identifying any sexual dysfunction by performing a thorough assessment. Assessment guidelines for sexual dysfunction are discussed in the Nursing Care section.

Geriatric Health Considerations

The reproductive system slows down with aging. The climacteric (change of life) in the male is not as dramatic as in the female since changes are more gradual. Most experts say there is no true climacteric in the male. They believe the decline in male sexual desire is related to less physical strength and aging of all the body tissues (Porth, 2002). Although testosterone levels decline with age, the ability to remain fertile may extend into old age.

FACTORS AFFECTING SEXUAL RESPONSE

Sexuality may be far more broadly defined by older adults. Their definition may include touching, hugging, romantic gestures (e.g., giving or receiving roses), comfort, warmth, dressing up, joy, spirituality, and beauty. Interest in sexual activity is not lost as men age. However, more time is needed to achieve an erection and to ejaculate. The volume of ejaculated fluid decreases. The intensity of contractions with orgasm may decrease, and the refractory period after orgasm is longer.

Older women remain capable of multiple orgasms and may experience an increase in sexual desire after menopause. Vaginal lubrication and elasticity decrease with menopause due to decreased estrogen levels. Use of water-soluble lubri-

cants will help make intercourse more comfortable (and water-soluble lubricants will not cause condoms to break like petroleum-based lubricants). The phases of the sexual response cycle may take longer to occur. There is a possibility of pain during sexual activity and intercourse (**dyspareunia**) related to vaginal dryness or chronic health conditions such as diabetes or arthritis. Lack of privacy may be a concern for older adults who live with family or in a rehabilitation or nursing home facility.

Personal values can influence sexuality in the older adult. Cultural and religious guidelines define acceptable behavior, forbidden behavior, and the consequences of breaking sexual rules (Box 15-8 ■). For example, many groups hold virginity before marriage to be important. Some cultures view forms of sexual expression other than male with female intercourse as wrong and unnatural. Cultural and religious values determine taboos. Many societies believe that sexual preferences are a personal and private matter as long as both adults are comfortable and freely consent to the type of sex practiced.

Health issues often interfere with sex and sexuality. Heart disease, diabetes, degenerative joint disease, STIs, cerebrovascular accidents, and disorders that cause mental deterioration may interfere with sexuality. Heart disease frequently influences sexual expression. Older adults are at risk for myocardial infarction and are often anxious about their sexuality and sexual activity. Concerns about the effect of sexual activity on the heart may cause people to restrict or avoid intercourse. Education by health professionals can alleviate client fears following heart surgery or hospitalization for alterations in heart function. Clients can be taught

---

BOX 15-8	CULTURAL PULSE POINTS

Factors That Increase Risk of HIV

Puerto Rico has the highest HIV infection of any U.S. state or territory. In the United States, Puerto Ricans have the highest incidence of HIV when compared to other ethnic groups. In some states, AIDS is the leading cause of death for Puerto Rican women ages 25 to 44 (Centers for Disease Control and Prevention CDC MMWR Weekly. February 28, 2003). These women become HIV positive mostly through heterosexual contact and/or intravenous drug use (National Center for Health Statistics, 2002).

Puerto Ricans abide by many socioeconomic and culturally supported gender roles, such as *machismo* and submissive women's roles. These roles foster high-risk behaviors that impede the prevention and increase the transmission of HIV. In traditional Puerto Rican culture, most men are given free will over sexual practices, including the approval and initiation of sex before marriage and extramarital affairs with other women. Some men may perceive that sexual intercourse with males is a sign of virility and sexual power rather than a homosexual behavior. This practice is not viewed positively by Puerto Rican women.

Knowledge about HIV, beliefs about health and illness, and beliefs and practices related to condom use are common difficulties encountered by healthcare providers in the prevention and transmission of HIV.

Lack of condom use is perhaps one of the most significant risk behaviors that needs immediate attention and intervention from healthcare providers. Issues such as embarrassment, cost, gender/power struggles, and abuse are among some of the barriers encountered by Puerto Rican women. Some men fear that if they use condoms they portray a less *macho* image, have decreased sexual satisfaction, or convey that they have an STI or HIV. Additionally, Catholicism, lower educational levels, lower socioeconomic status, and acculturation are significant variables related to the high rates of AIDS and HIV among Puerto Ricans and other Hispanics. Healthcare providers must be aware of these barriers, assess individual perceptions of high-risk behaviors, and intervene with programs designed to meet the particular needs of clients who are at high risk for HIV infection or other STIs.

to resume sexual activity based on reactions to exercise. They can be told to avoid sexual intercourse after large meals or consumption of alcoholic beverages. They can be taught safe positions to assume (client on bottom since it requires less cardiac work). Partners need to be aware of signs of distress and how to deal with these symptoms.

Men with long-term diabetes mellitus may develop erectile dysfunction. Women who have diabetes may experience orgasmic dysfunction, difficulty experiencing arousal, or loss of vaginal lubrication. Frequent vaginal yeast infections cause itching and irritation, which affect sexuality. Clients on long-term antibiotics or steroids are also likely to develop yeast infections.

Surgical procedures have the potential to alter a person's body image, especially when the surgery involves mutilating, removing, or altering parts of the body. Examples include amputations, radical neck surgery, excision of large portions of the lower jaw, and ostomies. The impact is even greater when the surgery alters or removes body parts linked directly with sexual functioning. Such surgeries include mastectomy and hysterectomy in women and **orchiectomy** (removal of the testicles due to cancer) and penectomy in men. Feelings of ugliness and loss of masculinity or femininity are common after these surgeries. These surgeries are more common among older adults and directly affect their sexuality. Allow clients to talk about their feelings regarding these procedures. Talking is part of the grieving and healing process. There are many support groups such as the American Cancer Society's Reach for Recovery program for women who experience breast cancer surgery. Additional support groups can be found locally in the telephone book or on the Internet. Both partners should be involved in this grief and healing process. Joint disease may indirectly affect sexual function because of pain, stiffness, loss of joint motion, and fatigue. Chronic pain often decreases sexual motivation. Altered positions for coitus may be necessary, and alternative ways to express sexual stimulation may need to be explored.

STIs affect all age groups. These include gonorrhea, chlamydia, syphilis, genital herpes, trichomoniasis, HIV/AIDS, and genital warts. Many older adults lack knowledge in this area, thinking they are exempt from STIs. Anyone, regardless of age, who practices unprotected sex is at risk for an STI. A new partner may have had multiple partners and acquired an STI. The STI chlamydia often has no symptoms and is easy to transfer to another person. Multiple partners create multiple risks for STIs regardless of age.

Another problem that can occur with the older adult population is altered mental status. Because mind and thought are both involved in sexual functioning, any impairment of the mind may affect sexual expression. For example, depression lowers libido and can affect both the depressed client and the partner. Some clients with mental disorders or brain injury may behave in an inappropriate sexual manner, such as touching their genitals, removing their clothing, or seeking frequent sexual activity. Clients with Alzheimer's disease may not remember any previous sexual contact with their partners.

Many geriatric clients take prescription medications that have side effects that affect sexual functioning. Older adults may need medications to enhance sexual motivation. With the introduction of drugs such as Viagra, there is increasing awareness of alternatives for men with these problems. There is also increased risk for injury if drugs such as Viagra are taken by clients who take nitroglycerin for poor heart circulation. Viagra taken with nitroglycerin can cause heart attacks and death. Drug interactions can be dangerous, so client teaching is very important. Drug labels must be read and client teaching included in their plan of care.

NURSING CARE

ASSESSING

When assessing a client for sexual concerns, the nurse should be aware of the person's developmental level. It is important to speak in clear, understandable terms to clients of any age, and to use the proper names for body parts and sexual activities. The nurse may need to ask specifically about any concerns or problems related to sexuality.

The nurse can assist the client in identifying any sexual dysfunction by performing a thorough assessment. An example of assessment guidelines is provided in Box 15-9 ■.

DIAGNOSING, PLANNING, AND IMPLEMENTING

Nursing diagnoses that might be seen in clients with sexual health issues are *Sexual Dysfunction, Ineffective Sexuality Patterns, Deficient Knowledge* (contraceptive methods), *Rape-Trauma Syndrome,* or *Interrupted Family Processes.*

Outcomes for clients with concerns about sexuality might include:

- Client seeks consultation with urologist about enlarged prostate.
- Client verbalizes the need to discuss dyspareunia with spouse and to use lubricants during intercourse.
- Client plans visit to gynecologist to obtain Pap smear and to learn about possible insertion of IUD.
- Client states that rape was not her fault.
- Mother states that she will nap when the baby naps for the next 4 weeks.

BOX 15-9 | **ASSESSING**

Sexual Health History

Women

- When did your menstrual periods first begin, and when did you have your last menstrual period?
- What is the usual length of your period in days and usual amount of bleeding?
- Do you have any concerns about the amount or regularity of your menstrual flow?
- If periods are irregular, problematic, or have stopped: Have you been evaluated for this change or done anything yourself to deal with it?
- Are you having any burning with urination, any vaginal itching or discharge, midcycle spotting, pain with intercourse, or any other problems?
- Have you ever been pregnant? (Explore number and outcome of pregnancies, including miscarriages and induced abortions.)
- How often do you do breast self-examination?
- Is there a history of breast or ovarian cancer in your family?
- When did you have your last Pap test and mammogram?

Men

- Are you having any difficulty with initiating urination, urinary frequency, or frequent urination at night?
- Are you having any itching or discharge from your penis?
- How often do you do testicular self-examination?
- Is there a history of testicular cancer in your family?

Men and Women

- Are you currently sexually active?
- What do you do to protect yourself from infection when you are sexually active?
- Have you ever had a sexually transmitted infection?
- Has any disease, injury, surgery, medication, or other situation affected your sexual health and happiness or your feelings about yourself as a woman or man?
- Do you have any questions about your sexual health or functioning, or is there anything else we have discussed that you would like clarified or explained?

Nurses can assist clients to deal with problems related to sexuality if they first resolve some of their own feelings about the issue. Nurses should take time to clarify their own views on sexuality, sex, and sexual relationships. Many ethical issues are related to sexuality, including:

- Contraception
- Abortion
- Sexual preference
- Types of sexual activity.

Education and emotional support are two important aspects of nursing care related to sexuality and reproductive concerns. The nurse can teach the importance of communicating with a spouse or sexual partner, and adapting to physical changes as part of life. The nurse should provide guidelines for safer sex for clients with high-risk behavior and multiple sexual partners (see Box 15-2). State facts clearly and simply using correct anatomic terms.

clinical ALERT

No matter what the nurse's upbringing and value system, it is important to approach the client with the client's needs in mind.

EVALUATING

The nurse reviews client outcomes related to specific sexual concerns. Physical and emotional aspects of the client's concerns are reassessed. The nurse may request referrals for specialized care.

NURSING PROCESS CARE PLAN
Client with Ineffective Sexuality Patterns

Jeffery Stevens is a 55-year-old carpet installer who is hospitalized with a myocardial infarction. He has been moved from the cardiac care unit (CCU) to the medical floor. He has had several episodes of chest pain relieved by medication. He has repeatedly made inappropriate sexual comments and gestures to the nursing staff.

Assessment. Mary Jennings, Mr. Stevens' night shift nurse, reported to the night charge nurse that Mr. Stevens stated, "Why don't you crawl up in here with me to keep me warm?" She states Mr. Stevens also stated, "A little heart attack can't keep me down." He stated, "My wife will be too afraid after what happened the other night when I came into the hospital to ever have sex again."

Ms. Jennings notes on the nurse's notes that Mr. Stevens had chest pain at 2200 relieved by Nitroglycerin gr 1/150 × 1 sublingual and that shortness of breath was also noted at this time. He has had no arrhythmias on the telemetry since moving to the floor. His BP was 134/82, P 64, R 22.

Nursing Diagnosis. The following important nursing diagnoses (among others) are established for this client:

- *Ineffective Sexuality Patterns* related to altered self-concept
- *Deficient Knowledge* related to absence of sexual teaching
- *Ineffective Sexuality Patterns* related to fear of chest pain

Expected Outcomes. The expected outcomes specify that Mr. Stevens will:

- Identify factors contributing to altered self-concept.
- Gain knowledge about sexual activity following a myocardial infarction.
- Experience decreased pain with sexual activity.

Planning and Implementation. The following nursing interventions are planned and implemented:

- Question to identify or clarify reasons for sexual comments and actions.
- Consistently refocus inappropriate sexual comments and actions to client's underlying fears and concerns.
- Allow expression of concern about sexual functioning or identity.
- Acquire information on usual sexual pattern and expectations.
- Identify limitations on sexual activity caused by myocardial infarction with cardiac rehabilitation team.
- Explain appropriate modifications in sexual practices in response to these limitations, including engaging in sexual activity after rest after a period of 4 to 8 weeks (when physician advises).
- Instruct client to terminate sexual activity if chest pain or dyspnea occurs.
- Teach client to take nitroglycerin as prescribed by the physician before sexual activity if angina occurs during sexual activity (and that Viagra-type medications could be very dangerous).
- Advise client to avoid intercourse 1 to 2 hours after a heavy meal or after alcohol consumption.
- Instruct client to avoid sexual activity when stressed.
- Advise client to position himself on the bottom during sexual activity to reduce cardiac workload.

Evaluation. By the end of the shift, Ms. Jennings was able to determine that Mr. Stevens normally had sexual activity two to three times a week with his wife and that they were engaging in sexual activity when he experienced his myocardial infarction. Mr. Stevens had stated he and his wife had been married for 27 years and he was afraid he would not be able to maintain the previous sexual relationship they had experienced. He also stated the chest pain he was continuing to have made him worry he would never be able to have sexual activity again without pain. Ms. Jennings was able to give Mr. Stevens information on sexual activity following a myocardial infarction; it was included in his cardiac rehabilitation notebook provided to him on discharge.

Critical Thinking in the Nursing Process

1. Why was Mr. Stevens making inappropriate sexual comments and gestures?
2. What other information would have been helpful in this situation?
3. Who else should be included in teaching Mr. Stevens about sexual activity during the cardiac rehabilitation process?

Note: Discussion of Critical Thinking questions appears in Appendix I.

Note: The references and resources for this and all chapters have been compiled at the back of the book.

Chapter Review

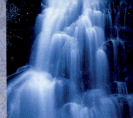

 KEY TERMS by Topic

Use the audio glossary feature of either the CD-ROM or the Companion Website to hear the correct pronunciation of the following key terms.

Sex versus Sexuality
sex, sexuality

Pediatric and Adolescent Considerations
puberty, menstruation, dysmenorrhea, sexual abuse, rape, date rape, circumcision, infibulation, sexually transmitted infections (STIs)

Maternal and Infant Considerations
hermaphroditism, infertility

Adult Health Considerations
sexual orientation, intercourse, coitus, sexual dysfunction, erectile dysfunction, impotence, orgasmic dysfunction

Geriatric Health Considerations
dyspareunia, orchiectomy

KEY Points

- Sexuality is important to all ages throughout the life span. It is not just gender or the sex act, but a whole dimension of personality.

- Puberty is a key time in the development of sexuality. Children need to be educated about the changes in their bodies and about the reproductive process. Parents should be the primary educators in this area, but many times children learn about sexual matters from their peers.

- Different cultures view sexuality and sexual activities differently. It is important to recognize one's own values about sexuality and to respect the client's values when giving client care. The focus should always be on client needs.

- Suspected sexual abuse must always be reported. Victims of abuse should be reminded that they are not to blame for being abused.

- The adult's sexuality evolves through sexual experiences. A person's sexual identity consists of biologic sex, gender identity, and sexual orientation.

- Inappropriate comments or actions by a client may signal a concern the client wishes to discuss. However, it is important to address the inappropriate actions immediately and state appropriate expectations clearly.

- Older adults continue to function sexually despite physical changes. They learn to adapt sexual activity to physical limitations.

 EXPLORE MediaLink

Additional interactive resources for this chapter can be found on the Companion Website at www.prenhall.com/ramont. Click on Chapter 15 and "Begin" to select the activities for this chapter.

For chapter-related NCLEX®-style questions and an audio glossary, access the accompanying CD-ROM in this book.

Animations/Videos
- Gender Identity: Sexual Preference
- HIV
- Sexual and Physical Abuse

⌒ **FOR FURTHER** Study

For additional information about cultural values, see Chapter 2.

For further study about client self-concept, see Chapter 14.

For more information about physical assessment, see Chapter 19.

Critical Thinking Care Map

Caring for a Client with Altered Sexuality
NCLEX-PN® Focus Area: Psychosocial Integrity

Case Study: Nancy Johnson is a 43-year-old who had a mastectomy 4 days ago for cancer of the breast. She states "I'll never be the same" as the LVN makes her morning rounds. She also states her husband has been very attentive assisting her but that he deserves more.

Nursing Diagnosis: Ineffective Sexuality Patterns

COLLECT DATA

Subjective	Objective
_____	_____
_____	_____
_____	_____
_____	_____
_____	_____
_____	_____
_____	_____

Would you report this data? Yes/No

If yes, to: _____

What would you report? _____

Nursing Care

_____
_____
_____
_____
_____
_____
_____
_____
_____
_____
_____

How would you document this? _____
_____
_____
_____

Compare your documentation to the sample provided in Appendix I.

Data Collected
(use those that apply)

- Client works as an administrative assistant in a large law firm
- States she will never be the same
- Medicated with Vicodin 2 tablets at 0800 and 1200
- States husband deserves more
- Reach for Recovery visited on the first and second postop days
- Looks down when speaking
- Holds robe tightly around chest
- Dressing on left breast clean/dry/intact
- Husband noted to be at bedside since returned from surgery and has not left the hospital
- Stayed in bed with face covered all morning
- Jackson–Pratt drain in place ×2
- Refused to ambulate in the hall
- Looked through mail brought to room by volunteer
- Ate 10% of breakfast and lunch

Nursing Interventions
(use those that apply; list in priority order)

- Instruct in the importance of communication with husband to work through feelings toward acceptance.
- Discuss with client importance of Reach for Recovery follow-up.
- Encourage client to express feelings about the way she feels about sexuality related to loss of the breast.
- Discuss the usual feelings of clients who are postoperative mastectomy and ways to cope.
- Encourage client to discuss sexuality issues with the primary healthcare provider.
- Discuss available support groups in the community and obtain necessary contacts for follow-up (American Cancer Society).

NCLEX-PN® Exam Preparation

1 The school nurse has been working with a group of adolescents helping them to identify myths and common misconceptions about sexuality. If the school nurse's teaching has been effective, which of the following statements will the students identify as a myth or common misconception about sexuality?

1. Masturbation is harmless.
2. Conceiving is unrelated to orgasm.
3. Sexual desire decreases little after middle age.
4. Alcohol is a sexual stimulant.

2 During a bath procedure, a client asks the nurse which sexual position is the correct position during sexual intercourse. The best answer by the nurse would be which of the following answers?

1. "The position that offers the most pleasure and is acceptable to both partners."
2. "A position in which both partners are able to see the face of the other partner."
3. "It is improper for you to ask this question and we need to focus on your bath."
4. "A variety of positions with frequent change of position is accepted as correct."

3 A parent informs the nurse that his son, who is in early adolescence, has had an increase in the size of the testes and scrotum, with the skin over the scrotum becoming darker. The nurse recognizes these signs as most likely being related to which of the following causes?

1. testicular cancer
2. normal growth and development
3. excessive masturbation
4. late phase of testicular herniation

4 While working with a child, the nurse finds the child has symptoms associated with sexual abuse of a child. The nurse most needs to do which of the following things?

1. Ask the child if she has been sexually abused.
2. Confront the parent(s) or caregivers about having sexually abused the child.
3. Report suspected child sexual abuse to the state agency dealing with child abuse.
4. Discuss the findings with other healthcare professionals.

5 Anyone in the United States who does an infibulation on a child under age 18 is considered by the courts to be doing which of the following things?

1. practicing procedures acceptable in some cultures
2. practicing medicine without a license to do so
3. committing a federal criminal offense
4. committing a misdemeanor

6 In educating teenagers about sexually transmitted infections, the nurse will explain that a person is more at risk of cervical cancer if she has which of the following problems or diagnoses?

1. human papillomavirus
2. trichomoniasis
3. herpes-zoster virus
4. candidiasis

7 When teaching clients about prevention of unwanted pregnancies, the nurse will point to which of the following methods of contraception as most ineffective?

1. diaphragm
2. coitus interruptus
3. birth control pills
4. intrauterine devices

8 A parent asks the nurse when gender determination can be made in the developing fetus. The nurse will explain that gender determination can be made by which of the following weeks of gestation?

1. 3 to 6 weeks
2. around 7 weeks
3. around 9 weeks
4. 11 to 14 weeks

9 When working with a female client who has orgasmic dysfunction, the nurse will explore a number of possible causes with the client, but will keep in mind that the majority of cases of orgasmic dysfunction have which of the following underlying causes?

1. alcohol or other drugs
2. aging
3. psychological causes
4. anatomic abnormalities

10 The nurse working with an older client who has had heart surgery or who has been hospitalized for alterations in heart function will most likely need to teach the client to avoid which of the following things?

1. having orgasm with sexual intercourse
2. sexual intercourse after large meals or drinking alcohol
3. having sexual intercourse more than once a month
4. sexual intercourse just before going to sleep

Answers and Rationales for Review Questions, as well as discussion of Care Plan and Critical Thinking Care Map questions, appear in Appendix I.

Chapter 16

Stress and Coping

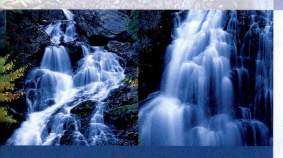

BRIEF Outline

Concept of Stress
Sources of Stress
Models of Stress
Indicators of Stress
Coping
Stress Management for Nurses

LEARNING Outcomes

After completing this chapter, you will be able to:

1. Discuss the three main models of stress.
2. Describe the three stages of Selye's general adaptation syndrome.
3. Identify physiological and psychological indicators of stress.
4. Differentiate four levels of anxiety.
5. Identify behaviors related to specific defense mechanisms.
6. Discuss types of coping and coping strategies.
7. Describe interventions to help clients minimize and manage stress.
8. Describe warning signs of job-related stress or burnout for the nurse.

HISTORICAL Perspectives

The term stress, *can be found as early as the 14th century. It first achieved technical importance in the 17th century in the work of physicist-biologist Robert Hooke. Hooke was concerned with how man-made structures must be designed to carry heavy loads and resist buffeting by natural forces that could destroy them. Hooke's analysis influenced early 20th century models of stress in physiology, psychology, and sociology. The theme that survives is the idea of stress as an external load or demand on a biological, social, or psychological system. During World War II there was interest in emotional breakdown in response to the "stresses" of combat. After World War II, it became evident that many conditions of ordinary life could produce effects comparable to those of combat. This led to a growing interest in stress as a cause of human distress and dysfunction.*

Stress is a universal phenomenon. All people experience it. It can be described as tension between two opposing forces. Not all stress is harmful. Limited stress can raise energy levels, which may be an asset when faced with certain tasks, such as a test. Excessive stress may cause physical illness and/or psychological distress.

Concept of Stress

Stress is a condition that requires a response. Stress has numerous consequences (Figure 16-1 ■):

- *Physiological*—Can threaten a person's physiological homeostasis.
- *Emotional*—Can produce negative or unconstructive feelings about the self.
- *Intellectual*—Can influence a person's perceptual and problem-solving abilities.
- *Social*—Can alter a person's relationships with others.
- *Spiritual*—Can challenge one's beliefs and values.

An individual is considered to be mentally healthy if he or she is able to love (form relationships), work, and cope

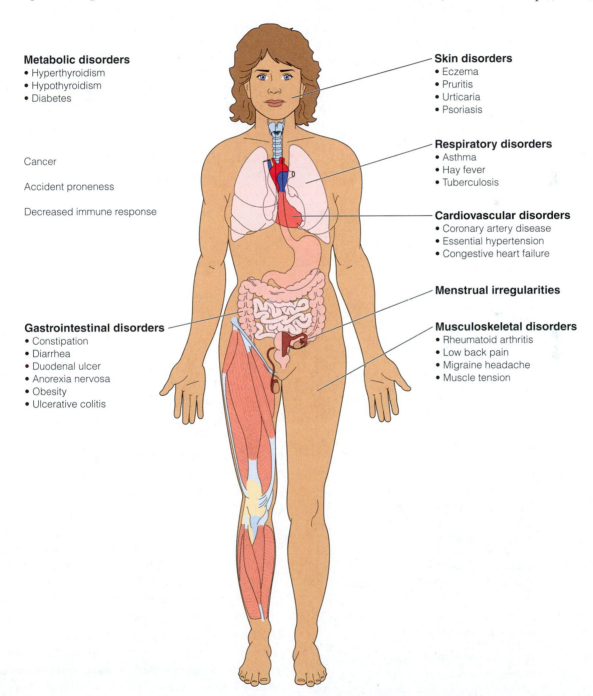

Metabolic disorders
- Hyperthyroidism
- Hypothyroidism
- Diabetes

Cancer

Accident proneness

Decreased immune response

Gastrointestinal disorders
- Constipation
- Diarrhea
- Duodenal ulcer
- Anorexia nervosa
- Obesity
- Ulcerative colitis

Skin disorders
- Eczema
- Pruritis
- Urticaria
- Psoriasis

Respiratory disorders
- Asthma
- Hay fever
- Tuberculosis

Cardiovascular disorders
- Coronary artery disease
- Essential hypertension
- Congestive heart failure

Menstrual irregularities

Musculoskeletal disorders
- Rheumatoid arthritis
- Low back pain
- Migraine headache
- Muscle tension

Figure 16-1. ■ Some disorders that can be caused or aggravated by stress. (*Source:* Adapted from G. Edlin and E. Golanty, *Health and Wellness: A Holistic Approach*, 4th ed., Boston: Jones and Bartlett, 1992, p. 210.)

simultaneously. Coping with stress then becomes an important factor in maintaining mental homeostasis or emotional balance.

Sources of Stress

Sources of stress can be broadly classified as either internal or external **stressors**. They may also be developmental or situational stressors, or both. Internal stressors originate within a person. Examples are receiving a diagnosis of cancer or experiencing feelings of depression. External stressors originate outside the individual. Examples are moving to another city, experiencing a death in the family, or feeling pressure from peers. Developmental stressors occur at predictable times throughout an individual's life. Examples of these are shown in Table 16-1 ■. Within each developmen-

TABLE 16-1

Selected Stressors Associated with Developmental Stages

DEVELOPMENTAL STAGE	STRESSORS
Child	Conflict between independence and dependence
	Beginning school
	Establishing peer relationships and adjustments
	Peer competition
Adolescent	Changing physique
	Developing relationships involving sexual attraction
	Achieving independence
	Choosing a career
Young adult	Getting married
	Leaving home
	Managing a home
	Getting started in an occupation
	Continuing one's education
	Rearing children
Middle adult	Physical changes of aging
	Maintaining social status and standard of living
	Teenage children becoming independent
	Adjusting to aging parents
Older adult	Decreasing physical abilities and health
	Changes in residence
	Retirement and reduced income
	Death of spouse and friends

tal stage, certain tasks must be achieved to prevent or reduce stress. Situational stressors are unpredictable and may occur at any time during life. Situational stress may be positive or negative. Examples of this type of stress include:

- Death of a family member
- Marriage or divorce
- Birth of a child
- New job
- Illness.

Models of Stress

The three main models used to explain the effects of stress are the stimulus-based, response-based, and transaction-based models. Nurses use knowledge of these models to help clients use healthy coping responses and change unhealthy, unproductive responses.

STIMULUS-BASED MODELS

In the **stimulus**-based model, stress is defined as a life event, or a set of circumstances that arouses physiological and/or psychological reactions that may increase the individual's vulnerability to illness. Holmes and Rahe (1967) created a scale that assigned a numerical value to 43 life changes or events. Similar scales have since been developed, but all such scales require caution because the degree of stress an event presents can be highly individual.

The scale of stressful life events is used to document a person's relatively recent experiences, such as divorce, pregnancy, and retirement. In this view, both positive and negative events are considered stressful. Research has shown that people who have a high level of stress are often more prone to illness. They also have a lowered ability to cope with an illness and subsequent stress.

RESPONSE-BASED MODELS

Stress may also be considered as a **response** to illness. Hans Selye, a recognized authority in the field of stress, observed:

> Whether a man suffers from severe blood loss, an infection or advanced cancer; he loses his appetite, strength, and ambition; usually he also loses weight and even his facial expression betrays his illness. I felt that the syndrome of "Just being sick," which is essentially the same no matter what disease we have, could be analyzed and expressed scientifically. (Selye, 1976, p. 12)

Selye realized that changes in the body occurred in the presence of stress, and this became the basis of his identification of the **general adaptation syndrome (GAS)**. He proposed three stages in this syndrome (1976, p. 38): alarm reaction, resistance, and exhaustion. Refer to Figures 16-1 and 16-2 ■. See Box 16-1 ■ for a description

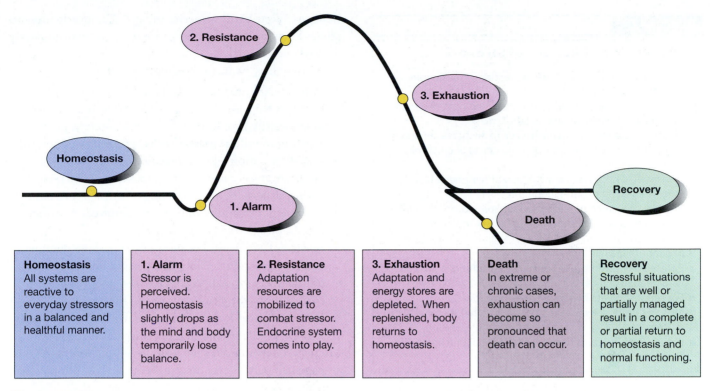

Homeostasis	1. Alarm	2. Resistance	3. Exhaustion	Death	Recovery
All systems are reactive to everyday stressors in a balanced and healthful manner.	Stressor is perceived. Homeostasis slightly drops as the mind and body temporarily lose balance.	Adaptation resources are mobilized to combat stressor. Endocrine system comes into play.	Adaptation and energy stores are depleted. When replenished, body returns to homeostasis.	In extreme or chronic cases, exhaustion can become so pronounced that death can occur.	Stressful situations that are well or partially managed result in a complete or partial return to homeostasis and normal functioning.

Figure 16-2. ■ The three stages of adaptation to stress: the alarm reaction, the stage of resistance, and the stage of exhaustion. (*Note:* From Wellness: Concepts and Application, 6th ed. (p. 298) by D. J. Anspaugh, M. Hamrick, and F. D. Rosato, 2005, New York: McGraw-Hill. Reprinted with permission.)

of these stages. Selye's general adaptation syndrome encompasses a range of physiological responses to stressors in the body as a whole.

TRANSACTION-BASED MODELS

The **transactional** view was developed by Richard Lazarus (1965). It focuses on individual differences in response to stress, rather than to events or reactions. The transactional view attempts to answer the following: Which factors lead some persons and not others to respond effectively to stress-ful events? Why are some persons more sensitive and vulnerable to stressful events? And why are some persons able to adapt better than others over longer periods to stressful events?

The Lazarus transactional stress theory includes cognitive, affective, and adaptive (coping) responses. This theory states that the person and the environment are inseparable; each affects and is affected by the other. Stress "refers to any event in which environmental demands, internal demands, or both tax or exceed the adaptive resources of an individual, social system, or tissue system" (Monat & Lazarus, 1991, p. 3). The individual responds to perceived environmental changes by adaptive (coping) responses. See the Coping section later in this chapter.

Indicators of Stress

Indicators of an individual's stress may be physiological or psychological.

PHYSIOLOGICAL INDICATORS

Responses to stress vary depending on the individual's perception of events. The physiological signs and symptoms of stress result from the activation of the sympathetic and neuroendocrine systems of the body. The autonomic nervous system reacts to a perceived threat by releasing large amounts of epinephrine (adrenaline) and cortisone into the

---

BOX 16-1

General Adaptation Syndrome Stages

Stage 1: Alarm reaction—This is the immediate reaction to stress or a stressor. A fight-or-flight response occurs. This response can diminish the effectiveness of the immune system, decreasing resistance.

Stage 2: Stage of resistance—As the stress continues, the body adapts to the stressors. The body changes at different levels in order to reduce the effects of stress.

Stage 3: Stage of exhaustion—The stress has been continuous; the body's resistance is lowered or can fail. People experiencing long-term stress may have severe physical manifestations such as a heart attack or severe immunodeficiencies.

BOX 16-2

Physiological Indicators of Stress

- Pupils dilate to increase visual perception when serious threats to the body arise.
- Sweat production (*diaphoresis*) increases to control elevated body heat due to increased metabolism.
- The heart rate increases, which leads to an increased pulse rate to transport nutrients and by-products of metabolism more efficiently.
- Skin is pallid because of constriction of peripheral blood vessels, an effect of norepinephrine.
- The rate and depth of respirations increase because of dilation of the bronchioles, promoting hyperventilation.
- Urinary output decreases.
- The mouth may be dry.
- Peristalsis of the intestines decreases, resulting in possible constipation and flatus.
- For serious threats, mental alertness improves.
- Muscle tension increases to prepare for rapid motor activity or defense.
- Blood sugar increases because of release of glucocorticoids and gluconeogenesis.

body. The person is then ready for "fight or flight." The **fight-or-flight response** can be described as a generalized response to an emergency situation. This includes internal stimulation of the sympathetic nervous system and the adrenal glands. The heart rate, respiratory rates, blood pressure, and blood flow to the muscles are increased. This response prepares the body to either flee or fight (Jacobs, 2001). See Box 16-2 ■ for physiological indicators of stress.

PSYCHOLOGICAL INDICATORS

Anxiety

A common reaction to stress is anxiety. **Anxiety** can be described as a state of mental uneasiness, apprehension, dread, or foreboding. It can also be a feeling of helplessness related to an unidentified threat to self or significant relationships. Anxiety can be experienced at the conscious, subconscious, or unconscious levels. It differs from fear in four ways:

- The source of anxiety may not be identifiable; the source of fear is identifiable.
- Anxiety is related to the future, that is, to an anticipated event. Fear is related to the present.
- Anxiety is vague, whereas fear is definite.
- Anxiety is the result of psychological or emotional conflict; fear is the result of a physical or psychological reality.

All people experience anxiety to some degree most of the time. Mild or moderate anxiety helps people accomplish developmental tasks and meet goals. In this sense, anxiety is an effective coping strategy. For example, mild anxiety motivates students to study. Excessive anxiety,

however, often has destructive effects. The overly anxious student may be unable to sleep or to eat, and may do poorly on a test as a result.

Anxiety may be manifested on four levels:

1. Mild anxiety produces a slight arousal state that enhances perception, learning, and productive abilities. Most healthy people experience mild anxiety, perhaps as a feeling of mild restlessness that prompts a person to seek information and ask questions.
2. Moderate anxiety increases the arousal state to a point where the person expresses feelings of tension, nervousness, or concern. Perceptual abilities are narrowed. Attention is focused on a particular aspect of a situation.
3. Severe anxiety consumes most of the person's energies and requires intervention. The person, unable to focus on what is really happening, focuses on only one specific detail of the situation causing the anxiety.
4. Panic is an overpowering, frightening level of anxiety that causes the person to lose control. It is less frequently experienced than other levels of anxiety. A panicked person may distort events as a result of altered perception.

See Table 16-2 ■ for indicators of these anxiety levels.

Fear

Fear is an emotion or feeling of apprehension aroused by impending danger, pain, or other perceived threat. People may fear something that has already occurred, a current threat, or something they believe will happen. The fear may or may not be based in reality. For example, beginning nursing students may fear their first experience in a client care setting. They may be worried that clients will not want to be cared for by students or that they might inadvertently harm the clients. The nursing students' feelings of fear are real and will probably elicit a stress response. However, the instructor arranges the students' first client assignment so that the students' feared outcomes are unlikely to occur.

Anger

Anger is an emotional state that includes feelings of animosity or strong displeasure. Many people feel guilty when they feel anger because they have been taught that to feel angry is wrong. When anger is expressed in a nonalienating verbal manner, it is considered a positive emotion. Anger can be a sign of emotional maturity when growth and positive interactions result from it.

A verbal expression of anger is a signal of internal psychological discomfort and a call for assistance to deal with perceived stress. Anger, hostility, violence, and aggression differ.

TABLE 16-2

Indicators of Levels of Anxiety

CATEGORY	LEVEL OF ANXIETY			
	MILD	MODERATE	SEVERE	PANIC
Verbalization changes	Increased questioning	Voice tremors and pitch changes	Communication difficult to understand	Communication may not be understandable
Motor activity changes	Mild restlessness Sleeplessness	Tremors, facial twitches, and shakiness Increased muscle tension	Increased motor activity, inability to relax Fearful facial expression	Increased motor activity, agitation Unpredictable responses Trembling, poor motor coordination
Perception and attention changes	Feelings of increased arousal and alertness Uses learning to adapt	Narrowed focus of attention Able to focus but selectively inattentive Learning slightly impaired	Inability to focus or concentrate Easily distracted Learning severely impaired	Perception distorted or exaggerated Unable to learn or function
Respiratory and circulatory changes	None	Slightly increased respiratory and heart rates	Tachycardia, hyperventilation	Dyspnea, palpitations, choking, chest pain or pressure
Other changes	None	Mild gastric symptoms, e.g., "butterflies in the stomach"	Headache, dizziness, nausea	Feeling of impending doom Paresthesia, sweating

Sources: Carpenito, L. J. (1997). *Nursing Diagnosis: Application to Clinical Practice* (7th ed.). Philadelphia: Lippincott; Fontaine, K. L., & Fletcher, J. S. (1999). *Essentials of Mental Health Nursing* (4th ed.). Menlo Park, CA: Addison-Wesley.

- *Hostility* is usually marked by antagonism and harmful or destructive behavior.
- *Violence* is the exertion of physical force to injure or abuse.
- *Aggression* is an unprovoked attack or a hostile, injurious, or destructive action or outlook.

Verbally expressed anger is not the same as hostility, aggression, or violence. However, if anger persists unabated, it can lead to destructiveness and violence.

When an angry person tells another person about the anger and carefully identifies the source, this is constructive. Clear communication gets the anger out into the open so it can be dealt with appropriately. The angry person "gets it off the chest" and an emotional buildup is prevented.

Depression

Depression is a common reaction to overwhelming or negative events. The signs and symptoms of depression vary with the client. Emotional symptoms can include feelings of tiredness, sadness, emptiness, or numbness. Behavioral signs of depression include irritability, inability to concentrate, difficulty making decisions, loss of sexual desire, crying, sleep disturbance, and social withdrawal. Physical signs of depression may include loss of appetite, weight loss, constipation, headache, and dizziness. Most people experience short periods of depression in response to overwhelming stressful events, such as the death of a loved one or loss of a job. When depression is prolonged, it is a cause for concern and may require treatment.

Coping

Coping means dealing with problems and situations successfully. A coping strategy (coping mechanism) is an inborn or learned way of responding to a changing environment, specific problem, or situation. Two types of coping strategies are problem-focused and emotion-focused coping. Problem-focused coping involves taking action to improve a situation. Emotion-focused coping involves using thoughts and actions to relieve emotional distress. Emotion-focused coping does not improve the situation but may help alleviate anxiety.

Coping can also be adaptive or maladaptive. Adaptive coping helps the person to deal effectively with stressful events and minimizes distress associated with them. Maladaptive coping can result in unnecessary distress for the person. Effective coping results in adaptation; ineffective

Factors Influencing the Effectiveness of Coping

- The number, duration, and intensity of the stressors
- Past experiences of the individual
- Support systems available to the individual
- Personal qualities of the person

coping results in maladaptation. When clients exhibit appropriate behavior, nurses should remember that clients are attempting to cope through such behavior.

How well a person copes is influenced by a number of factors, as listed in the Box 16-3 ■. If a person is under stress beyond the ability to cope, he or she will become exhausted and be at risk for developing health problems. Family members who undertake the care of a person in the home for a long period develop long-term stress called caregiver burden. Responses such as chronic fatigue, sleeping difficulties, and high blood pressure are common in caregivers. When coping strategies or defense mechanisms become ineffective, the individual may experience interpersonal problems, work difficulties, and inability to meet basic human needs. Sometimes, prolonged stress can result in mental illness. See Table 16-3 ■.

TABLE 16-3

Examples of the Effects of Stress on Basic Human Needs

NEEDS	EXAMPLES
Physiological	Altered elimination pattern
	Change in appetite
	Altered sleep pattern
Safety and security	Expresses nervousness and feelings of being threatened
	Focuses on stressors and inattention to safety measures
Love and belonging	Isolated and withdrawn
	Becomes overly dependent
	Blames others for own problems
Self-esteem	Fails to socialize with others
	Becomes a workaholic
	Draws attention to self
Self-actualization	Preoccupied with own problems
	Shows lack of control
	Unable to accept reality

DEFENSE MECHANISMS

Adaptive mechanisms may be conscious or unconscious. Unconscious ego defense mechanisms are psychological adaptive mechanisms. Sigmund Freud (1946) described them as mental mechanisms that develop as the personality attempts to defend itself, establish compromises among conflicting impulses, and allay inner tensions. **Defense mechanisms** are the unconscious mind working to protect the person from anxiety. They can be considered precursors to conscious cognitive coping mechanisms that will ultimately solve the problem. Like some verbal and motor responses, defense mechanisms release tension. Table 16-4 ■ describes these mechanisms and lists examples of their adaptive and maladaptive use.

Stress Management for Nurses

Nurses, like clients, are susceptible to experiencing anxiety and stress. Nursing practice involves many stressors related to both clients and the work environment: understaffing and increasing client care assignments and adjusting to various work shifts. Although most nurses cope effectively with the physical and emotional demands of nursing, in some situations nurses become overwhelmed and develop *burnout,* a complex syndrome of behaviors that can be likened to the exhaustion stage of the general adaptation syndrome. The nurse with burnout has little physical and emotional energy, has a negative attitude and self-concept, and experiences feelings of helplessness and hopelessness.

Nurses can prevent burnout by using the stress management techniques discussed earlier in this chapter. Nurses must first recognize their stress. They must recognize feelings of being overwhelmed, fatigue, angry outbursts, physical illness, and increases in coffee drinking, smoking, or other substance abuse as responses to overwhelming stress. Nurses then need to identify which situations cause the strongest responses so that steps can be taken to reduce these stressors. Suggestions for reducing stress that can lead to burnout are:

- Plan a daily relaxation program with meaningful quiet times to reduce tension (e.g., read a novel, listen to music, soak in a hot tub, or meditate).
- Establish a regular exercise program to direct energy outward (e.g., jog, play badminton, or join an aerobics dance class).
- Develop assertiveness techniques to overcome feelings of powerlessness in relationships with others. Learn to say no.
- Learn to accept failures—your own and others—and make it a constructive learning experience. Recognize that most people do the best they can. Learn to ask for help, to show your feelings with colleagues, and to support your colleagues in times of need.
- Accept what cannot be changed. There are certain limitations in every situation. Get involved in constructive

TABLE 16-4

Defense Mechanisms

DEFENSE MECHANISM	EXAMPLE(S)	USE/PURPOSE
Compensation Covering up weaknesses by emphasizing a more desirable trait or by overachievement in a more comfortable area.	A high school student too small to play football becomes the star long-distance runner for the track team.	Allows a person to overcome weakness and achieve success.
Denial An attempt to screen or ignore unacceptable realities by refusing to acknowledge them.	A woman, though told her father has metastatic cancer, continues to plan a family reunion 18 months in advance.	Temporarily isolates a person from the full impact of a traumatic situation.
Displacement The transferring or discharging of emotional reactions from one object or person to another object or person.	A husband and wife are fighting, and the husband becomes so angry he hits a door instead of his wife. A student gets a C on a paper she worked hard on and goes home and yells at her family.	Allows for feelings to be expressed through or to less dangerous objects or people.
Identification An attempt to manage anxiety by imitating the behavior of someone feared or respected.	A student nurse imitating the nurturing behavior she observes one of her instructors using with clients.	Helps a person avoid self-devaluation.
Intellectualization A mechanism by which an emotional response that normally would accompany an uncomfortable or painful incident is evaded by the use of rational explanations that remove from the incident any personal significance and feelings.	The pain over a parent's sudden death is reduced by saying, "He wouldn't have wanted to live with that disability."	Protects a person from pain and traumatic events.
Introjection A form of identification that allows for the acceptance of others' norms and values into oneself, even when contrary to one's previous assumptions.	A 7-year-old tells his little sister, "Don't talk to strangers." He has introjected this value from the instructions of parents and teachers.	Helps a person avoid social retaliation and punishment; particularly important for the child's development of superego.
Minimization Not acknowledging the significance of one's behavior.	A person says, "Don't believe everything my wife tells you. I wasn't so drunk I couldn't drive."	Allows a person to decrease responsibility for own behavior.
Projection A process in which blame is attached to others or the environment for unacceptable desires, thoughts, shortcomings, and mistakes.	A mother is told her child must repeat a grade in school, and she blames this on the teacher's poor instruction. A husband forgets to pay a bill and blames his wife for not giving it to him earlier.	Allows a person to deny the existence of shortcomings and mistakes; protects self-image.
Rationalization Justification of certain behaviors by faulty logic and ascription of motives that are socially acceptable but did not in fact inspire the behavior.	A mother spanks her toddler too hard and says it was all right because he couldn't feel it through the diaper anyway.	Helps a person cope with the inability to meet goals or certain standards.
Reaction Formation A mechanism that causes people to act exactly opposite to the way they feel.	An executive resents his bosses for calling in a consulting firm to make recommendations for change in his department, but verbalizes complete support of the idea and is exceedingly polite and cooperative.	Aids in reinforcing repression by allowing feelings to be acted out in a more acceptable way.
Regression Resorting to an earlier, more comfortable level of functioning that is characteristically less demanding and responsible.	An adult throws a temper tantrum when he does not get his own way. A critically ill client allows the nurse to bathe and feed him.	Allows a person to return to a point in development when nurturing and dependency were needed and accepted with comfort.

(continued)

TABLE 16-4

Defense Mechanisms (*continued*)

DEFENSE MECHANISM	EXAMPLE(S)	USE/PURPOSE
Repression An unconscious mechanism by which threatening thoughts, feelings, and desires are kept from becoming conscious; the repressed material is denied entry into consciousness.	A teenager, seeing his best friend killed in a car crash, becomes amnesic about the circumstances surrounding the accident.	Protects a person from a traumatic experience until he or she has the resources to cope.
Sublimation Displacement of energy associated with more primitive sexual or aggressive drives into socially acceptable activities.	A person with excessive, primitive sexual drives invests psychic energy into a well-defined religious value system.	Protects a person from behaving in irrational, impulsive ways.
Substitution The replacement of a highly valued, unacceptable, or unavailable object by a less valuable, acceptable, or available object.	A woman wants to marry a man exactly like her dead father and settles for someone who looks a little bit like him.	Helps a person achieve goals and minimizes frustration and disappointment.
Undoing An action or words designed to cancel some disapproved thoughts, impulses, or acts in which the person relieves guilt by making reparation.	A father spanks his child and the next evening brings home a present for him. A teacher writes an exam that is far too easy, then constructs a grading curve that makes it difficult to earn a high grade.	Allows a person to appease guilty feelings and atone for mistakes.

Source: Fontaine, K. L. & Fletcher, J. S. (1999). *Essentials of Mental Health Nursing* (4th ed.). Menlo Park, CA: Addison-Wesley Longman, pp. 9–10. Reprinted with permission.

change efforts if organizational policies and procedures cause stress.

■ Develop support groups to deal with feelings and anxieties generated in the work setting.

NURSING CARE

ASSESSING

When assessing a client's stress and coping patterns, the nurse takes a nursing history and examines the client for indicators of stress (e.g., nail biting, nervousness, weight changes) or stress-related health problems (e.g., hypertension, dyspnea). When obtaining the nursing history of any client, the nurse asks about stressful incidents in the client's life. The nurse also discusses signs and symptoms of stress, and coping strategies used in the past. During the physical examination, the nurse observes for verbal, motor, cognitive, or other physical manifestations of stress. The nurse should be aware of expected developmental transitions (see Table 16-1). This knowledge helps the nurse identify additional stressors that may be present and the client's response to them. Questions about the client's stress and coping patterns are shown in Box 16-4 ■.

BOX 16-4

Assessment Interview: Stress and Coping Patterns

■ On a scale of 1 to 10, how would you rate the stress you are experiencing in the following areas?

  a. Home
  b. Work or school
  c. Finance
  d. Recent illness or loss of loved one
  e. Your health
  f. Family responsibilities
  g. Ethnic or cultural group
  h. Religion
  i. Relationships with friends
  j. Relationship with parents or children
  k. Relationship with partner
  l. Recent hospitalization
  m. Other (specify).

■ How long have you been dealing with these stressor(s)?
■ How do you usually handle stressful situations?

  a. Cry
  b. Get angry
  c. Become verbally abusive
  d. Talk to someone (Who?)
  e. Withdraw from the situation
  f. Structure and control others or situation
  g. Go for a walk or physical exercise
  h. Try to arrive at a solution
  i. Pray for wisdom and courage
  j. Laugh, joke, or use some other expression of humor
  k. Meditate or use some other relaxation technique such as yoga or guided imagery

■ How well does your usual coping strategy work?

DIAGNOSING, PLANNING, AND IMPLEMENTING

The North American Nursing Diagnosis Association (NANDA) includes several diagnostic labels related to stress, adaptation, and coping. Examples of these are *Anxiety, Ineffective Coping,* and *Fear.*

Examples of desired outcomes would be:

- Describes causes of anxiety as appropriate.
- Identifies personal strengths.
- Describes usual coping patterns.

Clients with varying levels of anxiety are found in the acute hospital setting. Acute and chronic physical illness are stress producing. Illness coupled with necessary adjustments to an unfamiliar environment can manifest itself as behaviors such as anger, agitation, fear, or withdrawal. The nurse can help the client adjust in several ways:

- Provide compassionate, consistent care.
- Do not take the client's reactions personally.
- Keep the client informed.

Encouraging Health Promotion Strategies

Healthcare professionals at all levels should be role models for health promotion strategies. Physical exercise, optimal nutrition, adequate rest and sleep, and time management are all ways to promote health and reduce stress.

Exercise

Regular exercise promotes both physical and emotional health. Physiological benefits include improved muscle tone, increased cardiopulmonary function, and weight control. Psychological benefits include relief of tension, a feeling of well-being, and relaxation. In general, health guidelines recommend exercise at least three times a week for 60 to 90 minutes.

Nutrition

Optimal nutrition is essential for health and in increasing the body's resistance to stress. To minimize the effects of a stress response (e.g., irritability, hyperactivity, anxiety), people need to avoid excessive caffeine, salt, sugar, fat, and deficiencies in vitamins and minerals. Guidelines for a well-balanced, healthy diet are detailed in Chapter 25 ⚭.

Rest and Sleep

Rest and sleep restore the body's energy levels and are an essential aspect of stress management. To ensure adequate rest and sleep, clients may need comfort measures such as pain management. Nurses may need to teach techniques that promote peace of mind and relaxation. Rest and sleep are discussed further in Chapter 32 ⚭.

BOX 16-5

Relaxation Techniques

- Breathing exercises
- Massage
- Progressive relaxation
- Imagery
- Biofeedback
- Yoga
- Meditation
- Therapeutic touch
- Music therapy
- Humor and laughter

Relaxation Techniques

Several relaxation techniques can be used to quiet the mind, release tension, and counteract the fight-or-flight response of GAS discussed, earlier in this chapter. Nurses can teach these techniques to clients and encourage their use during and after hospitalization. Relaxation tapes can be purchased if desired. Some clients make their own recordings. Specific relaxation techniques that may be used are summarized in Box 16-5 ■.

Time Management

People who manage their time effectively usually experience less stress because they feel more in control of their circumstances. Feeling overwhelmed may indicate the need to prioritize tasks and make modifications in role demands. Responding appropriately to the demands of others is also an important aspect of effective time management. Since all requests made by others cannot always be met, individuals must decide which requests they can honor without undue stress, which ones can be negotiated, and which ones need to be declined. Another way to manage time effectively is to schedule daily or weekly times to do specific tasks. When people feel overwhelmed, they need to reexamine the "should, ought, and must" approach to their actions and develop more realistic self-expectations.

Minimizing Anxiety

Nurses have always carried out measures to minimize clients' anxiety and stress. For example, nurses encourage clients to take deep breaths before an injection, explain procedures before they are implemented including sensations likely to be experienced during the procedure, administer a back or neck rub to help the client relax, and offer support to clients and families during times of illness.

Mediating Anger

Often nurses find clients' anger difficult to handle. Caring for the client who is angry is difficult for two reasons:

- Clients rarely state, "I feel angry or frustrated," and rarely indicate the reason for their anger. Instead, they

---

BOX 16-6

Strategies for Dealing with Anger

Fontaine and Fletcher (2003) recommend the following strategies for dealing with clients' anger:

- Know and understand your own response to the feelings and expressions of anger.
- Accept the client's right to be angry; feelings are real and cannot be discounted or ignored.
- Ask the client in what way you may have contributed to the anger.
- Help the client "own" the anger—do not assume responsibility for her or his feelings.

BOX 16-7

Common Characteristics of Crises

- All crises are experienced as sudden. The person is usually not aware of a warning signal, even if others could "see it coming." The individual or family may feel that they have little or no preparation for the event or trauma.
- The crisis is often experienced as ultimately life threatening, whether this perception is realistic or not.
- Communication with significant others is often decreased or cut off.
- There may be perceived or real displacement from familiar surroundings or loved ones.
- All crises have an aspect of loss, whether actual or perceived. The losses can include an object, a person, a hope, a dream, or any significant factor for that individual.

---

may refuse treatment, become verbally abusive or demanding, threaten violence, or become overly critical. Their complaints rarely reflect the cause of their anger.

- Anger from clients can elicit fear and anger in the nurse, who may respond in a manner that intensifies the client's anger, even to the point of violence. The majority of nurses respond in a way that reduces their own stress rather than the client's stress. See Box 16-6 ■ for strategies for dealing with clients' anger.

Specific relaxation techniques that may be used are summarized in Box 16-5.

Intervening in Crisis Situations

A **crisis** is an acute, time-limited state of emotional imbalance resulting from sources of stress. It can be defined as a turning point in a person's life—a point at which usual resources and coping skills are no longer effective. A person in crisis is temporarily unable to cope with or adapt to the stressor by using previous methods of problem solving. People in crisis generally see a stressor as overwhelming. They often do not have adequate situational support, and do not have adequate coping mechanisms. Common characteristics of crises are shown in Box 16-7 ■.

Because a state of emotional imbalance is so uncomfortable, a crisis is self-limiting. However, a person experiencing a crisis alone has more difficulty handling the situation than a person working through a crisis with help.

Nurses in acute care or short-term care settings may not see the long-term effects of their crisis interventions. Typically, nurses in these settings will assess the crisis, and begin implementing a crisis intervention plan.

EVALUATING

The desired outcomes developed during the planning stage will be evaluated by collecting data about the client's

current status. To determine if the outcome has been achieved the nurse will ask questions such as these:

- How does the client perceive the problem?
- Is there an underlying problem that has not been identified?
- How does the client perceive the effectiveness of the new coping strategies?
- Have family members and significant others provided effective support?

Although stress is part of daily life, it is also highly individual. One person may be stressed by a situation that would not concern another person. Some methods for reducing stress will be effective for one person; other methods will be appropriate for a different person.

CONTINUING CARE

Clients who are experiencing stress may require ongoing nursing support or referral to community agencies after discharge. The determination of how much and what type of planning and home care follow-up is required is based in great part on the nurse's knowledge of how the client and family have coped with previous stressors and the nature of the present stressor. Box 16-8 ■ describes data to be gathered for home care or follow-up.

NURSING PROCESS CARE PLAN
Caring for a Client with Stress

Ms. Levitt is a 37-year-old divorced mother of three, ages 8, 11, and 14. In addition to her full-time job, she transports her children to numerous school and extracurricular activities, is active in her synagogue, and is attending school part time in order to obtain a better paying job. Ms. Levitt's ex-husband

---

BOX 16-8

Home Care Considerations: Stress and Coping

Client

- *Knowledge:* client's understanding of the nature of the stressors
- *Current coping strategies:* effectiveness of current coping strategies and willingness to learn new stress management techniques
- *Self-care abilities:* physical, emotional, social, and financial ability to minimize associated stressors
- *Role expectations:* client's perception of the need to return to prior roles and possible stressors associated with these roles

Family

- *Knowledge:* family members' and significant others' understanding of the nature of the client's stressors and their own relationship with client stressors
- *Family coping strategies:* effectiveness of family members' and significant others' coping strategies and willingness to learn new stress management techniques

- *Role expectations:* family members' and significant others' perception of the need for the client to return to family and work roles
- *Support people's availability and skills:* family members' and significant others' sensitivity to the client's emotional and physical needs and ability to provide a supportive environment

Community

- *Resources:* availability of and familiarity with possible sources of assistance for stress management such as massage therapists, religious or spiritual centers, physical care providers, and support groups
- Let clients talk about their anger.
- After the interaction is completed, take time to process your feelings and your responses to the client with your colleagues.

---

left the state years ago and does not financially assist with the care of the children. Ms. Levitt is brought to the employee clinic by a coworker for evaluation to rule out a heart attack.

Assessment. VS: T 98.6, P 102, R 30, BP 134/78. Pale, diaphoretic. C/o chest pain rated as 5/10; hold chest and rubbing arm. Wt 189 lbs (admits to a 20-lb weight gain over last year). Began smoking again 6 months ago, after 7 years of not smoking. C/o frequent feelings of nausea, her heart "pounding," headaches, and unusual fatigue of 3 weeks duration. ECG—normal. Client states, "I thought I was having a heart attack, but I am too young." Evaluation by nurse practitioner does not reveal any CVS disorder. It is determined that Mrs. Levitt is experiencing a panic attack.

Nursing Diagnosis. The following important nursing diagnoses (among others) are established for this client:

- *Anxiety* related to to situational crisis
- *Ineffective Coping* related to personal vulnerability
- *Risk for Powerlessness* related to ineffective coping skills
- *Compromised Family Coping* related to lack of available support for client.

Expected Outcomes. The expected outcomes of the plan of care specify that Mrs. Levitt will:

- Have vital signs that reflect baseline or decreased sympathetic stimulation.
- Verbalize ability to cope and ask for help when needed.
- Identify factors that are uncontrollable.
- Verbalize internal resources to help deal with family situation.

Planning and Implementation. The following interventions are planned and implemented:

- Assess client's level of anxiety and physical reaction to anxiety (e.g., tachycardia, tachypnea, nonverbal expression of anxiety).
- Explore coping skills previously used by the client to relieve anxiety; reinforce these skills and explore other outlets.
- Encourage use of appropriate community resources.
- Provide client and family members with information to help distinguish between a panic attack and serious physical illness.
- Teach client and family to problem solve.
- Teach relaxation techniques.
- Encourage moderate aerobic exercise.
- Observe for causes of ineffective coping such as poor self-concept, lack of problem-solving skills, lack of support, or changes in life situation.
- Teach stress reduction, relaxation, and imagery.
- Teach cognitive activities, such as self-talk.
- Help client practice assertive communication technique.
- Refer to support group, pastoral care, or social services.
- Observe for causative and contributing factors.
- Note other stressors (e.g., financial, job related).

Evaluation. Mrs. Levitt returns to the clinic in 1 week. VS are within normal limits. She reports that she had one additional episode during the last week. She has been practicing stress relieving relaxation and worked out at the company gym 2× during the week.

Critical Thinking in the Nursing Process

1. Speculate about the stressors that Ms. Levitt is experiencing.
2. From the data provided, how do you think Ms. Levitt is responding to the stressors you identified?
3. Explore anger as a possible cause of Ms. Levitt's symptoms.
4. What cues would alert you that Ms. Levitt is adapting to the stressors in her life in a positive and healthy manner?

Note: Discussion of Critical Thinking questions appears in Appendix I.

Note: The references and resources for this and all chapters have been compiled at the back of the book.

Chapter Review

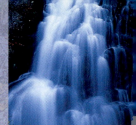

 KEY TERMS by Topic

Use the audio glossary feature of either the CD-ROM or the Companion Website to hear the correct pronunciation of the following key terms.

Introduction
stress

Sources of Stress
stressors

Models of Stress
stimulus, response, general adaptation syndrome (GAS), transactional

Indicators of Stress
fight-or-flight response, anxiety, anger

Coping
coping, defense mechanisms

Nursing Care
crisis

KEY Points

- Stress is a state of physiological and psychological tension that affects the whole person—physically, emotionally, intellectually, socially, and spiritually.

- Physiological responses to stress are described by the general adaptation syndrome (GAS).

- There are physiological and psychological indicators of stress.

- Common psychological indicators are anxiety, fear, anger, and depression. Anxiety, the most common response, has four levels: mild, moderate, severe, and panic.

- Unconscious ego defense mechanisms such as denial, rationalization, compensation, and sublimation protect individuals from anxiety.

- Prolonged stress and ineffective coping interfere with the meeting of basic needs and can affect physical and mental health.

- Nursing interventions for clients who are stressed are aimed at encouraging health promotion strategies (exercise, balanced diet, adequate rest, and time management), minimizing anxiety, mediating anger, teaching about specific relaxation techniques, and implementing crisis interventions as needed.

- Because nursing practice involves many stressors related to both clients and the work environment, nurses are susceptible to anxiety and in some cases burnout. Like clients, they need to implement stress reduction measures.

 EXPLORE Media Link

Additional interactive resources for this chapter can be found on the Companion Website at www.prenhall.com/ramont. Click on Chapter 16 and "Begin" to select the activities for this chapter.

For chapter-related NCLEX®-style questions and an audio glossary, access the accompanying CD-ROM in this book.

FOR FURTHER Study

Guidelines for a well-balanced, healthy diet are detailed in Chapter 25.

Rest and sleep are discussed further in Chapter 32.

Critical Thinking Care Map

Caring for a Client with Myocardial Infarction

NCLEX-PN® Focus Area: Psychosocial Integrity Coping and Adaptation

Case Study: Darryl Johnson, a 47-year-old accountant, was admitted to the emergency department with a heart attack. He says, "I'm scared about this. My dad died of a heart attack when he was forty-eight years old." He appears restless, questions everything that is going on, and is hyperventilating.

Nursing Diagnosis: Anxiety Related to Change in Health Status and Threat of Dying

COLLECT DATA

Subjective	Objective
_____	_____
_____	_____
_____	_____
_____	_____
_____	_____
_____	_____
_____	_____

Would you report this data? Yes/No

If yes, to: _____

What would you report? _____

Nursing Care

_____
_____
_____
_____
_____
_____
_____
_____
_____
_____
_____
_____
_____

How would you document this? _____
_____
_____
_____

Compare your documentation to the sample provided in Appendix I.

Data Collected
(use those that apply)

- Alert and oriented to time, place, and person
- VS: T 99.6, P 88, R 28, BP 140/82
- Peripheral pulse strong and equal
- Capillary refill less than 3 seconds
- Lungs clear
- Pale; skin cool and diaphoretic
- Nail bed pink
- ECG—normal sinus rhythm
- Severe chest pain

Nursing Interventions
(use those that apply; list in priority order)

- Assess for subtle signs of denial.
- Validate observations by asking client, "Are you feeling anxious now?
- Avoid confrontation.
- Allow and reinforce client's personal reaction to or expression of pain, discomfort, or threat to well-being.
- Provide back rub to decrease anxiety.
- Encourage realistic and achievable goal setting.
- Explore coping skills previously used by the client to relieve anxiety; reinforce these skills and explore other outlets.
- Explain all activities, procedures, and issues that involve the client; use nonmedical terms and calm, slow speech. Do this in advance of procedures when possible, and validate client's understanding.
- Assess source of fear with client.
- Assess client's level of anxiety and physical reaction to anxiety.

1 Mentally healthy individuals:
1. can cope with all crises.
2. demonstrate difficulty in solving complex problems.
3. frequently experience work-related difficulty.
4. work, form relationships, and cope.

2 The nurse is caring for a client who had a myocardial infarction 2 days ago. The client has been on bed rest, being allowed up in the chair for meals. When you enter the room, the client is sitting on the floor doing sit-ups. This is an example of the defense mechanism known as:
1. repression.
2. sublimation.
3. identification.
4. denial.

3 A client who was driving when involved in a motor vehicle crash has just learned that the passenger in the vehicle has died. The police are attempting to obtain information from the survivor, but the client is unable to recall even being in the car. The nurse on duty realizes that this is an example of:
1. dissociation.
2. denial.
3. regression.
4. transference.

4 Anxiety can manifest itself on four levels. Of the following levels, which one produces a slight arousal state that enhances perception, learning, and productive abilities?
1. mild
2. moderate
3. severe
4. panic

5 A client on your medical unit is experiencing dyspnea. You also sense that the client is anxious. As the nurse caring for this client, you:
1. ignore the anxiety, since it will probably go away when the client is breathing better.
2. notify the doctor immediately.
3. reassure the client that this is only temporary.
4. remain with the client and be supportive of the situation.

6 In order for a nurse to prevent burnout, first he or she must:
1. identify which situations cause the strongest responses.
2. recognize his or her stress.
3. decrease use of substances such as coffee, alcohol, and tobacco.
4. take steps to reduce stress.

7 Physiological responses to stress are described by:
1. coping responses.
2. local adaptation syndrome.
3. general adaptation syndrome.
4. stimulus-based stress model.

8 Stress manifests itself differently in different developmental ages. Of the following stages, which one is associated with accepting a changing physique and developing relationships involving sexual attraction?
1. adolescent
2. young adult
3. middle adult
4. older adult

9 The autonomic nervous system reacts to a perceived threat with release of adrenaline. This is known as:
1. a crisis.
2. stress.
3. fight or flight.
4. anxiety.

10 A male college student who is overweight and unable to participate in competitive sports becomes the life of the party and drives a new sporty car. He is displaying:
1. compensation.
2. reaction formation.
3. transference.
4. identification.

Answers and Rationales for Review Questions, as well as discussion of Care Plan and Critical Thinking Care Map questions, appear in Appendix I.

Chapter 17

Loss, Grieving, and Death

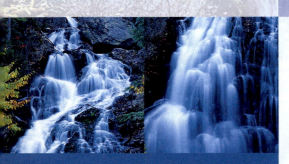

BRIEF Outline

Chronic Illness
Terminal Illness
Grief, Death, and Dying
Legal Issues
Death-Related Religious and Cultural Practices
Nurse's Response to Death

LEARNING Outcomes

After completing this chapter, you will be able to:

1. Define *chronic illness*.
2. Explain factors that influence chronic illness.
3. Describe the role of the nurse in caring for the chronically ill.
4. Discuss the roles of the client and nurse in rehabilitation.
5. Define *palliative care* and *hospice*.
6. Discuss the relationship between loss and grief.
7. Identify stages and clinical symptoms of grieving and factors that affect a grief response.
8. Identify measures to assist the grieving process.
9. List clinical signs of impending and actual death.
10. Describe the role and legal responsibilities of the nurse in caring for the dying client.
11. Describe essential aspects of the Patient Self-Determination Act.
12. Describe nursing measures for care of the body after death.
13. Describe the role of the nurse in working with families or caregivers of dying clients.

HISTORICAL Perspectives

The profile of diseases contributing most heavily to death, illness, and disability among Americans changed dramatically during the last century. Today, chronic diseases—such as cardiovascular disease (primarily heart disease and stroke), cancer, and diabetes—are among the most prevalent, costly, and preventable of all health problems. Seven of every 10 Americans who die each year, or more than 1.7 million people, die of a chronic disease.

The term hospice *(from the same linguistic root as* hospitality*) can be traced back to medieval times when it referred to a place of shelter and rest for weary or ill travelers on a long journey. The name was first applied to specialized care for dying patients in 1967 by physician Dame Cicely Saunders, who founded the first modern hospice—St. Christopher's Hospice in a residential suburb of London.*

In the last several decades, life expectancy in the United States has improved dramatically due to medical advances. This means both that healthy people are living longer, and that people with chronic or terminal conditions are living longer. Practical and vocational nurses play an active role in the long-term care of these groups of people.

Chronic Illness

A **chronic illness** has certain characteristics:

1. It is caused by disease that produces signs and symptoms within a variable period of time.
2. It develops slowly and runs a long course.
3. It allows only partial recovery.
4. It can impose an enormous financial burden on a family.

Some examples of chronic diseases are chronic obstructive pulmonary disease (COPD), cardiovascular disease (primarily heart disease and stroke), cancer, muscular dystrophy, diabetes mellitus, and lupus erythematosus.

Although the symptoms and general reactions caused by chronic disease may subside with proper treatment and care, the disease remains. The period during which the disease is controlled and symptoms are not obvious is known as **remission**. Reactivation of the disease and increase in severity of symptoms is known as an **exacerbation**. Exacerbations of chronic disease often cause the client to seek medical attention and may lead to hospitalization.

Several predisposing risk factors influence chronic illness. The first factor is age. Chronic illness can occur at any age, but the elderly are more likely to have long, drawn-out chronic diseases.

Other factors include genetics. Sometimes, an inherited trait or gene puts a person at greater risk for developing a certain disease. *Behavioral factors* may include, but not be limited to:

- *Lifestyle.* Sometimes the way we live and work can put us at risk for developing certain diseases.
- *Stress.* There are many different types of stress that can put one at risk of developing chronic high blood pressure, chronic depression, and headaches. Stress can be physical, psychological, or emotional.
- *Poor nutrition.* A poor diet can contribute to chronic disease and increase the risk of high blood pressure and high cholesterol.
- *Physical inactivity.* Insufficient or low physical activity can increase the risk for developing chronic disease.
- *Tobacco and alcohol use.* The use of tobacco, most often cigarette smoking, and overconsumption of alcohol contribute to several chronic problems and also increase the risk of developing chronic disease.

Physiological factors may include high blood pressure, high blood cholesterol, and obesity.

Environmental factors, such as pollution or exposure to pesticides, may put us at greater risk for developing a chronic disease such as cancer.

Race and ethnicity also are factors that influence chronic illness. There is an association between disease occurrence and race (called *race-specific rates*). Not only are some health problems more common among nonwhites, research also indicates that many nonwhites fail to receive necessary care.

PREVENTION OF CHRONIC ILLNESS

Because chronic disease evolves over time and pathologic changes may become irreversible, the goal is to detect risk factors as early as possible. Generally, *prevention* means interrupting or stopping the development of a disease before it occurs. **Primary prevention** refers to health promotion and specific protection against diseases. An example of a primary prevention activity would be giving a talk on how to prevent colon cancer. **Secondary prevention** refers to early detection of disease and prompt intervention to halt disease progression. An example of secondary prevention is doing fecal occult blood tests and screening colonoscopies to screen for colon cancers. **Tertiary prevention** refers to rehabilitation (appropriate to the stage of disability), preventing further complications, and restoring independent functioning to the highest possible level. An example of tertiary prevention would be dietary and lifestyle changes to prevent further cancers from developing.

REHABILITATION

Rehabilitation is the process of restoring a person's ability to return to a former capacity following an injury or illness. Rehabilitation assists individuals to achieve maximum performance and independence. It is an active process and is very different from "maintenance" care. A rehabilitation plan is made after a thorough assessment of a client's disabilities and capabilities. It is based on the potential for improving the client's condition and offers assistance with the learning or relearning of skills needed to perform activities of daily living (ADLs). If improvement cannot be made, then care is directed toward maintaining the client in the current condition and preventing further disability. When rehabilitation reaches a point at which no further progress is possible, then the focus of care changes to maintaining that optimal level. The purpose or extent of rehabilitation ranges from employment or reemployment for someone with a disability to the more limited achievement of providing one's own daily self-care. Rehabilitation involves a multidisciplinary approach. Members of the healthcare team use different areas of knowledge and skill to

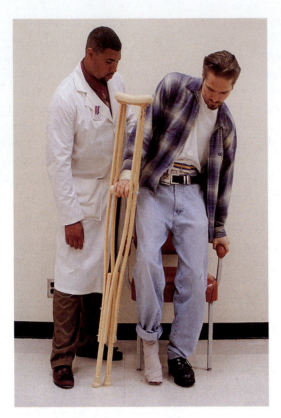

Figure 17-1. ■ The healthcare team works together to restore the client's optimal function.

contribute to the client's comprehensive plan of care (Figure 17-1 ■). Rehabilitation occurs in a variety of settings and is directed at an individualized plan of care that can optimize healing.

Role of the Nurse in Rehabilitation

Nurses have two major responsibilities when working with clients who have disabilities. Their first is to see that disability from disease is limited as much as possible. This is done by:

- Preventing complications through early recognition of symptoms
- Frequently reviewing the signs and symptoms with the client and family members
- Preventing deformities by maintaining client's proper body alignment, positioning limbs to prevent contractures, turning the client frequently to prevent skin breakdown (see Chapter 23 ⚭), and providing adequate nutrition and fluid intake (see Chapters 25 and 26 ⚭).

The second responsibility is to support the nursing plan and to implement an appropriate rehabilitation program. This is accomplished by determining the client's own goals for rehabilitation and by using appropriate nursing interventions based on mutually agreed-on goals. Nursing interventions should encourage the client to assume responsibility for his or her own ADLs as soon as possible. Short-term, realistic, measurable goals give the client the most opportunity for success. Assistive devices (Figure 17-2 ■) can enable a client to bathe or dress even when range of motion and muscle strength are compromised. Positive feedback from the nurse reinforces client progress. The nurse works with other team members to provide a consistent, coordinated plan.

Role of the Client in Rehabilitation

Clients themselves make the most important contributions to their rehabilitation. The client, physician, nurse, social worker, occupational therapist, physical therapist, and others can arrive at an ideal plan. However, only the client's attitude, acceptance, and motivation will make that ideal plan work. If the client cannot adjust to the disability, attempts at rehabilitation are hindered. The client's day-to-day behavior is the first indication of positive motivation, so self-care is always encouraged.

When you work with clients who are chronically ill, you will see that life has meaning for the individual, even though it may not be apparent to others. Nurses look for what motivates each client. For example, a woman who was a classical pianist developed severe arthritis in her hands. She needed to exercise those joints even though it was extremely painful. She decided that every day she would practice Mozart. Because she loved the music so much, she was able to focus on the music, not the pain, until her joints loosened up. When looking for ways to help clients with chronic illnesses, nurses can ask about what clients love to do. This knowledge can help them to support and motivate the client in meeting goals.

FACILITIES FOR CONTINUING CARE

As described in Chapter 35 ⚭, different types of healthcare institutions include long-term care facilities, assisted living facilities, and home care. With hospital stays being shorter than in the past, a great deal of care of clients with chronic illnesses takes place in long-term care facilities, outpatient facilities, and the home.

NURSING CARE

ASSESSING

Before a plan of care can be devised for someone who has a chronic illness, a thorough assessment of needs and capabilities is carried out. The assessment includes the individual's physical, psychological, social, and financial status.

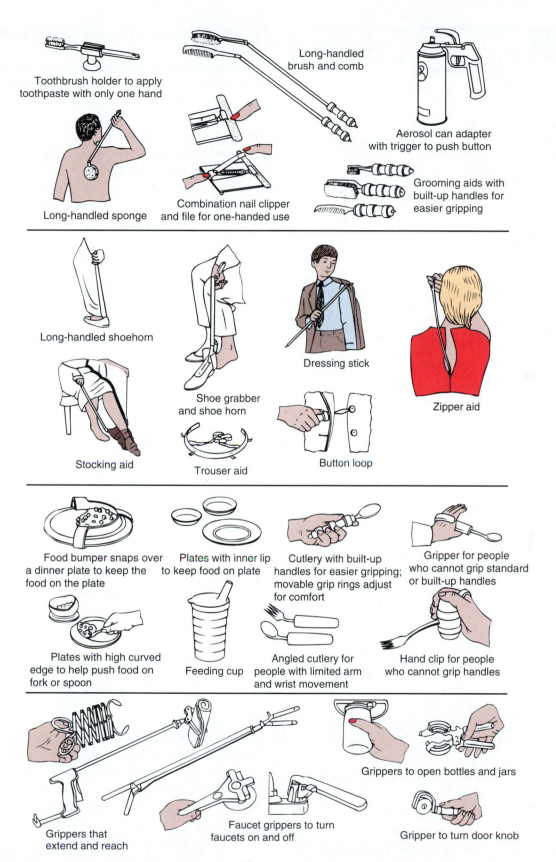

Toothbrush holder to apply toothpaste with only one hand

Long-handled brush and comb

Aerosol can adapter with trigger to push button

Long-handled sponge

Combination nail clipper and file for one-handed use

Grooming aids with built-up handles for easier gripping

Long-handled shoehorn

Shoe grabber and shoe horn

Dressing stick

Zipper aid

Stocking aid

Trouser aid

Button loop

Food bumper snaps over a dinner plate to keep the food on the plate

Plates with inner lip to keep food on plate

Cutlery with built-up handles for easier gripping; movable grip rings adjust for comfort

Gripper for people who cannot grip standard or built-up handles

Plates with high curved edge to help push food on fork or spoon

Feeding cup

Angled cutlery for people with limited arm and wrist movement

Hand clip for people who cannot grip handles

Grippers that extend and reach

Faucet grippers to turn faucets on and off

Grippers to open bottles and jars

Gripper to turn door knob

Figure 17-2. ■ Assistive/adaptive devices.

BOX 17-1

Nursing Diagnoses Related to Clients' Disorders

- *Anxiety*
- *Constipation*
- *Ineffective Breathing Pattern*
- *Impaired Verbal Communication*
- *Compromised Family Coping*
- *Impaired Home Maintenance*
- *Hopelessness*
- *Impaired Urinary Elimination*
- *Impaired Physical Mobility*
- *Imbalanced Nutrition*
- *Pain*
- *Powerlessness*
- *Self-Care Deficit*
- *Ineffective Role Performance*
- *Sexual Dysfunction*
- *Impaired Skin Integrity*
- *Impaired Social Interaction*

Some of the most common nursing diagnoses for the person with a chronic illness are:

- *Activity Intolerance*
- *Impaired Adjustment*
- *Ineffective Health Maintenance*
- *Risk for Injury*
- *Deficient Knowledge*
- *Disturbed Body Image*

DIAGNOSING, PLANNING, AND IMPLEMENTING

Nursing diagnoses are determined from all the data gathered about the client. Clients with chronic illnesses may have a long list of nursing diagnoses related to their disorders (Box 17-1 ■).

Prevention and Reduction of Disability

In caring for people with chronic illnesses, the nurse has three important goals:

- To prevent and reduce disability.
- To enable the client to remain active physically and mentally to the extent recommended by the rehabilitation team.
- To clarify healthcare goals and offer encouragement when progress occurs.

Many of the difficulties that limit those who are chronically ill may not have been caused by the disease itself. Instead, they may have developed because of immobility during the acute phase of illness. Keeping the person's body in good alignment, maintaining joint range of motion and strength, and preventing decubitus ulcers are physical measures that must be assessed continually. Careful planning

for rest and activity will help preserve the client's physical resources.

As mentioned earlier, recognizing what is meaningful to the individual is a primary step toward developing self-care. Physical needs become paramount to clients who are chronically ill (see Maslow's hierarchy of needs, Figure 5-4 ⬥). By meeting clients' physical needs, nurses can convey an interest in their progress and welfare. However, it is important to encourage clients to perform as much of their own care as possible. Clients who have been independent in self-care before hospitalization should not be allowed to regress in their abilities if at all possible.

Concerns

Care of the client who is chronically ill requires patience, understanding, and an ability to develop a trusting relationship. It is important to adapt to the client's routine as much as possible and be consistent. Very often the caring and concerned nurse can help a client become motivated and stay motivated. It may be time consuming to listen to the same questions and to say the same things over and over, but the nature of chronic illness may require this attention. Active listening and responding with warmth and interest is an important nursing intervention.

Identification of Coping Methods

Chronic pain, ongoing medical costs, and difficulty carrying out ADLs all challenge the coping skills of clients with chronic illnesses. Nurses can ask clients to identify their usual coping methods and explore alternative approaches if necessary. Success in learning to adjust to a disability depends on what the person's personality, total life experience, and family relationships were before the illness. It also depends on the client's current behavior and motivation. The nurse can assist greatly by helping clients to recognize their past strengths and to focus on the positive choices they can make in their lives.

EVALUATING

How can we know if the client's plan of care was a success? Outcomes for specific chronic diseases are reviewed and adjusted as necessary. The nurse asks the client which interventions have been helpful. The nurse also asks about ongoing support for rehabilitation or maintenance therapy. Success can be defined by the client and/or the client's caregiver. Professional caregivers have a responsibility to define these goals and evaluate if the desired outcome was achieved. Did the client benefit from the treatment provided? It is especially important to note if the client experienced enhanced quality of life.

CONTINUING CARE

Clients with chronic conditions require extra support and must plan for the long term. Generally, before discharge from the hospital, clients with chronic disease or their family members should be able to do the following:

- Demonstrate or explain measures that must be taken to avoid further preventable disability.
- Demonstrate or explain self-care activities they can perform.
- Identify activities for which they need help.
- Explain who will be available to help them with those activities and on what basis that help will be available.
- Explain what community resources are available and how to access support services.
- Discuss in reasonable detail their plans for follow-up care and reevaluation.
- Begin discussion regarding end-of-life care.

Terminal Illness

Dying will always be a part of life. When we interact with persons who are known to have a life-threatening disease, we are directly confronted with their dying and with our own mortality. This confrontation can evoke anxiety if we are not comfortable with the normal process of dying. The purpose of this section is to offer general guidelines that will assist the nurse in caring for people who are dying and in helping family members who are sharing the experience.

PALLIATIVE CARE

The term **palliative care** or *palliative management* involves a shift in treatment goals from treating a disease process to treating symptoms of the disease. Palliative care is also called comfort care. Relief of suffering in dying clients goes beyond identifying and treating physical symptoms. End-of-life care involves treating the physical, emotional, and spiritual needs of the client and family. Palliative care includes the following principles:

- The overall goal of treatment is to optimize quality of life; that is, the hopes and desires of the client are fulfilled as much as possible.
- Death is regarded as a natural process, to be neither hastened nor prolonged.
- Diagnostic tests and other invasive procedures are minimized, unless they are likely to alleviate symptoms.
- Use of "heroic" treatment measures is discouraged.
- When using narcotic analgesics, the right dose is the dose that provides pain relief without unacceptable side effects.
- The client is the "expert" on whether pain and symptoms are adequately relieved.
- Clients eat if they are hungry and drink if they are thirsty. Feeding and fluids are offered but not forced.
- Care is individualized and is based on the goals of the client and family.

HOSPICE

Hospice is not a "place"; rather, it is a "philosophy of care." Hospice care incorporates the holistic concepts of palliative care. Nursing care is aimed directly at treating symptoms of the disease, not the disease itself, and eliminates the suffering that may accompany the dying process. The hospice movement was founded in 1967 by Dame Cicely Saunders, a London physician, and was later extended to the United States. It grew rapidly after the enactment of the Medicare hospice benefit in 1983. The Medicare benefit outlines systematically how hospice care is to be delivered. It is important to note that palliative hospice care can occur in a hospital; however, the client's home is the most common and preferred setting. Care can also be provided in a long-term care or other residential facility. Independent hospice and hospital-based palliative care units are also becoming more available. Regardless of the setting, hospice care is always delivered by a team of healthcare professionals in order to ensure a holistic approach to care.

Entrance or admission into a hospice program requires a physician referral. Referral can occur in several ways. It may be initiated by the physician who finds that curative medical treatment no longer enhances the quality of life. A family member or caregiver may also initiate the hospice referral. Typically, the referring physician will discuss the referral with the client and family. The physician contacts the hospice team, the discharge planner, or the social worker to assist with the transition.

The Medicare coverage for hospice care is available only if:

- The client is eligible for Medicare Part A
- Two physicians certify that the client is terminally ill with a life expectancy of 6 months or less
- The client signs an informed consent choosing palliative care
- The client receives care from a Medicare-certified hospice program.

When a Medicare beneficiary elects to receive hospice care, he or she is entitled to receive care for two 90-day benefit periods followed by an unlimited amount of 60-day periods. The Medicare benefit covers the following services:

- Nursing
- Physician
- Home health aide
- Chaplain
- Medical social worker
- Bereavement coordinator
- Volunteer
- Medical equipment, medications, medical supplies related to the hospice diagnosis
- Short-term inpatient and respite care

- Continuous care for symptom management
- Physical, occupational, and speech therapy
- Dietary counseling.

Hospice programs that are not Medicare certified cannot provide services under Medicare Part A; they may, however, provide services free of charge. Many commercial insurance providers include a hospice benefit. Clients may revoke the hospice benefit for an extended prognosis or personal choice at any time.

Grief, Death, and Dying

Loss describes a real or potential situation in which something that is valued is gone, is unavailable, or is changed. People can experience a loss in many different ways. Loss of a family member, loss of a job, and loss of body image are a few examples. **Grief** is the whole range of feelings, thoughts, and behaviors related to loss. It is associated with overwhelming distress and sorrow. **Bereavement** is the normal grieving period experienced by the surviving loved ones. **Mourning** involves the process and rituals through which grief is eventually resolved. It is influenced by culture, beliefs, and customs. Normal ways of expressing grief include sorrow and a change in sleep patterns, eating habits, activity level, or communication patterns. This type of grieving is called **anticipatory grieving**. **Dysfunctional grieving** describes grief that is characterized by an extended period of denial, depression, severe physiological symptoms, or suicidal thoughts.

Grief can have negative effects on health. Survivors may experience such manifestations as depression, anxiety, fatigue, headaches, chest pain, dyspnea, dizziness, palpitations, or menstrual irregularities. Unresolved grief can lead to continued physical and emotional problems. To achieve mental and physical health, survivors must work through and resolve their grief.

STAGES AND MANIFESTATIONS OF GRIEF

Many authors have described the process of grief. The most famous is Dr. Elisabeth Kübler-Ross, who described five stages. Nurses can observe clinical signs to determine a person's stage of grieving:

1. **Denial**. The client refuses to believe that the loss is happening and is not ready to deal with practical problems, such as use of prosthesis after loss of a leg. The client may assume artificial cheerfulness to prolong denial. This stage is important and necessary and can assist to cushion the impact of the client's awareness.

2. **Anger**. The client or family may direct anger at the nurse or staff about matters that normally would not bother them. The client resents the fact that others will remain healthy and alive while he or she must die.

3. **Bargaining**. The client promises a change in behavior to avoid loss and may express feelings of guilt or fear of punishment for past sins, real or imagined. The client promises to be good in exchange for prolonged time.

4. **Depression**. The client grieves over what has happened and what cannot be. The client may talk freely (e.g., remembering past losses such as money or job) or may withdraw. The client then enters a state of "prepatory grief" getting ready for the arrival of death.

5. **Acceptance**. The client comes to terms with loss and may have decreased interest in physical surroundings and support people. The client may wish to begin making plans (e.g., will, prosthesis, altered living arrangements).

Note that not everyone goes through these stages of grief in the exact order listed. Also, individuals may move back and forth between stages. The amount of time one remains in each stage differs from person to person. Some individuals may never reach the acceptance stage.

Many factors affect a person's grieving responses. Some of these factors are described briefly in Table 17-1 ■.

PRIORITIES IN NURSING CARE

When caring for clients who are terminally ill, focus your care on meeting physiological needs, managing pain, and providing emotional support. Keep the client's skin clean, warm, and dry. Assist to positions of comfort. Offer food and fluids, but be aware that the terminally ill client may refuse them. Take every measure available to manage pain. If a patient-controlled analgesia (PCA) pump is in use, remind the client to push the button, if necessary. Administer ordered pain medications promptly and report breakthrough pain not managed by analgesics.

Allow the client to talk about dying if he or she wishes to do so. Expect the client to decrease contact with others gradually until only a few significant people are allowed in. Be supportive of family and friends, allowing them to verbalize their feelings about the client's illness and prognosis. Sometimes during the grieving process, clients and/or families will seem angry and hostile toward nursing staff. Remain supportive and know this response is caused by the anger and helplessness they feel about the client's illness.

TABLE 17-1	
Factors Affecting a Person's Grieving Response	
FACTOR	**MEANING OF LOSS AND GRIEF RESPONSE**
Age	Children differ from adults in their understanding of death and how they are affected by the loss of others. Skillful work with bereaved children is especially important because the experience of a significant loss in childhood can have serious lifelong effects emotionally. As adults, death and loss become part of normal development. For example, the middle-aged person may consider the loss of an elderly parent a normal occurrence when compared to the death of a younger person.
Culture	Customs about grieving vary. Some cultures value social support and expression of loss within the group. Others view the grieving period as a private matter to be dealt with internally.
Spiritual beliefs	Most religious affiliations have some practices that are related to death. For example, administration of the last rites by a Catholic priest is important to Catholics. To provide support at the time of death, nurses need to ask about the client's beliefs and practices.
Gender	Gender role expectations can influence the grieving process. For example, U.S. society generally expects men to "be strong" and show little emotion. Women are expected to express grief by crying.
Socioeconomic status	A person who is confronted with both a severe loss and economic hardship can have a more difficult time coping than a wealthy person who has financial stability.
Support systems	Studies have shown that people with available support systems cope much better with loss. If family or close friends are not comfortable with loss, the need for ongoing support may not be met. This may create a need for a support group or counselor.
Cause of loss or death	Some diseases evoke more compassion than others. A disease that is considered "unclean" or "brought on by themselves" (such as drug use) may be viewed with less sympathy than one that was accidental (such as a car crash).

NURSING CARE

Physical comfort is important to a dying person and the family. Some of the common signs and symptoms the dying client can have are:

- Nausea and vomiting due to slowing of GI tract processes
- Pain due to the disease process or skin breakdown (emotional and spiritual pain may also be present)
- Decreased appetite and thirst due to the slowing of GI tract processes
- Agitation, confusion, and restlessness due to the disease process or medications
- Fever due to the brain's inability to regulate temperature
- External hemorrhaging due to certain disease processes
- Skin wounds due to immobility and loss of body tissue
- Dyspnea (shortness of breath) due to the disease process, fluid buildup, or weakness and inability to cough
- Incontinence of bowel and bladder due to weakness of muscles.

ASSESSING

During the routine health care of a client, the nurse poses questions about previous losses and coping techniques. If there is a current or recent loss, greater detail is needed.

Clients do not always associate physical ailments with emotional responses such as grief. The nurse may need to ask specific questions to help identify possible loss-related stresses. If the client reports significant losses, it is important to understand how the client usually copes with loss and what resources are available to assist the client to cope. This information is gathered to help determine a plan of care. Box 17-2 ■ lists interview questions nurses may ask about loss and grief.

In collecting data on the client's response to a current loss, the nurse may identify dysfunctional grief. This is best treated by a healthcare professional who is expert in assisting such clients. If the observation reveals severe physical or psychological signs and symptoms, the client should be referred to an appropriate care provider.

DIAGNOSING, PLANNING, AND IMPLEMENTING

Some of the most common nursing diagnoses related to grieving are *Anticipatory Grieving* and *Dysfunctional Grieving*. When clients lose a body function or a body part, there are two crucial client goals:

- Adjusting to the changed ability
- Redirecting both physical and emotional energy into rehabilitation.

BOX 17-2 **ASSESSING**

Interview for Loss and Grieving

Previous Losses

- Have you ever lost someone or something very important to you?
- Have you or your family ever moved your home?
- What was it like for you when you first started school? Moved away from home? Got a job? Retired?
- Are you physically able to do all the things you like to do? Used to do?
- Do you think there will be any losses in your life in the near future?

Previous Grieving

- Tell me about (the loss). What was losing _____ like for you?
- Did you have trouble sleeping? Eating? Concentrating?
- What kinds of things did you do to make yourself feel better when something like that happened?
- Are there spiritual or cultural practices you observed when you had a loss like that?
- Who was a person you could turn to if you were very upset about (the loss)?
- How long did it take you to feel more like yourself again and go back to your usual activities?

Current Loss

- What have you been told about (the loss)? Is there anything else you would like to know or don't understand?
- What changes do you think this (illness, surgery) will cause in your life? What do you think it will be like without (the lost object)?
- Have you ever experienced a loss like this before?
- Can you think of anything good that might come out of this?
- What kind of help do you think you will need? Who is going to be helping you with this loss?
- Are there any people or organizations in your community that might be able to help?

Current Grieving

- Are you having trouble sleeping? Eating? Concentrating? Breathing?
- Do you have any pain or other new physical problems?
- Are you taking any drugs or medications to help you cope with this loss?
- What are you doing to help you deal with this loss?

When clients receive a diagnosis of terminal illness, goals are:

- To keep the client comfortable
- To help the client and family accept death.

When clients lose a loved one, priority outcomes are:

- Remembering that person without feeling intense pain
- Redirecting emotional energy into one's own life
- Adjusting to the actual or impending loss.

The nurse can help the client find specific ways of reaching these outcomes. Many times, the best intervention nurses can offer is their caring attention. Learn to listen.

Teach the Client about the Grieving Process

It is often helpful for clients to know more about the process of grieving. For example, nurses can inform clients of the grief stages they can expect to experience over time. They can prepare survivors for feelings of guilt that may arise as they recover from the initial impact of a loss. They can emphasize that holidays and other significant dates may be especially stressful for them. For some people, events and/or anniversaries will trigger painful feelings of loss long after the loss occurred. These feelings

can be alarming to someone who thought they had "gotten over it."

Whenever possible, nurses provide clients with resources to use in the future. They can teach clients that many people go back and forth through the stages of grief at different times. Preparing clients for these times and providing information about support groups and counseling are important aspects of teaching. They can also inform family and friends when the signs of approaching death occur (Box 17-3 ■).

BOX 17-3

Signs of Approaching Death

- Changes in level of consciousness
- Coolness, mottling, and cyanosis of the extremities
- Decreased sensation, taste, and smell
- Decreased, irregular, or *Cheyne-Stokes respirations* (deep to shallow breathing pattern, with periods of apnea)
- Decreasing blood pressure
- Difficulty talking or swallowing
- Nausea, flatus, abdominal distention
- Restlessness, agitation
- Urinary and/or bowel incontinence, constipation
- Weak, slow, and/or irregular pulse

Maintain Physical Comfort

The nurse can help the dying client maintain a level of comfort in several ways:

- Place a castor oil–soaked cloth on the abdomen. Administer antiemetics such as Compazine, Ativan, or Reglan, on schedule as prescribed. *The castor oil compress can act as a naturopathic control for nausea and vomiting. Antiemetics help promote comfort.*

- Apply cold moist compresses to specific painful sites. Provide natural pain relief measures such as relaxation and imagery. Administer prescription medications such as morphine, oxycodone, Dilaudid, and Duragesic around the clock as well as when needed for breakthrough pain. If the client has use of a PCA machine (Figure 17-3 ■), ensure that it is working. *Cold compresses can help to lessen localized pain. Pain medications are most effective when they are administered regularly to maintain a therapeutic level. Having a PCA device gives the client some control over the pain and so reduces anxiety.*

- Explain to the family that decreased circulation of body fluids can cause bloating and swelling. Fluids and food will be offered but never forced. *Decreased fluid and dietary intake can be distressing to the family (who may say the facility is "starving the client"). However, forcing food or fluids by feeding tubes and IVs can make the client more uncomfortable.*

- If a client is agitated, a warm sheet or blanket can be wrapped around the client for short periods of time. Medications such as Ativan, Xanax, Haldol, and Valium (if ordered) also help lessen agitation. *Client safety must always be maintained. Warm wraps can help reduce restlessness and agitation.*

- Provide frequent tepid sponge baths and frequent linen changes for clients with fever. Dress client in light, cotton clothing. Sometimes the fevers will respond to acetaminophen or aspirin as well. *High fevers can be very uncomfortable as the client perspires. Tepid baths and frequent changes of linens and light clothing can promote comfort.*

- If there is external hemorrhaging, put direct pressure and application of ice packs over the bleeding areas. Remain calm. Provide comfort and reassurance. *External hemorrhaging can be very frightening to all present.*

- Provide frequent turning and repositioning to prevent skin breakdown and pain. If skin breakdown already exists, provide dressing changes and good skin care along with pain medication. *Skin breakdown can cause infections as well as increase pain. The best intervention is to prevent skin breakdown. However, as a client enters into the active labor of dying, complete body care may become too uncomfortable. If the client is unable to speak, observe nonverbal communication such as facial expressions for grimacing, or moaning, and even breathing pattern changes.*

- Administer medications such as morphine and Ativan if ordered. Nurses who have been trained can perform chest percussion to help break up fluid collection in the lungs. *Both of these interventions help to ease dyspnea and help the client relax.*

- If client becomes incontinent of bowel and bladder, place a Foley catheter and provide frequent linen changes with extra padding added to the linen. *Incontinence can be distressing and can contribute to skin breakdown. Extra padding can make linen changes easier.*

Encourage Positive Coping

The nurse can assist the person to work through grief. Interventions would include the following:

- Provide opportunities for the client to participate in decision making about daily activities. *Involvement in decision making is empowering and helps the client begin to organize the experience.*

- Encourage the client to share loss with significant others. *This will assist with acceptance of loss.*

- Encourage the client to get increasingly involved in usual activities. *This will help the client establish a routine and help with closure.*

- Encourage the client to get enough sleep and adequate nutrition. *This will help keep the client from getting ill.*

- Encourage the client to seek out support services and resources available to assist during difficult episodes. *This will help promote healthy grieving. An objective listener can sometimes help a person get past an emotional barrier.*

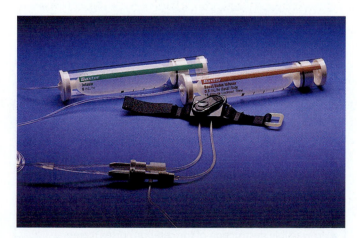

Figure 17-3. ■ PCA units allow the client to self-manage severe pain. Units can be portable or mounted on intravenous poles. (*Source:* Courtesy of Baxter Healthcare Corporation.)

- Encourage the client to verbalize positive expectations for the future. *This will help promote a positive focus.*
- Practice active and attentive listening, open and closed questioning, paraphrasing, clarifying and reflecting feelings, and summarizing. *These communication techniques allow clients to explore their own feelings. It is less helpful to clients for the nurse to respond by giving advice and evaluating, by interpreting and analyzing, or by giving empty reassurances. (See also Chapter 12 ⦾.)*

Communication with grieving clients needs to be appropriate to their stage of grief. For example, denial or depression can affect how a client hears a message or how the nurse interprets the client's comments. Box 17-4 ■ describes specific interventions nurses can perform as they relate to Kübler-Ross's five stages of grieving.

EVALUATING

Evaluating the effectiveness of nursing care of the grieving client is difficult because of the long-term nature of this life transition. Criteria for evaluation must be based on goals set by the client and family.

Client goals and desired outcomes for a grieving client depend on the characteristics of the loss and the client. For example, the nurse might ask about a client's participation in rehabilitation therapy sessions, or about whether the client is now sleeping through the night. Weight gain is an observable outcome in someone who has had no appetite during the first months of grief.

If outcomes are not achieved, the nurse needs to help the team explore why the plan was unsuccessful and adjust the plan as appropriate

Definitions and Signs of Death

Traditionally, clinical signs of death were cessation of the apical pulse, respirations, and blood pressure, also referred to as *heart-lung death*. However, since artificial means were developed to maintain respirations and blood circulation, it has become more difficult to identify death. Now, if a person is connected to life support equipment, death is determined by an absence of brain wave activity (measured by electroencephalogram) for at least 24 hours. Some would also include *cerebral death* (irreversible damage to the cerebral cortex) within the definition of death, even though a person might still be able to breathe. In this case, an irreversible state of unconscious (*vegetative state* or *coma*) becomes a defining factor. Box 17-5 ■ lists indications of death.

BOX 17-4	NURSING CARE CHECKLIST

Assisting Client in Different Stages of Grief

Denial Stage

☑ Verbally support client but do not reinforce denial.

☑ Examine your own behavior to ensure that you do not share in client's denial.

Anger Stage

☑ Help client understand that anger is a normal response to feelings of loss and powerlessness.

☑ Avoid withdrawal or retaliation; do not take anger personally.

☑ Deal with client's needs that underlie any angry reaction.

☑ Provide structure and continuity to promote feelings of security.

☑ Allow clients as much control as possible over their lives.

Bargaining Stage

☑ Listen attentively, and encourage client to talk to relieve guilt and irrational fear.

☑ If appropriate, offer spiritual support.

Depression Stage

☑ Allow client to express sadness.

☑ Communicate nonverbally by sitting quietly without expecting conversation.

☑ Convey caring by touch.

Acceptance Stage

☑ Help family and friends understand client's decreased need to socialize.

☑ Encourage client to participate as much as possible in the treatment program.

BOX 17-5	

Indications of Death

- Total lack of response to external stimuli
- No muscular movement, especially breathing
- No reflexes
- Flat encephalogram

For People on Artificial Support

- Absence of electric currents from the brain (measured by an electroencephalogram) for at least 24 hours
- Irreversible destruction of the cerebral cortex (cerebral death or higher brain death); the client may still be able to breathe but is irreversibly unconscious.

Legal Issues

The nurse's roles in legal issues related to death are determined by the laws of the region and the policies of the healthcare institution. For example, in some states a nasogastric feeding tube cannot be removed from a person in a coma without a prior directive from the client. In other states, the removal is allowed at the family's request or on a physician's order. These legal issues raise strong ethical concerns. The nurse may need support from other team members in understanding issues and providing appropriate care to clients facing death.

ADVANCE DIRECTIVES

The Patient Self-Determination Act, implemented in 1991, requires all healthcare facilities receiving Medicare and Medicaid reimbursement to do the following:

- Recognize advance directives.
- Ask clients whether they have advance directives.
- Provide educational materials advising clients of their rights to declare their personal wishes regarding treatment decisions, including the right to refuse medical treatment.

There are two types of advance medical directives: the living will and the healthcare proxy or surrogate. The **living will** provides specific instructions about what medical treatment the client chooses to omit or refuse in the event that the client becomes unable to make those decisions. Treatments that are commonly included are cardiopulmonary resuscitation (CPR), intubation, and ventilatory (breathing) support.

The healthcare proxy document (also called a **durable power of attorney for health care**) is a written statement appointing someone else to manage healthcare treatment decisions when the client is unable to do so (Figure 17-4 ■). The healthcare proxy is often a relative or trusted friend.

The proxy document is often used for specific clients who are in a coma, are having life-sustaining procedures, or are receiving artificial nutrition or hydration.

DO-NOT-RESUSCITATE ORDERS

Physicians may order "no code" or **Do-not-resuscitate (DNR)** orders for clients who are in a stage of terminal, irreversible illness or expected death. A DNR order is generally written when the client or surrogate has asked for no resuscitation to take place in the event of a respiratory or cardiac arrest. A *comfort measures only* order is written to indicate that the goal of treatment is a comfortable, dignified death and that further life-sustaining measures are not indicated.

LABELING OF THE DECEASED

Nurses have a duty to handle the deceased with dignity and respect and to label the body appropriately. Mishandling can cause emotional distress to survivors. It can also create legal problems if the body is inappropriately identified and prepared incorrectly for funeral services. In the hospital, the deceased's wrist identification tag is left on, and another tag is tied to the client's ankle or toe, in case one of the tags becomes detached. A third tag is attached to the shroud. All identification tags should include the client's name, hospital number, and physician's name. In most hospitals this is provided on the Addressograph plate or hospital card, which has the appropriate information already on it. Refer to Procedure 17-1 ■ on page 321 for postmortem care.

AUTOPSY

An **autopsy** or postmortem examination is an examination of the body after death. It is performed to learn more about the cause of death, to learn more about a disease, or to assist in gathering statistical data.

ORGAN DONATION

The Uniform Anatomical Gift Act and the National Organ Transplant Act in the United States, and the Human Tissue Act in Canada, are acts governing organ donation. Under these acts, people who are 18 years of age or older and of sound mind may become organ donors. They make a gift of all or any part of their own bodies for the following purposes: medical or dental education, research, advancement of medical or dental science, therapy, or transplantation.

Nurses may serve as witnesses for people consenting to donate organs or revoking the organ donor designation. In many states, healthcare workers are required to ask survivors for consent to donate the deceased's organs. Organ donation can be an emotional issue for the bereaved.

Death-Related Religious and Cultural Practices

Cultural and religious traditions and practices help people cope with death, dying, and the grieving process. They give crucial comfort to survivors. Nurses are often present through the dying process and at the moment of death. Knowledge of the client's religious and cultural beliefs helps nurses provide individualized care to clients and their families, even though they may not participate in the family's rituals.

Nurses also need to be knowledgeable about the client's death-related rituals, such as last rites, administration of Holy Communion, or chanting at the bedside (Box 17-6 ■). There may be ritual procedures for washing, dressing, positioning, and shrouding the dead. Certain immigrants may wish to retain their native customs, in which family members of the same sex wash and prepare the body for burial and

POWER OF ATTORNEY FOR HEALTH CARE

(1) DESIGNATION OF AGENT: I designate the following individual as my agent to make health care decisions for me: _____

_____
(Name of individual you choose as agent)

_____
(address) (city) (state) (zip code)

_____
(home phone) (work phone)

OPTIONAL: If I revoke my agent's authority or if my agent is not willing, able, or reasonably available to make a health-care decision for me, I designate as my first alternate agent:

_____
(Name of individual you choose as first alternate agent)

_____
(address) (city) (state) (zip code)

_____
(home phone) (work phone)

OPTIONAL: If I revoke the authority of my agent and first alternate agent or if neither is willing, able, or reasonably available to make a health care decision for me, I designate as my second alternate agent:

_____
(Name of individual you choose as second alternate agent)

_____
(address) (city) (state) (zip code)

_____
(home phone) (work phone)

(2) AGENT'S AUTHORITY: My agent is authorized to make all health care decisions for me, including decisions to provide, withhold, or withdraw artificial nutrition and hydration, and all other forms of health care to keep me alive, **except** as I state here:

(3) WHEN AGENT'S AUTHORITY BECOMES EFFECTIVE: My agent's authority becomes effective when my primary physician determines that I am unable to make my own health care decisions unless I mark the following box. If I mark this box [ ], my agent's authority to make health care decisions for me takes effect immediately.

(4) AGENT'S OBLIGATION: My agent shall make health care decisions for me in accordance with this power of attorney for health care, any instructions I give below, and my other wishes to the extent known to my agent. To the extent my wishes are unknown, my agent shall make health care decisions for me in accordance with what my agent determines to be in my best interest. In determining my best interest, my agent shall consider my personal values to the extent known to my agent.

(5) AGENT'S POSTDEATH AUTHORITY: My agent is authorized to make anatomical gifts, authorize an autopsy, and direct disposition of my remains, except as I state here or elsewhere in this form:

INSTRUCTIONS FOR HEALTH CARE
Strike any wording you do not want.

(6) END-OF-LIFE DECISIONS: I direct that my health care providers and others involved in my care provide, withhold, or withdraw treatment in accordance with the choice I have marked below: **(Initial only one box)**
[ ] (a) **Choice NOT To Prolong Life**
I do not want my life to be prolonged if (1) I have an incurable and irreversible condition that will result in my death within a relatively short time, (2) I become unconscious and, to a reasonable degree of medical certainty, I will not regain consciousness, or (3) the likely risks and burdens of treatment would outweigh the expected benefits, **OR**
[ ] (b) **Choice To Prolong Life**
I want my life to be prolonged as long as possible within the limits of generally accepted health care standards.

(7) RELIEF FROM PAIN: Except as I state in the following space, I direct that treatment for alleviation of pain or discomfort should be provided at all times even if it hastens my death:

DONATION OF ORGANS AT DEATH
(8) Upon my death: (mark applicable box)
[ ] (a) I give any needed organs, tissues, or parts,
OR
[ ] (b) I give the following organs, tissues, or parts only: _____
[ ] (c) My gift is for the following purposes:
(strike any of the following you do not want)
(1) Transplant
(2) Therapy
(3) Research
(4) Education

(9) EFFECT OF COPY: A copy of this form has the same effect as the original.

(10) SIGNATURE: Sign and date the form here:

_____   _____
(date)   (sign your name)

_____   _____
(address)   (print your name)

_____   _____
(city)   (state)

(11) WITNESSES: This advance health care directive will not be valid for making health care decisions unless it is either: (1) signed by two (2) qualified adult witnesses who are personally known to you and who are present when you sign or acknowledge your signature; or (2) acknowledged before a notary public.

Figure 17-4. ■ Sample of power of attorney for health care.

BOX 17-6   **CULTURAL PULSE POINTS**

Supporting Death Rituals

Death rituals are as varied as the number of cultures and religions in any given locale. Differences in these rituals involve the client's beliefs and actions as well as the mourning rituals of the family. Throughout the dying process, the healthcare team should make every effort to provide the time and privacy necessary to carry out the rituals that will show respect for the client. Allow spiritual counselors private time with the client and family. If death is imminent, provide care as unobtrusively as possible so as to not interfere with death rituals. Some cultures use music, drums, and incense. If this is the case, it might be necessary to remove other clients from the area so as to allow the client to be cared for in a culturally sensitive way while not disturbing other clients.

cremation. Muslims also customarily turn the body toward Mecca. Nurses need to ask family members about their preferences and verify who will carry out these activities. The nurse must ensure that any ritual items that were brought to the institution be given to the family or to the funeral home at the time of death to prevent such items from being lost.

PRIORITIES IN NURSING CARE

When caring for clients who are dying, focus your care on meeting physiological needs and supporting the family. Sometimes nurses avoid caring for dying clients because they do not want to "bother" the client. Give personal care as you would to any client to keep them clean and comfortable. Always speak to the client and explain what you are doing. Dying clients are able to hear, even if they are unable to respond. Include the client's family in the care as much as possible. It is a helpless feeling to stand by and watch someone you love as they die. When family members can help with care, it often helps relieve their anxiety. Give the family information about vital signs and other indicators of the client's status. Show kindness and empathy, even if the family seems angry or hostile. They may be angry because their loved one is leaving them or angry at the staff for being unable to save the client. Again, understand that the anger is not meant for you personally. Offer tissues, coffee, and a private area for the family to grieve.

NURSING CARE

ASSESSING

When gathering data to assess a dying client, the nurse must pay attention to the level of awareness of the client and the family. The type of awareness must be considered when planning care and communicating with caregivers. There are three basic types of awareness:

- *Closed awareness.* The client and family are unaware of impending death. They may not completely understand why the client is ill. They believe the client will recover.
- *Mutual pretense.* The client, family, and health personnel know that the prognosis is terminal. However, they do not talk about it and they try not to raise the subject.
- *Open awareness.* Both client and others know about the impending death and feel comfortable discussing it, even though it is difficult.

Nursing care includes collecting data to make accurate assessment of the signs of approaching death. In addition to signs related to the client's specific disease, the four main physical signs of impending death are:

- Loss of muscle tone
- Slowing of the circulation
- Changes in respirations
- Sensory impairment.

See Box 17-3 for additional signs of approaching death.

Various consciousness levels can occur just before death. Some clients are alert. Others are drowsy, stuporous, or comatose. However, hearing is always thought to be the last of the five senses lost. Loved ones may be comforted by knowing that they can talk to the dying loved one and say all the things they want to tell them.

DIAGNOSING, PLANNING, AND IMPLEMENTING

Common priority nursing diagnoses identified for the dying client include *Fear, Hopelessness, Powerlessness, Risk for Caregiver Role Strain,* and *Interrupted Family Processes.*

Maintaining comfort and dignity are two major goals for the dying client. When planning care with these clients, the Dying Person's Bill of Rights can be a useful guide (Figure 17-5 ■). The major nursing responsibility for clients who are dying is to assist the client to a peaceful death.

More specific responsibilities include the following:

- To provide relief from loneliness, fear, and depression (Figure 17-6 ■). *This can be achieved by active listening, therapeutic touch, or just your presence.*
- To maintain the client's sense of security, self-confidence, dignity, and self-worth. *Allowing the client to make treatment decisions and to maintain self-care duties is a way of reinforcing self-worth.*

The Dying Person's Bill of Rights

As we face death, what are our rights as human beings? This bill of rights was created at a workshop on "The Terminally Ill Patient and the Helping Person," sponsored by the Southwestern Michigan Insurance Education Council and conducted by Amelia J. Barbus.

- I have the right to be treated as a living human being until I die.
- I have the right to maintain a sense of hopefulness, however changing its focus may be.
- I have the right to be cared for by those who can maintain a sense of hopefulness, however changing this might be.
- I have the right to express my feelings and emotions about my approaching death in my own way.
- I have the right to participate in decisions concerning my care.
- I have the right to expect continuing medical and nursing attention even though "cure" goals must be changed to "comfort" goals.
- I have the right not to die alone.
- I have the right to be free from pain.
- I have the right to have my questions answered honestly.
- I have the right not to be deceived.
- I have the right to have help from and for my family in accepting my death.
- I have the right to die in peace and dignity.
- I have the right to retain my individuality and not be judged for my decisions which may be contrary to beliefs of others.
- I have the right to discuss and enlarge my religious and/or spiritual experiences, whatever these may mean to others.
- I have the right to expect that the sanctity of the human body will be respected after death.
- I have the right to be cared for by caring, sensitive, knowledgeable people who will attempt to understand my needs and will be able to gain some satisfaction in helping me face my death.

Figure 17-5. ■ The Dying Person's Bill of Rights.

- To maintain hope. This can be achieved by helping clients to think positively about the future. *When recovery is not possible, people can still make peace with their death.*
- To help the client accept losses. *Allowing grief to be expressed encourages healthy grieving.*
- To provide physical comfort. *Healing touch, a back rub, and a warm bath are physical ways to express your concern for the client's well-being.*

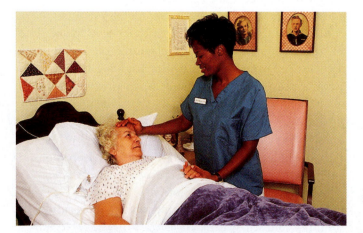

Figure 17-6. ■ The touch of your hand may be the dying person's last memory.

Meeting Physiological Needs of the Dying Client

Dying clients experience a slowing of body processes and homeostatic imbalances. Nursing interventions address the need to provide comfort and dignity to the dying person:

- Assist client to breathe by positioning client in Fowler's position and suctioning client as needed. *This helps mobilize secretions.*
- Help control pain by administering both scheduled and/or as-needed medications on time. Also use non-pharmacological techniques that are effective for the client. *These will help the client relax.*
- Assist with ADLs such as bathing and dressing. *This will help the client feel better physically and will comfort both client and family.*
- Assist with position changes or transfers. *This will promote comfort and decrease skin breakdown.*
- Support client's nutritional needs. Prevent constipation by administering prescribed laxatives or stool softeners. *This will decrease skin breakdown and prevent constipation.*
- Support urinary elimination by supplying easy access to water and juices as appropriate to client. *This will support intake as desired by client.*

- Monitor for sensory deficit or overload by adjusting television or radio volume. *This supports a more comfortable environment and shows respect for client preferences.*

Providing Spiritual Support

Not all clients have a specific religious faith or belief. However, most people need a sense of meaning in their lives, especially when they know they have a terminal illness. The nurse's responsibilities include seeing that the client's spiritual needs are met. This can be done by direct participation or by arranging access to individuals who can provide spiritual care.

Supporting the Family

The most important intervention the nurse can provide to the family members of a dying client is therapeutic communication. Refer to Chapter 12 ⚭ for a full discussion on therapeutic communication. No intervention can reverse the inevitable dying process, but the nurse can provide a caring presence. The nurse can present a calm and patient demeanor and allow client and family to express their grief. When grieving family members have not absorbed some information that they were told, the nurse can reinforce what is happening or what the family can expect. Some clients or families may need to have information repeated several times.

Family members should be allowed and encouraged to participate in the physical care of the dying person if they want to and are able. The nurse can suggest they assist with bathing, speak or read to the client, and hold hands. The nurse must realize, however, that every family member's desire and ability to help may be different. Those who feel unable to be with the dying person also require support from the nurse and from other family members. They should be shown to a quiet waiting area if they just wish to stay nearby. Close contact among several generations may help the survivors cope with the loss.

Providing Postmortem Care

After death, some characteristic physical changes occur. **Rigor mortis** is the stiffening of the body that occurs about 2 to 4 hours after death. It results from a lack of adenosine triphosphate (ATP). ATP is necessary for muscle fiber relaxation. Without it the muscles contract, which makes the joints rigid. Rigor mortis starts in the involuntary muscles (heart, bladder, etc.), then progresses to the head, neck, and trunk, and finally reaches the extremities. Rigor mortis usually leaves the body about 96 hours after death.

Algor mortis is the gradual decrease of the body's temperature after death. When blood circulation terminates and the hypothalamus ceases to function, body temperature falls about 1°C (1.8°F) per hour until it reaches room temperature. Simultaneously, the skin loses its elasticity and can easily be broken when dressings and adhesive tape are removed.

After blood circulation has ceased, the red blood cells break down, releasing hemoglobin, which discolors the surrounding tissues. This discoloration, referred to as **livor mortis**, appears in the lower (most *dependent*) areas of the body.

Tissues after death become soft, and bacterial fermentation eventually liquefies them. The hotter the temperature, the more rapid the change. Bodies are often stored in cool places to delay this process. Embalming prevents the process through injection of chemicals into the body to destroy the bacteria.

The nurse must be familiar with institutional policies and procedures about care of a body after death. Postmortem care should be carried out according to the policy of the institution. Because care of the body may be influenced by religious law, the nurse should check the client's religion and make every attempt to comply. If the deceased's family or friends wish to view the body, it is important to make the environment as clean and pleasant as possible and to make the body appear natural and comfortable. All equipment, soiled linen, and supplies should be removed from the bedside. Some institutions require that all tubes in the body remain in place. In other institutions, tubes may be cut to within 2.5 cm (1 in.) of the skin and taped in place. In still others, all tubes may be removed.

Normally the body is placed in a supine position with the arms either at the sides, palms down, or across the abdomen. One or two pillows are placed under the head and shoulders, or the head of the bed is elevated 30 degrees, to prevent blood from discoloring the face by settling in it. The eyelids are closed and held in place for a few seconds. Often, the eyes and mouth do not remain closed and require the intervention of a *mortician* (an undertaker or funeral director; a person trained in care of the dead).

Soiled areas of the body are washed. However, a complete bath is not necessary, because the body will be washed by the mortician. Absorbent pads are placed under the buttocks to capture any feces and urine released because of relaxation of the sphincter muscles. A clean gown is placed on the client, and the hair is brushed and combed. All jewelry is removed, except a wedding band in some instances, which is taped to the finger. The top bed linens are adjusted neatly to cover the client to the shoulders. Soft lighting and chairs should be provided for the family to make the surroundings as peaceful as possible.

In the hospital, after the body has been viewed by the family, additional identification tags are applied. The body is wrapped in a *shroud,* a large piece of plastic or cotton material used to enclose a body after death. Identification is placed on the outside of the shroud. The body is then taken to the morgue if arrangements have not been made to have a mortician pick it up from the client's room. Again, the nurse will need to be familiar with the institutional polices and procedures in order to make these events go as smoothly as possible for the family.

EVALUATING

The nurse evaluates care of the dying client by observing the client's relationship with significant others and by listening to the client directly. Ask about the client's feelings and thoughts. Is the client as physically comfortable as possible? Is pain sufficiently relieved? Does the client find the treatment plan acceptable? Is the client satisfied with visitation of family and support people?

NURSING PROCESS CARE PLAN
Client in Denial

Mrs. Smith is a 52-year-old smoker with a diagnosis of COPD. She has been smoking a pack of cigarettes a day for 32 years. She was admitted to the hospital for shortness of breath. Her condition has worsened during the last 5 years. She has more periods of shortness of breath and less quality of life. She needs continuous oxygen therapy. Her primary physician has begun speaking to her and her family about hospice care. Mrs. Smith explains to her physician that she does not want to go somewhere to die. She believes she will get better and she continues to go outside the hospital and smoke.

Assessment. She has several crisis episodes in which skin color is dusky and her nail beds are blue despite being on continuous oxygen therapy. Her physician speaks to her again about palliative care and hospice. This time Mrs. Smith agrees to hospice but she is very angry at her physician for "giving up." The physician writes the order for the social worker and discharge planning nurse to make the hospice referral.

Nursing Diagnosis. The following important nursing diagnoses (among others) are established for this client:

- *Powerlessness* related to terminal illness
- *Grieving* related to terminal illness.

Expected Outcomes. The expected outcomes specify that Mrs. Smith will:

- Participate in self-care activities as much as she is able.
- Make choices related to care and treatment.
- Maintain physiological comfort.

- Share values and personal meaning of life.
- Gain acceptance of the terminal state of her illness.

Planning and Implementation. The following nursing interventions are planned and implemented:

- Teach client and family about hospice and its philosophy.
- Reinforce to the client and family that hospice care is not about "giving up."
- Allow client to verbalize feelings.
- Identify support systems available to client and family.
- Allow client to participate in decision making about daily activities.
- Encourage client in self-care activities.
- Teach the client and family about appropriate grieving responses.

Evaluation. After 3 months in home hospice, Mrs. Smith's symptoms are under control with medications and oxygen. Her appetite has significantly decreased and she sleeps most of the time. After the fourth month in home hospice, Mrs. Smith dies peacefully at home.

Critical Thinking in the Nursing Process

1. Why is it important to allow Mrs. Smith to participate in self-care activities and decision making?
2. Why has Mrs. Smith's appetite decreased?
3. In order to control Mrs. Smith's pain, a combination fast-acting and long-acting narcotic is used. Why is this combination of medications ordered for terminally ill clients?

Note: Discussion of Critical Thinking questions appears in Appendix I.

Nurse's Response to Death

When working with clients who are chronically and terminally ill, it is natural for a nurse to form a bond with them. A nurse's personal views about death and dying and his or her personal coping techniques can affect how the nurse handles the death of a client. Nonetheless, it can still be hard to lose someone to whom you have become close. Some things you can do to promote your own healthy grieving are to recognize your grief and to cry if necessary. Some nurses attend memorial services or funeral services in order to provide the closure they need. Some units may hold their own special services or rituals to remember those who have died.

Note: The references and resources for this and all chapters have been compiled at the back of the book.

PROCEDURE 17-1   Performing Postmortem Care

Purpose

- To clear and prepare the body of a deceased client for family visitation and for transport to mortuary.

Equipment

- Bathing supplies
- Morgue packet
- Identification tags
- Rolled gauze and abdominal pads
- Plastic bag for client's personal belongs
- Gurney or morgue cart
- Clean gloves

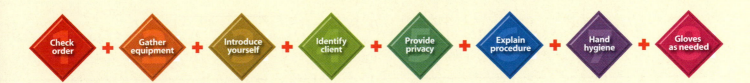

Interventions

1. If there are other clients or visitors in the room, temporarily remove them if possible *to provide privacy.*

2. Collect necessary equipment.

3. Follow facility procedures for notification of personnel and other departments:
   a. Follow the client's advance directives on file at the hospital for donor instructions.
   b. Determine if the client has a donor card and/or has made a decision to donate any organs.
   c. Notify appropriate hospital personnel or local procurement organization for assistance with organ donation.
   d. Follow specific procedures for organ transplants according to hospital policy.

4. Maintain proper alignment of the body. Raise the head of the bed 30 degrees. Maintain head elevation throughout care and transport to the morgue. *This prevents pooling of fluids in the head or face.*

5. Don gloves.

6. Do not replace dentures. *As facial muscles relax, dentures can fall out and be lost.* Leave dentures in denture cup and send with client to the morgue.

7. Remove any external objects causing pressure or injury to the skin (e.g., oxygen mask).

8. Convert all IV lines to intermittent infusion devices. *Removing catheter and IV lines can cause fluid to leak into tissues and cause edema and discoloration.* Hospital policy may supersede this action; if so, follow hospital policy.

9. Cleanse the body as needed. *Partial bath may be required to remove secretions, wound drainage, stains.*

10. Close the eyes, if necessary, using paper tape or gauze pads. You may do this after the family has visited the deceased.

11. Place protective incontinent pad under the buttocks and between the legs diaper fashion.

12. If the family is to visit the deceased, provide clean linen and gown for client.

13. Remove equipment used for cleaning the client.

14. If previously determined or requested by client or family, notify the appropriate clergy or religious support person.

15. After the family and clergy have visited, label the body, attaching ID tags to the great toe, wrist, and morgue bag or as determined by standard procedure.

16. Place arms and hands loosely at side or on abdomen. *Prevents discoloration of hands.*

17. Place the body in the shroud or morgue bag.

18. Label all personal belongings and place in bag.

19. Remove gloves and wash hands.

20. Close doors to client's room, clear hallways in preparation to transfer the body to the morgue.

21. Transfer the body to the morgue on a gurney or morgue cart. Keep client's head elevated.

22. Place client's personal belongings in the appropriate place determined by the facility.

23. Support family members as needed.

clinical ALERT

Inform the funeral home if the client has any infectious disease so that appropriate care can be taken to prevent contamination of personnel or the environment.

SAMPLE DOCUMENTATION

[date]
[time]   Without pulse or spontaneous respirations at 0600 assessment. Dr. Smitts notified at 0610. Pronounced by Dr. Owens at 0620. Family notified at 0630. Postmortem care provided. Family and clergy visited. Personal belongings signed for and taken by John Marsh (son). Peace Brothers Mortuary notified. Body transported to the morgue.

_____L. Anderson, LPN

Chapter Review

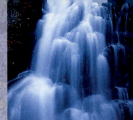

 ## KEY TERMS by Topic

Use the audio glossary feature of either the CD-ROM or the Companion Website to hear the correct pronunciation of the following key terms.

Chronic Illness
chronic illness, remission, exacerbation, primary prevention, secondary prevention, tertiary prevention, rehabilitation

Terminal Illness
palliative care

Grief, Death, and Dying
loss, grief, bereavement, mourning, anticipatory grieving, dysfunctional grieving, denial, anger, bargaining, depression, acceptance

Legal Issues
living will, durable power of attorney for health care, do-not-resuscitate (DNR), autopsy

Postmortem Nursing Care
rigor mortis, algor mortis, livor mortis

KEY Points

- Nurses help clients deal with all types of chronic illnesses. They educate clients on how to prevent chronic illnesses, and they also help clients live with their chronic illnesses.

- Nurses have two big roles in helping clients with chronic disease processes in rehabilitation. The first is to see that disability is limited as much as possible. The second is to plan and implement a rehabilitation program appropriate for the client.

- The most important contribution to a client's rehabilitation is made by clients themselves.

- Nurses help clients deal with all kind of losses, such as loss of body image, loss of limbs, loss of function, and death.

- Palliative care or palliative management shifts treatment goals from curative to comfort.

- Hospice care is based on the holistic concepts of palliative care and emphasizes quality of life.

- Grieving is a normal, subjective emotional response to loss. It is essential for mental and physical health.

- Knowledge of different stages of grieving can help the nurse understand the responses and needs of the client.

- How an individual deals with loss is related to the individual's stage of development, personal resources, and social support.

- Caring for the dying and bereaved is one of the nurse's most challenging responsibilities.

- Nurses must know their responsibilities with regard to legal and policy issues surrounding death.

- Dying clients and their families require open communication and physical, emotional, and spiritual support to achieve a peaceful and dignified death.

 ## EXPLORE MediaLink

Additional interactive resources for this chapter can be found on the Companion Website at www.prenhall.com/ramont. Click on Chapter 17 and "Begin" to select the activities for this chapter.

For chapter-related NCLEX®-style questions and an audio glossary, access the accompanying CD-ROM in this book.

Animations/Videos
- Care of the Dying
- Terminally Ill Patients

FOR FURTHER Study

See Figure 5-4 for Maslow's hierarchy of needs.

Refer to Chapter 12 for a full discussion on therapeutic communication.

See Chapters 23 for positioning limbs to prevent contractures and additional information on preventing skin breakdown.

Refer to Chapters 25 and 26 for information on adequate nutrition and fluid intake.

See Chapter 35 for a description of different types of health-care facilities.

Critical Thinking Care Map

Caring for a Client with Anticipatory Grieving

NCLEX-PN® Focus Area: Psychosocial Integrity

Case Study: Mr. Morris is at the end stages of advanced stage IV lung cancer. He has been admitted to an inpatient hospice setting because the family is having difficulty taking care of him at home.

Nursing Diagnosis: Anticipatory Grieving

COLLECT DATA

Subjective	Objective
_____	_____
_____	_____
_____	_____
_____	_____
_____	_____
_____	_____
_____	_____

Would you report this? Yes/No

If yes, to: _____

What would you report? _____

Nursing Care

_____
_____
_____
_____
_____
_____
_____
_____
_____
_____
_____
_____
_____

How would you document this? _____
_____
_____

Compare your documentation to the sample provided in Appendix I.

Data Collected
(use those that apply)

- Reports poor appetite
- Easily fatigued
- Skin color pink
- Skin color dusky
- Increased appetite
- Drowsy
- BP 90/40
- States pain is 9 on scale of 1 to 10

Nursing Interventions
(use those that apply; list in priority order)

- Auscultate breath sounds with RN.
- Position client for comfort.
- Encourage client to take a shower.
- Encourage client to eat.
- Set up for a bed bath.
- Moisten client's lips as needed.
- Administer oxygen as needed.
- Use therapeutic touch and encourage family communication.
- Administer pain medications as ordered around the clock.
- Observe family responses to grieving and offer appropriate support.

1 Both a client in end-stage renal failure and her family are aware of the signs of approaching death, but they do not talk about it. They are manifesting which state of awareness?

1. closed awareness
2. mutual pretense
3. open awareness
4. undisclosed pretense

2 A client diagnosed with inoperable lung cancer states, "Please get my discharge papers ready. We had vacation plans before I got this cold, and I feel well enough to go." The client is experiencing which stage of the grief process?

1. denial
2. anger
3. bargaining
4. acceptance

3 An unmarried adult is admitted following a motor vehicle crash. He is unresponsive and has been placed on life support. His mother and domestic partner arrive. His mother states, "I can't bear to take him off life support. I know he would want everything to be done." The domestic partner produces a notarized Durable Power of Attorney for Health Care that states no life support is to be used and that gives control to the partner. The physician must consider:

1. the mother's wishes.
2. the domestic partner's wishes.
3. the instructions outlined in the document.
4. the ER physician's assessment.

4 Following the death of a client, the nursing assistant leaves the room quickly and is found sobbing in the utility room. Which action would be the most supportive?

1. Sending the nursing assistant home for the rest of the shift
2. Reassigning the nursing assistant to an area where it is unlikely that a client may die
3. Sitting with her and allowing her to express how she feels
4. Insisting that she perform postmortem care for the client

5 A terminally ill client is alert but death seems imminent. He does not want any measures to prolong his life. What is your most important nursing action at this time?

1. Sit quietly and hold the dying client's hand.
2. Move the client to the hall so he can be observed.
3. Place him in a single room near the nursing stations.
4. Tell him to put on his call light if he needs anything.

6 The parents of a stillborn infant wish to see the body. The nurse should:

1. Show them the baby but not allow them to touch the baby.
2. Wash and clean the baby and wrap it in a soft baby blanket prior to allowing the parents to see and hold the baby.
3. Request that only the mother see the baby.
4. Not allow the mother to remove the blanket from the baby.

7 A client has terminal cancer and the physician has recommended hospice care to the family. The most appropriate explanation of hospice is:

1. "Hospice nurses give better care than the hospital nurses."
2. "Hospice care is cheaper than hospital care."
3. "Hospice allows terminal clients to be cared for at home."
4. "Hospice uses specialized equipment not available in the hospital."

8 Which of the following criteria must be met in order for the physician to pronounce the client on life support dead?

1. The family must agree to discontinuance of life support.
2. Absence of brain activity for at least 24 hours.
3. The client may still be able to breathe but is irreversibly unconscious.
4. A court order to discontinue life support.

9 A widower reports headache, loss of appetite, and inability to sleep following his wife's death. He related that his symptoms increased on his wife's birthday. He states he would just like to die and be with her. The most appropriate nursing diagnosis is:

1. *Anticipatory Grief*
2. *Compromised Family Coping*
3. *Dysfunctional Grieving*
4. *Compromised Individual Coping*

10 An 11-year-old child's grandfather has just died. Of the following statements, which is most developmentally appropriate?

1. "Grampa will get better and come home soon."
2. "I got mad because my grandfather would not buy me a video game. That is why he got sick."
3. "What happens after someone dies? Will Grampa's body go to heaven or just his heart?"
4. "When people die they go to live with God. I'm sad but Grampa isn't sick anymore, so that is good."

Answers and Rationales for Review Questions, as well as discussion of Care Plan and Critical Thinking Care Map questions, appear in Appendix I.

Thinking Strategically About...

You have been assigned your first case as an LPN working for a community hospice agency. The client is a 68-year-old Hispanic woman whose breast cancer has metastasized to her spine. The RN completed the intake interview with the family yesterday at the hospital. The client has been discharged to her home. You have reviewed her discharge plan and see that no additional treatment has been recommended because of her rapidly advancing disease.

When you arrive at home, the client's daughter meets you in the driveway and asks you to remove your name badge, which indicates you are from the hospice organization. She states, "Mother doesn't know how sick she is. We want her last days to be happy. We don't want her to think about dying." The daughter asks you to say that the doctor sent you to help with her bath and to see if all the equipment arrived.

You observe that the family relationship is very close and loving, but that there seems to be an underlying strain. You adhere to the daughter's request during that visit, but when you return to the agency you ask to have a conference with the RN and the social worker.

CULTURAL COMPETENCY

- Do you think that keeping the terminal diagnosis from the client has any relationship to culture?

- How can a nurse who adheres to values of honesty and individualism maintain integrity while honoring this client's culture?

CRITICAL THINKING

- What legal and ethical issues occur when a client's "right to know" is not addressed?
- What are the implications of this for healthcare institutions and workers?

COMPASSIONATE CARING

- How can you help the client to obtain a sense of closure if the family refuses to talk about the impending death?
- What tools are available that do not violate the family's specific request?

COMMUNITY CARE STRATEGIES

Arrange a visit to a family support group for people in hospice. Observe how the facilitator works with families to draw them out. List communication strategies used in these settings to allow people to face the death of a loved one and to cope with their grief.

Promoting Physiological Health

UNIT IV

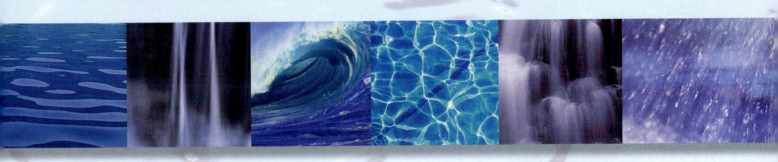

Chapter 18

Introduction to the Body

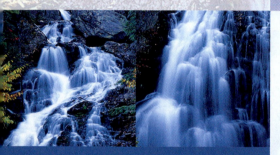

BRIEF Outline

Levels of Organization
Tissues
Body Systems
Anatomic Positions
Body Cavities

HISTORICAL Perspectives

Henry Gray was an English anatomist and surgeon and was elected a fellow of the Royal Society at the young age of 25. On May 6, 1845, he entered as a perpetual student at St. George's Hospital, London, and he is described by those who knew him as a most painstaking and methodical worker, and one who learned his anatomy by the slow but invaluable method of making dissections for himself.

In 1858, Gray published the first edition of his Anatomy, *which covered 750 pages and contained 363 figures. Students continue to use Gray's Anatomy today, which is now in its thirty-ninth edition.*

LEARNING Outcomes

After completing this chapter, you will be able to:

1. Define the terms *anatomy* and *physiology*.
2. Describe the levels of organization of the human body from the very simple to the very complex.
3. Describe the structure of a cell.
4. Understand the functions of the cell organelles.
5. Describe and understand the forms of cell division: mitosis and meiosis.
6. Describe the four main tissue classifications.
7. Explain the difference between exocrine and endocrine glands.
8. List the major body systems and describe the general function of each.
9. List and define the directional terms for the body.
10. List and define the three planes used to divide the body.
11. List the different body cavities and the organs found in each.

The study of the human body or, more specifically, **anatomy** and **physiology**, is absolutely essential for those considering a career in the health sciences. In fact, anyone can benefit from this knowledge. With rapid advances being made in the fields of biology and health care, people are being asked to make important decisions about their health and the health of their families. A basic understanding of anatomy and physiology can help people to make informed decisions.

So what exactly is meant by the terms *anatomy* and *physiology*? Anatomy is the study of the structure of the body, including its size, shape, and composition. Physiology is the study of how the body and its parts function separately and as a whole. These two fields of study form the basis for the study of medicine.

Levels of Organization

In the study of anatomy and physiology, it is readily apparent that the body's structure and functions are organized in increasing levels of complexity. The levels of organization begin with chemicals and progress to cells, tissues, organs, and organ systems and ultimately the organism as a whole. We will begin our study at the chemical level.

CHEMICAL LEVEL

Broken down to its most basic level, the human body is simply a collection of chemicals that combine to form increasingly complex structures. These structures in turn combine to form the basic unit of life, the cell.

CELL STRUCTURE

From the simplest microorganism to the complex human being, all living things share one common characteristic: They are made of cells. The **cell** is the basic unit of all life (Figure 18-1 ■). It is the simplest structure that possesses all the characteristics of life: organization, metabolism, responsiveness, **homeostasis**, growth, and reproduction.

The human body consists of trillions of individual cells. Although they do not all have the same functions and characteristics, they do share certain basic elements. The following are some of the shared characteristics.

Like the body, cells have a "skin." This "skin" is more properly known as the cell membrane or plasma membrane. The **cell membrane** functions as the boundary between the internal or intracellular environment and the external or extracellular environment of cells. Structurally it is a selectively permeable, double-layered membrane that is composed of phospholipids (fats or fatlike substances containing phosphorus), cholesterol, and proteins. The lipid nature of the cell membrane allows fat-soluble materials to enter and exit the cells through a process known as diffusion. The presence of *cholesterol* strengthens the cell membrane and helps to maintain its flexibility.

The different proteins found in the cell membrane generally fall into one of the following five functional categories:

1. **Receptors**—points of attachment for certain materials such as hormones on the surface of the cell membrane
2. **Enzymes**—proteins that catalyze the chemical reactions that occur at the cell membrane
3. **Channels**—openings or pores that permit the passage of certain materials into or out of the cell
4. **Transporters**—proteins that actively move materials that are too big for the channels through the cell membrane in both directions
5. **Antigens**—markers that identify the type of cell and help the immune system determine whether the cell should be present within the organism or whether it is foreign to the organism

Cytoplasm

The main substance filling the inside of the cell is a *colloidal* (jelly-like) suspension known as **cytoplasm**. This suspension consists of minerals, nutrients, and enzymes in water. Many of the cell's chemical reactions occur in the cytoplasm. Most of the organelles are found there.

Organelles

Within the cell are structures, often bound in their own membranes, known as *organelles* (meaning "little organs"). These are special subdivisions, similar to the human body's organs, which carry out many of the functions of the cell.

NUCLEUS.   The most prominent organelle is the **nucleus**. All cells in the human body (except for mature red blood cells) possess a nucleus. The nucleus is bound by a double-layered nuclear membrane and is the location of the genetic

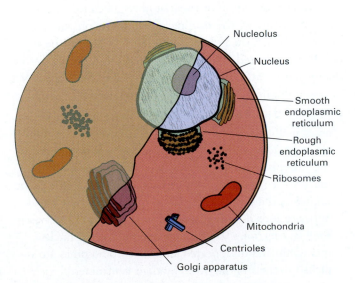

Nucleolus

Nucleus

Smooth endoplasmic reticulum

Rough endoplasmic reticulum

Ribosomes

Mitochondria

Centrioles

Golgi apparatus

Figure 18-1. ■ Human cell. (*Source:* Drawing by Thomas Ramont.)

material or deoxyribonucleic acid (DNA) of the cell. The DNA combined with proteins form the 46 chromosomes associated with human cells and can be thought as the instruction manual for assembling all of the proteins of the body. It is because of this that the nucleus is often referred to as the control center of the cell.

NUCLEOLUS AND RIBOSOMES.

Within the nucleus is a small sphere known as the nucleolus, which is composed of DNA, ribonucleic acid (RNA), and protein. The nucleolus is where organelles known as ribosomes are assembled. After assembly, the ribosomes travel from the nucleus into the cytoplasm. Some of the ribosomes continue to float freely within the cytoplasm. Others attach themselves to the endoplasmic reticulum. This structure is referred to as rough endoplasmic reticulum. Once the ribosomes leave the nucleus they serve as the sites of protein synthesis.

ENDOPLASMIC RETICULUM.

The **endoplasmic reticulum (ER)** is a network of membrane-bound tubules that extends from the cell membrane to the nuclear membrane. The ER functions as a transport system for the lipids and proteins needed for cell function. The endoplasmic reticulum comes in two forms. If ribosomes are present on its surface it is known as *rough ER;* if ribosomes are not present, the endoplasmic reticulum is referred to as *smooth ER.* Smooth ER serves as the site of lipid and cholesterol synthesis and drug detoxification. Rough ER is responsible for the transport of proteins produced by the ribosomes on its surface to the Golgi apparatus and other sites of the cell.

MITOCHONDRIA.

Mitochondria are large organelles surrounded by a double membrane. Often referred to as "power plants," they are the site of the aerobic phase of cellular respiration where **adenosine triphosphate (ATP)** is produced. Because ATP is the energy compound of cells, large numbers of mitochondria are found in cells that require large amounts of energy, such as muscle cells.

GOLGI APPARATUS.

The **Golgi apparatus** consists of layers of flat, membranous sacs. Its principal function is to package and modify proteins received from the endoplasmic reticulum. Once modified, these proteins may be secreted from the cell, become part of the plasma membrane, or be packaged into membranous sacs called lysosomes and remain in the cell.

LYSOSOMES.

Lysosomes are small membranous sacs that contain digestive enzymes. Their functions include breaking down waste and foreign materials, and helping to destroy bacteria engulfed by white blood cells known as phagocytes.

PEROXISOMES.

Peroxisomes are small membranous sacs that contain oxidase enzymes. These enzymes are used to detoxify harmful substances such as alcohol and to neutralize highly reactive compounds known as free radicals.

CENTRIOLES.

A pair of rod-shaped structures known as *centrioles* is located outside the nucleus. They provide attachment points for the spindle fibers that help separate the chromosomes during cell division.

CILIA AND FLAGELLA.

Some cells contain small projections known as cilia and flagella. **Cilia** are hairlike projections on the surface of some cells. Their function is to sweep back and forth, creating movement around the cell. Cells with cilia can be found in the respiratory and reproductive tracts. In contrast, a **flagellum** is a long, whiplike extension from a cell that is used to move the cell itself. The only human cells with flagella are sperm cells.

CELL DIVISION

In order for an organism to grow, repair damage, and reproduce, its cells must be able to increase their numbers through a process known as *cell division.* The two forms of cell division, mitosis and meiosis, serve very different purposes.

Mitosis

We all started life as a single fertilized egg cell. By the time adulthood is reached, the average human body contains approximately 75 trillion cells. In addition, our cells experience constant wear and tear. Because the average cell does not live as long as a person, a process is needed to produce more cells for growth and repair. This process consists of two events, mitosis and cytokinesis, that result in the production of two daughter cells that are genetically identical to the parent cell.

Mitosis or nuclear division is a four-stage process that results in the formation of two daughter nuclei that contain the same genes as the original nucleus. Before the parent nucleus divides, the genetic material (DNA) must be replicated or duplicated. This replication of DNA occurs during a stage in the cell's life known as interphase. Once the DNA has been duplicated, mitosis can begin (Figure 18-2 ■).

■ *Prophase.* The chromosomes coil up so tightly that they are actually visible as short rods if viewed through a microscope. Due to the DNA replication that occurred during interphase, each chromosome consists of two strands known as chromatids that are connected at a single point known as the centromere. The centrioles move toward opposite ends of the cell and spindle fibers form between the two centrioles. By the end of prophase the nuclear membrane has disappeared and the chromosomes are attached to the spindle fibers by their centromeres.

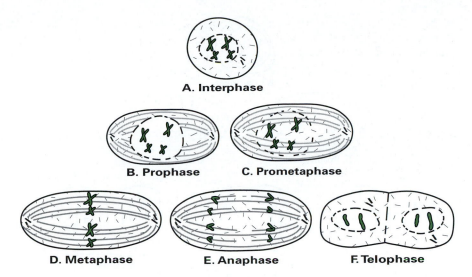

Figure 18-2. ■ Steps in cell mitosis. (*Source:* Drawing by Thomas Ramont.)

■ *Prometaphase.* The nuclear membrane dissolves, making the beginning of prometaphase. Protein attack to the centromeres creating the kinetochores. Microtubules attack at the kinetochores and the chromosomes begin moving.
■ *Metaphase.* The chromosomes line up across the equator of the cell.
■ *Anaphase.* The duplicated chromosomes separate and are pulled toward opposite ends of the cell by the spindle fibers.
■ *Telophase.* The chromosomes at each end of the cell uncoil and a nuclear membrane forms around each set of chromosomes.

In addition to division of the nucleus, the cytoplasm of the parent cell must also be divided. This event is known as cytokinesis. It begins during anaphase and is completed by the end of telophase. As the chromosomes move toward opposite ends of the cell, the cell begins to pinch in the middle and continues until the parent cell divides into two daughter cells. The daughter cells are smaller than the original cell, but otherwise they are genetically identical to the parent cell. The daughter cells will grow and carry out the same functions as the parent cell until they divide.

While all the cells in the human body are capable of mitosis, the rate at which it occurs varies widely. For example, skin cells and the cells of the stomach lining are in almost constant mitosis due to the continuous stress they are under. At the opposite extreme are nerve cells (neurons) and most muscle cells. In an adult, these cells do not experience mitosis. If they are damaged, they are not repaired. This is why, when a person's spinal cord is severed, permanent paralysis occurs below the point of injury.

There is also a general tendency for mitosis to occur more slowly as a person ages. As a result, bone fractures and lacerations take longer to heal in the elderly than in a young person.

Meiosis
Unlike mitosis, which results in two cells that are genetically identical to their parent cell, **meiosis** produces sex cells or **gametes** (sperm and egg cells) that have only half the number of chromosomes as the other cells found in the body. This means that in humans the gametes contain 23 chromosomes while the other cells of the body possess 46 chromosomes. This ensures that when an egg cell is fertilized by a sperm cell, the resulting zygote has only 46 chromosomes (Figure 18-3 ■). Meiosis in men occurs in the testes and is known as spermatogenesis, while in women it is known as oogenesis and takes place in the ovaries.

Tissues
Just as it takes a variety of materials to construct a building, so it is with **tissue** and the human body. While the cell is the basic unit of life, there is not one cell in the human body capable of carrying out all of the functions necessary to keep the body alive. Instead, the cells become specialized so that they can perform different functions. For example, liver cells only perform those functions associated with the liver. Muscle cells only do those things associated with muscles. Cells with similar structure and function group together and are referred to as tissues. There are four main classifications of tissue: epithelial, connective, muscle, and nervous tissue.

EPITHELIAL TISSUE
Epithelial tissue or epithelium is the tissue that forms a covering, lines a body cavity or passage, or forms glands. Some

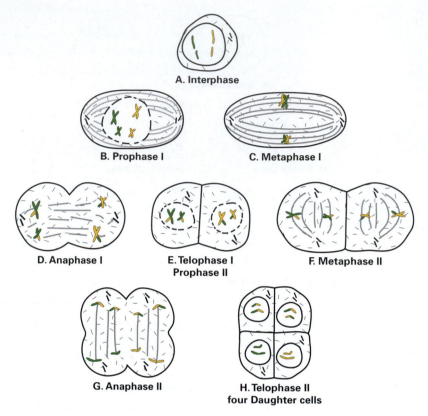

Figure 18-3. ■ Steps in cell meiosis. (*Source:* Drawing by Thomas Ramont.)

places that epithelium can be found are the outer layer of the skin; the lining of the respiratory, intestinal, and urinary tracts; blood vessels; and various glands of the body.

Functions of **epithelium** include protection, absorption, filtration, and secretion. The epithelium tissue of the skin acts as a barrier to protect against bacteria entering the body. In the digestive tract, epithelium allows for the absorption of nutrients. Filtration is performed by the epithelial tissue of the kidneys. Glandular epithelium produces different secretions such as mucus, digestive enzymes, and hormones.

To help in identifying the different epithelial tissue of the body, a two-part classification system is used. The first part is based on the number of cell layers and the second on the general shape of the cells in the tissue. *Simple epithelium* is the term used to indicate one layer of cells. *Stratified epithelium* is the term for more than one cell layer. For cell shape one of three terms is used:

■ *Squamous* cells are thin, flat, and irregular in shape.
■ *Cuboidal* cells are square or cube shaped.
■ *Columnar* cells are longer than they are wide.

The terms to indicate the number of layers and general cell shape are used together to describe or classify the epithelium. For example, the outer layer of the skin consists of many layers of thin, flat cells. Thus, the term *stratified squa-*

mous describes the epithelium in the outer portion of the skin.

There is one type of epithelial tissue that does not fit into this classification system. *Transitional epithelium* varies in shape from squamous to round and tends to be stratified. This tissue is found in the urinary bladder and the ureters. These cells change shape depending on the bladder's fullness.

Several types of epithelia are capable of producing secretions. When tissue produces some form of secretion it is referred to as a gland. **Glands** are divided into two categories: exocrine and endocrine glands. **Exocrine glands** have ducts that carry the secretions away from the gland. Examples include sweat, sebaceous (oil), and lacrimal (tear) glands. **Endocrine glands** do not have ducts. Their secretions, known as **hormones**, are transported away from the gland by blood flowing through the gland. The pituitary, thyroid, and adrenal glands are examples of endocrine glands.

CONNECTIVE TISSUE

Connective tissue is the supporting fabric of the body. It can be found everywhere and is the most abundant body tissue type. As its name implies, connective tissue is responsible for connecting different body tissues together. However, connective tissue is not limited to that one function. Additional functions include cushioning, insulation, support, protection, transportation, and storage.

There are several types of connective tissue. They vary greatly in appearance and function. They do however share three basic characteristics: (1) the presence of protein fibers, (2) specialized connective tissue cells, and (3) a nonliving extracellular matrix.

In many ways, the extracellular **matrix** is responsible for the unique properties associated with each type of connective tissue. The three main components of extracellular matrix are (1) ground substance, (2) protein fibers, and (3) fluid that consists of water. The ground substance usually consists of nonfibrous proteins and polysaccharide molecules. The nonfibrous proteins act like a glue in that they allow the connective tissue cells to attach themselves to the extracellular matrix. The polysaccharide molecules are a principal component in the relative hardness of the different connective tissues. As the number of polysaccharide molecules increases, the extracellular matrix becomes firmer or harder.

Three different protein fibers are associated with connective tissue. They are collagen, elastic, and reticular fibers. Collagen fibers are the most abundant and strongest of the three fibers. Elastic fibers possess the ability to stretch and return to their original shape. Reticular fibers often form the internal framework of soft organs such as the liver and spleen.

The following descriptions of the different connective tissues are arranged from softest to hardest and include liquid connective tissue, loose connective tissue, dense connective tissue, cartilage, and bone.

Liquid Connective Tissue

Blood and lymph fluid are liquid connective tissue. They consist of cells suspended in a liquid matrix. The matrix in blood is plasma. The specialized cells are red blood cells, white blood cells, and platelets. The protein fibers are usually soluble and only become visible during clotting. The matrix in lymph is tissue fluid and soluble protein fibers, while the cells are predominantly lymphocytes and some macrophages. Both of these tissues serve as transport medium in their respective body systems.

Loose Connective Tissue

Loose connective tissue serves as the filler material of the body. It can be found around organs, between muscles, and under the skin. The different forms are areolar tissue, adipose tissue, and reticular connective tissue.

Areolar tissue is the most widely distributed connective tissue. The matrix consists of tissue fluid, collagen, and elastic fibers. The specialized cells are fibroblasts. Areolar tissue works to hold the internal organs in place and is capable of soaking up excess tissue fluid.

Adipose tissue or fat is structurally similar to areolar tissue, but includes specialized cells. These cells are known as adipocytes and they contain droplets of oil. Adipose tissue is used by the body to store excess energy as fat, retain heat (insulator), and to cushion and protect organs and joints.

Reticular connective tissue consists of a network of interwoven reticular fibers. The predominant cells are reticular cells. This tissue is found in the liver, spleen, lymph nodes, and bone marrow. Its function is to provide a supporting framework to the organs in which it is found.

Dense Connective Tissue

While all connective tissue contains some fibers, dense connective tissue contains a greater proportion of fibers than the other connective tissues. The predominant fiber type is collagen fibers, although elastic fibers may be present. The fibers are produced by cells called fibroblasts. There are three types of dense connective tissue: (1) dense regular connective tissue, (2) dense irregular connective tissue, and (3) elastic connective tissue.

In dense regular connective tissue, the collagen fibers are arranged in bundles that run parallel to each other. This provides the tissue with great strength. Examples of dense regular connective tissue include tendons (which connect muscles to bones) and ligaments (which connect bones to other bones). Ligaments contain more elastic fibers than tendons and are capable of stretching more than tendons.

Dense irregular connective tissue varies from the regular form in that the collagen fiber bundles do not run parallel to each other. Instead, the bundles run in more than one direction giving the tissue strength in more than one direction. Dense irregular connective tissue is often arranged in sheets and can be found in the layer of the skin known as the dermis and in the fibrous coverings around such organs as the kidneys and bones.

Elastic connective tissue contains a greater proportion of elastic fibers than the other two varieties of dense connective tissue. These elastic fibers give the tissue the ability to stretch and return to its original shape and length. Locations of elastic connective tissue include in lung tissue, in the vocal cords, and in the walls of many arteries.

Cartilage

Cartilage is a flexible and tough tissue containing cells known as chondrocytes, a firm matrix consisting of collagen and elastic fibers, a gel-like ground substance, and a large amount of water. Unlike other connective tissues, cartilage does not have its own blood vessels. This means that cartilage heals very slowly after an injury and in some cases may not heal at all. The different forms of cartilage in the body are hyaline cartilage, fibrocartilage, and elastic cartilage.

Hyaline cartilage is the most abundant form of cartilage in the body. It is used by the body to reduce friction between moving parts such as bones, to attach the ribs to the sternum (breastbone), and to form the structure of the larynx. Additionally the fetal skeleton starts out as hyaline cartilage and is eventually replaced by bone.

Fibrocartilage has a matrix that contains more collagen fibers than the other forms of cartilage. This increased collagen fiber content gives fibrocartilage a highly compressible nature, allowing it to act like a shock absorber. Fibrocartilage is found in the disks between the vertebrae of the spinal column and in the cartilage pads of the knees.

Elastic cartilage is the most flexible form of cartilage. This is due to the greater number of elastic fibers found in its matrix. Elastic cartilage makes up the external ear structure.

Bone

Bone or *osseous* tissue is the hardest of all the connective tissues. This characteristic allows bone to both protect and support body structures. The living cells in mature bone are osteocytes, and the matrix consists of collagen fibers impregnated with calcium and phosphorous salts, which give bone its characteristic hardness. In addition to providing the framework of the body, bone is the site of blood cell production.

MUSCLE TISSUE

Movement of material in the body and of the body itself is generally due to the contraction of muscle tissue. There are three types of muscle tissue: skeletal, smooth, and cardiac.

Skeletal muscle is attached to the bones of the skeleton by tendons. When a skeletal muscle contracts, it pulls on the bone it is attached to, producing body movement. This movement can be limited to just part of the body or movement of the body as a whole. Because movement of the body usually results from a conscious effort, skeletal muscle is sometimes referred to as voluntary muscle. At the cellular level, skeletal muscle has large, cylinder-shaped cells with striations (parallel stripes) and multiple nuclei.

Smooth (visceral) muscle is found in the walls of the digestive organs, in tubular structures such as blood vessels, and at the base of each body hair. Because this type of muscle contracts without conscious thought, it is said to be *involuntary.* Some functions include moving food and waste through the digestive tract and regulating blood pressure by contracting and relaxing blood vessels. The cells of smooth muscle are small and tapered, have no striations, and contain a single nucleus for each cell.

Cardiac muscle, as the name implies, involves the heart. It forms the walls of the chambers of the heart and is also known as myocardium. Involuntary in nature, cardiac muscle's primary function is to pump blood throughout the body. Its contractions produce what we refer to as heartbeats. Cardiac muscle is characterized by branching cells, slight striations, and a single nucleus per cell.

NERVOUS TISSUE

Nervous tissue is a highly specialized tissue capable of generating and transmitting electrochemical impulses. These impulses allow different parts of the body to communicate and the central nervous system (brain and spinal cord) to control the different body systems. The cells that generate and conduct these impulses are known as neurons or nerve cells (Figure 18-4 ■). They consist of a cell body, an axon, and dendrites. The central portion of the neuron is the cell body, which contains the nucleus and regulates the function of the neuron. The axon is a single fiber that carries impulses or information away from the cell body. Dendrites, on the other hand, are fibers that receive impulses and carry them to the nerve cell body.

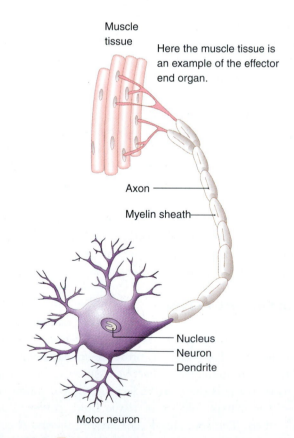

Muscle tissue

Here the muscle tissue is an example of the effector end organ.

Axon

Myelin sheath

Nucleus
Neuron
Dendrite

Motor neuron

Figure 18-4. ■ Neuron.

In addition to neurons, there are a number of support cells known as neuroglia in nervous tissue. The neuroglia do not generate impulses but rather protect, support, insulate, and nourish the neurons.

Body Systems

When organs function together for the same general purpose, they are said to be part of an **organ system**. The human body contains 11 major organ systems: integumentary, skeletal, muscular, nervous, endocrine, circulatory, lymphatic, respiratory, digestive, urinary, and reproductive.

INTEGUMENTARY SYSTEM

The skin is the body's largest organ and the only organ that can be inspected in its entirety without special equipment or surgery. The skin and its associated structures (including the hair, nails, oil and sweat glands, blood vessels, nerves, and sensory organs) make up the **integumentary system** (Figure 18-5 ■). Nursing care of the integumentary system is discussed in detail in Chapter 23 ◗◗. The primary functions of this system are the following:

1. Protect the body from infection by preventing pathogens from entering.
2. Protect against dehydration by preventing fluid loss.
3. Regulate body temperature. This involves dilation and constriction of blood vessels and perspiration.
4. Collect sensory information by special receptors. This information includes pain, touch, pressure, and temperature.

SKELETAL SYSTEM

There are 206 bones in the human body. Together, they form the skeletal system (Figure 18-6 ■).

The skeleton serves five major functions:

1. Serves as the body's framework.
2. Protects delicate structures like the brain and spinal cord.
3. Works with muscles as levers to produce movement.
4. Acts as a storehouse for calcium that can be used if calcium levels in the blood drop too low. Calcium is a very important component in muscle contractions and blood clotting.

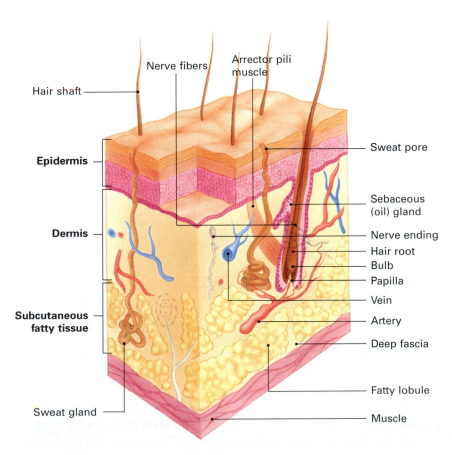

Figure 18-5. ■ Cross section of skin.

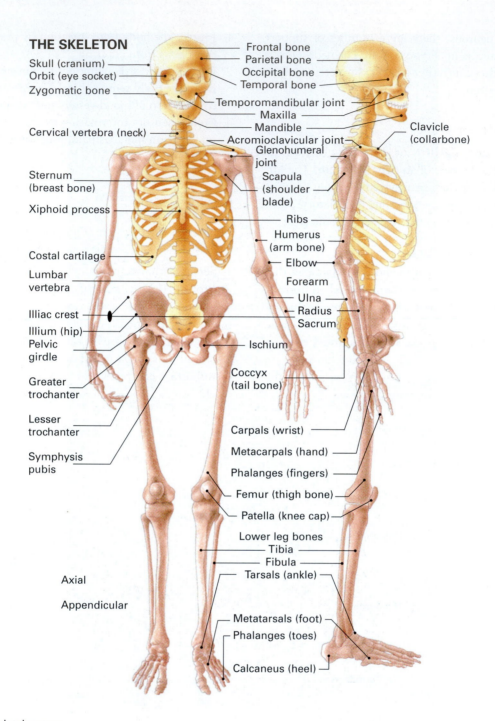

THE SKELETON

Skull (cranium)
Orbit (eye socket)
Zygomatic bone

Frontal bone
Parietal bone
Occipital bone
Temporal bone

Cervical vertebra (neck)

Temporomandibular joint
Maxilla
Mandible
Acromioclavicular joint
Glenohumeral joint

Clavicle (collarbone)

Sternum (breast bone)

Xiphoid process

Scapula (shoulder blade)

Ribs
Humerus (arm bone)
Elbow
Forearm
Ulna
Radius
Sacrum

Costal cartilage

Lumbar vertebra

Illiac crest
Illium (hip)
Pelvic girdle

Ischium

Greater trochanter

Coccyx (tail bone)

Lesser trochanter

Symphysis pubis

Carpals (wrist)
Metacarpals (hand)
Phalanges (fingers)
Femur (thigh bone)
Patella (knee cap)
Lower leg bones
Tibia
Fibula
Tarsals (ankle)

Axial

Appendicular

Metatarsals (foot)
Phalanges (toes)

Calcaneus (heel)

Figure 18-6. ■ Skeletal system.

5. Bones produce the blood cells in the red bone marrow. The cells produced are red blood cells, white blood cells, and platelets.

MUSCULAR SYSTEM

The primary function of the muscular system is to produce body movement (Figure 18-7 ■). This occurs when skeletal muscles contract and pull on the bones of the body. Additional functions include maintaining posture and producing heat that helps to keep the body warm.

NERVOUS SYSTEM

In order for the systems of the body to work together, there has to be a control center and a method of sending and re-

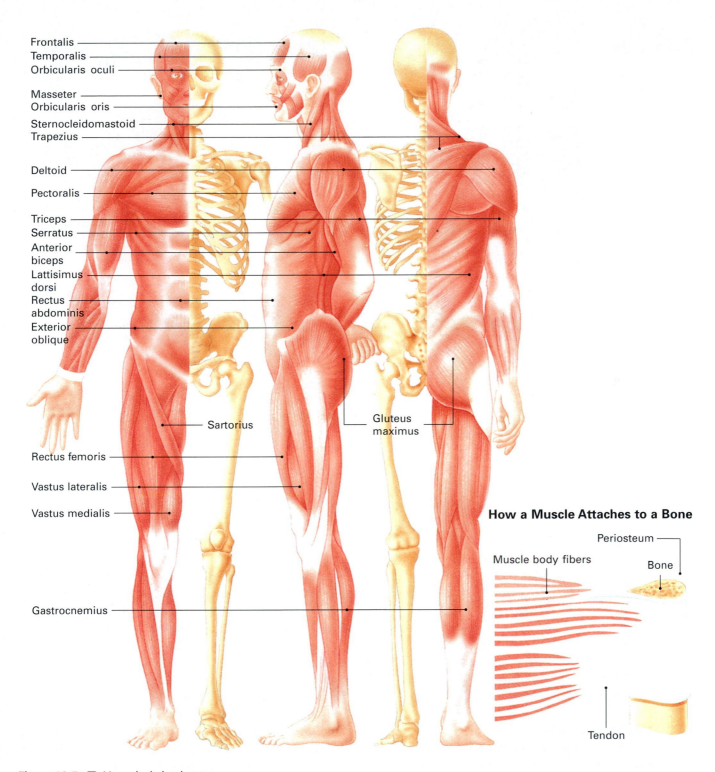

Frontalis
Temporalis
Orbicularis oculi
Masseter
Orbicularis oris
Sternocleidomastoid
Trapezius
Deltoid
Pectoralis
Triceps
Serratus
Anterior biceps
Lattisimus dorsi
Rectus abdominis
Exterior oblique
Sartorius
Rectus femoris
Vastus lateralis
Vastus medialis
Gastrocnemius
Gluteus maximus

How a Muscle Attaches to a Bone

Muscle body fibers
Periosteum
Bone
Tendon

Figure 18-7. ■ Musculoskeletal system.

ceiving information. This is accomplished by the nervous system (Figure 18-8 ■). The human nervous system consists of two divisions: the central nervous system (CNS) and the peripheral nervous system (PNS). The central nervous system includes the brain and spinal cord. This is where in-

formation or stimuli are analyzed and responses are generated. The CNS is also the site of thought, reasoning, and memory.

The information that the CNS receives comes from the PNS, which consists of all nervous tissue not included in the

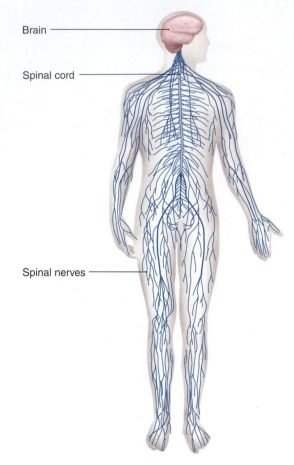

Brain

Spinal cord

Spinal nerves

Figure 18-8. ■ Nervous system.

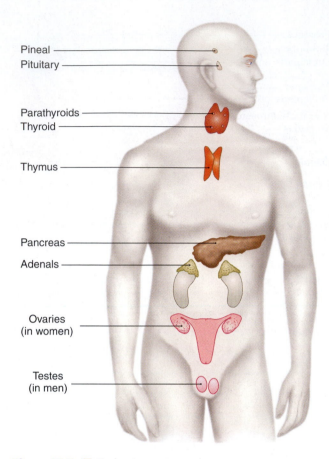

Pineal
Pituitary

Parathyroids
Thyroid

Thymus

Pancreas
Adenals

Ovaries
(in women)

Testes
(in men)

Figure 18-9. ■ Endocrine system.

CNS. The PNS has a vast number of receptors, which are used to gather information pertaining to the outside world.

ENDOCRINE SYSTEM

The endocrine system (Figure 18-9 ■) is made up of all the hormone secreting glands used by the body to regulate such activities as growth, metabolism, and reproduction. The endocrine system works in conjunction with the nervous system to regulate the body's systems.

CIRCULATORY SYSTEM

The body's tissues need a steady supply of oxygen and nutrients. In addition, the waste products of metabolism must be removed from these same tissues. These materials are transported by the blood, which is pumped throughout the body by the heart (Figure 18-10 ■). The circulatory system includes the heart and all the vasculature that carries oxygenated blood to, and deoxygenated blood away from, the body.

LYMPHATIC SYSTEM AND IMMUNITY

The tissues of the body contain a large amount of fluid. This fluid needs to be removed from the tissues so it does not

accumulate and cause the tissues to swell. The lymphatic system works to remove the fluid from the tissues and return it to the blood (Figure 18-11 ■). A second function of the lymphatic system is to protect the body from pathogens. When fluid enters the lymphatic system, it is filtered through lymph nodes. There, foreign materials are removed and destroyed by white blood cells.

RESPIRATORY SYSTEM

The respiratory system (Figure 18-12 ■) consists of the lungs and the passages that lead to them. The purpose of this system is to bring oxygen into the body so that it can enter the blood and be transported to all tissues of the body. Additionally, the respiratory system removes carbon dioxide, a waste product of cellular metabolism, from the body. See Chapter 24 ⌘.

DIGESTIVE SYSTEM

The cells of the human body need a constant supply of energy in order to function properly. This energy comes from the food we eat. Since food cannot directly enter the bloodstream, it needs to be broken down by the digestive system

MAJOR ARTERIES

MAJOR VEINS

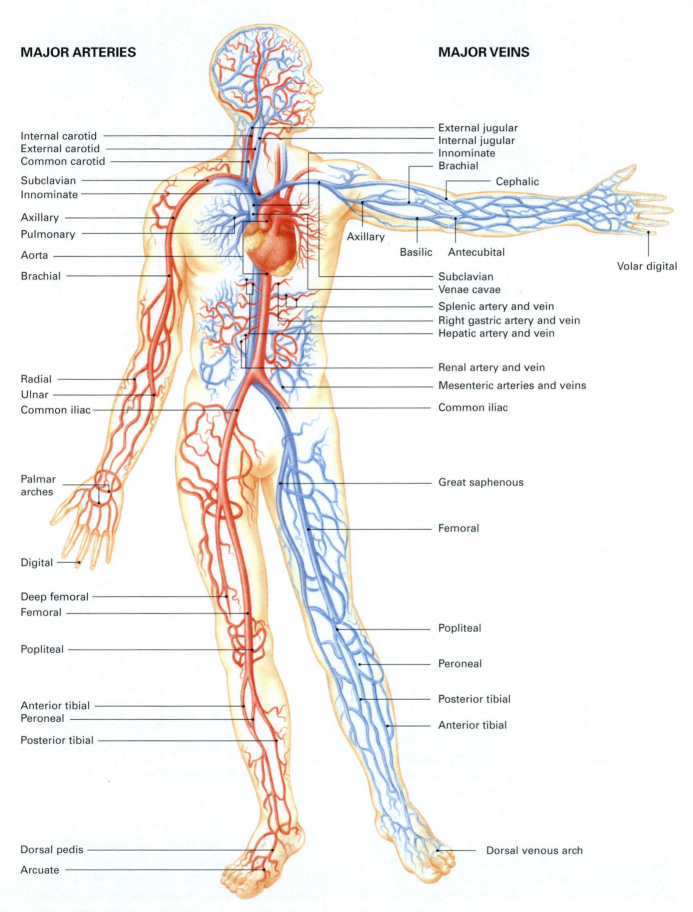

Internal carotid
External carotid
Common carotid
Subclavian
Innominate
Axillary
Pulmonary
Aorta
Brachial

External jugular
Internal jugular
Innominate
Brachial
Cephalic
Axillary
Basilic   Antecubital
Volar digital

Subclavian
Venae cavae
Splenic artery and vein
Right gastric artery and vein
Hepatic artery and vein
Renal artery and vein
Mesenteric arteries and veins
Common iliac

Radial
Ulnar
Common iliac

Palmar arches

Great saphenous

Femoral

Digital

Deep femoral
Femoral

Popliteal

Popliteal

Peroneal

Anterior tibial
Peroneal

Posterior tibial
Anterior tibial

Posterior tibial

Dorsal pedis
Arcuate

Dorsal venous arch

Figure 18-10. ■ Circulatory system.

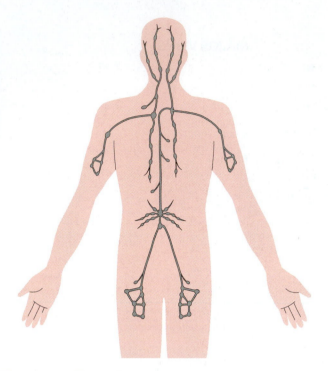

Figure 18-11. ■ Lymphatic system in torso.

(Figure 18-13 ■). Food is broken down through mechanical and chemical processes into a form that can enter the blood. The organs of the digestive system include the mouth, pharynx, esophagus, stomach, small intestine, and large intestine. Additionally, the salivary glands, liver, gallbladder, and pancreas play accessory roles in the process of digestion. See Chapters 25 and 28 ⬭.

URINARY SYSTEM

The main purpose of the urinary system is to eliminate waste products and excess water from the body (Figure 18-14 ■). The organs of this system include the kidneys, ureters, urinary bladder, and the urethra. Additionally, the urinary system aids in acid–base balance and electrolyte composition of body fluids. See Chapter 27 ⬭.

REPRODUCTIVE SYSTEM

The purpose of the male and female reproductive systems (Figure 18-15 ■) is to produce offspring to allow for continuation of the human species. Both male and female systems produce gametes. When an egg cell is fertilized by a sperm cell, the resulting zygote becomes implanted in the woman's uterus and stays there until it is sufficiently developed to survive outside the womb.

Despite obvious differences between males and females, the reproductive organs of each system can be divided into two groups: primary and accessory organs.

The *primary reproductive organs* (gonads) are responsible for producing the gametes. The gonads of the male are the testes and of the female are the ovaries.

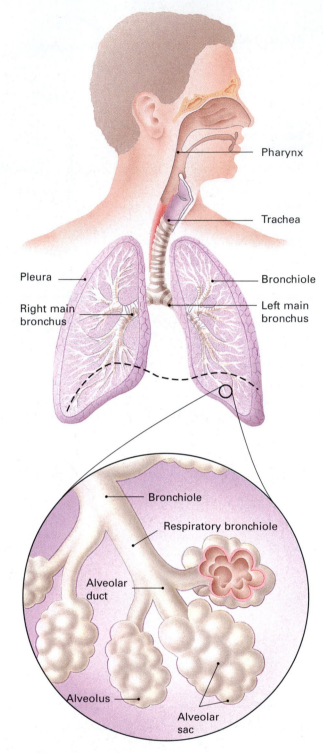

Figure 18-12. ■ Respiratory system.

The *accessory reproductive organs* are those structures that transport, protect, and nourish the gametes after they leave the gonads. In the male, the accessory organs include the epididymis, ductus deferens, seminal vesicles, prostate gland, bulbourethral glands, scrotum, and penis. In the female they are the uterine tubes (fallopian tubes), uterus, vagina, and vulva.

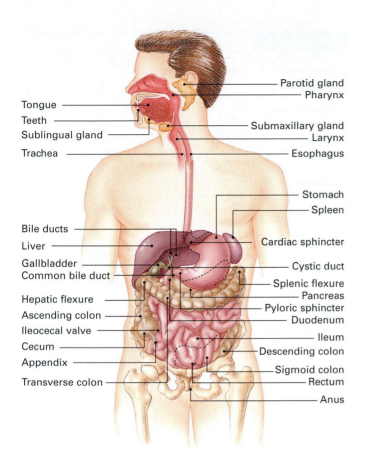

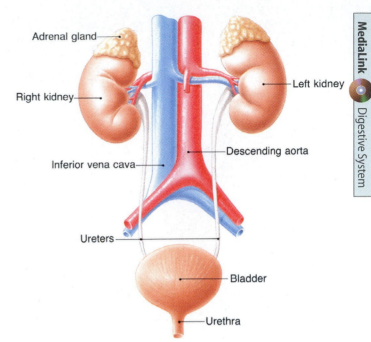

Figure 18-13. ■ Digestive system.

Figure 18-14. ■ Urinary system.

Hormones control the production of gametes in both the male and female. In males, follicle-stimulating hormone (FSH) and interstitial cell-stimulating hormone (which stimulates the testes to produce testosterone) are the major hor-mones. Testosterone is also responsible for the development of **secondary sex characteristics** (traits associated with gender but not directly necessary for reproduction in males). These characteristics include a deeper voice, broader shoulders, more muscle mass, and more body hair than in females.

The hormones that control the female reproductive cycle are FSH, estrogen, luteinizing hormone, and progesterone. If fertilization occurs, the embryo produces a hormone known as human chorionic gonadotropin. (See also Chapter 15 ⬤⬤.)

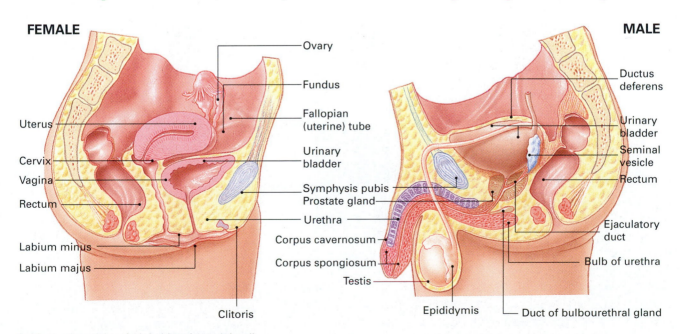

Labium minus (singular), Labia minora (plural)
Labium majus (singular), Labia majora (plural)

Figure 18-15. ■ Reproductive system.

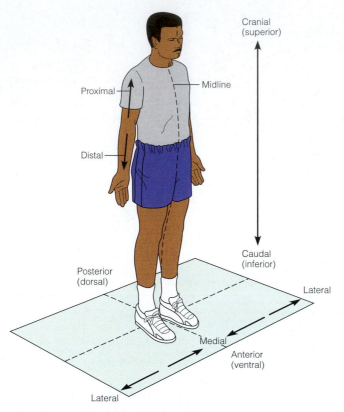

Figure 18-16. ■ Anatomic position.

Anatomic Positions

When discussing the human body, it is important to use terminology that accurately identifies the area that is being viewed. This section provides basic terminology.

BOX 18-1

Anatomic Terms for Direction

- **Anterior** or ventral—toward the front of the body or the belly
- **Posterior** or dorsal—toward the back of; opposite of ventral
- **Superior**—above or in a higher position
- **Inferior**—a point lower than or below a reference point
- **Superficial**—a point that is pertaining to or situated near the surface of an object
- **Deep**—a point or area that is below the surface of an object
- **Medial**—closer to the middle of the body
- **Lateral**—the opposite of medial, or toward the side
- **Proximal**—a point nearer the origin of a structure
- **Distal**—farther away from the origin of a structure

The starting position is known as the **anatomic position**. In this position, the body is upright with the face front, arms at the sides with the palms facing forward, and feet parallel (Figure 18-16 ■). Anatomic terms for direction are listed in Box 18-1 ■. For example, the hand is farther from the shoulder than is the elbow. Using the shoulder as the point of origin, the term that describes the hand in relation to the shoulder would be *distal* (farther away), while the elbow would be *proximal* (nearer).

BODY PLANES

When studying anatomy, it is often necessary to picture the body as being divided by planes. A **plane** is an imaginary flat surface that divides a structure into two portions. Three planes are used most often in anatomy (Figure 18-17 ■):

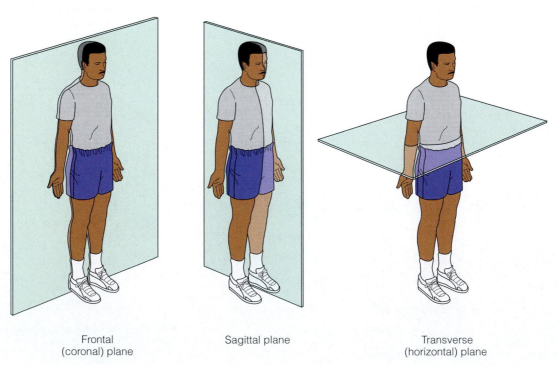

| Frontal (coronal) plane | Sagittal plane | Transverse (horizontal) plane |

Figure 18-17. ■ Body planes (frontal or coronal, sagittal, and transverse or horizontal).

- The **frontal plane** runs from one side of the body to the other, separating the body into front and back portions.
- The **sagittal plane** runs from front to back, separating the body into left and right portions. If the portions are equal, the plane is said to be **midsagittal plane**.
- The **transverse plane** cuts the body horizontally, creating a *superior* (higher) and *inferior* (lower) portion.

Body Cavities

The body contains two large internal spaces or cavities in which various organs are located. These spaces are the dorsal and ventral cavities (Figure 18-18 ■).

The dorsal cavity can be divided into the cranial and spinal cavities. The cranial cavity is the space inside the skull and is where the brain is located. The spinal cavity is where the spinal cord is housed. These two cavities form one continuous space.

The ventral cavity is much larger than the dorsal cavity. The ventral cavity can be divided into two smaller cavities, the thoracic and abdominopelvic cavities. The muscle known as the diaphragm divides the two cavities. The abdominopelvic cavity is sometimes further divided into the upper (abdominal) cavity and the lower (pelvic) cavity.

The thoracic cavity, above the diaphragm, contains the heart, lungs, and the major blood vessels that are attached to the heart. The organs located in the thoracic cavity are protected by the rib cage.

The abdominal portion of the abdominopelvic cavity is located below the diaphragm and extends downward to the top of the hipbones. Contained within the abdominal cavity are the stomach, kidneys, liver, spleen, gallbladder, and most of the intestines. Unlike the thoracic cavity, there is no protective skeletal structure over the abdominal cavity.

The pelvic cavity is below the abdominal cavity and contains the urinary bladder, rectum, and internal parts of both the male and female reproductive systems.

Because the abdominal cavity is so large, it is often divided even further to clarify which region is being discussed. This is especially helpful if a client reports "abdominal pain." It is very difficult to diagnose the cause of the pain if a region is not specified.

There are two methods of subdividing the abdominal cavity. The first method divides the cavity into nine regions. The upper three regions begin below the sternum and include the right hypochondriac region, epigastric region, and the left hypochondriac region. The middle three regions cover the navel and the area of the abdomen to the right and left of the navel. They are called the right lumbar region, umbilical region, and the left lumbar region. The final three regions cover the pelvis and are known as the right iliac region, hypogastric region, and the left iliac region. See Figure 18-19 ■ for proper placement of these regions.

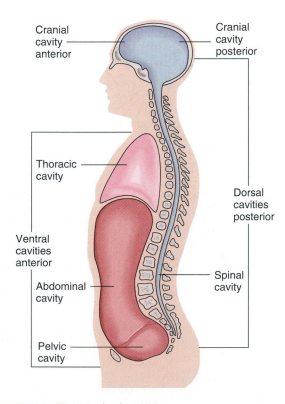

Figure 18-18. ■ Major body cavities.

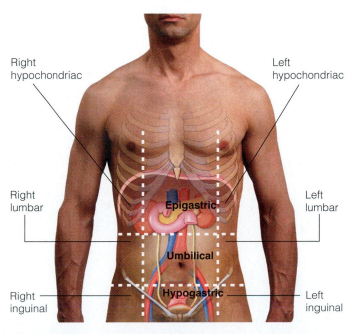

Figure 18-19. ■ Nine abdominal regions: *1*, epigastric; *2, 3*, left and right hypochondriac; *4*, umbilical; *5, 6*, left and right lumbar; *7*, suprapubic and hypogastric; *8, 9*, left and right inguinal or iliac.

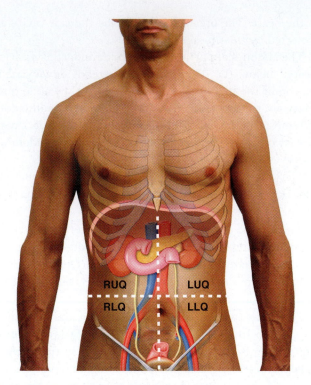

Figure 18-20. ■ The four abdominal quadrants and the underlying organs: *1,* right upper quadrant; *2,* left upper quadrant; *3,* right lower quadrant; *4,* left lower quadrant.

A simpler method and the one most often used in the medical community is to divide the abdominal cavity into quadrants. The quadrants are named according to their positions: the right upper quadrant (RUQ), the left upper quadrant (LUQ), the right lower quadrant (RLQ), and the left lower quadrant (LLQ). Figure 18-20 ■ shows the placement of these quadrants.

Note: The references and resources for this and all chapters have been compiled at the back of the book.

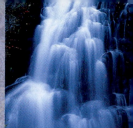

Chapter Review

 KEY TERMS by Topic

Use the audio glossary feature of either the CD-ROM or the Companion Website to hear the correct pronunciation of the following key terms.

Introduction
anatomy, physiology

Cell Structure
cell, homeostasis, cell membrane, receptors, enzymes, channels, transporters, antigens, cytoplasm, nucleus, endoplasmic reticulum (ER), mitochondria, adenosine triphosphate (ATP), Golgi apparatus, cilia, flagellum, mitosis, meiosis, gametes

Tissues
tissue, epithelium, glands, exocrine glands, endocrine glands, hormones, connective tissue, matrix

Body Systems
organ system, integumentary system, secondary sex characteristics

Anatomic Positions
anatomic position, plane, frontal plane, sagittal plane, midsagittal plane, transverse plane

KEY Points

- Anatomy is the study of body structures, while physiology is the study of body functions.

- The cell is the basic unit of life. It consists of a limiting boundary known as a plasma membrane, a nucleus surrounded by cytoplasm, and numerous structures called organelles.

- There are two types of cell division: mitosis and meiosis. Mitosis is involved in growth and repair of an organism. Meiosis is responsible for sperm and egg cells.

- The four main classifications of tissue are epithelial, connective, muscle, and nervous tissue.

- The human body consists of 11 major organ systems: integumentary, skeletal, muscular, nervous, endocrine, circulatory, lymphatic, respiratory, digestive, urinary, and reproductive.

- The anatomic position is achieved when the body is upright, face front, arms at the sides, palms facing forward, and the feet parallel.

- The planes of division of the body are sagittal, frontal, and transverse.

- The two main body cavities are the dorsal and ventral cavities.

 EXPLORE Media Link

Additional interactive resources for this chapter can be found on the Companion Website at www.prenhall.com/ramont. Click on Chapter 18 and "Begin" to select the activities for this chapter.

For chapter-related NCLEX®-style questions and an audio glossary, access the accompanying CD-ROM in this book.

Animations/Videos
- Digestive System
- Endocrine System
- Heart and Major Vessels
- Lymphatic System
- Respiratory System
- Urinary System

FOR FURTHER Study

For more information on sexuality, see Chapter 15.

Nursing care of the integumentary system is discussed in detail in Chapter 23.

Further information about the cardiovascular and respiratory systems is provided in Chapter 24.

For more about the digestive system, see Chapters 25 and 28.

For further study of the urinary system, see Chapter 27.

NCLEX-PN® Exam Preparation

1   The basic unit of all living organisms is the:
   1. respiratory system.
   2. brain.
   3. cell.
   4. heart.

2   In a cell, the organelle that is responsible for cholesterol synthesis is the:
   1. mitochondria.
   2. smooth endoplasmic reticulum.
   3. rough endoplasmic reticulum.
   4. Golgi apparatus.

3   The ventral cavity has two subdivisions. They are:
   1. cranial and spinal.
   2. superior and inferior.
   3. thoracic and cranial.
   4. thoracic and abdominopelvic.

4   The main body system that provides oxygen to and carries carbon dioxide away from the body is the:
   1. respiratory system.
   2. urinary system.
   3. skeletal system.
   4. nervous system.

5   The correct order of the stages in mitosis is:
   1. prophase, anaphase, metaphase, telophase.
   2. metaphase, anaphase, prophase, telophase.
   3. prophase, telophase, anaphase, metaphase.
   4. prophase, metaphase, anaphase, telophase.

6   The body plane that divides the body into left and right portions is the:
   1. frontal plane.
   2. sagittal plane.
   3. transverse plane.
   4. coronal plane.

7   A band of connective tissue that connects bone to bone is:
   1. a ligament.
   2. a tendon.
   3. cartilage.
   4. a fascia.

8   The term for many layers of cells is:
   1. squamous.
   2. columnar.
   3. stratified.
   4. simple.

9   Endocrine glands are often referred to as ductless glands and they secrete:
   1. oil.
   2. hormones.
   3. tears.
   4. blood.

10 Within the cell, ribosomes are attached to the:
   1. Golgi apparatus.
   2. lysosomes.
   3. endoplasmic reticulum.
   4. centrioles.

Answers and Rationales for Review Questions, as well as discussion of Care Plan and Critical Thinking Care Map questions, appear in Appendix I.

Chapter 19

Health Assessment

BRIEF Outline

Physical Health Assessment
Methods of Examination

LEARNING Outcomes

After completing this chapter, you will be able to:

1. Discuss the LPN's/LVN's role in health assessment.
2. Identify the purposes of the physical health examination.
3. List three types of physical assessment.
4. Discuss preparation of client and environment.
5. Explain the three methods of examination.
6. Explain the significance of selected physical findings.
7. Describe suggested sequencing to conduct a physical health assessment in an orderly fashion.
8. Discuss variations in assessment techniques that are appropriate for clients of different ages.

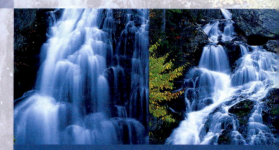

HISTORICAL Perspectives

An important responsibility of the nurse in any nursing situation is that of observation. It begins with the first contact with a patient and continues for as long as the patient is under the nurse's care. Observation means more than just looking. It is questioning, listening, and sometimes touching as well. Skill in observation is a continuous learning process. The more astute the nurse becomes, the more valuable is her or his contribution to the patient's welfare. (Fuerst & Wolff, 1964)

Assessing a client's health status is a major component of nursing care. There are two aspects of assessment: the nursing health history and the physical examination. The physical examination or assessment is the focus of this chapter. A **physical assessment** can be any of three types:

1. A complete assessment
2. A focused assessment by body systems (Figure 19-1 ■)
3. A focused assessment of a body part. Box 19-1 ■ on page 350 provides some guidelines for assessment by body systems.

Physical Health Assessment

COMPLETE ASSESSMENT

A complete assessment is conducted by an RN when the client is admitted to the healthcare facility. The LPN/LVN may be asked to collect some data for this. It includes a full head-to-toe assessment as well as information that pertains to the client's level of functioning. Information collected may include allergies; client's level of ambulation; personal property brought to the facility by the client, and people with whom any valuables are sent home; chronic health conditions and any medications taken for these conditions; past medical history; fall risk assessment; dietary habits; and impairments and disabilities (see Figure 10-1 ⚭). This complete assessment should remain in the client's chart so that all staff involved in the client's care may refer to it. This assessment also provides baseline information about the client to all staff members.

FOCUSED ASSESSMENT

A focused assessment may be conducted by the LPN/LVN at the beginning and end of the shift. It may be conducted in several ways. One efficient method is to start at the head and proceed in a systematic manner downward to the toes. The procedure can vary according to the age of the individual,

the severity of the illness, the method preferences of the nurse, the location of the examination, and the agency's priorities and required procedures. Regardless of what type of procedure is used, the client's energy and time need to be considered. The physical health assessment is always conducted in a systematic and efficient manner that requires the fewest position changes for the client.

The sequence of the assessment differs with children and adults. Box 19-2 ■ on page 351 discusses age-related differences and considerations. Frequently, nurses assess a specific system's body part or area instead of the entire body. These specific (or focused) assessments are made in relation to client complaints, the nurse's own observation of problems, the client's presenting problem, the nursing interventions provided, and medical therapies. Examples of these situations and assessments are presented in Table 19-1 ■.

PREPARING THE CLIENT

Most clients need an explanation of the physical health assessment. Explain when and where it will take place, why it is important, and what will happen during the assessment. Assist the client as needed to undress and put on an examination gown.

Clients should be instructed to empty their bladders before the examination. Doing so helps them feel more relaxed and facilitates palpation of the abdomen and pubic area. If a urinalysis is required, the urine should be collected at this time. Often, clients are anxious about what the nurse will find. They can be reassured during the assessment by explanations at each step.

clinical ALERT

Health assessments are usually painless. However, it is important to determine, in advance, any positions that are contraindicated for a particular client.

TABLE 19-1
Selected Client Situations and Focused Assessments

SITUATION	PHYSICAL ASSESSMENT
Client complains of abdominal pain.	Inspect, auscultate, and palpate the abdomen; assess vital signs and levels of pain.
Client is admitted with a head injury.	Assess level of consciousness using Glasgow Coma Scale (see Table 19-2); assess pupils for reaction to light and accommodation; assess vital signs.
The nurse prepares to administer a cardiotonic drug to a client.	Assess apical pulse and compare with baseline data.
The nurse administers postural drainage.	Auscultate lungs before and after the procedure.
The client has just had a cast applied to the lower leg.	Assess peripheral perfusion of toes, capillary blanch test, pedal pulse if able, and vital signs.
The client's fluid intake is minimal.	Assess tissue turgor, fluid intake and output, and vital signs.

PeaceHealth

ST. JOHN MEDICAL CENTER
LONGVIEW, WASHINGTON

MED / SURG / TELE / ONC - DAILY CARE RECORD

Symbol Key
Empty box = Not assessed
✓ = Assessment matches normal parameters
X = Variation, describe in Comments
→ = Variations same as last assessment
* = See progress notes
Initial each assessment block on line
Use right box for reassessment or daily care (dc) assessment

Date:	NOC - Time: /	DAY - Time: /	EVE - Time: /
SYSTEMS ASSESSMENTS	Comments Reassess ☐ D/C ☐	Comments Reassess ☐ D/C ☐	Comments Reassess ☐ D/C ☐
Pain If other than 0-10 scale used, check appropriate box: ☐ APP ☐ Faces	Intensity _____ If > 0, see Focused Assessment section	Intensity _____ If > 0, see Focused Assessment section	Intensity _____ If > 0, see Focused Assessment section
Neurological LEVEL OF CONSCIOUSNESS: alert SPEECH: coherent, clearly understandable speech, symmetry of facial expression SWALLOWING: handles oral secretions ORIENTATION: aware of time, place, person; short-term memory intact BEHAVIOR: interactions appropriate to situation	☐ _____ _____ ☐	☐ _____ _____ ☐	☐ _____ _____ ☐
Cardiovascular VITAL SIGNS: HR reg, BP & temp WNL for pt. RADIAL PULSE: easily palpated and regular SKIN: warm, dry, natural color for patient CIRCULATION: no peripheral edema or calf pain	☐ _____ _____ ☐	☐ _____ _____ ☐	☐ _____ _____ ☐
Respiratory RATE: regular pattern, rate WNL for patient EFFORT: unlabored at rest on room air BREATH SOUNDS: no audible wheeze, stridor, rattles or other adventitious sounds COUGH: none reported or observed SPUTUM: absent or reported clear	☐ _____ _____ ☐	☐ _____ _____ ☐	☐ _____ _____ ☐
Gastrointestinal PALPATION: soft, non-tender AUSCULTATION: normally active bowel sounds INTAKE: tolerating at least half of prescribed diet without nausea/vomiting BM: continent of soft, formed stool within past 48°	☐ _____ _____ ☐	☐ _____ _____ ☐	☐ _____ _____ ☐
Genitourinary URINATION: observed/reported continent voiding of clear urine in sufficient quantity; no dysuria BLADDER DISTENTION: none visible GENITALIA: no observed/reported genital discharge or swelling	☐ _____ _____ ☐	☐ _____ _____ ☐	☐ _____ _____ ☐
Musculoskeletal EXTREMITIES: functional, non-painful ROM x4 MOVEMENT: independent gait, transfers and ambulates without use of assistive devices	☐ _____ _____ ☐	☐ _____ _____ ☐	☐ _____ _____ ☐
Integumentary/Wounds PRESSURE: no blanching or redness at boney prominences. No skin breakdown. HYDRATION: normal skin turgor; moist mucosa WOUND: well-approximated edges, no redness, swelling, drainage OR dressing clean, dry, intact	☐ _____ _____ ☐	☐ _____ _____ ☐	☐ _____ _____ ☐
Psych/Soc SUPPORT: fam/soc support sys evident/ reported AFFECT: calm, cooperative, normal eye contact (within cultural context) SLEEP PATTERNS: able to sleep at night if undisturbed; absence of unusual fatigue	☐ _____ _____ ☐	☐ _____ _____ ☐	☐ _____ _____ ☐
IV Site Assessment No redness Dressing CD&I No swelling Site < 72 hr old No pain	☐ Site #1 _____ ☐ Site #2 _____ ☐ Site #3 _____	☐ Site #1 _____ ☐ Site #2 _____ ☐ Site #3 _____	☐ Site #1 _____ ☐ Site #2 _____ ☐ Site #3 _____
If Site > 72 hr old, reason not DC'd			
Site care	☐ Site #1 _____	☐ Site #2 _____	☐ Site #3 _____

Figure 19-1. ■ Focused assessment by body system. (*Source:* Courtesy of PeaceHealth St. John Medical Center, Longview, WA. Used with permission.)

BOX 19-1 · NURSING CARE CHECKLIST

Assessment by Body Systems

Neurologic

☑ LOC (level of consciousness):
- A/O × 3 (alert and oriented to name, time, and place)

☑ Verbal response:
- Clear
- Incoherent, rambling, slurred, stuttering
- Dysphasia, aphasia

☑ Motor response (<, = bilaterally, >):
- Grips (note strength)
- Obeys commands, localizes pain, withdrawal, flexion, extension, none
- Pain—sharp, burning, intense, sudden, agonizing, throbbing, stabbing
- Pain level 1–10

☑ Assess pupils:
- Note shape
- Pupils equally round and react to light, and accommodate (PERRLA)
  1. 1 mm after surgery
  2. 2–3 mm normal
  3. 6–9 mm "blown"; if permanent, possible herniation

Integumentary

☑ General appearance:
- Pale, flushed, cyanotic, discolored, freckled
- Moist, diaphoretic, clammy
- Hot, warm, cold
- Dry, scaly, oily
- Rash, abrasion, laceration, incisions, broken, sores, lesions, scars, calloused, contusions
- Tanned, glossy, tattoos
- Swollen, coarse or fine texture

☑ Turgor:
- Normal
- Loose
- Tight
- Tenting

☑ Integrity:
- Intact
- Impaired

☑ Mucous membranes:
- Color
- Condition

Cardiovascular (normal pulse 60–100)

☑ Ap, B/P, radial PP (present <, = bilaterally, >):
- Rate/rhythm
  - Regular
  - Irregular

- Strong
- Rapid
- Weak
- Absent
- Thready
- Intensity (force of blood flow felt at pulse site)
  - 1, 2 (hypo)
  - 3, 4 (hyper or bounding)
- Doppler

☑ Skin—pale, flushed, cyanotic, discolored, moist, cold, clammy

☑ Edema—pitting, nonpitting

☑ Capillary refilling time < 3 seconds

☑ Homans' sign +/2

Respiratory (18–20 normal respirations)

☑ Breathing:
- Dyspnea
- Apnea
- Deep/shallow

☑ SOB (shortness of breath):
- With which activities?

☑ Chest:
- Excursion symmetrical/asymmetrical (Respiratory sounds seems to move from usual course or location in chest to another area.)

☑ Lung sounds (audible all lobes):
- Rales (Sound is created by air passing over airway secretions; term used synonymously with crackles.)
- Crackles
- Rhonchi (A continuous musical sound heard with a stethoscope; it occurs in asthma, croup, hayfever, and can also result from tumor or obstruction.)
- Wheezes

☑ Sputum:
- Clear
- Thin/thick
- Tenacious
- Note color

☑ Measure O$_2$ saturation:
- Pulse oximeter

Gastrointestinal

☑ Abdomen:
- Soft, firm, rigid, tender, sensitive to touch
- Enlarged, distended, flat, round
- Note any rebound tenderness

☑ Bowel sounds (listen all four quadrants—2 to 5 minutes):
- Normal, faint, hypo, absent, hyper

☑ BM size (sm, med, lg)

☑ N/V (nausea/vomiting)—amount/color/frequency:
  - Milliters; small, large
  - Blood tinged, fecal
  - Projectile

☑ Diarrhea (amt/color/freq)

☑ Appetite (tolerance to prescribed diet):
  - Percentage

Genitourinary (30 mL/h normal output)

☑ Urination: independent, catheter, incontinent:
  - Amount
  - Color—yellow, amber, bloody, brown, dark red
  - Appearance—clear, cloudy, sediment
  - Odor—offensive, foul, musty, aromatic, ammonia-like, odorless

☑ I/O (intake/output)—all fluids should be balanced with output

☑ Bladder distention:
  - Check, feel, palpate

Musculoskeletal

☑ ROM (range of motion)

☑ Gait

☑ Deformities

Psychosocial

☑ Mental and spiritual:
  - Moods, affect, judgment, abilities, lifestyle, patterns, age

---

BOX 19-2	POPULATION FOCUS

Assessment Differences by Age or Condition

Infants and Children

Skin

- Jaundice (yellowish skin) possible in newborns for several weeks after birth.
- May have increased pigmentation in sacral area of infants and young children of dark-skinned races.
- Possible milia (whiteheads) over the nose and face, and vernix caseosa (white, greasy, protective material) on skin of newborns.

Head

- Shape altered by delivery for about 1 week in most newborns.
- Posterior fontanel (soft spot) generally closes by 8 weeks and anterior fontanel by 18 months.
- Voluntary head control by 6 months of age.

Eyes, Ears, Nose, Mouth

- Horizontal line from eye to top of the ear is normal. Auricle should angle no more than 10 degrees from vertical. (*Note:* Variation may indicate mental retardation or renal abnormalities.)
- Infants may blink at a sharp sound. (*Note:* To assess gross hearing, ring a bell from behind the infant or have the parent call the child's name to check for a response. At 3 to 4 months, the infant will turn head and eyes toward the sound.)
- Tooth development should be appropriate for age; permanent teeth are darker than deciduous teeth.
- Inspect the palate for a cleft.

Chest, Heart, and Lungs

- Infants and children up to age 6 tend to breathe more from abdomen than from chest.
- Chest circumference measurements at delivery and up to 9 months rule out birth injuries, congenital anomalies, or other dysfunction.
- Auscultated sounds are louder and harsher because of thinner chest wall.
- A third heart sound, best heard at the apex, is present in about one-third of all children.
- Palpation of pulses in the lower extremities (particularly the femoral pulses) can be used to screen for certain heart abnormalities.

Gastrointestinal

- Abdomen of the newborn and infant is round. Characteristic "pot belly" appearance of toddlers persists until about age 5.
- Peristaltic waves usually more visible than in adults.
- Children may not be able to pinpoint areas of tenderness. Observe facial expressions to determine areas of maximum tenderness.
- Liver is relatively larger than in adults, and can be palpated 1 to 2 cm below the right costal margin.

Musculoskeletal

- Lordosis (swayback) is common in young children.
- Pronation (in-turning) of the feet is common between 12 and 30 months of age.
- Genu varum (bowleg) is normal for 1 year after beginning to walk.
- Asymmetric gluteal folds, asymmetric abduction of the legs, or apparent shortening of the femur suggest developmental dysplasia of the hip (congenital dislocation).

Pregnant Women

- Breast, areola, and nipple size increase.

(continued)

- Areolae and nipples darken. Nipples may become more erect. Areolae contain small, scattered, elevated Montgomery's glands.
- Superficial veins become more prominent. Stretch marks may develop.
- Colostrum (thick yellow fluid) may be expressed from the nipples after the first trimester.

Older Adults

Skin, Hair, and Nails

- Skin loses elasticity, appears thin, translucent, more wrinkled.
- Skin often dry and flaky, takes longer to return to its natural shape after being tented between the thumb and finger.
- Increased number of discolorations and skin lesions.
- Scalp and facial hair grays.
- Toenails grow more slowly and thicken.
- Longitudinal bands commonly develop on fingernails in older adults, and the nails tend to split.

Eyes, Ears, Nose, and Mouth

- Ears may appear dry, with increased coarse hair growth.
- Tympanic membrane is more translucent and less flexible.
- Earwax is drier.
- Hearing loss (presbycusis) occurs.
- Oral mucosa may be drier because of decreased salivary gland activity or dehydration.
- Gums recede, giving an appearance of increased toothiness.
- Taste sensations diminish due to atrophy of the taste buds and a decreased sense of smell.
- Tooth loss may occur as a result of gum disease.

Chest, Heart, and Lungs

- Anteroposterior diameter of the chest deepens, giving the person barrel-chested appearance due to loss of skeletal muscle strength in the thorax and diaphragm and constant lung inflation (from excessive expiratory pressure on the alveoli).
- Breathing rate and rhythm are unchanged at rest; heart rate after activity may take longer to return to the resting rate.
- Inspiratory muscles become less powerful, and depth of respiration decreases.
- Expiration may require the use of accessory muscles. The amount of air remaining in the lungs at the end of a normal breath increases.
- Cilia in the airways become fewer and are less effective in removing mucus.
- Heart size remains the same (if no disease is present).
- Cardiac output and strength of contraction decrease, so activity tolerance is less.
- Sudden emotional and physical stresses may result in cardiac arrhythmias and heart failure.
- Overall effectiveness of blood vessels decreases; lower extremities are more likely to show signs of impairment.
- Systolic and diastolic blood pressures may increase.

clinical ALERT

Clients with a blood pressure reading above 140/90 should be referred for follow-up assessments.

- Peripheral edema is frequently observed.

Gastrointestinal

- Abdomen may appear round due to increase in adipose (fatty) tissue and decreased muscle tone. Abdominal wall is slacker and thinner, so palpation is easier and more accurate.
- Side effects of drugs are often manifested by nausea, vomiting, and diarrhea.
- Pain threshold is often higher; major abdominal problems such as appendicitis or other acute emergencies may therefore go undetected.
- Gastrointestinal pain needs to be differentiated from cardiac pain. (*Note:* Gastrointestinal pain may be located in the chest or abdomen, whereas cardiac pain is usually located in the chest. Factors aggravating gastrointestinal pain are usually related to either ingestion or lack of food intake; gastrointestinal pain is usually relieved by antacids, food, or an upright position. Common factors that can aggravate cardiac pain are activity or anxiety; cardiac pain is relieved by rest or nitroglycerin.)
- Emptying time of the stomach is slower because gastric acid secretion is decreased, resulting in indigestion and intolerance of certain foods. Decreases in the production of pancreatic enzymes also contribute to complaints of indigestion and anorexia.
- Stool passes through the intestines at a slower rate, and the perception of stimuli that produce the urge to defecate often diminishes.
- Fecal incontinence may occur in older adults who are confused or neurologically impaired.

clinical ALERT

Absence of a daily bowel movement does not signify constipation. When assessing for constipation, the nurse must consider the client's diet, activity, and medications; the characteristics of feces and ease or difficulty in defecating; and the frequency of bowel movements.

- Decreased absorption of oral medications.
- In the liver, impaired metabolism of certain drugs may occur.

Musculoskeletal

- Muscle mass decreases progressively with age, but there are wide variations among individuals.
- Decreases in speed, strength, resistance to fatigue, reaction time, and coordination occur.
- Bones become more fragile. Osteoporosis leads to a loss of total bone mass, predisposition to fractures, and compressed vertebrae.
- Osteoarthritic changes in joints may be observed.

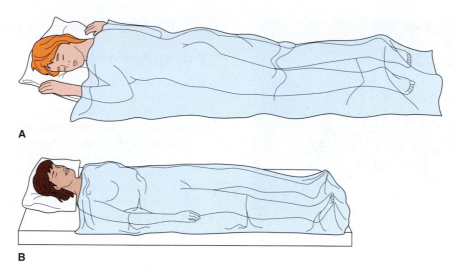

Figure 19-2. ■ Two most common client positions for assessment in bed: **A.** prone; **B.** supine.

Positioning

Frequently, several positions are required during the physical assessment. It is important to consider the client's ability to assume a position. The client's physical condition, energy level, and age should also be taken into consideration. The assessment is organized so that several body areas can be assessed in one position. The LPN/LVN most frequently assesses the client in (1) the prone or supine position in bed (Figure 19-2 ■) or (2) sitting in bed or in a chair.

Draping

Drapes, usually the client's bed linens, should be arranged so that the area to be assessed is exposed while other body areas are covered. Exposure of the body is frequently embarrassing to clients. Drapes provide not only privacy but also warmth.

PREPARING THE ENVIRONMENT

It is important to prepare the environment before starting the assessment. The time for the physical assessment should be convenient for both the client and the nurse. The environment should be well lit and the equipment organized for use.

Providing privacy is important. Curtains should be drawn. Most people are embarrassed if others can overhear or view them during the assessment. Family and friends should not be present during the examination unless the client specifically requests their presence.

The room temperature should be warm enough to be comfortable for the client. A well-prepared environment affects the client's response to the examination. The client who is physically relaxed usually experiences little discomfort.

Methods of Examination

Three primary techniques used by the LPN/LVN in the physical examination are inspection, auscultation, and palpation. A fourth technique, percussion, is learned in later

training and is used in specific procedures. These techniques are defined and discussed throughout this chapter as they apply to each body system.

INSPECTION

Inspection is visual examination, that is, assessing by using the sense of sight. Inspection should be deliberate, purposeful, and systematic. In addition to visual observations, olfactory (smelling) and auditory (hearing) cues are noted. Nurses frequently use visual inspection to assess moisture, color, and texture of body surfaces, as well as shape, position, size, color, and symmetry of the body. Lighting must be sufficient for the nurse to see clearly; either natural or artificial light can be used. When using the auditory senses, it is important to have a quiet environment for accurate hearing. Inspection can be combined with the other assessment techniques.

AUSCULTATION

Auscultation is the process of listening to sounds produced within the body. Auscultation may be direct or indirect. Direct auscultation is the use of the unaided ear, for example, to listen to a respiratory wheeze or the grating of a moving joint. Indirect auscultation (shown in Procedure 19-1 ■ on page 362) is done with the use of a stethoscope. The stethoscope amplifies the sounds and conveys them to the nurse's ears. A stethoscope is used primarily to listen to sounds from within the body, such as bowel sounds in the abdomen or valve sounds of the heart.

PALPATION

Palpation is the examination of the body using the sense of touch. The pads of the fingers are used because their concentration of nerve endings makes them highly sensitive and able to detect small differences or changes. Palpation is used to determine (1) texture (e.g., of the hair); (2) temperature (e.g., of a skin area); (3) vibration (e.g., of a joint); (4) position,

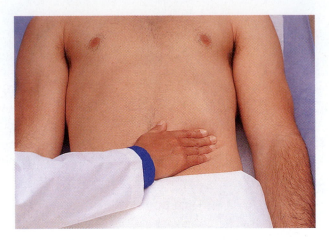

Figure 19-3. ■ The position of the hand for light palpation.

size, consistency, and mobility of organs or masses; (5) distention (e.g., of the urinary bladder); (6) pulsation; and (7) the presence of pain upon pressure.

There are two types of palpation: light and deep. The LPN/LVN is trained in light palpation (Figure 19-3 ■). Deep palpation is not usually done by the LPN/LVN, because pressure can damage internal organs. It is usually avoided in clients who have acute abdominal pain or who have pain that is not yet diagnosed.

PERCUSSION

Percussion is the act of striking a body part with short, sharp blows (1) to help gather data about internal organs, (2) to assist in massage, or (3) to help a client to clear the respiratory tract.

NURSING CARE

ASSESSING

General Survey

Physical **assessment** begins with a general survey that involves observation of the client's general appearance and behavior, and measurement of vital signs, height, and weight.

Many components of the general survey are assessed when the RN takes the client's health history, such as the client's body build, posture, hygiene, and mental status. Variations that relate to racial or ethnic background may occur (Box 19-3 ■). These data can be used by the LPN/LVN as a baseline with which to compare future assessment findings. Procedure 19-1 describes how to perform a focused physical assessment by body system.

The general appearance and behavior of an individual must be assessed in relationship to current circumstances. For example, an individual who has recently experienced a

personal loss may appropriately appear depressed. Also, the client's age, sex, and race are useful factors in interpreting findings that suggest increased risk for known conditions.

Neurologic Status

Level of Consciousness

Level of consciousness (LOC) can lie anywhere along a continuum from a state of alertness to coma. A fully alert client responds to questions spontaneously; a comatose client may not respond at all to verbal stimuli. The Glasgow Coma Scale (Table 19-2 ■) was originally developed to predict recovery from a head injury; however, it is used by

TABLE 19-2

Levels of Consciousness: Glasgow Coma Scale

FACULTY MEASURED	RESPONSE	SCORE
Eye response	Spontaneous	4
	To verbal command	3
	To pain	2
	No response	1
Motor response	To verbal command	6
	To localized pain	5
	Flexes and withdraws	4
	Flexes abnormally	3
	Extends abnormally	2
	No response	1
Verbal response	Oriented, converses	5
	Disoriented, converses	4
	Uses inappropriate words	3
	Makes incomprehensible sounds	2
	No response	1

many professionals to assess LOC. It is a practical and standardized system for assessing the degree of consciousness impairment. It tests in three major areas: eye response, motor response, and verbal response. An assessment totaling 15 points indicates the client is alert and completely oriented. A comatose client scores 7 or less. The Glasgow Coma Scale was developed in 1974 to provide a way for healthcare professionals to arrive at the same conclusion regarding patients' status. It saves time because the ratings are done numerically rather than with descriptions.

Orientation

The nurse determines the client's orientation to time, place, and person by tactful questioning. **Orientation** is easily assessed by asking the client the city and state of residence, time of day, date, day of the week, duration of illness, and names of family members. More direct questioning may be necessary for some people; for example, "Where are you now?" "What day is it today?" Most people readily respond and accept these questions. The nurse listens for quantity of speech (amount and pace), quality (loudness, clarity, and inflection), and organization (coherent thought, connection to what was asked, overgeneralization, or vagueness).

Pupil Reaction

Pupils are normally black, are equal in size (about 3 to 7 mm in diameter), and have round, smooth borders. Cloudy pupils often indicate cataracts. Unequal pupils (anisocoria) may result from a central nervous system disorder; however, slight variations may be normal. The reactions a nurse must check are discussed in Procedure 19-1. They include:

1. **Direct response**—In a semi-darkened room, a pupil should constrict or close when a bright light is shone into the eye.
2. **Consensual response**—When the bright light is shone on the same pupil a second time, the pupil of the other eye should also constrict.
3. **Accommodation**—A person alternates looking from a near object (about 10 cm or 4 in from the bridge of the nose) to a distant object (such as a point on the far wall). Accommodation is the alternating change in pupil size (constricts when looking at the near object, dilates when looking at the distant one).

A normal assessment of the pupils is recorded using the abbreviation **PERRLA** (pupils equally round and react to light and accommodation).

Skull

The skull of an adult client is not usually directly assessed. However, if the client has had head trauma or a procedure involving this area, the skull is assessed.

Part A of Procedure 19-1 focuses on assessing general appearance and mental status.

Vital Signs

Vital signs are measurements of temperature, pulse, respirations, and blood pressure. They are measured (1) to establish baseline data against which to compare future measurements and (2) to detect actual and potential health problems. Normal adult vital signs are T 98.6°F (37°C); P 60 to 100 per minute, average 80 beats per minute; R 12 to 20 per minute, average 16 per minute; BP 120/80. See Chapter 20 for full information and instructions related to taking vital signs.

Height and Weight

In adults, the ratio of weight to height provides a general measure of health. It is also important that the nurse and client be aware of any significant unintentional weight gain or loss. The height and weight are usually measured when a client is admitted to a healthcare agency. Measurement of height and weight is discussed in Chapter 25 .

Weight may also be measured regularly, for example, each morning before breakfast. When accuracy is essential, the nurse should use the same scale each time (because every scale weighs differently). The weight should be measured at the same time each day, making sure the client wears the same kind of clothing and no shoes. The client usually stands on a platform, and the weight is read from a digital display panel or a balancing arm. Clients who cannot stand are weighed on bed or chair scales.

Integumentary System

The integumentary system includes the skin, hair, and nails. In most documentation paperwork, condition of hair would be documented as a narrative note only in the event of a problem. Examination begins with a generalized inspection using a good source of lighting, preferably indirect natural daylight.

Skin

Assessment of the skin involves inspection and palpation. The nurse may also need to use the nose (olfactory sense) to detect unusual skin odors. These odors are usually most evident in the skin folds or in the axillae. Pungent body odor is frequently related to poor hygiene, hyperhidrosis (excessive perspiration), or bromhidrosis (foul-smelling perspiration). The entire skin surface may be assessed at one time or as each aspect of the body is assessed.

Pallor occurs when there is too little circulating blood or hemoglobin, which results in reduced amounts of oxygen being carried to body tissues. It is usually characterized by the absence of underlying red tones in the skin and may be most readily seen in the buccal mucosa. In brown-skinned clients, pallor may appear as a yellowish brown tinge; in black-skinned clients, the skin may appear ashen gray. When assessing clients with darker skin color, look for changes in skin color such as purple, brown, or bluish tones

TABLE 19-3		
Assessment of the Feet		
METHOD	NORMAL FINDINGS	DEVIATIONS FROM NORMAL
Inspect all skin surfaces, particularly between the toes, for cleanliness, odor, dryness, inflammation, swelling, abrasions, or other lesions.	Intact skin Absence of swelling or inflammation	Excessive dryness Areas of inflammation or swelling (e.g., corns, calluses) Fissures Scaling and cracking of skin (e.g., athlete's foot) Plantar warts
Palpate anterior and posterior surfaces of ankles and feet for edema.	No swelling	Swelling or pitting edema (see Procedure 19-1)
Palpate dorsalis pedis pulse on dorsal surface of foot.	Strong, regular pulses in both feet	Weak or absent pulses
Compare skin temperatures of the two feet.	Warm skin temperature	Cool skin temperature in one or both feet

that are darker than surrounding skin. It is usually best to assess darker skin in natural or halogen light. Fluorescent light casts a blue color, making skin assessment more difficult and less accurate. Pallor in all people is usually most evident in areas with the least pigmentation such as the conjunctiva, oral mucous membranes, nail beds, palms of the hand, and soles of the feet. Pallor may be seen in patients with anemia and in decreased blood flow as in fainting or insufficient arterial blood flow.

The integument can also be characterized as cyanotic, erythematous, or edematous. **Cyanosis** (a bluish tinge) is most evident in the nail beds, lips, and buccal mucosa. Common causes of cyanosis include advanced lung disease, congenital heart disease, and abnormal hemoglobins. Bruised areas normally blanch when pressure is applied. Cyanotic skin does not blanch to the same degree as bruised skin.

Jaundice is a yellowish color of skin, sclera, palms of hands, and oral mucous membranes. Jaundice is usually indicative of liver disease, pancreatic disease, or common bile duct obstruction. In the dark-skinned client, jaundice usually presents as yellowish-green and is most obviously seen in the sclera of the eye. Do not confuse jaundice with yellow pigmentation in palms of hands and soles of feet, which is typical in the healthy dark-skinned client.

Erythema is a redness associated with a variety of rashes. **Edema** is the presence of excess interstitial fluid (see Procedure 19-1B). Elasticity or **turgor** (fullness) of the skin is also observed.

A skin **lesion** is an alteration in a client's normal skin appearance. Nurses are responsible for describing skin lesions accurately in terms of location (e.g., face), distribution (i.e., body regions involved), and configuration (the arrangement or position of several lesions). They also note the color, shape, size, firmness, texture, and characteristics of individual lesions.

Assessment of the feet is an important consideration. This is especially important for clients with diabetes, peripheral vascular disease, or patients in traction from musculoskeletal injury or surgery (see Table 19-3 ■).

Nails

Nails are inspected for nail plate shape, nail texture, nail bed color, the intactness of the tissues around the nails, and the angle between the nail and the nail bed (Figure 19-4 ■).

Nail texture is normally smooth. Excessively thick nails can appear in the elderly, in the presence of poor circulation, or in relation to a chronic fungal infection. A bluish or pur-

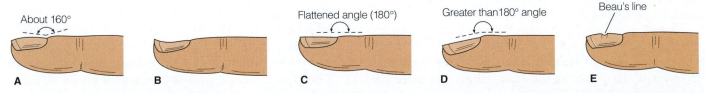

Figure 19-4. ■ **A.** A normal nail, showing the convex shape and the plate angle of about 160 degrees. **B.** A spoon-shaped nail, which may be seen in clients with iron-deficiency anemia. **C.** Early clubbing. **D.** Late clubbing (may be caused by long-term oxygen lack). **E.** Beau's line on nail (may result from severe injury or illness).

plish tint to the nail bed may reflect cyanosis. Pallor in the nail bed may reflect poor arterial circulation.

A blanch test can be carried out to test the **capillary refilling** time (the time the nail bed takes to return to its usual color after being pressed), to assess peripheral circulation. Normal nail bed capillaries blanch when pressed but quickly turn pink or their usual color when pressure is released. A capillary refill rate of more than 3 seconds may indicate circulatory problems.

Procedure 19-1, Part B, describes how to assess the skin and nails.

Cardiovascular System

Heart

In every physical assessment, it is important to listen to and count the apical **pulse** (heartbeat) for 1 full minute. Note pulse quality (bounding, normal, thready). Also note extra or skipped beats.

Associated with these sounds are systole and diastole. **Systole** is the period in which the ventricles contract. It begins with the first heart sound and ends at the second heart sound. Systole is normally shorter than diastole. **Diastole** is the period in which the ventricles relax. It starts with the second sound and ends at the following first sound. Both sounds are low in pitch and heard best at the apical site, with the bell of the stethoscope, and with the client lying on the left side. Palpation and or auscultation of an irregular rhythm reliably indicates atrial fibrillation. To accurately determine all other irregular patterns, an electrocardiogram is needed to identify the arrhythmia.

Peripheral Vascular System

The **peripheral vascular system** includes all of the blood vessels that carry oxygenated blood to body tissues and organs and return deoxygenated blood to the heart and lungs. When palpating peripheral pulses, note quality of pulses; document as bounding (palpable, forceful), normal, weak (difficult to palpate and easily stopped by pressure), or absent (not palpable). Assessing the peripheral vascular system also includes measuring the blood pressure; inspecting, palpating, and auscultating the carotid pulse; inspecting the jugular and peripheral veins; and inspecting the skin and tissues to determine **perfusion** (blood supply to an area) to the extremities. The force of the pulse indicates the strength of the heart's stroke volume and is recorded using a three-point scale: 3+, full bounding; 2+, normal; and 1+, weak, thready. Certain aspects of peripheral vascular assessment are often incorporated into other parts of the assessment procedure. For example, blood pressure is usually measured at the beginning of the physical examination (see Chapter 20 ⚭, the section on pulse sites and Procedure 20-2 ⚭; see also Procedure 20-4 ⚭ on assessing blood pressure). Procedure 19-1, Part C, describes how to assess the cardiovascular and peripheral vascular systems.

Respiratory System

Thorax and Lung Assessment

Abnormal breath sounds, called adventitious breath sounds, occur when air passes through narrowed airways or airways filled with fluid or mucus, or when pleural linings are inflamed. **Adventitious breath sounds**—crackles (referred to as **rales** or crepitations), gurgles, pleural friction rub, and **wheezes**—are often superimposed over normal sounds. Table 19-4 ■ describes normal sounds and adventitious breath sounds. Absence of breath sounds over some lung areas is also a significant finding; it is associated with collapsed and surgically removed lobes. Oxygenation is discussed in depth in Chapter 24 ⚭.

Assessing the lungs is frequently critical to assessing the client's air exchange status. Changes in the respiratory system can come about slowly or quickly. In clients with chronic obstructive pulmonary disease (COPD), such as chronic bronchitis, emphysema, and asthma, changes often occur gradually as the body attempts to increase lung expansion.

Auscultation

To hear the breath sounds accurately, the nurse performs auscultation with the stethoscope on the skin, not through clothing. For efficiency, the nurse usually examines the posterior chest first, then the anterior chest. For posterior and lateral chest examinations, the client is uncovered to the waist and is in a sitting position. A sitting or lying position may be used for anterior chest examination. The sitting position is preferred because it maximizes chest expansion. However, if the client is unable to sit up, the examination can be performed with the client lying on his or her side.

Ask the client to take slow, deep breaths through the mouth while the exam is performed. This allows the client to move a greater amount of air through the lungs, which helps the nurse detect abnormal sounds. It can sometimes be helpful to have the client cough two or three times before the nurse begins auscultation. Coughing helps to clear the lung fields, which in turn clears airway secretions in the healthy lower respiratory track. If crackles, rhonchi, or wheezes can be heard following patient cough, then these adventitious lung sounds need further evaluation.

To auscultate the anterior chest, begin just above the clavicle starting on the client's right side. Move to the left side. Move to each lobe in a right-to-left pattern. When auscultating the anterior chest of a female client, it may be necessary to have her lie down so that her breasts fall to the side, allowing more accurate auscultation of the lung fields.

Respirations should also be counted at this time. Respirations normally range from 18 to 20 breaths per minute in an adult. Respirations should be described as present, absent, deep, shallow, and with or without difficulty. A procedure called pulse oximetry is frequently conducted on

TABLE 19-4

Normal and Adventitious Breath Sounds

TYPE/NAME	DESCRIPTION	CHARACTERISTICS/CAUSES	LOCATION
NORMAL BREATH SOUNDS			
Vesicular	Soft-intensity, low-pitched, "gentle sighing" sounds created by air moving through smaller airways (bronchioles and alveoli)	Best heard on inspiration, which is about 2.5 times longer than the expiratory phase (5:2 ratio)	Over peripheral lung; best heard at base of lungs
Bronchovesicular	Moderate-intensity and moderate-pitched "blowing" sounds created by air moving through larger airways (bronchi)	Equal inspiratory and expiratory phases (1:1 ratio)	Between the scapulae and lateral to the sternum at the first and second intercostal spaces
Bronchial (tubular)	High-pitched, loud, "harsh" sounds created by air moving through the trachea	Louder than vesicular sounds; have a short inspiratory phase and long expiratory phase (1:2 ratio)	Anteriorly over the trachea; not normally heard over lung tissue
ADVENTITIOUS BREATH SOUNDS			
Crackles (rales)	Fine, short, interrupted crackling sounds; alveolar rales are high-pitched. Sound can be simulated by rolling a lock of hair near the ear. Best heard on inspiration but can be heard on both inspiration and expiration. May not be cleared by coughing.	Air passing through fluid or mucus in any air passage	Most commonly heard in the bases of the lower lung lobes
Gurgles (rhonchi)	Continuous, low-pitched, coarse, gurgling, harsh, louder sounds with a moaning or snoring quality. Best heard on expiration but can be heard on both inspiration and expiration. May be altered by coughing.	Air passing through narrowed air passages as a result of secretions, swelling, tumors	Loud sounds can be heard over most lung areas but predominate over the trachea and bronchi
Friction rub	Superficial grating or creaking sounds heard during inspiration and expiration. Not relieved by coughing.	Rubbing together of inflamed pleural surfaces	Heard most often in areas of greatest thoracic expansion (e.g., lower anterior and lateral chest)
Wheeze	Continuous, high-pitched, squeaky musical sounds. Best heard on expiration. Not usually altered by coughing.	Air passing through constricted bronchi as a result of secretions, swelling, tumors	Heard over all lung fields

clients with respiratory impairment (see Procedure 24-1 ⚭ for an explanation of use of an oximeter).

The nurse should also note any sputum, its appearance, and amount. See Box 19-1 for description of sputum. It is also important to note if the client is short of breath and which activity, if any, produces shortness of breath. Procedure 19-1, Part D, describes how to assess the lungs.

Gastrointestinal System

Upper GI

When assessing the mouth and oropharynx, the nurse should observe for the following: inflammation of the tongue and oral mucosa; accumulation of food, microorgan-

isms, and epithelial elements on the teeth and gums (referred to as sordes); or bleeding of the gums (which may be due to disease process or medication). Note that cancer of the lip and cancer of the tongue are the most common cancers of the mouth. Any persistent nodule or ulcer should be suspect and should be further evaluated.

The mouth is the beginning of the gastrointestinal system (digestive system) and should be assessed carefully. The Centers for Disease Control and Prevention (CDC) recommends that nurses wear gloves when in contact with the buccal mucosa (Figures 19-5A and B ■). A tongue blade can be used to aid inspection.

The nurse should note any difficulty swallowing and obtain further information about the cause. The nurse also

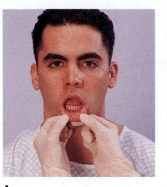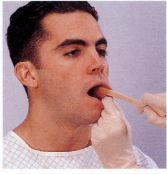

A   B

Figure 19-5. ■ **A.** Inspecting the mucosa of the lower lip.
B. Inspecting the buccal mucosa using a tongue blade.

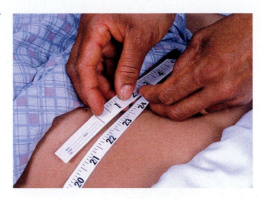

Figure 19-6. ■ Measuring abdominal girth at the level of the umbilicus. (Al Dodge, Pearson Education/PH.)

notes any subjective indications of discomfort or nausea and records the client's statement of when these manifestations began and how long they have persisted. Frequent vomiting along with macerated knuckles, swollen salivary glands, and dental caries may indicate an eating disorder. Any abnormal findings or change in client condition should be reported to the team leader.

Abdomen

To assist in obtaining valid observations and to enhance client comfort, as mentioned previously, the nurse asks the client to urinate before beginning the assessment. If necessary, the nurse assists the client to a supine position, with arms placed comfortably at the sides. The nurse also places small pillows beneath the knees and the head. This position and an empty bladder prevent tension in the abdominal muscles. By contrast, the abdominal muscles tense when the client is sitting or when the client is supine with knees and arms extended and hands clasped behind the head.

The nurse exposes only the client's abdomen from chest line to the pubic area to avoid chilling and shivering, which can also tense the abdominal muscles.

The nurse locates and describes abdominal findings in a client by dividing the abdomen into quadrants, imagining a vertical line from the xiphoid process to the pubic symphysis, and a horizontal line across the umbilicus (see Figure 18-20 ⚭). These quadrants are labeled (1) right upper quadrant (RUQ), (2) left upper quadrant (LUQ), (3) right lower quadrant (RLQ), and (4) left lower quadrant (LLQ). Assessment of the abdomen involves all four methods of examination (inspection, auscultation, palpation, and percussion). As mentioned already, inspection, auscultation, and light palpation are the skills first practiced by LPNs/LVNs.

The nurse performs inspection first, followed by auscultation, and palpation last. Auscultation is done before palpation because palpation causes movement or stimulation of the bowel. This can increase bowel motility and heighten bowel sounds, creating false results.

Thus, the order of abdominal assessment should be:

1. *Look.* While standing at the side of the supine client, inspect the abdomen for contour and symmetry. Is it flat, rounded, or concave? If rounded, is it distended (stretched out)? When distention is present, measure the abdominal girth by placing a tape around the abdomen at the level of the umbilicus (Figure 19-6 ■). Look for movement associated with peristalsis or pulsations.
2. *Listen.* Place the diaphragm of your stethoscope lightly on the client's abdomen and listen for bowel sounds in all four quadrants (see Figure 18-20 ⚭). Landmarks for identifying abdominal areas are shown in Figure 19-7 ■. Are sounds normal, increased, decreased, or absent? If you suspect absent bowel sounds, listen for 5 minutes. Be sure that the client's bladder is empty before reporting absent bowel sounds. A full bladder may obscure sounds.
3. *Feel.* Light palpation is used mainly for determining areas of tenderness. Palpate in all four quadrants (Figure 19-8 ■). The best indicator of tenderness is the client's facial expression. Pain with pressure, such as in palpation or percussion, in the costovertebral angle may suggest kidney infection or a musculoskeletal cause. In either case, further and more focused assessment should be conducted. Tenderness and rigidity 1 to 2 inches above

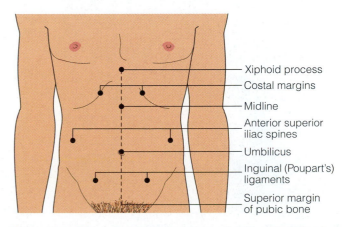

- Xiphoid process
- Costal margins
- Midline
- Anterior superior iliac spines
- Umbilicus
- Inguinal (Poupart's) ligaments
- Superior margin of pubic bone

Figure 19-7. ■ Landmarks commonly used to identify abdominal areas.

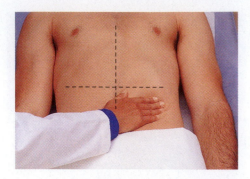

Figure 19-8. ■ Light palpation used in all four quadrants to check for areas of tenderness.

the anterosuperior spine of the right ilium and the umbilicus (McBurney's point) are indicative of appendicitis. Caution should be used when palpating this area of the abdomen if there is complaint of pain. Voluntary or involuntary guarding may be present.

Procedure 19-1, Part E, describes how to assess the abdomen.

Genitourinary System

Note whether the client is continent or incontinent of urine or if an indwelling catheter is present. The amount, color, frequency, and odor of the urine should be described. This is a good opportunity to check the client's intake and output.

In some clients, it may be necessary to palpate the bladder to determine whether the client has emptied it completely (Figure 19-9 ■). Locate the edge of the bladder by pressing in the midline about 1 to 2 inches above the symphysis pubis. If the bladder is palpable, the nurse will feel a smooth, firm, slightly bouncy area. The client may indicate the urge to empty the bladder when it is palpated. During the postpartum period, the bladder can be easily palpated by first identifying the fundus of the uterus and then creeping the fingers down toward the symphysis pubis.

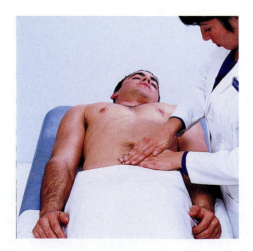

Figure 19-9. ■ Palpating the bladder.

Procedure 19-1, Part F, describes how to assess the bladder and urine.

Musculoskeletal System

The musculoskeletal system encompasses the muscles, bones, and joints (see Figure 18-7 ⬭).

Range of Motion

There are two types of range of motion (ROM): active and passive. In **active range of motion**, the extremities and joints are moved by the client through a systematic series of movements. The nurse asks the client to move each joint through a full range of motion. The nurse notes the degree and type of pain or weakness, or any limitation of movement. Each movement is compared with the same movement on the other side. The nurse proceeds to passive ROM if the client is unable to perform active ROM.

In **passive range of motion**, the client's extremities and joints are supported and moved by the nurse. The same series of movements are made as in active ROM. Any pain or increased limitation of movement is noted, and each movement is compared with the other side. If a client is able to stand or walk, observe his or her ability. Also describe any deformities. (See Procedure 32-1 ⬭ for passive ROM exercises.) The nurse should be especially alert to signs of inflammation and arthritis in joints.

■ *Swelling:* May indicate synovitis; swelling may involve the synovial membrane, effusion from excess synovial fluid within the joint space, or soft-tissue injury.
■ *Warmth:* May be indicative of arthritis, tendonitis, bursitis, or osteomyelitis.
■ *Tenderness:* Usually indicative of arthritis or infection.
■ *Redness:* Usually indicative of septic or gouty arthritis or rheumatoid arthritis.

Procedure 19-1, Part G, describes how to assess the extremities, joints, and movement.

Psychosocial Status

Psychosocial status should be considered. The client's mental and spiritual status can have significant effects on physical recovery. Much can be discovered about the client through an assessment of mood, affect, judgment, abilities, and lifestyle patterns. Refer to Chapters 2, 11, 14, and 16 ⬭ for more about psychosocial aspects of care.

Variations in the Geriatric Assessment

The elderly client should be kept warm and comfortable during the physical assessment. Loss of subcutaneous fat in the elderly decreases their ability to stay warm. It may be necessary to adapt assessment and positioning to physical limitations. Perform as much of the assessment as possible in the position most comfortable for the client.

The elderly client's skin is fragile and care should be used when assessing the skin and or helping the client change positions. Use care when removing tape and bandages to prevent skin tears.

Sensory deficits (loss of hearing, sight, touch) can occur in the elderly. Provide a quiet environment with minimal distractions.

Avoid using vigorous assessment techniques such as hopping on one foot or doing deep knee bends when doing musculoskeletal assessments of the elderly. Elderly clients have limited range of motion and decreased balance.

DIAGNOSING, PLANNING, AND IMPLEMENTING

Data from focused assessments are used to shape the plan of care and provide appropriate interventions to suit the client's needs. The nurse learns to assess using all of the senses and is always alert to changes in the client's condition.

An accurate picture of the client's health can be achieved by thorough, organized assessment of all the body systems and by regular communication of all findings to the team leader. Assessment serves as a tool to all members of the healthcare team who care for the client.

EVALUATING

The LPN/LVN performs the focused assessment as ordered. A focused assessment is usually done at the end of a shift. The results are then shared in an end-of-shift report. During a shift, changes in status are reported to the charge nurse as needed and according to institutional policy.

NURSING PROCESS CARE PLAN
Client with Postpartum Bleeding

Stephanie Franklin is a 35-year-old lawyer who gave birth to her first baby 3 hours ago. Her labor and delivery were uneventful and she is now on the postpartum floor. Her vaginal bleeding has increased during the past hour.

Assessment. Janet Rodriguez, Ms. Franklin's day shift nurse, assists her to the bathroom and notices that she has bled through two pads in the past hour. Ms. Franklin passes an orange-sized, bright red clot of blood; she complains of dizziness. Ms. Rodriguez assists Ms. Franklin back to bed. On palpation of the uterus, Ms. Rodriguez notes that it is boggy. Two more orange-sized blood clots are expressed as Ms. Rodriguez firmly massages the fundus (top of the uterus). Ms. Rodriguez continues fundal massage; however, the bleeding remains heavy. Ms. Rodriguez collects the following assessment data: T 98.6, BP 80/50, P 120, quick hemoglobin and hematocrit (HemoCue) result 6. Complains of dizziness and nausea. Increased blood loss is discussed with RN and reported to physician.

Nursing Diagnosis. The following important nursing diagnoses (among others) are established for this client:

- *Risk for Deficient Fluid Volume* related to blood loss
- *Activity Intolerance* related to dizziness secondary to blood loss
- *Risk for Infection* related to possible retained placenta
- *Risk for Interrupted Family Processes*.

Expected Outcomes. The expected outcomes specify that Ms. Franklin will:

- Regain fluid balance as evidenced by normal BP and pulse, and experience no further drop in hemoglobin level.
- Be able to ambulate without dizziness.
- Maintain a normal temperature.
- Have a fluid intake of at least 2000 mL/day.
- Breast feed baby according to baby's feeding needs.

Planning and Implementation. The following nursing interventions are planned and implemented:

- Monitor vital signs according to doctor's orders.
- Monitor condition of fundus every 30 minutes.
- Encourage fluid intake.
- Provide perineal care every 2 hours.
- Bring baby to mother for feedings and remain with mother and baby throughout feeding.
- Measure intake and output every 4 hours.

Evaluation. After being transported to the labor and delivery unit for manual removal of remaining placenta, Ms. Franklin is returned to the postpartum unit. At the end of the shift, Ms. Franklin is sitting up in bed, breastfeeding her baby. She complains of "a little dizziness if I sit up too fast." BP 110/68, Temp 98.5, HemoCue remains at 6; 1000 mL urine output in 4 hours. Oral intake 400 mL, IV intake 1000 mL in 4 hours.

Critical Thinking in the Nursing Process

1. Why was Ms. Franklin's blood pressure low and pulse elevated?
2. Why did Ms. Franklin complain of dizziness?
3. Why would the nursing diagnosis *Risk for Interrupted Family Processes* with baby be appropriate?

Note: Discussion of Critical Thinking questions appears in Appendix I.

Note: The references and resources for this and all chapters have been compiled at the back of the book.

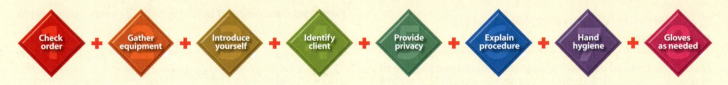

PROCEDURE 19-1   Focused Physical Assessment by Body Systems*

Purposes

- To obtain measurements to compare to baseline data
- To obtain information to assess effect of medications
- To determine health and comfort status of the client before or after a procedure or at the end of shift

Equipment

- Stethoscope or Doppler Ultrasound (DUS)
- Penlight or flashlight
- Thermometer
- Sphygmomanometer and cuff

Check order + Gather equipment + Introduce yourself + Identify client + Provide privacy + Explain procedure + Hand hygiene + Gloves as needed

Part A: General Appearance and Mental Status

General Appearance

INSPECTION

1. Observe body build, height, and weight in relation to the client's age, lifestyle, and health.

2. Observe the client's posture and gait, standing, sitting, and walking.

3. Observe the client's overall hygiene and grooming. Relate these to the person's activities prior to the assessment.

4. Note body and breath odor in relation to activity level.

5. Observe for signs of distress in posture (e.g., bending over because of abdominal pain) or facial expression (e.g., wincing or labored breathing).

6. Note obvious signs of health or illness (e.g., in skin color or breathing).

BEHAVIOR

1. Assess the client's attitude.

2. Note the client's affect/mood; assess the appropriateness of the client's response and level of orientation to time, place, and persons.

3. Listen for quantity of speech (amount and pace), quality (loudness, clarity, inflection), and organization (coherence of thought, overgeneralization, vagueness).

4. Listen for relevance and organization of thoughts.

Normal Findings

- Varies with lifestyle
- Relaxed, erect posture; coordinated movement

- Clean, neat
- No body odor or minor body odor relative to work or exercise; no breath odor
- Healthy appearance
- Cooperative
- Appropriate to situation
- Understandable, moderate pace
- Exhibits thought association
- Logical sequence
- Makes sense; has sense of reality

Deviations from Normal

- Excessively thin or obese
- Tense, slouched, bent posture; uncoordinated movement; tremors
- Dirty, unkempt
- Foul body odor; ammonia odor; acetone breath odor; foul breath
- Pallor; weakness; obvious illness
- Negative, hostile, withdrawn
- Inappropriate to situation
- Rapid or slow pace
- Uses generalizations; lacks association
- Illogical sequence
- Flight of ideas; confusion

Neurologic

LEVEL OF CONSCIOUSNESS (LOC)

1. Ask client to give name, present location, and date or time of day.

---

* This is an abbreviated assessment that can be conducted by the LPN/LVN at the beginning and/or the end of the shift. A complete physical assessment is done by the RN on admission.

Normal Findings

- Alert and oriented ×3: able to give correct name, location, and/or time of day or date.

Deviations from Normal

- Inability to correctly name one or more items.

VERBAL RESPONSE

1. Assess how the client communicates rather than what is communicated, through normal conversation.

Normal Findings

- Clear
- Rate consistent with overall psychomotor status
- Volume audible, normal conversational tone
- Modulation and flow—fluid and expressive
- Production—able to produce words

Deviations from Normal

- Incoherent, rambling, slurred, stuttering
- Monotone
- Dysphasia, aphasia

Assessing Motor Response

GRIPS

1. Ask the client to grasp your index and middle finger while you try to pull the fingers out.

PUSHES/PULLS

1. Have the client hold arm up and resist while you try to push it down.
2. Have the client fully extend each arm and try to flex it while you attempt to hold arm in extension.
3. Have the client resist while you attempt to dorsiflex the foot and again while you attempt to flex the foot.

WALKING GAIT

1. Ask the client to walk across the room and back with eyesight focused ahead; assess the client's gait.

Normal Findings

- Bilateral/equal 100% normal strength; normal full movement; against gravity and against full resistance
- Has upright posture and steady gait with opposing arm swing; walks unaided, maintaining balance

Deviations from Normal

- Unequal strength
- 10% of normal strength; no movement, contraction of muscle is palpable or visible
- Has poor posture and unsteady, irregular, staggering gait with wide stance; bends legs only from hips; has rigid or no arm movements

Assessing Pupil Reactions

DIRECT AND CONSENSUAL REACTION TO LIGHT

1. Partially darken the room.
2. Ask the client to look straight ahead.
3. Using a penlight or flashlight and approaching from the side, shine a light on the pupil.
4. Observe the response of the illuminated pupil. It should constrict (direct response).
5. Shine the light on the pupil again, and observe the response of the other pupil. It should also constrict (consensual response).

REACTION TO ACCOMMODATION

1. Hold an object (a penlight or pencil) about 10 cm (4 in.) from the bridge of the client's nose.
2. Ask the client to look first at the top of the object and then at a distant object (e.g., the far wall) behind the penlight. Alternate the gaze from the near to the far object.
3. Observe the pupil response. The pupils should constrict when looking at the near object and dilate when looking at the far object.
4. Next, move the penlight or pencil toward the client's nose. The pupils should converge.
5. To record normal assessment of the pupils, use the abbreviation PERRLA (pupils equally round and react to light and accommodation).
6. Assess each pupil's reaction to accommodation.

Normal Findings

- Pupils constrict when looking at near object; pupils dilate when looking at far object; pupils converge when near object is moved toward nose

Deviations from Normal

- One or both pupils fail to constrict, dilate, or converge

Part B: Integumentary Assessment

Assessing the Skin

1. Inspect skin color (best assessed under natural light and on areas not exposed to the sun).
2. Inspect uniformity of skin color.
3. Assess edema, if present (i.e., location, color, temperature, and the degree to which the skin remains indented or pitted when pressed by a finger). See Figure 19-10 ■.
4. Inspect and describe skin lesions.

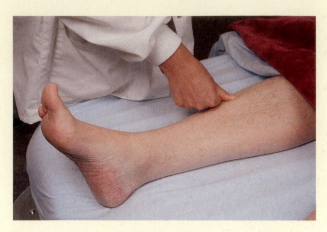

Figure 19-10. ■ Assess edema by pressing your finger firmly against client's skin for several seconds (especially in ankle area). After removing your finger, observe for lasting impression or indentation.

clinical ALERT

Assess skin turgor over the sternum in older adults. Loss of subcutaneous tissue in aging makes the skin of the arms a less reliable indicator of fluid status.

5. Observe and palpate skin moisture.

6. Palpate skin temperature. Compare the two feet and the two hands, using the backs of your fingers. Backs of fingers pick up temperature differences more readily.

7. Note skin turgor (fullness or elasticity) by lifting and pulling the skin on an extremity into a tent position.

Normal Findings

■ Varies from light to deep brown; from ruddy pink to light pink; from yellow overtones to olive
■ Generally uniform except in areas exposed to the sun; areas of lighter pigmentation (palms, lips, nail beds) in dark-skinned people
  Scale for Describing Edema
  1 = Barely detectable
  2 = Indentation of less than 5 mm
  3 = Indentation of 5 to 10 mm
  4 = Indentation of more than 10 mm.
■ Freckles, some birthmarks, some flat and raised nevi (moles); no abrasions or other lesions
■ Moisture in skin folds and the axillae (varies with environmental temperature and humidity, body temperature, and activity)
■ Uniform; within normal range
■ When tented, skin springs back to previous state

Deviations from Normal

■ Pallor, cyanosis, jaundice, erythema
■ Areas of either hyperpigmentation or hypopigmentation (e.g., vitiligo, albinism, edema)
■ Various interruptions in skin integrity
■ Excessive moisture (e.g., in hyperthermia); excessive dryness (e.g., in dehydration)
■ Generalized hyperthermia (e.g., in fever); generalized hypothermia (e.g., in shock); localized hyperthermia (e.g., in infection); localized hypothermia (e.g., in arteriosclerosis)
■ Skin stays tented or moves back slowly (e.g., in dehydration)

Assessing Mucous Membranes

1. Inspect and palpate the inner lips and buccal mucosa for color, moisture, texture, and the presence of lesions. Uniform pink color (darker, e.g., bluish hue, in dark-skinned clients).

Normal Findings

■ Soft, moist, smooth texture
■ Uniform pink color (freckled brown pigmentation in dark-skinned clients)
■ Moist, smooth, soft, glistening, and elastic texture

Deviations from Normal

■ Pallor; cyanosis
■ Blisters; generalized or localized swelling; fissures, crusts, or scales (may result from excessive moisture, nutritional deficiency, or fluid deficit)
■ Inability to purse lips (indicative of facial nerve damage)
■ Pallor; white patches (leukoplakia)
■ Excessive dryness

Assessing Teeth and Gums

1. Inspect the teeth and gums while examining the inner lips and buccal mucosa.

Normal Findings

■ 32 adult teeth
■ Smooth, white, shiny tooth enamel
■ Pink gums (bluish or dark patches in dark-skinned clients)
■ Moist, firm texture to gums
■ No retraction of gums (pulling away from the crown of the tooth)

Deviations from Normal

■ Missing teeth
■ Ill-fitting dentures
■ Brown or black discoloration of the enamel (may indicate staining or the presence of caries)

- Excessively red gums
- Spongy texture; bleeding; tenderness (may indicate periodontal disease)
- Receding, atrophied gums; swelling that partially covers the teeth
- Dry, furry tongue (associated with fluid deficit)
- Nodes, ulcerations, discolorations (white or red areas); areas of tenderness
- Restricted mobility
- Swelling, ulceration
- Swelling, nodules
- Inflammation (redness and swelling)
- Discoloration (e.g., jaundice or pallor)
- Palates the same color
- Irritations
- Bony growths (exostoses) growing from the hard palate

- Deviation to one side from tumor or trauma; immobility (may indicate damage to trigeminal [fifth cranial] nerve or vagus [tenth cranial] nerve)
- Reddened or edematous; presence of lesions, plaques, or exudate
- Inflamed
- Presence of discharge
- Swollen
- Sordes (accumulation of brown crusts on teeth and lips; may be related to mild elevated temperature)

Assessing the Nails

1. Note the color of the nail bed. Bluish nails suggest cyanosis.
2. Perform a capillary refill test if necessary. A capillary refill time of more than 3 seconds may indicate circulatory problems.

Part C: Cardiovascular Assessment
Assessing Heart Sounds

1. Auscultate the heart in all four anatomic sites: aortic, pulmonic, tricuspid, and apical (mitral). Auscultation need not be limited to these areas. However, the nurse may need to move the stethoscope to find the most audible sounds for each client.
2. Eliminate all sources of room noise. *Heart sounds are of low intensity, and other noise hinders the nurse's ability to hear them.*
3. Keep the client in a supine position with head elevated 30 to 45 degrees.
4. Use both the flat-disk diaphragm and the bell-shaped diaphragm to listen to all areas.
5. In every area of auscultation, distinguish both S_1 and S_2 sounds.
6. When auscultating, concentrate on one particular sound at a time in each area: the first heart sound, followed by systole, then the second heart sound, then diastole. Systole and diastole are normally silent intervals.
7. Later, reexamine the heart while the client is in the upright sitting position. *Certain sounds are more audible in this position.*

Normal Findings

- S_1: Usually heard at all sites. Usually louder at the apical and tricuspid areas
- S_2: Usually heard at all sites. Usually louder at base of heart and aortic and pulmonic areas
- Systole: Silent interval. Slightly shorter duration than diastole at normal heart rate (60–90 bpm)
- Diastole: Silent interval. Slightly longer duration than systole at normal heart rates
- S_3 in children and young adults

- S_4 in many older adults

Deviations from Normal

- Increased or decreased intensity
- Varying intensity with different beats
- Increased intensity at aortic area
- Increased intensity at pulmonic area
- Sharp-sounding ejection clicks
- S_3 in older adults
- S_4 may be a sign of hypertension

Assessing the Peripheral Vascular System
PERIPHERAL PULSES

1. Palpate the peripheral pulses (except the carotid pulse) on both sides of the client's body simultaneously and systematically to determine the symmetry of pulse volume. *This method helps to determine the symmetry of pulse volume.*
2. Assess radial pulses and compare. Check capillary refill. Ask client to wiggle fingers. Ask client not to look at his or her feet. Touch the client's feet one at a time, asking the client if he or she is able to feel your touch. *This will determine level of touch perception.*
3. Assess pedal pulses and compare one side to the other. Note strength of pulse. If pedal pulses are not palpable, palpate posterior tibial pulse and compare one side to the other. Check capillary refill in toes. Ask client to wiggle toes. Ask the client if he or she experiences numbness or tingling in extremities or sensation of cold. *Tibial pulse should be more palpable because it is closer to the heart.*

4. Palpate skin temperature. Compare the two feet and the two hands, using the backs of your fingers. *Coolness may indicate lack of tissue perfusion.*

5. Note color of feet and toes and edema of the lower extremities.

6. Check for Homans' sign. To perform this test, the nurse supports the leg while flexing the foot in dorsiflexion. Ask the client if pain is felt as foot is flexed. Palpate muscles of calf for tender, hot areas. *A positive Homans' sign indicates venous thrombosis (blood clots).*

Normal Findings

- Symmetric pulse volumes
- Full pulsations
- In dependent position, distention and nodular bulges at calves are present
- When limbs are elevated, veins collapse (veins may appear tortuous or distended in older people)
- Limbs not tender
- Symmetric in size

Deviations from Normal

- Asymmetric volumes (indicate impaired circulation)
- Absence of pulsation (indicates arterial spasm or occlusion)
- Decreased, weak, thready pulsations (indicate impaired cardiac output)
- Increased pulse volume (may indicate hypertension, high cardiac output, or circulatory overload)
- Distended veins in the anteromedial part of thigh and/or lower leg or on posterolateral part of calf from knee to ankle
- Tenderness on palpation
- Pain in calf muscles with passive dorsiflexion of the foot (Homans' sign)
- Warmth and redness over vein
- Swelling of one calf or leg

PERIPHERAL PERFUSION

1. Inspect the skin of the hands and feet for color, temperature, edema, and skin changes. These factors can identify poor blood perfusion.

---

clinical ALERT

Report

If signs of arterial insufficiency occur, report findings to charge nurse.

---

2. Assess the adequacy of arterial flow if arterial insufficiency is suspected.

Normal Findings

- Natural skin color
- Skin temperature not excessively warm or cold
- No edema
- Skin texture resilient and moist
- Buerger's test: original color returns in 10 seconds; veins in feet or hands fill in about 15 seconds
- Capillary refill test: Immediate return of color

Deviations from Normal

- Cyanosis, pallor
- Skin cool
- Marked edema
- Skin thin and shiny or thick, waxy, shiny, and fragile, reduced hair, ulceration
- Delayed color return or mottled appearance; delayed venous filling; marked redness of arms or legs (indicates arterial insufficiency)
- Delayed return of color (arterial insufficiency)

Part D: Respiratory Assessment
Assessing the Thorax and Lungs

POSTERIOR THORAX

1. Inspect the shape and symmetry of the thorax from posterior and lateral views.

2. Palpate the posterior thorax.

3. For clients who have no respiratory complaints, rapidly assess the temperature and integrity of all chest skin.

4. For clients who do have respiratory complaints, palpate all chest areas for bulges, tenderness, or abnormal movements. Do not perform deep palpation. Observe caution when palpating (lightly). *If rib is fractured, deep palpation could lead to displacement of the bone fragment against the lungs.*

Normal Finding

- Chest symmetric

Deviations from Normal

- Chest asymmetric
- Bulges, tenderness, or abnormal movements in chest area

ANTERIOR THORAX

1. Auscultate the chest using the flat-disk diaphragm of the stethoscope. *The flat-disk side is best for transmitting the high-pitched breath sounds. Use the systematic zigzag procedure used in percussion (Figure 19-11 ■). This ensures that no areas are missed.*

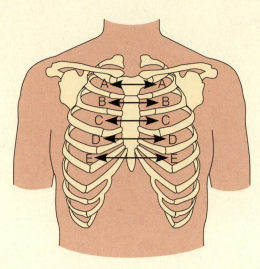

Figure 19-11. ■ Systematic zigzag pattern.

2. Ask the client to take slow, deep breaths through the mouth. Listen at each point to the breath sounds during a complete inspiration and expiration. Compare findings at each point with the corresponding point on the opposite side of the chest. *Slow, deep breaths move more air and allow abnormalities to be heard.*

Normal Findings

- Quiet, rhythmic, and effortless respirations
- Full, symmetric respiratory effort

Deviations from Normal

- Adventitious breath sounds (e.g., crackles, rhonchi, wheezes, friction rub)
- Absence of breath sounds (associated with collapsed and surgically removed lung lobes)
- Asymmetric and/or decreased respiratory exchange

Part E: Abdominal Assessment
Inspection

1. Inspect the abdomen for skin integrity (refer to the discussion of skin assessment earlier in this chapter).

2. Inspect the abdomen for contour and symmetry.

3. Observe the abdominal contour (profile line from the rib margin to the pubic bone) while standing at the client's side when the client is supine.

4. Ask the client to take a deep breath and to hold it (makes any abnormality such as an enlarged liver or spleen more obvious).

5. Assess the symmetry of contour while standing at the foot of the bed.

6. If distention is present, measure the abdominal girth by placing a tape around the abdomen at the level of the umbilicus. *Distention may indicate hidden fluid imbalances.*

Normal Findings

- Unblemished skin
- Uniform color
- Silver-white striae or surgical scars
- Flat, rounded (convex), or scaphoid (concave or boat shaped)
- No evidence of enlargement of liver or spleen
- Symmetric contour

Deviations from Normal

- Presence of rash or other lesions
- Tense, glistening skin (may indicate ascites, edema)
- Purple striae (associated with Cushing's disease)

- Generalized distention (associated with gas retention, obesity, ascites, or tumors)
- Lower abdominal distention (may indicate bladder distention, pregnancy, or ovarian mass)
- Markedly *scaphoid* (concave or boat-shaped) abdomen (associated with malnutrition)
- Evidence of enlargement of liver or spleen
- Asymmetric contour, such as localized protrusions around umbilicus, inguinal ligaments, or scars (possible hernia or tumor)

Auscultation

1. Auscultate the abdomen for bowel sounds and vascular sounds.

2. Warm the hands and the stethoscope diaphragms. *Cold hands and a cold stethoscope may cause the client to contract the abdominal muscles, and these contractions may be heard during auscultation.*

FOR BOWEL SOUNDS

1. Use the flat-disk diaphragm (Figure 19-12 ■). *Intestinal sounds are relatively high pitched and best accentuated by the flat-disk diaphragm. Light pressure with the stethoscope is adequate to detect sounds.*

2. Ask when the client last ate. *The frequency of sounds relates to the state of digestion or the presence of food in the gastrointestinal tract. Shortly after or long after eating, bowel sounds may normally increase. They are loudest when a meal is long overdue. Four to 7 hours after a meal, bowel sounds in the RLQ may be heard continuously over the ileocecal valve area while the digestive contents from the small intestine empty through the valve into the large intestine.*

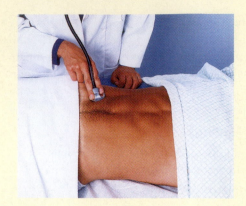

Figure 19-12. ■ Auscultating the abdomen for bowel sounds.

3. Place the flat-disk diaphragm of the stethoscope in each of the four quadrants of the abdomen (see Figure 18-20 ⟲⟳). Many nurses begin in the lower right quadrant in the area of the cecum.

4. Listen for active bowel sounds—irregular gurgling noises occurring about every 5 to 20 seconds. *The duration of a single sound may range from less than a second to more than several seconds.*

5. Normal bowel sounds are described as audible. Alterations in sounds are described as absent or hypoactive, that is, extremely soft and infrequent (e.g., one per minute), and hyperactive or increased, that is, high-pitched, loud, rushing sounds that occur frequently (e.g., every 3 seconds) also known as borborygmi. *Absence of sounds indicates a cessation of intestinal motility. Hypoactive sounds indicate decreased motility and are usually associated with manipulation of the bowel during surgery, inflammation, paralytic ileus, or late bowel obstruction. Hyperactive sounds indicate increased intestinal motility and are usually associated with diarrhea, an early bowel obstruction, or the use of laxatives.*

FOR ABSENT, HYPOACTIVE, OR HYPERACTIVE BOWEL SOUNDS

1. If bowel sounds appear to be absent, listen for 3 to 5 minutes before concluding that they are absent. *Because bowel sounds are so irregular, a longer time and more sites are used to confirm absence of sounds.*

Normal Finding

■ Audible bowel sounds

Deviations from Normal

■ Limited movement due to pain or disease process
■ Visible peristalsis in nonlean clients (with bowel obstruction)

PALPATION

1. Perform light palpation first to detect areas of tenderness and/or muscle guarding. Systematically explore all four quadrants. *Palpation is used to detect tenderness, the presence of masses or distention, and the outline and position of abdominal organs (e.g., the liver, spleen, and kidneys). Two types of palpation are used: light and deep. In some practice settings, palpation is limited to light abdominal palpation to assess tenderness and bladder palpation to assess for distention.*

2. Before palpation, ensure that the client's position is appropriate for relaxation of the abdominal muscles, and warm the hands. *Cold hands can cause muscle tension and thus impede palpatory evaluation.*

3. For light palpation, hold the palm of your hand slightly above the client's abdomen, with your fingers parallel to the abdomen.

4. Depress the abdominal wall lightly, about 1 cm or to the depth of the subcutaneous tissue, with the pads of your fingers (Figure 19-13 ■).

5. Move the finger pads in a slight circular motion.

6. Note areas of slight tenderness or superficial pain, large masses, and muscle guarding. To determine areas of tenderness, ask the client to tell you about them, watch for changes in the client's facial expressions, and note areas of muscle guarding.

Normal Findings

■ No tenderness; relaxed soft abdomen with smooth, consistent tension; pain free

Deviations from Normal

■ Tenderness and hypersensitivity
■ Superficial masses
■ Localized areas of increased tension
■ Generalized or localized areas of tenderness

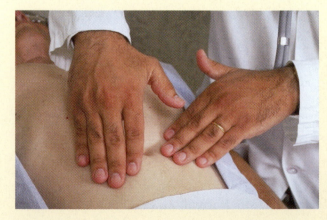

Figure 19-13. ■ For light palpation of the abdomen, depress the abdominal wall lightly, about 1 cm or to the depth of the subcutaneous tissue, with the pads of your fingers.

Part F: Genitourinary Assessment
Urination

1. Assess client for continence and independent urination.

Normal Finding

- Continent

Deviation from Normal

- Incontinent

INDWELLING CATHETER

1. Assess amount, color, odor, clarity, sediment, and frequency.

Normal Findings/Deviations from Normal

- Refer to Table 27-3 for normal characteristics of urine.

PALPATION OF THE BLADDER

1. Palpate the area above the pubic symphysis if the client's history indicates possible urinary retention.

Normal Finding

- Not palpable

Deviation from Normal

- Distended and palpable as smooth, round, tense mass (indicates urinary retention)

Part G: Musculoskeletal System Assessment
Muscles

1. Inspect the muscles for size. Compare the muscles on one side of the body (e.g., of the arm, thigh, and calf) to the same muscle on the other side. For any discrepancies, measure the muscles with a tape.
2. Inspect the muscles and tendons for contractures (shortening).
3. Inspect the muscles for fasciculations and tremors. Inspect any tremors of the hands and arms by having the client hold the arms in front of the body.

Bones

1. Inspect the skeleton for normal structure and deformities.
2. Examine for scoliosis in persons over age 12. Client stands facing away from the nurse and bends over to touch the toes.

Joints

1. Inspect the joints for swelling.
2. Palpate each joint for tenderness, smoothness of movement, swelling, crepitation, presence of nodules.
3. Assess joint range of motion.

Normal Findings

- Equal size on both sides of the body
- No contractures
- No fasciculations or tremors
- Normally firm
- Smooth coordinated movements
- Equal strength on each body side
- No deformities
- Straight spine
- No tenderness, swelling, crepitation, or nodules
- Joints move smoothly
- Varies to some degree in accordance with person's genetic makeup and degree of physical activity

Deviations from Normal

- Atrophy (a decrease in size) or hypertrophy (an increase in size)
- Malposition of body part (e.g., a foot fixed in dorsiflexion)
- Presence of fasciculation or tremor
- Atonic (lacking tone)
- Flaccidity (weakness or laxness) or spasticity (sudden involuntary muscle contraction)
- 25% or less of normal strength
- Bones misaligned
- A hump in the thoracic spine indicating a lateral curve
- Presence of tenderness or swelling (may indicate fractures, neoplasms, or osteoporosis)
- One or more swollen joints
- Presence of tenderness, swelling, crepitation, or nodules
- Limited range of motion in one or more joints

SAMPLE DOCUMENTATION

[date] [time] Client alert and oriented ×3, eyes PERRLA, I&O 700 mL in 6 h; BP 130/80; R 16; P 80; breath sounds clear; bowel sounds present and active in all quadrants. Abdominal incision open to air, without redness or swelling, staples intact. Complained of incision pain with a stated pain level of 7. PRN Pain meds given 1100. Pain level 1 at 1145.
_____Barbara Cook, LPN

Chapter Review

 KEY TERMS by Topic

Use the audio glossary feature of either the CD-ROM or the Companion Website to hear the correct pronunciation of the following key terms.

Introduction
physical assessment

Methods of Examination
inspection, auscultation, palpation, percussion, assessment, level of consciousness (LOC), orientation, direct response, consensual response, accommodation, PERRLA, vital signs, pallor,

cyanosis, erythema, edema, turgor, lesion, capillary refill, pulse, systole, diastole, peripheral vascular system, perfusion, adventitious breath sounds, rales, wheezes, active range of motion, passive range of motion

KEY Points

- The health examination is conducted to assess the function and integrity of the client's body parts.

- The health examination may entail a complete head-to-toe assessment or focused assessment of one or more body systems or a body part. If the head-to-toe assessment is performed during the admission process, it is carried out by the RN. Findings by the LPN/LVN during the focused assessment should be brought to the attention of the RN.

- The health assessment is conducted in a systematic manner that requires the fewest position changes for the client.

- Aspects of the physical assessment procedures should be incorporated in the assessment, intervention, and evaluation phases of the nursing process.

- Data obtained in the physical health examination are reported to the team leader. They are used to help establish nursing diagnoses and are helpful to all nursing staff in planning the client's care and evaluating nursing care outcomes.

- Initial assessment findings provide baseline data about the client's functional abilities. Subsequent assessment findings are compared to them.

 EXPLORE Media Link

Additional interactive resources for this chapter can be found on the Companion Website at www.prenhall.com/ramont. Click on Chapter 19 and "Begin" to select the activities for this chapter.

For chapter-related NCLEX®-style questions and an audio glossary, access the accompanying CD-ROM in this book.

Animations/Videos
- Various Breath Sounds

FOR FURTHER Study

Refer to Chapters 2, 11, 14, and 16 for more about psychosocial aspects of care.

Chapter 10 provides more information about collecting health history data.

Figure 18-7 illustrates the musculoskeletal system, and Figure 18-20 shows the four quadrants of the abdominal cavity.

See Chapter 20, Procedures 20-1 through 24-4 for detailed instructions related to measuring vital signs (body temperature, pulse, respirations, and blood pressure).

See Chapter 24 for more discussion of oxygenation and assessing respirations.

See Procedure 24-1 for using a pulse oximeter.

See Chapters 25 and 26 for additional information on measurement of height and weight, and for more about fluid balance.

See Table 27-3 for characteristics of urine.

See Procedure 32-1 for passive range-of-motion exercises.

Critical Thinking Care Map

Caring for a Client with Activity Intolerance
NCLEX-PN® Focus Area: Physiological Integrity

Case Study: Theresa Harris, 88, was admitted from a long-term care facility yesterday to rule out pneumonia. Theresa states, "I get dizzy when I get out of bed." Theresa has a history of cerebrovascular accident with some residual weakness of the left hand.

Nursing Diagnosis: Activity Intolerance

COLLECT DATA

Subjective	Objective
_____	_____
_____	_____
_____	_____
_____	_____
_____	_____
_____	_____

Would you report this? Yes/No

If yes, to: _____

What would you report? _____

Nursing Care

_____
_____
_____
_____
_____
_____
_____
_____
_____
_____
_____
_____

How would you document this? _____
_____
_____
_____

Compare your documentation to the sample provided in Appendix I.

Data Collected
(use those that apply)

- Weight 135 lbs
- BP 128/80—110/72—90/50; lying/sitting/standing
- Pulse 89
- Respiratory rate at rest 18 and shallow; 26 and shallow on exertion
- Temp 99.0°F
- Skin is pale and client is diaphoretic
- Complains of dizziness on standing
- Skin dry and flaky
- Oral mucosa dry
- Taking oral antibiotics every 4 hours
- Pitcher of water is on the left side of the bed and is full
- Family not present, uninvolved in care of client
- Saline lock in place and patent
- Complains of loss of appetite over the past week
- Crackles noted in lower lobes of lungs, bilaterally
- Nonproductive cough
- Blood oxygen level 98%
- Client unmotivated to get better
- Pupils PERRLA

Nursing Interventions
(use those that apply; list in priority order)

- Place water pitcher on client's right side, within reach.
- Determine cause of activity intolerance: physical, psychological, motivational.
- State, "You need to eat your meals to get better."
- Encourage client to change positions slowly.
- Instruct client to sit up in bed for a few minutes before standing.
- Put a bed alarm in place according to agency policy.
- Slow pace of care, allowing client extra time.
- Check orders for IV fluid administration and discuss with RN.
- When mobilizing client, monitor for orthostatic hypotension accompanied by dizziness/fainting.
- Encourage client to deep breathe and cough.
- Encourage client to increase clear fluid intake.
- Instruct client to call for assistance before ambulating.
- Use a walking belt when ambulating client.

NCLEX-PN® Exam Preparation

1 You are assigned to care for a 19-year-old female client who has been brought to the hospital by her parents. They are concerned that she may be seriously ill because of noticeable weight loss and frequent vomiting and diarrhea. The physician suspects that she may have an eating disorder. Which of the following signs would help to confirm a diagnosis of an eating disorder?

1. headaches, confusion, and lack of concentration
2. dental caries and skin excoriations on knuckles
3. yellow skin and sclera
4. excessive bruising and petechiae

2 The nurse's observation of the problem, the client's presenting problem, nursing interventions provided, and medical therapies are specific assessments made in relationship to:

1. the nursing diagnosis.
2. the client's complaints.
3. physician's orders.
4. nursing orders.

3 A client is admitted through the emergency department with a complaint of severe right lower quadrant abdominal pain of 5 hours' duration. Lab work reveals elevated WBCs; vital signs are T 101.2, P 98, R 24, BP 120/78. Which of the following data collected during the focused assessment would help to confirm a diagnosis of appendicitis?

1. a palpable mass in the right upper quadrant
2. report of black tarry stools
3. rebound tenderness at McBurney's point
4. projectile vomiting

4 You are setting up for a focused assessment for a client with tonsillitis. Of the following choices, which pieces of equipment would be required?

1. stethoscope and sphygmomanometer
2. tongue depressor and flashlight
3. ophthalmoscope and split-lamp
4. thermometer and scale

5 Your primary nurse requests that you assess peripheral perfusion of toes, capillary blanch test, pedal pulse if able, and vital signs. This assessment would be carried out for a client with which of the following conditions?

1. deep venous thrombosis (DVT)
2. hip fracture with Buck's traction application
3. femur fracture with long leg cast
4. total knee replacement leg in continuous passive motion (CPM) machine

6 You have been assigned to take a client's blood pressure. The reading is 100/60. Which would be the most appropriate action for you to take?

1. Retake the blood pressure in 1 hour.
2. Chart the blood pressure reading.
3. Report the findings immediately.
4. Administer antihypertensive medication immediately.

7 Breath sounds that are continuous, low-pitched, coarse, gurgling, harsh, louder sounds with a moaning or snoring quality, which may be altered by coughing, are known as:

1. crackles (rales).
2. gurgles (rhonchi).
3. friction rub.
4. wheezes.

8 You are assigned to assist with the admission assessment of a client who has been living alone and is unable to provide for his own hygiene needs. As you examine the integumentary system, you notice numerous red lesions, which appear as "red tracks" under the skin. Which of the following would be an appropriate nursing action?

1. Don gloves prior to continuing your assessment.
2. Postpone your assessment until the nursing assistant has bathed the client.
3. Place the client in isolation.
4. Proceed with the assessment but do not touch the client.

9 You are assigned to work the night shift. As you are completing your assessment for a client who had surgery today, the client begins to yell, "Get them off of me! There are rats crawling all over the bed." Your best nursing action would be to:

1. turn on the light and tell her there are no rats.
2. stop the pain medication.
3. check her chart for a history of mental illness.
4. inform the charge nurse or the physician immediately.

10 Moods, affect, judgment, abilities, and lifestyle are part of what type of assessment?

1. history and physical
2. psychosocial assessment
3. focus assessment
4. family health history

Answers and Rationales for Review Questions, as well as discussion of Care Plan and Critical Thinking Care Map questions, appear in Appendix I.

Chapter 20

Vital Signs

BRIEF Outline

Body Temperature
Pulse
Respirations
Blood Pressure

LEARNING Outcomes

After completing this chapter, you will be able to:

1. Describe factors that affect the vital signs and their accurate measurement.
2. Identify normal ranges for each vital sign and variations by age.
3. Describe ways in which the body produces and loses heat.
4. Describe the body's temperature-regulating system.
5. Discuss the advantages and disadvantages of oral, tympanic, rectal, and axillary methods for measuring body temperature.
6. Describe appropriate nursing care for alterations in body temperature.
7. Identify nine sites commonly used to assess the pulse and state the reasons for their use.
8. Explain how to measure the apical pulse and apical–radial pulse.
9. Describe the mechanics of breathing and identify the characteristics that should be included in a respiratory assessment.
10. Differentiate systolic from diastolic blood pressure and describe five phases of Korotkoff's sounds.
11. Describe various methods and sites used to measure blood pressure.

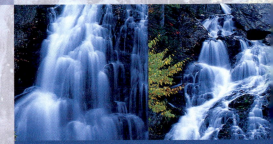

HISTORICAL Perspectives

The inventor of the stethoscope was Rene Theophile-Hyacinthe Laënnec. One day, when he needed to examine an obese young woman, Laënnec hesitated to put his head to her chest. Remembering that you can hear a pin scraping one end of a plank by putting your ear to the other end, he came up with the idea for a stethoscope prototype. He rolled a stack of paper into a cylinder, pressed one end to the patient's chest, and held his ear to the other end.

"I was surprised and pleased to hear the beating of the heart much more clearly than if I had applied my ear directly to the chest," Laënnec said in 1816.

TABLE 20-1

Variations in Normal Vital Signs by Age

AGE	TEMPERATURE IN DEGREES CELSIUS	AVERAGE PULSE (RANGES)	AVERAGE RESPIRATIONS (RANGES)	BLOOD PRESSURE (MM HG)
Newborns	36.8 (axillary)	130 (80–180)	35 (30–80)	73/55
1–3 years	37.7 (rectal)	120 (80–140)	30 (20–40)	90/55
6–8 years	37 (oral)	100 (75–120)	20 (15–25)	95/57
10 years	37 (oral)	70 (50–90)	19 (15–25)	102/62
Teen years	37 (oral)	70 (50–90)	18 (15–20)	120/80
Adult	37 (oral)	80 (60–100)	16 (12–20)	120/80
Older adult (>70 years)	36 (oral)	80 (60–100)	16 (15–20)	Possible increased diastolic

Together, the vital or cardinal signs—body temperature, pulse, respirations, and blood pressure—reflect changes in function that otherwise might not be observed. Monitoring a client's vital signs should be a thoughtful, scientific assessment. Vital signs must be evaluated with reference to the client's present and prior health status and be compared to accepted normal standards. (See Table 20-1 ■.) The "fifth vital sign," pain, is discussed in Chapter 21 ⚭.

Some medical facilities have policies about how often to take the clients' vital signs. Physicians may also order a vital sign (e.g., "blood pressure every 2 hours") to be taken at specific times. Ordered assessments, however, should be considered the minimum. A nurse should measure vital signs more often if the client's health status requires it. Vital signs are routinely assessed in the following order: temperature first; pulse and respirations are taken while the thermometer is in place, if possible. Respirations should be assessed while your fingers are still touching the pulse point, so that the client will be unaware and not alter the breathing pattern. The blood pressure should follow the other vital signs.

Body Temperature

Body temperature reflects the balance between the heat produced and the heat lost from the body, measured in heat units called degrees.

The normal body temperature (temperature of deep tissues of the body) is actually a range of temperatures. When measured orally, the average body temperature of an adult is between 36.7°C (98°F) and 37°C (98.6°F) (Figure 20-1 ■). Rectal temperature is one degree higher, 37.5°C (99.6°F); axillary is one degree lower, 35.4°C (97.6°F); and tympanic is 37.6°C (99.7°F).

The body continually produces heat as a by-product of metabolism. When the amount of heat produced by the body exactly equals the amount of heat lost, the person is in heat balance.

A number of factors affect the body's heat production. The most important are these five:

1. *Basal metabolic rate.* The **basal metabolic rate (BMR)** is the rate of energy utilization in the body required to maintain essential activities such as breathing. Metabolic rates decrease with age. In general, the younger the person, the higher the BMR.
2. *Muscle activity.* Muscle activity, including shivering, increases the metabolic rate.

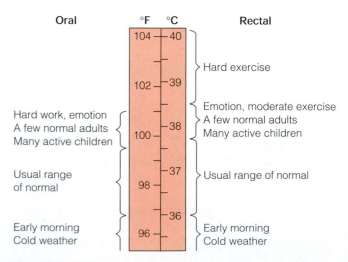

Figure 20-1. ■ Estimated ranges of body temperatures in normal persons. (*Source:* E. F. DuBois, *Fever and the regulation of body temperature,* Springfield, IL: Charles C. Thomas, 1948. Courtesy of Charles C. Thomas, Publisher.)

3. *Thyroxine output.* Increased thyroxine output increases the rate of cellular metabolism throughout the body and increases heat.
4. *Epinephrine, norepinephrine, and sympathetic stimulation.* These hormones immediately increase the rate of cellular metabolism in many body tissues.
5. *Fever.* Fever increases the cellular metabolic rate and thus increases the body's temperature further.

REGULATION OF BODY TEMPERATURE

When the skin becomes chilled over the entire body or when cold sensors in the brain are stimulated, three physiological processes take place to increase the body temperature:

1. *Shivering* increases heat production.
2. *Sweating* is inhibited to decrease heat loss.
3. *Vasoconstriction* decreases heat loss.

When the sensors in the hypothalamus of the brain detect heat, they send out signals intended to reduce the temperature. The body decreases heat production and increases heat loss by:

1. Sweating, which increases evaporation and cooling
2. Peripheral vasodilation, which facilitates cooling.

Also, when sensors are stimulated, the person consciously makes appropriate adjustments, such as putting on additional clothing in response to cold or turning on a fan in response to heat.

Factors Affecting Body Temperature

Nurses should be aware of the factors that can affect a client's body temperature. They should recognize normal temperature variations and understand the significance of body temperature measurements that deviate from normal. Among the factors that affect body temperature are the following:

- *Age.* The infant is greatly influenced by the temperature of the environment and must be protected from extreme changes. Children's temperatures continue to fluctuate more than those of adults until puberty. Older people, particularly those over 75 years of age, are sensitive to extremes in temperature, and are at risk of hypothermia (temperatures below 36°C [96.8°F]). Some of the reasons for this include inadequate diet, loss of subcutaneous fat, lack of activity, and reduced efficiency of the temperature-regulating system (see Table 20-1).
- *Diurnal variations (circadian rhythms).* Body temperatures normally change throughout the day, varying as much as 1.0°C (1.8°F) between the early morning and the late afternoon. The point of highest body temperature is usually reached between 1600 and 2000 hours (4:00 P.M. and 8 P.M.), and the lowest point is reached during sleep between 0400 and 0600 hours (4:00 A.M. and 6:00 A.M.) (Figure 20-2 ■).

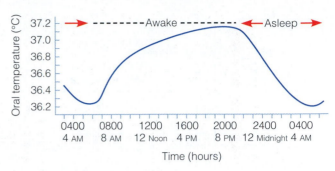

Figure 20-2. ■ Range of oral temperatures during 24 hours for a healthy young adult.

- *Exercise.* Hard work or strenuous exercise can increase body temperature to as high as 38.3° to 40°C (101° to 104°F) measured rectally.
- *Hormones.* Women usually experience more hormonal fluctuations than men. In women, progesterone secretion at the time of ovulation raises body temperature by about 0.3° to 0.6°C (0.5° to 1.0°F) above basal temperature.
- *Stress.* Stimulation of the sympathetic nervous system can increase the production of epinephrine and norepinephrine, thereby increasing metabolic activity and heat production. Nurses may anticipate that a highly stressed or anxious client could have an elevated body temperature for that reason.
- *Environment.* Extremes in environmental temperatures can affect a person's temperature-regulating systems. If the temperature is assessed in a very warm room, the temperature may be elevated. Similarly, if the client has been outside in extremely cold weather without suitable clothing, the body temperature may be low.

ALTERATIONS IN BODY TEMPERATURE

Pyrexia

A body temperature above the usual range is called **pyrexia**, **hyperthermia**, or fever. A very high fever, such as 41°C (105.8°F), is called *hyperpyrexia* (Figure 20-3 ■). The client who has a fever is referred to as *febrile;* one who does not have a fever is referred to as **afebrile**.

Four common types of fevers are intermittent, remittent, relapsing, and constant. During an *intermittent fever,* the body temperature alternates at regular intervals between periods of fever and periods of normal or subnormal temperatures. During a *remittent fever,* a wide range of temperature fluctuations (more than 2°C [3.6°F]) occurs over a 24-hour period, all of which are above normal. In a *relapsing fever,* short febrile periods of a few days are interspersed with periods of 1 or 2 days of normal temperature. During a *constant fever,* the body temperature fluctuates minimally but always remains above normal. The manifestations of

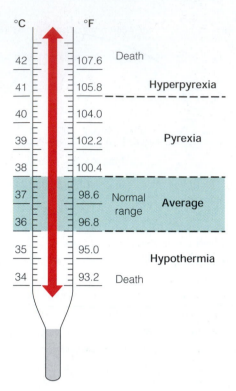

Figure 20-3. ■ Terms used to describe alterations in body temperature (oral measurements) and ranges in Celsius (centigrade) and Fahrenheit scales.

| BOX 20-1 | MANIFESTATIONS OF FEVER |

Onset (Cold or Chill Stage)
- Increased heart rate
- Increased respiratory rate and depth
- Shivering
- Pallid, cold skin
- Complaints of feeling cold
- Cyanotic nail beds
- "Gooseflesh" appearance of the skin
- Cessation of sweating

Course
- Absence of chills
- Skin that feels warm
- Photosensitivity
- Glassy-eyed appearance
- Increased pulse and respiratory rates
- Increased thirst

Mild to severe dehydration
- Drowsiness, restlessness, delirium, or convulsions
- Herpetic lesions of the mouth
- Loss of appetite (if the fever is prolonged)
- Malaise, weakness, and aching muscles

Defervescence (Fever Abatement)
- Skin that appears flushed and feels warm
- Sweating
- Decreased shivering
- Possible dehydration

fever vary with the onset, course, and abatement stages of the fever (Box 20-1 ■).

Very high temperatures, such as 41° to 42°C (106° to 108°F), damage cells throughout the body, particularly in the brain where destruction of neuronal cells is irreversible. Damage to the liver, kidneys, and other body organs can also be great enough to disrupt functioning and eventually cause death.

When the cause of the high temperature is suddenly removed, the body's thermostat is reduced to a lower value, perhaps even back to the original normal level. In this instance, the hypothalamus now attempts to lower the temperature to 37°C (98.6°F). Heat loss responses cause a reduction of the body temperature to occur; manifestations are excessive sweating and a hot, flushed skin due to sudden vasodilation. This sudden change of events is known as the **crisis** of a pyrexic condition. A more gradual return of the body temperature to normal is referred to as a *resolution by lysis.* Nursing interventions for a client who has a fever are designed to support the body's normal physiological processes, provide comfort, and prevent complications. During the course of fever, the nurse needs to monitor the client's vital signs closely (Box 20-2 ■).

Nursing measures during the chill phase are designed to help the client decrease heat loss and raise the core body temperature. During flushing or the crisis phase, body processes are attempting to lower the core temperature to normal. At this time, the nurse takes measures to increase heat loss and decrease heat production.

Hypothermia

Hypothermia is core body temperature below the lower limit of normal. The three physiological mechanisms of hypothermia are (1) excessive heat loss, (2) inadequate heat production to counteract the heat loss, and (3) impaired hypothalamic temperature regulation. The manifestations of hypothermia are given in Box 20-3 ■.

Hypothermia may be accidental or induced. Accidental hypothermia can occur as a result of (1) exposure to a cold environment (i.e., below 16°C [60.8°F]), (2) immersion in cold water, and (3) lack of adequate clothing, shelter, or heat. In older people the problem can be compounded by a decreased metabolic rate and the use of sedatives, which depress the metabolic rate further.

BOX 20-2	NURSING CARE CHECKLIST

Clients with Fever

☑ Monitor vital signs.

☑ Assess skin color and temperature.

☑ Monitor white blood cell count, hematocrit value, and other pertinent laboratory reports for indications of infection or dehydration.

☑ Remove excess blankets when the client feels warm, but provide extra warmth when the client feels chilled.

☑ Provide adequate nutrition and fluids (e.g., 2500 to 3000 mL per day) to meet the increased metabolic demands and prevent dehydration. Clients who sweat profusely can become dehydrated.

☑ Measure intake and output.

☑ Reduce physical activity to limit heat production, especially during the flush stage.

☑ Administer antipyretics (drugs that reduce the level of fever) as ordered.

☑ Provide oral hygiene to keep the mucous membranes moist. They can become dry and cracked as a result of excessive fluid loss.

☑ Provide a tepid sponge bath to increase heat loss through conduction.

☑ Provide dry clothing and bed linens.

Managing the hypothermia involves removing the client from the cold and rewarming the client's body. For the client with mild hypothermia, the body is rewarmed by applying blankets. For the client with severe hypothermia, a hyperthermia blanket (an electronically controlled blanket that provides a specified temperature) is applied, and warm intravenous fluids are given. Wet clothing, which increases heat loss because of the high conductivity of water, should

BOX 20-3	MANIFESTATIONS OF HYPOTHERMIA

- Decreased body temperature, pulse, and respirations
- Severe shivering (initially)
- Feelings of cold and chills
- Pale, cool, waxy skin
- Hypotension
- Decreased urinary output
- Lack of muscle coordination
- Disorientation
- Drowsiness progressing to coma

BOX 20-4	NURSING CARE CHECKLIST

Clients with Hypothermia

☑ Provide a warm environment (room temperature).

☑ Provide dry clothing.

☑ Apply warm blankets.

☑ Keep limbs close to body.

☑ Cover the client's scalp with a cap or turban.

☑ Supply warm oral or intravenous fluids.

☑ Apply warming pads.

be replaced with dry clothing. See Box 20-4 ■ for nursing interventions for clients who have hypothermia.

Induced hypothermia is the deliberate lowering of the body temperature to decrease the need for oxygen by the body tissues. Induced hypothermia can involve the whole body or a body part. It is sometimes indicated prior to surgery (e.g., cardiac and brain surgery).

TEMPERATURE ASSESSMENT METHODS

The four most common sites for measuring body temperature are oral, rectal, axillary, and the tympanic membrane. Each of the sites has advantages and disadvantages (Table 20-2 ■).

The tympanic membrane (see Figure 20-22 in Procedure 20-1 on page 393), is becoming the preferred site for taking body temperature. Tympanic membrane temperature readings average 1.1 to 1.5°F higher than oral temperature readings. Like the sublingual oral site, the tympanic membrane has an abundant arterial blood supply. The tympanic infrared method is quickly becoming the method of choice in clients over 3 months of age. The oral site is an equally preferred site. This method reflects changing body temperature more quickly than the rectal method. Rectal temperature readings are considered to be the most accurate. The axilla is the preferred site for measuring temperature in newborns because it is accessible and offers no possibility of rectal perforation. Nursing students should check facility protocol when taking the temperature of newborns, infants, toddlers, and children. Clients for whom the axillary method of temperature assessment is appropriate include adult clients with oral inflammation or wired jaws, clients recovering from oral surgery, clients who are breathing through their mouths (e.g., following nasal surgery), irrational clients, and clients for whom other temperature sites are contraindicated.

In addition to the four common sites for measuring temperature, the forehead may also be used. Body temperature is measured by using a chemical thermometer. Forehead temperature measurements are most useful for infants and

TABLE 20-2

Comparison of Four Sites for Measuring Body Temperature

SITE	ADVANTAGES	DISADVANTAGES
Oral	Most accessible and convenient	Mercury-in-glass thermometers can break if bitten; therefore they are contraindicated for children under 6 years and clients who are confused or who have convulsive disorders. Inaccurate if client has just ingested hot or cold food or fluid or smoked. Could injure the mouth following oral surgery.
Rectal	Most reliable measurement	Inconvenient and more unpleasant for clients; difficult for client who cannot turn to the side. Could injure the rectum following rectal surgery. Placement of the thermometer at different sites within the rectum yields different temperatures, yet placement at the same site each time is difficult. A rectal glass thermometer does not respond to changes in arterial temperatures as quickly as an oral thermometer, a fact that may be potentially dangerous for febrile clients because misleading information may be acquired. Presence of stool may interfere with thermometer placement. If the stool is soft, the thermometer may be embedded in stool rather than against the wall of the rectum. If the stool is impacted, the depth of the thermometer insertion may be insufficient. In newborns and infants, insertion of the rectal thermometer has resulted in ulcerations and rectal perforations. Many agencies advise against using rectal thermometers on neonates.
Axillary	Safest and most noninvasive	The thermometer must be left in place a long time to obtain an accurate measurement.
Tympanic membrane	Readily accessible; reflects the core temperature; very fast	Can be uncomfortable and involves risk of injuring the membrane if the probe is inserted too far. Repeated measurements may vary. Right and left measurements can differ. Presence of cerumen can affect the reading.

children where a more invasive measurement is not necessary. If the forehead indicates a temperature elevation, a glass or electronic thermometer should be used to obtain a more accurate measurement.

Types of Thermometers

Traditionally, body temperatures have been measured using mercury-in-glass thermometers. Oral thermometers may have long, slender tips or short, rounded tips (Figure 20-4 ■). The rounded thermometer can be used at the rectal as well as other sites. In some medical facilities, thermometers may be color coded (red thermometers for rectal temperatures, silver blue for oral and axillary temperatures).

Many facilities have discontinued the use of mercury-in-glass thermometers due to breakage and potential for hazardous contamination from spilled mercury.

Electronic thermometers offer another method of assessing body temperatures. They can provide a reading in only

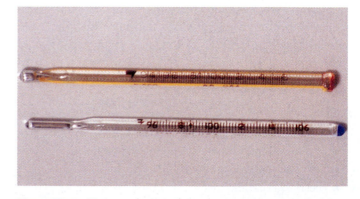

Figure 20-4. ■ Two types of thermometer tips for glass thermometers. (Photographer: Elena Dorfman.)

2 to 60 seconds, depending on the model. The equipment consists of a battery-operated portable electronic unit, a probe that the nurse attaches to the unit, and a probe cover, which is usually disposable (Figure 20-5 ■).

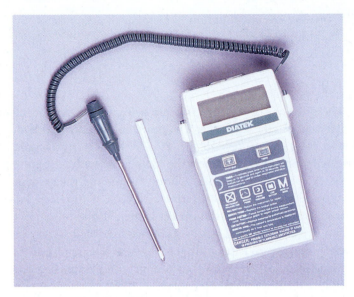

Figure 20-5. ■ An electronic thermometer. Note the probe and probe cover. (Photographer: Elena Dorfman.)

Chemical disposable thermometers are also used to measure body temperatures. Chemical thermometers using liquid crystal dots, bars, or heat-sensitive tape or patches applied to the forehead change color to indicate temperature. Some of these are single use and others may be reused several times. One type that has small chemical dots at one end is shown in Figure 20-6 ■. To read the temperature, the nurse notes the highest reading among the dots that have changed color.

Temperature-sensitive tape may also be used to obtain a general indication of body surface temperature. The tape contains liquid crystals that change color according to temperature. When applied to the skin, usually of the forehead or abdomen, the temperature digits on the tape respond by changing color (Figure 20-7 ■). The skin area should be dry. After the length of time specified by the manufacturer (e.g., 15 seconds), a color appears on the tape. The tape is removed and discarded after the color has been compared to the scale provided by the manufacturer. This method is particularly useful at home and for infants whose temperatures are to be monitored for any reason.

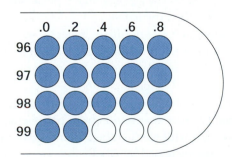

Figure 20-6. ■ A chemical thermometer showing a reading of 99.2°F.

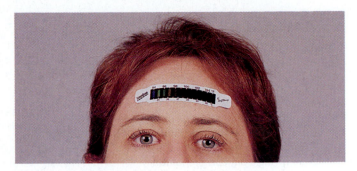

Figure 20-7. ■ A temperature-sensitive skin tape. (Photographer: Jenny Thomas.)

Temperature Scales

The body temperature is measured in degrees on two scales: Celsius (centigrade) and Fahrenheit. On a glass thermometer, the Celsius scale normally extends from 34.0° to 42.0°C. The Fahrenheit scale usually extends from 94° to 108°F. Body temperatures rarely extend beyond these scales (see Figure 20-3).

Sometimes a nurse needs to convert a Celsius reading to Fahrenheit, or vice versa. To convert from Fahrenheit to Celsius, deduct 32 from the Fahrenheit reading and then multiply by the fraction 5/9, that is:

$$C = (\text{Fahrenheit temperature} - 32) \times 5/9$$

For example, when the Fahrenheit reading is 100:

$$C = (100 - 32) \times 5/9 = (68) \times 5/9 = 37.7$$

To convert from Celsius to Fahrenheit, multiply the Celsius reading by the fraction 9/5 and then add 32; that is:

$$F = (\text{Celsius temperature} \times 9/5) + 32$$

For example, when the Celsius reading is 40:

$$F = (40 \times 9/5) + 32 = (72) + 32 = 104$$

NURSING CARE

ASSESSING

Times for assessing vital signs are listed in Box 20-5 ■. See Box 20-1 for manifestations of fever and Box 20-3 for manifestations of hypothermia. Refer to Table 20-1 for temperature variation by age.

DIAGNOSING, PLANNING, AND IMPLEMENTING

The most common nursing diagnosis for clients with alterations of temperature beyond normal limits is *Ineffective Thermoregulation*. Refer to Table 20-2 for selecting an appropriate site for measuring body temperature. Procedure 20-1 on page 393 explains how to measure body temperature.

BOX 20-5

Times to Assess Vital Signs

- On admission to a healthcare agency to obtain baseline data
- When a client has a change in health status or reports symptoms such as chest pain or feeling hot or faint
- Before and after surgery or an invasive procedure
- Before and/or after the administration of a medication that could affect the respiratory or cardiovascular systems (e.g., before giving a digitalis preparation)
- Before and after any nursing intervention that could affect the vital signs (e.g., ambulating a client who has been on bed rest)

EVALUATING

The temperature measurement is compared to baseline data or normal range. Client's age, time of day, and any other influencing factors are considered. Temperature readings are reviewed in relation to other vital signs.

Safety Precautions

Safety is a major consideration when assessing temperature due to the disadvantages of the various sites and equipment. Never force any type of thermometer into place. If it does not enter easily, reassess the site and consider using a different location or type of thermometer.

The oral site should not be used if the client cannot cooperate or there is a risk that he or she may bite a glass thermometer. The rectal thermometer should always be held in place and never be left unattended. Severe injury could occur if the client rolled onto the thermometer. Glass thermometers must be handled carefully since they pose a safety hazard if broken. If a glass thermometer does not shake down easily or has any signs of cracks, it should be disposed of according to facility policy.

Electronic thermometers and other electrical equipment should not be used if damaged, since malfunctioning equipment can present a shock hazard to both the client and the nurse.

CONTINUING CARE

- Teach the client accurate use and reading of the type of thermometer to be used. Reinforce the importance of reporting the site and type of thermometer used and the value of using one consistently. Provide a recording chart or table if indicated.
- Discuss means of keeping the thermometer clean, such as warm water and soap, and avoiding cross-contamination.
- Ensure that the client has water-soluble lubricant if using a rectal thermometer.
- Have the client or family member demonstrate use of the thermometer so proper technique can be reinforced.

- Instruct the client or family member to notify the healthcare provider if the temperature is 37.7°C (100°F) or higher.

Pulse

The **pulse** is a wave of blood created by contraction of the left ventricle of the heart. The heart is a pulsating pump, and the blood enters the arteries with each contraction, causing pressure pulses or pulse waves. Generally, the pulse wave represents the stroke volume output and the amount of blood that enters the arteries with each ventricular contraction. *Compliance* of the arteries is their ability to contract and expand. When a person's arteries lose their ability to expand, as can happen in old age, greater pressure is required to pump the blood into the arteries because the rigid arterial walls offer resistance.

When an adult is resting, the heart pumps about 5 liters of blood each minute. This volume is called the cardiac output.

In a healthy person, the pulse reflects the heartbeat. In other words, the pulse rate is the same as the rate of the ventricular contractions of the heart. However, in some types of cardiovascular disease, the heartbeat and pulse rates can differ. For example, a client's heart may produce very weak or small pulse waves that are not detectable in a peripheral pulse far from the heart. In these instances, the nurse should assess the heartbeat and the peripheral pulse. See the section on assessing the apical pulse later in this chapter. A **peripheral pulse** is a pulse located in the periphery of the body, for example, in the foot, hand, or neck. The **apical pulse,** in contrast, is a central pulse; that is, it is located at the apex of the heart.

FACTORS AFFECTING PULSE RATE

The rate of the pulse is expressed in beats per minute (bpm). A pulse rate varies according to a number of factors. The nurse should consider each of the following factors when assessing a client's pulse:

- *Age.* As age increases, the pulse rate gradually decreases. See Table 20-1 for specific variations in pulse rates from birth to adulthood.
- *Sex.* After puberty, the average male's pulse rate is slightly lower than the female's.
- *Exercise.* The pulse rate normally increases with activity. The rate of increase in the professional athlete is often less than in the average person because of greater cardiac size, strength, and efficiency.
- *Fever.* The pulse rate increases (1) in response to the lowered blood pressure that results from peripheral vasodilation associated with elevated body temperature and (2) because of the increased metabolic rate.
- *Medications.* Some medications decrease the pulse rate, and others increase it. For example, cardiotonics

(e.g., digitalis preparations) decrease the heart rate, whereas epinephrine causes an increase.

- *Hemorrhage.* Loss of blood from the vascular system (hemorrhage) normally increases pulse rate. In adults the loss of a small amount of blood (e.g., 500 mL, the amount lost after a blood donation) results in a temporary adjustment of the heart rate as the body compensates for the lost blood volume. An adult has about 5 liters of blood in the system and can usually lose up to 10% without adverse effects.
- *Stress.* In response to stress, sympathetic nervous stimulation increases the overall activity of the heart. Stress increases the rate as well as the force of the heartbeat. Fear and anxiety as well as the perception of severe pain stimulate the sympathetic system.
- *Position changes.* When a person assumes a sitting or standing position, blood usually pools in dependent vessels of the venous system. Pooling results in a transient decrease in the venous blood return to the heart and a subsequent reduction in blood pressure and increase in heart rate.

PULSE SITES

A pulse is commonly taken in any of nine sites (Figure 20-8 ■):

1. *Temporal,* where the temporal artery passes over the temporal bone of the head. The site is superior (above) and lateral to (away from the midline of) the eye.

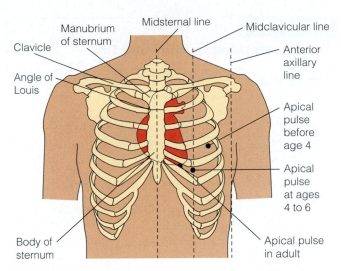

Figure 20-9. ■ Location of the apical pulse for a child under 4 years, a child 4 to 6 years, and an adult.

2. *Carotid,* at the side of the neck where the carotid artery runs between the trachea and the sternocleidomastoid muscle. Never press both carotids at the same time because this can cause a reflex drop in blood pressure or pulse rate.
3. *Apical,* at the apex of the heart. In an adult, this is located on the left side of the chest, no more than 8 cm (3 in.) to the left of the sternum (breastbone) and at the fourth, fifth, or sixth intercostal space (area between the ribs). For a child 7 to 9 years of age, the apical pulse is located at the fourth or fifth intercostal spaces. Before 4 years of age, it is left of the midclavicular line (MCL); between 4 and 6 years, it is at the MCL (Figure 20-9 ■).
4. *Brachial,* at the inner aspect of the biceps muscle of the arm (especially in infants) or medially in the antecubital space (elbow crease).
5. *Radial,* where the radial artery runs along the radial bone, on the thumb side of the inner aspect of the wrist.
6. *Femoral,* where the femoral artery passes alongside the inguinal ligament.
7. *Popliteal,* where the popliteal artery passes behind the knee. This point is difficult to find, but it can be palpated if the client flexes the knee slightly (see Figure 20-8).
8. *Posterior tibial,* on the medial surface of the ankle where the posterior tibial artery passes behind the medial malleolus.
9. *Pedal (dorsalis pedis),* where the dorsalis pedis artery passes over the bones of the foot. This artery can be palpated by feeling the *dorsum* (upper surface) of the foot on an imaginary line drawn from the middle of the ankle to the space between the big and second toes.

The radial site is most commonly used. It is easily found in most people and is readily accessible. The reasons for use of each site are given in Table 20-3 ■.

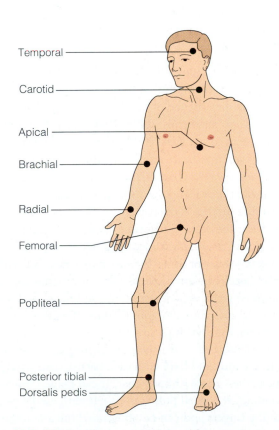

Figure 20-8. ■ Nine sites commonly used for assessing a pulse.

TABLE 20-3

Reasons for Using Specific Pulse Sites

PULSE SITE	REASONS FOR USE
Radial	Readily accessible
Temporal	Used when radial pulse is not accessible
Carotid	Used for infants Used in cases of cardiac arrest Used to determine circulation to the brain
Apical	Routinely used for infants and children up to 3 years of age Used to determine discrepancies with radial pulse Used in conjunction with some medications
Brachial	Used to measure blood pressure Used during cardiac arrest for infants
Femoral	Used in cases of cardiac arrest Used for infants and children Used to determine circulation to a leg
Popliteal	Used to determine circulation to the lower leg
Posterior tibial	Used to determine circulation to the foot
Pedal	Used to determine circulation to the foot

NURSING CARE

ASSESSING

A pulse is commonly assessed by palpation (feeling) or auscultation (hearing). The middle three fingertips are used for palpating all pulse sites except the apex of the heart. A stethoscope is used for assessing apical pulses and fetal heart tones. A Doppler ultrasound stethoscope (DUS; Figure 20-10 ■) is used for pulses that are difficult to

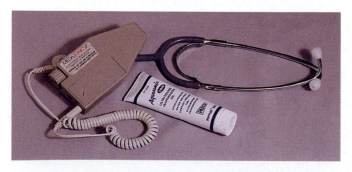

Figure 20-10. ■ An ultrasound (Doppler or DUS) stethoscope. (Photographer: Elena Dorfman.)

assess. The DUS headset has earpieces similar to standard stethoscope earpieces, but it has a long cord attached to a volume-controlled audio unit and an ultrasound transducer. The DUS detects movement of red blood cells through a blood vessel. In contrast to the conventional stethoscope, it excludes environmental sounds. It cannot detect blood flow in deep vessels or in blood vessels underlying bone, such as the vessels in the abdomen, thorax, or skull.

A pulse is normally palpated by applying moderate pressure with the three middle fingers of the hand. The pads on the most distal aspects of the finger are the most sensitive areas for detecting a pulse. With excessive pressure one can obliterate a pulse, whereas with too little pressure one may not be able to detect it. Before the nurse assesses the resting pulse, the client should assume a comfortable position. The nurse should also be aware of the following:

- Whether the client has taken any medication that could affect the heart rate.
- Whether the client has been physically active. If so, wait 10 to 15 minutes until the client has rested and the pulse has slowed to its usual rate.
- Whether any baseline data exist about the normal heart rate for the client. For example, a physically fit athlete may have a heart rate below 60 bpm.
- Whether the client should assume a particular position (e.g., sitting). In some clients, the rate changes with the position because of changes in blood flow volume and autonomic nervous system activity.

When assessing the pulse, the nurse collects the following data: the rate, rhythm, volume, arterial wall elasticity, and presence or absence of bilateral equality. The normal pulse rates are shown in Table 20-1. An excessively fast heart rate (e.g., more than 100 bpm in an adult) is referred to as *tachycardia*. A heart rate in an adult of 60 bpm or less is called *bradycardia*. If a client has either tachycardia or bradycardia, the apical pulse should be assessed.

The pulse rhythm is the pattern of the beats and the intervals between the beats. Equal time elapses between beats of a normal pulse. A pulse with an irregular rhythm is referred to as a *dysrhythmia* or *arrhythmia*. It may consist of random, irregular beats or a predictable pattern of irregular beats. When a dysrhythmia is detected, the apical pulse should be assessed. An electrocardiogram (ECG or EKG) is necessary to define the dysrhythmia further.

Pulse volume, also called the pulse strength or amplitude, refers to the force of blood with each beat. Usually, the pulse volume is the same with each beat. It can range from absent to bounding. A normal pulse can be felt with moderate pressure of the fingers and can be obliterated (unable to be felt) with greater pressure. A forceful or full blood volume that is

TABLE 20-4

Scale for Measuring Pulse Volume

SCALE	DESCRIPTION OF PULSE
0	Absent, not discernible
1	Thready or weak, difficult to feel
2	Normal, detected readily, obliterated by strong pressure
3	Bounding, difficult to obliterate

obliterated only with difficulty is called a *full* or *bounding pulse.* A pulse that is readily obliterated with pressure from the fingers is referred to as weak, feeble, or *thready.* A pulse volume is usually measured on a scale of 0 to 3 (Table 20-4 ■).

The elasticity of the arterial wall reflects its ability to expand or its deformities. A healthy, normal artery feels straight, smooth, soft, and pliable. Older people often have inelastic arteries that feel twisted (*tortuous*) and irregular on palpation.

When assessing a peripheral pulse to determine the adequacy of blood flow to a particular area of the body, the nurse should also assess the corresponding pulse on the other side of the body. The second assessment gives the nurse data with which to compare the pulses. For example, when assessing the blood flow to the right foot, the nurse assesses the right dorsalis pedis pulse and then the left dorsalis pedis pulse. If the client's right and left pulses are the same, the client's dorsalis pedis pulses are said to be *bilaterally equal.*

Peripheral Pulse Assessment

A peripheral pulse, usually the radial pulse, is assessed by palpation in all individuals except:

- Newborns and children up to 2 or 3 years. Apical pulses are assessed in these clients.
- Very obese or elderly clients, whose radial pulse may be difficult to palpate. Doppler equipment may be used for these clients, or the apical pulse is assessed.
- Individuals with a heart disease, who require apical pulse assessment.
- Individuals in whom the circulation to a specific body part must be assessed; for example, following leg surgery, the pedal (dorsalis pedis) pulse is assessed.

Apical–Radial Pulse Assessment

An apical–radial pulse may need to be assessed for clients with certain cardiovascular disorders. Normally, the apical and radial rates are identical. An apical pulse rate greater than a radial pulse rate can indicate that the thrust of the blood from the heart is too feeble for the wave to be felt at the peripheral pulse site, or it can indicate that vascular disease is

preventing impulses from being transmitted. Any differences between the two pulse rates (called a **pulse deficit**) needs to be reported promptly. In no instance is the radial pulse greater than the apical pulse.

An apical–radial pulse can be taken by two nurses or one nurse, although the two-nurse technique may be more accurate.

DIAGNOSING, PLANNING, AND IMPLEMENTING

A possible nursing diagnosis would be *Decreased Cardiac Output.* Refer to Table 20-3 for selection of an appropriate site. Procedure 20-2 ■ on page 395 provides guidelines for various methods of assessing pulse.

EVALUATING

Evaluate pulse in relationship to baseline data or normal range for age of client, relationship of pulse rate and volume to other vital signs, and health status. Compare peripheral pulses; equality, rate, and volume in corresponding extremities.

CONTINUING CARE

- Teach the client or family member to monitor the pulse prior to taking medications that affect the heart rate.
- Tell the client to report any notable changes in heart rate or rhythm (regularity) to the healthcare provider.
- Ensure that the client or family member is aware of which pulse findings should be reported and to whom.

NURSING PROCESS CARE PLAN
Client with Left-Sided Heart Failure

Naomi Munson, a 75-year-old female, has been a resident at Knight's Bridge Road Retirement Center since her husband died 6 months ago. She was admitted through the ED for left-sided heart failure. Mrs. Munson expresses a dislike for her low-sodium diet. She admits to taking no medication except "natural" therapy prescribed by her herbalist.

She is presently taking multivitamins and dried English hawthorne to decrease her blood pressure and decrease her oxygen needs. She states, "I don't want to take drugs because they gave them to my husband and he died anyway."

Assessment. VS: T 97.4, apical pulse 102 and irregular, 28 and labored, BP 148/90, pulse ox 94%; orthopnea; inspiratory crackles and wheezes base of lungs; nonproductive cough; states "I have to sleep sitting up in a chair." +3 edema ankles bilaterally, abdomen distended. ECG–atrial fib.; chest x-ray revealed cardiomegaly.

Nursing Diagnosis. The following important nursing diagnoses (among others) are established for this client:

- *Excess Fluid Volume* related to impaired excretion of sodium and water
- *Activity Intolerance* related to weakness, fatigue
- *Powerlessness* related to illness-related regimen

Expected Outcomes. The expected outcomes specify that Mrs. Munson will:

- Maintain clear lung sounds, no evidence of dyspnea or orthopnea.
- Express an understanding of need to balance rest and activity.
- Participate in planning care; makes decision regarding care and treatments when possible.

Planning and Implementation. The following nursing interventions are planned and implemented:

- Monitor location and extent of edema; use a millimeter tape in the same area at the same time each day to measure edema in extremities and abdomen.
- Monitor lung sounds for crackles; monitor respirations for effort and determine the presence and severity of orthopnea.
- Recognize that the presence of risk factors for excessive fluid volume is particularly serious in the elderly.
- Slow the pace of care. Allow client extra time to carry out activities.
- Encourage family and/or caretaker to help/allow elder to be independent in whatever activities possible.
- Refer client to physical therapy to help increase activity level and strength.
- Establish therapeutic relationship by listening; give the client choices and accept her statement of limitations.
- Help client identify factors not under her control.
- Validate client's feelings regarding the impact of health status on current lifestyle.

Evaluation. Mrs. Munson is being discharged to the skilled nursing center in her retirement community, after 4 days of hospitalization. Her respirations are unlabored at rest and edema in ankles reduced to +2. Lungs clear, able to sleep in low Fowler's position. Mrs. Munson referred to dietitian at the care facility to develop an eating plan that she can live with; stated "I will take my meals in the dining room after I return to my own apartment so that I can follow my prescribed diet." Participating in PT 3 days per week, can ambulate 25 feet without difficulty or shortness of breath. Taking Lasix 20 mg every day and still refusing other medications. BP 140/80. Mrs. Munson expresses fear of having a stroke.

Critical Thinking in the Nursing Process

1. Mrs. Munson expressed a wish to return to her own apartment as soon as possible. Design an activity program that will help her regain her strength and mobility
2. Mrs. Munson wants to continue her natural medicine. What would be your response to her desire?
3. Mrs. Munson is fearful that she may have a stroke. What warning signs should she be aware of, and what actions should she take if they occur?

Note: Discussion of Critical Thinking questions appears in Appendix I.

Respirations

Respiration is the act of breathing. **External respiration** refers to the interchange of oxygen and carbon dioxide between the alveoli of the lungs and the pulmonary blood. **Internal respiration** is the interchange of these same gases between the circulating blood and the cells of the body tissues.

Inhalation or inspiration refers to the intake of air into the lungs. *Exhalation* or expiration refers to breathing out or the movement of gases from the lungs to the atmosphere. *Ventilation* is also used to refer to the movement of air in and out of the lungs. Hyperventilation refers to very deep, rapid respirations; hypoventilation refers to very shallow respirations.

There are two types of breathing. *Costal* (thoracic) breathing involves external intercostal and accessory muscles. It can be observed by the movement of the chest upward and outward. Diaphragmatic (abdominal) breathing involves contraction and relaxation of the diaphragm. The abdomen moves with the diaphragm's contraction and downward movement.

MECHANICS AND REGULATION

During inhalation, the diaphragm contracts, the ribs move upward and outward, and the sternum moves outward (Figure 20-11 ■). During exhalation, the diaphragm relaxes, the ribs move downward and inward, and the sternum moves inward, decreasing the size of the thorax as the lungs are compressed. Normal breathing is automatic and effortless. An inspiration lasts 1 to 1.5 seconds, and an expiration lasts 2 to 3 seconds.

Respiration is controlled by (1) respiratory centers in the medulla oblongata and the pons of the brain and (2) by chemoreceptors located centrally in the medulla and peripherally in the carotid and aortic bodies. These centers and

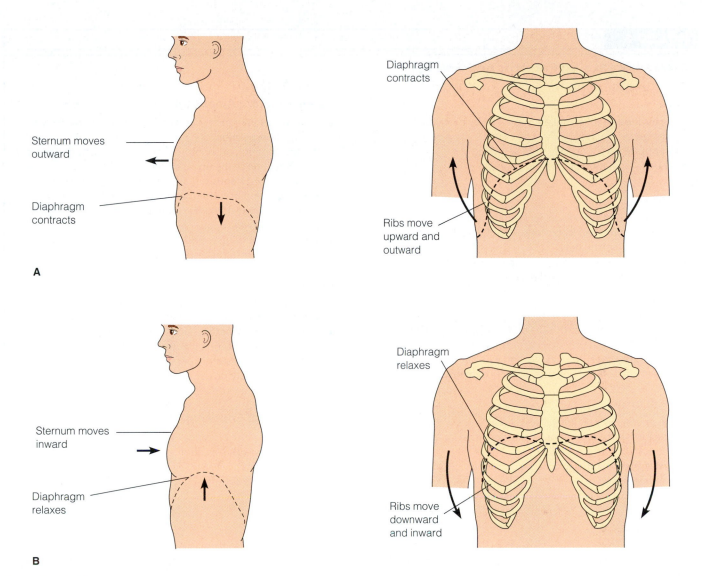

Sternum moves
outward

Diaphragm
contracts

A

Diaphragm
contracts

Ribs move
upward and
outward

Sternum moves
inward

Diaphragm
relaxes

B

Diaphragm
relaxes

Ribs move
downward
and inward

Figure 20-11. ■ **A.** Respiratory inhalation: *left:* lateral view; *right:* anterior view. **B.** Respiratory exhalation: *left:* lateral view; *right:* anterior view.

receptors respond to changes in the concentrations of oxygen (O_2), carbon dioxide (CO_2), and hydrogen (H) in the arterial blood. See Chapter 24 for details.

NURSING CARE

ASSESSING

Resting respirations should be assessed when the client is relaxed. Both exercise and anxiety affect respiratory rate and depth. Respirations may also need to be assessed after exercise to identify the client's tolerance to activity. Before assessing a client's respirations, a nurse should be aware of:

■ The client's normal breathing pattern
■ The influence of health problems on respirations

■ Any medications or therapies that might affect the client's respirations
■ Relationship of respirations to cardiovascular function.

The rate, depth, rhythm, and special characteristics of respirations should always be assessed. Box 20-6 ■ provides terms for breathing patterns, sounds, and movements. For the respiratory rates for different age groups, see Table 20-1. Several factors influence respiratory rate; major factors are listed in Table 20-5 ■.

The depth of a person's respirations can be established by watching the movement of the chest. Respiratory depth is generally described as normal, deep, or shallow. During a normal inspiration and expiration, an adult takes in about 500 mL of air. Body position also affects the amount of air that can be inhaled. People in a supine position experience two physiological processes that suppress respiration: an increase in the volume of blood inside the thoracic cavity

BOX 20-6

Altered Breathing Patterns and Sounds

Breathing Patterns

Rate

- **Tachypnea**—rapid respiration marked by quick, shallow breaths
- **Bradypnea**—abnormally slow breathing
- **Apnea**—cessation of breathing

Volume

- **Hyperventilation**—an increase in the amount of air in the lungs characterized by prolonged and deep breaths; may be associated with anxiety
- **Hypoventilation**—a reduction in the amount of air in the lungs, characterized by shallow respirations

Rhythm

- **Cheyne–Stokes breathing**—rhythmic waxing and waning of respirations, from very deep to very shallow breathing and temporary apnea; often associated with cardiac failure, increased intracranial pressure, or brain damage

Ease or Effort

- **Dyspnea**—difficult and labored breathing during which the individual has a persistent, unsatisfied need for air and feels distressed
- **Orthopnea**—ability to breathe only in upright sitting or standing positions

Breath Sounds

Audible without Amplification

- **Stridor**—a shrill, harsh sound heard during inspiration with laryngeal obstruction
- **Stertor**—snoring or sonorous respiration, usually due to a partial obstruction of the upper airway
- **Wheeze**—continuous, high-pitched musical squeak or whistling sound occurring on expiration and sometimes on inspiration when air moves through a narrowed or partially obstructed airway
- **Bubbling**—gurgling sounds heard as air passes through moist secretions in the respiratory tract

Chest Movements

- **Intercostal retraction**—indrawing between the ribs
- **Substernal retraction**—indrawing beneath the breastbone
- **Suprasternal retraction**—indrawing above the clavicles
- **Flail chest**—the ballooning out of the chest wall through injured rib spaces; results in paradoxical breathing, during which the chest wall balloons on expiration but is depressed or sucked inward on inspiration

Secretions and Coughing

- **Hemoptysis**—the presence of blood in the sputum
- **Productive cough**—a cough accompanied by expectorated secretions
- **Nonproductive cough**—a dry, harsh cough without secretions

---

and compression of the chest. So, clients lying on their back have poorer lung aeration. This predisposes them to the stasis of fluids and subsequent infection. Certain medications also affect the respiratory depth. For example, barbiturates in large doses depress the respiratory centers in the brain, thereby depressing the respiratory rate and depth.

TABLE 20-5

Major Factors Influencing Respiratory Rate

FACTOR	INFLUENCE
Exercise: increases metabolism	Increase
Stress: readies the body for "fight or flight"	Increase
Environment: increased temperature	Increase
Environment: decreased temperature	Decrease
Increased altitude: lower oxygen concentration	Increase
Certain medications (e.g., narcotic, analgesic)	Decrease
Increased intracranial pressure	Decrease

Respiratory rhythm or pattern refers to the regularity of expirations and inspirations. Normally, respirations are evenly spaced. Respiratory rhythm can be described as regular or irregular. An infant's respiratory rhythm may be less regular than an adult's.

Respiratory quality or character refers to those aspects of breathing that are different from normal, effortless breathing. Two of these are the amount of effort a client must exert to breathe and the sound of breathing. Usually, breathing does not require noticeable effort; some clients, however, breathe only with decided effort, referred to as *labored breathing*.

The sound of breathing is also significant. Normal breathing is silent. Many sounds occur as a result of the presence of fluid in the lungs, and are most clearly heard with a stethoscope (see Box 20-6).

The effectiveness of respirations is measured in part by the uptake of oxygen from the air into the blood and the release of carbon dioxide from the blood into expired air. The amount of hemoglobin in arterial blood that is saturated with oxygen can be measured indirectly through pulse oximetry. (See Chapter 24 for an illustration of a pulse oximeter.)

DIAGNOSING, PLANNING, AND IMPLEMENTING

A common nursing diagnosis for clients with respiratory difficulty is *Ineffective Breathing Pattern*. Procedure 20-3 ■ on page 399 provides guidelines for assessing respirations.

EVALUATING

Respirations are evaluated in relationship to the client's baseline data or normal range for age. The nurse documents the rate, volume, rhythm, and effort of respirations.

Blood Pressure

Arterial **blood pressure** is a measure of the pressure exerted by the blood as it flows through the arteries. Because the blood moves in waves, there are two blood pressure measurements. The **systolic pressure** is the pressure of the blood as a result of contraction of the ventricles (the pressure of the height of the blood wave). The **diastolic pressure** is the pressure when the ventricles are at rest; it is the lower pressure that is present at all times within the arteries. The difference between the diastolic and the systolic pressures is called the *pulse pressure.*

Blood pressure is measured in millimeters of mercury (mm Hg) and recorded as a fraction. The systolic pressure is written over the diastolic pressure. The average blood pressure of a healthy adult is 120/80 mm Hg. A number of conditions are reflected by changes in blood pressure.

DETERMINANTS OF BLOOD PRESSURE

Arterial blood pressure is the result of several factors: the pumping action of the heart, the *peripheral vascular resistance* (the resistance supplied by the blood vessels through which the blood flows), and the blood volume and viscosity.

Pumping Action of the Heart

Cardiac output is the volume of blood pumped into the arteries by the heart. When the pumping action of the heart is weak, less blood is pumped into arteries, and the blood pressure decreases. When the heart's pumping action is strong and the volume of blood pumped into the circulation increases, the blood pressure increases.

Peripheral Vascular Resistance

Peripheral resistance can increase blood pressure. The diastolic pressure especially is affected. Some factors that create resistance in the arterial system are the size of the arterioles and capillaries, the compliance of the arteries, and the viscosity of the blood.

The size of the arterioles and the capillaries determines in great part the peripheral resistance to the blood in the body. A lumen is a channel within a tube. The smaller the lumen of a vessel, the greater the resistance. Normally, the arterioles are in a state of partial constriction. Increased vasoconstriction raises the blood pressure, whereas decreased vasoconstriction lowers the blood pressure.

The arteries account for most of the peripheral resistance. The major factor reducing arterial compliance is pathologic change affecting the arterial walls. When elastic and muscular tissues of the arteries are replaced with fibrous tissue, the arteries lose much of their compliance. This condition, most common in middle-aged and elderly adults, is known as *arteriosclerosis.*

Blood Volume

When the blood volume decreases (e.g., from hemorrhage or dehydration), the blood pressure decreases because of decreased fluid in the arteries. When the volume increases (e.g., with an intravenous infusion), the blood pressure increases because of the greater fluid volume within the circulatory system.

Blood Viscosity

Viscosity is a physical property that results from friction of molecules in a fluid. In a viscous (or "thick") fluid, there is a great deal of friction among the molecules as they slide by each other. The blood pressure is higher when the blood is highly viscous, that is, when the proportion of red blood cells to the blood plasma is high. This proportion is referred to as the *hematocrit.* The viscosity increases markedly when the hematocrit is more than 60% to 65%.

FACTORS AFFECTING BLOOD PRESSURE

Among the factors influencing blood pressure are:

- *Age.* Newborns have a mean systolic pressure of about 75 mm Hg. The pressure rises with age, reaching a peak at the onset of puberty, and then tends to decline somewhat. One quick way to determine the normal systolic blood pressure of a child is to use the following formula:

  Normal systolic BP = 80 + (2 × child's age in years)

  In older people, elasticity of the arteries is decreased—the arteries are more rigid and less yielding to the pressure of the blood. This produces an elevated systolic pressure. Because the walls no longer retract as flexibly with decreased pressure, the diastolic pressure is also higher. (See Table 20-1.)
- *Exercise.* Physical activity increases the cardiac output and the blood pressure. So, 20 to 30 minutes of rest following exercise is indicated before the resting blood pressure can be reliably assessed.
- *Stress.* Stimulation of the sympathetic nervous system increases cardiac output and vasoconstriction of the arterioles, increasing the blood pressure reading. However, severe pain can decrease blood pressure greatly and

TABLE 20-6

Follow-up Recommendations for Blood Pressure Measurement for Adults Older Than 18 Years

INITIAL SCREENING BLOOD PRESSURE (MM HG)[a]		
SYSTOLIC	DIASTOLIC	FOLLOW-UP RECOMMENDED[b]
<130	<85	Recheck in 2 years.
130–139	85–89	Recheck in 1 year.[c]
140–159	90–99	Confirm within 2 months.
160–179	100–109	Evaluate or refer to source of care within 1 month.
180–209	110–119	Evaluate or refer to source of care within 1 week.
≥210	≥120	Evaluate or refer to source of care immediately.

[a]If the systolic and diastolic categories are different, follow recommendation for the shorter time to follow up (e.g., 160/85 mm Hg should be evaluated or referred to source of care within 1 month).
[b]The scheduling of follow-up should be modified by reliable information about past blood pressure measurements, other cardiovascular risk factors, or target-organ disease.
[c]Consider providing advice about lifestyle modifications.
Source: From the fifth report of the Joint National Committee for the Detection, Evaluation, and Treatment of High Blood Pressure, National Heart, Lung, and Blood Institute, National Institutes of Health, 1993, *Archives of Internal Medicine, 329,* 1912.

cause shock by inhibiting the vasomotor center and producing vasodilation.

- *Race.* African American males over 35 years of age have higher blood pressures than European American males of the same age. (Box 20-7.)
- *Obesity.* Pressure is generally higher in some overweight and obese people than in people of normal weight.
- *Sex.* After puberty, females usually have lower blood pressures than males of the same age; this difference is thought to be due to hormonal variations. Women generally have higher blood pressures after menopause than before.
- *Medications.* Many medications may increase or decrease the blood pressure; nurses should be aware of the specific medications a client is receiving and consider their possible impact when interpreting blood pressure readings.
- *Diurnal variations.* Pressure is usually lowest early in the morning, when the metabolic rate is lowest, then rises throughout the day and peaks in the late afternoon or early evening.
- *Disease process.* Any condition affecting the cardiac output, blood volume, blood viscosity, or compliance of the arteries has a direct effect on the blood pressure.

HYPERTENSION

A blood pressure that is persistently above normal is called *hypertension.* It is usually asymptomatic and is often a contributing factor to myocardial infarctions (heart attacks). An elevated blood pressure of unknown cause is called *primary hypertension.* An elevated blood pressure of known cause is called *secondary hypertension.* Hypertension is a widespread health problem. The diagnosis is made when the average of two or more diastolic readings on two visits following the initial assessment is 90 mm Hg or higher, or when the average of multiple systolic blood pressure readings is higher than 140 mm Hg. Categories of hypertension have been identified and are described in Table 20-6 ■. Factors associated with hypertension include thickening of the arterial walls, which reduces the size of the arterial lumen; inelasticity of the arteries; and lifestyle factors such as cigarette smoking, obesity, heavy alco-

hol consumption, lack of physical exercise, high blood cholesterol levels, and continued exposure to stress. Follow-up care should include lifestyle changes conducive to lowering the blood pressure as well as monitoring the pressure itself.

HYPOTENSION

Hypotension is a blood pressure that is below normal (a systolic reading consistently between 85 and 110 mm Hg in an adult). **Orthostatic hypotension** is a blood pressure that falls when the client sits or stands. It is usually the result of peripheral vasodilation in which the blood flow leaves the central body organs, especially the brain, and moves to the periphery, often causing the person to feel faint. Hypotension can also be caused by analgesics such as meperidine hydrochloride (Demerol), bleeding, severe burns, and prolonged diarrhea and vomiting. It is important to monitor hypotensive clients carefully to prevent falls. See Box 20-8 ■ for instructions for measuring blood pressure for clients with orthostatic hypotension.

BLOOD PRESSURE EQUIPMENT

Blood pressure is measured with a blood pressure cuff, a sphygmomanometer, and a stethoscope. The blood pressure cuff consists of a rubber bag that can be inflated with air. It

BOX 20-8

Measuring Blood Pressure for Orthostatic Hypotension

When measuring the blood pressure of a client who has orthostatic hypotension:

- Place the client in a supine position for 2 to 3 minutes. This allows the blood pressure and pulse to stabilize in this position.
- Record the client's pulse and blood pressure.
- Assist the client to sit or stand slowly. Support the client in case of faintness.
- After 1 minute in the upright position, recheck the client's pulse and blood pressure in the same sites as previously.

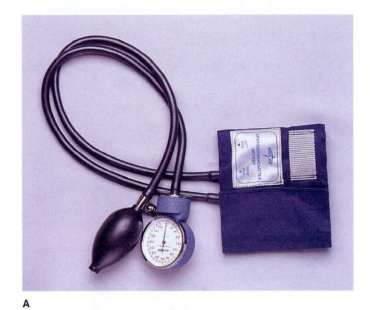

A

is called the *bladder* (Figure 20-12 ■). It is covered with cloth and has two tubes attached to it. One tube connects to a rubber bulb that inflates the bladder. A small valve on the side of this bulb releases the air in the bladder. When the valve is closed, air pumped into the bladder remains there. The other tube is attached to a sphygmomanometer.

The sphygmomanometer indicates the pressure of the air within the bladder. There are two types of sphygmomanometers: aneroid and mercury (Figure 20-13 ■). The aneroid sphygmomanometer is a calibrated dial with a needle that points to the calibrations.

The mercury sphygmomanometer is a calibrated cylinder filled with mercury. The pressure is indicated at the point to which the rounded curve (the base) of the meniscus (the curved top of a column of liquid in a small tube) rises (Figure 20-14 ■). The blood pressure reading should be made with the eye at the level of the rounded curve in order

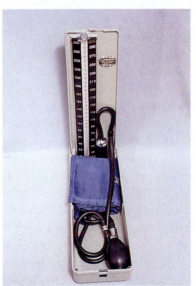

B

Figure 20-13. ■ Blood pressure equipment: **A.** aneroid manometer and cuff; **B.** mercury manometer and cuff.

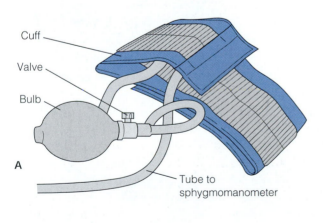

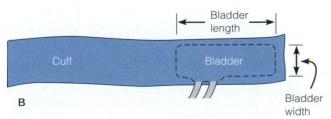

Figure 20-12. ■ **A.** Blood pressure cuff and bulb; **B.** bladder inside the cuff.

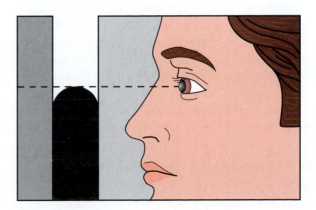

Figure 20-14. ■ To obtain an accurate reading from a mercury manometer, position the meniscus at eye level.

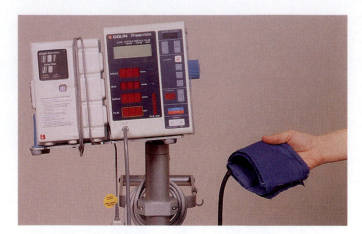

Figure 20-15. ■ Electronic blood pressure monitors automatically register systolic, diastolic, and mean blood pressures. (Photographer: Jenny Thomas.)

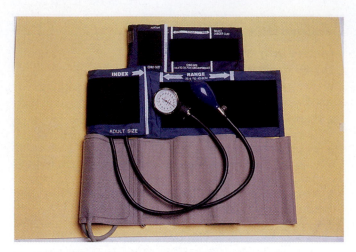

Figure 20-16. ■ Three standard cuff sizes: a small cuff for an infant, small child, or frail adult; a normal adult-size cuff; and a large cuff for measuring the blood pressure on the leg or on the arm of an obese adult. (Photographer: Elena Dorfman.)

to be accurate. If the eye is looking up or down, a distortion in the reading can occur. A distortion that occurs as a result of the angle of view is called *parallax.*

Some medical facilities use electronic sphygmomanometers (Figure 20-15 ■), which eliminate the need to listen to the sounds of the client's systolic and diastolic blood pressures through a stethoscope. Electronic blood pressure devices should be calibrated against a mercury sphygmomanometer to check accuracy. Automated electronic devices have been shown to give higher values than manual cuffs.

Doppler ultrasound stethoscopes are also used to assess blood pressure (see Figure 20-10). These are of particular value when blood pressure sounds are difficult to hear, such as in infants, obese clients, and clients in shock. A systolic blood pressure assessed with a DUS is recorded with a large D, for example, 85D. Systolic pressure may be the only blood pressure obtainable with some ultrasound models.

Blood pressure cuffs come in various sizes because the bladder must be the correct width and length for the client's arm (Figure 20-16 ■). If the bladder is too narrow, the blood pressure reading will be erroneously elevated; if it is too wide, the reading will be erroneously low. The arm circumference, not the age of the client, should always be used to determine bladder size (Figure 20-17 ■).

The length of the bladder also affects the accuracy of measurement. The bladder should be sufficiently long to cover at least two-thirds of the limb's circumference.

Blood pressure cuffs are made of nondistensible material so that an even pressure is exerted around the limb. Most cuffs are held in place by hooks, snaps, or Velcro.

BLOOD PRESSURE ASSESSMENT SITES

The blood pressure is usually assessed in the client's arm using the brachial artery and a standard stethoscope. If the arm is very large or grossly misshapen and the conventional

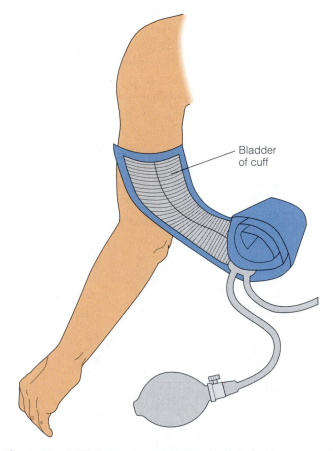

Bladder of cuff

Figure 20-17. ■ To ensure an accurate reading, the nurse must determine that the bladder of a blood pressure cuff is 40% of the arm circumference or 20% wider than the diameter of the midpoint of the limb. To do this, the nurse lays the cuff lengthwise at the midpoint of the upper arm, holding the outermost side of the bladder edge laterally on the arm. With the other hand, the nurse wraps the width of the cuff around the arm to ensure that it covers 40% of the arm's circumference.

cuff cannot be properly applied, leg or forearm measurements can be taken. See Procedure 20-4 ■ on page 400 for directions for measuring blood pressure on the thigh.

Assessing the blood pressure on a client's thigh is usually indicated in these situations:

- The blood pressure cannot be measured on either arm (e.g., because of burns or other trauma).
- The blood pressure in one thigh is to be compared with the blood pressure in the other thigh.

Blood pressure is not measured on a client's arm or thigh in the following situations:

- The shoulder, arm, or hand (or the hip, knee, or ankle) is injured or diseased.
- A cast or bulky bandage is on any part of the limb.
- The client has had removal of axillary (or hip) lymph nodes on that side.
- The client has an intravenous infusion in that limb.
- The client has an arteriovenous fistula (e.g., for renal dialysis) in that limb.

To obtain a forearm blood pressure, apply an appropriate-sized cuff to the forearm 14 cm (5 in.) below the elbow. Blood pressure sounds can then be heard from the radial artery.

BLOOD PRESSURE ASSESSMENT METHODS

Blood pressure can be assessed directly or indirectly. Direct (invasive monitoring) measurement involves the insertion of a catheter into the brachial, radial, or femoral artery. Arterial pressure is represented as wavelike forms displayed on an oscilloscope. With correct placement, this pressure reading is highly accurate.

Two noninvasive indirect methods of measuring blood pressure are the auscultatory and palpatory methods. The auscultatory method is most commonly used in hospitals, clinics, and homes. When carried out correctly, the auscultatory method is relatively accurate.

When taking a blood pressure using a stethoscope, the nurse identifies five phases in the series of sounds called Korotkoff's sounds (Figure 20-18 ■). Box 20-9 ■ describes Korotkoff's phases.

NURSING CARE

ASSESSING

The palpatory method is sometimes used when Korotkoff's sounds cannot be heard and electronic equipment to amplify the sounds is not available, or when an auscultatory gap occurs. An *auscultatory gap,* which occurs particularly in hypertensive clients, is the temporary disappearance of sounds normally heard over the brachial artery when the

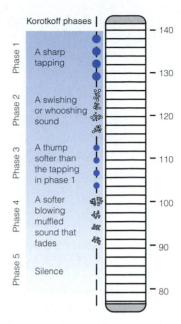

Figure 20-18. ■ Korotkoff's sounds can be differentiated into five phases. In the illustration, the blood pressure is 138/90 or 138/102/90.

BOX 20-9

Korotkoff's Sounds

- **Phase 1:** The pressure level at which the first faint, clear tapping or thumping sounds are heard. These sounds gradually become more intense. To ensure that they are not extraneous sounds, the nurse should identify at least two consecutive tapping sounds. The first tapping sound heard during deflation of the cuff is the systolic blood pressure.
- **Phase 2:** The period during deflation when the sounds have a muffled, whooshing, or swishing quality.
- **Phase 3:** The period during which the blood flows freely through an increasingly open artery and the sounds become crisper and more intense and again assume a thumping quality but softer than in phase 1.
- **Phase 4:** The time when the sounds become muffled and have a soft, blowing quality.
- **Phase 5:** The pressure level when the last sound is heard. This is followed by a period of silence. The pressure at which the last sound is heard is the diastolic blood pressure in adults.[a]

---

[a]For children, the American Heart Association (2005, p. 4) recommends that the onset of phase 4, where the sounds become muffled, be considered the diastolic pressure. In agencies in which the fourth phase is considered the diastolic pressure of adults, three measures are recommended (systolic pressure, diastolic pressure, and phase 5). These may be referred to as systolic, first diastolic, and second diastolic pressures. The phase 5 (second diastolic pressure) reading may be zero; that is, the muffled sounds are heard even when there is no air pressure in the blood pressure cuff. In some instances, muffled sounds are never heard, in which case a dash is inserted where the reading would normally be recorded (e.g., 190/–/110).

cuff pressure is high followed by the reappearance of the sounds at a lower level. This temporary disappearance of sounds occurs in the latter part of phase 1 and phase 2 and may cover a range of 40 mm Hg. Instead of listening for the blood flow sounds, the nurse palpates the pulsations of the artery as the pressure in the cuff is released. The systolic pressure is read from the sphygmomanometer when the first pulsation is felt. A single whiplike vibration, felt in addition to the pulsations, identifies the point at which the pressure in the cuff nears the diastolic pressure. This vibration is no longer felt when the cuff pressure is below the diastolic pressure. To palpate the diastolic pressure, the nurse applies light to moderate pressure over the pulse point.

Common Errors in Assessing Blood Pressure

The importance of the accuracy of blood pressure assessments cannot be overemphasized. Many judgments about a client's health are made on the basis of blood pressure. It is an important indicator of the client's condition and is used extensively as a basis for nursing interventions. Some reasons for erroneous blood pressure readings are given in Table 20-7 ■.

DIAGNOSING, PLANNING, AND IMPLEMENTING

A frequent nursing diagnosis for clients with problems of blood pressure is *Ineffective Therapeutic Regimen Management.* Procedure 20-4 gives guidelines for assessing blood pressure.

Vital signs are documented in a flow sheet (see Figure 6-5) or in graphic form in most facilities. This type of documentation provides easy access for the physician and other members of the healthcare team. Occasionally, a nurse will insert vital signs in a nurse's note. See Box 20-10 ■ for an example of this.

EVALUATING

Vital signs individually as well as in combination tell the nurse and ultimately the physician what is happening with the client. The nurse knows that a low blood pressure (hypotension) in the presence of a rapid pulse (tachycardia) can be signs of hemorrhage and impending shock. Widening pulse pressure—a separation of more than 40 mm Hg between the systolic and diastolic blood pressure readings—should alert the nurse to possible increased intracranial pressure. In the presence of pain, vital signs may also be elevated. It is important to consider not only the vital sign readings, but also the whole assessment. The data obtained from vital signs measurement will aid you in making sound judgments regarding the client's care.

Note: The references and resources for this and all chapters have been compiled at the back of the book.

TABLE 20-7

Blood Pressure Assessment Errors

ERROR	EFFECT
Bladder cuff too narrow	Erroneously high
Bladder cuff too wide	Erroneously low
Arm unsupported	Erroneously high
Insufficient rest before the assessment	Erroneously high
Repeating assessment too quickly	Erroneously high systolic or low diastolic readings
Cuff wrapped too loosely or unevenly	Erroneously high
Deflating cuff too quickly	Erroneously low systolic and high diastolic readings
Deflating cuff too slowly	Erroneously high diastolic reading
Failure to use the same arm consistently	Inconsistent measurements
Arm above level of the heart	Erroneously low
Assessing immediately after a meal or while client smokes or has pain	Erroneously high
Failure to identify auscultatory gap	Erroneously low systolic pressure and erroneously low diastolic pressure

clinical ALERT

Because BP varies among individuals, the nurse must know a client's baseline BP. If a client's usual BP is 180/100 mm Hg, but after surgery is 120/80 mm Hg, report this drop in pressure to the physician.

BOX 20-10

Sample Nurse's Notes Containing Vital Signs

Focus

CVS	D	0835	VS 99.8/100/24 158/90 c/o chest pain 5/10. Sitting in chair.
	A		PRN ms given as prescribed. Assisted to return to bed. K. Turner LVN
	R	0915	Client resting comfortably; chest pain resolved. 0/10. VS 98.8/86/20 140/88. K. Turner LVN

PROCEDURE 20-1 · Assessing Body Temperature

Purposes

- To establish baselinedata for follow-up evaluation
- To identify whether the core temperature is within normal range
- To monitor clients at risk for change in temperature (e.g., clients at risk for infection or diagnosis of infection; those who have been exposed to temperature extremes; those with a leukocyte count below 5,000 or above 12,000)

Equipment

- Oral, rectal, axillary thermometer
- Towel, if the axillary site is used
- Lubricant and tissue, if the rectal site is used
- Disposable gloves, if the rectal site is used

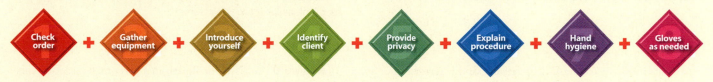

Check order ➕ Gather equipment ➕ Introduce yourself ➕ Identify client ➕ Provide privacy ➕ Explain procedure ➕ Hand hygiene ➕ Gloves as needed

Interventions

1. Prepare client.

For an Oral Temperature

- Determine the time the client last took hot or cold food or fluids or smoked. *To obtain an accurate oral temperature reading, allow 15 to 30 minutes to elapse between a client's intake or smoking and the measurement.*

For a Rectal Temperature

- Assist the client to assume a lateral position. Place newborn in a lateral or prone position. Place a young child in a lateral position with knees flexed, or prone across the lap.

For Comfort and Safety

- Provide privacy before folding the bedclothes back to expose the buttocks. *Privacy is essential because exposure of the buttocks embarrasses most people.*

For an Axillary Temperature

- Expose the client's axilla. If the axilla is moist, dry it with the towel, using a patting motion. *Friction created by rubbing can raise the temperature of the axilla.*

2. Prepare the equipment.
- Remove the thermometer from its storage container, and check the temperature reading on the thermometer.
- Shake down the mercury (if necessary) by holding the thermometer between the thumb and forefinger at the end farthest from the bulb. Snap the wrist downward. Repeat until the mercury is below 35°C (95°F). *For Accurate Assessment of Subnormal Temperature*
- Place the thermometer in a plastic sheath according to agency policy. *Disposable sheaths prevent spread of infections.*

3. Take the temperature.

For an Oral Temperature

- Place the thermometer or probe at the base of the tongue to the right or left of the frenulum, in the posterior sublingual pocket (Figure 20-19 ■). *The thermometer needs to reflect the core temperature of the blood in the larger blood vessels of the posterior pocket.*
- Ask the client to close the lips, not the teeth, around the thermometer. *A client who bites a glass thermometer can break it and injure the mouth.*
- Leave the thermometer in place a sufficient time for the temperature to register or for the length of time recommended by the agency. *The recommended time is generally 2 minutes.*

For a Rectal Temperature

- Place some lubricant on a piece of tissue. Then apply lubricant to the thermometer. *The lubricant facilitates insertion of the thermometer without irritating the mucous membrane.*
- Put on disposable gloves. With the nondominant hand, raise the client's upper buttock to expose the anus.

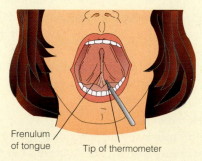

Frenulum of tongue — Tip of thermometer

Figure 20-19. ■ The tip of the oral thermometer is placed beside the frenulum below the tongue.

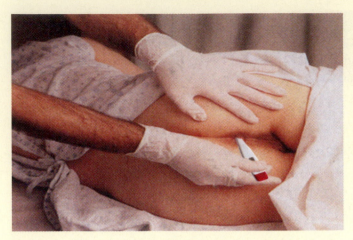

Figure 20-20. ■ Inserting a rectal thermometer. (Patrick Watson.)

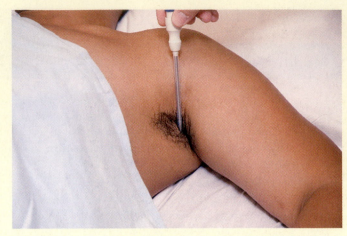

Figure 20-21. ■ Placing the bulb of the thermometer in the center of the axilla. (Patrick Watson.)

■ Ask the client to take a deep breath, and insert the thermometer into the anus anywhere from 1.5 to 4 cm (0.5 to 1.5 in.), depending on the age and size of the client (for example, 1.5 cm [0.5 in.] for an infant, 2.5 cm [0.9 in.] for a child, and 3.7 cm [1.5 in.] for an adult) (Figure 20-20 ■). *Taking a deep breath often relaxes the external sphincter muscle, thus easing insertion.*

■ Do not force insertion of the thermometer. *Inability to insert the thermometer into a newborn could indicate the rectum is not patent.*

■ Hold the thermometer in place for 3 minutes or for the length of time recommended by the agency. For neonates, hold the thermometer in place for 5 minutes or according to agency protocol. Hold the young child firmly while the probe is in the rectum. *The thermometer may become displaced inside or outside the anus if not held in place.*

For an Axillary Temperature

■ Place the thermometer in the center of the client's axilla (Figure 20-21 ■). *This allows the thermometer to come in contact with the axillary blood supply.*

■ Assist the client to place the arm tightly across the chest to keep the thermometer in place. *This maintains the proper position.*

■ Leave the thermometer in place for 9 minutes or according to agency protocol. For infants and children, leave the thermometer in place 5 minutes. *Device must stay in position long enough to ensure an accurate temperature.*

■ Remain with the client, and hold the thermometer in place if the client is irrational or very young. *This provides safety for the client and prevents breakage.*

4. Remove the thermometer.

■ Remove the plastic sheath, or if a sheath is not used, wipe the thermometer with a tissue. Wipe in a rotating manner toward the bulb. *The thermometer is wiped from the area of least contamination to that of greatest contamination.*

■ Discard the tissue or sheath in a receptacle used for contaminated items. *This prevents spread of infection.*

5. Read the temperature.

■ Hold the thermometer at eye level and rotate it until the mercury column is clearly visible. The upper end of the mercury column registers the client's body temperature. On the Fahrenheit thermometer, each long line reflects 1 degree, and each short line 0.2 degree. On the Celsius (centigrade) thermometer, each long line reflects 0.5 degree, and each short line 0.1 degree.

6. Clean and shake down the thermometer.

■ Wash the thermometer in tepid, soapy water. Rinse the thermometer in cold water, dry it, and store it dry. *Organic material, such as mucus, must be removed before the thermometer can be stored. Organic materials on the thermometer can harbor microorganisms. Hot water expands the mercury and may break the thermometer.*

■ Shake down the thermometer and return it to its container or discard it. *Some agencies also have special equipment for spinning down the mercury levels.*

■ If the thermometer is to be disinfected before storage, follow agency policy.

7. Document the temperature.

■ Record the temperature to the nearest indicated tenth (for example, 37.1°C, 98.4°F,) on a designated flow sheet. See Figure 6-5. *Recording the temperature immediately ensures it is not forgotten.*

VARIATION: USING AN ELECTRONIC THERMOMETER

■ Remove the electronic unit from the battery charging area.

■ Remove the temperature probe. If the probe is not attached, attach it to the appropriate circuit (oral, rectal, or axillary) in models that have separate circuits for each.

- Place a disposable cover securely on the probe.
- Warm up the machine by switching it on if removal of the probe does not automatically prepare the machine for functioning.
- Take the temperature as indicated in step 3.
- Listen for a sound indicating that the maximum measurement has been reached, and read the temperature on the dial or readout.
- Remove the thermometer.
- Record the temperature.
- Remove and discard the probe cover.
- Return the unit to the charging base.

VARIATION: USING A TYMPANIC (INFRARED) THERMOMETER

- Apply a disposable sheath to the probe. Different sheaths fit adults and infants. They can be applied without being touched.
- Select the ear opposite the side on which the client may have been lying. The ear against a surface can build up heat.
- Use your right hand to hold the thermometer when using the client's right ear, left hand for the left ear. This helps achieve the proper angle for a good seal.
- Gently pull the pinna upward and back for children over age 3 and adults (Figure 20-22 ■), straight back for children under age 3. This straightens the ear canal.
- Place the probe tip into the outer position of the ear canal just at the opening. The probe tip seals the opening of the canal.

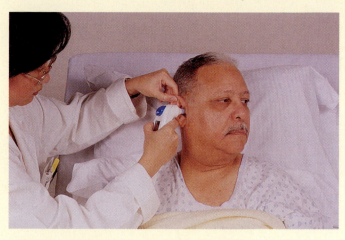

Figure 20-22. ■ Pull the pinna of the ear up and back while inserting the tympanic thermometer.

- Press the button on the electronic thermometer. Do not wait too long to do this. The presence of the probe can "draw down" the temperature reading.
- Remove the thermometer.
- Read the temperature on the screen. In 1 to 2 seconds, the temperature is displayed on the screen.
- Remove and discard the probe cover. Covers can be ejected without being touched.
- Return the unit to the charging base.

SAMPLE DOCUMENTATION

See Figure 6-5 for a common documentation of temperature.

PROCEDURE 20-2 | **Assessing Pulse**

Purposes

- To establish baseline data for subsequent evaluation
- To identify whether the pulse rate is within normal range
- To determine whether the pulse rhythm is regular and the pulse volume is appropriate
- To compare the equality of corresponding peripheral pulses on each side of the body
- To monitor and assess changes in the client's health status
- To monitor clients at risk for pulse alterations (e.g., those with a history of heart disease or experiencing

cardiac arrhythmias, hemorrhage, acute pain, infusion of large volumes of fluids, fever)
- To obtain the heart rate of newborns, infants, and children 2 to 3 years old or of an adult with an irregular peripheral pulse
- To determine whether the cardiac rate is within normal range and the rhythm is regular
- To monitor clients with cardiac disease and those receiving medications to improve heart action
- To determine adequacy of peripheral circulation or presence of pulse deficit

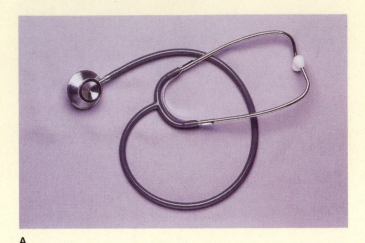

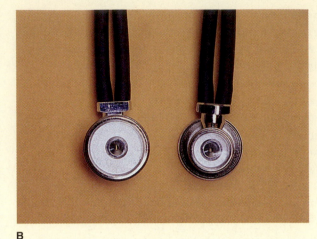

A

B

Figure 20-23. ■ **A.** Stethoscope with both a bell-shaped and flat-disk amplifier. **B.** Close-up of a flat-disk amplifier (*left*) and a bell amplifier (*right*). (Photographer: Elena Dorfman.)

Equipment

- Watch with a second hand or indicator
- If using Doppler ultrasound stethoscope, the transducer in the DUS probe, a stethoscope headset, and transmission gel

- Antiseptic wipes
- Stethoscope with a bell-shaped or flat disk (Figure 20-23 ■)
- Stethoscope

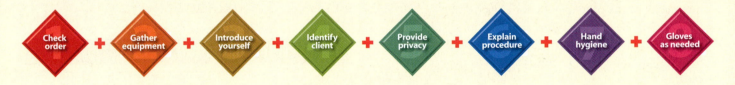

Check order ◆ Gather equipment ◆ Introduce yourself ◆ Identify client ◆ Provide privacy ◆ Explain procedure ◆ Hand hygiene ◆ Gloves as needed

Part A: Peripheral Pulse

Interventions

1. Prepare the client.
   - Select the pulse point. *Normally, the radial pulse is taken unless it cannot be exposed or circulation to another body area is to be assessed.*
   - Assist the client to a comfortable resting position. When the radial pulse is assessed, the client's arm can rest alongside the body, the palm facing downward. Or the forearm can rest at a 90-degree angle across the chest with the palm downward. For the client who can sit, the forearm can rest across the thigh, with the palm of the hand facing downward or inward. Position a child comfortably in the parent's arms, or have the parent remain close by. *Having the parent close or holding the child may decrease anxiety and yield more accurate results.*

2. Palpate and count the pulse (Figure 20-24 ■).
   - Place two or three middle fingertips lightly and squarely over the pulse point (Figure 20-24B). *Using the thumb is contraindicated because the thumb has a pulse that the nurse could mistake for the client's pulse.*

- If the pulse is regular, count for 30 seconds and multiply by 2. If it is irregular, count for 1 minute. When taking a client's pulse for the first time or obtaining baseline data, count the pulse for a full minute. *An irregular pulse requires a full minute's count for a correct assessment and indicates the need to take the apical pulse.*

3. Assess the pulse rhythm and volume.
   - Assess the pulse rhythm by noting the pattern of the intervals between the beats. *A normal pulse has equal time periods between beats.* If this is an initial assessment, assess for 1 minute.
   - Assess the pulse volume. *A normal pulse can be felt with moderate pressure, and the pressure is equal with each beat. A forceful pulse volume is full; an easily obliterated pulse is weak.*

4. Document and report to the nurse in charge pertinent assessment data.
   - Record the pulse rate, rhythm, and volume on the appropriate records.
   - Report to the nurse in charge pertinent data such as (1) pale skin color and cool skin temperature; (2) a pulse rate faster

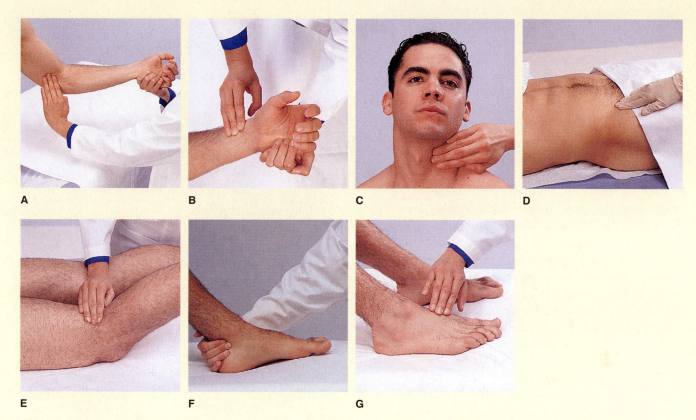

Figure 20-24. ■ Assessing the pulses: **A.** brachial; **B.** radial; **C.** carotid; **D.** femoral; **E.** popliteal; **F.** posterior tibial; **G.** pedal (dorsalis pedis).

or slower than normal for the client; (3) a full, bounding, or weak pulse volume; and (4) an irregular pulse rhythm.

VARIATION: USING A DUS

- Plug the stethoscope headset into one of the two output jacks located next to the volume control. DUS units may have two jacks so that a second person can listen to the signals (see Figure 20-10).
- Apply transmission gel either to the probe at the narrow end of the plastic case housing the transducer or to the client's skin. Ultrasound beams do not travel well through air. *The gel makes an airtight seal, which then promotes optimal ultrasound wave transmission.*
- Press the "on" button.
- Hold the probe against the skin over the pulse site. Use light pressure, and keep the probe in contact with the

skin. *Too much pressure can stop the blood flow and obliterate the signal.*

- Distinguish artery sounds from vein sounds. The artery sound (signal) is distinctively pulsating and has a pumping quality. The venous sound is intermittent and varies with respirations. *Both artery and vein sounds are heard simultaneously through the DUS because major arteries and veins are situated close together throughout the body.*
- If arterial sounds cannot be easily heard, reposition the probe.
- After assessing the pulse, remove all gel from the probe to prevent damage to its surface. Clean the transducer with aqueous solutions. *Alcohol or other disinfectants may damage the face of the transducer.* Remove all gel from the client.

Part B: Apical Pulse

Interventions

1. Prepare client. Position the client appropriately.
   - Assist an adult or young child to a comfortable supine position or to a sitting position.
   - Place a baby in a supine position, and offer a pacifier if the baby is crying or restless. *Crying and physical ac-*

tivity will increase the pulse rate. Take the apical pulse rate of infants and small children before assessing body temperatures.
   - Demonstrate the procedure to the child using a stuffed animal or doll, and allow the child to handle the stethoscope before beginning the procedure. *This will decrease anxiety and promote cooperation.*

■ Expose the area of the chest over the apex of the heart. *Clothing may interfere with ability to assess heartbeat.*

2. Locate the apical impulse.
   ■ This is the point over the apex of the heart where the apical pulse can be most clearly heard. It is also referred to as the point of maximal impulse (PMI).
   ■ Palpate the angle of Louis (the angle between the manubrium, the top of the sternum, and the body of the sternum). It is palpated just below the suprasternal notch and is felt as a prominence (see Figure 20-9).
   ■ Slide your index finger just to the left of the client's sternum, and palpate the second intercostal space.
   ■ Place your middle or next finger in the third intercostal space, and continue palpating downward until you locate the apical impulse, usually about the fifth intercostal space if the client is an adult or a child 7 years or older. If the client is a young child, palpate downward to the fourth intercostal space. *The apex of the heart is normally located in the fifth intercostal space in individuals who are 7 years of age and over; it is in the fourth intercostal space in young children, and one or two spaces above the adult apex during infancy.*
   ■ Palpate the apical impulse. If the client is an adult, move your index finger laterally along the fifth intercostal space to the MCL. *Normally, the apical impulse is palpable at or just medial to the MCL.* For a young child, move your finger along the fourth intercostal space to a position between the MCL and the anterior axillary line (see Figure 20-9).

3. Auscultate and count heartbeats.
   ■ Use antiseptic wipes to clean the earpieces and diaphragm of the stethoscope if their cleanliness is in doubt. *The diaphragm needs to be cleaned and disinfected if soiled with body substances.*
   ■ Warm the diaphragm of the stethoscope by holding it in the palm of the hand for a moment. *The metal of the diaphragm is usually cold and can startle the client when placed immediately on the chest.*
   ■ Insert the earpieces of the stethoscope into your ears in the direction of the ear canals, or slightly forward. *This facilitates hearing.*
   ■ Tap your finger lightly on the diaphragm to be sure it is the active side of the head. If necessary, rotate the head to select the diaphragm side.
   ■ Place the diaphragm of the stethoscope over the apical impulse (Figure 20-25 ■) and listen for the normal S_1 and S_2 heart sounds, which are heard as "lub-dub." Each

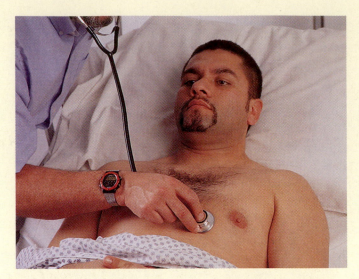

Figure 20-25. ■ Taking an apical pulse using the flat disk of the stethoscope. Note how the amplifier is held against the chest.

lub-dub is counted as one heartbeat. The heartbeat is normally loudest over the apex of the heart. The two heart sounds are produced by closure of the valves of the heart. The S_1 heart sound (lub) occurs when the atrioventricular valves close after the ventricles have been sufficiently filled. The S_2 heart sound (dub) occurs when the semilunar valves close after the ventricles empty.
   ■ If the rhythm is regular, count the heartbeats for 30 seconds and multiply by 2. If the rhythm is irregular or if the apical impulse is being taken on an infant or child, count the beats for 60 seconds. *A 60-second count provides a more accurate assessment of an irregular pulse than a 30-second count.*

4. Assess the rhythm and the strength of the heartbeat.
   ■ Assess the rhythm of the heartbeat by noting the pattern of intervals between the beats. *A normal pulse has equal time periods between beats.*
   ■ Assess the strength (volume) of the heartbeat. *Normally, the heartbeats are equal in strength and can be described as strong or weak.*

5. Document and report pertinent assessment data.
   ■ Record the pulse site and rate, rhythm, and volume on the appropriate records.
   ■ Report to the nurse in charge any pertinent data such as pallor, cyanosis, dyspnea, tachycardia, bradycardia, irregular rhythm, and reduced strength of the heartbeat.

Part C: Apical–Radial Pulse

Interventions

1. Position the client appropriately.
   ■ Assist the client to assume the physiological position described for taking the apical pulse (on page 397).
   ■ If previous measurements were taken, determine what position the client assumed and use the same position. *This ensures an accurate comparative measurement.*

2. Locate the apical and radial pulse sites.

3. Count the apical and radial pulse rates.

Two-Nurse Technique

- In the two-nurse technique, one nurse locates the apical impulse by palpation or with the stethoscope while the other nurse palpates the radial pulse site.
- Place the watch where both nurses can see it. The nurse who is taking the radial pulse may hold the watch.
- Decide on a time to begin counting. *A time when the second hand is on 12, 3, 6, or 9 is usually selected to help in obtaining an accurate reading.* The nurse taking the radial pulse says "Start" at the designated time. *This ensures that simultaneous counts are taken.*
- Each nurse counts the pulse rate for 60 seconds. Both nurses end the count when the nurse taking the radial pulse says "Stop." *A full 60-second count is necessary for accurate assessment of any differences between the two pulse sites.*
- The nurse who assesses the apical rate also assesses the apical pulse rhythm and volume (i.e., whether the heartbeat is strong or weak). If the pulse is irregular, note whether the irregular beats come at random or predictable times.
- The nurse assessing the radial pulse rate also assesses the radial pulse rhythm and volume.

One-Nurse Technique (Not Recommended for Clients with Irregular Heartbeat)

- Assess the apical pulse for 60 seconds.
- Assess the radial pulse for 60 seconds.

4. Document and report pertinent assessment data.

- Promptly report any notable changes from previous measurements or any difference between the two pulses.
- Document the apical and radial (AR) pulse rates, rhythm, volume, and any pulse deficit.
- Record any other pertinent observations, such as pallor, cyanosis, or dyspnea.
- Check the physician's orders for any directions related to a difference in the AR pulse rates.

SAMPLE DOCUMENTATION

[date]	Apical-radial pulse taken: 80 apical,
[time]	65 radial at left wrist and weak.
	Edema left arm +3.
	_____ S. Markham, LPN

PROCEDURE 20-3 Assessing Respirations

Purposes

- To acquire baseline data against which future measurements can be compared
- To monitor abnormal respirations and respiratory patterns and identify changes
- To assess respirations before the administration of a medication such as morphine (an abnormally slow respiratory rate may warrant withholding the medication)
- To monitor respirations following the administration of a general anesthetic or any medication that influences respirations
- To monitor clients at risk for respiratory alterations (e.g., those with fever, pain, acute anxiety, chronic obstructive pulmonary disease, respiratory infection, pulmonary edema or emboli, chest trauma or constriction, brainstem injury)

Equipment

- Watch with a second hand or indicator

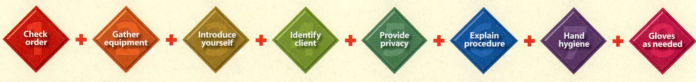

Check order + Gather equipment + Introduce yourself + Identify client + Provide privacy + Explain procedure + Hand hygiene + Gloves as needed

Interventions

1. Determine the client's activity schedule.

- Choose a suitable time to monitor the respirations. *A client who has been exercising will need to rest for a few minutes to permit the accelerated respiratory rate to return to normal. An infant or child who is crying will have an abnormal respiratory rate and will need quieting before respirations can be accurately assessed.*

2. Observe or palpate and count the respiratory rate.

- Place a hand against the client's chest to feel the client's chest movements, or place the client's arm across the chest and observe the chest movements while appearing to take the radial pulse. Because young children are diaphragmatic breathers, observe the rise and fall of the abdomen. *Awareness of respiratory rate assessment could cause the client voluntarily to alter the respiratory pattern.*

■ Count the respiratory rate for 30 seconds and multiply by 2 if the respirations are regular. Count for 60 seconds if they are irregular. An inhalation and an exhalation count as one respiration.

3. Observe the depth, rhythm, and character of respirations.

■ Observe the respirations for depth by watching the movement of the chest. *During deep respirations, a large volume of air is exchanged; during shallow respirations, a small volume is exchanged.*

■ Observe the respirations for regular or irregular rhythm. *Normally, respirations are evenly spaced.*

■ Observe the character of respirations—the sound they produce and the effort they require. *Normally, respirations are silent and effortless.*

4. Document and report pertinent assessment data.

■ Document the respiratory rate, depth, rhythm, and character on the appropriate records.

■ Report:

a. Respiratory rate significantly above or below the normal range and any notable change in respirations from previous assessments

b. Irregular respiratory rhythm

c. Inadequate respiratory depth

d. Abnormal character of breathing—orthopnea, wheezing, stridor, or bubbling

e. Any complaints of dyspnea.

SAMPLE DOCUMENTATION

[date]	Client c/o difficulty breathing. R 26.
[time]	Wheezing noted. Encouraged huff coughing. Expelled thick yellow sputum.
R 20.	Resting in semi-Fowler.
	_____ Erin McClellan, LVN

PROCEDURE 20-4 | **Assessing Blood Pressure**

Purposes

■ To obtain a baseline measure of arterial blood pressure for subsequent evaluation

■ To determine the client's hemodynamic status (e.g., stroke volume of the heart and blood vessel resistance)

■ To identify and monitor changes in blood pressure resulting from a disease process and medical therapy (e.g., presence or history of cardiovascular disease, renal disease, circulatory shock, or acute pain; rapid infusion of fluids or blood products)

Equipment

■ Stethoscope or DUS

■ Blood pressure cuff of the appropriate size (newborn, infant, child, small adult, adult, large adult, thigh)

■ Sphygmomanometer

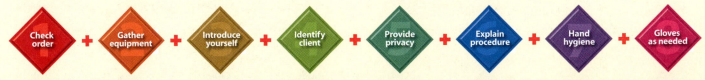

Check order + Gather equipment + Introduce yourself + Identify client + Provide privacy + Explain procedure + Hand hygiene + Gloves as needed

Interventions

1. Prepare and position the client appropriately.

■ Make sure that the client has not smoked or ingested caffeine within 30 minutes prior to measurement. *Nicotine and caffeine can elevate BP.*

■ Make sure that the bladder of the cuff encircles at least two-thirds of the arm and that the width of the cuff is appropriate (see Figure 20-17). *Inappropriate size can result in altered readings.*

■ Position the client in a sitting position unless otherwise specified. The elbow should be slightly flexed with the palm of the hand facing up and the forearm supported at heart level. *Readings in any other position should be specified. The blood pressure is normally similar in sitting, standing, and lying positions, but it can vary significantly by position in certain people. The blood pressure increases when the arm is below heart level and decreases when the arm is above heart level.*

■ Expose the upper arm.

2. Wrap the deflated cuff evenly around the upper arm.

■ Locate the brachial artery (Figure 20-26 ■).

■ Apply the center of the bladder directly over the artery. *The bladder inside the cuff must be directly over the artery to be compressed if the reading is to be accurate.*

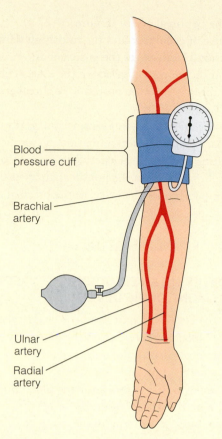

Figure 20-26. ■ Location of the brachial artery and application of the cuff.

■ For an adult, place the lower border of the cuff approximately 2.5 cm (1 in.) above the antecubital space. The lower edge can be closer to the antecubital space of an infant.

■ If this is the client's initial examination, perform a preliminary palpatory determination of systolic pressure. *The initial estimate tells the nurse the maximal pressure to which the manometer needs to be elevated in subsequent determinations. It also prevents underestimation of the systolic pressure or overestimation of the diastolic pressure should an auscultatory gap occur.*

■ Palpate the brachial artery with the fingertips.

■ Close the valve on the pump by turning the knob clockwise.

■ Pump up the cuff until you no longer feel the brachial pulse. *At that pressure the blood cannot flow through the artery.*

■ Note the pressure on the sphygmomanometer at which the pulse is no longer felt. *This gives an estimate of the maximum pressure required to measure the systolic pressure.*

■ Release the pressure completely in the cuff, and wait 1 to 2 minutes before making further measurements. *A waiting period gives the blood trapped in the veins time to be released.*

3. Position the stethoscope appropriately.

■ Clean the earpieces with alcohol or recommended disinfectant. *Infection control measures are necessary unless a nurse is using a personal stethoscope.*

■ Insert the ear attachments of the stethoscope in your ears so that they tilt slightly forward. *Sounds are heard more clearly when the ear attachments follow the direction of the ear canal.*

■ Ensure that the stethoscope hangs freely from the ears to the diaphragm. *Rubbing the stethoscope against an object can obliterate the sounds of the blood within an artery.*

■ Place the bell side of the stethoscope (see Figure 20-23) over the brachial pulse. *Because the blood pressure is a low-frequency sound, it is best heard with the bell-shaped diaphragm* (Bates, 1995, p. 278). Hold the diaphragm with the thumb and index finger.

4. Auscultate the client's blood pressure.

■ Pump up the cuff until the sphygmomanometer registers about 30 mm Hg above the point where the brachial pulse disappeared.

■ Release the valve on the cuff carefully so that the pressure decreases at the rate of 2 to 3 mm Hg per second. *If the rate is faster or slower an error may occur.*

■ As the pressure falls, identify the manometer reading at each of the five phases.

■ Deflate the cuff rapidly and completely.

■ Wait 1 to 2 minutes before making further determinations. *This permits blood trapped in the veins to be released.*

■ Repeat the preceding steps once or twice as necessary to confirm the accuracy of the reading.

5. Remove the cuff.

■ Wipe the cuff with an approved disinfectant. *Cuffs can become significantly contaminated.*

■ If this is the client's initial examination, repeat the procedure on the client's other arm.

■ There should be a difference of no more than 5 to 10 mm Hg between the arms.

■ The arm found to have the higher pressure should be used for subsequent examinations.

6. Document and report pertinent assessment data.

■ Document the blood pressure according to agency policy. Record two pressures in the form "130/80" where "130" is the systolic (phase 1) and "80" is the diastolic (phase 5) pressure. Record three pressures in the form "130/110/90," where "130" is the systolic, "110" is the first diastolic (phase 4), and "90" is the second diastolic (phase 5) pressure. Use the abbreviations RA for right arm and LA for left arm. Record a difference of greater than 10 mm Hg in the arms.

■ Report any significant change in the client's blood pressure. Also report these findings:
   a. Systolic blood pressure (of an adult) above 140 mm Hg
   b. Diastolic blood pressure (of an adult) above 90 mm Hg
   c. Systolic blood pressure (of an adult) below 100 mm Hg

VARIATION: TAKING A THIGH BLOOD PRESSURE

■ Help the client to assume a prone position. If the client cannot assume this position, measure the blood pressure

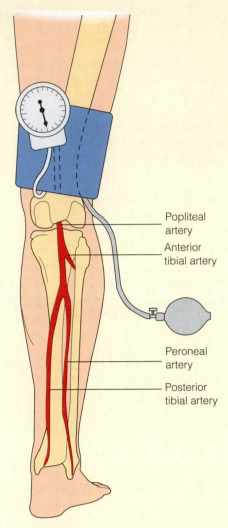

Figure 20-27. ■ Location of the popliteal artery and application of the cuff.

while the client is in a supine position with the knee slightly flexed. *Slight flexing of the knee will facilitate placing the stethoscope on the popliteal space.*

■ Expose the thigh, taking care not to expose the client unduly.

■ Locate the popliteal artery (Figure 20-27 ■).
■ Wrap the cuff evenly around the midthigh with the compression bladder over the posterior aspect of the thigh and the bottom edge above the knee. The bladder must be directly over the posterior popliteal artery if the reading is to be accurate.
■ If this is the client's initial examination, perform a preliminary palpatory determination of systolic pressure by palpating the popliteal artery (see Figure 20-24E). The systolic pressure in the popliteal artery is usually 20 to 30 mm Hg higher than that in the brachial artery because of use of a larger bladder; the diastolic pressure is usually the same.
■ Auscultate the pressure as for the arm.

VARIATION: USING AN ELECTRONIC INDIRECT BLOOD PRESSURE MONITORING DEVICE

■ Unplug the electronic unit from the electrical outlet.
■ Place the blood pressure cuff on the extremity according to the manufacturer's guidelines.
■ Turn on the blood pressure switch.
■ When the device has determined the blood pressure reading, note the digital results.
■ Record the blood pressure according to agency policy.

SAMPLE DOCUMENTATION

[date]	T 38 rectal, P 95, R 22, BP 145/95.
[time]	Client confused, not oriented to time and place. Team leader notified.
	_____ J. Lopez, LPN

Chapter Review

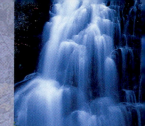

 ## KEY TERMS by Topic

Use the audio glossary feature of either the CD-ROM or the Companion Website to hear the correct pronunciation of the following key terms.

Body Temperature
body temperature, basal metabolic rate (BMR), pyrexia, hyperthermia, afebrile, crisis, hypothermia

Pulse
pulse, peripheral pulse, apical pulse, pulse deficit

Respirations
respiration, external respiration, internal respiration

Blood Pressure
blood pressure, systolic pressure, diastolic pressure, cardiac output, viscosity, orthostatic hypotension

KEY Points

- Vital signs reflect changes in body function that otherwise might not be observed.

- Various sites and methods can be used to assess vital signs. The nurse selects the site and method that is safe for the client and that will provide the most accurate measurement possible.

- The most accurate values are obtained when the client is at rest and comfortable.

- Changes in one vital sign can trigger changes in other vital signs.

- Vital signs are assessed when a client is admitted to a healthcare agency to establish baseline data and when there is a change or possibility of a change in the client's condition.

- Data obtained from measurements of vital signs are used to plan and implement appropriate nursing interventions and to evaluate a client's response to these interventions or prescribed medical therapy.

- Body temperature is the balance between heat produced by the body and heat lost from the body.

- Knowledge of factors affecting heat production and heat loss helps the nurse to implement appropriate interventions when the client has a fever or hypothermia.

- Factors affecting body temperature include age, diurnal variations, exercise, hormones, stress, and environmental temperatures.

- Pyrexia (fever) is a common sign of disease. Four common types of fever are intermittent, remittent, relapsing, and constant. Clinical signs of fever vary during the onset, course, and abatement stages.

- Hypothermia involves three mechanisms: excessive heat loss, inadequate heat production by body cells, and increasing impairment of hypothalamic temperature regulation.

- Body temperature can be measured orally, tympanically, rectally, or by axilla. The nurse selects the most appropriate site according to the client's age and condition.

- Normally a peripheral pulse reflects the client's heartbeat, but it may differ from the heartbeat in clients with certain cardiovascular diseases; in these instances, the nurse takes an apical pulse and compares it to the peripheral pulse.

- Many factors affect a person's pulse rate: age, sex, exercise, presence of fever, certain medications, hemorrhage, stress, and (in some situations) position changes.

- Respirations are normally quiet, effortless, and automatic and are assessed by observing respiratory rate, depth, rhythm, and sound.

- Blood pressure reflects cardiac output, peripheral vascular resistance, blood volume, and blood viscosity. Peripheral vascular resistance varies according to the size of the arterioles and capillaries, and the elasticity of the arteries.

 ## EXPLORE MediaLink

Additional interactive resources for this chapter can be found on the Companion Website at www.prenhall.com/ramont. Click on Chapter 20 and "Begin" to select the activities for this chapter.

For chapter-related NCLEX®-style questions and an audio glossary, access the accompanying CD-ROM in this book.

FOR FURTHER Study

See Figure 6-5 for documenting vitals signs on a graphic flow sheet.

See Chapter 21 for an in-depth discussion of pain.

See Chapter 24 for more information about regulation of breathing and about pulse oximetry.

Critical Thinking Care Map

Caring for a Client after a Heart Attack
NCLEX–PN® Focus Area: Physiological Adaptation

Case Study: Edgar Wilson, a 50-year-old African American, was brought to the ED after chest pain of 1 hour's duration. He was admitted to rule out myocardial infarction (MI). The pain radiating to his back and down his left arm is 9/10. After receiving morphine sulfate 4 mg IV × 3, his pain is now 5/10. He has a history of hypertension (treated with Verapamil) and a family history of cardiovascular disease. His father died of a heart attack at 56. His mother had a disabling stroke at age 60.

Vital signs: BP 158/90, P 100, R 24, T 99.8 oral. Height 5'10", weight 295 lbs. Cardiac monitoring showed sinus tachycardia with occasional PVC. Twelve-lead ECG and cardiac enzymes obtained in ED.

Mr. Wilson was in a MVC 1 week ago in which he sustained a head injury. He lives with his wife; a son lives nearby. He is a history teacher at a local community college. Mr. Wilson states, "I probably won't live to an old age. I have bad genes for heart attack and stroke."

Nursing Diagnosis: Health-Seeking Behaviors Related to Lack of Knowledge

---

COLLECT DATA

Subjective	Objective
_____	_____
_____	_____
_____	_____
_____	_____
_____	_____
_____	_____

Would you report this data? Yes/No

If yes, to: _____

What would you report? _____

Nursing Care

_____
_____
_____
_____
_____
_____
_____

How would you document this?_____
_____
_____

Compare your documentation to the sample provided in Appendix I.

Data Collected
(use those that apply)

- 50-year-old African American male
- Chest pain, radiating to back and left arm 9/10. Morphine sulfate 4 mg IV × 3; pain now 5/10
- Verapamil ED. 180 mg bid for hypertension
- Father died of a heart attack age 56
- Mother stroke at 60; now 69, disabled
- VS: T 99.8 BP 158/90, P 100, R 24
- Height 5'10", weight 295 lbs
- Diet: "I normally eat fast food for lunch. My wife does make healthy dinners."
- Sinus tachycardia with occasional PVC
- 12-lead ECG and cardiac enzymes obtained in ED (no report)
- MVC 1 week ago sustained a head injury
- Lives with wife; one son nearby
- History teacher at local college
- "I probably won't live to an old age. I have bad genes for heart attack and stroke."

Nursing Interventions
(use those that apply; list in priority order)

- Assess client's feelings, values, and reasons for not following prescribed plan of care.
- Discuss client's beliefs about health and his ability to maintain health.
- Identify barriers and benefits to being healthy.
- Help client to choose healthy lifestyle and to have appropriate diagnostic tests.
- Compare client's height and weight to standards for age and height.
- Encourage client to eat a diet with fresh foods, low saturated fat, and no added salt.
- Teach stress-relieving techniques.
- Assess for the influences of culture and values on the client's beliefs about health.
- Identify support groups related to the disease process.

NCLEX-PN® Exam Preparation

1 You are assigned to take morning vital signs on several clients on a medical surgical unit. Of the following vital signs, which would you report immediately to the RN?

1. 99.6 (R), 86, 24, 140/88
2. 97.2 (O), 110, 18, 110/78
3. 101.8 (A), 72, 18, 90/60
4. 98 (O), 100, 26, 148/80

2 Your assigned client has a history of mastectomy of right breast, 1 year ago. She has been admitted with a fracture of her left humerus. You need to assess her blood pressure. Using your knowledge of her condition and your critical thinking skills, what method would you use to assess the blood pressure?

1. Apply the cuff to her right arm, being careful not to pump it up above 150 mm.
2. Obtain a large cuff and assess her blood pressure using her thigh.
3. Place the cuff below her left elbow and palpate her radial pulse.
4. Take her other vital signs and chart that you were unable to assess the blood pressure.

3 It is important to use the appropriate size of cuff when assessing blood pressure. When a cuff that is too narrow is used, you expect the result to be a blood pressure that is an:

1. erroneously high reading.
2. erroneously low reading.
3. erroneously low diastolic reading.
4. erroneously high systolic.

4 Phase 5 of Korotkoff's sounds is considered to be:

1. the systolic blood pressure.
2. the diastolic blood pressure in an adult.
3. the diastolic blood pressure in a child.
4. the period of silence at the end of the blood pressure.

5 Your primary nurse tells you that your client needs to have Tylenol administered for a fever. The temperature is recorded as 38.6°C. The physician has written an order for Tylenol for a temperature above 101°F. You will need to convert the temperature to Fahrenheit in order to determine if the client should be medicated. Of the following readings, which is closest to 38.6°C?

1. 100.6
2. 104
3. 103.2
4. 101.5

6 You are assigned to admit clients in the pediatric urgent care unit. Using your knowledge of the cardiovascular system, which of the peripheral pulse sites would you normally select for a 30-month-old child?

1. radial
2. carotid
3. brachial
4. apical

7 Your neighbor asks you what is the normal blood pressure for her 6-year-old child. Which of the following would be the most appropriate answer?

1. systolic blood pressure of 92
2. 100/70
3. diastolic blood pressure of 80
4. 72/40

8 Standing, sitting, and lying blood pressures are taken to assess for:

1. orthostatic hypotension.
2. orthostatic hypertension.
3. pulse deficit.
4. auscultatory gap.

9 Your client has a physician's order for digoxin. Prior to administering the medication the nurse should:

1. assess the blood pressure and give medication if systolic pressure is greater than 140.
2. assess the radial pulse and hold if it is greater than 100.
3. assess the apical pulse and hold if less than 60.
4. assess the apical pulse and give if less than 60.

10 Your client is being discharged home. The physician has ordered MS Contin for pain control. Of the following discharge instructions, which one should be considered when administering morphine?

1. take blood pressure prior to administration.
2. take blood pressure 20 minutes after administration.
3. assess respirations following administration.
4. assess apical pulse prior to administration.

Answers and Rationales for Review Questions, as well as discussion of Care Plan and Critical Thinking Care Map questions, appear in Appendix I.

Chapter 21

Pain: The Fifth Vital Sign

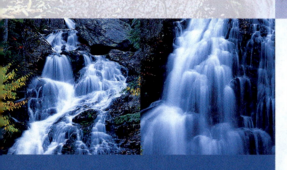

BRIEF Outline

Types of Pain
Concepts Associated with Pain
Physiology of Pain
Key Factors in Pain Management
Barriers to Pain Management

HISTORICAL Perspectives

In the 20th century, beginning with the International Congress of 1912, many of the world's nations placed severe restrictions on the use of opium and its derivatives; these sanctions failed to end narcotic smuggling and abuse but contributed to the demonization of these drugs. By the 1950s, fears of addiction led many physicians and nurses to limit opioid use despite its great value in relieving the suffering of patients in severe and chronic pain.

LEARNING Outcomes

After completing this chapter, you will be able to:

1. Identify types and categories of pain according to location, etiology, and duration.
2. Differentiate pain threshold from pain tolerance.
3. Describe pain transmission, perception, interpretation, and modulation.
4. Describe the gate control theory and its application to nursing care.
5. Describe pharmacologic interventions for pain.
6. Describe the World Health Organization's three-step ladder approach to cancer pain.
7. Identify rationales for using various analgesic delivery routes.
8. Describe nonpharmacologic pain control interventions.
9. Identify barriers to effective pain management.
10. Define tolerance, dependence, and addiction.
11. Identify subjective and objective data to collect and analyze when assessing pain.
12. Identify examples of nursing diagnoses for clients with pain.
13. State outcome criteria by which to evaluate a client's response to interventions for pain.

Pain is a highly unpleasant and very personal sensation. Pain can consume a person's thoughts and take over daily activities. Yet pain is a difficult concept for a client to communicate. A nurse can neither feel nor see a client's pain.

No two people experience pain in exactly the same way. Because of the differences in how individuals perceive and react to pain, as well as the many causes of pain, the nurse is faced with a complex situation when developing a plan to relieve pain and provide comfort. Effective pain management is an important aspect of care.

As we have learned more about pain, we have seen a shift in focus toward pain control and pain management independent of the cause of the pain. Severe pain is now being viewed as an emergency situation deserving anticipation and prompt treatment. Pain is more than a symptom of a problem; it is a high-priority problem in itself. Pain presents both physiological and psychological dangers to health and recovery. Pain increases morbidity and mortality. Unresolved pain has been shown to prolong hospital stays, delay the healing process, and contribute to depression.

Types of Pain

Although pain is a universal experience, its exact nature remains a mystery. There are a number of definitions of pain. **Pain** is sensation that is highly subjective and individual; it is one of the body's defense mechanisms indicating that a problem exists.

McCaffery (1979, p. 11) defines pain as "whatever the experiencing person says it is, existing whenever he (or she) says it does." The most vital part of this definition is the care provider's willingness to believe that the client is experiencing pain and that the client is the real authority about that pain.

Pain may be described in terms of its duration, location, or etiology. When pain lasts only through the expected recovery period, it is described as **acute pain**, whether it has a sudden or slow onset and regardless of the intensity. **Chronic pain** lasts beyond the typical healing time period. Pain is generally labeled chronic after 3 to 6 months. Chronic pain can be further classified as chronic malignant pain, when associated with cancer or other life-threatening conditions, or as chronic nonmalignant pain when the etiology is a nonprogressive disorder, such as damage from trauma. Chronic pain that persists despite therapeutic interventions is classified as **intractable pain**. Acute and chronic pain result in different physiological and behavioral responses, shown in Table 21-1 ■.

Pain can be categorized according to its origin as cutaneous, deep somatic, or visceral. **Cutaneous pain** originates in the skin or subcutaneous tissue. A paper cut causing a sharp pain with some burning is an example of cutaneous pain. **Somatic pain** arises from ligaments, tendons, bones, blood vessels, and nerves. It is diffuse and tends to last longer than cutaneous pain. An ankle sprain is an example of deep somatic pain. **Visceral pain** results from stimulation of pain receptors in the abdominal cavity, cranium, and thorax. Visceral pain tends to appear diffuse and often feels like deep somatic pain, that is, burning, aching, or creating a feeling of pressure. Visceral pain is frequently caused by stretching of the tissues, ischemia, or muscle spasms. For example, an obstructed bowel will result in visceral pain.

TABLE 21-1	
Comparison of Acute and Chronic Pain	
ACUTE PAIN	**CHRONIC PAIN**
Mild to severe	Mild to severe

Sympathetic nervous system responses:
    Increased pulse rate
    Increased respiratory rate
    Elevated blood pressure
    Diaphoresis
    Dilated pupils
	Parasympathetic nervous system responses:
	    Vital signs normal
	    Dry, warm skin
	    Pupils normal or dilated

Related to tissue injury; resolves with healing.	Continues beyond healing.
Client appears restless and anxious.	Client appears depressed and withdrawn.
Client reports pain.	Client often does not mention pain unless asked.
Client exhibits behavior indicative of pain: crying, rubbing area, holding area.	Pain behavior often absent.

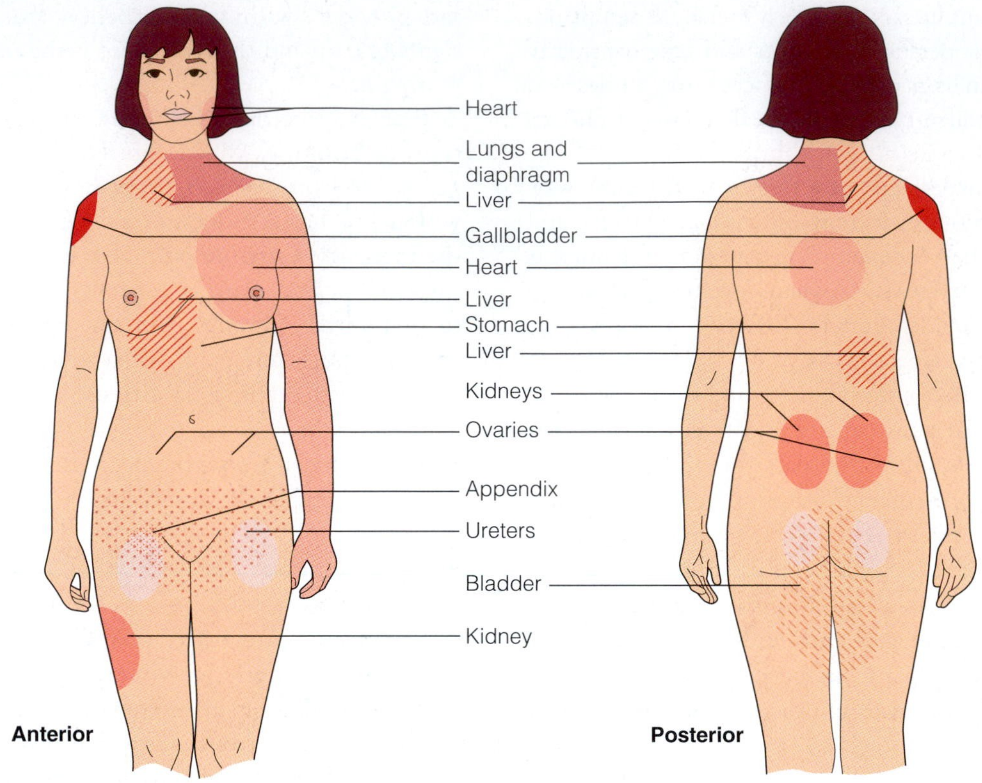
Heart
Lungs and diaphragm
Liver
Gallbladder
Heart
Liver
Stomach
Liver
Kidneys
Ovaries
Appendix
Ureters
Bladder
Kidney
Anterior
Posterior

Figure 21-1. ■ Common sites of referred pain from various body organs.

Pain may also be described according to where it is experienced in the body. **Radiating pain** is perceived at the source of the pain and extends to nearby tissues. For example, cardiac pain may be felt not only in the chest but also along the left shoulder and down the arm. **Referred pain** is pain felt in a part of the body that is considerably removed from the tissues causing the pain. The pain is felt along the nerve pathways for the tissue of origin. For example, pain from one part of the abdominal viscera may be perceived in an area of the skin remote from the organ causing the pain (Figure 21-1 ■).

Intractable pain is pain that is highly resistant to relief. One example is the pain from an advanced malignancy. Often, nurses are challenged to use a number of methods, such as imagery and patient-controlled analgesia (PCA), to provide a client with pain relief.

Neuropathic pain is the result of a disturbance of the nerve pathways either from past or continuing tissue damage that results in pain. Neuropathic pain is described as shooting or stabbing and is often severe. Clients with conditions such as AIDS and diabetes often suffer from neuropathic pain.

Phantom pain, which is a painful sensation perceived in a body part that is missing (e.g., an amputated leg) or paralyzed by a spinal cord injury, is also an example of neuropathic pain. This can be distinguished from phantom sensation, that is, the feeling that the missing body part is still present.

Concepts Associated with Pain

When an individual perceives pain from injured tissue, the pain threshold is reached. An individual's **pain threshold** is the amount of pain stimulation a person requires in order to feel pain. People's pain threshold is generally fairly uniform; however, it can change. For example, the same stimuli that once produced mild pain can at another time produce intense pain.

Two additional terms used in the context of pain are pain reaction and tolerance. **Pain reaction** includes the autonomic nervous system and behavioral responses to pain. The *autonomic nervous system response* is the automatic reaction of the body that often protects the individual from further harm, such as the automatic withdrawal of the hand from a hot stove. The *behavioral response* is a learned response used as a method of coping with the pain. Behavioral responses can be related to the anticipation of pain, the sensation of pain, or the aftermath of pain. For example, explaining to a client what he or she will feel prior to administering an injection may reduce the behavioral reaction to the injection.

Pain tolerance is the maximum amount and duration of pain that an individual is willing to endure. Some clients are unable to tolerate even the slightest pain, whereas others are willing to endure severe pain rather than be treated for it. Thus, pain tolerance varies greatly among people and is widely influenced by psychological and sociocultural factors. Pain tolerance may increase with age.

Physiology of Pain

How pain is transmitted and perceived is still incompletely understood. Whether pain is perceived and to what degree depend on the interaction between the body's analgesia system and the nervous system's transmission and interpretation of stimuli.

TRANSMISSION AND PERCEPTION

The peripheral nervous system includes primary sensory neurons specialized to detect tissue damage and to evoke the sensation of touch, heat, cold, pain, and pressure. **Nociceptor** is related to a pain receptor, whereas proprioceptor is a response to stimuli within the body of pressure, position, or stretch, including pacinian corpuscles which includes sensory nerve endings. (Figure 21-2 ■). These pain receptors or nociceptors can be excited by mechanical, thermal, or chemical stimuli (Table 21-2 ■). When there are sufficient noxious stimuli, biochemical mediators are released that sensitize or activate the nociceptors. These chemicals cause the cardinal signs and symptoms we see when tissue damage has occurred. The release of inflammatory chemicals causes vasodilation (redness) and increased capillary permeability (swelling); it also contributes to the conduction of nociception. (See also Chapter 23 ∞.)

Pain impulses are transmitted via two types of fibers. The A-delta (large-diameter) fibers are *myelinated* (they con-

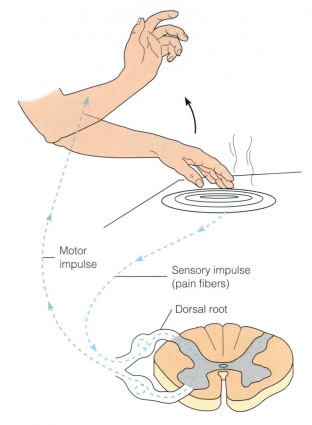

Figure 21-2. ■ Proprioceptive reflex to a pain stimulus.

Motor impulse

Sensory impulse (pain fibers)

Dorsal root

duct electrical impulses rapidly). These fibers are associated with the sensation of sharp, pricking pain. The C fibers (small-diameter, unmyelinated fibers) transmit the impulse more slowly and mediate long-lasting, burning pain. The fast A fibers primarily conduct impulses from mechanical and thermal pain. The slow, type C fibers conduct impulses from mechanical, thermal, and chemical stimuli.

TABLE 21-2	
Types of Pain Stimuli	
STIMULUS TYPE	**PHYSIOLOGICAL BASIS OF PAIN**
Mechanical	
1. Trauma to body tissues (e.g., surgery)	Tissue damage; direct irritation of the pain receptors; inflammation
2. Alterations in body tissues (e.g., edema)	Pressure on pain receptors
3. Blockage of a body duct	Distention of the lumen of the duct
4. Tumor	Pressure on pain receptors; irritation of nerve endings
5. Muscle spasm	Stimulation of pain receptors (also see chemical stimuli)
Thermal	
Extreme heat or cold (e.g., burns)	Tissue destruction; stimulation of thermosensitive pain receptors
Chemical	
1. Tissue ischemia (e.g., blocked coronary artery)	Stimulation of pain receptors because of accumulated lactic acid (and other chemicals, such as bradykinin and enzymes) in tissues
2. Muscle spasm	Tissue ischemia secondary to mechanical stimulation (see above)

As pain impulses stimulate the brain, nerve fibers conduct impulses from the brain to the spinal cord, where the pain impulses are inhibited in the spinal cord by the release of endogenous opioids. The three classes of **endogenous opioids** are enkephalins, dynorphins, and beta endorphins. These substances bind to opiate receptor sites in the central and peripheral nervous system, decreasing or blocking any pain impulse. The opiate binding sites are the same sites where **exogenous opioid analgesics** (e.g., morphine) bind to provide pain relief.

GATE CONTROL THEORY

In 1965, Melzack and Wall proposed the **gate control theory**. According to this theory, peripheral nerve fibers carrying pain to the spinal cord can have their message modified at the spinal cord level before transmission to the brain. Synapses in the spinal cord act as gates that close to keep messages from reaching the brain or open to permit messages to ascend to the brain.

According to the gate control theory, small-diameter nerve fibers carry pain stimuli through a gate, but large-diameter nerve fibers going through the same gate can inhibit the transmission of those pain messages—that is, close the gate (Figure 21-3 ■). Because a limited amount of sensory information can reach the brain at any given time, certain cells can interrupt the pain messages. The brain also appears to influence whether the gate is open or closed. For example, previous experiences with pain are known to affect how an individual responds to pain. The involvement of the brain helps explain why painful stimuli are interpreted differently by people. Although the gate control theory is not unanimously

accepted, it does help explain why electrical and mechanical interventions as well as heat and pressure can relieve pain. The gate control theory, simply put, suggests that a nerve pathway can only carry a few messages at a time. To inhibit the pain message, we must send another message on the nerve pathway for the brain to interpret. For example, a back massage may stimulate impulses in large nerves, which in turn close the gate to back pain allowing only the message of tactile stimulation to reach the brain, not the message of pain.

RESPONSES TO PAIN

The body's response to pain is a complex process rather than a specific action. It involves physiological and psychosocial aspects. Initially the sympathetic nervous system responds, resulting in the fight-or-flight response. As pain continues, the body adapts; the parasympathetic nervous system takes over, reversing many of the initial physiological responses. This adaptation to the pain occurs after several hours or days of pain. The actual pain receptors adapt very little and continue to transmit the pain message. This serves the purpose of keeping the person continually aware of the damaging stimuli causing the pain (Guyton & Hall, 2000). The person may learn to cope with the pain through cognitive and behavioral activities, such as diversions, imagery, and excessive sleeping. The individual may respond to pain by seeking out physical interventions to manage the pain, such as analgesics, massage, and exercise.

FACTORS AFFECTING THE PAIN EXPERIENCE

Numerous factors can affect a person's perception of and reaction to pain. These include the person's ethnic and cultural values, developmental stage, environment and support people, previous pain experiences, and the meaning of the current pain, as well as anxiety and stress (Box 21-1 ■).

COLLABORATIVE CARE

Pharmacologic Management

Pharmacologic pain management involves the use of opioids (narcotics), nonopioids or nonsteroidal anti-inflammatory drugs (NSAIDs), and adjuvants, or coanalgesic drugs.

WHO THREE-STEP LADDER APPROACH. The World Health Organization (WHO) recommends a sequential or three-step ladder approach to manage cancer pain (Figure 21-4 ■). This approach may also apply to pain resulting from causes other than cancer. Therapy begins with a nonopioid/NSAID (step 1). If the client receives the maximum recommended dose of nonopioids and continues to experience pain, a weak opioid is given (step 2). The dose of the weak opioid is increased until the ceiling dose is reached. If the client continues to experience pain, a stronger opioid is given (step 3). Adjuvant drugs may also be given at any stage of therapy.

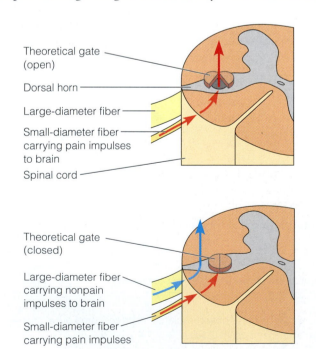

Figure 21-3. ■ A schematic illustration of the gate control theory.

Theoretical gate (open)
Dorsal horn
Large-diameter fiber
Small-diameter fiber carrying pain impulses to brain
Spinal cord

Theoretical gate (closed)
Large-diameter fiber carrying nonpain impulses to brain
Small-diameter fiber carrying pain impulses

BOX 21-1

Factors Affecting the Pain Experience

Ethnic and Cultural Values

- Ethnic background and cultural heritage. Behavior related to pain is a part of the socialization process.
- There appears to be little variation in pain threshold, but cultural background can affect the level of pain that an individual is willing to tolerate. In some Middle Eastern and African cultures, self-infliction of pain is a sign of mourning or grief. In other groups, pain may be anticipated as part of the ritualistic practices, and therefore tolerance of pain signifies strength and endurance. Additionally, studies have shown that individuals of northern European descent tend to be more stoic and less expressive of their pain than people from southern European backgrounds.

Developmental Stage

- Behavioral observation is recommended for pain assessment in infants since physiological responses vary greatly.
- Children are less able to articulate their experience or needs related to pain; therefore, their pain is often undertreated.
- The prevalence of pain in the older population is generally higher due to both acute and chronic disease conditions.
- Pain threshold does not appear to change with aging, although the effect of analgesics may increase due to physiological changes related to drug metabolism.

Environment and Support People

- A strange environment such as a hospital, with its noises, lights, and activity, can compound pain.
- A person who is without a support network may perceive pain as severe, whereas the person who has supportive people around may perceive less pain.
- Some people prefer to withdraw when they are in pain, whereas others prefer the distraction of people and activity around them.
- Family caregivers can be a significant support for a person in pain. With the increase in outpatient and home care, families are assuming an increased responsibility for the management of pain.
- Education related to the assessment and management of pain can positively affect the perceived quality of life for both clients and their caregivers.
- Expectations of significant others can affect a person's perceptions of and responses to pain (e.g., girls may be permitted to express pain more openly than boys).
- Family role can also affect how a person perceives or responds to pain (e.g., a single mother supporting three children may ignore pain because of her need to stay on the job).

- The presence of support people often changes a client's reaction to pain (e.g., toddlers often tolerate pain more readily when supportive parents or nurses are nearby).

Past Pain Experiences

- Previous pain experiences alter a client's sensitivity to pain. People who have personally experienced pain or who have been exposed to the suffering of someone close are often more threatened by anticipated pain than people without a pain experience.
- The success or lack of success of pain relief measures influences a person's expectations for relief (e.g., a person who has tried several pain relief measures without success may have little hope about the helpfulness of nursing interventions).

Meaning of Pain

- Some clients may accept pain more readily than others, depending on the circumstances and the client's interpretation of its significance.
- A client who associates the pain with a positive outcome may withstand the pain amazingly well (e.g., a woman giving birth to a child or an athlete undergoing knee surgery to prolong his career may tolerate pain better because of the benefit associated with it).
- Clients with unrelenting chronic pain may suffer more intensely. They may respond with despair, anxiety, and depression because they cannot attach a positive significance or purpose to the pain. In this situation, the pain may be looked upon as a threat to body image or lifestyle and as a sign of possible impending death.

Anxiety and Stress

- Anxiety often accompanies pain. Threat of the unknown and the inability to control the pain or the events surrounding it often augment the pain perception. See Chapter 16 ⚭ for more on effects of stress.
- Fatigue also reduces a person's ability to cope, thereby increasing pain perception. When pain interferes with sleep, fatigue and muscle tension often result and increase the pain; thus, a cycle of pain, fatigue, pain develops.
- People in pain who believe that they have control of their pain have decreased fear and anxiety, which decreases their pain perception.
- A perception of lacking control or a sense of helplessness tends to increase pain perception.
- The expression of pain to an attentive listener and the participation in pain management decisions can increase the sense of control.

OPIOID ANALGESICS. Opioid (narcotic) analgesics include opium derivatives, such as morphine and codeine. Narcotics relieve pain and provide a sense of euphoria largely by binding to opiate receptors and activating endogenous pain suppression in the central nervous system.

When administering any analgesic, the nurse must review side effects. All opioids result in some initial drowsiness when first administered, but with regular administration, this side effect tends to decrease. Opioids also may cause nausea, vomiting, constipation, and respiratory depression. The

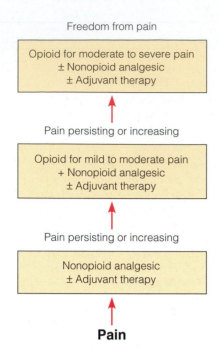

Freedom from pain

Opioid for moderate to severe pain
± Nonopioid analgesic
± Adjuvant therapy

Pain persisting or increasing

Opioid for mild to moderate pain
+ Nonopioid analgesic
± Adjuvant therapy

Pain persisting or increasing

Nonopioid analgesic
± Adjuvant therapy

Pain

Figure 21-4. ■ The WHO three-step analgesic ladder. (*Source:* World Health Organization.)

most common and most troubling side effect of opioids is constipation. If a client requires long-term opioid therapy, a laxative should be prescribed along with the opioid.

clinical ALERT

Before administering narcotics, the nurse needs to assess a client's level of alertness and respiratory rate for baseline data. An increased sedation level can be an early warning sign of impending respiratory depression.

Opioids must be used cautiously in clients with respiratory problems. If the client experiences significant respiratory depression (e.g., a drop from 18 to 12) or is overly sedated, the dosage is excessive. See the sedation rating scale in Box 21-2 ■. Often clients will manifest an increase in sedation be-

BOX 21-2

Sedation Rating Scale

S = sleeping, easily aroused; requires no action

1 = awake and alert; requires no action

2 = occasionally drowsy, easy to arouse; requires no action

3 = frequently drowsy, arousable, drifts off to sleep during conversation; decrease the opioid dose

4 = somnolent, minimal or no response to stimuli; discontinue opioid and consider use of naloxone (Narcan)

Source: McCaffery, M., & Pasero, C. (1999). *Pain clinical manual,* p. 267. St. Louis, MO: Mosby. Reprinted by permission.

fore they manifest a decrease in respiratory rate and depth. The nurse should assess and document the client's level of sedation at the same time that respiratory status is checked. Early recognition of an increasing level of sedation or respiratory depression will enable the nurse to implement appropriate measures promptly (e.g., obtaining an order to decrease the opioid dosage). Healthcare providers should never allow the fear of respiratory depression to inhibit adequate pain control. Box 21-3 ■ provides common side effects of, and preventive measures for, opioid analgesics.

BOX 21-3

Common Opioid Side Effects and Preventive Measures

Constipation

■ Increase fluid intake (e.g., to 8 glasses daily).

■ Increase fiber and bulk-forming agents in the diet (e.g., fresh fruits and vegetables).

■ Increase exercise regimen.

■ Administer stool softeners and provide a mild laxative if necessary.

Nausea and Vomiting

■ Inform client that tolerance to this emetic effect generally develops after several days of opiate therapy.

■ Provide an antiemetic as required.

■ Change the analgesic as indicated.

Sedation

■ Inform client that tolerance usually develops over 3 to 5 days.

■ Administer a stimulant, such as dextroamphetamine sulfate (Dexedrine) or methylphenidate hydrochloride (Ritalin) each morning to clients who receive opiate therapy for chronic pain and do not develop tolerance.

Respiratory Depression

■ Administer an opioid antagonist, such as naloxone hydrochloride (Narcan) until respirations return to an acceptable rate. Administer the medication slowly by intravenous route with 10 mL of saline. Monitor the client, and repeat the procedure as required.

■ If the client is receiving intravenous PCA, stop or slow the infusion.

Pruritus

■ Apply cool packs, lotion, and diversional activity.

■ Administer an antihistamine (e.g., diphenhydramine hydrochloride [Benadryl]).

■ Inform the client that tolerance also develops to pruritus.

Urinary Retention

■ May need to catheterize client.

■ Administer narcotic antagonist (naloxone hydrochloride [Narcan]).

Older clients are particularly sensitive to the analgesic properties of opioids and often require less medication than younger clients. This sensitivity may be related to reduced excretion of the drug in elderly clients.

NONOPIOIDS/NSAIDS. Nonopioids (non-narcotic analgesics) include NSAIDs such as aspirin and ibuprofen. These analgesics have anti-inflammatory, analgesic, and antipyretic effects. (Acetaminophen has only analgesic and antipyretic effects.) They relieve pain by acting on peripheral nerve endings at the injury site and decreasing the level of inflammatory mediators generated at the site of injury.

Individual drugs in this category vary widely in their analgesic properties, metabolism, excretion, and side effects. In addition, the analgesic activity of these drugs has a ceiling effect—the level at which increasing the dose results in no further increase in analgesia.

The most common side effect of nonopioid analgesics is indigestion, which can be prevented by taking the medication with antacid or food. Stomach ulcers and gastric bleeding have also been reported. NSAIDs reduce the dose of opioids needed when the drugs are given together and provide better pain relief than use of either type separately. These drugs must be ordered by the physician; they all have a maximum daily dose limit.

Pharmacologic management of mild to moderate pain should begin with NSAIDs, unless there is a specific contraindication (Pinnell, 1996, p. 646). NSAIDs are contraindicated, for example, in clients with impaired blood clotting, gastrointestinal bleeding or ulcer risk, renal disease, thrombocytopenia, and possibly infection (because NSAIDs will obscure fever).

ADJUVANT ANALGESICS. Adjuvant analgesics are medications that were developed for uses other than analgesia but have been found to reduce certain types of chronic pain in addition to their primary action. For example, mild sedatives or tranquilizers, such as diazepam (Valium), may help reduce painful muscle spasms as well as anxiety, stress, and tension so that the client can obtain a good night's sleep. Antidepressants, such as amitriptyline hydrochloride (Elavil), are used to treat underlying depression or mood disorders but may also enhance other pain strategies. Anticonvulsants, such as carbamazepine (Tegretol) and clonazepam (Klonopin), usually prescribed to treat seizures, can be useful in controlling painful neuropathies such as herpes zoster (shingles) and diabetic neuropathies.

Nonpharmacologic Pain Management

Nonpharmacologic pain management consists of a variety of physical and cognitive–behavioral pain management strategies. Physical interventions include cutaneous stimulation, immobilization, transcutaneous electrical nerve stimulation (TENS), and acupuncture. Mind–body (cognitive–behavioral) interventions include distraction activities, relaxation techniques, imagery, meditation, biofeedback, hypnosis, and therapeutic touch. See Box 21-4 ■ for a detailed description of these interventions.

Key Factors in Pain Management

ACKNOWLEDGING AND ACCEPTING

Basic to all strategies for reducing pain is that nurses convey to clients that they believe the client is having pain. Four ways of communicating this belief follow:

1. Verbally acknowledge the presence of the pain: "I understand your leg is very painful. How do you feel about the pain?"
2. Listen attentively to what the client says about the pain.
3. Convey that you are assessing the client's pain to understand it better, not to determine whether the pain is real, for example, "How does your pain feel now?" or "Tell me how it feels compared to an hour ago."
4. Attend to the client's needs promptly.

ASSISTING SUPPORT PERSONS

Support persons often need assistance to respond positively to the client experiencing pain. Enlisting the aid of support persons in the provision of pain relief to the client, such as massaging the client's back, may diminish his or her feelings of helplessness and foster a more positive attitude toward the client's pain experience. Support persons also may need the nurse's verbal recognition of their concern and participation in the client's care.

REDUCING MISCONCEPTIONS ABOUT PAIN

Reducing a client's misconceptions about the pain and its treatment will often avoid intensifying the pain. The nurse should explain to the client that pain is a highly individual experience and that it is only the client who really experiences the pain, although others can understand and empathize. Misconceptions are also dealt with when nurse and client discuss why the pain has increased or decreased at certain times. For example, a client whose pain increases in the evening may mistakenly think this is the result of eating dinner rather than the result of fatigue.

REDUCING FEAR AND ANXIETY

It is important to help relieve the emotional component, that is, anxiety or fear, associated with the pain. When clients have no opportunity to talk about their pain and associated fears, their perceptions and reactions to the pain can be intensified.

MediaLink

Pain Management

BOX 21-4

Nonpharmacologic Pain Interventions

Cutaneous Stimulation

Cutaneous stimulation can provide effective temporary pain relief. It distracts the client and focuses attention on the tactile stimuli, away from the painful sensations, thus reducing pain perception. Cutaneous stimulation can be applied directly to the painful area, proximal to the pain, distal to the pain, and contralateral (opposite side) to the pain. Cutaneous stimulation techniques include the following:

Massage

Massage is a comfort measure that can aid relaxation, decrease muscle tension, and may ease anxiety. Massage can also decrease pain intensity by increasing superficial circulation to the area. Massage can involve the back and neck, hands and arms, or feet. The use of ointments or liniments may provide localized pain relief with joint or muscle pain.

Heat and Cold Applications

A warm bath, heating pads, ice bags, ice massage, hot or cold compresses, and warm or cold sitz baths in general relieve pain and promote healing of injured tissues.

Acupressure

Acupressure developed from the ancient Chinese healing system of acupuncture. The therapist applies finger pressure to points that correspond to many of the points used in acupuncture.

Contralateral Stimulation

Contralateral stimulation can be accomplished by stimulating the skin in an area opposite to the painful area (e.g., stimulating the left knee if the pain is in the right knee). The contralateral area may be scratched for itching, massaged for cramps, or treated with cold packs or analgesic ointments. This method is particularly useful when the painful area cannot be touched because it is hypersensitive, inaccessible by a cast or bandages, or when the pain is felt in a missing part (phantom pain).

Transcutaneous Electrical Nerve Stimulation

TENS is a method of applying low-voltage electrical stimulation directly over identified pain areas, at an acupressure point, along peripheral nerve areas that innervate the pain area, or along the spinal column. The TENS unit consists of a portable, battery-operated device with lead wire and electrode pads that are applied to the chosen area of skin. Cutaneous stimulation from the TENS unit is thought to activate large-diameter fibers that modulate the transmission of the nociceptive impulse in the peripheral and central nervous system (closing the pain "gate"), resulting in pain relief. This stimulation may also cause a release of endorphins from the central nervous system centers.

Distraction

Distraction draws the person's attention away from the pain and lessens the perception of pain. In some instances, distraction can make a client completely unaware of pain. For example, a client recovering from surgery may feel no pain while watching a football game on television, yet feel pain again when the game is over.

Visual Distraction
- Reading or watching TV
- Watching a baseball game
- Guided imagery

Auditory Distraction
- Humor
- Listening to music

Tactile Distraction
- Slow, rhythmic breathing
- Massage
- Holding or stroking a pet or toy

Intellectual Distraction
- Crossword puzzles
- Card games (e.g., bridge)
- Hobbies (e.g., stamp collecting, writing a story)

Nonpharmacologic Invasive Therapies

A nerve block is a chemical interruption of a nerve pathway, effected by injecting a local anesthetic into the nerve. Nerve blocks are widely used during dental work. The injected drug blocks nerve pathways from the painful tooth, thus stopping the transmission of pain impulses to the brain. Nerve blocks are often used to relieve the pain of whiplash injury, lower back disorders, bursitis, and cancer.

Pain conduction pathways can be interrupted surgically. Because this disruption is permanent, surgery is performed only as a last resort, generally for intractable pain. Several surgical procedures may be performed and depend on area of pain origin.

The client may become angry or complain about the nurse's care when the problem really is a belief that the pain is not being attended to. If the nurse is honest and sincere and promptly attends to the client's needs, the client is much more likely to know that the nurse does believe the client is in pain.

By providing accurate information, the nurse can also reduce many of the client's fears, such as a fear of addiction or a fear that the pain will always be present. It also helps many clients to have privacy when they are experiencing pain.

PREVENTING PAIN

A preventive approach to pain management involves the provision of measures to treat the pain before it occurs or before it becomes severe. **Preemptive analgesia** is the administration of analgesics prior to an invasive or operative procedure. Nurses can also use a preemptive approach by providing analgesic around-the-clock (ATC), rather than as needed (prn). For clients who routinely feel pain, for example, with diseases such as cancer, administering pain medication at scheduled intervals maintains the level of analgesia without allowing the peaks and valleys associated with metabolism of the medication given on a prn basis. PCA pumps allow clients to self-administer medication to lessen breakthrough pain (Figure 21-5 ■).

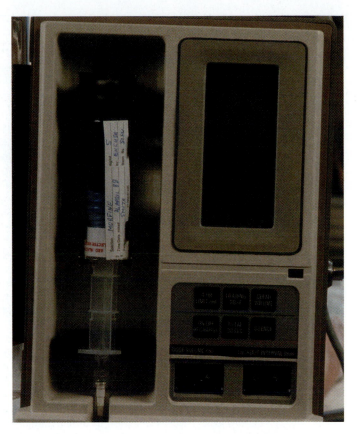

Figure 21-5. ■ A continuous, subcutaneous PCA infusion device.

ROUTES FOR OPIATE DELIVERY

Opioids have traditionally been administered by oral, subcutaneous, intramuscular, and intravenous routes. In addition, newer methods of delivering opiates have been developed to circumvent potential obstacles that occur with these traditional routes. Examples are transnasal and transdermal drug therapy, continuous subcutaneous infusions, and intraspinal infusion. See Table 21-3 ■ for routes and their benefits.

TABLE 21-3

Routes of Administration for Pain Medications and Their Benefits

ROUTE OF ADMINISTRATION	BENEFITS
Oral	Oral administration of opiates remains the preferred route of delivery because of ease of administration. Because the duration of action of most opiates is approximately 4 hours, people with chronic pain have had to awaken several times during the night to medicate themselves for pain. To circumvent this problem, long-acting forms of morphine with a duration of 8 or more hours have been developed. Two examples of long-acting morphine are MS Contin and Oramorph SR. Clients receiving long-acting morphine also may need prn rescue doses of immediate-release analgesics (e.g., short-acting morphine) for acute breakthrough pain. Another new method of oral opiate delivery is high-concentration liquid morphine. This formulation enables clients who can swallow only small amounts to continue taking the drug orally.
Nasal	Transnasal administration has the advantage of rapid action of the medication because of direct absorption through the vascular nasal mucosa. A commonly used agent is butorphanol (Stadol) for acute headaches.
Transdermal	Transdermal drug therapy is advantageous in that it delivers a relatively stable plasma drug level and is noninvasive. Fentanyl (Duragesic) is an opioid currently available as a skin patch with various dosages. It provides drug delivery for up to 72 hours.
Rectal	Several opiates are now available in suppository form. The rectal route is particularly useful for clients who have dysphagia (difficulty swallowing) or nausea and vomiting. Oral analgesics, with the exception of sustained-release analgesics, may be crushed, dissolved in water, and given rectally (McCaffery & Beebe, 1989, p. 92).

(continued)

TABLE 21-3

Routes of Administration for Pain Medications and Their Benefits (*continued*)

ROUTE OF ADMINISTRATION	BENEFITS
Subcutaneous	Although the subcutaneous (SC) route has been used extensively to deliver opioids, a new technique uses subcutaneous catheters and infusion pumps to provide continuous subcutaneous infusion (CSCI) of narcotics. CSCI is particularly helpful for clients (1) whose pain is poorly controlled by oral medications, (2) who are experiencing dysphagia or gastrointestinal obstruction, or (3) who have a need for prolonged use of parenteral narcotics. CSCI involves the use of a small, light, battery-operated pump that administers the drug through a 23- or 25-gauge butterfly needle. The needle can be inserted into the anterior chest, the subclavicular region, the abdominal wall, the outer aspects of the upper arms, or the thighs. Client mobility is maintained with the application of a shoulder bag or holster to hold the pump. The frequency of site change ranges from 3 to 7 days.
Intramuscular	The intramuscular (IM) route is the least desirable route for opioid administration because of variable absorption, pain involved with administration, and the need to repeat administration every 3 to 4 hours.
Intravenous	The intravenous (IV) route provides rapid and effective pain relief with few side effects. The analgesic can be administered by IV bolus or by continuous infusion controlled by the client using a PCA machine at the bedside.
Intraspinal	Another recent method of delivery is the infusion of opiates into the epidural or intrathecal (subarachnoid) space. Intraspinal analgesics act directly on opiate receptors in the spinal cord. Two commonly used medications are preservative-free morphine sulfate and fentanyl. The major benefit of intraspinal drug therapy is that it exerts a lesser sedative effect than do systemic opiates. The epidural space is most commonly used because the dura mater acts as a protective barrier against infection, including meningitis.
Patient-controlled analgesia	PCA is the self-administration of an analgesic by a client who has been instructed regarding the process (Carr et al., 1992). The physician prescribes the analgesic dose, route, and frequency, with the client administering the medication. With parenteral routes, an infusion pump is used to deliver the medication. Whether in an acute hospital setting, an ambulatory clinic, or with home care, the nurse is responsible for the initial instruction regarding use of the PCA and for the ongoing monitoring of the therapy. The client's pain must be assessed at regular intervals and analgesic use is documented in the client's record. PCA can be effectively used for clients with acute pain related to a surgical incision, traumatic injury, or labor and delivery, and for chronic pain, as with cancer. In some settings, PCAs are used even if the client is unable to initiate a dose by pushing the button, as long as a caregiver is willing to accept the responsibility, for example, when the client is an infant or toddler or is physically or cognitively impaired (Pasero & McCaffery, 1996). The benefits of this mode of administration include: ■ Self-control over pain relief ■ More stable analgesic blood level for sustained pain relief ■ Tendency for the client to need less medication for pain relief. PCA pumps usually have a chamber or cartridge that contains the analgesic, a mechanism for setting the ordered dose, and a control for client activation (see Figure 21-5). When clients want a dose of analgesic, they can push a button attached to the infusion pump and the preset dose is delivered. A programmable lockout interval (usually 10 to 15 minutes) follows the dose, when an additional dose cannot be given even if the client activates the button. It is also possible to program the maximum dose that can be delivered over a period of hours (usually 4). Many pumps are capable of delivering a low continuous infusion, or basal rate, to provide sustained analgesia during times of rest and sleep.

Barriers to Pain Management

Misconceptions and biases can affect pain management. Some of these involve attitudes of the nurse or the client as well as knowledge deficits. Clients respond to pain experiences based on their culture (Box 21-5 ■), personal experiences, and the meaning the pain has for them. For many people, pain is expected and accepted as a normal aspect of illness. Clients and families may lack knowledge of the adverse effects of pain and may have misinformation regarding the use of analgesics. Clients may not report pain because they

BOX 21-5 CULTURAL PULSE POINTS

Pain Experiences and Culture

The meaning and expression of pain are influenced by people's cultural backgrounds. Pain is not just a physiological response to tissue damage. Not everyone in a culture conforms to a set of expected behaviors or beliefs, so cultural stereotyping can lead to inadequate assessment and treatment of pain. Healthcare professionals need to be aware of their own values and perceptions because they affect how they evaluate the patient's response to pain and ultimately how pain is treated. Even subtle cultural and individual differences, particularly in nonverbal, spoken, and written language, between healthcare providers and patient can impact care.

reassessed at an interval appropriate for the intervention. For example, following the intravenous administration of morphine, the severity of pain should be reassessed in 20 to 30 minutes.

clinical ALERT

A quick pain assessment rubric is:

P—Precipitation/Palliation: What causes your pain? What relieves (or helps) your pain?

Q—Quality: What does your pain feel like (sharp, dull, shooting, etc.)?

R—Region/Radiation: Where did the pain start? Does it radiate (travel to another location)?

S—Severity: How bad is the pain on a pain scale with zero meaning no pain and ten meaning the worst pain imaginable?

T—Timing: When did the pain start? How long does it last?

expect nothing can be done, they think it is not severe enough, or because they feel it would distract or prejudice the healthcare provider. Other common misconceptions are shown in Table 21-4 ■.

NURSING CARE

ASSESSING

Accurate pain assessment is essential for effective pain management. Because pain is subjective and experienced uniquely by each individual, nurses need to assess all factors affecting the pain experience—physiological, psychological, behavioral, emotional, and sociocultural.

Pain is considered the fifth vital sign, and should be assessed at least every 4 hours. Pain is also assessed following pain management interventions. Pain intensity should be

Because many people will not voice their pain unless asked about it, pain assessments *must* be initiated by the nurse. Some of the many reasons clients may be reluctant to report pain are listed in Box 21-6 ■. Nurses must listen to and rely on the client's perceptions of pain. Believing the person experiencing and conveying the perceptions is crucial in establishing a sense of trust. (See Chapter 12 ⊂⊃.)

Pain assessments consist of a pain history to obtain facts from the client and direct observation of behavioral and physiological responses of the client. The goal of assessment is to gain an objective understanding of a subjective experience.

While taking pain histories, the nurse must provide an opportunity for clients to express in their own words how they view the pain and the situation. This will help the nurse understand what the pain means to the client and

TABLE 21-4

Common Misconceptions about Pain

MISCONCEPTION	CORRECTION
Clients experience severe pain only when they have had major surgery.	Even after minor surgery, clients can experience intense pain.
The nurse and other healthcare professionals are the authorities about a client's pain.	The person who experiences the pain is the only authority about its existence and nature.
Administering analgesics regularly for pain will lead to addiction.	Clients are unlikely to become addicted to an analgesic provided to treat pain.
The amount of tissue damage is directly related to the amount of pain.	Pain is a subjective experience, and the intensity and duration of pain vary considerably among individuals.
Visible physiological or behavioral signs accompany pain and can be used to verify its existence.	Even with severe pain, periods of physiological and behavioral adaptation can occur.

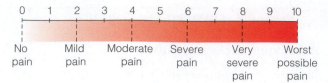

Figure 21-6. ■ A 10-point pain intensity scale with word modifiers.

Why Clients May Be Reluctant to Report Pain

- Unwillingness to trouble staff who are perceived as busy
- Fear of the injectable route of analgesic administration (children in particular)
- Belief that pain is to be expected as part of the recovery process
- Belief that pain is a normal part of aging or a necessary part of life (older adults in particular)
- Belief that expressions of pain reveal weakness
- Difficulty expressing personal discomfort
- Concern about risks associated with opioid drugs (e.g., addiction)
- Fear about the cause of pain or that reporting pain will lead to further tests and expenses
- Concern about unwanted side effects, especially of opioid drugs
- Concern that use of drugs now will render the drug inefficient if or when the pain becomes worse

---

how the client is coping with it. Remember that each person's pain experience is unique and that the client is the best interpreter of the pain experience. The initial pain assessment for someone in severe acute pain may consist of only a few questions before intervention occurs, such as location, intensity, and quality. For the person with chronic pain, the nurse may focus on the client's coping mechanisms, effectiveness of current pain management, and ways in which the pain has affected activities of daily living (ADLs).

Location

To identify the specific location of the pain, ask the individual to point to the site of the discomfort. A chart consisting of drawings of the body can assist in identifying pain locations. The client marks the location of pain on the chart. This tool can be especially effective with clients who have more than one source of pain.

When assessing the location of a child's pain, the nurse needs to understand the child's vocabulary. For example, "tummy" might mean the abdomen or part of the chest. Asking the child to point to the pain helps clarify the child's word usage to identify location. Again, the use of figure drawings can assist in identifying pain locations. (See also Chapter 33 ⬭.) Parents can also be helpful in interpreting the meaning of a child's words.

Intensity

The single most important indicator of the intensity of pain is the client's report of pain. Studies have shown that healthcare providers may underrate or overrate the pain intensity. The use of pain intensity scales is an easy and reliable method of deter-

mining pain intensity. Such scales provide consistency for nurses to communicate with the client and other healthcare providers. Most scales use either a 0-to-5 or 0-to-10 range with 0 indicating "no pain" and the highest number indicating the "worst pain possible" for that individual. A 10-point rating scale is shown in Figure 21-6 ■. It is important for the nurse to understand that the pain scale is intended to compare the client to himself or herself, not to other individuals. A nurse should never compare one client's rating of pain with another client's rating of pain. The scale is intended to gauge the amount of relief or distress the client is in at any given time. It should not be used to compare levels of pain perception.

When noting pain intensity, it is important to determine any related factors that may be affecting the pain. When the intensity changes, the nurse needs to consider the possible cause. For example, the abrupt cessation of acute abdominal pain may indicate a ruptured appendix. Several factors affect the perception of intensity: (1) the amount of distraction, or the client's concentration on another event; (2) the client's state of consciousness; (3) the level of activity; and (4) the client's expectations.

Not all clients can understand or relate to numerical pain intensity scales. These include children who are unable to communicate discomfort verbally, elderly clients with impairments in cognition or communication, and people who do not speak English. For these clients, the Wong/Baker Faces Rating Scale (Figure 21-7 ■) may be easier to use (Pasero, 1997b). The face scale includes a number scale in relation to each expression so that the pain intensity can be documented. When it is not possible to use any kind of rating scale with a client, the nurse must rely on observation of behavior and the physiological cues discussed later in this section. The input of the client's significant others, such as parents or caregivers, can assist the nurse in interpreting the observations. An objective description of the behavior and the physiological data are then documented.

For effective use of pain rating scales, clients need to not only understand the use of the scale but also be educated about how the information will be used to determine changes in their condition and the effectiveness of pain management interventions. Clients should also be asked to indicate what level of comfort is acceptable so that they can perform specific activities. This will ensure that adequate pain management is achieved.

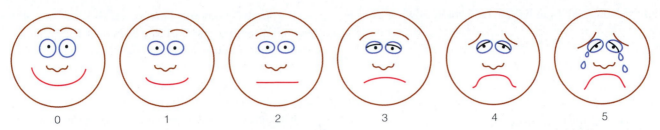

<table>
| 0 | 1 | 2 | 3 | 4 | 5 |
</table>

1. Explain to the child that each face is for a person who feels happy because he or she has no pain (hurt, or whatever word the child uses) or feels sad because he or she has some or a lot of pain.

2. Point to the appropriate face and state, "This face..." :
   0—"is very happy because he (or she) doesn't hurt at all."
   1—"hurts just a little bit."
   2—"hurts a little more."
   3—"hurts even more."
   4—"hurts a whole lot."
   5—"hurts as much as you can imagine, although you don't have to be crying to feel this bad."

3. Ask the child to choose the face that best describes how he or she feels. Be specific about which pain (e.g., "shot" or incision) and what time (e.g., Now? Earlier before lunch?).

Figure 21-7. ■ The Wong/Baker Faces Rating Scale. (*Source:* Wong, D. L. (2001). *Wong's Essentials of Pediatric Nursing* (6th ed.). St. Louis, MO: Mosby. Reprinted with permission.)

Quality

Descriptive adjectives help people communicate the quality of pain. A headache may be described as "hammer-like" or an abdominal pain as "piercing like a knife." Sometimes clients have difficulty describing pain because they have never experienced any sensation like it. Terms commonly used to describe pain can be classified as sensory words and affective words. Examples of sensory words are *searing, scalding, sharp, piercing, drilling, wrenching, shooting, splitting, crushing, penetrating, numb, radiating, dull, aching,* and *cramping.* Examples of affective words are *unbearable, killing, intense, torturing, agonizing, terrifying, grueling, suffocating, frightful, punishing, miserable, annoying, nagging, tiring,* and *troublesome.*

Nurses need to record the exact words clients use to describe pain. A client's words are more accurate and descriptive than an interpretation in the nurse's words. Exact information can be significant in both the diagnosis of the pain etiology and in the treatment choices made. For example, pain described as hot, electrical, and sharp tends to be neuropathic in origin and will be more responsive to anticonvulsants (e.g., Tegretol) than to an opioid (e.g., morphine).

Pattern

The pattern of pain includes time of onset, duration, and recurrence or intervals without pain. The nurse therefore determines when the pain began; how long the pain lasts; whether it recurs and, if so, the length of the interval without pain; and when the pain last occurred.

Precipitating Factors

Certain activities sometimes precede pain; for example, physical exertion may precede chest pain, or abdominal pain may occur after eating. These observations can help prevent pain and determine its cause.

Environmental factors such as extreme cold or heat and extremes of humidity can affect some types of pain. For example, sudden exercise on a hot day can cause muscle spasm.

Physical and emotional stressors can also precipitate pain. Emotional tension frequently brings on a migraine headache. Intense fear or physical exertion can cause angina.

Alleviating Factors

Nurses must ask clients to describe anything that they have done to help alleviate the pain (e.g., home remedies such as herbal teas, or medications, rest, applications of heat or cold, prayer, or distractions such as watching TV). It is important to explore the effect any of these measures had on the pain, whether or not relief was obtained, or whether the pain became worse.

Associated Symptoms

Also included in the clinical appraisal of pain are other associated symptoms, such as nausea, vomiting, dizziness, and diarrhea. These symptoms may relate to the onset of the pain or they may result from the presence of the pain.

Effect on Activities of Daily Living

When caring for clients with chronic pain, knowing how ADLs are affected helps the nurse understand the client's perspective on the pain's severity. The nurse asks the client to describe how the pain has affected the following aspects of life:

- Sleep
- Appetite
- Concentration
- Work/school
- Interpersonal relationships
- Marital relations/sex
- Home activities
- Driving/walking
- Leisure activities
- Emotional status (mood, irritability, depression, anxiety).

A rating scale of none, a little, or a great deal or another range can be used to determine the degree of alteration.

Coping Resources

Each individual will exhibit personal ways of coping with pain. Strategies may relate to past pain experiences or the specific meaning of the pain; some may reflect religious or cultural influences. Nurses can encourage and support the client's use of methods known to have helped in modifying pain. Strategies may include withdrawal, use of distraction, prayer or other religious practices, and support from significant others.

Affective Responses

Affective responses vary according to the situation, the degree and duration of pain, the interpretation of it, and many other factors. The nurse needs to explore the client's feelings—for example, anxiety, fear, exhaustion, depression, or a sense of failure. Because many people with chronic pain become depressed and potentially suicidal, it may also be necessary to assess the client's suicide risk. In such situations, the nurse needs to ask the client, "Do you ever feel so bad that you want to die? Do you feel that way now?"

Observation of Behavioral and Physiological Responses

There are wide variations in nonverbal responses to pain. For clients who are very young, aphasic, confused, or disoriented, nonverbal expressions may be the only means of communicating pain. Facial expression is often the first indication of pain, and it may be the only one. Clenched teeth, tightly shut eyes, open somber eyes, biting of the lower lip, and other facial grimaces may be indicative of pain. Vocalizations such as moaning and groaning or crying and screaming are also associated with pain.

Immobilization of the body or a part of the body may also indicate pain. The client with chest pain often holds the left arm across the chest. A person with abdominal pain may assume the position of greatest comfort, often with the knees and hips flexed, and move reluctantly.

Purposeless body movements can also indicate pain—for example, tossing and turning in bed or flinging the arms about. Involuntary movements such as a reflexive jerking away from a needle inserted through the skin indicate pain. An adult may be able to control this reflex; however, a child may be unable or unwilling to do so.

Rhythmic body movements or rubbing may indicate pain. An adult or child may assume a fetal position and rock back and forth when experiencing abdominal pain. During labor a woman may massage her abdomen rhythmically with her hands.

It is important to note that behavioral responses can be controlled and so may not be very revealing. When pain is chronic, there are rarely overt behavioral responses because the individual develops personal coping styles for dealing with pain, discomfort, or suffering. Therefore, it is imperative that nurses believe clients when they report they are in pain. It is unacceptable for the nurse to doubt a client who reports pain because "he did not look like he was hurting."

Physiological responses vary with the origin and duration of the pain. Early in the onset of acute pain, the sympathetic nervous system is stimulated, resulting in increased blood pressure, pulse rate, respiratory rate, pallor, diaphoresis, and pupil dilation. However, in clients with chronic pain, the sympathetic nervous system adapts to the stimulus, making the physiological responses less evident or even absent. When people experience visceral pain, signs of parasympathetic stimulation may be observed, such as decreased blood pressure and pulse rate, pupil constriction, and warm, dry skin.

Daily Pain Diary

For clients who experience chronic pain, a daily diary may help the client and nurse identify pain patterns and factors that exacerbate or mediate the pain experience. In home care, the family or other caregiver can be taught to complete the diary. The record can include time or onset of pain, activity before pain, pain-related positions or behaviors, pain intensity level, use of analgesics or other relief measures, duration of pain, and time spent in relief activities. Recorded data can provide the basis for developing or modifying the plan for care. For this tool to be effective, it is important that the nurse educate the client and family about the value and use of the diary in achieving effective pain control. Determining the client's abilities to use the diary is essential.

DIAGNOSING, PLANNING, AND IMPLEMENTING

The North American Nursing Diagnosis Association (NANDA) includes the following diagnostic labels for clients experiencing pain or discomfort:

- *Acute Pain*
- *Chronic Pain.*

TABLE 21-5

Selected Nursing Interventions by Developmental Level

DEVELOPMENTAL LEVEL	SELECTED NURSING INTERVENTIONS
Infant	Give a glucose pacifier.
	Use tactile stimulation. Play music or tapes of a heartbeat.
Toddler/preschooler	Distract the child with toys, books, pictures. Involve the child in blowing bubbles as a way of "blowing away the pain."
	Appeal to the child's belief in magic by using a "magic" blanket or glove to take away pain.
	Hold the child to provide comfort.
	Explore misconceptions about pain.
School-age child	Use imagery to turn off "pain switches."
	Provide a behavioral rehearsal of what to expect and how it will look and feel.
	Provide support and nurturing.
Adolescent	Provide opportunities to discuss pain.
	Provide privacy.
	Present choices for dealing with pain.
	Encourage music or TV for distraction.
Adult	Deal with any misconceptions about pain.
	Focus on the client's control in dealing with the pain.
	Allay fears and anxiety when possible.
Older adult	Spend time with the client, and listen carefully.
	Clarify misconceptions.
	Encourage independence whenever possible.

Goals and interventions for clients should be individualized for the client, the particular pain process, and developmental level (Table 21-5 ■).

Because the presence of pain can affect so many areas of a person's functioning, pain may be the etiology of other nursing diagnoses. Examples of such nursing diagnoses follow:

- *Ineffective Airway Clearance* related to postoperative incisional chest pain
- *Powerlessness* related to past experiences of poor control of pain (See also Chapter 17 ⬤⬤.)
- *Ineffective Coping* related to prolonged continuous back pain, ineffective pain management, and inadequate support systems
- *Impaired Physical Mobility* related to arthritic pain in knee and ankle joints
- *Disturbed Sleep Pattern* related to increased pain perception at night.

Preventing Pain

Review the section Key Factors in Pain Management on pages 413–416. As mentioned, the nurse provides measures to treat the pain before it occurs or before it becomes severe.

Preemptive analgesia is appropriate before an invasive or operative procedure. It is often appropriate for clients with chronic pain. Administering pain medication at scheduled intervals maintains the level of analgesia without allowing the peaks and valleys in pain relief. Box 21-7 ■ lists guidelines for individualizing care for clients with pain.

Supporting the Client and Significant Others

Nurses assist the client who is in pain by assessing pain regularly. Open-ended questions that allow the client to describe the type, location, or level of pain are much more useful than closed questions. For example, "How is your side feeling now?" encourages the client to answer more fully than "Did that medication work?" An attentive attitude and prompt attention to the client's needs help to build trust and reduce the anxiety that often accompanies severe or unremitting pain. The nurse can also help the client analyze when and why the pain worsens. Understanding more about the pain can sometimes help the client feel more in control.

The nurse's attitude of respect for the client in pain is important. Nurses can help family members by giving them accurate information about medications and about expected

---

BOX 21-7 | **NURSING CARE CHECKLIST**

Individualizing Care for Clients with Pain

☑ Establish a trusting relationship. Convey your concern, and acknowledge that you believe that the client is experiencing pain. A trusting relationship promotes expression of the client's thoughts and feelings and enhances effectiveness of planned pain therapies.

☑ Consider the client's ability and willingness to participate actively in pain relief measures. Some clients who are excessively fatigued, are sedated, or have altered levels of consciousness (LOC) are less able to participate actively. For example, a client with an altered LOC or altered thought processes may not be able to deal with PCA. In contrast, a fatigued client may express a willingness to use pain relief measures that require little effort, such as listening to music or performing relaxation techniques.

☑ Use a variety of pain relief measures. It is thought that using more than one measure has an additive effect in relieving pain. Two measures that should always be part of any pain relief plan are (1) establishing a client–nurse relationship and (2) client teaching. Because a client's pain may vary throughout a 24-hour period, different types of pain relief are often indicated during that time.

☑ Provide measures to relieve pain before it becomes severe. For example, providing an analgesic before the onset of pain is preferable to waiting for the client to complain of pain, when a larger dose may be required.

☑ Use pain-relieving measures that the client believes are effective. It has been recognized that clients are usually the au-

thorities about their own pain. Thus, incorporating the client's measures into a pain relief plan is sensible unless they are harmful.

☑ Base the choice of pain relief measure on the client's report of the severity of the pain. If a client reports mild pain, an analgesic such as aspirin may be indicated, whereas a client who reports severe pain often requires a more potent relief measure.

☑ If a pain relief measure is ineffective, encourage the client to try it once or twice more before abandoning it. Anxiety may diminish the effects of a pain measure, and some approaches, such as distraction strategies, require practice before they are effective.

☑ Maintain an unbiased attitude (open mind) about what may relieve the pain. New ways to relieve pain are continually being developed. It is not always possible to explain pain relief measures; however, measures should be supported unless they are harmful.

☑ Keep trying. Do not ignore a client because pain persists in spite of measures. In these circumstances, reassess the pain, and consider other relief measures.

☑ Prevent harm to the client. Pain therapy should not increase discomfort or harm the client. Some pain relief measures may have adverse untoward effects, such as fatigue, but they should not disable the client.

☑ Educate the client and support people about pain. Clients and support people need to be informed about possible causes of pain, precipitating and alleviating factors, and alternatives to drug therapy. Misconceptions also need to be corrected.

---

resolution of pain (e.g., period of recovery after surgery). Explaining when pain is likely to be the worst, when pain medication begins to take effect, and when the effect of medication wears off will enable support persons to organize their time and efforts to help the client. Providing accurate information about possible side effects, as well as reassurance that medications used appropriately will not cause addiction, is also a part of client teaching. The nurse can encourage family to participate in client care and to provide distractions they know the client would enjoy.

Chronic pain is debilitating and frustrating. When chronic pain exists, the nurse can serve an important role in reminding support people that only the client really knows the pain. The client is the source about the client's pain. However, family and significant others can provide caring, encouragement, distraction, and empathy, all of which support the client.

EVALUATING

The nurse reviews client goals and outcomes to determine whether they have been achieved. Both subjective data (phys-

ical stance and facial expression) and objective data (heart rate and respirations) are collected to evaluate client comfort.

To assist in the evaluation process, flow sheet records or a client diary may be helpful. A weekly log or diary can be structured in a similar fashion for the individual client. For example, columns including day, time, onset of pain, activity before pain, pain relief measure, and duration of pain can be devised to help the client and nurse determine the effectiveness of pain relief strategies.

If outcomes are not achieved, the nurse and client might consider the following:

- Would the client benefit from a change in dose or in the time interval between doses?
- Did the client understate the pain experience for some reason?
- Did the client and support people understand the instructions about pain management techniques?
- Is the client receiving adequate support from significant others?
- Has the client's physical condition changed?

NURSING PROCESS CARE PLAN
Client with Pain

Mrs. Lundahl underwent abdominal surgery approximately 6 hours ago. She has a 21-cm midline incision that is covered with a dry and intact surgical dressing.

Assessment. Mrs. Lundahl is perspiring, lying in a rigid position, holding her abdomen, and grimacing. Her blood pressure is 150/90, heart rate 100, and respiratory rate 32. When asked to rate her pain on a scale of 1 to 10, Mrs. Lundahl rates her pain as 5.

Nursing Diagnosis. The following important nursing diagnosis (among others) is established for this client:

- *Acute Pain* related to surgical incision.

Expected Outcomes The expected outcomes specify that Mrs. Lundahl will:

- State postoperative discomfort is relieved "to a pain level of (whatever level client has identified as acceptable)" within 20 to 30 minutes of verbalized pain.
- Practice one relaxation technique for relief of pain by end of second postop day.
- Turn, cough, and deep breathe with minimum of discomfort by second postop day.

Planning and Implementation. The following interventions are planned and implemented for Mrs. Lundahl:

- Teach Mrs. Lundahl about her medications, as well as side effects and how to treat them.

- Encourage Mrs. Lundahl to request prn analgesics before pain becomes unmanageable.
- Teach Mrs. Lundahl relaxation and distraction techniques.

Evaluation. Mrs. Lundahl c/o dizziness following 2 tabs Vicodin ES; 1 tab adequately relieved pain without noticeable side effects in 30 minutes. Able to space prn pain meds to 5 to 6 hours by using relaxation technique (deep breathing and muscle group relaxation). Mrs. Lundahl using pillow to splint during coughing, able to change position and transfer to chair from bed without discomfort.

Critical Thinking in the Nursing Process

1. What conclusions, if any, can be drawn about Mrs. Lundahl's pain status?
2. Does Mrs. Lundahl's rating her pain as 5 mean that she is not experiencing pain severe enough to warrant intervention?
3. What type of pain is Mrs. Lundahl experiencing?
4. What interventions, in addition to pain medication, may be useful in reducing Mrs. Lundahl's pain?
5. How will you know if your interventions have been effective in reducing Mrs. Lundahl's pain?

Note: Discussion of Critical Thinking questions appears in Appendix I.

Note: The references and resources for this and all chapters have been compiled at the back of the book.

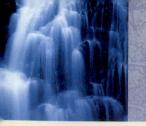

Chapter Review

 KEY TERMS by Topic

Use the audio glossary feature of either the CD-ROM or the Companion Website to hear the correct pronunciation of the following key terms.

Types of Pain
pain, acute pain, chronic pain, intractable pain, cutaneous pain,

somatic pain, visceral pain, radiating pain, referred pain, neuropathic pain, phantom pain

Concepts Associated with Pain
pain threshold, pain reaction, pain tolerance

Physiology of Pain
nociceptor, endogenous opioids, exogenous opioids analgesics, gate control theory

Key Factors in Pain Management
preemptive analgesia

KEY Points

- Pain is a subjective sensation. Pain can directly impair health and prolong recovery from surgery, disease, and trauma.

- Ethnic and cultural values, age, environment and support people, anxiety, and stress all influence a person's perception and reaction to pain.

- The overall client goal is to increase a client's functional capacity by preventing, modifying, or eliminating pain.

- The most reliable indicator of the presence or intensity of pain is the client's self-report.

- Nurses must acknowledge and convey belief in the client's report of pain and reduce fear and anxiety associated with the pain. Nurses should also assist support people and reduce misconceptions about pain.

- Do not allow fear of potential side effects to inhibit full and aggressive treatment of a client's pain.

- The nurse's evaluation of the client's pain therapy is multifaceted and should include the response of the client, changes in the pain, and the client's perceptions of the effectiveness of therapy.

 EXPLORE Media Link

Additional interactive resources for this chapter can be found on the Companion Website at www.prenhall.com/ramont. Click on Chapter 21 and "Begin" to select the activities for this chapter.

For chapter-related NCLEX®-style questions and an audio glossary, access the accompanying CD-ROM in this book.

Animations/Videos
- Pain Management

FOR FURTHER Study

For more information about communicating effectively with clients, see Chapter 12.

For effects of anxiety and stress, see Chapter 16.

For more about helplessness in relation to pain, see Chapter 17.

For more information on incessinal or wound pain, see Chapter 23.

For further discussion of listening skills, see Chapters 33 and 37.

Critical Thinking Care Map

Caring for a Client with Postoperative Pain

NCLEX-PN® Focus Area: Physiological Adaptation

Case Study: Mr. Lee Chin is a 57-year-old Chinese businessman who was admitted to the surgical unit for treatment of a possible strangulated inguinal hernia. Two days ago he had a partial bowel resection.

Nursing Diagnosis: Acute Pain Related to Surgical Incision

COLLECT DATA

Subjective

_____

_____

_____

_____

_____

_____

Objective

_____

_____

_____

_____

_____

_____

Would you report this data? Yes/No

If yes, to: _____

What would you report? _____

Nursing Care

_____

_____

_____

_____

_____

_____

_____

_____

_____

_____

_____

_____

How would you document this? _____

_____

_____

_____

Data Collected
(use those that apply)

- Height: 188 cm (6'3")
- Weight: 90.0 kg (200 lbs)
- Temperature: 37°C (98.6°F)
- Pulse: 90 bpm
- Respirations: 24/min
- Blood pressure: 158/82 mm Hg
- Lying in dorsal recumbent position with legs drawn up
- Skin pale and moist, pupils dilated
- NPO, intravenous infusion of $D_5\frac{1}{2}NS$ at 125 mL/h left arm, nasogastric tube to low intermittent suction
- Restless
- Complaint of pain (7 on a scale of 1–10)
- "I am cold and tired, I wish I could sleep."
- Complaint of being thirsty
- Midline abdominal incision, sutures dry and intact
- Chest x-ray and urinalysis negative
- WBC 12,000
- Complaint of nausea but no vomiting

Nursing Interventions
(use those that apply; list in priority order)

- Medicate before an activity to increase participation.
- Teach client to use incentive spirometer.
- Evaluate the effectiveness of the pain control measures used through ongoing assessment.
- Assess wound drainage at each dressing change.
- Provide extra blanket for warmth.
- Determine analgesic selections (narcotic, non-narcotic, or NSAID) based on type and severity of pain.
- Institute safety precautions as appropriate if receiving narcotic analgesics.
- Encourage coughing and deep breathing.
- Instruct client to request prn pain medication before the pain is severe.
- Create a quiet, nondisruptive environment with dim lights and comfortable temperature when possible.

Compare your documentation to the sample provided in Appendix I.

NCLEX-PN® Exam Preparation

1 The nurse is faced with a complex situation when developing a plan to relieve pain and provide comfort because:

1. most clients have very low pain tolerance and request medication too frequently.
2. physicians are reluctant to order adequate pain control.
3. pain is a sensation that is highly subjective and individual.
4. the client does not have enough knowledge to be an authority about pain.

2 You are assigned to do postsurgical checks on a client returning to the surgical unit. The client is complaining of incisional pain. Which of the following statements by the nurse would be most effective in determining the severity of the pain?

1. "Can you describe your pain for me?"
2. "Please rate your pain on a scale of zero to ten, with ten being the worst pain."
3. "Your facial expression appears pained. Are you in pain?"
4. "Would you describe your pain as mild, moderate, or severe?"

3 Pain that lasts only through the expected recovery period, regardless of its intensity, is described as:

1. chronic pain.
2. intractable pain.
3. referred pain.
4. acute pain.

4 The most common and most troubling side effect of opioids is:

1. constipation.
2. respiratory depression.
3. rash.
4. anaphylaxis.

5 Pain described as hot, electrical, and sharp tends to be neuropathic in origin and will be more responsive to a(n):

1. nonsteroidal anti-inflammatory.
2. nonopioid analgesic.
3. anticonvulsant.
4. opioid.

6 Time of onset, duration, and recurrence or intervals without pain are known as the pain:

1. intensity.
2. pattern.
3. duration.
4. severity.

7 Fentanyl (Duragesic) is an opioid analgesic available as a skin patch. It provides drug delivery for up to 72 hours. Which of the following is the appropriate label for the form of this drug?

1. patient-controlled analgesic
2. intraspinal analgesic
3. transdermal analgesic
4. intravenous analgesic

8 Level 4 of the sedation rating scale is characterized by:

1. easily arousable sleep.
2. being awake and alert.
3. frequent drowsiness, arousability, drifting off to sleep during conversation.
4. minimal or no response to stimuli.

9 Which of the following is a chemical type of pain stimuli?

1. trauma to body tissues (e.g., surgery)
2. tissue ischemia
3. blockage of a body duct
4. tumor

10 Your client it requesting an injection for pain; from the list below prioritize the order of your interventions.

1. Prepare injection.
2. Check physician's order.
3. Assess client's pain level.
4. Don gloves.
5. Document medication administration.
6. Administer medication.
7. Establish time of last injection.
8. Reassess client.
9. Wash hands.

Answers and Rationales for Review Questions, as well as discussion of Care Plan and Critical Thinking Care Map questions, appear in Appendix I.

Chapter 22

Hygiene

BRIEF Outline

Skin, Foot, and Nail Care
Hair Care
Mouth Care
Eye Care
Ear Care
Nose Care
Supporting a Hygienic Environment

LEARNING Outcomes

After completing this chapter, you will be able to:

1. Describe the kinds of hygienic care the LPN/LVN provides to clients.
2. Identify factors influencing personal hygiene.
3. Identify normal and abnormal findings obtained during inspection and palpation of the skin, feet, nails, mouth, hair, eyes, ears, and nose.
4. Describe nursing interventions for the skin, feet, nails, mouth, hair, eyes, ears, and nose.
5. Explain specific ways in which the LPN/LVN assists clients with self-care deficits in maintaining personal hygiene.
6. Describe methods of making an unoccupied and an occupied bed.
7. Identify safety and comfort measures that are part of bed-making procedures.

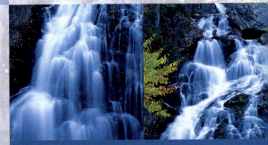

HISTORICAL Perspectives

After the Crimean war broke out in 1854, Florence Nightingale was moved by reports about the primitive sanitation methods and inadequate nursing facilities at the large barracks-hospital in Turkey. She dispatched a letter to the British minister of war, volunteering her services. Nightingale set out for Turkey accompanied by 38 nuns and lay nurses. They found that the military hospitals lacked supplies, the wounded soldiers were unwashed, and disease was rampant. Under Nightingale's supervision, efficient nursing departments were established. Through her tireless efforts, the death rate among the sick and the wounded was greatly reduced.

Hygiene is the science of health and its maintenance. Personal hygiene is the self-care by which people attend to such functions as bathing, toileting, general body hygiene, and grooming. Hygiene is a highly personal matter determined by individual values and practices. Culture plays a role in how often a person bathes and how much privacy a person needs when bathing (Box 22-1 ■). Economics also plays a role, because access to warm water, soap, shampoo, and so on may be limited.

Hygiene involves care of the skin (including perineal and genital areas), hair, nails, teeth, oral and nasal cavities, eyes, and ears. Nursing assistance with hygiene also includes bed-making and changing clients' clothes.

It is important for the LPN/LVN to know exactly how much assistance a client needs for hygienic care. Clients may require help after urinating or defecating, after vomiting, and whenever they become soiled, such as from wound drainage or profuse perspiration. Box 22-2 ■ lists factors that influence hygiene practices.

The following terms are commonly used to describe types of hygienic care. **Early morning care** is provided to clients as they awaken in the morning. This care consists of providing a urinal or bedpan to the client confined to bed, washing the face and hands, and giving oral care. **Morning care** is provided after clients have breakfast. It usually includes the provision of a urinal or bedpan (to clients who are not ambulatory), a bath or shower, perineal care, back massages, and oral, nail, and hair care. It also includes making the client's bed. **Afternoon care** often includes providing a bedpan or urinal, washing the hands and face, and assisting with oral care to refresh clients' mouths. **Hour of sleep (HS) care** is provided to clients before they retire for the night. It usually involves providing for elimination needs, washing face and hands, giving oral care, and giving a back massage. **As-needed (prn) care** is provided as required by the client. For example, a

---

BOX 22-1   **CULTURAL PULSE POINTS**

Bathing and Body Odor

Personal hygiene is a cultural issue. The dominant North American culture seems to have an obsession with minimizing natural body odors. Daily bathing and use of deodorant, mouthwash, and perfumes is the norm. However, a client may have been raised in an area where water was limited and bathing was restricted. Or, the client may follow religious or cultural practices that prohibit bathing during the menstrual cycle or following childbirth. You may be called on to care for clients from cultures that are not bothered by body odor and do not cover up natural smells. It is important not to prejudge the person because of different values.

BOX 22-2   **POPULATION FOCUS**

Factors Influencing Individual Hygienic Practices

Culture: As mentioned in Box 22-1, North American culture places a high value on cleanliness. Many North Americans bathe or shower once or twice a day, whereas people from some other cultures bathe once a week. Some cultures consider privacy essential for bathing, whereas others practice communal bathing. Body odor is offensive in some cultures and accepted as normal in others.

Religion: Ceremonial washings are practiced by some religions.

Environment: Finances may affect the availability of facilities for bathing. For example, homeless people may not have warm water available; soap, shampoo, shaving lotion, and deodorants may be too expensive for people who have limited resources.

Developmental level: Children learn hygiene in the home. Practices vary according to the individual's age; for example, preschoolers can carry out most tasks independently with encouragement.

Health and energy: Ill people may not have the motivation or energy to attend to hygiene. Some clients who have neuromuscular impairments may be unable to perform hygienic care.

Personal preferences: Some people prefer a shower to a tub bath.

---

client who is *diaphoretic* (sweating profusely) may need frequent bathing and changes of clothes and linen.

Skin, Foot, and Nail Care

The skin is the largest organ of the body. As described in Chapter 23 ⚭, the skin protects underlying tissues from injury. It regulates body temperature. (See Chapter 20 ⚭ for a detailed discussion of body heat losses and gains). Skin secretes an oily substance called **sebum** that softens and lubricates the hair and skin. Sebum decreases water loss from the skin when the external humidity is low. Fat is a poor conductor of heat, so sebum lessens the amount of heat lost from the skin. Sebum also has a *bactericidal* (bacteria-killing) action. Skin transmits sensations through nerve receptors, which are sensitive to pain, temperature, touch, and pressure. It also produces and absorbs vitamin D in conjunction with ultraviolet rays from the sun. The normal skin of a healthy person has transient and resident microorganisms that are not usually harmful. (See Table 9-1 ⚭.) Elderly clients exhibit skin changes that need to be considered when bathing. Their skin loses its elasticity, vascular changes occur, and many times nutritional deficiencies are present. See Box 23-2 ⚭ for factors that inhibit wound healing in older adults.

TYPES OF BATHS

Two categories of baths are given to clients: cleaning and therapeutic. **Cleaning baths** are given chiefly for hygiene purposes and include these types:

- *Complete bed bath.* The LPN/LVN washes the entire body of a dependent client in bed.
- *Self-assist bed bath.* Clients confined to bed are able to bathe themselves with assistance for the back and perhaps the feet.
- *Partial bath.* Only the parts of the client's body that might cause discomfort or odor, if neglected, are washed: the face, hands, axillae, perineal area, and back. Omitted are the arms, chest, abdomen, legs, and feet. The LPN/LVN provides this care for dependent clients and assists self-sufficient clients confined to bed by washing their backs. Some ambulatory clients prefer to take a partial bath at the sink. The client can be assisted with washing the back.
- *Bag bath.* Required equipment consists of a plastic bag, 10 to 12 washcloths, and a cleaner and water mixture that doesn't require rinsing. The solution and washcloths are placed in a warmer. Each area of the body is cleaned with a different cloth and then air dried. Because the body is not rubbed dry, the emollient in the solution remains on the skin. Some agencies may provide commercially prepared, disposable bag baths. Each pack usually contains enough wipes to bathe the entire body. These are warmed in the warmer according to directions on the packaging.
- *Tub bath.* Tub baths are preferred to bed baths because it is easier to wash and rinse in a tub. Tubs are also used for therapeutic baths. The amount of assistance offered depends on the abilities of the client. Specially designed tubs are available for dependent clients. These tubs greatly reduce the work and potential for injury in lifting clients in and out of the tub and offer greater benefits than a sponge bath in bed.
- *Shower.* Many ambulatory clients are able to use shower facilities and require only minimal assistance.

Therapeutic baths are given for physical effects, such as to soothe irritated skin or to treat an area (e.g., the perineum). Medications may be placed in the water. A therapeutic bath is generally taken in a tub one-third or one-half full, about 114 L (30 gal). The client remains in the bath for a designated time, often 20 to 30 minutes. If the client's back, chest, and arms are to be treated, these areas need to be immersed in the solution. The bath temperature is generally included in the order; 37.7° to 46°C (100° to 115°F) may be ordered for adults, and 40.5°C (105°F) is usually ordered for infants. Procedure 22-1 ■ on page 448 provides guidelines for bathing clients.

Purposes of Baths

Bathing removes accumulated oil, perspiration, dead skin cells, and some bacteria. The uppermost layer of the epidermis is composed of dead cells that are continuously being shed by the millions and replaced.

Excessive bathing, however, can interfere with the intended lubricating effect of the sebum, causing dryness of the skin. This is an important consideration, especially for older adults, who produce less sebum.

In addition to cleaning the skin, bathing stimulates circulation. A warm or hot bath dilates superficial arterioles, bringing more blood and nourishment to the skin. Vigorous rubbing has the same effect. Rubbing with long smooth strokes from the distal to proximal parts of extremities (from the point farthest from the body to the point closest) is particularly effective in facilitating venous blood flow.

Bathing also produces a sense of well-being. It is refreshing and relaxing and frequently improves morale, appearance, and self-respect. Some people take a morning shower for its refreshing, stimulating effect. Others prefer an evening bath because it is relaxing. These effects are more evident when a person is ill. For example, it is not uncommon for clients who have had a restless or sleepless night to feel relaxed, comfortable, and sleepy after a morning bath.

Bathing offers an excellent opportunity for the LPN/LVN to assess ill clients. During the bath, it is easy to observe the condition of the client's skin and physical conditions such as sacral edema or rashes. While assisting a client with a bath, the LPN/LVN can also assess the client's psychosocial needs, such as orientation to time and ability to cope with the illness. Learning needs, such as a diabetic client's need to learn foot care, can also be assessed.

FEET

The feet are essential for ambulation. They need attention even when people are confined to bed. Children's feet are easily damaged by tight, binding stockings and ill-fitting shoes. They should be well supported, and the bony structure and the feet should grow without restrictions. Feet are not fully grown until about age 20. Healthy feet remain relatively unchanged during life. However, the elderly often require special attention for their feet. Reduced blood supply and accompanying arteriosclerosis can make a foot prone to infection following trauma. Common foot problems include calluses, corns, unpleasant odors, plantar warts, fissures between the toes, and fungal infections such as athlete's foot.

NAILS

Nails are normally present at birth. They continue to grow throughout life and change very little until people are elderly. At that time, the nails tend to be tougher, more brittle, and in some cases thicker. The nails of an older person normally grow less quickly than those of a younger person and may be ridged and grooved.

NURSING CARE

ASSESSING

The LPN/LVN checks the nursing history for the client's skin care practices, self-care abilities, and past or current skin problems. Data about the client's skin care practices enable the LPN/LVN to incorporate the client's needs and preferences as much as possible in the plan of care and to determine necessary learning needs. Clients may have difficulty performing bathing activities. They may not be able to wash the body or certain body parts, to obtain or get to a water source, or to regulate water temperature or flow. Clients may also have difficulties in dressing and grooming. They may not be able to obtain, put on, take off, fasten, or replace articles of clothing; and to maintain appearance at a satisfactory level. They may have difficulties with toileting, such as getting to the toilet or commode, or sitting on and rising from it. Also, clients may have trouble manipulating their clothes for toileting, cleaning themselves after using the toilet, flushing the toilet, or emptying the *commode* (portable toilet, often used at the bedside by people who have limited mobility).

The client's self-care abilities determine the amount of nursing assistance and the kind of bath (bed, tub, or shower) the client requires. The client's balance, coordination, and strength are important factors. The confused or very ill client will lack the motivation and energy to provide self-care. It is important to determine the client's functional level, so the nurse can maintain and promote as much client independence as possible. This also enables the LPN/LVN to identify the client's potential for growth and rehabilitation.

A physical assessment of the skin is performed, and clients who are at risk for developing skin impairment are identified (Box 22-3 ■). The presence of past or current skin problems alerts the LPN/LVN to specific nursing interventions or referrals the client may require. Common skin problems and implications for nursing interventions are shown in Table 22-1 ■. Refer to Chapter 23 ◯◯ for types and descriptions of skin lesions.

BOX 22-3	RISK FACTORS FOR SELF-CARE DEFICIT

- Visual impairment
- Activity intolerance or weakness
- Pain or discomfort
- Mental impairment
- Neuromuscular or skeletal impairment
- Psychological or motivation impairment
- Medically prescribed restriction
- Therapeutic procedure restraining mobility (e.g., intravenous infusion, cast)
- Environmental barriers

TABLE 22-1

Common Skin Problems and Nursing Implications

PROBLEM AND APPEARANCE	NURSING IMPLICATIONS
Abrasion Superficial layers of the skin are scraped or rubbed away. Area is reddened and may have localized bleeding or serous weeping.	1. Prone to infection; therefore, wound should be kept clean and dry. 2. Do not wear rings or jewelry when providing care to avoid causing abrasions to clients. 3. Lift, do not pull, a client across a bed. See Chapter 32 ◯◯.
Excessive Dryness Skin can appear flaky and rough.	1. Prone to infection if the skin cracks; therefore, provide alcohol-free lotions to moisturize the skin and prevent cracking. 2. Bathe client less frequently; use no soap, or limit use of nonirritating soap. Rinse skin thoroughly because soap can be irritating and drying. 3. Encourage increased fluid intake if health permits to prevent dehydration.
Ammonia Dermatitis (Diaper Rash) Caused by skin bacteria reacting with urea in the urine. The skin becomes reddened and is sore.	1. Keep skin dry and clean by applying protective ointments containing zinc oxide to areas at risk. (Ointments may require a physician's order.)
Acne Inflammatory condition with papules and pustules.	1. Keep the skin clean to prevent secondary infection. 2. Treatment varies widely.
Erythema Redness associated with a variety of conditions, such as rashes, exposure to sun, elevated body temperature.	1. Wash area carefully to remove excess microorganisms. 2. Apply antiseptic spray or lotion to prevent itching, promote healing, and prevent skin breakdown.
Hirsutism Excessive hair on a person's body and face, particularly in women.	1. Remove unwanted hair by using depilatories, shaving, electrolysis, or tweezing. 2. Enhance client's self-concept. See Chapter 14 ◯◯.

Physical assessment of the skin, feet and nails, which involves inspection and palpation, is discussed in Chapter 19 ⊙⊙ (see Table 19-3 and Figures 19-4 and 19-13) and described further in Chapter 23 ⊙⊙. A systematic head-to-toe assessment includes collection of data about skin color, uniformity of color, texture, turgor, temperature, intactness, and lesions.

Attention is paid to risk factors for foot problems (such as diabetes) and foot discomfort. The feet are assessed at the beginning and end of each shift, unless otherwise ordered. Changes are reported to the RN.

DIAGNOSING, PLANNING, AND IMPLEMENTING

For clients who have problems performing hygiene care, *Self-Care Deficit* diagnoses are used in collaboration with the LPN/LVN. Three *Self-Care Deficit* diagnoses are discussed in this chapter:

- *Self-Care Deficit: Bathing/Hygiene*
- *Self-Care Deficit: Dressing/Grooming*
- *Self-Care Deficit: Toileting*

Associated diagnoses commonly include *Deficient Knowledge* (e.g., related to lack of experience with skin condition and treatment) and *Risk for Situational Low Self-Esteem* (e.g., related to body odor). The diagnoses *Risk for Impaired Skin Integrity* and *Impaired Skin Integrity* are discussed in Chapter 23 ⊙⊙.

In planning care, the LPN/LVN identifies nursing interventions that will assist the client to maintain or improve skin cleanliness, maintain circulation to the skin, and improve or maintain a sense of well-being. Nursing activities for hygiene include assisting dependent clients with bathing, skin and nail care, and perineal care; providing back massages to promote circulation (discussed in Chapter 32 ⊙⊙); and providing instruction to clients about ways to promote good hygiene and prevent skin lesions.

When planning to assist a client with personal hygiene, the nurse considers the client's personal preferences, health, and limitations; the best time to give the care; and the equipment, facilities, and personnel available. A client's personal preferences about when and how to bathe should be followed as long as they are compatible with the client's health and the equipment available. The LPN/LVN provides whatever assistance the client requires, either directly or by delegating this task to other nursing personnel.

Examples of desired outcomes for clients with self-care deficits might be:

- Client bathes in tub twice weekly with assistance.
- Client participates in self-care (foot hygiene) to optimal level of capacity (specify).

| BOX 22-4 | NURSING CARE CHECKLIST |

Skin Care Guidelines

Dry Skin

- ☑ Use cleansing creams to clean the skin rather than soap or detergent, which cause drying and, in some cases, allergic reactions.
- ☑ Use bath oils, but take precautions to prevent falls caused by slippery tub surfaces.
- ☑ Thoroughly rinse soap or detergent (if used) from the skin.
- ☑ Bathe less frequently when environmental temperature and humidity are low.
- ☑ Increase fluid intake.
- ☑ Humidify the air with a humidifier.
- ☑ Use moisturizing or emollient creams that contain lanolin, petroleum jelly, or cocoa butter to retain skin moisture.

Skin Rashes

- ☑ Keep the area clean by washing it with a mild soap. Rinse the skin well, and pat it dry.
- ☑ To relieve itching, try a tepid bath or soak. Some over-the-counter preparations, such as Caladryl lotion, may help but should be used with full knowledge of the product.
- ☑ Avoid scratching the rash to prevent inflammation, infection, and further skin lesions.
- ☑ Choose clothing carefully. Too much can cause perspiration and aggravate a rash.

Acne

- ☑ Wash the face frequently with mild soap or detergent and water to remove oil and dirt.
- ☑ Avoid using oily creams, which aggravate the condition.
- ☑ Avoid using cosmetics that block the ducts of the sebaceous glands and the hair follicles.
- ☑ Never squeeze or pick at the lesions. This increases the potential for infection and scarring.

- Client reports satisfaction with appearance.
- Client demonstrates nail care as instructed.

Nursing guidelines for providing skin care to clients are listed in Box 22-4 ■.

Bathing

Sponge baths are suggested for the newborn to prevent hypothermia. An infant's ability to regulate body temperature has not yet fully developed. Body surface area is very large in relation to body mass, contributing to heat loss. Infants perspire minimally, and shivering starts at a lower temperature. Therefore, significant heat loss occurs before shivering begins. After the bath, the infant should be immediately dried and wrapped (swaddled) for warmth.

BOX 22-5 **NURSING CARE CHECKLIST**

Changing a Hospital Gown for a Client with an IV Infusion

☑ Slip the gown completely off the arm without the infusion and onto the tubing connected to the arm with the infusion.

☑ Holding the container above the client's arm, slide the sleeve up over the container to remove the used gown.

☑ Place the clean gown sleeve for the arm with the infusion over the container as if it were an extension of the client's arm, from the inside of the gown to the sleeve cuff.

☑ Rehang the container. Slide the gown carefully over the tubing toward the client's hand.

☑ Guide the client's arm and tubing into the sleeve, taking care not to pull on the tubing.

☑ Assist the client to put the other arm into the second sleeve of the gown, and fasten as usual.

☑ Count the rate of flow of the infusion to make sure it is correct before leaving the bedside. Immediately report an incorrect rate of flow to RN.

Caution is needed when bathing clients who are receiving intravenous therapy. Easy-to-remove gowns that have Velcro or snap fasteners along the sleeves may be used. If a special gown is not available, the LPN/LVN must pay special attention when changing the client's gown after the bath (or whenever the gown becomes soiled). These guidelines are provided in Box 22-5 ■. These guidelines do not apply if the client has an IV pump or controller. In this situation, use a special gown or do not put the sleeve of a gown over the client's involved arm.

The water for a bath should feel comfortably warm to the client. People vary in their sensitivity to heat; generally, the temperature should be 43° to 46°C (110° to 115°F). Most clients can verify a comfortable temperature. The water for a bed bath should be changed at least once.

Perineal-Genital Care

Perineal-genital care is also referred to as perineal care or peri-care. Perineal care as part of the bed bath is embarrassing for many clients. LPNs/LVNs also may find it embarrassing initially, particularly with clients of the opposite sex. Most clients who require a bed bath are able to clean their own genital areas with minimal assistance. The LPN/LVN may need to hand a moistened washcloth and soap to the client, rinse the washcloth, and provide a towel.

Because some clients are unfamiliar with terminology for the genitals and perineum, it may be difficult to explain what is expected. Most clients, however, understand what is meant if the LPN/LVN simply says, "I'll give you a

washcloth to finish your bath." Older clients may be familiar with the term "private parts." Whatever expression is used, it needs to be one that the client understands and one that is comfortable for the LPN/LVN to use.

The LPN/LVN needs to provide perineal care efficiently and matter-of-factly. Nurses wear gloves while providing this care, both for the comfort of the client and to protect themselves from infection. Part B of Procedure 22-1 explains how to provide perineal-genital care.

Foot

Interventions may include teaching the client about correct nail and foot care, proper footwear, and ways to prevent potential foot problems (e.g., infection, injury, and decreased circulation). For clients with self-care difficulties, the LPN/LVN plans a schedule for soaking the client's feet and assisting with regular cleaning and trimming of nails (if not contraindicated and within agency policy). Foot and nail care is often provided during the client's bath but may be provided at any time in the day to accommodate the client's preference or schedule. The frequency of foot care is determined by the LPN/LVN and client. It is based on objective assessment data and the client's specific problems. For some clients, the feet need to be bathed daily; for those whose feet perspire excessively, bathing more than once a day may be necessary.

Part C of Procedure 22-1 describes how to provide foot care. (See also discussion of nails.) During these procedures, the LPN/LVN has the opportunity to teach the client appropriate methods for foot care (see Continuing Care on page 433). Clients with reduced peripheral circulation to the feet, such as clients with diabetes or peripheral vascular disease, may require specialized care by a physician or podiatrist. These clients should be discouraged from attempting some aspects of personal foot care and cautioned about "commercial" pedicures, such as at salons or spas.

Nails

One hand or foot is soaked, if needed, and dried. Then the nail is cut or filed straight across beyond the end of the finger or toe (Figure 22-1 ■). Avoid trimming or digging

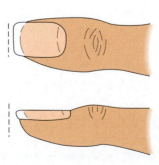

Figure 22-1. ■ Fingernails are trimmed straight across.

BOX 22-6	CLIENT TEACHING

Teaching for Discharge: Foot Care

- Wash the feet daily, and dry them well, especially between the toes.
- When washing, inspect the skin of the feet for breaks or red or swollen areas. Use a mirror if needed to visualize all areas.
- To prevent burns, check the water temperature before immersing the feet.
- Use creams or lotions to moisten the skin, or soak the feet in warm water with Epsom salts to avoid excessive drying of the skin of the feet. Lotion will also soften calluses. A lotion that reduces dryness effectively is a mixture of lanolin and mineral oil.
- To prevent or control an unpleasant odor due to excessive foot perspiration, wash the feet frequently and change socks and shoes at least daily. Special deodorant sprays or absorbent foot powders are also helpful.
- File the toenails rather than cutting them to avoid skin injury. File the nails straight across the ends of the toes. If the nails are too thick or misshapen to file, consult a podiatrist.
- Wear clean stockings or socks daily. Avoid socks with holes or darns that can cause pressure areas.
- Wear correctly fitting shoes that neither restrict the foot nor rub on any area; rubbing can cause corns and calluses. Check worn shoes for rough spots in the lining. Break in new shoes gradually by increasing the wearing time 30 to 60 minutes each day.
- Avoid walking barefoot, because injury and infection may result. Wear slippers in public showers and in change areas to avoid contracting athlete's foot or other infections.
- Several times each day exercise the feet to promote circulation. Point the feet upward, point them downward, and move them in circles.
- Avoid wearing constricting garments such as knee-high elastic stockings and avoid sitting with the legs crossed at the knees, which may decrease circulation.
- When the feet are cold, use extra blankets and wear warm socks rather than using heating pads or hot water bottles, which may cause burns. Test bathwater before stepping into it.
- Wash any cut on the foot thoroughly, apply a mild antiseptic, and notify the physician.
- Avoid self-treatment for corns or calluses. Pumice stones and some callus and corn applications are injurious to the skin. Consult a podiatrist or physician first.
- Notify the physician if you notice abnormal sores or drainage, pain, or changes in temperature, color, and sensation of the foot.

into nails at the lateral corners. (This predisposes the client to ingrown toenails.) File rather than cut the nails of clients who have diabetes or circulatory problems. Inadvertent injury to tissues can occur if scissors are used. After the initial cut or filing, file the nail to round the corners, and clean under the nail. Push the cuticle back gently, taking care not to injure it. Care for the next finger or toe in the same manner. Record and report any abnormality, such as inflammation of the tissue around the nail, to the RN.

EVALUATING

Using data collected during care, the LPN/LVN judges whether desired outcomes have been achieved, and documents changes in self-care. The nurse determines whether the client maintains skin cleanliness, reports satisfaction with appearance, states that feet are not as sore, and so on. If the outcomes are not achieved, the LPN/LVN explores reasons why. For example:

- Did the LPN/LVN overestimate the client's functional abilities (physical, mental, emotional) for self-care?
- Were provided instructions not clear?
- Were appropriate assistive devices or supplies not available to the client?
- Did the client's condition change?
- Were required analgesics provided before hygienic care?

- What currently prescribed medications and therapies could affect the client's abilities or tissue integrity?
- Is the client's fluid and food intake adequate or appropriate to maintain skin and mucous membrane moisture and integrity?

CONTINUING CARE

To provide for continuity of care when a client is to be discharged, the nurse assesses the client's and family's abilities for care. Referrals and home health services may be required. Also, the nurse determines the client's learning needs and provides written or verbal instructions as needed. Use the guidelines listed in Box 22-4 to provide client teaching on general skin care. Clients with impaired circulation or diabetes are especially in need of teaching about foot care (Box 22-6 ■).

NURSING PROCESS CARE PLAN
Client with Diabetes

Gerard Bucholz is a 52-year-old, divorced man who was admitted to the hospital with a nonhealing cut on his left, great toe. The cut occurred when Mr. Bucholz trimmed his toenails a month ago. He is an insulin-dependent diabetic and was diagnosed 6 years ago. It has taken him most of the 6 years to begin managing his diabetes well and to comply with his prescribed diet. Although his blood sugars have been in good control over the last 1.5 years, the high blood sugar in the past has resulted in poor peripheral circulation. His lower extremities are mainly affected, but he does complain of decreased sensation in his fingertips. Mr. Bucholz states, "Nobody ever told me I shouldn't cut my nails."

Assessment. T 98.6, P 72, R 18, BP 130/72. Pedal pulses weak, bilaterally, radial pulses palpable. Feet cold to touch; client denies feeling in toes when touched. Hands cool; client states he has feeling in the tips when touched. Ulcerated area on left, great toe, approximately 2 cm by 2 cm. Skin around and inside ulcer is black; client denies pain. The bone is visible.

Nursing Diagnosis. The following important nursing diagnoses (among others) are established for this client:

- *Impaired Skin Integrity* related to non-healing skin injury
- *Deficient Knowledge* (diabetic nail care) related to possible lack of exposure to information.

Expected Outcomes. The expected outcomes for the plan of care are that Mr. Bucholz will:

- Demonstrate proper nail care.
- Will have no further injuries to the extremities as a result of improper nail care.

Planning and Implementation. The following nursing interventions are implemented for Mr. Bucholz:

- Discuss with client the relationship between diabetes and decreased peripheral circulation.
- Discuss with client other activities that may cause impaired skin integrity, for example, possible burn related to use of a heating pad on areas with impaired circulation, going without proper footwear outside.
- Demonstrate proper nail care techniques to client.
- Supply client with handouts explaining proper nail care techniques and encourage him to keep them in an accessible area at home.

Evaluation. Mr. Bucholz is able to repeat information given to him regarding proper nail care. He has made a monthly appointment with a podiatrist near his home.

Critical Thinking in the Nursing Process

1. What might have helped Mr. Bucholz to avoid cutting himself in the first place?
2. Why is it important to note in the evaluation that Mr. Bucholz has contacted a podiatrist and has a standing appointment?
3. What is the possible consequence of untreated foot injuries for clients with poor peripheral circulation?

Note: Discussion of Critical Thinking questions appears in Appendix I.

Hair Care

The appearance of the hair often reflects a person's feelings or general state of health. A person who feels ill may neglect grooming. Changes in hair texture and volume can result from disease or medication. For example, hypothyroidism may cause excessively thin, dry, or brittle hair. Chemotherapy or radiation to treat cancer often causes hair loss (**alopecia**).

Newborns may have **lanugo** (the fine hair on the body of the fetus, also referred to as down or woolly hair) over their shoulders, back, and sacrum. This generally disappears, and the hair distribution on the eyebrows, head, and eyelashes of young children becomes noticeable. Some newborns have hair on their scalps. Others grow hair over the scalp during the first year.

Pubic hair usually appears in early puberty followed in about 6 months by the growth of axillary hair. Boys develop facial hair in later puberty. In adolescence, sebaceous glands activity increases. Hair follicle openings enlarge to accommodate increased sebum, which can make the adolescent's hair more oily.

In older adults, the hair is generally thinner, grows more slowly, and loses its color as a result of aging tissues and diminishing circulation. Men often lose their scalp hair and may become completely bald. Male baldness is influenced by genetics; it may occur even when a man is relatively young. The older person's hair also tends to become drier. Axillary and pubic hair becomes finer and scanter, but eyebrows become bristly and coarse. Many women develop some facial hair.

NURSING CARE

ASSESSING

During the nursing history, data about usual hair care, self-care abilities, history of hair or scalp problems, and conditions (such as hypothyroidism) that affect the hair are obtained. Questions about medications, hair dyes, and curling or straightening preparations can provide more information to assess dry and brittle hair. Common hair problems follow.

Often accompanied by itching, **dandruff** appears as a diffuse scaling of the scalp. In severe cases, it involves the auditory canals and the eyebrows. Dandruff can usually be treated effectively with a commercial shampoo. In severe or persistent cases, the client may need the advice of a physician.

Hair loss and growth are continual processes. By middle age, some permanent thinning of hair normally occurs.

Baldness, common in men, is thought to be a hereditary problem. Hairpieces, surgical hair transplantation, and various medications address the issue of baldness.

Ticks are small, gray-brown parasites that bite into tissue and suck blood. Ticks transmit several diseases to people, including Rocky Mountain spotted fever, Lyme disease, babesiosis, and tularemia. Ticks should never be forcibly pulled from the skin because the sucking apparatus remains and may become infected. To ease removal, cover the tick with mineral oil or a lubricating jelly such as petroleum jelly. This deprives the tick of oxygen, and allows it to be removed more easily.

Lice are parasitic insects that infest mammals. They are very small, grayish white, and difficult to see. The crab louse in the pubic area has red legs. Lice may be contracted from infested clothes and direct contact with an infested person. Infestation with lice is called **pediculosis**. Hundreds of varieties of lice infest humans. Three common kinds are *Pediculus capitis* (the head louse), *Pediculus corporis* (the body louse), and *Pediculus pubis* (the crab louse).

Pediculus capitis tends to stay hidden in scalp hair; similarly, *Pediculus pubis* stays in pubic hair. Head and pubic lice lay their eggs on the hairs. The eggs are oval, similar to dandruff, and they cling to the hair. Bites and pustular eruptions may be noticed at the hair line and behind the ears. *Pediculus corporis* tends to cling to clothing, so when a client undresses, the lice may not be seen on the body. These lice suck blood from the person and lay their eggs on the clothing. The nurse can suspect their presence in the clothing if (1) the person habitually scratches, (2) there are scratches on the skin, and (3) there are hemorrhagic spots on the skin where the lice have sucked blood.

Gamma benzene hexachloride (Kwell) was widely used for treatment of pediculosis, but serious side effects and parasite resistance with its use were reported. It is more common now to use an over-the-counter preparation such as pyrethrin shampoo. If the client has head lice, the hair is washed with the shampoo and the bed linens are changed. This treatment is repeated 12 to 24 hours later if needed. A client with pubic or body lice takes a bath or shower, dries, and applies the lotion or cream—to the entire body surface for body lice, and to the pubic area and adjacent areas for pubic lice. After 12 to 24 hours the lotion is washed off, and clean clothing and linens are supplied.

Scabies is a contagious skin infestation by the itch mite. The characteristic lesion is the burrow produced by the female mite as it penetrates into the upper layers of the skin. Burrows are short, wavy, brown or black thread-like lesions, usually seen between the webs of the fingers and the folds of the wrists and elbows. The mites cause intense itching. Itching is more pronounced at night,

because the increased warmth of the skin stimulates the parasites. Secondary lesions caused by scratching include vesicles, papules, pustules, excoriations, and crusts. Treatment involves thorough cleansing of the body with soap and water to remove scales and debris from crusts, and then an application of a scabicide lotion. All bed linens and clothing are washed in very hot or boiling water.

> ### clinical ALERT
>
> Because some conditions of the scalp are highly contagious, the nurse should always don gloves for the initial physical assessment of the scalp and hair.

The growth of excessive body hair is called **hirsutism**. The acceptance of body hair in the axillae and on the legs is largely dictated by culture. In North America media, well-groomed women are depicted with no hair on the legs or under axillae. In many other cultures, it is customary for women not to remove this hair. Excessive facial hair on a woman is thought unattractive in most Western and Asian cultures.

The cause of excessive body hair is not always known. Older women may have some on their faces, and women in menopause may also experience the growth of facial hair. These conditions may be due to hormonal changes. Heredity also influences the pattern of hair distribution and the production of androgens by the adrenal glands.

Inflammation, flaking, and itching may also be produced by a fungal infection of the skin. When it appears on the upper body, it is sometimes called "ringworm." When it appears in the groin it is commonly called "jock itch." A fungal infection of the feet produces redness, peeling, and cracking of the skin and is commonly known as "athlete's foot."

DIAGNOSING, PLANNING, AND IMPLEMENTING

Nursing diagnoses related to hair hygiene and hair and scalp problems include:

- *Self-Care Deficit: Grooming*
- *Impaired Skin Integrity*
- *Risk for Infection*
- *Disturbed Body Image.*

Factors such as imposed immobility (bed rest), pain in upper extremities, and insect bite can contribute to these diagnoses.

Examples of desired outcomes might be:

- Client performs hair grooming with assistance (specify).
- Client has reduced or absent scalp lesions or infestations.
- Client takes preventive measures for specific hair problem (e.g., dandruff).

Plans for assisting the client should take into account the client's personal preferences, health, and energy resources as well as the time, equipment, and personnel available. Often, clients like to receive hair care after a bath, before receiving visitors, and before retiring. At some agencies, shampoos can be given to clients only after a physician's order.

Shampooing the Hair

Hair should be washed as often as needed to keep it clean. There are several ways to shampoo clients' hair, depending on their health, strength, and age. The client who is well enough to take a shower can shampoo there. The client who is unable to shower may be given a shampoo while sitting on a chair in front of a sink. The client who must remain in bed can be given a shampoo with water brought to the bedside. Shampoo basins to catch the water and direct it to the washbasin or other receptacle are usually made of plastic or metal. A pail or large washbasin can be used to catch the shampoo water. If possible, the receptacle should be large enough to hold all of the shampoo water so that it does not have to be emptied during the shampoo.

Water used for the shampoo should be 40.5°C (105°F) for an adult or child to be comfortable and not injure the scalp. Usually the client will supply a liquid or cream shampoo. If the shampoo is being given to destroy lice, a medicated shampoo should be used. Dry shampoos are also available. They will remove some of the dirt, odor, and oil. Their main disadvantage is that they dry the hair and scalp.

How often a person needs a shampoo is highly individual, depending largely on the person's activities and the amount of sebum secreted by the scalp. Oily hair tends to look stringy and dirty, and it feels unclean to the person.

Another option available for shampoo for bed rest clients is commercial "bag shampoo." The shampoo solution is in a shower cap that can be warmed in the microwave or a warming device and then used in the same manner as the "bag bath" discussed earlier. After warming, the cap is placed on the client's head for 20 minutes. The nurse massages the client's head through the cap prior to removing. The hair is towel dried and styled. Part A of Procedure 22-2 ■ on page 453 explains how to provide a shampoo for a client confined to bed.

Brushing and Combing Hair

To be healthy, hair needs to be brushed daily. Brushing stimulates the circulation of blood in the scalp, distributes the oil along the hair shaft, and helps to arrange the hair.

For clients confined to bed, hair should be combed and brushed at least once a day to prevent matting. A brush with stiff bristles provides the best stimulation to the scalp, but bristles should not be sharp enough to injure the client's scalp. A comb with dull, even teeth is advisable. Some clients are pleased to have their hair tied neatly in the

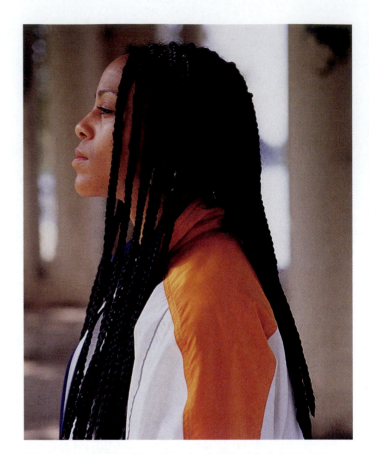

Figure 22-2. ■ An African American's hair styled with braids. (Photographer: Elena Dorfman.)

back or braided until other assistance is available or until they feel better and can look after it themselves.

African American people often have thicker, drier, curlier hair than many Caucasian people. Spiraled or very curly hair may stand out from the scalp and has less strength than straight hair. If straightened, it tends to tangle and mat easily, especially at the back and the sides if the client is confined to bed. Some African Americans style their hair in small braids (Figure 22-2 ■). These braids do not have to be unbraided for shampooing and washing. The LPN/LVN should obtain the client's permission before any such unbraiding. Some people with spiraled hair need to oil their hair daily to prevent hair strands from breaking and the scalp from becoming too dry.

Procedure 22-2, Part B, describes how to provide hair care for African American clients.

Beard and Mustache Care

Beards and mustaches also require daily care. The most important aspect of the care is to keep them clean. Food particles tend to collect in beards and mustaches, and they need washing and combing periodically. Clients may also wish a beard or mustache trim to maintain a well-groomed appearance. A beard or mustache should not be shaved off without the client's consent.

BOX 22-7 | NURSING CARE CHECKLIST

Using a Safety Razor to Shave Facial Hair

☑ Don gloves in case there are facial nicks and contact with blood.

☑ Check client's medication record for drugs in which shaving with a blade is contraindicated (i.e., anticoagulants).

☑ Apply shaving cream or soap and water to soften the bristles and make the skin more pliable.

☑ Hold the skin taut, particularly around creases, to prevent cutting the skin.

☑ Hold the razor so that the blade is at a 45-degree angle to the skin, and shave in short, firm strokes in the direction of hair growth.

☑ After shaving the entire area, wipe the client's face with a wet washcloth to remove any remaining shaving cream and hair.

☑ Dry the face well, then apply aftershave lotion or powder as the client prefers.

☑ To prevent irritating the skin, pat on the lotion with the fingers and avoid rubbing the face.

Male clients often shave or are shaved after a bath. Frequently clients supply their own electric or safety razors. See Box 22-7 ■ for the steps involved in shaving facial hair with a safety razor.

EVALUATING

The nurse collects data to determine whether desired outcomes have been reached.

Mouth Care

Teeth begin to appear 5 to 8 months after birth, and by age 2 years, children usually have all 20 temporary teeth (Figure 22-3A ■). These are gradually replaced by the 32 permanent teeth (Figure 22-3B) by age 25.

The incidence of periodontal disease increases during pregnancy. Many pregnant women experience more bleeding during brushing and increased redness and swelling of the **gingiva** (the gums).

Older adults may lose permanent teeth; some have dentures. Loss of permanent teeth is usually due to periodontal disease (gum disease) rather than dental **caries** (cavities). However, caries are also common in middle-aged adults.

Some receding of the gums and a brownish pigmentation of the gums occur with age. Saliva production decreases with age, so dryness of the oral mucosa is a common finding in older people.

Poor oral hygiene, dry mouth, and poor nutrition are common causes of oral problems. Poor oral hygiene may be the result of a lack of knowledge or illness. Confused, depressed,

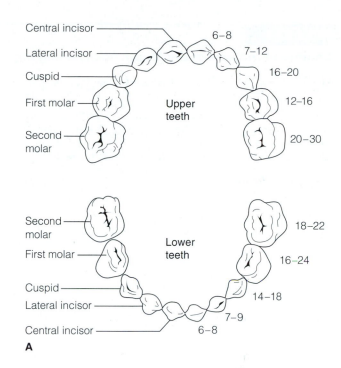
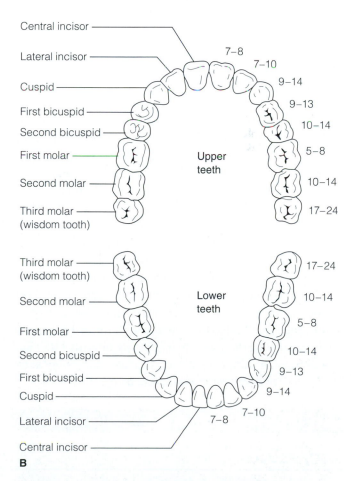

Figure 22-3. ■ A. Temporary teeth and their times of eruption (stated in months). **B.** Permanent teeth and their times of eruption (stated in years).

TABLE 22-2

Common Problems of the Mouth and Nursing Implications

PROBLEM	DESCRIPTION	NURSING IMPLICATIONS
Halitosis	Bad breath	Teach or provide regular oral hygiene.
Glossitis	Inflammation of the tongue	As above
Gingivitis	Inflammation of the gums	As above
Periodontal disease	Gums appear spongy and bleeding	As above; advise client to see a dentist
Reddened or excoriated mucosa		Check for ill-fitting dentures.
Excessive dryness of the buccal mucosa		Increase fluid intake as health permits.
Cheilosis	Cracking of lips	Lubricate lips; use antimicrobial ointment to prevent infection.
Dental caries	Teeth have darkened areas, may be painful	Advise client to see a dentist.
Sordes	Accumulation of foul matter (food, microorganisms, and epithelial elements) in the mouth	Teach or provide regular cleaning.
Stomatitis	Inflammation of the oral mucosa	Teach or provide regular cleaning.
Parotitis	Inflammation of the parotid salivary glands	Teach or provide regular oral hygiene.

physically weak, or comatose clients generally have poor oral hygiene. Clients who have nasogastric tubes, are on oxygen, or breathe through their mouths experience increased oral dryness. Dry mouth is also caused by aging and medication. Older adults experience decreased saliva production and thinning of the oral mucosa. Medications that cause dry mouth include diuretics, laxatives (if used excessively), tranquilizers such as chlorpromazine (Thorazine) and diazepam (Valium), and chemotherapeutic agents to treat cancer. Dry mouth is aggravated by anxiety, poor fluid intake (dehydration), high salt intake, and smoking. Current medications being used to stimulate saliva production include Salagen (pilocarpine HCl) and Evoxac (cevimeline). Poor eating habits, such as excessive intake of salt and refined sugars, can erode tooth enamel, increasing risk. Recent mouth injury or surgery increases the risk of infection. Clients with impaired immune systems (such as those on chemotherapy or with HIV) and those who wear dental appliances (such as retainers) are at increased risk of developing mouth lesions.

NURSING CARE

ASSESSING

Assessment of the client's mouth and hygiene practices includes (1) a nursing history, (2) physical assessment of the mouth, and (3) identification of clients at risk for developing oral problems.

During the nursing history, data are obtained about the client's oral hygiene practices, including dental visits, self-care abilities, and past or current mouth problems. Learning needs and client preferences are also determined. Clients whose hand coordination is impaired, whose cognitive function is impaired, whose illness alters energy levels and motivation, or whose therapy imposes restrictions on activities will need assistance.

Common problems of the mouth and nursing implications are detailed in Table 22-2 ■. For more information about mouth assessment, see also Chapter 19 ⬭.

DIAGNOSING, PLANNING, AND IMPLEMENTING

Three nursing diagnoses related to problems with oral hygiene and the oral cavity are *Self-Care Deficit, Impaired Oral Mucous Membrane,* and *Deficient Knowledge.* NANDA includes oral hygiene in the diagnostic label *Self-Care Deficit: Bathing/Hygiene.* In this book, the diagnosis *Self-Care Deficit: Oral Hygiene* is used for clients who cannot perform oral care independently. This includes the inability to brush or floss teeth or clean dentures.

The diagnosis *Impaired Oral Mucous Membrane* refers to the state in which an individual experiences disruptions in the tissue layers of the oral cavity. Manifestations include a coated tongue; dry mouth; dental caries; **halitosis** (bad breath); gingivitis; oral plaque, pain, discomfort, erythema, lesions or ulcers; and lack of or decreased salivation. These may be the result of inadequate oral hygiene; physical injury or drying effect (e.g., mouth breathing, oxygen therapy); mechanical trauma (e.g., surgery, injury from oral tube, broken teeth or ill-fitting dentures); chemical trauma (e.g., side effects of medications); or radiation injury. The diagnosis *Deficient Knowledge* is discussed in detail in Chapter 33 👁️.

A major goal for clients with oral hygiene or oral problems is to maintain or restore the integrity of the oral tissues and to prevent associated risks. Examples of desired outcomes include:

- Gums are firm, well hydrated, uniform in color, and do not bleed.
- Brushes and flosses teeth after meals and at bedtime.
- Mucosa, tongue, and lips are pink, moist, and intact.

Good oral hygiene includes daily stimulation of the gums, mechanical brushing and flossing of the teeth, and flushing of the mouth. The LPN/LVN is often in a position to help people maintain oral hygiene by helping or teaching them to clean the teeth and oral cavity, and by inspecting whether clients (especially children) have done so. They can provide special oral hygiene for clients who are debilitated, unconscious, or have lesions of the mucous membranes or other oral tissues. (See Procedure 22-2.) The LPN/LVN can also be instrumental in identifying problems that require the intervention of a dentist or oral surgeon and in arranging a referral. These problems should be discussed with the RN before conferring with the physician.

Promoting Oral Health through the Life Span

A major role of the LPN/LVN in promoting oral health is to teach clients about specific oral hygiene measures. Most dentists recommend that dental hygiene should begin when the first tooth erupts and be practiced after each feeding. Cleaning can be accomplished by using a wet washcloth or a cotton ball or small gauze moistened with water.

Dental caries (cavities) occur frequently during the toddler period, often as a result of the excessive intake of sweets or a prolonged use of the bottle during naps and at bedtime. The LPN/LVN should give parents the following instructions to promote and maintain dental health:

- Beginning at about 18 months of age, brush the child's teeth with a soft toothbrush. Use only a toothbrush moistened with water. Introduce toothpaste later; use one that contains fluoride.
- Give a fluoride supplement daily or as recommended by the physician or dentist, unless the drinking water is fluoridated.
- Schedule an initial dental visit for the child at about 2 or 3 years of age, as soon as all 20 primary teeth have erupted.

- Some dentists recommend an inspection type of visit when the child is about 18 months old to provide an early pleasant introduction to the dental examination.
- Seek professional dental attention for any problems such as discoloring of the teeth, chipping, or signs of infection such as redness and swelling.

Because deciduous teeth guide the entrance of permanent teeth, dental care for preschoolers and school-age children is essential to keep these teeth in good repair. Abnormally placed or lost deciduous teeth can cause misalignment of permanent teeth. Fluoride helps prevent dental caries. Preschoolers need to be taught to brush their teeth after eating, and parents should limit the child's intake of refined sugars. Regular dental checkups are required during these years when permanent teeth appear.

Proper diet and mouth care should be taught to adolescents and adults.

Care of Teeth

Brushing and Flossing the Teeth

Thorough brushing of the teeth is important in preventing tooth decay. The mechanical action of brushing removes food particles that can harbor and incubate bacteria. It also stimulates circulation in the gums, maintaining their healthy firmness. Fluoride toothpaste is often recommended because of its antibacterial protection. An effective toothpaste can also be made by combining two parts table salt to one part baking soda. (However, this paste is not to be used by clients on sodium-restricted diets.) Part A of Procedure 22-3 ■ on page 455 provides instruction in brushing and flossing the client's teeth

Caring for Dentures

Dentures (a "plate" of artificial teeth for one jaw) may be worn to replace upper or lower teeth or both. When only a few artificial teeth are needed, a "bridge" may be worn. Bridges may be fixed or removable. Clients should always be encouraged to wear their dentures (or other oral prostheses) to prevent gum shrinkage and further tooth loss.

Like natural teeth, dentures collect microorganisms and food. They need to be cleaned at least once a day. Dentures may be removed, scrubbed with a toothbrush, rinsed, and reinserted. Some people use toothpaste; others use commercial cleaning compounds or soaking solutions for plates. Always rinse dentures thoroughly before inserting into the mouth, especially after soaking. Procedure 22-3B describes how to clean dentures.

Assisting Clients with Oral Care

When providing mouth care for partially or totally dependent clients, the LPN/LVN should wear gloves. Required equipment includes a curved basin that fits snugly under the client's chin (e.g., a kidney basin) to receive the rinse water and a towel to protect the client and the bedclothes (see Procedure 22-3A). Foam swabs are often used in health-care agencies to clean the mouths of dependent clients. These swabs are convenient and effective in removing excess debris from the teeth and mouth but should be used infrequently and for short periods (i.e., less than 3 days); foam swabs are not as effective as a toothbrush in removing plaque from "sheltered" areas of the teeth and gingival crevices.

Most people prefer privacy when they take their artificial teeth out to clean them. Many do not like to be seen without their teeth. One of the first requests of many postoperative clients is "May I have my teeth in, please?"

For the client who is debilitated or unconscious or who has excessive dryness, sores, or irritations of the mouth, it may be necessary to clean the oral mucosa and tongue in addition to the teeth. Agency practices differ in regard to special mouth care and the frequency with which it is provided. Depending on the health of the client's mouth, special care may be needed every 2 to 8 hours. Mouth care for unconscious or debilitated people is important because their mouths tend to become dry and consequently predisposed to infections. Dryness occurs because the client cannot take fluids by mouth, is often breathing through the mouth, or may be receiving oxygen, which tends to dry the mucous membranes. The nurse can request an order for humidified oxygen to decrease dryness for the client.

The LPN/LVN can use commercially prepared applicators of lemon oil juice and oil glycerin to clean the mucous membranes. If these are unavailable, a gauze square wrapped around a tongue blade and dipped into lemon juice and oil or into mouthwash usually suffices. Note, however, that most commercial mouthwashes contain alcohol, which can lead to further dryness of the mucosa. An alcohol-free mouthwash is usually available from agency pharmacies or central supply units. Mineral oil is contraindicated because aspiration could cause an infection. Hydrogen peroxide is not recommended for use in oral care, because it irritates healthy oral mucosa and may alter the microflora of the mouth (Tombes & Gallucci, 1993). Normal saline solution is recommended for oral hygiene for the dependent client.

Procedure 22-3C focuses on oral care for the unconscious client but may be adapted for conscious clients who are seriously ill or have mouth problems.

EVALUATING

To evaluate care of the mouth, data are collected on the status of oral mucosa, lips, tongue, and teeth. The nursing team determines whether desired outcomes have been achieved. If they are not achieved, the RN, LPN/LVN, and client explore the reasons. The care plan may be modified.

Eye Care

Normally eyes require no special hygiene, because *lacrimal fluid* (tears) continually washes the eyes, and because the eyelids and lashes prevent the entrance of foreign particles. However, special interventions are needed for unconscious clients and for clients recovering from eye surgery or having eye injuries, irritations, or infections. In unconscious clients, the blink reflex may be absent, and excessive drainage may accumulate along eyelid margins. In clients with eye trauma or eye infections, excessive discharge or drainage is common. Excessive secretions on the lashes need to be removed before they dry on the lashes as crusts. Clients who wear eyeglasses, contact lenses, or an artificial eye also may require instruction and care by the LPN/LVN.

NURSING CARE

ASSESSING

During the nursing history, the RN obtains data about the client's eyeglasses or contact lenses, recent examination by an ophthalmologist, and any history of eye problems and related treatments. In the physical assessment, all external eye structures are inspected for signs of inflammation, excessive drainage, encrustations, or other obvious abnormalities. Inspection of the external eye structures is detailed in Chapter 19 ∞.

DIAGNOSING, PLANNING, AND IMPLEMENTING

Nursing diagnoses related to eye problems may include

- *Self-Care Deficit* (such as contact lens insertion, removal, and cleaning)
- *Risk for Infection* (as with accumulation of secretions on eyelids)
- *Risk for Injury* (for example, related to absence of the blink reflex associated with unconsciousness).

Nursing activities are identified that will assist the client in maintaining the integrity of the eye structures or a prosthesis and in preventing eye injury and infection. Nursing activities may include teaching clients about how to insert, clean, and remove contact lenses or a prosthesis, and ways to protect the eyes from injury and strain. Examples of desired outcomes to evaluate the effectiveness of nursing interventions follow:

- Eyelids free of secretions
- No eye discomfort
- Demonstrates appropriate methods of caring for contact lenses.

Eye Care for the Comatose Client

When a comatose client's corneal reflex is impaired, eye care is essential to keep moist the areas of the cornea that are exposed to air.

- ☑ Administer moist compresses to cover the eyes every 2 to 4 hours.
- ☑ Clean the eyes with saline solution and cotton balls. Wipe from the inner to outer canthus. This prevents debris from being washed into the nasolacrimal duct.
- ☑ Use a new cotton ball for each wipe. This prevents extending infection in one eye or to the other eye.
- ☑ Instill ophthalmic ointment or artificial tears into the lower lids as ordered. This keeps the eyes moist.
- ☑ If the client's corneal reflex is absent, keep the eyes moist with artificial tears and protect the eye with a protective shield. These should be ordered by a physician.
- ☑ Monitor the eyes for redness, exudate, or ulceration.

Eye Care

When giving eye care, always wear clean gloves. Dried secretions that have accumulated on the lashes need to be softened and wiped away. Soften dried secretions by placing a sterile cotton ball moistened with sterile water or normal saline over the lid margins. Wipe the loosened secretions from the inner canthus of the eye to the outer canthus to prevent the particles and fluid from draining into the lacrimal sac and nasolacrimal duct.

If the client is unconscious and lacks a blink reflex or cannot close the eyelids completely, drying and irritation of the cornea must be prevented. Lubricating eye drops may be ordered. See the Box 22-8 ■ for eye care for the comatose client.

Eyeglass Care

It is essential to exercise caution when cleaning eyeglasses to prevent breaking or scratching the lenses. Glass lenses can be cleaned with warm water and dried with a soft tissue that will not scratch the lenses. Plastic lenses are more easily scratched; they may require special cleaning solutions and drying tissues. When not being worn, all glasses should be placed in a case that is labeled appropriately. They should be stored in the client's bedside table drawer.

Contact Lens Care

Contact lenses, thin curved disks of hard or soft plastic, fit on the cornea of the eye directly over the pupil. They float on the tear layer of the eye. For some people, contact lenses offer several advantages over eyeglasses. They cannot be seen and thus have cosmetic value. They are highly effective in correcting some astigmatisms. They are safer than glasses for some physical activities. They do not fog, as eyeglasses do. They provide better vision in many cases.

Contact lenses may be either hard or soft or a compromise between the two types—gas-permeable (GP) lenses. Hard contact lenses are made of a rigid, unwettable, airtight plastic that does not absorb water or saline solutions. They usually cannot be worn for more than 12 to 14 hours and are rarely recommended for first-time wearers.

Soft contact lenses cover the entire cornea. Because they are more pliable and soft, they mold to the eye for a firmer fit. The duration of extended wear varies by brand from 1 to 30 days or more. Eye specialists recommend that long-wear brands be removed and cleaned at least once a week. These lenses require very careful care and handling.

GP lenses are rigid enough to provide clear vision but are more flexible than the traditional hard lens. They permit oxygen to reach the cornea, thus providing greater comfort, and will not cause serious damage to the eye if left in place for several days.

Most clients normally care for their own contact lenses. In general, each lens manufacturer provides detailed cleaning instructions. Depending on the type of lens and cleaning method, warm tap water, normal saline, or special rinsing or soaking solutions may be used.

clinical ALERT

Never substitute saline marked "for injection" as a wetting or cleansing solution. Injectable saline may harm soft lenses or the client's eye.

All users should have a special container for their lenses. Each lens container has a slot with a label indicating whether it is for the right or left lens. Lenses must be stored in the appropriate slot so that they are placed in the correct eye.

Removing Contact Lenses

Hard contact lenses must be positioned directly over the cornea for proper removal. If the lens is displaced, the LPN/LVN asks the client to look straight ahead, and gently exerts pressure on the upper and lower lids to move the lens back onto the cornea. Figures 22-4A–C ■ show the steps needed to remove a hard lens. To avoid lens mixups, always place the first lens in its designated storage cup before removing the second lens.

Soft lenses can be removed in two ways. First, after separating the eyelids with the nondominant hand, move the lens down to the inferior part of the sclera using the pad of

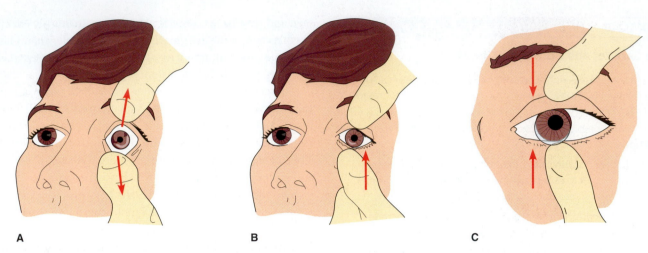

Figure 22-4. ■ Removing hard contact lenses: **A.** Separate the eyelids until they are beyond the edge of the lens. **B.** Hold the top eyelid stationary at the edge to the lens, and lift the bottom edge of the contact lens by pressing the lower lid at its margin. **C.** After the lens is slightly tipped, slide the lens out of the eye by moving both eyelids toward each other.

the dominant index finger (Figure 22-5A ■). This reduces the risk of damage to the cornea. Second, remove the lens by gently pinching it between the pads of the thumb and index finger of your dominant hand (Figure 22-5B). Pinching causes the lens to double up, so that air entering under the lens overcomes the suction and allows removal. Use the pads of the fingers to prevent scratching the eye or the lens with the fingernails.

Inserting Contact Lenses

Seriously ill clients whose contact lenses have been removed do not need them reinserted until they become more active in their care and require the lenses to see properly. Contact lenses need to be lubricated in a sterile, nonirritating wetting solution (usually a saline solution) before they are in-

serted. The wetting solution helps the lens glide over the cornea and reduces the risk of injury. Most clients, when well, will reinsert the lenses independently.

Artificial Eyes

Artificial eyes are usually made of glass or plastic. Some are permanently implanted; others are removed regularly for cleaning. Most clients who wear a removable artificial eye follow their own care regimen. Even for an unconscious client, daily removal and cleaning are not necessary.

To remove an artificial eye, the LPN/LVN dons clean gloves and uses the dominant thumb to pull the client's lower eyelid down over the infraorbital bone, exerting slight pressure below the eyelid to overcome the suction in the eye socket

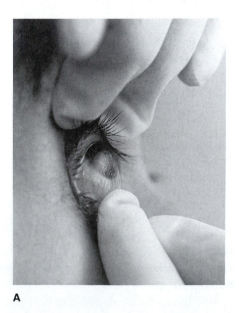

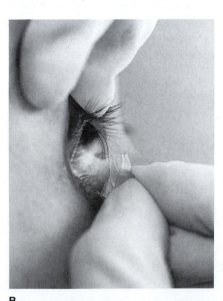

Figure 22-5. ■ **A.** Moving a soft lens down to the inferior part of the sclera. **B.** Removing a soft lens by pinching it between the pads of the thumb and index finger. (Photographer: William Thompson.)

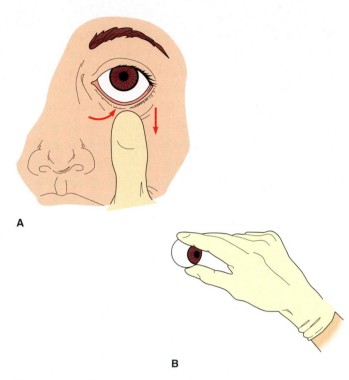

A

B

Figure 22-6. ■ A. Remove an artificial eye by retracting the lower eyelid and exerting slight pressure below the eyelid. **B.** Hold an artificial eye between the thumb and index finger for insertion.

(Figure 22-6A ■). An alternate method is to compress a small rubber bulb and apply the tip directly to the eye. As the pressure on the bulb is gradually released, the suction of the bulb counteracts the suction to draw the eye out of the socket.

The eye is cleaned with warm normal saline and placed in a container filled with water or saline solution. The socket and tissues around the eye are usually cleaned with cotton wipes and normal saline. To reinsert the eye, the thumb and index finger of one hand are used to retract the eyelids, exerting pressure on the supraorbital and infraorbital bones. The nurse holds the eye between the thumb and index finger of the other hand and slips the eye gently into the socket (Figure 22-6B).

EVALUATING

Evaluation of the eyes is part of a regular head-to-toe or body systems assessment. Any unusual redness, discharge, or pain should be documented and reported to the team leader. Changes in vision or unusual dryness should be noted.

CONTINUING CARE

Many clients may need to learn specific information about care of the eyes. The nurse can provide these general guidelines:

- Avoid home remedies for eye problems. Eye irritations or injuries at any age should be treated medically and immediately.

- If dirt or dust gets into the eyes, clean them copiously with clean, tepid water as an emergency treatment.
- Take measures to guard against eyestrain and to protect vision, such as maintaining adequate lighting for reading and obtaining shatterproof lenses for glasses.
- Schedule regular eye examinations, particularly after age 40, to detect problems such as cataracts and glaucoma.

Ear Care

Normal ears require minimal hygiene. Clients who have excessive **cerumen** (earwax) and dependent clients who have hearing aids may require assistance with hygiene tasks. Hearing aids are usually removed before surgery.

CLEANING THE EARS

The auricles of the ear are cleaned during the bed bath. The LPN/LVN or client removes excessive cerumen that is visible or that causes discomfort or hearing difficulty. Visible cerumen may be loosened and removed by retracting the auricle downward. If this measure is ineffective, irrigation is necessary (see the section on otic irrigation in Chapter 29 ⚭, Medications). Clients should be advised never to use bobby pins, toothpicks, or cotton-tipped applicators to remove cerumen. Bobby pins and toothpicks can injure the ear canal and rupture the tympanic membrane. Cotton-tipped applicators can cause wax to become impacted within the canal.

CARE OF HEARING AIDS

A **hearing aid** is a battery-powered, sound-amplifying device used by people with hearing impairments (Figures 22-7A and B ■). It consists of a microphone that picks up sound and converts it to electric energy, an amplifier that magnifies the electric energy electronically, a receiver that converts the amplified energy back to sound energy, and an earmold that directs the sound into the ear. There are several types of hearing aids. They may be positioned in or behind the ear or on the body.

Procedure 22-4 ■ on page 459 describes how to remove, clean, and insert a hearing aid.

Nose Care

The LPN/LVN usually does not need to provide special care for the nose. Clients can ordinarily clear nasal secretions by blowing gently into a soft tissue. When the external nares are encrusted with dried secretions, they should be cleaned with a cotton-tipped applicator or moistened with saline or water. The applicator should not be inserted beyond the length of the cotton tip; inserting it further may cause injury to the mucosa.

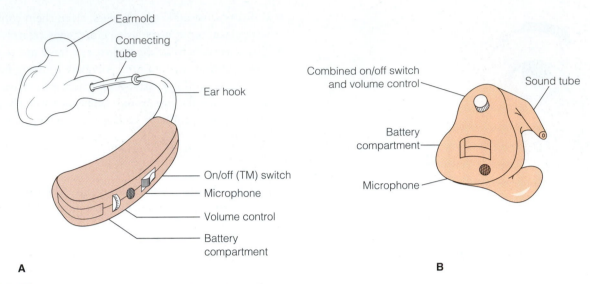

Earmold
Connecting tube
Ear hook
On/off (TM) switch
Microphone
Volume control
Battery compartment

Combined on/off switch and volume control
Sound tube
Battery compartment
Microphone

A

B

Figure 22-7. ▪ **A.** A behind-the-ear hearing aid. **B.** An in-the-ear hearing aid.

Supporting a Hygienic Environment

Because ill people are usually confined to bed, often for long periods, the bed becomes an important element in the client's life. A place that is clean, safe, and comfortable contributes to the client's ability to rest and sleep and to a sense of well-being. Basic furniture in a healthcare facility includes the bed, bedside table, overbed table, one or more chairs, and a storage space for clothing. Most bed units also have a call light, light fixtures, electric outlets, and hygienic equipment in the bedside table. Three types of equipment that are often installed in an acute care facility are a suction outlet for several kinds of suction, an oxygen outlet for most oxygen equipment, and a sphygmomanometer (blood pressure cuff and gauge) to measure the client's blood pressure. Some long-term care agencies also permit clients to have personal furniture, such as a television, a chair, and lamps, at the bedside. In the home, a client often has personal and medical equipment.

To provide a comfortable environment, it is important to consider the client's age, severity of illness, and level of activity. The very young, the very old, and the acutely ill frequently need a room temperature higher than normal. A room temperature between 20° and 23°C (68° and 74°F) is comfortable for most clients.

Good ventilation is important to remove unpleasant odors and stale air. For example, odors caused by urine, draining wounds, or vomitus can be offensive. Room deodorizers can help eliminate odors, but good hygienic practices are the best way to prevent offensive body and breath odors. Hospitals are required to restrict smoking. Hospitals often have an outside staff and visitors smoking area. Smoking in client rooms is prohibited; with a physician's order, a client may be taken outside to smoke.

Certain clients may benefit from specially ventilated rooms. Infection can be contained by using special rooms with different types of air pressure, depending on the type of infection. A negative-pressure room is used for clients with highly communicable disease. This negative pressure filters the contamination without allowing it to pass out of the room into other areas. Positive-pressure rooms keep the contamination out; they are used for clients who are vulnerable to infection, such as those who have just undergone transplant surgery.

Ill persons are usually sensitive to noise such as clanging of metal equipment, loud talking, and laughter. The nursing staff always tries to control noise in healthcare settings. (See Chapter 32 ⚭.)

HOSPITAL BEDS

The frame of a hospital bed is divided into three sections. This permits the head and the foot to be elevated separately. Most hospital beds have electric motors to operate the movable joints. The motor is activated by pressing a button or by moving a small lever, located either at the side of the bed, in the side rail, or on a small panel separate from the bed but attached to it by a cable, which the client can readily use. Common bed positions are described in Table 22-3 ▪.

Hospital beds are usually narrower than the usual bed, so that the nursing staff can reach the client from either side of the bed without undue stretching. The length is usually 1.9 m (6.5 ft). Some beds can be extended in length to accommodate very tall clients. Long-term care facilities for ambulatory clients usually have low beds to facilitate movement in and out of bed. Most hospital beds have "high" and "low" positions that can be adjusted either mechanically or electrically by a button or lever. The high position permits the nursing staff to reach the client without undue stretching or stooping. The low position allows the client to step easily to the floor.

TABLE 22-3		
Commonly Used Bed Positions		
POSITION	DESCRIPTION	INDICATIONS FOR USE
Flat	Mattress is completely horizontal.	Client sleeping in a variety of bed positions, such as back-lying, side-lying, and prone (face down)
		To maintain spinal alignment for clients with spinal injuries
		To assist clients to move and turn in bed
		Bed-making by LPN/LVN
Fowler's position	Semisitting position in which head of bed is raised to angle of at least 45°. Knees may be flexed or horizontal.	Convenient for eating, reading, visiting, watching TV
		Relief from lying positions
		To promote lung expansion for client with respiratory problem
		To assist a client to a sitting position on the edge of the bed
Semi-Fowler's position	Head of bed is raised only to 30° angle.	Relief from lying position
		To promote lung expansion
Trendelenburg's position	Head of bed is lowered and the foot raised in a straight incline.	To promote venous circulation in certain clients
		To provide postural drainage of basal lung lobes
Reverse Trendelenburg's position	Head of bed raised and the foot lowered. Straight tilt in direction opposite to Trendelenburg's position.	To promote stomach emptying and prevent esophageal reflux in client with hiatal hernia

Mattresses

Mattresses are usually covered with a water-repellent material that resists soiling and can be cleaned easily. Most mattresses have handles on the sides, called "lugs," by which the mattress can be moved. Many special mattresses are also used in hospitals to relieve pressure on the body's bony prominences, such as the heels. They are particularly helpful for clients confined to bed for a long time. For additional information about mattresses, see Chapter 23, Table 23-5 🔗.

Side Rails

Side rails, or safety sides, are used on both hospital beds and stretchers. They are of various shapes and sizes and are usually made of metal. Devices to raise and lower them differ. When side rails are being used, it is crucial that the client's bedside is never elevated while the rail is lowered. Some agencies have a release form that the client can sign if the use of side rails is refused.

Footboard or Footboot

Footboards are used to support the immobilized client's foot in a normal right angle to the legs to prevent plantar flexion contractures.

Bed Cradles

A **bed cradle**, sometimes called an Anderson frame, is a device designed to keep the top bedclothes off the feet, legs, and even abdomen of a client (e.g., a client with a skin condition in which contact with covers could cause pain or irritation). The bedclothes are arranged over the device and may be pinned in place. There are several types of bed cradles. One of the most common is a curved metal rod that fits over the bed. Part of the cradle fits under the mattress, and small metal brackets press down on each side of the mattress to keep the cradle in place. The frame of some cradles extends over half of the width of the bed, above one leg.

INTRAVENOUS RODS

Intravenous (IV) rods (poles, stands, standards), usually made of metal, support IV infusion containers while fluid is being administered to a client. These rods were traditionally freestanding on the floor beside the bed. Now, intravenous rods are often attached to the hospital beds. Some special care units have overhead hanging rods on a track for IVs.

MAKING BEDS

The LPN/LVN needs to be able to prepare hospital beds in different ways for specific purposes. In most instances, beds are made after the client receives certain care and when beds are unoccupied. However, at times it may be necessary to make an occupied bed or prepare a bed for a client who is having surgery (an anesthetic, postoperative, or surgical bed). No matter what type of bed equipment is available, whether the bed is occupied or unoccupied, or why the bed is being prepared, certain guidelines apply. The guidelines for bed-making are summarized in the Box 22-9 ■.

An unoccupied bed can be either closed or open. Generally the top covers of an *open bed* are folded back (thus the term open bed) to make it easier for a client to get in. Open and closed beds are made the same way, except that the top sheet, blanket, and bedspread of a *closed bed* are drawn up to the top of the bed and under the pillows.

A surgical or postoperative bed is similar to an open bed. The purpose is to be able to transfer the postoperative client into the bed easily. The top sheet is not tucked or mitered at the bottom of the bed. The top sheets can be folded low at the bottom to be pulled up over the client or folded lengthwise to be pulled across the client.

Beds are often changed after bed baths, although the linen is not usually changed unless it is soiled. Check the policy at each clinical agency. Unfitted sheets, blankets, and bedspreads are *mitered* at the corners of the bed. The purpose of mitering is to secure the bedclothes while the bed is occupied. Figure 22-8 ■ shows how to miter the corner of a bed.

Part A of Procedure 22-5 ■ on page 460 explains how to change an unoccupied bed.

BOX 22-9	NURSING CARE CHECKLIST

Bed-Making and Infection Control Issues

☑ Wash hands thoroughly after handling a client's bed linen. Linens and equipment that have been soiled with secretions and excretions harbor microorganisms that can be transmitted to others directly or by the LPN's/LVN's hands or uniform.

☑ Hold soiled linen away from uniform.

☑ Linen for one client is never (even momentarily) placed on another client's bed.

☑ Place soiled linen directly in a portable linen hamper or tucked into a pillowcase at the end of the bed before it is gathered up for disposal.

☑ Do not shake soiled linen in the air because shaking can disseminate secretions and excretions and the microorganisms they contain.

☑ When stripping and making a bed, conserve time and energy by stripping and making up one side as much as possible before working on the other side.

☑ To avoid unnecessary trips to the linen supply area, gather all linen before starting to strip a bed.

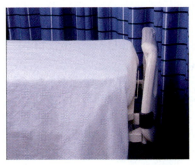

A

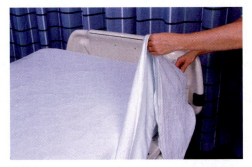

B

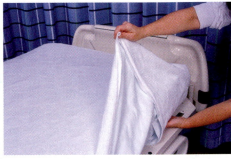

C

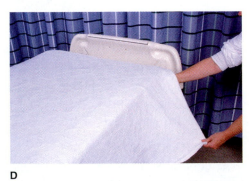

D

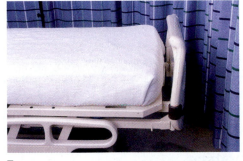

E

Figure 22-8. ■ Mitering the corner of a bed: **A.** Tuck in the bedcover (sheet, blanket, and/or spread) firmly under the mattress at the bottom or top of the bed. **B.** Lift the bedcover at point 1 so that it forms a triangle with the side edge of the bed and the edge of the bedcover is parallel to the end of the bed. **C.** Tuck the part of the cover that hangs below the mattress under the mattress while holding the cover against the side of the mattress. **D.** Bring point 1 down toward the floor while the other hand holds the fold of the cover against the side of the mattress. **E.** Remove the hand and tuck the remainder of the cover under the mattress, if appropriate. The side of the top sheet, blanket, and bedspread may be left hanging freely rather than tucked in. The bedspread is mitered separately and left hanging freely if the top sheet and blanket are tucked in.

Changing an Occupied Bed

Some clients may be too weak to get out of bed because of the nature of their illness. Others may be restricted in bed by the presence of traction or other therapies. When changing an occupied bed, the LPN/LVN works quickly and disturbs the client as little as possible. To conserve the client's energy, use the following guidelines:

- Maintain the client in good body alignment. Never move or position a client in a manner that is contraindicated by the client's health. Obtain help if necessary to ensure safety.

- Move the client gently and smoothly. Rough handling can cause the client discomfort and abrade the skin.
- Throughout the procedure, explain what you plan to do before you do it. Use terms that the client can understand.
- Use the bed-making time, like the bed bath time, to assess and meet the client's needs.

Part B of Procedure 22-5 describes how to change an occupied bed.

Note: The references and resources for this and all chapters have been compiled at the back of the book.

Bathing Clients

Purposes

- To remove transient microorganisms, body secretions and excretions, dead skin cells, and normal secretions and odors
- To stimulate circulation to the skin
- To produce a sense of well-being
- To promote relaxation and comfort
- To prevent or eliminate unpleasant body odors
- To maintain skin integrity

Equipment

- Bedpan or urinal
- Changing table
- Bath blanket
- Gloves (if giving perineal care)
- Washcloth
- Soap
- Washbasin
- Water between 43° and 46°C (110° and 115°F) for adults, 38° and 40°C (100° and 105°F) for children
- Two bath towels
- Additional bed linen and towels, if required
- Hygiene supplies such as lotion and deodorant
- Clean gown or pajamas as needed
- Cotton balls or swabs
- Solution bottle, pitcher, or container filled with warm water or a prescribed solution
- Bedpan to receive rinse water
- Moisture-resistant bag or receptacle for used cotton swabs
- Moisture-resistant disposable pad
- Pillow (optional)

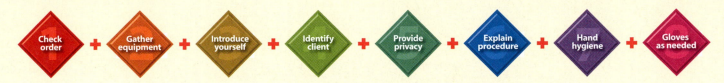

Check order + Gather equipment + Introduce yourself + Identify client + Provide privacy + Explain procedure + Hand hygiene + Gloves as needed

Part A: Bathing an Adult or Pediatric Client

Interventions

1. Prepare the client and the environment.
   - Invite a parent or family member to participate if desired.
   - Close the windows and doors to make sure that the room is free from drafts. *Air currents increase loss of heat from the body by convection.*
   - Provide privacy by drawing the curtains or closing the door. *Hygiene is a personal matter. Some agencies provide signs indicating the need for privacy.*
   - Offer the client a bedpan or urinal or ask whether the client wishes to use the toilet or commode. *The client will be more comfortable after voiding, and voiding before cleaning the perineum is advisable.*
   - During the bath, assess each area of the skin carefully.

FOR A BED BATH

2. Prepare the bed, and position the client appropriately.
   - Place the bed in the high position. Place an infant or small child on a changing table or elevated crib. *This avoids undue strain on the LPN's/LVN's back.*
   - Remove the top bed linen and replace it with the bath blanket. If the bed linen is to be reused, place it over the bedside chair. If it is to be changed, place it in the linen hamper.

- Assist the client to move near you. *This helps prevent undue reaching and straining.*
   - Remove the client's gown.

3. Make a bath mitt with the washcloth (Figure 22-9 ■). *A bath mitt retains water and heat better than a loosely held cloth.*
   - Triangular method: (1) Lay your hand on the washcloth; (2) fold the top corner over your hand; (3,4) fold the side corners over your hand; and (5) tuck the second corner under the cloth on the palmar side to secure the mitt.
   - Rectangular method: (1) Lay your hand on the washcloth and fold one side over your hand; (2) fold the second side over your hand; (3) fold the top of the cloth down; and (4) tuck it under the folded side against your palm to secure the mitt.

4. Wash the face.
   - Place one towel across the client's chest.
   - Wash the client's eyes with water only and dry them well. Use a separate corner of the washcloth for each eye. *Using separate corners prevents transmitting microorganisms from one eye to the other.* Wipe from the inner to the outer canthus. *Cleaning from the inner to the outer canthus prevents secretions from entering the nasolacrimal ducts.*

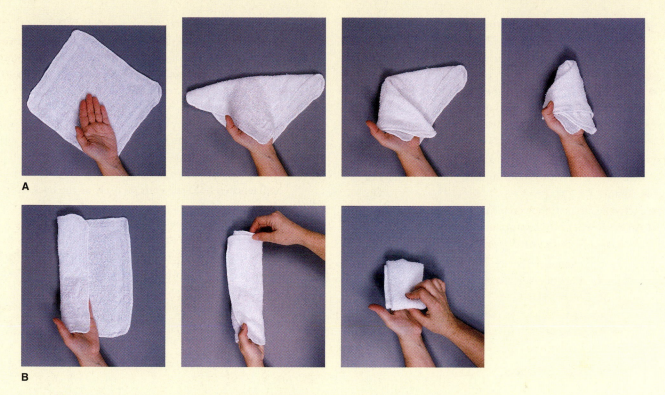

Figure 22-9. ■ Making a bath mitt: **A.** triangular method; **B.** rectangular method.

- Ask whether the client wants soap used on the face. *Soap has a drying effect, and the face, which is exposed to the air more than other body parts, tends to be drier.*
- Wash, rinse, and dry the client's face, neck, and ears.

5. Wash the arms and hands. (Omit the arms for a partial bath.)
   - Place the bath towel lengthwise under the arm. *It protects the bed from becoming wet.*
   - Wash, rinse, and dry the arm, using long, firm strokes from distal to proximal areas (from the point farthest from the body to the point closest). *Firm strokes from distal to proximal areas increase venous blood return.*
   - Wash the axilla well. Repeat for the other arm. Exercise caution if an intravenous infusion is present, and check its flow after moving the arm. Immediately report any problems with the IV to the RN.
   - Place a towel directly on the bed and put the basin on it. Place the client's hands in the basin. *Many clients enjoy immersing their hands in the basin and washing themselves. Assist the client as needed to wash, rinse, and dry the hands, paying particular attention to the spaces between the fingers.*

6. Wash the chest and abdomen. (Omit the chest and abdomen for a partial bath. However, the areas under a woman's breast may require bathing if they are irritated.)
   - Fold the bath blanket down to the client's pubic area, and place the towel alongside the chest and abdomen.
   - Wash, rinse, and dry the chest and abdomen, giving special attention to the skinfold under the breasts. Keep the chest and abdomen covered with the towel between the wash and the rinse.

- Replace the bath blanket when the areas have been dried. Avoid undue exposure when washing the chest and abdomen. For some clients, it may be preferable to wash the chest and the abdomen separately. In that case, place the bath towel horizontally across the abdomen first and then across the chest.

7. Wash the legs and feet. (Omit legs and feet for a partial bath.)
   - Wrap one of the client's legs and feet with the bath blanket, ensuring that the pubic area is well covered.
   - Place the bath towel lengthwise under the other leg, and wash that leg. Use long, smooth, firm strokes, washing from the ankle to the knee to the thigh. *Washing from distal to proximal areas stimulates venous blood flow.*
   - Rinse and dry that leg, reverse the coverings, and repeat for the other leg.
   - Wash the feet by placing them in the basin of water.
   - Dry each foot. Pay particular attention to the spaces between the toes. If you prefer, wash one foot after that leg, before washing the other leg.
   - Obtain fresh, warm bathwater now or when necessary. *Water may become dirty or cold. Because surface skin cells are removed with washing, the bathwater from dark-skinned clients may be dark; however, this does not mean the client is dirty.*

8. Wash the back and then the perineum.
   - Assist the client to turn to a prone position or side-lying position facing away from you, and place the bath towel lengthwise alongside the back and buttocks.

■ Wash and dry the back, buttocks, and upper thighs, paying particular attention to the gluteal folds. Avoid undue exposure of the client, as for the abdomen and chest in step 6.

■ Assist the client to the supine position, and determine whether the client can wash the perineal-genital area independently. If the client cannot do so, drape the client as shown in Figure 22-10 and wash the area. See also Procedure 22-1B.

9. Assist the client with grooming aids such as lotion or deodorant.

■ Help the client to put on a clean gown or pajamas.

■ Assist the client to care for hair, mouth, and nails. *Some people prefer or need mouth care prior to the bath.*

10. Document pertinent data.

■ Record assessments, such as excoriation in the folds beneath the breasts or reddened areas over bony prominences and report changes to the RN.

■ Record the type of bath given (i.e., complete, partial, or self-help). *This is usually recorded on a flow sheet.*

FOR A TUB BATH OR SHOWER

11. Prepare the client and the tub.

■ Fill the tub about one-third to one-half full of water at 43° to 46°C (110° to 115°F). *Sufficient water is needed to cover the perineal area.*

■ Cover all intravenous catheters or wound dressings with plastic coverings, and instruct client to prevent wetting these areas if possible.

■ Obtain assistance with holding a pediatric client as indicated. *Holding minimizes contamination of open skin areas.*

■ Apply a rubber bath mat or towel to the floor of the tub if safety strips are not on tub floor. *These prevent the client from slipping during the bath or shower.*

■ Use a small basin or large sink for a small child. *Smaller containers decrease the danger of slipping and possible drowning.*

12. Assist the client into the shower or tub.

■ Assist the client taking a standing shower with the initial adjustment of the water temperature and water flow pressure, as needed. *Some clients need a chair to sit in the shower because of weakness. Elderly people often feel faint under hot water.*

■ If the client requires considerable assistance with a tub bath, additional staff may be needed. To provide support as the client sits down in the tub, fold a towel lengthwise and place it around the chest under both axillae; then hold the ends securely at the back as the client sits. It may be helpful to seat the client on the edge of the tub or on a chair beside the tub before transferring the client into the tub.

■ Explain how the client can signal for help, leave the client for 2 to 5 minutes, and place an "occupied" sign on the door.

■ Never leave an infant or small pediatric client unattended in a tub. *Slippage and drowning can occur in a matter of seconds and in very little water.*

13. Assist the client with washing and getting out of the tub.

■ Wash the client's back, lower legs, and feet, if necessary.

■ Assist the client out of the tub. If the client is unsteady, place a bath towel over the client's shoulders and drain the tub of water before the client attempts to get out of it. *Draining the water first lessens the likelihood of a fall. The towel prevents chilling.*

14. Dry the client, and assist with follow-up care.

■ Follow step 9.

■ Assist the client back to the room.

■ Clean the tub or shower in accordance with agency practice, discard used linen in the laundry hamper, and place the "unoccupied" sign on the door.

15. Document pertinent data.

■ Follow step 10.

Part B: Providing Perineal-Genital Care

Interventions

1. Prepare the client.

■ Offer the client an appropriate explanation, being particularly sensitive to any embarrassment felt by the client.

■ Determine whether the client is experiencing any discomfort in the perineal-genital area.

■ Fold the top bed linen to the foot of the bed, and fold the gown up to expose the genital area.

■ Place a bath towel under the client's hips. *The bath towel prevents the bed from becoming soiled.*

2. Position and drape the client, and clean the upper inner thighs.

FOR FEMALES

■ Position the female in a back-lying position, with the knees flexed and spread well apart (abducted).

■ Cover her body and legs with the bath blanket. Drape the legs by tucking the bottom corners of the bath blanket under the inner sides of the legs (Figure 22-10 ■). *Minimum exposure lessens embarrassment and helps to provide*

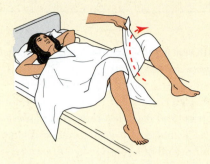

Figure 22-10. ■ Draping the client for perineal-genital care.

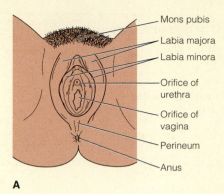

A

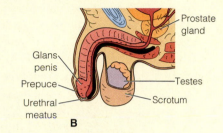

B

Figure 22-11. ■ **A.** Female genitals; **B.** male genitals.

warmth. Bring the middle portion of the base of the blanket up over the pubic area.

■ Don gloves, and wash and dry the upper inner thighs.

FOR MALES

■ Position the male client in a supine position with knees slightly flexed and hips slightly externally rotated.

■ Don gloves, and wash and dry the upper inner thighs.

3. Inspect the perineal area.

■ Note particular areas of inflammation, excoriation, or swelling, especially between the labia in females and the scrotal folds in males.

■ Also note excessive discharge or secretions from the orifices and the presence of odors.

4. Wash and dry the perineal-genital area.

FOR FEMALES

■ Clean the labia majora. Then spread the labia to wash the folds between the labia majora and the labia minora (Figure 22-11A ■). *Secretions that tend to collect around the labia minora facilitate bacterial growth.*

■ Use separate quarters of the washcloth for each stroke, and wipe from the pubis to the rectum. For menstruating women and clients with indwelling catheters, use disposable wipes, cotton balls, or gauze. Use a clean ball for each stroke. *Using separate quarters of the washcloth or new cotton balls or gauzes prevents the transmission of microorganisms from one area to the other.* Wipe from the area of least contamination (the pubis) to that of greatest (the rectum).

■ Rinse the area well. You may place the client on a bedpan and use a periwash or solution bottle to pour warm water over the area. Dry the perineum thoroughly, paying particular attention to the folds between the labia. *Moisture supports the growth of many microorganisms.*

FOR MALES

■ Wash and dry the penis, using firm strokes. *Handling the penis firmly may prevent an erection.*

■ If the client is uncircumcised, retract the prepuce (foreskin) to expose the glans penis (the tip of the penis) for cleaning. Replace the foreskin after cleaning the glans penis (Figure 22-11B). *Retracting the foreskin is necessary to remove the smegma that collects under the foreskin and facilitates bacterial growth.*

■ Wash and dry the scrotum. The posterior folds of the scrotum may need to be cleaned in step 6 with the buttocks. *The scrotum tends to be more soiled than the penis because of its proximity to the rectum; thus it is usually cleaned after the penis.*

5. Inspect perineal orifices for intactness.

■ Inspect particularly around the urethra in clients with indwelling catheters. *A catheter may cause excoriation around the urethra.*

6. Clean between the buttocks.

■ Assist the client to turn onto the side facing away from you.

■ Pay particular attention to the anal area and posterior folds of the scrotum in males. Clean the anus with toilet tissue before washing it, if necessary.

■ Dry the area well.

■ For postdelivery or menstruating females, apply a perineal pad as needed from front to back. *This prevents contamination of the vagina and urethra from the anal area.*

7. Document any assessments (redness, swelling, discharge) and report findings to RN.

Part C: Providing Foot Care

Interventions

1. Prepare the equipment and the client.
   - Fill the washbasin with warm water at about 40° to 43°C (105° to 110°F). *Warm water promotes circulation, comforts, and refreshes.*
   - Assist the ambulatory client to a sitting position in a chair, or the bed client to a supine or semi-Fowler's position.
   - Place a pillow under the bed client's knees. *This provides support and prevents muscle fatigue.*
   - Place the washbasin on the moisture-resistant pad at the foot of the bed for a bed client or on the floor in front of the chair for an ambulatory client.
   - For a bed client, pad the rim of the washbasin with a towel. *The towel prevents undue pressure on the skin.*

2. Wash the foot and soak it as required (Figure 22-12 ■).
   - Place one of the client's feet in the basin, and wash it with soap, paying particular attention to the interdigital areas. *Prolonged soaking is generally not recommended for diabetic clients or individuals with peripheral vascular disease. Prolonged soaking may remove natural skin oils, thus drying the skin and making it more susceptible to cracking and injury.*
   - Rinse the foot well to remove soap. *Soap irritates the skin if not properly removed.*

   - Rub callused areas of the foot with the washcloth. *This helps remove dead skin layers.*
   - If the nails are brittle or thick and require trimming, replace the water and allow the foot to soak for 10 to 20 minutes. *Soaking softens the nails and loosens debris under them.* Clean the nails as required with an orange stick or the blunt end of a toothpick. *This removes excess debris that harbors microorganisms.*
   - Remove the foot from the basin and place it on the towel.

3. Dry the foot thoroughly and apply lotion or foot powder.
   - Blot the foot gently with the towel to dry it thoroughly, particularly between the toes. *Harsh rubbing can damage the skin. Thorough drying reduces the risk of infection.*
   - Apply lotion or lanolin cream. *This lubricates dry skin.*

4. *If agency policy permits,* trim the nails of the first foot while the second foot is soaking.
   - See the discussion on nails for the appropriate method to trim nails. Note that in many agencies, toenail trimming requires a physician's order or is contraindicated for clients with diabetes mellitus, toe infections, and peripheral vascular disease, unless performed by a podiatrist or general practice physician.

5. Document any foot problems observed and report them to the RN.
   - Foot care is not generally recorded unless problems are noted.
   - Record any signs of inflammation, infection, breaks in the skin, corns, troublesome calluses, bunions, and pressure areas. *This is of particular importance for clients with peripheral vascular disease and diabetes.*

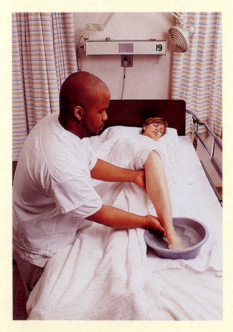

Figure 22-12. ■ Soaking a foot in a basin.
(Photographer: Jenny Thomas.)

SAMPLE DOCUMENTATION

[date]	Self-help, bed bath given. Client
[time]	tolerated bath without complaint. Client able to complete bath with assistance only for back. Skin intact, no redness or inflammation noted.
	_____ Lisa Patel, LPN

| PROCEDURE 22-2 | # Providing Hair Care |

Purposes

- To stimulate blood circulation to the scalp through massage
- To clean the hair and increase the client's sense of well-being
- To distribute hair oils and provide a healthy sheen
- To assess or monitor hair or scalp problems (e.g., matted hair or dandruff)

Equipment

- Comb and brush
- Plastic sheet or pad
- Two bath towels

- Shampoo basin
- Washcloth or pad
- Bath blanket
- Receptacle for the shampoo water
- Cotton balls (optional)
- Pitcher of water
- Bath thermometer
- Liquid or cream shampoo
- Hair dryer
- Large, open-toothed or long-toothed comb (a pick)
- Lubricant (optional)

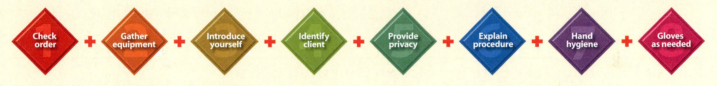

Check order + Gather equipment + Introduce yourself + Identify client + Provide privacy + Explain procedure + Hand hygiene + Gloves as needed

Part A: Shampooing the Hair

Interventions

1. Verify agency policy and the physician's order.
   - Determine whether a physician's order is needed before a shampoo can be given. *Some agencies require an order.*
   - Determine the type of shampoo to be used (e.g., medicated shampoo).

2. Prepare the client.
   - Determine the best time of day for the shampoo. Discuss this with the client. *A person who must remain in bed may find the shampoo tiring.* Choose a time when the client is rested and can rest after the procedure.
   - Assist the client to the side of the bed from which you will work.
   - Remove pins and ribbons from the hair, and brush and comb it to remove any tangles.

3. Arrange the equipment.
   - Put the plastic sheet or pad on the bed under the head. *The plastic keeps the bedding dry.*
   - Remove the pillow from under the client's head, and place it under the shoulders. *This hyperextends the neck.*
   - Tuck a bath towel around the client's shoulders. *This keeps the shoulders dry.*
   - Place the shampoo basin under the head (Figure 22-13 ■), putting a folded washcloth or pad where the client's neck rests on the edge of the basin. *If the client is on a stretcher, the neck can rest on the edge of the sink with the washcloth as padding. Padding supports the muscles of the neck and prevents undue strain and discomfort.*

- Fanfold the top bedding down to the waist, and cover the upper part of the client with the bath blanket. *The folded bedding will stay dry, and the bath blanket, which can be discarded after the shampoo, will keep the client warm.*

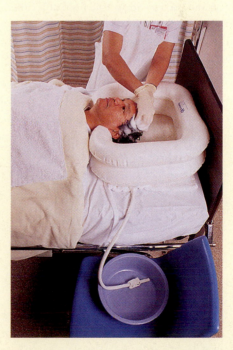

Figure 22-13. ■ Shampooing the hair of a client confined to bed. Note the shampoo basin and the receptacle below. (Photographer: Jenny Thomas.)

- Place the receiving receptacle on a table or chair at the bedside. Put the spout of the shampoo basin over the receptacle.
4. Protect the client's eyes and ears.
   - A damp washcloth may be placed over the client's eyes. *The washcloth protects the eyes from soapy water. A damp washcloth will not slip.*
   - Place cotton balls in the client's ears if indicated. These keep water from collecting in the ear canals.
5. Shampoo the hair.
   - Wet the hair thoroughly with the water.
   - Apply shampoo to the scalp. Make a good lather with the shampoo while massaging the scalp with the pads of your fingertips. Massage all areas of the scalp systematically, for example, starting at the front and working toward the back of the head. *Massaging stimulates the blood circulation in the scalp. The pads of the fingers are used so that the fingernails will not scratch the scalp.*

- Rinse the hair briefly, and apply shampoo again.
- Make a good lather and massage the scalp as before.
- Rinse the hair thoroughly this time to remove all the shampoo. *Shampoo remaining in the hair may dry and irritate the hair and scalp.*
- Squeeze as much water as possible out of the hair with your hands.
6. Dry the hair thoroughly.
   - Rub the client's hair with a heavy towel.
   - Dry the hair with the dryer. Set the temperature at "warm."
   - Continually move the dryer to prevent burning the client's scalp.
7. Ensure client comfort.
   - Assist the person confined to bed to a comfortable position.
   - Arrange the hair using a clean brush and comb.
8. Document the shampoo and any assessments.
   - Report any problems noted to the RN.

Part B: Providing Hair Care for African American Clients

Interventions

1. Position and prepare the client appropriately.
   - Assist the client who can sit to move to a chair. *Hair is more easily brushed and combed when the client is in a sitting position.* If health permits, assist a client confined to a bed to a sitting position by raising the head of the bed. Otherwise, assist the client to alternate side-lying positions, and do one side of the head at a time.
   - If the client remains in bed, place a clean towel over the pillow and the client's shoulders. Place it over the sitting client's shoulders. *The towel collects any removed hair, dirt, and scaly material.*

- Remove any pins or ribbons in the hair.
2. Comb the hair.
   - Apply a lubricant as the client indicates or as needed.
   - Using a large and open-toothed comb, start at the neckline and lift and fluff the hair outward, moving upward toward the forehead (Figure 22-14 ■).
   - Continue fluffing the hair outward and upward until all of the hair is combed on half of the head. Repeat the procedure for the other half.
3. Remove tangles gradually.
   - After the hair has been lubricated, weave and lift your opened fingers through the hair to ease the tangles free.

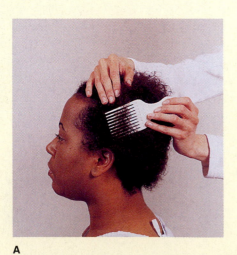

A

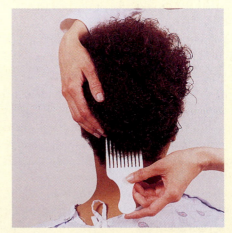

B

Figure 22-14. ■ **A.** Removing tangles with a long open-toothed comb. **B.** Using a long open-toothed comb to comb an African American client's hair from the neck line upward toward the forehead. (Photographer: Jenny Thomas.)

or

Support the hair securely at the base of the scalp, if possible, to prevent pulling and discomfort. Insert a long-toothed comb into the ends of the hair and carefully comb out the ends of the tangles (Figure 22-14**A**).

- Repeat this step, each time working the comb farther up the hair shaft toward the scalp, until the hair is untangled.

4. Document assessments and special nursing interventions.
   - Daily combing and brushing of hair are not normally recorded.
   - Record problems such as excessive dandruff, very dry or very oily hair, or the presence of lice.

PROCEDURE 22-3   # Providing Oral Care

Purposes

- To remove food particles and microorganisms from around and between the teeth and artificial teeth
- To remove dental plaque
- To enhance the client's feelings of well-being
- To prevent sordes and infection of the oral tissues
- To maintain the continuity of the lips, tongue, and mucous membranes of the mouth
- To clean and moisten the membranes of the mouth and lips

Equipment

- Towel
- Disposable gloves
- Curved basin (emesis basin)
- Toothbrush (or stiff-bristled brush for dentures)
- Cup of tepid water
- Toothpaste or denture cleaner
- Mouthwash
- Dental floss, at least two pieces 20 cm (8 in.) in length
- Floss holder (optional)
- Tissue or piece of gauze
- Denture container
- Clean washcloth
- Bite-block to hold the mouth open and teeth apart
- Rubber-tipped bulb syringe
- Suction catheter with suction apparatus (optional)
- Applicators and cleaning solution for cleaning the mucous membranes
- Petroleum jelly (Vaseline)

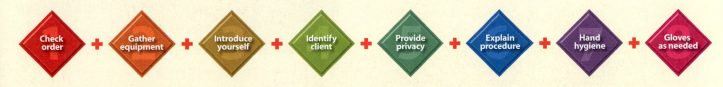

Check order + Gather equipment + Introduce yourself + Identify client + Provide privacy + Explain procedure + Hand hygiene + Gloves as needed

Part A: Brushing and Flossing the Teeth

Interventions

1. Prepare the client.
   - Explain the procedure.
   - Assist the client to a sitting position in bed, if health permits. If not, assist the client to a side-lying position with the head on a pillow so that the client can spit out the rinse water.

2. Prepare the equipment.
   - Place the towel under the client's chin.
   - Don gloves. *Wearing gloves while providing mouth care prevents the LPN/LVN from acquiring infections. Gloves also prevent transmission of microorganisms to the client.*
   - Moisten the bristles of the toothbrush with tepid water, and apply the toothpaste to the toothbrush.

- Use a soft toothbrush (a small one for a child) and the client's choice of toothpaste. For the person who does not have toothpaste, use a mixture of salt and baking soda.
- For the client who must remain in bed, place or hold the curved basin under the client's chin, fitting the small curve around the chin or neck.
- Inspect the mouth and teeth.

3. Brush the teeth.
   - Hand the toothbrush to the client, or brush the client's teeth as follows:
     a. Hold the brush against the teeth with the bristles at a 45-degree angle (Figure 22-15 ■). The tips of the outer bristles should rest against and penetrate under the gingival sulcus (Figure 22-15B). *The brush will clean under the sulcus of two or three teeth at one time. This sulcular technique removes plaque and cleans under the gingival margins.*
     b. Move the bristles back and forth using a vibrating or jiggling motion, from the sulcus to the crowns of the teeth.
     c. Repeat until all outer and inner surfaces of the teeth and sulci of the gums are cleaned.
     d. Clean the biting surfaces by moving the brush back and forth over them in short strokes (Figure 22-15C).
     e. If the tongue is coated, brush it gently with the toothbrush. *Brushing removes accumulated materials and coatings. A coated tongue may be caused by poor oral hygiene and low fluid intake. Brushing gently and carefully helps prevent gagging or vomiting.*
   - Hand the client the water cup or mouthwash to rinse the mouth vigorously. Then ask the client to spit the water and excess toothpaste into the basin. Some agencies supply a standard mouthwash. Alternatively, a mouth rinse of normal saline can be an effective cleaner and moisturizer. *Vigorous rinsing loosens food particles and washes out already loosened particles.*
   - Repeat the preceding steps until the mouth is free of toothpaste and food particles.
   - Remove the curved basin, and help the client wipe the mouth.

4. Floss the teeth.
   - Assist the client to floss independently, or floss the teeth as follows. Waxed floss is less likely to fray than unwaxed floss; particles between the teeth attach more readily to unwaxed floss than to waxed floss. Some believe that waxed floss leaves a residue on the teeth and that plaque then adheres to the wax.
     a. Wrap one end of the floss around the third finger of each hand (Figure 22-16 ■).
     b. To floss the upper teeth, use your thumb and index finger to stretch the floss (Figure 22-16B). Move the floss up and down between the teeth from the tops of the crowns to the gum and along the gum lines as far as possible. Make a "C" with the floss around the

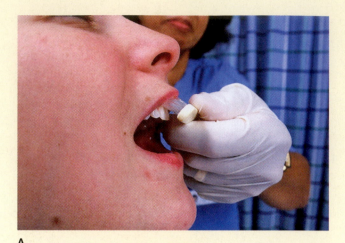

A

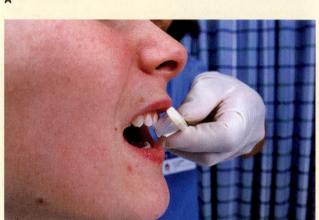

B

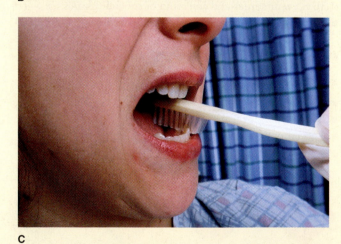

C

Figure 22-15. ■ **A.** The sulcular technique: placing the bristles at a 45-degree angle against the teeth. **B.** Brushing from the sulcus to the crown of the teeth. **C.** Brushing the biting surfaces. (Al Dodge, Pearson Education/PH.)

tooth edge being flossed. Start at the back on the right side and work around to the back of the left side, or work from the center teeth to the back of the jaw on either side.
   c. To floss the lower teeth, use your index fingers to stretch the floss (Figure 22-16C).

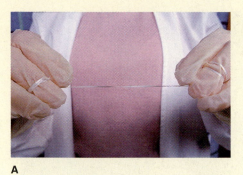
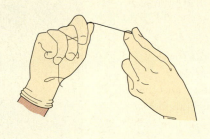
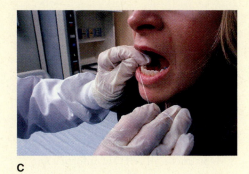

A   B   C

Figure 22-16. ■ A. Stretching the floss between the third finger of each hand. **B.** Flossing the upper teeth by using the thumbs and index fingers to stretch the floss. **C.** Flossing the lower teeth by using the index finger to stretch the floss.

- Give the client tepid water or mouthwash to rinse the mouth and a curved basin in which to spit the water.
- Assist the client in wiping the mouth.

5. Remove and dispose of equipment appropriately.
   - Remove and clean the curved basin.
   - Remove and discard the gloves.

6. Document assessment of the teeth, tongue, gums, and oral mucosa. Include any problems such as sores or inflammation and swelling of the gums and report findings to RN. *Brushing and flossing teeth are not usually recorded.*

Part B: Cleaning Dentures

Before beginning to clean dentures, determine (1) areas in the mouth that require ongoing assessment and (2) whether the client has upper and lower dentures.

Interventions

1. Place denture solution in denture container according to directions.

2. Prepare the client.
   - Assist the client to a sitting or side-lying position.

3. Remove the dentures.
   - Don gloves. *Wearing gloves protects the LPN/LVN and client from infection.*
   - If the client cannot remove the dentures, take the tissue or gauze, grasp the upper plate at the front teeth with your thumb and second finger, and move the denture up and down slightly (Figure 22-17 ■). The slight movement breaks the suction that holds the plate on the roof of the mouth.
   - Lower the upper plate, move it out of the mouth, and place it in the denture container.
   - Lift the lower plate, turning it so that the left side, for example, is slightly lower than the right, to remove the plate from the mouth without stretching the lips. Place the lower plate in the denture container.

4. Inspect the dentures and the mouth.
   - Observe the dentures for any rough, sharp, or worn areas that could irritate the tongue or mucous membranes of the mouth, lips, and gums.

- Inspect the mouth for any redness, irritated areas, or indications of infection.
- Assess the fit of the dentures. People who have them should see a dentist at least once a year to check the fit and the presence of any irritation to the soft tissues of the mouth. *Clients who need repairs to their dentures or new dentures may need a referral for financial assistance.*

5. Return the dentures to the mouth.
   - Offer some mouthwash and a curved basin to rinse the mouth. If the client cannot insert the dentures independently, insert the plates one at a time. Hold each

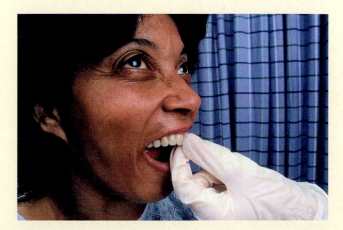

Figure 22-17. ■ Removing the top dentures by first breaking the suction.

plate at a slight angle while inserting it, to avoid injuring the lips (Figure 22-18 ■).

6. Assist the client as needed.
   - Wipe the client's hands and mouth with the towel.
   - If the client does not want to or cannot wear the dentures, store them in a denture container with water. Label the cup with the client's name and identification number.

7. Remove and discard gloves.

8. Document all relevant information.
   - Document all assessments, and include any problems, such as an irritated area on the mucous membrane and report findings to RN.
   - Once dentures are clean, replace them in client's mouth unless client prefers them to be left out.

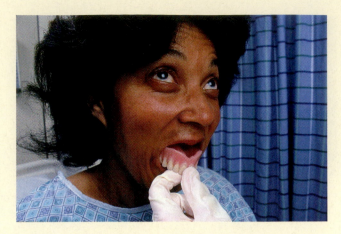

Figure 22-18. ■ Inserting the denture at a slight angle.

Part C: Providing Special Oral Care

Interventions

1. Prepare the client.
   - Position the unconscious client in a side-lying position, with the head of the bed lowered. *In this position, the saliva automatically runs out by gravity rather than being aspirated into the lungs. This position is the one of choice for the unconscious client receiving mouth care.* If the client's head cannot be lowered, turn it to one side. *The fluid will readily run out of the mouth or pool in the side of the mouth, where it can be suctioned.*
   - Place the towel under the client's chin.
   - Place the curved basin against the client's chin and lower cheek to receive the fluid from the mouth (Figure 22-19 ■).
   - Don gloves.

2. Clean the teeth and rinse the mouth.
   - If the client has natural teeth, brush the teeth as described in Procedure 22-3A. Brush gently and carefully to avoid injuring the gums. If the client has artificial teeth, clean them as described in Procedure 22-3B.
   - Rinse the client's mouth by drawing about 10 mL of water or mouthwash into the syringe and injecting it gently into each side of the mouth. *If the solution is injected with force, some of it may flow down the client's throat and be aspirated into the lungs.*
   - Watch carefully to make sure that all the rinsing solution has run out of the mouth into the basin. If not, suction the fluid from the mouth. See the section on oropharyngeal suctioning in Chapter 24 ⦵. *Fluid remaining in the mouth may be aspirated into the lungs.*
   - Repeat rinsing until the mouth is free of toothpaste, if used.

3. Inspect and clean the oral tissues.
   - If the tissues appear dry or unclean, clean them with the applicators or gauze and cleaning solution following agency policy.
   - Picking up one applicator, wipe the mucous membrane of one cheek. If no commercially prepared applicators are available, wrap a small gauze square around a tongue blade and moisten it. Discard the applicator or tongue blade in a waste container, and with a fresh one clean the next area. *Using separate applicators for each area of the mouth prevents the transfer of microorganisms from one area to another.*
   - Clean all the mouth tissues in an orderly progression, using separate applicators: the cheeks, roof of the mouth, base of the mouth, and tongue.
   - Observe the tissues closely for inflammation and dryness.

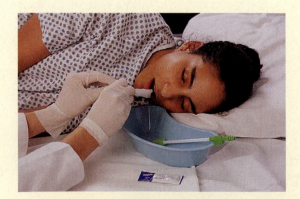

Figure 22-19. ■ Position of the client and placement of curved basin when providing special mouth care. (Photographer: Elena Dorfman.)

- Rinse the client's mouth as described in step 2.
- Remove and discard gloves.

4. Ensure client comfort.
   - Remove the basin, and dry around the client's mouth with the towel. Replace artificial dentures, if indicated.
   - Lubricate the client's lips with petroleum jelly. *Lubrication prevents cracking and subsequent infection.*

5. Document pertinent data.
   - Record special oral hygiene and pertinent observations.
   - Report problems to the RN in charge.

PROCEDURE 22-4 # Removing, Cleaning, and Inserting a Hearing Aid

Purpose

- To maintain proper hearing aid function

Equipment

- Client's hearing aid
- Soap, water, and towels or a damp cloth
- Pipe cleaner or toothpick (optional)
- New battery (if needed)

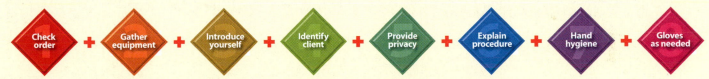

Check order + Gather equipment + Introduce yourself + Identify client + Provide privacy + Explain procedure + Hand hygiene + Gloves as needed

Interventions

1. Remove the hearing aid.
   - Turn the hearing aid off and lower the volume. The on/off switch may be labeled "O" (off), "M" (microphone), "T" (telephone), or "TM" (telephone/microphone). *The batteries continue to run if the aid is not turned off.*
   - Remove the earmold by rotating it slightly forward and pulling it outward.
   - If the aid is not to be used for several days, remove the battery. *Removal prevents corrosion of the aid from battery leakage.*
   - Store the hearing aid in a safe place. Avoid exposure to heat and moisture. *Proper storage prevents loss or damage.*

2. Clean the earmold.
   - Detach the earmold if possible. Disconnect the earmold from the receiver of a body hearing aid or from the hearing aid case of behind-the-ear and eyeglasses aids where the tubing meets the hook of the case. Do not remove the earmold if it is glued or secured by a small metal ring. *Removal facilitates cleaning and prevents inadvertent damage to the other parts.*
   - If the earmold is detachable, soak it in a mild soapy solution. Rinse and dry it well. Do not use isopropyl alcohol. *Alcohol can damage the hearing aid.*
   - If the earmold is not detachable or is for an in-the-ear aid, wipe the earmold with a damp cloth.
   - Check that the earmold opening is patent. Blow any excess moisture through the opening or remove debris (e.g., earwax) with a pipe cleaner or toothpick.
   - Reattach the earmold if it was detached from the rest of the hearing aid.

3. Insert the hearing aid.
   - Determine from the client if the earmold is for the left or the right ear.
   - Check that the battery is inserted in the hearing aid. Turn off the hearing aid, and make sure the volume is

turned all the way down. *A volume that is too loud is distressing.*

■ Inspect the earmold to identify the ear canal portion. Some earmolds are fitted for only the ear canal and concha; others are fitted for all the contours of the ear. *The canal portion, common to all, can be used as a guide for correct insertion.*

■ Line up the parts of the earmold with the corresponding parts of the client's ear.

■ Rotate the earmold slightly forward, and insert the ear canal portion.

■ Gently press the earmold into the ear while rotating it backward.

■ Check that the earmold fits snugly by asking the client if it feels secure and comfortable.

■ Adjust the other components of a behind-the-ear or body hearing aid.

■ Turn the hearing aid on, and adjust the volume according to the client's needs.

4. Correct problems associated with improper functioning.
■ If the sound is weak or there is no sound:
   a. Ensure that the volume is turned high enough.
   b. Ensure that the earmold opening is not clogged.
   c. Check the battery by turning the aid on, turning up the volume, cupping your hand over the earmold, and listening. A constant whistling sound indicates the battery is functioning. If necessary, replace the battery. Be sure that the negative ($-$) and positive ($+$) signs on the battery match those on the aid.

d. Ensure that the ear canal is not blocked with wax. *Wax can obstruct sound waves.*

■ If the client reports a whistling sound or squeal after insertion:
   a. Turn the volume down.
   b. Ensure that the earmold is properly attached to the receiver.
   c. Reinsert the earmold.

5. Document pertinent data.
■ The removal and the insertion of a hearing aid are not normally recorded.
■ Record any problems the client has with the hearing aid and report findings to the RN.

SAMPLE DOCUMENTATION

[date]
[time]   No wax buildup in external ear canal noted. Client denies ear discomfort. Hearing aid inserted and volume adjusted by client. Client denies discomfort upon insertion and states adequacy of hearing acuity.
_____ Alfred Donofrio, LPN.

PROCEDURE 22-5   Changing a Bed

Purposes

■ To promote the client's comfort
■ To provide a clean, neat environment for the client
■ To provide a smooth, wrinkle-free bed foundation, thus minimizing sources of skin irritation
■ To conserve the client's energy and maintain current health status

Equipment

■ Two large sheets (some agencies may use fitted bottom sheets)
■ Cloth draw sheet (optional)
■ One blanket
■ One bedspread (some agencies do not use bedspreads)
■ Waterproof draw sheet or waterproof pads (optional)
■ Pillowcase(s) for the head pillow(s)
■ Portable linen hamper, if available

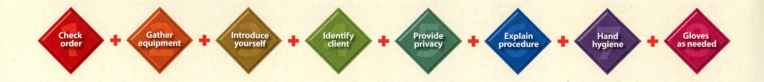

Part A: Changing an Unoccupied Bed

Interventions

1. Place the fresh linen on the client's chair or overbed table; do not use another client's bed. *This prevents cross-contamination (the movement of microorganisms from one client to another) via soiled linen.*

2. Assess and assist the client out of bed.
   - Make sure that this is an appropriate and convenient time for the client to be out of bed.
   - Assess the client's health status to determine that the person can safely get out of bed. *In some hospitals, it is necessary to have a written order if the client has been in bed continuously.*
   - Assess the client's pulse and respirations if indicated.
   - Assist the client to a comfortable chair.

3. Strip the bed.
   - Check bed linens for any items belonging to the client, and detach the call bell or any drainage tubes from the bed linen.
   - Loosen all bedding systematically, starting at the head of the bed on the far side and moving around the bed up to the head of the bed on the near side. *Moving around the bed systematically prevents stretching and reaching and possible muscle strain.*
   - Remove the pillowcases, if soiled, and place the pillows on the bedside chair near the foot of the bed.
   - Fold reusable linens, such as the bedspread and top sheet on the bed, into fourths. First, fold the linen in half by bringing the top edge even with the bottom edge, and then grasp it at the center of the middle fold and bottom edges (Figure 22-20 ■). *Folding linens saves time and energy when reapplying the linens on the bed.*
   - Remove the waterproof pad and discard it if soiled.
   - Roll all soiled linen inside the bottom sheet, hold it away from your uniform, and place it directly in the linen hamper. These actions are essential to prevent the transmission of microorganisms to the LPN/LVN and others.
   - Grasp the mattress securely, using the lugs if present, and move the mattress up to the head of the bed.

4. Apply the bottom sheet and draw sheet.
   - Place the folded bottom sheet with its center fold on the center of the bed. Make sure the sheet is hemside down for a smooth foundation. Spread the sheet out over the mattress, and allow a sufficient amount of sheet at the top to tuck under the mattress. The top of the sheet needs to be well tucked under to remain securely in place, especially when the head of the bed is elevated. Place the sheet along the edge of the mattress at the foot of the bed and do not tuck it in (unless it is a contour sheet).
   - If the bottom sheet is not fitted, miter the sheet at the top corner on the near side (see Figure 22-8) and tuck the sheet under the mattress, working from the head of the bed to the foot.
   - If a waterproof draw sheet is used, place it over the bottom sheet so that the center fold is at the center line of the bed and the top and bottom edges will extend from the middle of the client's back to the area of the midthigh or knee. Fan-fold the uppermost half of the folded draw sheet at the center or far edge of the bed and tuck in the near edge.
   - Lay the cloth draw sheet over the waterproof sheet in the same manner.
   - *Optional:* Before moving to the other side of the bed, place the top linens on the bed hemside up, unfold them, tuck them in, and miter the bottom corners. *Completing the entire side of the bed saves time and energy.*

5. Move to the other side and secure the bottom linens.
   - Tuck the bottom sheet in under the head of the mattress, pull the sheet firmly, and miter the corner of the sheet if a fitted sheet is not being used.
   - Pull the remainder of the sheet firmly so that there are no wrinkles. *Wrinkles can cause discomfort for the client. Tuck the sheet in at the side.*
   - Complete this same process for the draw sheet(s).

6. Apply or complete the top sheet, blanket, and spread.
   - Place the top sheet, hemside up, on the bed so that its center fold is at the center of the bed and the top edge is even with the top edge of the mattress.
   - Unfold the sheet over the bed.
   - *Optional:* Make a vertical or a horizontal toe pleat in the sheet to provide additional room for the client's feet.
     a. *Vertical toe pleat:* Make a fold in the sheet 5 to 10 cm (2 to 4 in.) perpendicular to the foot of the bed (Figure 22-21A ■).

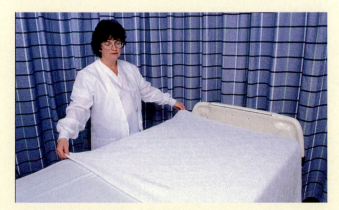

Figure 22-20. ■ Folding reusable linens into fourths when removing them from the bed. (Al Dodge, Pearson Education/PH.)

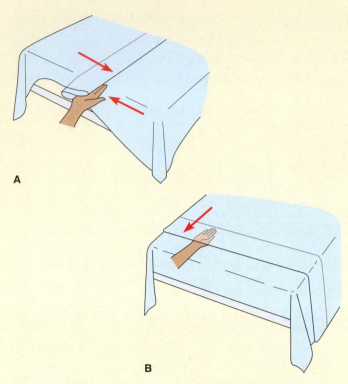

A

B

Figure 22-21. ■ **A.** A vertical toe pleat; **B.** a horizontal toe pleat.

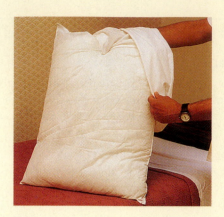

Figure 22-22. ■ Method for putting a clean pillowcase on a pillow.

b. *Horizontal toe pleat:* Make a fold in the sheet 5 to 10 cm (2 to 4 in.) across the bed near the foot (Figure 22-21B).
Loosening the top covers around the feet after the client is in bed is another way to provide additional space.

■ Follow the same procedure for the blanket and the spread, but place the top edges about 15 cm (6 in.) from the head of the bed to allow a cuff of sheet to be folded over them.

■ Tuck in the sheet, blanket, and spread at the foot of the bed, and miter the corner, using all three layers of linen. Leave the sides of the top sheet, blanket, and spread hanging freely unless toe pleats were provided.

■ Fold the top of the top sheet down over the spread, providing a cuff. *The cuff of sheet makes it easier for the client to pull the covers up.*

■ Move to the other side of the bed and secure the top bedding in the same manner.

7. Put clean pillowcases on the pillows as required.
■ Grasp the closed end of the pillowcase at the center with one hand.

■ Gather up the sides of the pillowcase and place them over the hand grasping the case. Then grasp the center of one short side of the pillow through the pillowcase (Figure 22-22 ■).

■ With the free hand, pull the pillowcase over the pillow.

■ Adjust the pillowcase so that the pillow fits into the corners of the case and the seams are straight. *A smoothly fitting pillowcase is more comfortable than a wrinkled one.*

■ Place the pillows appropriately at the head of the bed.

8. Provide for client comfort and safety.
■ Attach the signal cord so that the client can conveniently use it. Some cords have clamps that attach to the sheet or pillowcase. Others are attached by a safety pin.

■ If the bed is currently being used by a client, either fold back the top covers at one side or fan-fold them down to the center of the bed. *This makes it easier for the client to get into the bed.*

■ Place the bedside table and the overbed table so that they are available to the client.

■ Leave the bed in the high position if the client is returning by stretcher, or place in the low position if the client is returning to bed after being up.

9. Document and report pertinent data.
■ Bed-making is not normally recorded.

■ Record any nursing assessments, such as the client's physical status and pulse and respiratory rates before and after being out of bed, as indicated. Report any changes in client's status to the RN.

Part B: Changing an Occupied Bed

Interventions

1. Remove the top bedding.
■ Remove any equipment attached to the bed linen, such as a signal light.

■ Loosen all the top linen at the foot of the bed, and remove the spread and the blanket.

■ Leave the top sheet over the client (the top sheet can remain over the client if it is being changed and if it will provide sufficient warmth), or replace it with a bath blanket as follows:

    a. Spread the bath blanket over the top sheet.

    b. Ask the client to hold the top edge of the blanket.

    c. Reaching under the blanket from the side, grasp the top edge of the sheet and draw it down to the foot of the bed, leaving the blanket in place.

    d. Remove the sheet from the bed and place it in the soiled linen hamper.

2. Move the mattress up on the bed.

   ■ Place the bed in the flat position, if the client's health permits.

   ■ Grasp the mattress lugs and, using good body mechanics, move the mattress up to the head of the bed. Ask the client to assist, if permitted, by grasping the head of the bed and pulling as you push. If the client is heavy, you may need help from another staff member.

3. Change the bottom sheet and draw sheet.

   ■ Assist the client to turn on the side facing away from the side where the clean linen is.

   ■ Raise the side rail nearest the client. This protects the client from falling. If there is no side rail, have another staff member support the client at the edge of the bed.

   ■ Loosen the foundation of the linen on the side of the bed near the linen supply.

   ■ Fan-fold the draw sheet and the bottom sheet at the center of the bed (Figure 22-23 ■), as close to the client as possible. *Doing this leaves the near half of the bed free to be changed.*

   ■ Place the new bottom sheet on the bed, and vertically fan-fold the half to be used on the far side of the bed as close to the client as possible. Tuck the sheet under the near half of the bed and miter the corner if a fitted sheet is not being used.

   ■ Place the clean draw sheet on the bed with the center fold at the center of the bed. Fan-fold the uppermost

half vertically at the center of the bed and tuck the near side edge under the side of the mattress.

   ■ Assist the client to roll over toward you onto the clean side of the bed. The client rolls over the fan-folded linen at the center of the bed.

   ■ Move the pillows to the clean side for the client's use. Raise the side rail before leaving the side of the bed.

   ■ Move to the other side of the bed and lower the side rail.

   ■ Remove the used linen and place it in the portable hamper.

   ■ Unfold the fan-folded bottom sheet from the center of the bed.

   ■ Facing the side of the bed, use both hands to pull the bottom sheet so that it is smooth and tuck the excess under the side of the mattress.

   ■ Unfold the drawsheet fanfolded at the center of the bed and pull it tightly with both hands. Pull the sheet in three sections: (a) face the side of the bed to pull the middle section; (b) face the far top corner to pull the bottom section; and (c) face the far bottom corner to pull the top section.

   ■ Tuck the excess draw sheet under the side of the mattress.

4. Reposition the client in the center of the bed.

   ■ Reposition the pillows at the center of the bed.

   ■ Assist the client to the center of the bed. Determine what position the client requires or prefers and assist the client to that position.

5. Apply or complete the top bedding.

   ■ Spread the top sheet over the client and either ask the client to hold the top edge of the sheet or tuck it under the shoulders. *The sheet should remain over the client when the bath blanket or used sheet is removed.*

   ■ Complete the top of the bed.

6. Ensure continued safety of the client.

   ■ Raise the side rails. Place the bed in the low position before leaving the bedside.

   ■ Attach the signal cord to the bed linen within the client's reach.

   ■ Put items used by the client within easy reach.

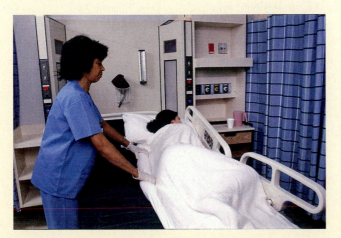

Figure 22-23. ■ Moving soiled linen as close to the client as possible. (Photographer: Alain McLaughlin.)

SAMPLE DOCUMENTATION

[date]   Bed linens changed with client occupy-

[time]   ing bed. Client able to turn in bed with assistance and denies discomfort during procedure. Indwelling catheter patent and draining. IV tubing patent. Client sitting up in bed with side rails up, call light within reach.

             _____ Tari Heiland, LPN.

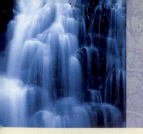# Chapter Review

 KEY TERMS by Topic

Use the audio glossary feature of either the CD-ROM or the Companion Website to hear the correct pronunciation of the following key terms.

Introduction
hygiene, early morning care, morning care, afternoon care, hour of sleep (HS) care, as-needed (prn) care

Skin, Foot, and Nail Care
sebum, cleaning baths, therapeutic baths

Hair Care
alopecia, lanugo, dandruff, pediculosis, scabies, hirsutism

Mouth Care
gingiva, caries, halitosis, dentures

Eye Care
contact lenses

Ear Care
cerumen, hearing aid

Supporting a Hygienic Environment
bed cradle

KEY Points

- Clients' hygienic practices are influenced to a large degree by their sociocultural background.

- When clients cannot meet their own hygiene needs, the LPN/LVN assists them.

- The major functions of the skin are to help regulate body temperature, to protect underlying tissues, to secrete sebum, and to contain nerve receptors that act in sensory perception.

- When planning hygiene care, the LPN/LVN must consider client preferences.

- The LPN/LVN provides perineal-genital care for clients who are unable to do so for themselves.

- The LPN/LVN can often teach clients how to prevent foot problems.

- Oral hygiene should include daily dental flossing and mechanical brushing of the teeth.

- Regular dental checkups and fluoride supplements are recommended to maintain healthy teeth.

- The LPN/LVN provides special oral care to clients who are helpless (e.g., unconscious) and who have oral problems.

- Hair care includes daily combing and brushing and regular shampooing.

- African American clients' hair may require special care.

- The LPN/LVN may need to assist clients with their artificial eyes, eyeglasses, and contact lenses.

- Clients with a hearing aid may require nursing assistance with the device.

- Changing bed linens is a part of maintaining hygiene.

- It is important to keep beds clean and comfortable for clients.

 EXPLORE Media Link

Additional interactive resources for this chapter can be found on the Companion Website at www.prenhall.com/ramont. Click on Chapter 22 and "Begin" to select the activities for this chapter.

For chapter-related NCLEX®-style questions and an audio glossary, access the accompanying CD-ROM in this book.

FOR FURTHER Study

Table 9-1 lists examples of normal flora found on the skin.

For more about enhancing a client's self-concept, see Chapter 14.

For detailed information about physical assessment, see Chapter 19.

For a detailed discussion of body heat losses and gains, see Chapter 20.

For discussion of skin integrity, skin impairment, skin lesions, and heat and cold applications, see Chapter 23.

Box 23-2 lists factors that inhibit wound healing in older adults, and Table 23-5 provides additional information about mattresses.

For additional information on medications, see Chapter 29.

Back massages to promote circulation are discussed in Chapter 32, as are ways to move a client in bed.

The diagnosis *Deficient Knowledge* is discussed in detail in Chapter 33.

Caring for a Client with Oral Cavity Problems

NCLEX-PN® Focus Area: Health Promotion and Maintenance: Prevention and Early Detection of Disease

Case Study: Joe Kwan, 46 years old, was admitted with a fractured femur. On bed rest and in Buck's traction; scheduled for an ORIF at 11:00 A.M. Maureen Stiffel, LVN, has been assigned to assist him with his bath and oral hygiene. NPO; Foley catheter in place. Intravenous 5% D/W in NSS in place and infusing at 100 mL/h. VS: T 99.2, P 78, R 20, BP 134/82; pulse ox 98% on room air.

Nursing Diagnosis: Impaired Oral Mucous Membrane

COLLECT DATA

Subjective	Objective
_____	_____
_____	_____
_____	_____
_____	_____
_____	_____
_____	_____
_____	_____

Would you report this data? Yes/No

If yes, to: _____

What would you report? _____

Nursing Care

_____

_____

_____

_____

_____

_____

_____

_____

_____

How would you document this? _____

_____

_____

Compare your documentation to the sample provided in Appendix I.

Data Collected
(use those that apply)

- Teeth stained from heavy smoking
- One large cavity evident in second lower left molar
- Tartar buildup along gum margins
- Pronounced halitosis
- Gums are reddened in some area and bleed when flossed
- States, "I can't remember when I last saw a dentist."

Nursing Interventions
(use those that apply; list in priority order)

- Thoroughly orient the client to environment. Place call light within reach and show how to call for assistance. Answer call light promptly.
- Use tap water or normal saline to provide oral care; do not use commercial mouthwash containing alcohol or hydrogen peroxide.
- Plan care activities around periods of greatest comfort whenever possible.
- Use foam sticks to moisten the oral mucous membrane, clean out debris, and swab while client is NPO.
- Keep lips well lubricated using petroleum jelly or a similar product.
- Encourage client to take deep breaths and cough at intervals.
- Inspect oral cavity at least once daily and note any discoloration, lesions, edema, bleeding, exudate, or dryness.
- Determine client's usual method of oral care and address any concerns related to oral care.
- Identify reasons client has not seen a dentist regularly.

NCLEX-PN® Exam Preparation

1 The client's primary nurse asks you if your assigned client has had early A.M. care. The primary nurse wants to know if you (or someone else) have done which of the following things with or for the client?

1. taken the client's vital signs
2. completed the initial assessment
3. helped the client with oral care and face and hand hygiene
4. given the client a shower or bath and ambulated the client

2 When working with a client who needs assistance with personal hygiene and who has a number of personal preferences about how and when it should be done, the best action on your part would be to do which of the following things?

1. Follow client's preferences as long as compatible with client's health and equipment is available.
2. Tell client you are a professional nurse and you will determine when and how to do these tasks.
3. Determine the most efficient way to carry out the personal hygiene tasks and do it this way.
4. Ignore the client's preferences and quietly do hygiene tasks the way you have been taught.

3 You are assigned to care for a client with impaired circulation of the lower extremities. You assess the client's feet and find that the skin is very dry and the heels have reddened areas. Of the following which are the appropriate interventions?

1. Be sure that the bottom sheet is taut and free of wrinkles.
2. Massage the feet with alcohol and allow to air dry.
3. After bathing the client, dry the client's feet briskly.
4. Tuck top sheet and blanket in tightly to keep feet warm.

4 The incidence of skin breakdown in the elderly in a long-term care facility can be reduced the most through which of the following actions on the part of the nursing staff?

1. offering a wider variety of pureed foods
2. restricting the use of caffeine drinks
3. offering water throughout the day
4. reducing the amount of pain medication

5 When doing oral hygiene on an unconscious client, the position of choice is which of the following positions?

1. head elevated
2. side-lying
3. prone
4. supine

6 The long-term care facility nursing staff has scheduled the elderly clients to be showered or bathed every other day. Younger clients are being showered or bathed daily. Which of the following reasons is the best reason for showering or bathing the elderly clients every other day?

1. Showering and bathing tires the elderly more.
2. It takes longer to shower or bathe the elderly.
3. There is not enough staff to give everyone daily showers or baths.
4. Less frequent bathing prevents removal of sebum from the skin of elderly clients.

7 When a client is not going to be using her hearing aid for several days, the nurse needs to do which of the following things?

1. Turn the volume down.
2. Plug hearing aid into a charger.
3. Remove the batteries.
4. Store hearing aid in refrigerator.

8 The school nurse is working with the physical education director and the students in physical education classes in order to prevent tinea pedis. The nurse will evaluate that a student is trying to prevent getting or spreading tinea pedis if the student demonstrates which of the following behaviors?

1. washing the body well with an antiseptic soap in the gym shower
2. wearing shower shoes in the shower and the dressing room
3. drying the feet well after leaving the shower room
4. wearing stockings and changing these stockings daily

9 You are bathing an unconscious client. Which of the following things do you most need to do in providing eye care?

1. Wipe from the outer to inner canthus.
2. Use a different cotton ball for each wipe.
3. Cover the eyes with an eye shield.
4. Use fresh water to cleanse the eyes.

10 When changing a client's bed linens, you most need to do which of the following things?

1. Shake each of the client's bed linens before putting it in the hamper.
2. Wrap soiled linen in bottom sheet, hold away from you, and put it in the hamper.
3. Put the dirty linen on the floor until you have finished changing the bed linens.
4. Take the dirty linen out of the room before putting the clean linen on the bed.

Answers and Rationales for Review Questions, as well as discussion of Care Plan and Critical Thinking Care Map questions, appear in Appendix I.

Chapter 23

Skin Integrity and Wound Care

BRIEF Outline

Skin Integrity
Types of Wounds
Wound Healing
Pressure Ulcers

LEARNING Outcomes

After completing this chapter, you will be able to:

1. Describe factors affecting skin integrity.
2. Describe the three phases of wound healing.
3. Describe factors that affect wound healing.
4. Discuss measures to prevent and treat pressure ulcer formation.
5. Identify purposes of commonly used dressing materials and binders.
6. Describe methods of applying dry and moist heat and cold.
7. Describe the four stages of pressure ulcer development.
8. Identify data pertinent to skin integrity, pressure sites, and wounds.
9. Identify essential steps of applying transparent and hydrocolloid dressings obtaining wound specimens, and irrigating a wound.

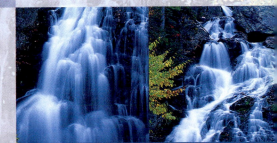

HISTORICAL Perspectives

Ambroise Pare (1510–1590) began his career as a barber surgeon and then became an army surgeon. He became an expert at treating battle wounds. Previously he had treated amputations with hot pitch or boiling elder oil, which he used to cauterize wounds to staunch the bleeding. One day he found his supplies diminished and he substituted egg, oil of roses, and turpentine which accomplished cauterization without subjecting the wounded to burns. He also introduced ligatures and found that his patients recovered far better than those treated in the conventional way. He resolved "never again to so cruelly burn the poor wounded by gunshot." Pare made false limbs for the amputees and also developed false eyes and false teeth.

The skin is the largest organ in the body. It protects the body and helps to maintain health. Factors that increase risk for impaired skin integrity are aging, restricted mobility, chronic illnesses, trauma, and invasive healthcare procedures. Nursing care of the skin includes maintaining skin integrity and promoting wound healing. Nurses must be aware of risk factors and specific measures that promote optimal skin conditions. They must also understand the physiology of wound healing.

Skin Integrity

Intact skin is normal skin and skin layers, uninterrupted by wounds. Genetics and heredity determine many aspects of a person's skin, including skin color (Box 23-1 ■), sensitivity to sunlight, and allergies. Age influences skin integrity in both young and elder populations. Aging skin is more fragile and susceptible to injury. Wounds tend to heal more rapidly in infants and children.

Many chronic illnesses and their treatments affect skin integrity. People with impaired peripheral arterial circulation may have loss of leg hair and skin on the legs that appears shiny and damages easily. Some medications, such as steroids, cause thinning of the skin and allow it to be much more readily harmed. Certain antibiotics increase sensitivity to sunlight and can predispose a person to severe sunburns. Poor nutrition can interfere with the appearance and function of normal skin, as well as with healing.

Types of Wounds

Body wounds may be intentional or unintentional. *Intentional traumas* occur during therapy. Operations and venipunctures are intentional traumas that break skin in-

---

BOX 23-1   **CULTURAL PULSE POINTS**

Assessing Changes in Skin Color

Numerous biocultural variations occur in the integumentary system. The range of normal skin color varies widely. It is important to establish a baseline color in order to be able to assess pertinent changes in a client.

The following skin assessment terms have different meanings for biocultural variations:

- *Cyanosis* is a difficult clinical sign to observe in clients with dark skin. In light-skinned individuals, it appears as a yellowish skin discoloration. In dark-skinned individuals, it may appear as a grayish tone. Because cyanosis can signal decreased oxygenation to the brain, other clinical signs rather than skin color should be assessed.
- *Jaundice* in both dark- and light-skinned clients can best be observed in the sclera, rather than the skin.

---

tegrity. *Unintentional wounds* are accidental; for example, a person may fracture an arm in an automobile collision. If the tissues are traumatized without a break in the skin, there is a *closed wound*. An *open wound* occurs when the skin or mucous membrane surface is broken.

Wounds are frequently described according to how they are acquired (Table 23-1 ■). They also can be described according to the likelihood and degree of wound contamination:

- *Clean wounds* are uninfected wounds in which minimal inflammation is encountered. Clean wounds are primarily closed wounds.
- *Contaminated wounds* include open, fresh, accidental wounds and surgical wounds involving a major break in sterile technique. Contaminated wounds show evidence of inflammation.

TABLE 23-1

Types of Wounds

TYPE	CAUSE	DESCRIPTION AND CHARACTERISTICS
Incision	Sharp instrument (e.g., knife or scalpel)	Open wound; painful; deep or shallow
Contusion	Blow from a blunt instrument	Closed wound, skin appears ecchymotic (bruised) because of damaged blood vessels
Abrasion	Surface scrape, either unintentional (e.g., scraped knee from a fall) or intentional (e.g., dermal abrasion to remove pockmarks)	Open wound involving the skin; painful
Puncture	Penetration of the skin and often the underlying tissues by a sharp instrument, either intentional or unintentional	Open wound
Laceration	Tissues torn apart, often from accidents (e.g., with machinery)	Open wound; edges are often jagged
Penetrating wound	Penetration of the skin and the underlying tissues, usually unintentional (e.g., from a bullet or metal fragments)	Open wound

- *Dirty* or *infected wounds* include old, accidental wounds containing dead tissue and wounds with evidence of a clinical infection, such as purulent drainage.

Wounds are also classified by depth, that is, the tissue layers involved in the wound. *Partial-thickness wounds* are confined to the skin (dermis and epidermis). *Full-thickness wounds* involve the dermis, epidermis, subcutaneous tissue, and possibly muscle and bone.

Pressure ulcers are a type of wound (usually preventable) that progress from closed to open. They are a great concern in hospitals, in long-term care facilities, and in work with any client with impaired mobility. Pressure ulcers are discussed separately later in this chapter.

Wound Healing

Wound healing is the regeneration (renewal) of tissues. The two types of healing are distinguished by the amount of tissue loss. *Primary intention healing* (or first intention healing) occurs where the tissue surfaces have been *approximated* (closed) and there is minimal or no tissue loss. It characteristically has minimal granulation tissue and scarring. A closed surgical incision is an example of primary intention healing (Figure 23-1 ■).

A wound that is extensive and involves considerable tissue loss, and in which the edges cannot or should not be

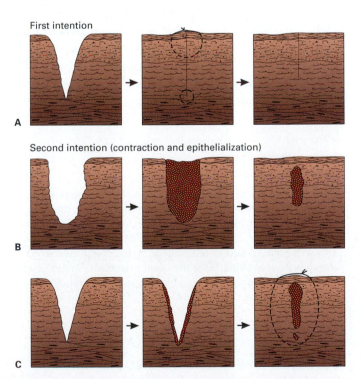

Figure 23-1. ■ Classification of wound healing: **A.** First intention: A clean incision is made with primary closure; there is minimal scarring. **B, C.** Second intention: The wound is left open so that granulation can result (B), or the wound is intentionally left open and later closed when there is no further evidence of infection (C).

approximated, heals by *secondary intention healing*. A pressure ulcer is an example of a wound that heals by secondary intention. Secondary intention healing differs from primary intention healing in three ways: (1) The repair time is longer, (2) the scarring is greater, and (3) the risk of infection is greater.

PHASES OF WOUND HEALING

The phases of healing are the steps in the body's natural processes of tissue repair. The rate of healing varies depending on factors such as the type of healing, wound location and size, and the health of the client. Wound healing can be broken down into three phases: inflammatory, proliferative, and maturation.

Inflammatory Phase

The inflammatory phase starts immediately after injury and lasts 3 to 6 days. Two major processes (hemostasis and phagocytosis) occur during this phase.

Hemostasis (the arrest or cessation of bleeding) results from vasoconstriction, *retraction* (drawing back) of injured blood vessels, the deposition of fibrin (connective tissue), and blood clot formation. The blood clots become the framework for cell repair. A scab, made of clots and dead or dying tissue, also forms on the surface of the wound. This scab aids hemostasis and helps prevent contamination of the wound by microorganisms.

During the inflammatory phase, vascular and cellular responses promote removal of foreign substances and dead or dying tissue. The blood supply to the wound increases, bringing with it substances and nutrients needed in the healing process. The area appears reddened and edematous as a result.

Macrophages (certain white blood cells) engulf microorganisms and cellular debris by a process known as **phagocytosis**. This inflammatory response is essential to healing. Measures that impair inflammation, such as use of steroid medications, can slow or prevent the healing process.

Proliferative Phase

The proliferative phase, the second phase in healing, extends from day 3 to about day 21 postinjury. *Fibroblasts* (connective tissue cells) migrate into the wound about 24 hours after injury. There they begin to synthesize collagen, a whitish protein substance that adds strength to the wound and gradually decreases the wound's chance of reopening.

Capillaries grow across the wound, increasing the blood supply, which brings oxygen and nutrients. Fibroblasts move from the bloodstream into the wound, depositing fibrin. As the capillary network develops, the tissue becomes a translucent red color. This tissue, called **granulation tissue**, is fragile and bleeds easily.

When the skin edges of a wound are not sutured, the area fills in with granulation tissue. If the wound does not close by *epithelialization* (skin formation), the area becomes covered with dried plasma proteins and dead cells. This is called **eschar** (scar tissue). Initially, wounds that heal by secondary intention seep blood-tinged (**serosanguineous**) drainage.

Maturation Phase

The maturation phase begins on about day 21 and can extend 1 or 2 years after the injury. Fibroblasts continue to synthesize collagen. The collagen fibers reorganize into a more orderly structure. During maturation, the wound is remodeled and contracted. The scar becomes stronger, but the repaired area is never as strong as the original tissue. In some individuals, particularly dark-skinned persons, an abnormal amount of collagen is laid down. This can result in a hypertrophic scar (or **keloid**).

KINDS OF WOUND DRAINAGE

Exudate is material, such as fluid and cells, that has escaped from blood vessels during the inflammatory process and is deposited in tissue or on tissue surfaces. The nature and amount of exudate vary according to the tissue involved, the intensity and duration of the inflammation, and the presence of microorganisms.

There are three major types of exudate: serous, purulent, and sanguineous (hemorrhagic). A **serous** *exudate* consists chiefly of serum (the clear portion of the blood) derived from blood. It looks watery and has few cells.

A *purulent exudate* is thicker than serous exudate because it contains pus. Pus consists of leukocytes, liquefied dead tissue debris, and dead and living bacteria. The process of pus formation is referred to as **suppuration**. Purulent exudates may have tinges of blue, green, or yellow. The color may depend on the causative organism. However, not all microorganisms are *pyogenic* (pus producing).

A **sanguineous** *(hemorrhagic) exudate* consists of large amounts of red blood cells. This type of exudate indicates damage to capillaries that allows escape of red blood cells from the plasma. It is frequently seen in open wounds. Nurses often need to distinguish whether the sanguineous exudate is dark or bright. A bright sanguineous exudate indicates fresh bleeding. Dark sanguineous exudate denotes older bleeding. Mixed types of exudates are often observed.

COMPLICATIONS OF WOUND HEALING

Hemorrhage

Some escape of blood from a wound is normal. However, **hemorrhage** (persistent bleeding) is abnormal. It may be caused by a dislodged clot, a slipped suture, or erosion of a blood vessel.

Internal hemorrhage may often be detected by swelling or distention in the area of the wound and or sanguineous drainage from a surgical drain. Some clients have a hematoma, a localized collection of blood underneath the skin that may appear as a reddish blue swelling.

External hemorrhage often either appears under a dressing or escapes from the dressing and pools under the client. The risk of hemorrhage is greatest during the first 48 hours after surgery. Hemorrhage is an emergency that requires the application of extra sterile pressure dressings to the area, monitoring the client's vital signs, and notifying the physician.

Infection

A wound can be infected with microorganisms at the time of injury, during surgery, or postoperatively during open wound healing (see Chapter 9 ⦻). Wounds that occur as a result of injury (bullet and knife wounds) are most likely to be contaminated at the time of injury. Surgery involving the intestines can also result in infection from the microorganisms inside the intestine. Surgical infection is most likely to become apparent 2 to 11 days postoperatively.

Dehiscence with Possible Evisceration

Dehiscence is the partial or total rupturing of a sutured wound. Dehiscence usually involves an abdominal wound in which the layers below the skin also separate. **Evisceration** is the protrusion of the internal viscera through an incision. A number of factors, including obesity, poor nutrition, multiple trauma, failure of suturing, excessive coughing, vomiting, and dehydration, heighten a client's risk of wound dehiscence.

clinical ALERT

Wound dehiscence is more likely to occur 4 to 5 days postoperatively. An increase in the flow of serosanguineous drainage into the wound dressing can indicate an impending dehiscence. When dehiscence or evisceration occurs, the wound should be quickly supported by large sterile dressings soaked in sterile normal saline. Place the client in bed with knees bent to decrease pull on the incision. The surgeon should be notified, because immediate surgical repair of the area is necessary.

FACTORS AFFECTING WOUND HEALING

Age and Lifestyle

Healthy children and adults often heal more quickly than older people. See Box 23-2 ■ for factors that inhibit wound healing in older adults.

People who exercise regularly tend to have good circulation. Because blood brings oxygen and nourishment to the wound, people who exercise are more likely to heal quickly. Smoking reduces the amount of functional hemoglobin in the blood, thus limiting the oxygen-carrying capacity of the blood.

Nutrition

Wound healing requires a diet rich in protein, carbohydrates, lipids, vitamins A and C, and minerals, such as iron, zinc, and copper. Malnourished clients may require time to improve their nutritional status before surgery. Obese clients are at increased risk of wound infection and slower healing because *adipose* (fatty) tissue usually has a minimal blood supply.

Medications

Anti-inflammatory drugs (e.g., steroids and aspirin), heparin, and antineoplastic agents interfere with healing. Prolonged use of antibiotics may make a person susceptible to wound infection by resistant organisms.

Contamination and Infection

Contamination of a wound surface with pathogenic microorganisms usually results in infection. These organisms compete with new cells for oxygen and nutrition and can impair wound healing. When the microorganisms multiply, infection occurs. Clients who are immunosuppressed are especially susceptible to wound infections.

COLLABORATIVE CARE

Wound Cleaning

Wound cleaning has traditionally involved the removal of *debris* (i.e., foreign materials, excess slough, necrotic tissue,

bacteria, and other microorganisms). Formerly, antimicrobial solutions such as povidone-iodine (Betadine), 3% hydrogen peroxide, 70% alcohol, and Dakin's solution were commonly used. However, these solutions have caustic effects on granulation tissue and the skin. The choices of cleaning agent and method depend largely on agency protocol and the physician's preference.

WOUND IRRIGATION AND PACKING. An *irrigation* (*lavage*) is the washing or flushing out of an area. Sterile technique is required for a wound irrigation, because there is a break in the skin integrity.

Using piston syringes instead of bulb syringes to irrigate a wound reduces the risk of aspirating drainage and provides safe, effective pressure. For deep wounds with small openings, a sterile straight catheter may also be necessary. Frequently used irrigation solutions are sterile normal saline, lactated Ringer's solution, and antibiotic solutions.

Gauze packing is placed in wounds to facilitate the formation of granulation tissue and healing by secondary intention. Generally, moistened 4×4 non–cotton-filled gauze dressings are used. Cotton fibers are contraindicated because they can pull loose and remain in the wound, encouraging bacterial growth and contamination.

The wet-to-damp technique is generally used to pack wounds. In this technique, moist gauzes are packed in the wound to absorb exudate, but they are not allowed to dry before removal.

Wound Dressings

Dressings are applied to wounds for the following purposes:

- To protect the wound from mechanical injury.
- To protect the wound from microbial contamination.
- To provide or maintain high humidity of the wound.
- To provide thermal insulation.
- To absorb drainage or debride a wound or both.
- To prevent hemorrhage (when applied as a pressure dressing or with elastic bandages).
- To splint or immobilize the wound site and thereby facilitate healing and prevent injury.
- To provide psychological comfort.

Various dressing materials are available to cover wounds. The type of dressing used depends on several factors:

- The location, size, and type of the wound
- The amount of exudate
- Whether the wound requires debridement, is infected, or has sinus tracts
- Such considerations as frequency of dressing change, ease or difficulty of dressing application, and cost.

TABLE 23-2			
Selected Types of Wound Dressings			
DRESSING	**DESCRIPTION**	**PURPOSE**	**EXAMPLES**
Transparent adhesive films/wound barriers	Adhesive plastic, semipermeable, nonabsorbent dressings that allow exchange of oxygen between the atmosphere and wound bed. They are impermeable to bacteria and water.	To provide protection against contamination and friction; to maintain a clean moist surface that facilitates cellular migration; to provide insulation by preventing fluid evaporation; and to facilitate wound assessment.	Op-Site, Tegaderm, Bio-occlusive, ACU-derm
Impregnated non-adherent dressings	Woven or nonwoven cotton or synthetic materials that are impregnated with petrolatum, saline, zinc-saline, antimicrobials, or other agents. Require secondary dressings to secure them in place, retain moisture, and provide wound protection.	To cover, soothe, and protect partial- and full-thickness wounds without exudate.	Vaseline gauze, CarraGauze, Dermagran Wet Dressing, Xeroform
Hydrocolloids	Waterproof adhesive wafers, pastes, or powders. Wafers, designed to be worn for up to 7 days, consist of two layers. The inner adhesive layer has particles that absorb exudate and form a hydrated gel over the wound; the outer film provides a seal.	To absorb exudate; to produce a moist environment that facilitates healing but does not cause maceration of surrounding skin; to protect the wound from bacterial contamination, foreign debris, and urine or feces; and to prevent shearing.	DuoDERM, Comfeel, Tegasorb, Restore, RepliCare
Hydrogels	Glycerin or water-based, nonadhesive, jelly-like sheets, granules, or gels that are oxygen permeable, unless covered by a plastic film. May require secondary occlusive dressing.	To liquefy necrotic tissue or slough, rehydrate the wound bed, and fill in dead space.	Aquasorb, ClearSite, Elasto-Gel, IntraSite, Vigilon
Polyurethane foams	Nonadherent hydrocolloid dressings that need to have their edges taped down or sealed. Require secondary dressings to obtain an occlusive environment. Surrounding skin must be protected to prevent maceration.	To absorb light to moderate amounts of exudate; to debride wounds.	LYOfoam, Allevyn, Nu-Derm, Flexzan
Exudate absorbers	Nonadherent dressings of powder, beads or granules, or paste that conform to the wound surface and absorb up to 20 times their weight in exudate; require a secondary dressing.	To provide a moist wound surface by interacting with exudate; to form a gelatinous mass; to absorb exudate; to eliminate dead space or pack wounds; and to support debridement.	Debrisan, Triad paste, Sorbsan

Table 23-2 ■ describes materials for dressing wounds. Common gauze dressings (Figure 23-2 ■) may be applied in several ways to achieve different goals. Other dressing materials are used for specific types and conditions of wounds. Methods of applying gauze dressings are described in Table 23-3 ■.

TRANSPARENT WOUND BARRIERS. Transparent dressings are often applied to wounds including ulcerated or burned skin areas (Figure 23-3 ■). These dressings offer several advantages:

- They act as temporary skin.
- They are nonporous, self-adhesive dressings that do not require daily changing as other dressings do.

- Because they are transparent, the wound can be assessed through them.
- Because they are occlusive, the wound remains moist and retains the serous exudate, which promotes epithelial growth, hastens healing, and reduces the risk of infection.
- Because they are elastic, they can be placed over a joint without disrupting the client's mobility.
- They adhere only to the skin area around the wound and not to the wound itself because they keep the wound moist.
- They allow the client to shower or bathe without removing the dressing.
- They can be removed without damaging wound tissues.

Part A of Procedure 23-1 ■ on page 489 describes how to apply a moist transparent wound barrier.

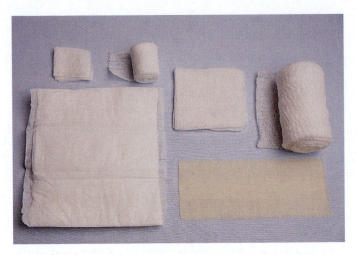

Figure 23-2. ■ Some frequently used dressing materials (clockwise from bottom left): surgipad or abdominal pad, 2 × 2 gauze, 2-in. roller gauze, 4 × 4 gauze, 4-in. roller. (Photographer: Elena Dorfman.)

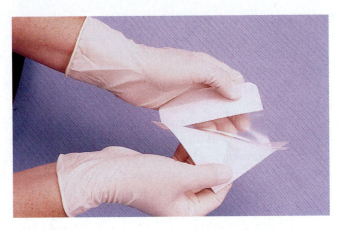

Figure 23-3. ■ A transparent wound dressing. (Photographer: Jenny Thomas.)

HYDROCOLLOID DRESSINGS. Hydrocolloid dressings (see Table 23-2) are frequently used over venous stasis leg ulcers and pressure ulcers. These dressings offer several advantages:

- They can last 5 to 7 days.
- They do not need a "cover" dressing and are water resistant.
- They can be molded to uneven body surfaces.
- They act as temporary skin and provide an effective bacterial barrier.
- They decrease pain and thus reduce the need for analgesics.
- They absorb some drainage and therefore can be used on draining wounds.
- They contain wound odor.

These dressings have certain limitations, however. Some of their disadvantages include the following:

- They are opaque and obscure wound visibility.
- They have a limited absorption.
- They can facilitate anaerobic bacterial growth.
- They can soften and wrinkle at the edges with wear and movement.
- They can be difficult to remove and may leave a residue on the skin.

Hydrocolloid dressings should not be used for infected wounds or those with deep tracts or **fistulas** (abnormal passage that develops between a hollow organ and the skin or between two hollow organs). Part B of Procedure 23-1 describes how to apply hydrocolloid dressings.

TABLE 23-3		
Methods of Applying Gauze Dressings		
DRESSING	**DESCRIPTION**	**PURPOSE**
Dry-to-dry	A layer of wide-mesh cotton gauze lies next to the wound surface. A second layer of dry absorbent cotton or Dacron is on top.	Protect the wound. If the wound is open or draining, necrotic debris and exudates are trapped in the interstices of the gauze layer and are removed when the dressing is removed.
Wet-to-dry	Next to the wound surface is a layer of wide-mesh cotton gauze saturated with saline or an antimicrobial solution. This layer is covered by a moist absorbent material that is moistened with the same solution.	Debride the wound. Necrotic debris is softened by the solution and then adheres to the mesh gauze as it dries. It is removed when the dressing is removed. Also, moisture helps dilute viscous exudates.
Wet-to-damp	A variation of the wet-to-dry dressing, this dressing is removed before it has completely dried.	The wound is debrided when the gauze is removed.
Wet-to-wet	A layer of wide-mesh gauze saturated with antibacterial solution lies next to the wound surface. Above is a second layer of absorbent material saturated with the same solution. The entire dressing is kept moist with a wetting agent.	The wound surface is continually bathed. Moisture dilutes viscous exudate.

NEGATIVE-PRESSURE WOUND THERAPY. Negative-pressure wound therapy (NPWT) is an advanced wound care method and treatment for chronic and acute wound types. Challenging cases of pressure ulcers, diabetic wounds, abdominal wounds, partial-thickness burns, trauma wounds, flaps, and grafts are being treated with NPWT. This therapy removes fluids and infectious materials; it helps promote perfusion, provides a moist healing environment, and aids in wound approximation. The action is a controlled application of subatmospheric pressure using a mechanized unit to intermittently or continuously convey negative pressure to a specialized wound dressing, promoting wound healing. The resilient and foam-like dressing assists in tissue granulation and is sealed with an adhesive drape that contains the subatmospheric pressure at the wound site. The technology used regulates pressure at the wound site. The system directs drainage to a designated receptacle, reducing exposure to exudate and infectious materials. It decreases the number of dressing changes and diminishes the risk of cross-contamination.

MEANS OF SECURING DRESSINGS. Dressings over wounds must cover the entire wound in order to protect it. They must also be secured so that they do not become dislodged, exposing the healing wound. The correct type of tape must be selected. For example, elastic tape can provide pressure; nonallergenic tape can be used when a client is allergic to other tape.

Montgomery straps (tie tapes) are commonly used for wounds that require frequent dressing changes (Figure 23-4 ■). These straps prevent skin irritation and discomfort caused by removing the adhesive each time the dressing is changed. The nurse can protect the skin by applying tincture of benzoin to the site where the adhesive is to be placed.

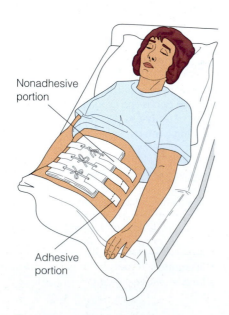

Nonadhesive portion

Adhesive portion

Figure 23-4. ■ Montgomery straps, or tie tapes, are used to secure large dressings that require frequent changing.

Supporting and Immobilizing Wounds

Bandages and binders serve various purposes:

- Supporting a wound (e.g., a fractured bone)
- Immobilizing a wound (e.g., a strained shoulder)
- Applying pressure (e.g., elastic bandages on the lower extremities to improve venous blood flow)
- Securing a dressing (e.g., for an extensive abdominal surgical wound)
- Retaining warmth (e.g., a flannel bandage on a rheumatoid joint).

Several types of bandages and binders are available, and they are applied in various ways. When correctly applied, they promote healing, provide comfort, and can prevent injury. Clinical guidelines for bandaging are discussed in the Nursing Care section starting on page 477.

BANDAGES. A *bandage* is a strip of cloth used to wrap some part of the body. Bandages are available in various widths, most commonly 1.5 to 7.5 cm (0.5 to 3 in.), and are usually supplied in rolls for easy application to a body part.

Many types of materials are used for bandages. Gauze is one of the most commonly used; it is light and porous and readily molds to the body. It is also relatively inexpensive, so it is generally discarded when soiled. Gauze is frequently used to retain dressings on wounds and to bandage the fingers, hands, toes, and feet. It supports dressings and at the same time permits air to circulate. It can also be saturated with petroleum jelly or other medications for application to wounds.

Many kinds of elasticized bandages are applied to provide pressure to an area. They are commonly used as tensor bandages or as partial stockings (TEDS). They provide support and improve the venous circulation in the legs.

The width of the bandage used depends on the size of the body part to be bandaged. The greater circumference of a part, the wider the bandage. Padding (e.g., abdominal pads and gauze squares) is frequently used to cover bony prominences (e.g., the elbow) or to separate skin surfaces (e.g., the fingers).

Before applying a bandage, the nurse needs to know its purpose and to assess the area requiring support. See Box 23-3 ■ for assessment guidelines. When bandages are used to secure dressings, the nurse wears gloves to prevent contact with body fluids.

BINDERS. A *binder* is a type of bandage designed for a specific body part; for example, the triangular binder (sling) fits the arm. Binders are used to support large areas of the body, such as the abdomen, arm, or chest.

A triangular arm binder or *sling* is usually applied as a full triangle to support the arm, elbow, and forearm of the client or to reduce or prevent swelling of a hand. Most agencies use commercial strap slings.

BOX 23-3	ASSESSING CLIENTS BEFORE APPLYING BANDAGES OR BINDERS

- Inspect and palpate the area for swelling.
- Inspect for the presence of and status of wounds (open wounds will require a dressing before a bandage or binder is applied).
- Note the presence of drainage (amount, color, odor, viscosity).
- Inspect and palpate for adequacy of circulation (skin temperature, color, and sensation). Pale or cyanotic skin, cool temperature, tingling, and numbness can indicate impaired circulation.
- Ask the client about any pain experienced (location, intensity, onset, quality).
- Assess the ability of the client to reapply the bandage or binder when needed.
- Assess the capabilities of the client regarding activities of daily living (e.g., to eat, dress, comb hair, bathe) and assess the assistance required during the convalescence period.

TABLE 23-4

Physiological Effects of Heat and Cold

HEAT	COLD
Vasodilation	Vasoconstriction
Increases capillary permeability	Decreases capillary permeability
Increases cellular metabolism	Decreases cellular metabolism
Relaxes muscles	Relaxes muscles
Increases inflammation; increases blood flow to an area	Slows bacterial growth; decreases inflammation
Decreases pain by relaxing muscles	Decreases pain by numbing the area, by slowing the flow of pain impulses, and by increasing the pain threshold
Sedative effect	Local anesthetic effect
Reduces joint stiffness by decreasing viscosity of synovial fluids	Decreases bleeding

Straight abdominal binders are used to support the abdomen. A straight binder is also used to support the chest. Chest binders often have shoulder straps.

Heat and Cold Applications

Heat and cold are applied to the body for local and systemic effects. They can be useful in the healing process for closed wounds.

EFFECTS OF HEAT AND COLD. Heat causes vasodilation and increases blood flow to the affected area, bringing oxygen, nutrients, antibodies, and leukocytes. Table 23-4 ■ describes the physiological effects of heat and cold. Application of heat promotes soft tissue healing and increases suppuration. Heat is often used for clients with musculoskeletal problems such as joint stiffness from arthritis, contractures, and low back pain.

A possible disadvantage of heat is that it increases capillary permeability, allowing extracellular fluid and substances such as plasma proteins to pass through the capillary walls. This may result in edema. Also, when heat is applied to a large body area, it may cause excessive peripheral vasodilation and a drop in blood pressure. A significant drop in blood pressure can cause fainting.

Cold lowers the temperature of the skin and underlying tissues and causes vasoconstriction, which reduces blood flow to the affected area. It reduces the supply of oxygen and metabolites, decreases the removal of wastes, and produces skin pallor and coolness. Cold applications are most often used for sports injuries (e.g., sprains, strains, fractures) to limit swelling and bleeding.

Prolonged exposure to cold results in impaired circulation, cell deprivation, and subsequent damage to the tissues from lack of oxygen and nourishment. The signs of tissue damage due to cold are a bluish purple mottled appearance of the skin, numbness, and sometimes blisters and pain.

Shivering is an initial, normal response to systemic cold, as the body attempts to warm itself (see also Chapter 20 ⬭). With extensive cold applications, a client's blood pressure can increase because vasoconstriction causes blood to be shunted from the cutaneous circulation to the internal blood vessels.

THERMAL TOLERANCE. Variables such as extremes of age, length of exposure, and intactness of the skin affect tolerance to heat and cold. Some body parts (like the back of the hand and the foot) are not very temperature sensitive. Others (the neck, the inside of the wrist, the perineal area) are very sensitive to temperature. Certain conditions require added caution in the use of hot or cold applications:

- *Neurosensory impairment.* People who cannot perceive heat or cold normally are at risk for burns or tissue injury.
- *Impaired mental status.* People who are confused or have an altered level of consciousness need monitoring during applications to ensure safe therapy.
- *Impaired circulation.* People with peripheral vascular disease, diabetes, or congestive heart failure lack the normal ability to dissipate heat via the blood circulation. This puts them at risk for tissue damage with heat and cold applications.

■ *Recent injury or surgery.* Immediately after injury or surgery, heat increases bleeding and swelling.

■ *Open wounds.* Cold can decrease blood flow to the wound, thereby inhibiting healing.

Methods for Applying Heat and Cold

Heat can be applied to the body in both dry and moist forms. Dry heat is applied locally by means of a hot water bottle, electric pad, aquathermia pad, or disposable heat pack. Moist heat can be provided by compress, hot pack, soak, or sitz bath. Guidelines for nurses to follow for local applications of heat or cold are discussed in the following Nursing Care section.

AQUATHERMIA PAD.   The aquathermia or Aquamatic pad (also referred to as a K-pad) is a pad constructed with tubes containing water. The pad is attached by tubing to an electrically powered control unit that has an opening for water and a temperature gauge (Figure 23-5 ■). Some aquathermia pads have an absorbent surface through which moist heat can be applied. The other surface of the pad is waterproof. These pads are disposable.

HOT AND COLD PACKS.   Commercially prepared packs provide heat or cold for a designated time. Directions on the package tell how to initiate the heating or cooling process, such as by striking, squeezing, or kneading the pack.

ICE BAGS, ICE GLOVES, AND ICE COLLARS.   Ice bags, ice gloves, and ice collars are filled either with ice chips or with an alcohol-based solution. They are applied to the body to provide cold to a localized area (e.g., a collar is often applied to the throat following a tonsillectomy).

COMPRESSES.   Compresses can be either warm or cold. A *compress* is a moist gauze dressing applied to a wound. When hot compresses are ordered, the solution is heated to the temperature indicated by the order or according to agency protocol, for example, 40.5°C (105°F). When there is a break in the skin or when the body part (e.g., an eye) is vulnerable to microbial invasion, sterile technique is necessary. Sterile gloves are needed to apply the compress, and all materials must be sterile.

SOAKS.   A *soak* refers to immersing a body part (e.g., an arm) in a solution or to wrapping a part in gauze dressings and then saturating the dressing with a solution. Sterile technique is generally indicated for open wounds, such as a burn or an unhealed surgical incision. Determine agency protocol regarding the temperature of the solution. Hot soaks are frequently done to soften and remove encrusted secretions and dead tissue.

SITZ BATH.   A **sitz bath** is used to soak a client's pelvic area. The client sits in a special tub or chair and is usually immersed from the midthighs to the iliac crests or umbilicus. Special tubs or chairs are preferred because then the legs are also immersed and because a regular bathtub decreases blood circulation to the perineum or pelvic area. Disposable sitz baths are also available.

The temperature of the water should be from 40° to 43°C (105° to 110°F), unless the client is unable to tolerate the heat. Determine agency protocol. Some sitz tubs have temperature indicators attached to the water taps. The duration of the bath is generally 15 to 20 minutes, depending on the client's health.

COOLING SPONGE BATH.   The purpose of a cooling sponge bath is to reduce a client's fever by promoting heat loss through conduction and vaporization. The bath consists of water or a combination of alcohol and water that is below body temperature. Alcohol evaporates at a low temperature and therefore removes body heat rapidly. However, alcohol-and-water sponge baths are less frequently used than in the past because alcohol has a drying effect on the skin. The temperatures for cooling sponge baths range from 18° to 32°C (65° to 90°F). A tepid sponge bath generally refers to one in which the water temperature is 32°C (90°F) throughout the bath.

The decision to give a tepid sponge bath is generally made only when a marked fever or a temperature increase is noted. Some agencies require a physician's order; others permit a decision by a nurse.

HYPERTHERMIA AND HYPOTHERMIA BLANKETS.   Hyperthermia and hypothermia blankets are used to increase or decrease a client's body temperature. The blanket has an associated control panel on which the desired temperature is set and the client's core temperature is registered. Follow institutional policy for further details.

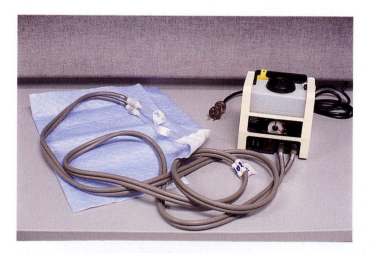

Figure 23-5. ■ An aquathermia heating unit.

Laboratory Data

Laboratory data often support the nurse's clinical assessment of the wound's progress in healing. A decreased leukocyte count can delay healing and increase the possibility of infection. Blood coagulation studies are also significant. Prolonged coagulation times can result in excessive blood loss and prolonged clot absorption. Serum protein analysis provides an indication of the body's nutritional reserves for rebuilding cells. Wound cultures can either confirm or rule out the presence of infection. Sensitivity studies are helpful in the selection of appropriate antibiotic therapy.

NURSING CARE

ASSESSING

The nurse examines the integument as part of a routine observation and assessment during regular care. During the review of systems as part of the nursing history, the nurse collects information about skin diseases, previous bruising, general skin condition, skin lesions, and usual healing of sores. Inspection and palpation of the skin focus on skin color distribution, skin turgor, presence of edema, and characteristics of any lesions. Box 23-4 ■ describes assessment of common pressure sites.

BOX 23-4	ASSESSING COMMON PRESSURE SITES

- Be sure there is good lighting, preferably natural or fluorescent.
- Regulate the environment before beginning the assessment so that the room is neither too hot nor too cold. Heat can cause the skin to flush; cold can cause the skin to blanch or become cyanotic.
- Inspect pressure areas for any whitish or reddened spots; discoloration can be caused by impaired blood circulation to the area. It should disappear in a few minutes when rubbing restores circulation.
- Inspect pressure areas for abrasions and excoriations. An abrasion (wearing away of the skin) can occur when skin rubs against a sheet (e.g., when the client is pulled). Excoriations (loss of superficial layers of the skin) can occur when the skin has prolonged contact with body secretions or excretions or with dampness in skinfolds.
- Palpate the surface temperature of the skin over the pressure areas. Normally, the temperature is the same as that of the surrounding skin. Increased temperature is abnormal and may be due to inflammation or blood trapped in the area.
- Palpate over bony prominences and dependent body areas for the presence of edema, which feels spongy.

Untreated Wounds

Untreated wounds usually are seen shortly after an injury (e.g., at the scene of an emergency or in an emergency center). The following steps are important when assessing an untreated wound:

- Note size and severity of wound and check for associated injuries. Call for help to treat severe wounds.
- Inspect the wound for foreign bodies (soil, glass, etc.).
- If wound is contaminated with foreign material, assess need for tetanus immunization or booster.

Treated Wounds

Treated wounds, or sutured wounds, are usually assessed to determine the progress of healing. These wounds may be inspected during a dressing change unless a transparent dressing has been applied. If the wound itself cannot be inspected directly, the dressing is inspected and other data regarding the wound (e.g., the presence of pain) are assessed. Many treated wounds are covered with a transparent occlusive dressing that permits observation of the wound without exposure to the air.

Assessment of a treated wound includes observation of its appearance, size, and drainage; the presence of swelling or pain; and status of drains or tubes.

DIAGNOSING, PLANNING, AND IMPLEMENTING

Nursing diagnoses that relate to clients who have skin wounds or who are at risk for skin breakdown are:

- *Risk for Impaired Skin Integrity*
- *Impaired Skin Integrity* (commonly applies to superficial wounds extending through the epidermis but not through the dermis)
- *Impaired Tissue Integrity* (applies to wounds extending into subcutaneous tissue, muscle, or bone)
- *Risk for Infection*
- *Pain* related to nerve involvement
- *Disturbed Body Image*.

In planning nursing care, the primary goals are maintaining skin integrity and avoiding potential risks. For clients with *Impaired Skin Integrity* or *Impaired Tissue Integrity,* the goal is to achieve progressive wound healing and regain intact skin.

Nursing interventions for maintaining skin integrity and providing wound care involve supporting wound healing, preventing pressure ulcers, treating pressure ulcers, cleaning and dressing wounds, supporting and immobilizing wounds, and applying heat and cold. Examples of nursing interventions for maintaining intact skin follow:

- Inspect skin at regular intervals.
- Keep skin clean, dry, and moisturized.
- Provide appropriate pressure-relieving devices and measures (Table 23-5 ■).

TABLE 23-5

Mechanical Devices for Reducing Pressure on Body Parts

DEVICE	DESCRIPTION/COMMENTS
Gel flotation pads	Polyvinyl, silicone, or Silastic pads are filled with a gelatinous substance similar to fat.
Sheepskins (natural and artificial)	Some manufacturers produce mixed natural and synthetic pads; artificial pads are less likely to be damaged by washing but are more likely to make the client hot than natural skins.
Pillows and wedges (foam, gel and air, foam and fluid)	Can raise a body part (e.g., heels) off the bed surface.
Heel protectors (sheepskin boots, padded splints, foam wedges)	Limit pressure on heels when the client is in bed.
Egg-crate mattress	Polyurethane foam mattress resembling an egg crate; some types are flammable.
Foam mattress	Foam molds to the body.
Alternating pressure mattress	Composed of a number of cells in which the pressure alternately increases and decreases; uses a pump.
Water bed	Special mattress filled with water; controls temperature of water.
Air-fluidized (AF) bed (static high air loss bed)	Forced temperature-controlled air is circulated around millions of tiny silicone-coated beads, producing a fluid-like movement. Provides uniform support to body contours. Decreases skin maceration by its drying effect. Moisture from the client penetrates the bed sheet and soaks the beads. Air flow forces the beads away from the client and rapidly dries the sheet. A major disadvantage is that the head of the bed cannot be elevated.
Static low air loss (LAL) bed	Consists of many air-filled cushions divided into four or five sections. Separate controls permit each section to be inflated to a different level of firmness; thus pressure can be reduced on bony prominences but increased under other body areas for support.
Active or second-generation LAL bed	Like the static LAL, but in addition gently pulsates or rotates from side to side, thus stimulating capillary blood flow and facilitating movement of pulmonary secretions.

For clients with untreated wounds, the nurse performs the following interventions:

- Control severe bleeding, apply direct pressure to the wound, and elevate the extremity.
- Prevent infection by cleansing or flushing abrasions or lacerations with water. Box 23-5 ■ provides guidelines for cleaning wounds.
- If bleeding is severe or if internal bleeding is suspected, assess the client and report any signs of shock (rapid thready pulse, cold clammy skin, pallor, lowered blood pressure).
- Cover the wound with a clean dressing (a sterile dressing is preferred). If the first layer of dressing becomes saturated with blood, apply a second layer. *Removing the first layer of dressing might disturb blood clots, resulting in more bleeding.*

Supporting Wound Healing

There are three major areas in which nurses can support wound healing: obtaining sufficient nutrition and fluids, preventing wound infections, and positioning the client properly.

- Assist the client to take in at least 2500 mL of fluids a day unless conditions contraindicate this amount. The nurse should ensure that clients receive sufficient protein; vitamins C, A, B_1, B_2; and zinc *although there is no evidence that excessive doses of vitamins or minerals enhance healing.*
- Provide excellent infection control: (1) Prevent microorganisms from entering the wound, and (2) prevent transmission of bloodborne pathogens to or from the client to others. (See Chapter 9 ⬭ for more information about infection control.)
- Obtain a wound culture whenever an infection is suspected. Procedure 23-2 ■ on page 491 provides guidelines for obtaining a specimen of wound drainage.
- Position clients to keep pressure off the wound. Changes of position and transfers must be accomplished without shear or friction damage.

BOX 23-5	NURSING CARE CHECKLIST

Cleaning Wounds

☑ Use physiological solutions, such as isotonic saline or lactated Ringer's solution, to clean or irrigate wounds. If antimicrobial solutions are used, make sure they are well diluted.

☑ When possible, warm the solution to body temperature before use. This prevents lowering of the wound temperature, which slows the healing process.

☑ If a wound is grossly contaminated by foreign material, bacteria, slough, or necrotic tissue, clean the wound at every dressing change. Foreign bodies and devitalized tissue act as a focus for infection and can delay healing.

☑ If a wound is clean, has little exudate, and reveals healthy granulation tissue, avoid repeated cleaning. Unnecessary cleaning can delay wound healing by traumatizing newly produced, delicate tissues, reducing the surface temperature of the wound, and removing exudate, which itself may have bactericidal properties.

☑ Use gauze squares. Avoid using cotton balls and other products that shed fibers onto the wound surface. The fibers become embedded in granulation tissue and can act as foci for infection. They may also stimulate "foreign body" reactions, prolonging the inflammatory phase of healing and delaying the healing process.

☑ Clean superficial noninfected wounds by irrigating them with normal saline. The hydraulic pressure of an irrigating stream of fluid dislodges contaminating debris and reduces bacterial colonization.

☑ To retain wound moisture, avoid drying a wound after cleaning it.

- Encourage the client to be as mobile as possible. *Activity enhances circulation*. If the client cannot move independently, implement range-of-motion exercises and a turning schedule.

Cleaning, Irrigating, and Dressing Wounds

- Wear gloves and follow standard precautions to prevent transmission of bloodborne pathogens.
- Wash hands before and after caring for wounds.
- Follow recommended guidelines for cleaning wounds (see Box 23-5). A major principle of cleaning wounds is always to clean from "clean to dirty."

- Touch an open or fresh surgical wound only when wearing sterile gloves or using sterile forceps. *Irrigate* (wash or flush out) the wound using sterile technique. *Sterile technique is required because of the break in skin integrity*. See Procedure 23-3 ■ on page 492 for the steps involved in irrigating a wound.
- Pack the wound as ordered. Clinical guidelines for applying wet-to-damp dressings are described in Box 23-6 ■.

Securing Dressings

- Ensure that the dressing covers the entire wound and select the appropriate tape to secure it.

BOX 23-6	NURSING CARE CHECKLIST

Applying Wet-to-Damp Dressings

☑ Open the packages of the sterile dressing set, fine-mesh gauze, and sterile solution container.

☑ Pour the ordered solution into the solution container.

☑ Place the fine-mesh gauze dressings into the solution container, and thoroughly saturate them with solution. The entire gauze must be moistened to enhance its absorptive abilities.

☑ If agency protocol indicates, clean the wound.

☑ Wring out the packing material so that it is slightly moist. Avoid packing that is too wet. An excessively wet wound bed increases the risk for bacterial growth and may macerate the surrounding skin.

☑ Pack the moistened dressings into all depressions and grooves of the wound, ensuring that all exposed surfaces are covered. If necessary, use forceps to feed the gauze gradually into deep depressed areas. Necrotic tissue is usually more prevalent in depressed wound areas and needs to be covered with gauze.

☑ Avoid applying packing too tightly. A tight application inhibits wound edges from contracting and compresses capillaries.

☑ To prevent maceration of the surrounding skin, pack only to the edge of the wound without overlapping the skin.

☑ If necessary, protect surrounding skin with a skin barrier (e.g., hydrocolloid dressing).

☑ Apply a secondary dressing (e.g., 4 × 4 gauze) over the wet dressings to absorb excess exudate.

☑ Cover all the dressings with a surgipad or abdominal pad. The pad protects the wound from external contaminants.

☑ Remove gloves inside out and discard them.

☑ To remove dressings, wear disposable gloves. If packing material adheres to any tissue during removal, soak it with normal saline. This facilitates removal and preserves new granulation tissue.

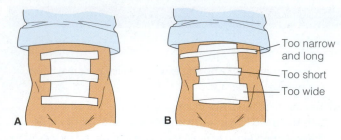

Figure 23-6. ■ The strips of tape should be placed at the ends of the dressing and must be sufficiently long and wide to secure the dressing. The tape should adhere to intact skin.

- Place the tape so that the dressing cannot be folded back to expose the wound. Place strips at the ends of the dressing, and space tapes evenly in the middle (Figure 23-6 ■).
- Ensure that the tape is long and wide enough to adhere to several inches of skin on each side of the dressing, but not so long or wide that the tape loosens with activity.
- Place the tape in the opposite direction from expected body action (Figure 23-7 ■).

Applying Bandages and Binders

General guidelines for bandaging include the following interventions:

- Bandage the part in its normal position, with the joint flexed slightly. *This avoids putting strain on the ligaments and muscles of the joint.*

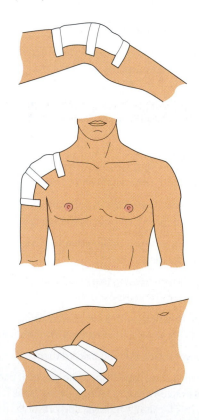

Figure 23-7. ■ Dressings over moving parts must remain secure in spite of the movement. Place the tape over a joint at a right angle to the direction the joint moves.

- Pad between skin surfaces and over bony areas. *This prevents friction and abrasion of the skin.*
- Bandage body parts from the distal to the proximal end. *This aids the return of venous blood.*
- If possible, leave the end of the body part (e.g., a toe) exposed. *This allows visual assessment of blood circulation to the extremity.*
- Cover the dressings with bandages at least 5 cm (2 in.) beyond the edges of the dressing. *This prevents the dressing and wound from becoming contaminated.*
- Face the client when applying the bandage. *This maintains uniform tension and alignment of the bandage.*

Circular turns are used chiefly to anchor bandages or to bandage certain areas, such as the proximal aspect of a finger or a wrist. Circular turns for roller bandages are done as follows:

- Apply the end of the bandage to the part of the body to be bandaged.
- Wrap the bandage around the body part a few times or as often as needed, each turn directly covering the previous turn (Figure 23-8 ■). This provides even support to the area.
- Secure the end of the bandage with tape, metal clips, or a safety pin over an uninjured area. Clips and pins can be uncomfortable when situated over an injured area.

Figure-eight turns are used to bandage an elbow, knee, or ankle, because they permit some movement after application. To apply a figure-eight turn with a roller bandage, follow these steps:

- Anchor the bandage with two circular turns.
- Carry the bandage above the joint, around it, and then below it, making a figure eight (Figure 23-9 ■).
- Continue above and below the joint, overlapping the previous turn by two-thirds the width of the bandage.

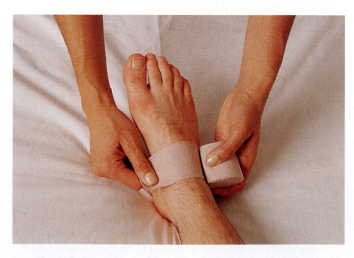

Figure 23-8. ■ Starting a bandage with two circular turns. (Photographer: Elena Dorfman.)

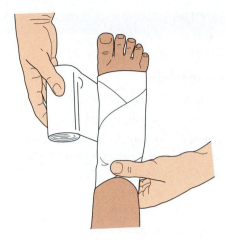

Figure 23-9. ■ Applying a figure-eight bandage.

■ End the bandage above the joint with two circular turns, and secure the end appropriately.

Binders are also sometimes called slings. To apply a large arm sling:

■ Place one end of the unfolded triangular binder over the shoulder of the uninjured side so that the binder falls down the front of the chest of the client with the point of the triangle (apex) under the elbow of the injured side.

■ Take the upper corner, and carry it around the neck until it hangs over the shoulder on the injured side (Figure 23-10 ■).

■ Bring the lower corner of the binder up over the arm to the shoulder of the injured side. Using a square knot, secure this corner to the upper corner at the side of the neck on the involved side.

■ Fold the sling neatly at the elbow, and secure it with safety pins or tape. It may be folded and fastened at the front.

Straight abdominal binders are also useful. To apply straight abdominal binders, follow these steps:

■ With the client in a supine position, place the abdominal binder smoothly under the client, with the upper

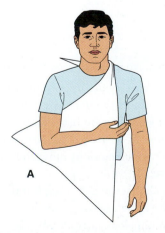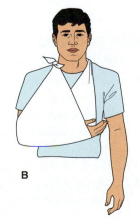

A   B

Figure 23-10. ■ Large arm sling.

border of the binder at the waist and the lower border at the level of the gluteal fold. *A binder placed above the waist can interfere with respiration. One placed too low can interfere with elimination and walking.*

■ Apply padding over the iliac crests if the client is thin.

■ For a straight abdominal binder, bring the ends around the client, overlap them, and secure them with pins or Velcro.

Heat and Cold Applications

Heat and cold applications can assist the healing process. Nursing care guidelines for selected heat and cold therapies are provided in Box 23-7 ■.

For all local applications of heat or cold, the following guidelines apply:

■ Determine the client's ability to tolerate the therapy.

■ Identify conditions that might contraindicate treatment (e.g., bleeding, circulatory impairment).

■ Explain the application to the client.

■ Assess the skin area to which the heat will be applied.

■ Ask the client to report any discomfort.

■ Return to the client 15 minutes after starting the heat, and observe the local skin area for any untoward signs (e.g., redness). Stop the heat if any problems occur.

■ Remove the equipment at the designated time, and dispose of it appropriately.

■ Examine the area to which the heat was applied, and record the client's response.

EVALUATING

To judge whether client outcomes have been achieved, the nurse uses data collected during care, such as skin status over bony prominences and perineal area, nutritional and fluid intake, mental status, and signs of healing if an ulcer is present. If outcomes are not achieved, the nurse should explore the reasons why:

■ Has the client's physical condition changed?

■ Were risk factors correctly identified?

■ Were appropriate lifting devices and techniques used?

■ Was the repositioning schedule adhered to?

■ Are the client's nutritional and fluid intake adequate?

CONTINUING CARE

Prior to discharge, the nurse must ensure that clients have an understanding of wound care. Clients should know how to change a dressing and how frequently. They should understand what normal healing looks like. They should be given a list of signs that might indicate an infection or other complication and when to notify the physician.

BOX 23-7	NURSING CARE CHECKLIST

Selected Heat and Cold Applications

Aquathermia Pad

☑ Fill the reservoir of the unit two-thirds full of distilled water.

☑ Set the desired temperature. Check the manufacturer's instructions. Most units are set at 40.5°C (105°F) for adults.

☑ Cover the pad and plug in the unit. Some manufacturers suggest warming the pad before applying it.

☑ Apply the pad to the body part. The treatment is usually continued for 10 to 15 minutes. Check orders and agency protocol.

Ice Bag, Glove, or Collar

☑ Always wrap the container in a cloth or towel before applying.

Sitz Bath

☑ Assist the client into the tub. Provide support for the client's feet; a footstool can prevent pressure on the backs of the thighs.

☑ Provide a bath blanket for the client's shoulders, and eliminate drafts to prevent chilling.

☑ Observe the client closely during the bath for signs of faintness, dizziness, weakness, accelerated pulse rate, and pallor.

☑ Maintain the water temperature.

☑ Following the sitz bath, assist the client out of the tub. Help the client to dry.

Cooling Sponge Bath

☑ Determine the client's vital signs (i.e., TPR).

☑ Protect the client's bed with moisture-proof material.

☑ Sponge the face, arms, legs, back, and buttocks. The chest and abdomen are not usually sponged. Each area is sponged slowly and gently. Rubbing may increase heat production.

☑ Leave each area wet, and cover with a damp towel.

☑ Place ice bags and cold packs, if used, or a cool cloth on the forehead for comfort and in each axilla and at the groin. These areas contain large superficial blood vessels that help the transfer of heat.

☑ Sponge one body part and then another. The sponge bath should take about 30 minutes. A bath given more quickly tends to increase the body's heat production by causing shivering.

☑ Discontinue the bath if the client becomes pale or cyanotic or shivers, or if the pulse becomes rapid or irregular.

☑ Pat each area dry.

☑ Reassess the vital signs at 15 minutes and after completing the sponge bath.

Pressure Ulcers

Pressure ulcers (also called *decubitus ulcers, pressure sores,* or *bedsores*) are lesions caused by unrelieved pressure that results in damage to underlying tissue. Pressure ulcers are a problem in both acute care settings and long-term care settings, including homes.

Pressure ulcers are caused by localized **ischemia**, a deficiency in the blood supply to the tissue. The tissue is caught between two hard surfaces, usually the surface of the bed and the bony skeleton. When blood cannot reach the tissue, the cells are deprived of oxygen and nutrients, and waste products accumulate in the cells. Prolonged, unrelieved pressure damages the small blood vessels, and the tissue eventually dies.

Pressure ulcers usually occur over bony prominences. After the skin has been compressed, it appears pale. When pressure is relieved, the skin takes on a bright red flush, called **reactive hyperemia**. The flush is due to vasodilation; extra blood floods to the area to compensate for the impeded blood flow. If the redness disappears, no tissue damage can be anticipated. If the redness does not disappear, then tissue damage has occurred.

Besides pressure, two other factors often produce pressure ulcers: friction and shearing force. **Friction** is a force acting parallel to the skin surface. For example, sheets rubbing against skin create friction. Friction can remove the superficial layers, making the skin more prone to breakdown.

Shearing force is a combination of friction and pressure. It occurs commonly when a client assumes a Fowler's position in bed. The body slides down toward the foot of the bed, but the skin over the sacrum tends not to move. The skin and superficial tissues are held by the bed surface, but the deeper tissues attached to the skeleton move downward. The shearing force occurs where the deeper tissues and the superficial tissues meet. The force damages blood vessels and tissues in this area.

RISK FACTORS

Several factors contribute to the formation of pressure ulcers:

- *Immobility.* Immobility and inactivity are important risk factors for pressure ulcers. Immobility refers to a reduction in the amount of movement a person has. Paralysis, extreme weakness, or any cause of decreased activity can hinder a person's ability to change positions independently and relieve the pressure.

- *Inadequate nutrition.* Nutritional factors are crucial in the development of pressure ulcers. Generally, prolonged inadequate nutrition causes weight loss, anemia, muscle atrophy, and the loss of subcutaneous tissue. Reduction in padding between the skin and the bones increases the risk of pressure sore development. Inadequate intake of protein, carbohydrates, fluids, and vitamin C specifically contributes to pressure ulcer formation.

- *Edema* (presence of excess fluid in the tissues) makes skin more prone to injury by decreasing its elasticity and resilience.
- *Fecal and urinary incontinence.* Moisture from incontinence promotes skin **maceration** (softening of tissue by prolonged wetting) and makes the epidermis susceptible to injury. Digestive enzymes in feces also contribute to skin excoriation. Any accumulation of secretions or excretions is irritating to the skin, harbors microorganisms, and makes an individual prone to skin breakdown and infection.
- *Decreased mental status.* Individuals with a reduced level of awareness and those who are unconscious or heavily sedated are at risk for pressure ulcers. They are less able to recognize and respond to pain associated with prolonged pressure.
- *Diminished sensation.* Paralysis, or other neurologic disease causing loss of sensation, reduces a person's ability to respond to damaging levels of heat and cold and to feel the tingling ("pins and needles") that signals loss of circulation.
- *Excessive body heat.* Body heat is another factor in the development of pressure sores. An elevated body temperature increases the body's metabolic rate, increasing the need for cellular oxygen. This increased need is severe in the cells of an area under pressure, which are already oxygen deficient. Severe infections with accompanying elevated body temperatures may affect the body's ability to deal with the effects of tissue compression.
- *Advanced age.* The aging process can make older people more prone to impaired skin integrity. Older adults may be prone to loss of lean body mass, generalized thinning and dryness of the epidermis, and decreased strength and elasticity of the skin. They may have diminished pain perception due to decreased sensation of pressure and light touch. (See also Box 23-2.)
- *Other factors.* Poor lifting techniques, incorrect positioning, repeated injections in the same area, hard support surfaces, and incorrect application of pressure-relieving devices also contribute to the formation of pressure sores.

STAGES OF PRESSURE ULCER FORMATION

The four stages in pressure ulcer formation relate to observable tissue damage (see Figures 23-11 ■ and 23-12 ■):

- *Stage I:* Nonblanchable erythema of intact skin.
- *Stage II:* Partial-thickness skin loss involving epidermis, dermis, or both. The ulcer is superficial and presents as an abrasion, blister, or shallow crater.

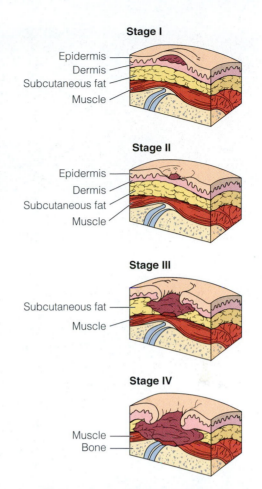

Figure 23-11. ■ Four stages of pressure ulcers. (*Source:* U.S. Department of Health and Human Services, PPPPUA, *Clinical Practice Guideline, Pressure Ulcers in Adults: Prediction and Prevention* AHCPR, Publication No. 92-0047, Rockville, MD: Public Health Service, 1992, p. 8.)

- *Stage III:* Full-thickness skin loss involving damage or necrosis of subcutaneous tissue that may extend down to, but not through, underlying fascia. The ulcer presents as a deep crater with or without undermining of adjacent tissue.
- *Stage IV:* Full-thickness skin loss with extensive destruction, tissue necrosis, or damage to muscle, bone, or supporting structures, such as a tendon or joint capsule. Undermining and sinus tracts may also be associated with stage IV pressure ulcers.

COLLABORATIVE CARE

Supportive Devices

For clients confined to bed, special support surfaces and positioning devices can be used to protect bony prominences. Three types of support surfaces can be used to relieve pressure. The overlay mattress or egg-crate mattress is applied on top of the standard bed mattress. A replacement

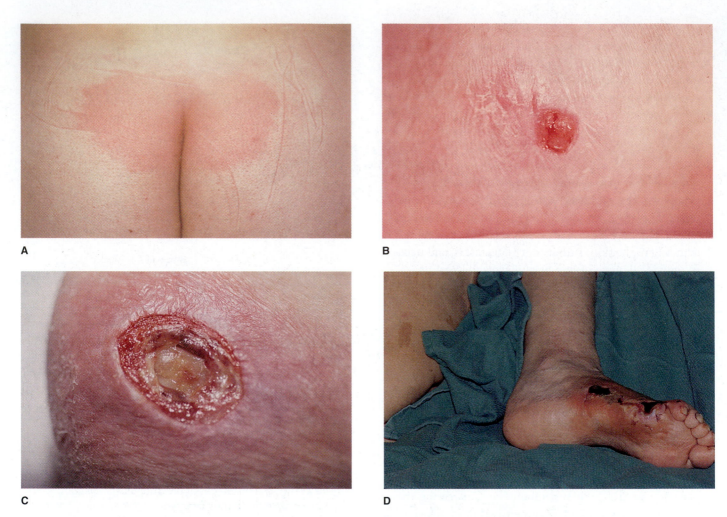

Figure 23-12. ■ The four stages of a decubitus ulcer: **A.** stage I—nonblanchable erythema signaling potential ulceration; **B.** stage II—abrasion, blister, or shallow crater involving the epidermis and possibly the dermis; **C.** stage III—deep ulcer exhibiting necrotic tissue and extending through the subcutaneous layer; **D.** stage IV—tissue necrosis and damage involving muscle, bone, or supporting structures. (**D.** © Caliendo/Custom Medical Stock Photo, Inc.)

mattress is a mattress that replaces the standard mattress; most are made of foam and gel combinations. Specialty beds replace hospital beds. They provide pressure relief, eliminate shearing and friction, and decrease moisture

Figure 23-13. ■ An alternating pressure mattress provides comfort and helps distribute body weight evenly. (Courtesy of Ease).

(Figure 23-13 ■). See Table 23-5 for selected mechanical devices for reducing pressure on body parts.

When a client is confined to bed or to a chair, pressure-reducing devices, such as pillows made of foam, gel, air, or a combination of these, can be used. When the client is sitting, weight should be distributed over the entire seating surface so that pressure does not center on just one area. To protect a client's heels in bed, supports such as wedges or pillows can be used to raise the heels completely off the bed. Doughnut-type devices should not be used (Panel for the Prediction and Prevention of Pressure Ulcers in Adults [PPPPUA], 1994).

Risk Assessment Tools

Several risk assessment tools are available to help the nurse identify clients at high risk for pressure ulcer development. Data collection includes the areas of immobility, incontinence, nutrition, and level of consciousness. Two validated assessment tools are the Braden scale (Figure 23-14 ■) and

BRADEN SCALE FOR PREDICTING PRESSURE SORE RISK

Patient's Name _____ Evaluator's Name _____ Date of Assessment

SENSORY PERCEPTION

Ability to respond meaningfully to pressure-related discomfort

1. Completely Limited:
Unresponsive (does not moan, flinch, or grasp) to painful stimuli, due to diminished level of consciousness or sedation,
OR
limited ability to feel pain over most of body surface.

2. Very Limited:
Responds only to painful stimuli. Cannot communicate discomfort except by moaning or restlessness,
OR
has a sensory impairment which limits the ability to feel pain or discomfort over 1/2 of body.

3. Slightly Limited:
Responds to verbal commands but cannot always communicate discomfort or need to be turned,
OR
has some sensory impairment which limits ability to feel pain or discomfort in 1 or 2 extremities.

4. No Impairment:
Responds to verbal commands. Has no sensory deficit which would limit ability to feel or voice pain or discomfort.

MOISTURE

Degree to which skin is exposed to moisture

1. Constantly Moist:
Skin is kept moist almost constantly by perspiration, urine, etc. Dampness is detected every time patient is moved or turned.

2. Moist:
Skin is often but not always moist. Linen must be changed at least once a shift.

3. Occasionally Moist:
Skin is occasionally moist, requiring an extra linen change approximately once a day.

4. Rarely Moist:
Skin is usually dry; linen requires changing only at routine intervals.

ACTIVITY

Degree of physical activity

1. Bedfast:
Confined to bed.

2. Chairfast:
Ability to walk severely limited or nonexistent. Cannot bear own weight and/or must be assisted into chair or wheelchair.

3. Walks Occasionally:
Walks occasionally during day but for very short distances, with or without assistance. Spends majority of each shift in bed or chair.

4. Walks Frequently:
Walks outside the room at least twice a day and inside room at least once every 2 hours during waking hours.

MOBILITY

Ability to change and control body position

1. Completely Immobile:
Does not make even slight changes in body or extremity position without assistance.

2. Very Limited:
Makes occasional slight changes in body or extremity position but unable to make frequent or significant changes independently.

3. Slightly Limited:
Makes frequent though slight changes in body or extremity position independently.

4. No Limitations:
Makes major and frequent changes in position without assistance.

NUTRITION

Usual food intake pattern

1. Very Poor:
Never eats a complete meal. Rarely eats more than 1/3 of any food offered. Eats 2 servings or less of protein (meat or dairy products) per day. Takes fluids poorly. Does not take a liquid dietary supplement,
OR
is NPO and/or maintained on clear liquids or IV's for more than 5 days.

2. Probably Inadequate:
Rarely eats a complete meal and generally eats only about 1/2 of any food offered. Protein intake includes only 3 servings of meat or dairy products per day. Occasionally will refuse a meal, but will usually take a supplement if offered,
OR
receives less than optimum amount of liquid diet or tube feeding.

3. Adequate:
Eats over half of most meals. Eats a total of 4 servings of protein (meat, dairy products) each day. Occasionally will refuse a meal, but will usually take a supplement if offered,
OR
is on a tube feeding or TPN regimen, which probably meets most of nutritional needs.

4. Excellent:
Eats most of every meal. Never refuses a meal. Usually eats a total of 4 or more servings of meat and dairy products. Occasionally eats between meals. Does not require supplementation.

FRICTION AND SHEAR

1. Problem:
Requires moderate to maximum assistance in moving. Complete lifting without sliding against sheets is impossible. Frequently slides down in bed or chair, requiring frequent repositioning with maximum assistance. Spasticity, contractures, or agitation leads to almost constant friction.

2. Potential Problem:
Moves feebly or requires minimum assistance. During a move skin probably slides to some extent against sheets, chair, restraints, or other devices. Maintains relatively good position in chair or bed most of the time but occasionally slides down.

3. No Apparent Problem:
Moves in bed and in chair independently and has sufficient muscle strength to lift up completely during move. Maintains good position in bed or chair at all times.

Total Score _____

Figure 23-14. ■ Braden Scale for Predicting Pressure Sore Risk. (*Source:* U.S. Department of Health and Human Services, *Clinical Practice Guideline, Pressure Ulcers in Adults: Prediction and Prevention,* Publication No. 92-0047, Rockville, MD: Public Health Service, 1992, pp. 16–17. Copyright © Barbara Braden and Nancy Bergstrom, 1988. Reprinted with permission.)

TABLE 23-6

Norton's Pressure Area Risk Assessment Form (Scoring System)

GENERAL PHYSICAL CONDITION		MENTAL STATE		ACTIVITY		MOBILITY		INCONTINENCE	
Good	4	Alert	4	Ambulatory	4	Full	4	Absent	4
Fair	3	Apathetic	3	Walks with help	3	Slightly limited	3	Occasional	3
Poor	2	Confused	2	Chairbound	2	Very limited	2	Usually urinary	2
Very bad	1	Stuporous	1	Bedfast	1	Immobile	1	Double	1

Source: D. Norton, R. McLaren, and A.N. Exton-Smith, *An Investigation of Geriatric Nursing Problems in Hospital* (Edinburgh: Churchill Livingstone, 1962). Reissued 1975. Used by permission.

---

the Norton scale (Table 23-6 ■). These scales include sub-scales and categories that are assigned points. Scores of 16 or lower may be indicators of potential risk.

NURSING CARE

ASSESSING

Particular attention is paid to skin condition in areas most likely to break down: in skinfolds (such as under the breasts), in areas that are frequently moist (such as the perineum), and in areas that receive extensive pressure (such as the coccyx and trochanters) (Figure 23-15 ■; see also Box 23-4 about assessing common pressure sites).

When a pressure ulcer is present, the nurse notes the following:

- Location of the lesion
- Size of lesion in centimeters (Measure length, width, and depth, beginning with length [head to toe] and then width [side to side]. To measure depth, gently insert a sterile swab at the deepest part of the wound, and then measure against a measuring guide.)
- Stage of the ulcer (see Figure 23-11)
- Color of the wound bed and location of necrosis or eschar
- Condition of the wound margins
- Integrity of surrounding skin
- Clinical signs of infection, such as redness, warmth, swelling, pain, odor, and exudate (note color of exudate).

DIAGNOSING, PLANNING, AND IMPLEMENTING

Nursing diagnoses that are common in clients with pressure ulcers are:

- *Impaired Skin Integrity* (commonly applies to stage I and II pressure ulcers)
- *Impaired Tissue Integrity* (applies to stage III and IV pressure ulcers)
- *Pain*.

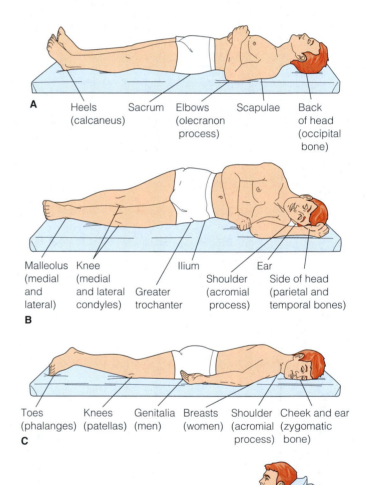

Figure 23-15. ■ Body pressure areas: **A.** supine position; **B.** lateral position; **C.** prone position; **D.** Fowler's position.

Preventing Pressure Ulcers

To prevent pressure ulcers, the LPN/LVN, in collaboration with the RN, implements meticulous skin care as described earlier in the chapter:

- Provide nutritional supplements for nutritionally compromised clients. *An inadequate intake of calories, protein, and iron is believed to be a risk factor for pressure ulcer development.*
- Keep the client's skin clean, dry, and free of irritation from urine, feces, and sweat. When bathing the client, avoid using hot water and apply minimal force and friction. Use mild cleansing agents that do not disrupt the skin's "natural barriers," and apply moisturizing lotions as needed. Also, minimize dryness by not exposing clients to cold and low humidity.
- Avoid massaging over bony prominences. *Nurses have used massage to stimulate blood circulation, with the intention of preventing pressure sores. Scientific evidence does not support this belief; in fact, massage may lead to deep tissue trauma.*
- Provide the client with a smooth, firm, and wrinkle-free foundation on which to sit or lie down. Position, transfer, and turn clients correctly. For bedridden clients, reduce shearing force by elevating the head of the bed to no more than 30 degrees, if this position is not contraindicated by the client's condition.
- Encourage or assist the client to shift weight every 15 to 30 minutes and, whenever possible, exercise or ambulate to stimulate blood circulation. *Frequent shifts in position, even if only slight, effectively change pressure points.*
- When lifting a client to change position, use a lifting device such as a trapeze rather than dragging the client across or up in bed. *The friction that results from dragging the skin against a sheet can cause blisters and abrasions, which may contribute to more extensive tissue damage.*
- At least every 2 hours, reposition any at-risk client who is confined to bed—even when a special support mattress is used. Establish a written schedule for turning and repositioning. This allows another body surface to bear the weight. Six body positions, can be used: prone, supine, right and left lateral (side-lying), and right and left Sims' positions.

Treating Pressure Ulcers

To treat clients with pressure ulcers, the following interventions are performed:

- Follow the agency protocols and the physician's orders, if any.
- Protect wounds (like those developing granulation tissue). Clean them gently, apply a topical antimicrobial agent, cover with a transparent film or hydrocolloid dressing, and disturb the dressing as infrequently as pos-

sible. *This will allow the healing process to continue uninterrupted.* Box 23-8 ■ provides guidelines for treating pressure ulcers.

- Clean wounds to remove drainage and nonviable tissue. See Irrigating a Wound section on page 479.
- Report any signs of infection and obtain a wound specimen with a physician's order (see Procedure 23-2).
- Provide supportive care of the client during removal of black (nonviable) tissue. Once the necrotic tissue has been removed (**debrided**), dress wound per physician orders.

BOX 23-8

Treating Pressure Ulcers

- Minimize direct pressure on the ulcer. Reposition the client at least every 2 hours. Use a schedule, and record position changes on the client's chart.
- Clean the pressure ulcer daily. The method of cleaning depends on the stage of the ulcer and agency protocol. For example, a whirlpool bath may be indicated for a stage I ulcer and a wound irrigation for a stage IV ulcer (see Procedure 23-3).
- Clean and dress the ulcer using surgical asepsis.
- If the pressure ulcer is infected, obtain a sample of the drainage for culture and sensitivity to antiseptic agents (see Procedure 23-2).
- If the client cannot keep weight off the pressure ulcer, use pressure-relieving devices such as an egg-crate mattress.
- Teach the client to move, if only slightly, to relieve pressure.
- Provide range-of-motion (ROM) exercises as the client's condition permits.

EVALUATING

Pressure sores are a challenge for nurses because of the number of variables involved (e.g., risk factors, types of ulcers, and degrees of impairment) and the many treatment measures that are advocated. Existing and potential infections are the most serious complications of pressure sores.

Evaluation of a client with pressure ulcers includes documentation of location, size, depth, stage, color, status of wound margins and surrounding skin, and specific signs of infection. Include care provided and client response to treatment.

CONTINUING CARE

Clients and their support people often need teaching in order to carry out measures to prevent pressure ulcers. The following information should be provided:

- Causes of pressure ulcers
- Skin care plan to keep the skin clean, lubricated, and protected from secretions and excretions

- Importance of maintaining or increasing correct activity level
- Avoidance of massage, doughnuts, and heat lamps
- Need to contact the physician when there is skin reddening, blister formation, or breakdown.

NURSING PROCESS CARE PLAN
Client with Pressure Ulcer

Jamie Lee, a 73-year-old female, was admitted to the hospital for a decubitus ulcer on her left hip. Jamie lives in a skilled nursing center and is being treated for diabetes. She takes insulin twice a day. Mrs. Lee is unhappy with the restrictions of her diabetic diet. The staff must remind her about the dangers of eating candy bars, which they frequently find in her bedside table. Her mobility is limited, and she complains when the staff encourages her to sit up. She favors her left side because she can watch the television from that angle easily.

Assessment. VS: T 99, apical P 76, R 22, BP 146/90. Blood sugar is 320; hemoglobin is 10; hematocrit is 36; and WBC count is 12,000. The decubitus ulcer is described as having full-thickness skin loss, measuring 2 × 2 across and 0.5 in. deep. No undermining noted.

Nursing Diagnosis. The following important nursing diagnoses (among others) are established for this client:

- *Impaired Skin Integrity*
- *Risk for Infection* related to decubitus ulcer
- *Activity Intolerance*
- *Powerlessness* related to illness related regimen
- *Deficient Knowledge* related to diabetes.

Expected Outcomes. The expected outcomes for the plan of care are:

- Skin integrity effectively managed.
- Wound is maintained without evidence of infection.
- Expresses an understanding of need to balance rest and activity.
- Participates in planning care; makes decisions regarding care and treatments when possible.

- Expresses a basic understanding of the principles in diabetes care and treatment.

Planning and Implementation. The following nursing interventions are implemented:

- Monitor wound healing; measurements and documentation taken when dressing is changed.
- Maintain glucose levels with insulin adjustments.
- Observe for signs and symptoms of infection.
- Encourage the client to be independent in activities when possible.
- Determine the client's perception of level and strength.
- Refer to physical therapy to help increase activity level and strength.
- Reinforce diabetes teaching and understanding to family and client.

Evaluation. Mrs. Lee returns to her skilled nursing center after 5 days of hospitalization. Her vital signs are stable and glucose level has steadily dropped to 150. Wound cultures are negative for infection. Granulation tissue is apparent as evidence of healing progresses. Dressing changes will continue with nursing supervision. The client expresses understanding about mobility and position changes. She has been sitting up three times for meals and extends the time with each sitting. The client and family members understand the diabetic diet calorie restriction and the need to control blood sugars. She states she has a better understanding of diabetes and how it affects healing. She wants to take a more active role in her care and management.

Critical Thinking in the Nursing Process

1. How will you reinforce Mrs. Lee's understanding of diabetes and wound healing?
2. Compare treatment for a stage III and stage IV decubitus ulcer.
3. Describe how nutrition can affect the healing process in pressure ulcers.

Note: Discussion of Critical Thinking questions appears in Appendix I.

Note: The references and resources for this and all chapters have been compiled at the back of the book.

Wound Dressings

Part A: Moist Transparent Barrier Dressing

Before applying or changing a moist transparent wound barrier, (1) verify the physician's order regarding frequency and type of dressing change, and (2) determine agency protocol about solutions used to clean the wound and whether clean or sterile technique is to be used. Many agencies recommend clean rather than sterile technique for chronic wounds such as a decubitus ulcer.

Assessment Focus   Appearance and size of the wound; the amount and character of exudate; complaints of discomfort; signs of systemic infection (e.g., elevated body temperature, diaphoresis, malaise; leukocytosis).

Purposes

- To provide a moist wound environment and promote wound healing
- To protect the wound from trauma and infectious agents
- To facilitate assessment of wound healing
- To prevent the entrance of microorganisms into the wound
- To minimize wound discomfort

- To promote autolysis of necrotic material by white blood cells
- To decrease the frequency of dressing changes

Equipment

- Disposable gloves
- Hair scissors or clippers
- Alcohol or acetone
- Moisture-proof bag
- Sterile gloves (optional)
- Sterile gauze and the wound-cleaning agents specified by the physician or agency (e.g., sterile saline)
- Wound barrier dressing
- Scissors
- Paper tape
- Dressing set
- Sterile normal saline or other cleaning agent used by the agency
- Hydrocolloid dressing at least 3 to 4 cm (1.5 in.) larger than wound on all four sides

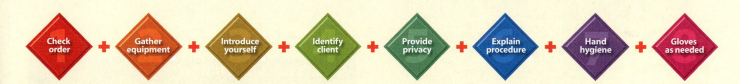

Check order + Gather equipment + Introduce yourself + Identify client + Provide privacy + Explain procedure + Hand hygiene + Gloves as needed

Interventions

1. Obtain assistance as needed.
   - If the size of the wound requires it, acquire the assistance of a coworker to help apply the dressing.

2. Thoroughly clean the skin area around the wound.
   - Put on disposable gloves.
   - Clean the skin well with normal saline or a mild cleansing agent. Always rinse the adjacent skin well prior to applying a dressing.
   - Clip the hair about 5 cm (2 in.) around the wound area if indicated.
   - If adherence of the dressing is a concern, clean the area adjacent to the wound with alcohol or acetone, and allow it to dry. *Alcohol or acetone defats the skin. Defatted, clean, dry skin ensures better adhesion of the dressing.*
   - Remove gloves, and dispose of them in the moisture-proof bag.

3. Clean the wound if indicated.
   - Put on clean disposable or sterile gloves in accordance with agency practice.
   - Clean the wound with the prescribed solution. Either (a) pour the sterile solution directly on the wound and collect drainage with an emesis basin, or (b) use a moist, sterile gauze and hold it so that the area that touches the wound remains sterile.
   - Dry the surrounding skin with a dry gauze.

4. Assess the wound.

5. Apply the wound barrier.
   - Remove part of the paper backing on the dressing. If you have an assistant, remove all of the paper backing; the two of you should hold the colored tabs attached to the dressing.
   - Apply the dressing at one edge of the wound site, allowing at least 2.5-cm (1-in.) coverage of the skin surrounding the wound.

- Gently lay or press the barrier over the wound. Keep it free of wrinkles, but avoid stretching it too tightly. *A stretched dressing restricts mobility.*
- Cut off the colored tabs after the wound is completely covered.
- Remove and dispose of gloves appropriately.

6. Reinforce the dressing only if absolutely needed.
   - Apply paper or other porous tape to the edges of the dressing.

7. Assess the wound at least daily.
   - Determine the extent of serous fluid accumulation under the dressing, wound healing, and the need to repair the dressing.
   - If excessive serum has accumulated, consider replacing the transparent wound barrier with a more absorbent type of dressing, such as hydrocolloid.
   - If the dressing is leaking, remove it and apply another dressing.

8. Document the procedure and all nursing assessments.

Part B: Hydrocolloid Dressing

A hydrocolloid dressing should be changed whenever it becomes dislodged, leaks, or develops an odor. If the wound has substantial drainage or yellow slough, the dressing may need to be changed every 24 to 72 hours. When drainage subsides, the dressing may be left in place for 3 to 7 days.

Interventions

1. Remove the old dressing.
   - Put on disposable gloves.
   - Pull the dressing off gradually in the direction of hair growth. *This minimizes skin irritation.*
   - Dispose of the soiled dressing in the moisture-proof bag.

2. Clean the skin area around the wound.
   - Gently wash the skin surrounding the wound with a mild cleansing agent or with normal saline and dry it thoroughly with gauze squares.
   - Leave the residue that is difficult to remove on the skin.
   - Remove gloves and dispose of them in the moisture-proof bag.

3. Clean the wound if indicated.
   - Open the sterile dressing supplies.
   - Pour saline or other cleaning agent into the sterile container.
   - Put on disposable or sterile gloves in accordance with agency protocol.
   - Clean the wound with the prescribed solution.

4. Assess the wound.
   - Observe the appearance and the size of the wound and the amount and character of exudate.
   - Determine presence of pain.

5. Apply the dressing.
   - Follow the manufacturer's instructions.
   - Remove and dispose of the gloves.
   - *Optional:* Tape all four sides of the dressing as required or according to agency protocol. *Taping prevents the dressing from sticking to bed linens and keeps the edges from lifting.*

6. Assess and change the dressing as indicated.
   - Inspect the dressing at least daily for leakage, dislodgement, odor, and wrinkling.
   - Change the dressing if any of these signs are present.

7. Document the technique and all nursing assessments.

SAMPLE DOCUMENTATION

[date]   Stage II superficial reddened wound
[time]   2 × 2 to coccyx cleansed with saline, hydrocolloid wafer applied and windowed with tape. Client complained of 3/10 on pain scale, medicated prior to procedure.
_____ D. Haus, LVN

PROCEDURE 23-2

Obtaining a Specimen of Wound Drainage

Purposes

- To identify the microorganisms potentially causing an infection and the antibiotics to which they are sensitive
- To evaluate the effectiveness of antibiotic therapy

Equipment

- Disposable gloves
- Sterile gloves
- Moisture-resistant bag
- Sterile dressing set
- Normal saline and irrigating syringe
- Culture tube with swab and culture medium (aerobic and anaerobic tubes are available) and/or sterile syringe with needle for anaerobic culture
- Completed labels for each container
- Completed requisition to accompany the specimens to the laboratory

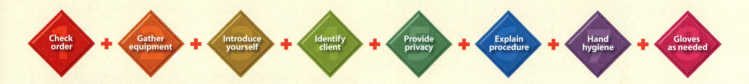

Check order + Gather equipment + Introduce yourself + Identify client + Provide privacy + Explain procedure + Hand hygiene + Gloves as needed

Interventions

1. Remove any dressings that cover the wound.
   - Put on disposable gloves.
   - Remove the dressing, observe any drainage on it. Hold the dressing so that the client does not see the drainage. *The appearance of the drainage could upset the client.*
   - Determine the amount of the drainage, for example, one 2 × 2 gauze saturated with pale yellow drainage.
   - Discard the dressing in the moisture-resistant bag. Handle it carefully so that the dressing does not touch the outside of the bag. *Touching the outside of the bag will contaminate it.*
   - Remove gloves and dispose of them properly.

2. Open the sterile dressing set using sterile technique.

3. Assess the wound.
   - Put on sterile gloves.
   - Assess the appearance of the tissues in and around the wound and the drainage. *Infection can cause reddened tissues with a thick discharge, which may be foul smelling, whitish, or colored.*

4. Clean the wound.
   - Irrigate the wound with normal saline until all visible exudate has been washed away. See Procedure 23-3.
   - After irrigating, apply a sterile gauze pad to the wound. *This absorbs excess saline.*
   - If a topical antimicrobial ointment or cream is being used to treat the wound, use a swab to remove it. *Residual antiseptic must be removed prior to culture.*
   - Remove and discard sterile gloves.

5. Obtain the culture.
   - Open a specimen culture tube and place the cap upside down on a firm, dry surface so that the inside will not become contaminated, or if the swab is attached to the lid, twist the cap to loosen the swab. Hold the tube in one hand, and take out the swab in the other (Figure 23-16 ■).
   - Rotate the swab back and forth over clean areas of granulation tissue from the sides or base of the wound. *Microorganisms most likely to be responsible for a wound infection reside in viable tissue.*
   - Do not use pus or pooled exudate to culture. *These secretions contain a mixture of contaminants that are not the same as those causing the infection.*
   - Avoid touching the swab to intact skin at the wound edges. *This prevents the introduction of superficial skin organisms into the culture.*

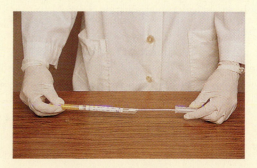

Figure 23-16. ■ A culture tube for a wound specimen.

- Return the swab to the culture tube, taking care not to touch the top or the outside of the tube.
- Crush the inner ampule containing the medium for organism growth at the bottom of the tube. *This ensures that the swab with the specimen is surrounded by culture medium.*
- Twist the cap to secure it.
- If a specimen is required from another site, repeat the preceding steps. Specify the exact site (e.g., inferior drain site or lower aspect of incision) on the label of each container. Be sure to put each swab in the appropriately labeled tube. *This ensures that tests can be carried out as intended.*

6. Dress the wound.
   - Apply any ordered medication to the wound.
   - Cover the wound with a sterile moist transparent wound dressing. See Procedure 23-1A.

7. Arrange for the specimen to be transported to the laboratory immediately. Be sure to include the completed requisition. *This prevents specimen from being lost or mislabeled.*

8. Document all relevant information.
   - Record on the client's chart the taking of the specimen and source.
   - Include the date and time; the examination requested; the appearance of the wound; the color, consistency, amount, and odor of any drainage; and any discomfort experienced by the client. *Complete documentation supports continuity of care.*

VARIATION: OBTAINING A SPECIMEN FOR ANAEROBIC CULTURE, USING A STERILE SYRINGE AND NEEDLE

- Insert a sterile 10-mL syringe (without needle) into the wound, and aspirate 1 to 5 mL of drainage into the syringe.
- Attach the #21 gauge needle to the syringe, and expel all air from the syringe and needle.
- Immediately inject the drainage into the anaerobic culture tube.
  or
  If a rubber stopper or cork is available, insert the needle into the rubber stopper or cork to prevent the entry of air.
- Label the tube or syringe appropriately.
- Send the syringe of drainage to the laboratory immediately. *This ensures that the specimen will be fresh when it reaches the laboratory.*

SAMPLE DOCUMENTATION

[date]	Anaerobic culture of lt. hip wound
[time]	obtained and sent to the lab.
	_____ D Haus, LVN

PROCEDURE 23-3 **Irrigating a Wound**

Before irrigating a wound, determine (a) the type of irrigating solution to be used, (b) the frequency of irrigations, and (c) the temperature of the solution.

Purposes

- To clean the area
- To apply heat and hasten the healing process
- To apply an antimicrobial solution

Equipment

- Sterile dressing equipment and dressing materials
- Sterile irrigating syringes (e.g., a 30- to 50-mL piston syringe) with a catheter of an appropriate size (e.g., #18 or #19) attached or a 250-mL squeezable bottle with irrigating tip
- Sterile basin for the irrigating solution
- Moisture-proof bag
- Sterile basin to receive the irrigation returns
- Irrigating solution, usually 200 mL (6.5 oz) of solution warmed to body temperature, according to the agency's or physician's choice
- Clean disposable gloves
- Sterile gloves
- Moisture-proof sterile drape
- Sterile straight catheter or irrigating tip, if needed

Check order ✚ Gather equipment ✚ Introduce yourself ✚ Identify client ✚ Provide privacy ✚ Explain procedure ✚ Hand hygiene ✚ Gloves as needed

Interventions

1. Verify the physician's order.
   - Confirm the type and strength of the solution.
2. Prepare the client.
   - Assist the client to a position in which the irrigating solution will flow by gravity from the upper end of the wound to the lower end and then into the basin.
   - Place the moisture-proof drape over the client and the bed.
   - Put on disposable gloves and remove and discard the old dressing.
   - Clean from the center of the wound outward, using circular strokes.
   - Use a separate swab for each stroke, and discard each swab after use. *This prevents the introduction of microorganisms to other wound areas.*
   - Assess the wound and drainage.
   - Remove and discard disposable gloves.
3. Prepare the equipment.
   - Open the sterile dressing set and supplies.
   - Pour the ordered solution into the solution container.
   - Put on sterile gloves.
   - Position the sterile basin below the wound to receive the irrigating fluid.
4. Irrigate the wound.
   - Instill a steady stream of irrigating solution into the wound. Make sure all areas of the wound are irrigated.
   - Use either a syringe with a catheter attached or a 250-mL squeezable bottle with irrigating tip to flush the wound. *Effective irrigation requires 4 to 15 pounds per square inch of pressure. These devices provide this pressure; bulb syringes do not.*
   - If you are using a catheter, insert the catheter into the wound until resistance is met. Do not force the catheter. *Forcing the catheter can cause tissue damage.*
   - Continue irrigating until the solution becomes clear (no exudate is present). *The irrigation washes away tissue debris and drainage so that later returns are clearer.*

   - Dry the area around the wound. *Moisture left on the skin promotes the growth of microorganisms and can cause skin irritation and breakdown.*
5. Assess and dress the wound.
   - Assess the appearance of the wound, noting in particular the type and amount of exudate and the presence and extent of granulation tissue.
   - Pack the wound if ordered.
   - Apply a sterile dressing to the wound as described in Procedure 23-1.
6. Document all relevant information.
   - Document the irrigation, the solution used, the appearance of the irrigation returns, and nursing assessments. Note the presence of any exudate and sloughing tissue.

SAMPLE DOCUMENTATION

[date] [time]	Lt. hip wound, stage IV measured 2 × 4, 1 in. in depth. Drainage consists of yellow purulent material, no necrosis noted. Wound irrigated with saline solution and packed with 0.5-in. gauze, covered with gauze dressing. No sinus tract detected. Client complained of minimal pain, 4/10 on pain scale. Client medicated prior to procedure.

_____ D. Haus, LVN

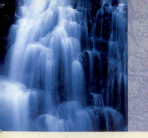

Chapter Review

KEY TERMS by Topic

Use the audio glossary feature of either the CD-ROM or the Companion Website to hear the correct pronunciation of the following key terms.

Wound Healing
hemostasis, phagocytosis, granulation

tissue, eschar, serosanguineous, keloid, exudate, serous, suppuration, sanguineous, hemorrhage, dehiscence, evisceration, fistulas, sitz bath

Pressure Ulcers
pressure ulcers, ischemia, reactive hyperemia, friction, shearing force, maceration, debride

KEY Points

- Skin integrity is the body's first line of defense.
- The wound healing process has three phases: inflammatory, proliferative, and maturation.
- Essential data for wounds include wound appearance, size, drainage, swelling, pain, and the presence of tubes and drains.
- Nurses are usually responsible for obtaining specimens of wound drainage for culture. Laboratory data support wound assessment.
- Nurses must wash hands before and after providing wound care to prevent infection and transmission of bloodborne pathogens.
- Major nursing responsibilities related to wound care include preventing infection, preventing further tissue damage, preventing hemorrhage, promoting healing, and preventing skin excoriation around draining wounds.
- Wound care may involve cleaning wounds, changing dressings, maintaining drains, irrigating, inserting packing, applying heat and cold, and applying bandages and binders.
- Nurses must use extra precautions when applying heat or cold to clients with neurosensory or circulatory impairment.
- Major types of wound exudate are serous, purulent, and sanguineous (hemorrhagic). The main complications of wound healing are hemorrhage, infection, dehiscence, and evisceration.
- A pressure ulcer is caused by unrelieved pressure resulting in damage to underlying tissues.
- Friction and shearing forces can also produce a pressure ulcer. Frequent change of position and care when moving a client can help prevent pressure ulcers.

- The nurse describes a pressure ulcer in terms of location, size, depth, stage, color, status of wound margins and surrounding skin, and specific signs of infection.
- Wound assessment continually requires visual inspection, palpation, and the sense of smell.

EXPLORE MediaLink

Additional interactive resources for this chapter can be found on the Companion Website at www.prenhall.com/ramont. Click on Chapter 23 and "Begin" to select the activities for this chapter.

For chapter-related NCLEX®-style questions and an audio glossary, access the accompanying CD-ROM in this book.

Animations/Videos
- Pressure Ulcers

FOR FURTHER Study

For more information about infection control, see Chapter 9.

For further information about the body's normal responses to heat and cold, see Chapter 20.

Caring for a Debilitated Client

NCLEX-PN® Focus Area: Physiological Integrity

Case Study: Mr. Johns is an 84-year-old client being treated for a urinary tract disorder. Mr. Johns suffered a cerebrovascular accident (stroke) 6 months ago and has difficulty ambulating and attending to his own needs because of right-sided weakness. While assessing Mr. Johns, you note that he is thin for his 6-foot frame, weighs 135 lbs, is incontinent of foul-smelling urine, and has deeply reddened areas on his right hip, coccyx, and entire perineal area. He is alert and oriented to person, place, and time, but he has decreased sensation on his entire right side. He spends most of his time in bed or sitting at his bedside chair due to his difficulty with ambulation.

Nursing Diagnosis: Risk for Impaired Skin Integrity

COLLECT DATA

Subjective	Objective
_____	_____
_____	_____
_____	_____
_____	_____
_____	_____
_____	_____
_____	_____

Would you report this? Yes/No

If yes, to: _____

What would you report? _____

Nursing Care

_____
_____
_____
_____
_____
_____
_____
_____
_____
_____
_____

How would you document this? _____
_____
_____

Compare your documentation to the sample provided in Appendix I.

Data Collected
(use those that apply)

- Difficulty ambulating
- Height: 6 ft
- Weight: 135 lbs
- Client states, "I'm not hungry most of the time."
- Weakened
- BP 150/88
- Incontinent of urine
- General malaise
- Deeply reddened coccyx, right hip, and perineal area
- Alert and oriented
- Decreased sensation to his entire right side
- Right-sided weakness
- Negative for fecal blood
- TSH 5 mcgIU/mL (microgram of international units/mL)

Nursing Interventions
(use those that apply; list in priority order)

- Monitor urine output.
- Monitor reddened area.
- Check vital signs every 2 hours.
- Turn client every 2 hours.
- Refer to dietitian.
- Steadily increase ambulation.
- Weigh daily.
- Offer urinal frequently.

NCLEX-PN® Exam Preparation

1. In some clients, pressure can cause the beginning of a decubitus ulcer within a matter of hours. When you observe the first sign of pressure, you should immediately do which of the following?
   1. Make sure the skin is warm and dry.
   2. Reposition and turn the client at least every 2 hours.
   3. Put client on an airflow mattress.
   4. Apply protective pads and adhesive dressings.

2. The purpose of a wet-to-damp dressing is:
   1. cooling.
   2. antipruritic.
   3. nevus removal.
   4. debridement.

3. When intact skin surface has been injured or broken, the client has lost some ability to:
   1. resist infection.
   2. take in vitamin D.
   3. eliminate waste products.
   4. lubricate the skin.

4. A client has a decubitus ulcer exposing the bone in the hip. The nurse identifies this type of ulcer as a:
   1. stage I ulcer.
   2. stage II ulcer.
   3. stage III ulcer.
   4. stage IV ulcer.

5. A danger seen in closed wet dressings is:
   1. maceration.
   2. frequent dressing changes.
   3. debridement.
   4. ischemia.

6. In the second phase of healing, a wound will show evidence of a red tissue that is fragile and bleeds easily. This tissue is called:
   1. granulation tissue.
   2. phagocytosis.
   3. necrosis.
   4. exudates.

7. Many factors are involved in the development of pressure ulcers. A combination of friction and pressure occurs when a client slides down in bed but the skin does not move. This is known as:
   1. evisceration.
   2. hematoma.
   3. reactive hyperemia.
   4. shearing force.

8. A surgical wound infection can be reduced primarily by:
   1. leaving incisions open to air.
   2. changing dressings using surgical technique.
   3. adhering to the principles of handwashing.
   4. cleansing incisions from the least contaminated to the most contaminated area.

9. Diabetes is a predisposing condition for decubitus ulcer formation. Which factor may be involved?
   1. peripheral vascular disease
   2. kidney disease
   3. immune disorder
   4. hepatic disease

10. A disadvantage of using alcohol as a cooling measure is:
    1. that it blisters the skin.
    2. that it dries the skin.
    3. maceration.
    4. suppuration.

Answers and Rationales for Review Questions, as well as discussion of Care Plan and Critical Thinking Care Map questions, appear in Appendix I.

Chapter 24

Oxygenation

BRIEF Outline

Structure and Function of the Respiratory System
Structure and Function of the Cardiovascular System
Treatment of Oxygenation Problems

LEARNING Outcomes

After completing this chapter, you will be able to:

1. Outline the structure and function of the respiratory system.
2. Describe the processes of breathing (ventilation) and gas exchange (respiration).
3. Identify factors influencing respiration and circulatory function.
4. Identify common signs of impaired respiratory function.
5. Outline the structure and function of the cardiovascular system.
6. Identify and describe nursing measures to promote cardiorespiratory function and oxygenation.
7. Explain the use of therapeutic measures such as artificial airways, medications, oxygen therapy, inhalation therapy, pharyngeal suction, and chest drainage to promote cardiorespiratory function and oxygenation.

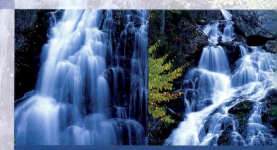

HISTORICAL Perspectives

Oxygen was discovered independently by the Swedish apothecary Karl W. Scheele in 1772 and by the English amateur chemist Joseph Priestley (1733–1804) in August 1774. In 1783, the French physician Caillens was the first doctor reported to have used oxygen therapy as a remedy.

Oxygen, a clear, odorless gas that constitutes about 21% of the air we breathe, is necessary for all living cells. The absence of oxygen can lead to death. Although the delivery of oxygen to body tissues is affected at least indirectly by all body systems, the respiratory system and the cardiovascular system are directly involved in this process. Impaired function of either system can significantly affect our ability to breathe, transport gases, and participate in everyday activities.

Respiration is the process of gas exchange between the individual and the environment. The process of respiration involves several components:

1. Pulmonary **ventilation** (breathing), which is the movement of air between the atmosphere and the alveoli of the lungs
2. Diffusion of oxygen and carbon dioxide between the alveoli and pulmonary capillaries
3. Transport of oxygen and carbon dioxide via the blood to and from tissues
4. Diffusion of oxygen and carbon dioxide between the capillaries and the cells of body tissues.

Structure and Function of the Respiratory System

The primary function of the respiratory system is gas exchange. Structures of the respiratory system function to move air, eliminate waste products, maintain acid–base balance, and protect the airway from infection.

STRUCTURE OF THE RESPIRATORY SYSTEM

The respiratory system (Figure 24-1A ■) is divided structurally into the upper respiratory system and the lower respiratory system. The mouth, nose, pharynx, and larynx compose the upper respiratory system. The lower respiratory system includes the trachea and lungs, with the bronchi, bronchioles, alveoli, pulmonary capillary network, and pleural membranes.

Air enters through the nose, where it is warmed, humidified, and filtered. Large particles in the air are trapped by the hairs at the entrance of the nares (nostrils), and smaller particles are filtered and trapped by the nasal turbinates and septum inside the nose. The sneeze reflex is initiated by irritants in nasal passages. During a sneeze, a large volume of air exits rapidly through the nose and mouth, helping to clear nasal passages.

Inspired air passes from the nose through the pharynx, commonly known as the throat. The pharynx is a shared pathway for air and food. It is richly supplied with lymphoid tissue that traps and destroys pathogens that enter with the air.

The larynx can be identified externally (the Adam's apple). In addition to its role in speech, the larynx is important for maintaining airway patency and protecting the lower airways from swallowed food and fluids. During swallowing, the inlet to the larynx (the **epiglottis**) closes, routing food to the esophagus. The epiglottis is open during breathing, allowing air to move freely into the lower airways.

Below the larynx, the trachea leads to the right and left main bronchi (primary bronchi) and the airways of the lungs. Within the lungs, the primary bronchi divide repeatedly into smaller and smaller bronchi, ending with the terminal bronchioles. Together these airways are known as the *bronchial tree*. The trachea and bronchi are lined with cells that produce a thin layer of mucus to trap pathogens and microscopic matter. These foreign particles are then swept upward toward the larynx and throat by *cilia*, tiny hairlike projections on the epithelial cells. The cough reflex is triggered by irritants in the larynx, trachea, or bronchi.

The respiratory zone of the lungs includes the respiratory bronchioles, the alveolar ducts, and the alveoli (Figure 24-1B). Until air enters the respiratory bronchioles and alveoli, no gas exchange occurs. Alveoli have very thin walls, composed of a single layer of epithelial cells covered by a thick mesh of pulmonary capillaries. The alveolar and capillary walls form the membrane where gas exchange occurs (see Figure 24-1B).

The outer surface of the lungs is covered by a thin, double layer of tissue known as the pleura. The pleura has two parts:

1. The parietal pleura lines the thorax and surface of the diaphragm.
2. The visceral pleura covers the external surface of the lungs.

Between these pleural layers is a space that contains a small amount of pleural fluid, a serous lubricating solution. This fluid prevents friction during the movements of breathing and keeps the layers adherent, much as a film of water can cause two glass slides to cling to each other.

PULMONARY VENTILATION

Ventilation (breathing) is accomplished through **inspiration** (inhalation) when air flows into the lungs and **expiration** (exhalation) when air moves out of the lungs. When inflammation, edema, and excessive mucous production occur, small airways become clogged, impairing ventilation of the alveoli.

The respiratory centers of the medulla and pons in the brainstem control breathing. Severe head injury or drugs that depress the central nervous system (e.g., opiates or barbiturates) can affect the respiratory centers, impairing the drive to breathe.

The degree of chest expansion during normal breathing is minimal and requires little energy. However, when a client has **chronic obstructive pulmonary disease (COPD)**

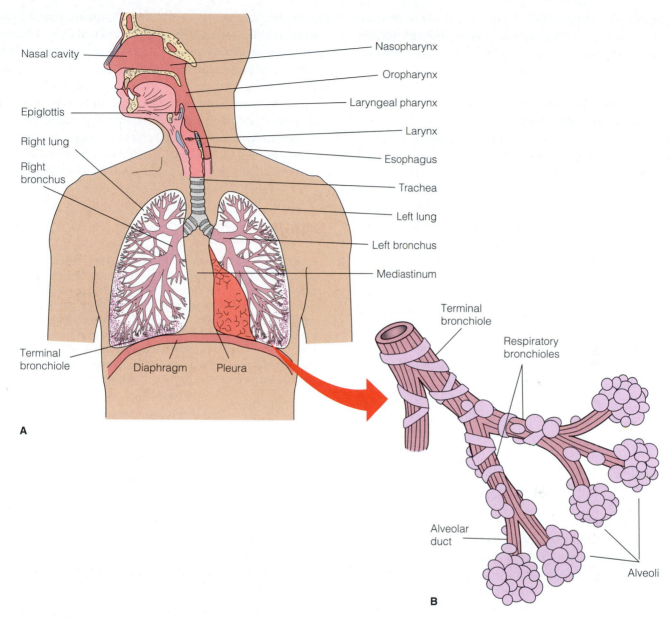

Figure 24-1. ■ **A.** Organs of the respiratory tract. **B.** Respiratory bronchioles, alveolar ducts, and alveoli.

(persistent obstruction of bronchial air flow), chest expansion requires greater effort. This client must use accessory muscles of respiration, including the anterior neck muscles, intercostal muscles, and muscles of the abdomen, to move air into and out of the chest.

When a client has diseases or trauma such as spinal cord injury that affect the muscles of respiration, the thoracic cavity may not be able to expand and contract effectively. When trauma occurs to the chest wall, the pressure within the chest cavity changes, causing the lung to collapse. If the thin, double-layered pleural membrane is disrupted by lung disease, surgery, or trauma, negative pressure between the pleural layers may be lost, and the lung may collapse. Air in the pleural space is known as a **pneumothorax**.

Blood (**hemothorax**) or fluid (**pleural effusion**) in the pleural space places pressure on lung tissue and also interferes with lung expansion.

ALVEOLAR GAS EXCHANGE

The second phase of the respiratory process is the diffusion of oxygen from the alveoli into the pulmonary blood vessels. **Diffusion** is the movement of gases or other particles from an area of greater pressure or concentration to an area of lower pressure or concentration.

Pressure differences in the gases on each side of the respiratory membrane affect diffusion. When the pressure of oxygen is greater in the alveoli than in the blood, oxygen diffuses into the blood. Likewise, when the pressure of carbon dioxide in venous blood is greater than the pressure of carbon dioxide in the alveoli, carbon dioxide diffuses from the blood into the alveoli, where it can be eliminated with expired air.

TRANSPORT OF OXYGEN AND CARBON DIOXIDE

The third part of the respiratory process involves the transport of respiratory gases. Oxygen needs to be transported from the lungs to the tissues, and carbon dioxide must be transported from the tissues back to the lungs. Normally 97% of the oxygen combines loosely with **hemoglobin** (an oxygen-carrying red pigment) in the red blood cells (RBCs). It is carried to the tissues as *oxyhemoglobin* (the compound of oxygen and hemoglobin). The remaining oxygen is dissolved and transported in the fluid of the plasma and cells.

Several factors affect the rate of oxygen transport from the lungs to the tissues; cardiac output, number of **erythrocytes** (RBCs), and exercise.

The amount of blood pumped by the heart is called **cardiac output**. Normally, it is approximately 5 L per minute. Any pathologic condition that decreases cardiac output (e.g., damage to the heart muscle, blood loss, or pooling of blood in the peripheral blood vessels) diminishes the amount of oxygen delivered to the tissues. The heart compensates for inadequate output by increasing its pumping rate. However, with severe damage or blood loss, this may not restore adequate blood flow and oxygen to the tissues.

Another factor influencing oxygen transport is the number of erythrocytes. **Hematocrit** is a measurement of the percentage of erythrocytes (RBCs) in the blood. (In men, the number of circulating erythrocytes normally averages about 5 million per cubic milliliter of blood, and in women, about 4.5 million per cubic milliliter. Normally the hematocrit is about 40% to 54% in men and 37% to 47% in women.) Excessive increases in the blood hematocrit raise the blood *viscosity* (thickness), reducing the cardiac output and oxygen transport. Excessive reductions in the blood hematocrit, such as occur in anemia, reduce oxygen transport

Exercise also has a direct influence on oxygen transport. In well-trained athletes, oxygen transport can be increased up to 20 times the normal rate, due in part to an increased cardiac output and to efficient use of oxygen by the cells.

RESPIRATORY REGULATION

Respiratory rate and depth are controlled by nerves and the concentration of certain gases in the blood. The brain regulates respirations to maintain correct concentrations of oxygen, carbon dioxide, and hydrogen ions in the body fluids.

An area in the medulla of the brain is highly responsive to increases in blood carbon dioxide (CO_2). When CO_2 or hydrogen ion concentration increases, the brain increases the rate and depth of respirations. In addition, special nerve receptors are sensitive to decreases in oxygen (O_2) concentration in the blood. When they sense decreases in the amount of oxygen in the arteries, they stimulate the respiratory center to increase respirations. Of the three blood gases (hydrogen, oxygen, and carbon dioxide), increased carbon dioxide concentration normally stimulates respiration most strongly.

clinical ALERT

In clients with certain lung ailments such as emphysema, oxygen concentration (not carbon dioxide) may determine regulation of respiration. For such clients, decreased oxygen concentration is the main stimulus for respiration. This is called the *hypoxic drive*. If the concentration of oxygen is increased, it will depress the respiratory rate, causing the client to go into respiratory distress. Oxygen must be administered to these clients only in low concentrations to avoid causing severe respiratory problems or death. See Box 24-1 ■ for oxygen therapy guidelines for clients with COPD.

ALTERATIONS IN RESPIRATORY FUNCTION

Respiratory function can be altered by conditions that affect:

- The movement of air into or out of the lungs
- The diffusion of oxygen and carbon dioxide between the alveoli and the pulmonary capillaries
- The transport of oxygen and carbon dioxide via the blood to and from the tissue cells.

Three major alterations in respiration are hypoxia, altered breathing patterns, and an obstructed or partially obstructed airway.

BOX 24-1 | POPULATION FOCUS

Oxygen Therapy for Clients with COPD

Low-flow oxygen systems are essential for clients with COPD. People with COPD may have a chronically high carbon dioxide level. Their stimulus to breathe is not high levels of carbon dioxide but low levels of oxygen (*hypoxemia*). High flows of oxygen can potentially relieve this hypoxemia, but they may also remove the stimulus to breathe. Low flows maintain a slightly hypoxemic state, thus maintaining the respiratory drive. Clients who have COPD and are receiving oxygen therapy should be observed carefully (especially when therapy is first initiated) for respiratory depression or arrest.

Hypoxia

Hypoxia is a condition of insufficient oxygen anywhere in the body. The inhaled air may lack enough oxygen, or an insufficient amount of oxygen may be delivered to the tissues. Hypoxia can be related to ventilation, diffusion of gases, or transport of gases by the blood. It can be caused by any condition that alters one or more parts of the respiratory process. An early sign of hypoxia is restlessness.

Hypoventilation, or inadequate alveolar ventilation, can lead to hypoxia. Hypoventilation may be due to respiratory diseases, drugs, decreased respiratory rate, or anesthesia and often causes carbon dioxide to accumulate in the blood. This is a condition called **hypercarbia** or **hypercapnia**.

Hypoxia can also develop when oxygen does not diffuse effectively into the arterial blood (as in pulmonary edema). Hypoxia can also result from problems in the delivery of oxygen to the tissues. This occurs with anemia, heart failure, and pulmonary embolism. The term *hypoxemia* refers to reduced oxygen in the blood. Box 24-2 ■ lists manifestations of hypoxia.

Cyanosis (bluish discoloration of the skin, nail beds, and mucous membranes due to reduced hemoglobin-oxygen saturation) may also be present. The brain can tolerate hypoxia for only 4 to 6 minutes before permanent damage occurs. The face of the acutely hypoxic person usually appears anxious, tired, and drawn. The person usually assumes a sitting position, often leaning forward slightly to permit greater expansion of the thoracic cavity.

With chronic hypoxia, the client often appears fatigued and is lethargic. The client's fingers and toes may be clubbed as a result of long-term lack of oxygen. With clubbing, the base of the nail becomes swollen and the ends of the fingers and toes increase in size. The angle between the nail and the base of the nail increases to more than 180 degrees (see Figure 19-4D ⚭).

Altered Breathing Patterns

Breathing patterns refer to the rate, volume, rhythm, and relative ease or effort of respiration. Normal respiration (**eupnea**) is quiet, rhythmic, and effortless. **Tachypnea** (rapid breathing rate) is seen with fevers, metabolic acidosis, pain, hypercapnia, or hypoxemia. **Bradypnea** is an abnormally slow respiratory rate, which may be seen in clients who have taken narcotics, who have metabolic alkalosis, or who have increased intracranial pressure (e.g., from brain injuries). **Apnea** is defined as periods of no breathing. (For further information, see Box 20-6. ⚭)

Hyperventilation is an increased rate and depth of respirations. In this situation, more CO_2 is eliminated than is produced. One particular type of hyperventilation that accompanies metabolic acidosis is called **Kussmaul's breathing** found in diabetic ketoacidosis, a diabetic complication. The body attempts to rid itself of excess body acids by blowing off the carbon dioxide through deep and rapid breathing. Hyperventilation often occurs as a response to stress.

Normal breathing is effortless, with evenly spaced respirations that vary little in depth. Abnormal respiratory rhythms create an irregular breathing pattern. Review the different respiratory rhythms in Box 20-6 ⚭.

Difficult or labored breathing is called **dyspnea**. The dyspneic person often appears anxious and may experience **shortness of breath (SOB)**, a feeling of being unable to get enough air. When a person is dyspneic, the nostrils may be flared because of the increased effort of inspiration. The skin may appear dusky; heart rate is increased. See Box 24-3 ■ for cultural issues.

Obstructed Airway

A completely or partially obstructed airway can occur anywhere along the upper or lower respiratory passageways. An obstruction of the nose, pharynx, or larynx is an *upper airway obstruction.* It can be caused by a foreign object such as food, by the tongue blocking the oropharynx when a person is unconscious, or by secretions collecting in the passageways. In the last instance, the respirations sound gurgly or bubbly as the air attempts to pass through the secretions. *Lower airway obstruction* involves partial or complete blockage of the passageways in the bronchi and lungs. This can be caused

---

BOX 24-2	MANIFESTATIONS OF HYPOXIA

- Rapid pulse
- Rapid, shallow respirations and dyspnea
- Increased restlessness or light-headedness
- Flaring of the nares
- Substernal or intercostal retractions
- Cyanosis

BOX 24-3	CULTURAL PULSE POINTS

Frequency of Asthma

Among adults, women of all races have higher rates of illness and death from asthma than do men. Death from asthma is two to six times more likely to occur among African Americans and Hispanics than among whites. Rates for African Americans hospitalized for asthma are almost triple those for whites. African Americans are four times more likely than whites to visit an emergency department because of asthma. Asthma clients in general, and high-risk inner-city clients in particular, need to be able to recognize the signs and symptoms of uncontrolled asthma and know how to respond appropriately

(U.S. Department of Health and Human Services, 2000).

by bronchospasm; increased production of secretions; thick, sticky secretions; or bronchial inflammation.

Maintaining an open (*patent*) airway is a nursing responsibility that requires immediate action. A low-pitched snoring sound during inhalation indicates partial obstruction of the upper airway. Complete obstruction is indicated by extreme inspiratory effort that produces no chest movement. *Intercostal retractions* (the drawing of skin and muscle against the ribs) indicate this extreme effort. Lower airway obstruction is not always as easy to observe. **Stridor** (a harsh, high-pitched sound) may be heard during inspiration. The client may have altered arterial blood gas (ABG) levels, restlessness, dyspnea, and *adventitious* (abnormal) breath sounds. See Chapter 19 🔗 on assessment and Box 20-6 🔗.

Structure and Function of the Cardiovascular System

The respiratory and cardiovascular systems are closely linked and depend on each other to deliver oxygen to the tissues of the body. Alterations in function of either system can affect the other and lead to hypoxia, or lack of oxygen.

The heart, blood vessels, and blood form the major transport system of the body, bringing oxygen and nutrients to the cells and removing wastes for disposal. The heart serves as the system pump, moving blood through the vessels to the tissues.

THE HEART

The heart is a hollow, cone-shaped organ about the size of a fist. It is located in the mediastinum (between the lungs and below the sternum). The heart is made of three layers:

1. The *endocardium* lines the inside of the heart's chambers and great vessels.
2. The *myocardium* is made up of cardiac muscle cells that form the bulk of the heart and contract with each beat.
3. The *epicardium* forms the outer layer. It is enclosed by a double-layered membrane known as the *pericardium.* The parietal, or outermost, pericardium protects the heart and anchors it to surrounding structures. The visceral pericardium adheres to the surface of the heart and forms the epicardium.

The heart contains four hollow chambers: two upper atria and two lower ventricles. They are separated by a septum, or wall, that forms two parallel pumps (Figure 24-2 ■). The atria and ventricles are separated from one another by the atrioventricular valves. The tricuspid valve is on the right, and the bicuspid or mitral valve is on the left. The ventricles, in turn, are separated from the *great vessels* (the pulmonary arteries and aorta) by the semilunar valves. The pulmonic valve is on the right, and the aortic valve is on the left. The valves direct the flow of blood from the atria to the ventricles, and the ventricles

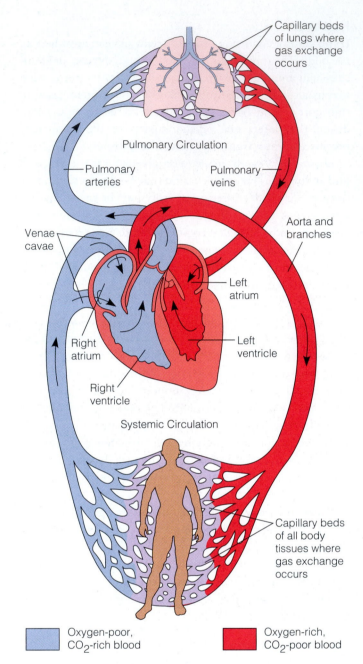

Figure 24-2. ■ The heart and blood vessels. The left side of the heart pumps oxygenated blood into the arteries. Deoxygenated blood returns via the venous system into the right side of the heart.

to the great vessels. The valves act as one-way doors, allowing the blood to flow in one direction and preventing backflow.

Deoxygenated blood returns to the heart from the veins. It enters the right atrium through the superior and inferior venae cavae. From there it flows into the right ventricle, which pumps it through the pulmonary artery into the lungs for gas exchange. Freshly oxygenated blood enters the pulmonary veins and returns to the left atrium. From here the blood enters the left ventricle to be pumped out through the aorta to the body.

Coronary Circulation

The heart pumps blood to the lungs and peripheral tissues but receives no oxygen or nourishment from the blood within its chambers. Instead, it is supplied by a network of vessels known as the coronary circulation. The coronary arteries originate at the base of the aorta, branching out to encircle and penetrate the myocardium. The coronary arteries bring oxygen-rich blood to the myocardium. If these arteries become clogged with **atherosclerotic plaque** (fat deposits within the blood vessels) or if the arteries are obstructed by a blood clot, oxygenated blood cannot reach the myocardium. The client may develop chest pain (**angina pectoris**) or experience a **myocardial infarction** or **MI** (heart attack).

Cardiac Output

Cardiac output, the amount of blood pumped by the ventricles in 1 minute, is an important indicator of how well the heart is functioning as a pump. If the cardiac output is poor, tissue perfusion suffers and oxygen and nutrients do not reach the cells as needed.

BLOOD VESSELS

With each cardiac contraction, blood is ejected into a closed system of blood vessels that transport blood to the tissues and return it to the heart. The heart supports two circulatory systems: the low-pressure pulmonary system and the higher pressure systemic circulatory system.

Pulmonary Circulation

Deoxygenated blood from the right ventricle enters the pulmonary vascular system through the pulmonary arteries. The pulmonary arteries subdivide into lobar arteries that branch out to form arterioles and the dense capillary networks that encompass the alveoli. Oxygen diffuses into the blood from the alveoli, and carbon dioxide diffuses into the alveoli from the blood. The blood then returns to the left side of the heart via venules and the pulmonary veins.

Systemic Circulation

The muscular left ventricle of the heart pumps oxygenated blood into the aorta. The blood then moves into major arteries that branch from the aorta, and into successively smaller arteries, arterioles, and finally the thin-walled capillary beds of organs and tissues. Capillary walls contain only one thin layer of cells. Gases and molecules can diffuse easily between the blood and the tissues. In the capillary beds, oxygen and nutrients are exchanged for metabolic waste products. The deoxygenated blood then returns to the heart through a series of venules and veins that become progressively larger until they empty into the superior and inferior venae cavae.

BLOOD

Blood transports oxygen via the lungs and nutrients from the gastrointestinal system to the cells. Blood is a mixture of blood cells suspended in fluid (plasma). Its primary functions are:

- Transporting oxygen, nutrients, and hormones to the cells
- Transporting metabolic wastes from the tissues for elimination through the lungs, liver, and kidneys
- Regulating body temperature, pH, and fluid volume
- Controlling infection and blood loss.

As previously noted, most oxygen is transported bound to hemoglobin. Hemoglobin is a major component of erythrocytes, the predominant cells present in blood. Hemoglobin binds easily with oxygen, releasing it in the body tissues. **Anemia** is a condition of too few RBCs that contain too little or abnormal hemoglobin. This condition interferes with oxygen delivery to the tissues, causing fatigue and activity intolerance.

ALTERATIONS IN CARDIOVASCULAR FUNCTION

Cardiovascular function can be altered by conditions that affect:

1. The function of the heart as a pump (cardiac output)
2. Blood flow to organs and peripheral tissues (tissue perfusion)
3. The composition of the blood and its ability to transport oxygen and carbon dioxide (blood alterations).

Decreased Cardiac Output

Although the heart normally is able to increase its rate and force of contraction to increase cardiac output during exercise, fever, or other times of need, some conditions interfere with these mechanisms. Heart attack (MI), congestive heart failure, and certain infections of the heart (*myocarditis*) cause damage to the heart muscle. When this occurs, the heart can no longer pump effectively.

Very irregular or excessively rapid or slow heart rates can decrease the cardiac output. Abnormalities of the heart rate and rhythm are known as **dysrhythmias** and can be identified on an electrocardiogram (ECG).

Alterations in the structure of the heart can affect cardiac output. Congenital heart defects and infectious heart disorders such as bacterial endocarditis and rheumatic fever can both cause decreased cardiac output.

Impaired Tissue Perfusion

Ischemia is a lack of blood supply to tissues and organs due to obstructed circulation. **Atherosclerosis** (narrowing and obstruction of circulatory vessels) is by far the most common cause of ischemia. Any artery in the body may be affected by atherosclerosis. Risk factors for atherosclerosis include:

- Cigarette smoking
- High fat intake
- Obesity
- Sedentary lifestyle
- Hypertension
- Uncontrolled diabetes mellitus.

Obstruction of the coronary arteries causes myocardial ischemia. Ischemia of the cerebral vessels may cause a *transient ischemic attack* or *cerebral vascular accident* (stroke). Peripheral vascular disease leads to ischemia of distal tissues such as the legs and feet. Gangrene and amputation may result.

Veins that do not function properly can cause impaired tissue perfusion. When heart valves do not open and close correctly, blood may pool in veins, causing edema and decreasing venous return to the heart. Veins also can become inflamed, reducing blood flow and increasing the risk of **thrombus** (clot) formation (see the Preventing Venous Stasis subsection in the Nursing Care section of this chapter). The thrombus may then break loose, becoming an **embolus** (plural: emboli). Emboli tend to travel as far as the pulmonary circulation, where they become trapped in small vessels (*pulmonary emboli*), occluding blood supply to the alveolar-capillary membrane. Although alveolar ventilation to the affected area often remains adequate, no gas exchange occurs there because of impaired blood flow.

Blood Alterations

When blood is unable to transport oxygen to tissues effectively, impaired tissue perfusion results. Lack of RBCs, low hemoglobin levels, or abnormal hemoglobin structure all affect tissue oxygenation. Anemia may be caused by acute or chronic bleeding, a diet deficient in iron or folic acid, malfunction in the formation of hemoglobin and RBCs, or disorders that cause RBCs to break down excessively. People with sickle cell disease produce an abnormal form of hemoglobin and may experience tissue ischemia during **exacerbations** (flare-ups) of the disease.

Blood volume also affects tissue oxygenation. If the blood volume is inadequate as in hemorrhage or severe dehydration (**hypovolemia**), the blood pressure and cardiac output fall, and tissues may become ischemic. **Hypervolemia** (excess blood volume) can result from fluid retention or kidney failure, and may lead to tissue ischemia.

Factors that Affect Oxygenation

In the healthy person, the cardiovascular and respiratory systems can provide sufficient oxygen to meet the body's needs. However, certain factors can affect oxygen delivery and oxygen entering the bloodstream:

- Diseases of the cardiovascular and/or respiratory systems (e.g., anemia).
- Medications. Narcotics such as morphine and meperidine (Demerol) depress the respiratory center in the medulla, causing decreased respiratory depth and rate.
- Stress. When stressed, some people hyperventilate. Oxygen levels in arterial blood rise, and carbon dioxide levels fall. This causes symptoms of dizziness, numbness of fingers and toes, and numbness around the mouth.
- Anger may be connected to heart disease. Recent studies indicate that people who repress their anger or become hostile appear to have a higher incidence of heart disease.
- Gender may affect cardiopulmonary function. Through middle adulthood (until menopause), estrogen has a protective effect in women, slowing the progress of atherosclerosis and reducing the risk of cardiovascular disease. This effect is lost at menopause, but hormone replacement therapy may be beneficial in reducing this risk later in life. Among people in their 40s and 50s, men have a higher incidence of hypertension than women.

Treatment of Oxygenation Problems

COLLABORATIVE CARE

Pulse Oximetry

A pulse oximeter is a noninvasive device that measures oxygen saturation (SpO_2 or O_2 sat). The pulse oximeter is connected to a sensor attached to the client's finger (Figure 24-3 ■), toe,

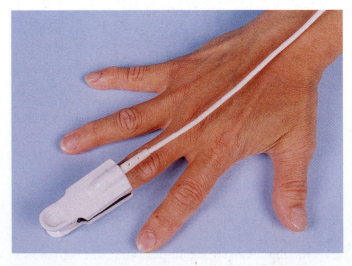

Figure 24-3. ■ A finger clip sensor for a pulse oximeter. (Photographer: Jenny Thomas.)

nose, earlobe, or forehead (or around the hand or foot of a neonate). The sensor detects hypoxemia before clinical signs and symptoms develop.

The pulse oximeter uses infrared light and a process known as spectrophotometry to measure the amount of oxygenated hemoglobin in arterial blood. Normal SpO_2 is 95% to 100%. An SpO_2 below 70% is life threatening. Measurement of SpO_2 may be taken intermittently, often as an aspect of vital sign measurement, but it also may be continuously monitored. The procedure for using a pulse oximeter is described in Procedure 24-1 ■ on page 515.

clinical ALERT

Pulse oximetry measures only the amount of hemoglobin that is bound with oxygen. Results can be misleading if the client's hemoglobin is bound to another substance, such as carbon monoxide.

Cardiac Monitoring

Cardiac monitoring allows continuous observation of the client's cardiac rhythm. It is used in many instances, such as during and after surgery, and in clients who have known or suspected cardiovascular disease. Electrodes placed on the client's chest may be attached to a monitor cable and bedside monitor. The monitor is equipped with alarms used to warn of potential problems such as very fast or very slow heart rates.

Diagnostic Studies

The physician may order various diagnostic tests to assess respiratory and cardiovascular status, function, and oxygenation. Included are sputum specimens, throat cultures, skin testing for allergies, venous and arterial blood specimens, pulmonary and cardiac function tests, and visualization procedures. Check the facility's policy for specimens that the LPN/LVN is responsible for collecting.

SPECIMENS. **Sputum** is the mucous secretion from the lungs, bronchi, and trachea. It is important to differentiate it from saliva, the clear liquid secreted by the salivary glands in the mouth, sometimes referred to as "spit."

Healthy individuals do not produce sputum. Clients need to cough to bring sputum up from the lungs, bronchi, and trachea into the mouth in order to expectorate it (spit it out) into a collecting container (Figure 24-4 ■).

A throat culture sample is collected from the mucosa of the oropharynx and tonsillar regions using a culture swab (Figure 24-5 ■). The sample is then cultured and examined for the presence of disease-producing microorganisms. Guidelines for obtaining a client's sputum sample and a throat culture are provided in Box 24-4 ■.

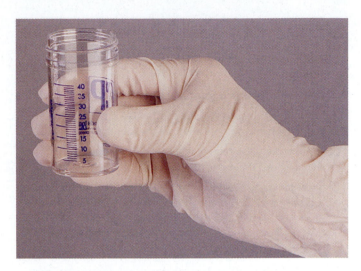

Figure 24-4. ■ Sputum container. (Photographer: Elena Dorfman.)

BLOOD TESTS. Specimens of venous blood are taken for a complete blood count (CBC), which includes hemoglobin and hematocrit measurements, erythrocyte (RBC) count, leukocyte (white blood cell or WBC), RBC indices, and a differential WBC count.

A number of other tests may be performed on blood serum (the liquid portion of the blood). These tests are often referred to as blood chemistries. Common chemistry examinations include serum electrolytes (sodium, potassium, chloride, calcium, and bicarbonate), cardiac enzymes, serum glucose, hormones such as thyroid hormone, metabolic waste products such as creatinine and blood urea nitrogen (BUN), and other substances such as cholesterol and triglycerides. These tests provide valuable diagnostic cues. Nurses often obtain venous blood samples for testing. Arterial blood gases (ABG) give information about oxygen levels, carbon dioxide levels, and pH of the blood. ABG samples are usually obtained by healthcare staff who have had additional training.

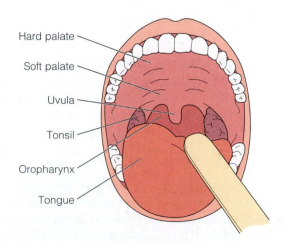

Figure 24-5. ■ Taking a throat culture.

BOX 24-4	NURSING CARE CHECKLIST

Collecting a Sputum Specimen and a Throat Swab Specimen

Collecting a Sputum Specimen

☑ Offer mouth care so that the specimen will not be contaminated with microorganisms from the mouth.

☑ Ask the client to breathe deeply and then cough up 15 to 30 mL (1 or 2 tablespoons) of sputum.

☑ Wear gloves to avoid direct contact with the sputum. Follow special precautions if tuberculosis is suspected, obtaining the specimen in a room equipped with a special airflow system or ultraviolet light, or outdoors. If these options are not available, wear a mask capable of filtering droplet nuclei.

☑ Ask the client to *expectorate* (spit out) the sputum into the specimen container (see Figure 24-4). Make sure the sputum does not contact the outside of the container. If the outside of the container does become contaminated, wash it with a disinfectant.

☑ Following sputum collection, offer mouthwash to remove any unpleasant taste.

☑ Document the amount of sputum collected, color, odor, consistency (thick, tenacious, watery), and presence of **hemoptysis** (blood in sputum).

Collecting a Throat Culture Specimen

☑ Don clean gloves.

☑ Insert the swab into the oropharynx and run the swab along the tonsils and areas on the pharynx that are reddened or contain exudate. (The gag reflex, active in some clients, may be decreased by having the client sit upright if health permits, open the mouth, extend the tongue, and say "ah," and by taking the specimen quickly.)

☑ If the posterior pharynx cannot be seen, use a light and depress the tongue with a tongue blade (see Figure 24-5).

☑ Carefully place the swab with culture into the culture container, being sure not to contaminate the outside of the container.

ELECTROCARDIOGRAPHY. Electrocardiography provides a graphic recording of the heart's electrical activity. Electrodes placed on the skin transmit the electrical impulses to an oscilloscope or graphic recorder. The ECG can then be examined to detect dysrhythmias and alterations in conduction indicative of myocardial damage, enlargement of the heart, or drug effects.

Stress electrocardiography uses ECGs to assess the client's response to an increased cardiac workload during exercise. As the body's demand for oxygen increases with exercising, the cardiac workload increases, as does the oxygen demand of the heart muscle itself. Clients with coronary artery dis-

ease may develop chest pain and characteristic ECG changes during exercise.

PULMONARY FUNCTION TESTS. Pulmonary function tests measure lung volume and capacity. Clients undergoing pulmonary function tests, which are usually carried out by a respiratory therapist, do not require an anesthetic. The client breathes into a tube attached to a machine and a computer. The tests are painless but often tiring, especially for clients with pulmonary or cardiac conditions. The test requires the client's full cooperation.

VISUALIZATION PROCEDURES. A number of visualization procedures can be done to examine the respiratory tract and cardiovascular system. X-ray, lung scan, endoscopy (bronchoscopy and laryngoscopy), angiography, and echocardiography are a few.

Oxygen Therapy

Clients who have difficulty ventilating all areas of their lungs, those whose gas exchange is impaired, or people with heart failure may require oxygen therapy to prevent hypoxia.

Oxygen therapy is prescribed by the physician, who specifies the concentration, method of delivery, and liter flow per minute. The nurse may initiate oxygen therapy in an emergency situation. For clients who have COPD, a low-flow oxygen system is essential. Safety precautions are essential during oxygen therapy. Box 24-5 ■ provides instructions for oxygen safety.

BOX 24-5	NURSING CARE CHECKLIST

Oxygen Therapy Safety Precautions

☑ Place cautionary signs reading "No Smoking: Oxygen in Use" on the client's door, at the foot or head of the bed, and on the oxygen equipment.

☑ Handle and store oxygen cylinders with caution, and strap them securely in wheeled transport devices or stands to prevent possible falls and outlet breakages. Place them away from traffic areas and heaters.

☑ Instruct the client and visitors about the hazard of smoking with oxygen in use. Teach family members and roommates to smoke only outside or in provided smoking rooms away from the client.

☑ Make sure that electric devices (such as razors, hearing aids, radios, televisions, and heating pads) are in good working order to prevent the occurrence of short-circuit sparks.

☑ Avoid materials that generate static electricity, such as woolen blankets and synthetic fabrics. Advise clients and caregivers to wear cotton fabrics and use cotton blankets.

☑ Avoid the use of volatile, flammable materials, such as oils, greases, alcohol, ether, and acetone (e.g., nail polish remover), near clients receiving oxygen.

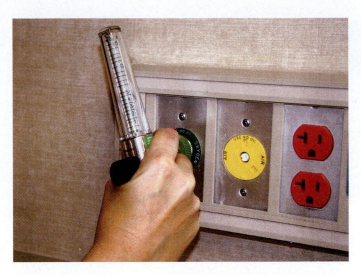

Figure 24-6. ■ An oxygen flow meter attached to a wall outlet.

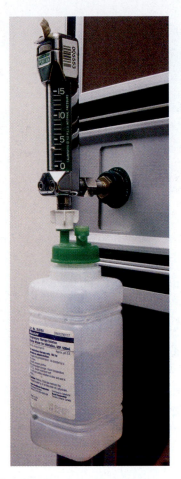

Figure 24-7. ■ An oxygen humidifier.

Because oxygen is colorless, odorless, and tasteless, people are often unaware of its presence. Although oxygen by itself will not burn or explode, it does facilitate combustion and burning. For example, a bed sheet ordinarily burns slowly when ignited in the atmosphere. However, if the sheet is saturated with oxygen and ignited by a spark, it will burn rapidly. The greater the concentration of the oxygen, the more rapidly fires start and burn, and the harder they are to extinguish.

Oxygen is supplied in several different ways. In hospitals and some long-term care facilities, it is usually piped into wall outlets at the client's bedside, making it readily available for use at all times (Figure 24-6 ■). Tanks or cylinders of oxygen under pressure are also frequently available for use when wall oxygen either is unavailable or impractical.

Clients who require oxygen therapy in the home or in facilities without piped-in oxygen may use small cylinders of oxygen, oxygen in liquid form, or an oxygen concentrator. Portable oxygen delivery systems are available to increase the client's independence. Home oxygen therapy services are readily available in most communities. These services generally supply the oxygen and delivery devices, training for the client and family, equipment maintenance, and emergency services should a problem occur.

Oxygen administered from a cylinder or wall-outlet system is dry. Dry gases dehydrate the respiratory mucous membranes. Humidifying devices that add water vapor to inspired air are thus an essential adjunct of oxygen therapy, particularly for liter flows over 2 L/min (Figure 24-7 ■). These devices provide 20% to 40% humidity. The oxygen passes through distilled water and then along a line to the device through which the moistened oxygen is inhaled (e.g., a nasal cannula or oxygen mask). Liter flows of 2 L/min or less by nasal cannula do not require humidification.

OXYGEN DELIVERY SYSTEMS. Oxygen is most often delivered via cannula or face mask. When it is important to regulate the percentage of oxygen received by the client more precisely, a Venturi mask may be used. Refer to Procedure 24-2 ■ on page 516 for descriptions of equipment and interventions.

Artificial Airways

Artificial airways are inserted to maintain a patent air passage for clients whose airway has become or may become obstructed. Here are four of the more common types of artificial airways:

■ Oropharyngeal and nasopharyngeal airways (Figures 24-8A and B ■) are used to keep the upper air passages open when they may become obstructed by secretions or the tongue. These airways are easy to insert and have a low risk of complications.

■ Endotracheal tubes (Figure 24-8C) are most commonly inserted for clients who have had general anesthetics or for those in emergency situations where mechanical ventilation is required. An endotracheal tube is inserted by the physician or RN with specialized education. Because an endotracheal tube passes through the

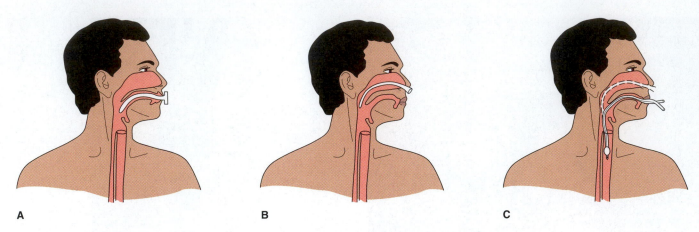

Figure 24-8. ■   **A.** An oropharyngeal airway. **B.** A nasopharyngeal airway. **C.** An endotracheal tube.

epiglottis and glottis, the client is unable to speak while it is in place.

■ Clients who need long-term airway support may have a **tracheostomy** (Figure 24-9 ■), a surgical incision in the trachea just below the larynx through which a tracheostomy tube is inserted.

Tracheostomy tubes may be either plastic or metal and are available in different sizes. Tracheostomy tubes (Figure 24-10 ■) have an outer *cannula* that is inserted into the trachea and a *flange* that rests against the neck and allows the tube to be secured in place with tape or ties. All tubes also have an *obturator;* it is used to insert the outer cannula and is then removed. The obturator is kept at the client's bedside in case the tube becomes dislodged and needs to be reinserted. Some tracheostomy tubes have an inner cannula that may be removed for periodic cleaning.

Cuffed tracheostomy tubes (Figure 24-11 ■) are surrounded by an inflatable cuff that produces an airtight seal between the tube and the trachea. Procedure 24-3 ■ on page 518 describes tracheostomy care.

Chest Tubes and Drainage Systems

Chest tubes may be inserted into the pleural cavity to restore negative pressure and drain collected fluid or blood. Because air rises, chest tubes for pneumothorax often are placed in the upper anterior thorax. Chest tubes used to drain blood or fluid are usually placed in the lower lateral chest wall.

When chest tubes are inserted, they must be connected to a sealed drainage system or a one-way valve that allows air and fluid to be removed from the chest cavity but prevents air from entering from the outside. Water-seal drainage systems are used to prevent outside air from entering the chest tube. Sterile disposable systems commonly are used. These systems typically have a closed collection chamber for drainage that is connected to the water-seal chamber (Figure 24-12 ■). When the client inhales, the water prevents air from entering the system from the atmosphere. During exhalation, however, air can exit the chest cavity, bubbling up through the water. Suction can be added to the system to facilitate the removal of air and secretions from the chest cavity.

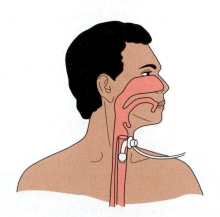

Figure 24-9. ■   A tracheostomy tube in place.

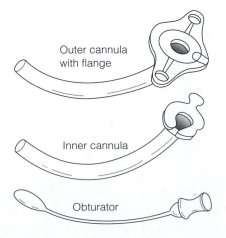

Outer cannula with flange

Inner cannula

Obturator

Figure 24-10. ■   Components of a tracheostomy tube.

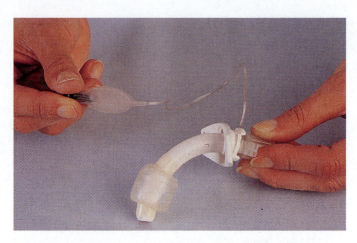

Figure 24-11. ■ A tracheostomy tube with a low-pressure cuff. (Photographer: Elena Dorfman.)

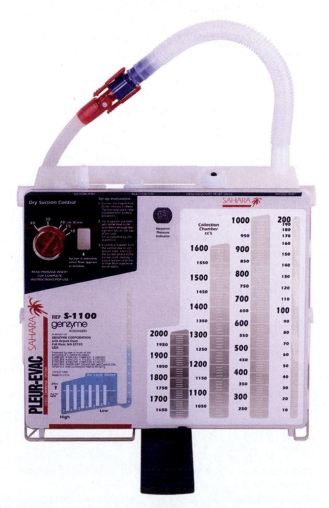

Figure 24-12. ■ A disposable chest drainage system. Fluid and blood collect in the white calibrated chambers. The red chamber provides the water seal, and the blue chamber is a suction-control chamber. (Pleur-evac® Chest Drainage System. Reprinted with permission from Genzyme Biosurgery, Cardiothoracic Division, Fall River, MA.)

NURSING CARE

ASSESSING

A nursing history and physical exam give valuable information about past health problems and current oxygenation status. During the physical exam, it is very important to evaluate the blood pressure in both arms to detect deficits (see Chapter 20 ⚭). There should be no more than 10 mm Hg difference between the arms.

Variations in the shape of the thorax may indicate adaptation to chronic respiratory conditions. For example, clients with emphysema frequently develop a barrel chest.

The nursing assessment specific to oxygenation includes pulse oximetry, cardiac monitoring, and the review of results of diagnostic tests. Nurses obtain sputum or throat swab cultures for culturing (see Box 24-4).

DIAGNOSING, PLANNING, AND IMPLEMENTING

Some of the NANDA diagnoses that may be appropriate for clients with oxygenation problems are:

- *Impaired Gas Exchange*
- *Ineffective Breathing Pattern*
- *Ineffective Tissue Perfusion.*

It is important to be familiar with the NANDA diagnoses; a complete list can be found in Appendix II ⚭.

Promoting Oxygenation

Respiratory Function

Most people in good health give little thought to their respiratory and cardiovascular functions. Changing position frequently, ambulating, and exercising usually maintain adequate ventilation, gas exchange, and cardiovascular function in healthy people.

When people become ill, however, pain and immobility may cause shallow respirations or inadequate chest expansion. Respiratory secretions may pool in the lungs and promote infection. This situation is often compounded when clients are given narcotics for pain.

Interventions by the nurse to maintain the normal respirations of clients include:

- Positioning the client in semi-Fowler's or high-Fowler's to allow for maximum chest expansion
- Encouraging or providing frequent changes in position, especially from side to side to promote lung expansion and mobilization of pulmonary secretions (The orthopneic position helps relieve pressure on the diaphragm from abdominal organs.)

- Encouraging ambulation
- Implementing measures that promote comfort, such as giving pain medications.

Cardiovascular Function

Immobility is detrimental to cardiovascular function. Without exercise of the calf and leg muscles, blood pools in the veins of the lower extremities and *thrombi* (blood clots) may form. Interventions by the nurse to maintain cardiovascular function in clients include:

- Positioning with the legs elevated to promote venous return to the heart
- Avoiding pillows under the knees or more than 15 degrees of knee flexion to improve blood flow to the lower extremities and reduce venous stagnation
- Encouraging leg exercises (such as flexion and extension of the feet, active contraction and relaxation of calf muscles) for a client on bed rest, and promoting ambulation as soon as possible
- Encouraging or providing frequent position changes.

Oxygenation

Deep breathing exercises and coughing help remove secretions from the lungs. Breathing exercises are frequently indicated for clients with restricted chest expansion, such as people with COPD or clients recovering from thoracic surgery.

Commonly employed breathing exercises are abdominal (diaphragmatic) breathing and pursed-lip breathing. Abdominal (diaphragmatic) breathing permits deep full breaths with little effort. Pursed-lip breathing helps the client develop control over breathing. The pursed lips create a resistance to the air flowing out of the lungs; it prolongs exhalation and prevents airway collapse by maintaining positive airway pressure. Box 24-6 ■ provides instructions for performing abdominal (diaphragmatic) and pursed-lip breathing.

BOX 24-7

Controlled and Huff Coughing

- After using a bronchodilator treatment (if prescribed), inhale deeply and hold your breath for a few seconds.
- Cough twice. The first cough loosens the mucus; the second expels secretions.
- For huff coughing, lean forward and exhale sharply with a huff sound. This technique helps keep your airways open while moving secretions up and out of the lungs.
- Inhale by taking rapid short breaths in succession (sniffing) to prevent mucus from moving back into smaller airways.
- Rest.
- Try to avoid prolonged episodes of coughing because these may cause fatigue and hypoxia.

Forceful coughing often is less effective than using controlled or huff coughing techniques. Instructions for coughing techniques are provided in Box 24-7 ■.

Incentive Spirometry

Incentive spirometers, also referred to as sustained maximal inspiration devices (SMIs), are used to:

- Improve pulmonary ventilation
- Counteract the effects of anesthesia or hypoventilation
- Loosen respiratory secretions
- Facilitate respiratory gaseous exchange
- Expand collapsed alveoli.

Incentive spirometers measure the flow of air inhaled through the mouthpiece. They therefore offer an incentive to improve inhalation (Figure 24-13 ■).

The client should be assisted into a position, preferably an upright sitting position in bed or a chair. This position facilitates maximum ventilation. Box 24-8 ■ lists instructions for clients in the use of incentive spirometers.

BOX 24-6   **CLIENT TEACHING**

Abdominal (Diaphragmatic) and Pursed-Lip Breathing Techniques

Teach client to:

- Assume a comfortable semi-sitting position in bed or on a chair or a lying position in bed with one pillow.
- Flex your knees to relax the muscles of the abdomen.
- Place one or both hands on your abdomen, just below the ribs.
- Breathe in deeply through the nose, keeping the mouth closed.
- Concentrate on feeling your abdomen rise as far as possible; stay relaxed and avoid arching your back. If you have difficulty raising your abdomen, take a quick, forceful breath through the nose.
- Then purse your lips as if about to whistle, and breathe out slowly and gently, making a slow whooshing sound without

puffing out the cheeks. This pursed-lip breathing creates a resistance to air flowing out of the lungs, increases pressure within the bronchi (main air passages), and minimizes collapse of smaller airways, a common problem for people with COPD.

- Concentrate on feeling the abdomen fall or sink, and tighten (contract) the abdominal muscles while breathing out to enhance effective exhalation. Count to 7 during exhalation.
- Use this exercise whenever feeling short of breath, and increase gradually to 5 to 10 minutes four times a day. Regular practice will help you do this type of breathing without conscious effort. The exercise, once learned, can be performed when sitting upright, standing, or walking.

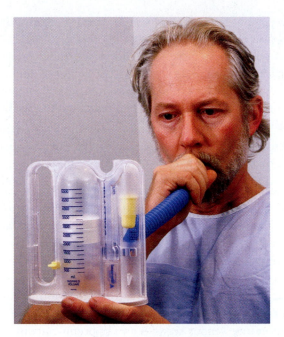

Figure 24-13. ■ Client using a plastic, disposable, volume-oriented incentive spirometer, or SMI. (Photographer: Richard Tauber.)

lizers (atomizers, devices for throwing spray) are used to deliver humidity and medications. They also are used with oxygen delivery systems to provide moistened air directly to the client. Their purposes are to prevent mucous membranes from drying and becoming irritated and to loosen secretions for easier expectoration.

Percussion, Vibration, and Postural Drainage

Percussion, vibration, and postural drainage are dependent nursing functions performed according to a physician's order. These procedures help loosen thick, tenacious secretions. The positions in postural drainage facilitate the removal of secretions. Nurses who work in areas where they are expected to assist with these procedures will receive additional training.

Suctioning

When clients have difficulty expectorating their secretions or when an airway is in place, suctioning may be necessary to clear air passages. **Suctioning** means aspirating secretions through a catheter connected to a suction machine or wall suction outlet. Even though the upper airways (the oropharynx and nasopharynx) are not sterile, sterile technique is recommended for all suctioning to avoid introducing pathogens into the airways.

Suction catheters may be either open tipped or whistle tipped (Figure 24-14 ■). The whistle-tipped catheter is less irritating to respiratory tissues, although the open-tipped catheter may be more effective for removing thick mucous plugs. Most suction catheters have a thumb port on the side to control the suction. The catheter is connected to suction

Hydration of Inspired Air

Adequate hydration maintains the moisture of the respiratory mucous membranes. Normally, respiratory tract secretions are thin and therefore moved readily by ciliary action. However, when the client is dehydrated or when the environment has a low humidity, the respiratory secretions can become thick and tenacious. Fluid intake should be as great as the client can tolerate.

Humidifiers are devices that add water vapor to inspired air. Room humidifiers provide cool mist to room air. *Nebu-*

BOX 24-8	**CLIENT TEACHING**

Using an Incentive Spirometer

- Hold or place the spirometer in an upright position. A tilted flow-oriented device requires less effort to raise the balls or disks; a volume-oriented device will not function correctly unless upright.
- Exhale normally.
- Seal the lips tightly around the mouthpiece.
- Take in a slow, deep breath to elevate the balls or cylinder, and then hold the breath for 2 seconds initially, increasing to 6 seconds (optimum), to keep the balls or cylinder elevated if possible.
- For a flow-oriented device, avoid brisk, low-volume breaths that snap the balls to the top of the chamber. Greater lung expansion is achieved with a very slow inspiration than with a brisk, shallow breath, even though it may not elevate the balls or keep them elevated while you hold your breath. Sustained

elevation of the balls or cylinder ensures adequate ventilation of the alveoli (lung air sacs).
- If you have difficulty breathing only through the mouth, a nose clip can be used.
- Remove the mouthpiece, and exhale normally.
- Cough after the incentive effort. Deep ventilation may loosen secretions, and coughing can facilitate their removal.
- Relax, and take several normal breaths before using the spirometer again.
- Do 5 to 10 repetitions. Repeat the procedure. Practice increases inspiratory volume, maintains alveolar ventilation, and prevents *atelectasis* (collapse of the air sacs).
- Clean the mouthpiece with water and shake it dry. Change disposable mouthpieces every 24 hours.

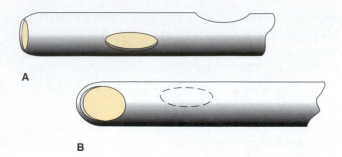

Figure 24-14. ■ Types of suction catheters: **A.** open tipped; **B.** whistle tipped.

tubing, which in turn is connected to a collection chamber and suction control gauge (Figure 24-15 ■).

Oropharyngeal or nasopharyngeal suctioning removes secretions from the upper respiratory tract. Refer to Procedure 24-4 ■ on page 521.

Monitoring Chest Tubes and Drainage Systems

Nurses are responsible for the care of clients with chest tubes and drainage systems in the pleural cavity. Nursing responsibilities regarding drainage systems include the following:

■ Assist with the insertion and removal of the tube.
■ Maintain the water seal and patency of the drainage system.
■ Assess the client's vital signs, cardiovascular status, and respiratory status.
■ Monitor the patency and integrity of the drainage system.
■ Always keep the drainage system below the level of the client's chest to prevent fluid and drainage from being drawn back into the chest cavity.

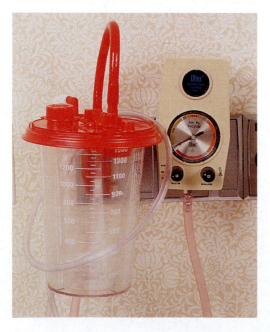

Figure 24-15. ■ A wall suction unit. (Photographer: Jenny Thomas.)

■ Keep rubber-tipped clamps and a sterile occlusive dressing near the client. The chest tube will need to be clamped quickly, close to the insertion site, if connections are broken or an air leak develops in the drainage system. If the chest tube is inadvertently pulled out, the wound should be immediately covered with a sterile occlusive dressing.

See Procedure 24-5 ■ on page 524 on the care and maintenance of chest tubes.

Preventing Venous Stasis

When clients have limited mobility or are confined to bed, venous return to the heart is impaired, and the risk of venous stasis increases. Immobility is a problem not only for ill or debilitated clients but also for some travelers who sit with legs dependent for long periods in a motor vehicle or an airplane. Venous stasis can lead to thrombus formation and edema of the extremities.

Preventing venous stasis is an important nursing intervention to reduce the risk of complications following surgery, trauma, or major medical problems. Positioning and leg exercises are discussed in Chapter 32 ⬤. Antiemboli stockings and sequential compression devices are additional measures to help prevent venous stasis.

Antiemboli Stockings

Antiemboli stockings are tight-fitting elastic hosiery that provide varying degrees of leg compression. They frequently are used for clients with limited mobility. When obtaining antiemboli stockings for a client, follow the manufacturer's recommendation for measuring and fitting the stockings.

Sequential Compression Devices

Clients who are undergoing surgery or who are immobilized because of illness or injury may benefit from a sequential compression device (SCD) to promote venous return from the legs. SCDs consist of plastic sleeves wrapped around the legs that inflate and deflate to promote venous return. The plastic sleeves are attached by tubing to an air pump that alternately inflates and deflates portions of the sleeve to a specified pressure. The ankle area inflates first, followed by the calf region, and then the thigh area. This sequential inflation and deflation assists the leg muscles in moving blood toward the heart.

Antiemboli stockings are worn under the SCD to provide added support and protect the skin from irritation by the plastic. The SCD is removed for ambulation and is usually discontinued when the client resumes activities. SCDs are useful in preventing thrombi and edema from venous stasis, but they are not used for clients who have arterial insufficiency, cellulitis, infection of the extremity, or preexisting venous thrombosis. Procedure 24-6 ■ on page 525 outlines how to apply a sequential compression device.

Cardiopulmonary Resuscitation

Cardiopulmonary resuscitation (CPR) is a combination of oral resuscitation (mouth-to-mouth breathing), which supplies oxygen to the lungs, and external cardiac massage (chest compression), which is intended to reestablish cardiac function and blood circulation. CPR is also referred to as basic life support. Training in CPR is provided by some facilities, the American Heart Association, and the Red Cross; see Box 8-5 ⚭ for a CPR overview.

A *cardiac arrest* is the cessation of cardiac function; the heart stops beating. Often a cardiac arrest is unexpected and sudden. When it occurs, the heart no longer pumps blood to any of the organs of the body. Breathing then stops and the person becomes unconscious and limp. Within 20 to 40 seconds of a cardiac arrest, the victim is clinically dead. After 4 to 6 minutes, the lack of oxygen supply to the brain causes permanent and extensive damage.

A *respiratory arrest* (pulmonary arrest) is the cessation of breathing. It often occurs as a result of a blocked airway, but it can occur following a cardiac arrest and for other reasons. A respiratory arrest may occur abruptly or be preceded by short, shallow breathing that becomes increasingly labored.

It is vital that all nurses be trained to perform CPR so that resuscitation measures can be initiated immediately when a cardiac or respiratory arrest occurs. Nurses also can be instrumental in increasing community awareness of the need for CPR training and ensuring its availability. Most healthcare agencies have established practices and policies governing CPR.

EVALUATING

Using the goals and desired outcomes identified in the planning stage of the nursing process, the nurse collects data to evaluate the effectiveness of interventions. If outcomes are not achieved, the nurse, client, and support person if appropriate need to explore the reasons before modifying the care plan. Outcomes for clients with alterations in oxygenation might include:

- Maintaining a patent airway with breath sounds clear/clearing and absence of dyspnea
- Demonstrating behaviors to improve airway clearance (e.g., cough effectively and expectorate secretions)
- Demonstrating improved ventilation and adequate oxygenation of tissues by ABGs within client's normal range and be free of symptoms of respiratory distress
- Establishing a normal/effective respiratory pattern within client's normal range
- Be free of cyanosis and other signs/symptoms of hypoxia.

CONTINUING CARE

The nurse provides client education regarding:

- Behaviors and lifestyle changes to regain and/or maintain appropriate weight
- Identifying interventions to prevent/reduce risk of infection
- Verbalization of condition/disease process and treatment
- Identification of relationship of current sign/symptoms to the disease process and correlation of these with causative factors.

NURSING PROCESS CARE PLAN
Client with Hemothorax

Jerry Markert, 21, was admitted to the acute care facility following a biking incident in which he received multiple injuries, including a hemothorax. He is receiving 6 L of oxygen by nasal cannula and has a chest tube connected to a closed drainage system.

Assessment. He is alert, stable, and progressing well. Pulse oximeter indicates an oxygen saturation level of 98 percent, BP 110/60; pulse 120. C/o difficulty breathing. Multiple bruises left side of torso, breath sounds decreased. Lacerations on forehead and legs, no evidence of extremity fracture. Chest x-ray revealed hemothorax.

Nursing Diagnosis. The following important nursing diagnoses (among others) are established for this client:

- *Impaired Gas Exchange*
- *Risk for Injury.*

Expected Outcomes. The expected outcomes specify that Mr. Markert will:

- Demonstrate improved ventilation and adequate oxygenation as evidenced by blood gases within client's normal parameters.
- Maintain clear lung fields and remain free of signs of respiratory distress.
- Remain free of injury as evidenced by chest tube in place and closed drainage system functioning properly.

Planning and Implementation. The following interventions are planned and implemented:

- Document vital signs, oxygen saturation, and respiratory status every 4 hours.
- Place in Fowler's position.
- Administer oxygen as ordered.
- Provide rest.
- Assess chest tube and drainage system at least every 2 hours.

- Secure chest tube to chest wall and prevent tension during care.
- Prevent kinking or occlusion of drainage or chest tube.
- Keep drainage system below chest when sitting or ambulating.
- Observe for redness, swelling, drainage, or pain at insertion site.
- If tube is inadvertently dislodged/removed, promptly seal with sterile occlusion dressing.

Evaluation. Chest tube in place connected to closed drainage, secured to chest wall. 200 mL of bloody drainage. SpO_2 98% on 2 L. Diminished breath sounds on left. Respirations 20, HR 86, BP 120/78.

Critical Thinking in the Nursing Process

1. If Mr. Markert is stable and progressing well, why is his oxygen saturation being monitored?
2. What precautions need to be taken when caring for Mr. Markert while his chest tube is in place?
3. Offer suggestions that would help Mr. Markert, or any person with a respiratory problem, to establish healthy breathing after his chest tube has been removed.

Note: Discussion of Critical Thinking questions appears in Appendix I.

Note: The references and resources for this and all chapters have been compiled at the back of the book.

| PROCEDURE 24-1 | # Using a Pulse Oximeter |

Purposes

- To measure the arterial blood oxygen saturation (SpO_2)
- To detect the presence of hypoxemia before visible signs develop

Equipment

- Pulse oximeter
- Nail polish remover as needed
- Sheet or towel

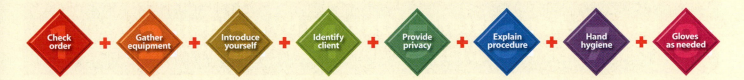

Interventions

1. Select an appropriate sensor.
   - Choose a sensor appropriate for the client's weight and size. *Because weight limits of infant, pediatric, and adult sensors overlap, a neonatal sensor could be used for an infant or a pediatric sensor for a small adult.* See the manufacturer's directions for weight limits.
   - If the client is allergic to adhesive, use a clip or reflectance sensor without adhesive.

2. Select an appropriate site.
   - Use a location appropriate for the type of sensor.
   - If using an extremity, assess the proximal pulse and capillary refill at the point closest to the site. *Decreased circulation can alter the SpO_2 measurements.*
   - If the client has low tissue perfusion due to peripheral vascular disease or therapy using vasoconstrictive medications, use a nasal sensor or a reflectance sensor on the forehead.
   - Avoid using lower extremities that have a compromised circulation and extremities that are used for infusions or other invasive monitoring.

3. Prepare the site.
   - Remove a female client's nail polish or acrylic nails. *These items can interfere with accurate measurements.*

4. Apply the sensor, and connect it to the pulse oximeter.
   - Make sure the LED and photodetector are accurately aligned, that is, opposite each other on either side of the finger, toe, nose, or earlobe. Many sensors have markings to facilitate correct alignment of the LED and photodetector. *Correct alignment is essential for accurate SpO_2 measurement.*
   - Attach the sensor cable to the connection outlet on the oximeter. Appropriate connection will be confirmed by an audible beep indicating each arterial pulsation. Turn on the machine according to the manufacturer's direc-

tions. Some devices have a wheel that can be turned clockwise to increase the signal volume and counterclockwise to decrease it.
   - Ensure that the bar of light or waveform on the face of the oximeter fluctuates with each pulsation and reflects the pulse volume or strength. *A signal that is too weak will not produce an accurate SpO_2 measurement.*

5. Set and turn on the alarm.
   - Check the preset alarm limits for high and low oxygen saturation and high and low pulse rates.
   - Change these alarm limits according to the manufacturer's directions as indicated.
   - Ensure that the audio and visual alarms are on before you leave the client. A tone will be heard and a number will blink on the faceplate.

6. Ensure client safety.
   - Inspect the location of an adhesive toe or finger sensor every 4 hours and a spring-tension sensor every 2 hours. Move it slightly or change the location as needed. *Movement prevents tissue necrosis due to prolonged pressure.*
   - Inspect the sensor site tissues for irritation from adhesive sensors.

7. Ensure the accuracy of measurement.
   - Minimize motion artifacts by using an adhesive sensor, or immobilize the client's monitoring site. *Movement of the client's finger or toe may be misinterpreted by the oximeter as arterial pulsations.*
   - Cover a sensor with a sheet or towel to block large amounts of light from external sources (e.g., sunlight, procedure lamps, or bilirubin lights in the nursery). *Large amounts of outside light may be sensed by the photodetector and alter the SpO_2 value.*

■ Verify that the client's hemoglobin level is normal. *An SpO_2 measurement may register normal when the client's hemoglobin is low because the available hemoglobin to carry oxygen is fully saturated.*

8. Document all relevant information.
   ■ Record the application of the pulse oximeter, its type and size, and all nursing assessments.

SAMPLE DOCUMENTATION

[date]   Oxygen saturation 91. Client complained of discomfort on rt. second finger. Moved tester
[time]   to rt. third finger. Expressed comfort. T 36°C, P 62, R 15, BP 128/85.
_____ R. Parks, LVN

PROCEDURE 24-2 · Administering Oxygen by Cannula or Face Mask

Purposes

■ To deliver a relatively low concentration of oxygen when only minimal O_2 support is required
■ To allow uninterrupted delivery of oxygen while the client ingests food or fluids
■ To provide moderate O_2 support and a higher concentration of oxygen and/or humidity than is provided by cannula

Equipment

■ Oxygen supply with a flow meter
■ Humidifier with sterile, distilled water or tap water according to agency protocol
■ Nasal cannula or prescribed face mask and tubing
■ Gauze pads as needed

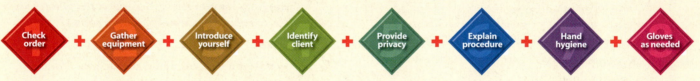

Check order + Gather equipment + Introduce yourself + Identify client + Provide privacy + Explain procedure + Hand hygiene + Gloves as needed

Interventions

1. Determine the need for oxygen therapy, and verify the order for the therapy.
   ■ Perform a respiratory assessment. *This determines the need for O_2 therapy and develops baseline data if not already available.*

2. Prepare the client and support people.
   ■ Assist the client to a semi-Fowler's position if possible. *This position permits easier chest expansion and breathing.*
   ■ Explain that oxygen is not dangerous when safety precautions are observed and that it will ease the discomfort of dyspnea. Inform the client and support people about the safety precautions connected with oxygen use.

3. Set up the oxygen equipment and the humidifier.

4. Turn on the oxygen at the prescribed rate, and ensure proper functioning.
   ■ Check that the oxygen is flowing freely through the tubing. *There should be no kinks in the tubing, and the connections should be airtight. There should be bubbles in the humidifier as the oxygen flows through the water. You should feel the oxygen at the outlets of the cannula or mask.*
   ■ Set the oxygen at the flow rate ordered, for example, 2 to 6 L/min.

5. Apply the appropriate oxygen delivery device.

Cannula

■ Put the cannula over the client's face, with the outlet prongs fitting into the nares and the elastic band around the head (Figure 24-16 ■). Some models have a strap to adjust under the chin.
■ If the cannula will not stay in place, tape it at the sides of the face.

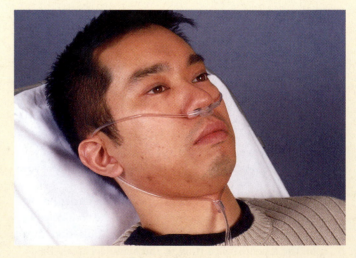

Figure 24-16. ■ Nasal cannula in place.

- Pad the tubing and band over the ears and cheekbones as needed. *This helps prevent skin breakdown.*

Face Masks (Figures 24-17A to D ■)

- Guide the mask toward the client's face, and apply it from the nose downward.
- Fit the mask to the contours of the client's face. *The mask should mold to the face so that very little oxygen escapes into the eyes or around the cheeks and chin.*

- Secure the elastic band around the client's head so that the mask is comfortable but snug.
- Pad the band behind the ears and over bony prominences. *Padding will prevent irritation from the mask.*

6. Assess the client regularly. *This allows early response to any changes or problems.*
   - Assess the client's level of anxiety, color, ease of respirations, and pulse oximeter reading (if available). Provide support while the client adjusts to the device.

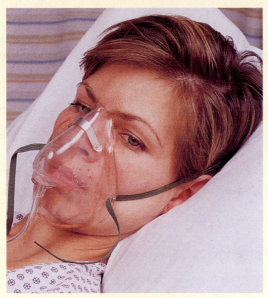

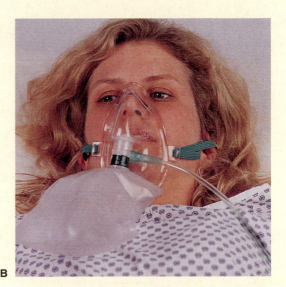

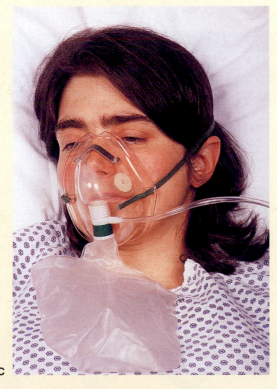

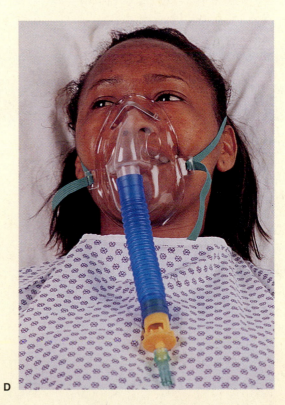

Figure 24-17. ■ **A.** A simple oxygen mask. (Photographer: Jenny Thomas.) **B.** A partial rebreather mask. (Photographer: Elena Dorfman.) **C.** A nonrebreather mask. (Photographer: Jenny Thomas.) **D.** A Venturi oxygen mask. (Photographer: Elena Dorfman.)

- Assess the client in 15 to 30 minutes, depending on the client's condition, and regularly thereafter. Assess vital signs, color, breathing patterns, and chest movements.
- Assess the client regularly for clinical signs of hypoxia, tachycardia, confusion, dyspnea, restlessness, and cyanosis. Obtain ABG results if available.

Cannula

- Assess the client's nares for encrustations and irritation. Apply a water-soluble lubricant as required. *Lubricants soothe the mucous membranes.*

Face Mask

- Inspect the facial skin frequently for dampness or chafing, and dry and treat it as needed.

7. Inspect the equipment on a regular basis.
   - Check the liter flow and the level of water in the humidifier in 30 minutes and whenever providing care to the client.
   - Maintain the level of water in the humidifier.
   - Make sure that safety precautions are being followed.

8. Document relevant data.
   - Record the initiation of the therapy and all nursing assessments.

SAMPLE DOCUMENTATION: FOCUS CHARTING

Date	Time	Data Action Response
[date]	[time]	**D:** Client is anxious, resp rate 32, labored and shallow. Use of accessory muscles noted. C/o SOB. O_2 Sat 86% on room air. No history of COPD. **A:** Assisted client to semi-Fowler's and applied O_2 @4 L/min via nasal cannula per MD order. Distilled water humidification added. Assured patency of tubing/O_2 flowing freely w/bubbling in humidifier. Nasal prongs positioned properly in nares; gauze placed under tubing on ears. _____ N. Nurse, LPN
[date]	[time]	**R:** Decreased anxiety, RR 26, resp less labored. O_2 sat 91% on 4 L/min. Client states "It's easier to breathe." _____ N. Nurse, LPN

PROCEDURE 24-3 **Providing Tracheostomy Care**

Purposes

- To maintain airway patency
- To maintain cleanliness and prevent infection at the tracheostomy site
- To facilitate healing and prevent skin excoriation around the tracheostomy incision
- To promote comfort

Equipment

- Sterile disposable tracheostomy cleaning kit or supplies including sterile containers, sterile nylon brush and/or pipe cleaners, sterile applicators, gauze squares
- Towel or drape to protect bed linens
- Hydrogen peroxide and sterile normal saline
- Sterile gloves (1 pair)
- Clean gloves
- Moisture-proof bag
- Commercially prepared sterile tracheostomy dressing or sterile 4 × 4 gauze dressing
- Cotton twill ties or commercially prepared self-closing ties
- Clean scissors
- Disposable inner cannula

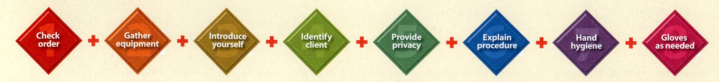

Check order + Gather equipment + Introduce yourself + Identify client + Provide privacy + Explain procedure + Hand hygiene + Gloves as needed

Interventions

1. Prepare the client and the equipment.
   - Assist the client to a semi-Fowler's or Fowler's position. *This promotes lung expansion.*
   - Explain the procedure to the client and provide for a means of communication, such as eye blinking or raising a finger to indicate pain or distress. *This reduces client anxiety.*
   - Suction tracheostomy prior to cleaning if indicated. (See Procedure 24-4 Part B.)
   - Don clean gloves and remove soiled tracheostomy dressing and discard the gloves and the dressing.
   - Open the tracheostomy kit or sterile basins. Pour sterile normal saline into both basins. Pour hydrogen peroxide into one basin only.
   - Establish a sterile field.
   - Don sterile gloves; place sterile towel on client's chest and under tracheostomy area.
   - Open other sterile supplies as needed, including sterile applicators and tracheostomy dressing.

2. Remove inner cannula.
   - Optional: Discard disposable inner cannula. *Many agencies are using disposable inner cannulas; eliminating cleaning steps.*
   - Using one part of a fully opened 4 × 4, stabilize the flange with one hand. With the other end of the 4 × 4, use the other gloved hand to unlock the inner cannula (if present) and remove it by gently pulling it out toward you in line with its curvature. Place the inner cannula in the hydrogen peroxide solution to soak. *This moistens and loosens dried secretions.*

3. Clean the incision site and tube flange.
   - Using sterile applicators or gauze dressings moistened with normal saline, clean the tracheostomy (stoma) site (Figure 24-18 ■). Use each applicator or gauze dressing only once, then discard. *This avoids contaminating a clean area with a soiled gauze dressing or applicator.*
   - The hydrogen peroxide/saline solution may be used to remove encrustations. Thoroughly rinse the cleaned area, using gauze squares moistened with sterile normal saline. *Hydrogen peroxide can be irritating to the skin and inhibit healing if not thoroughly removed.*

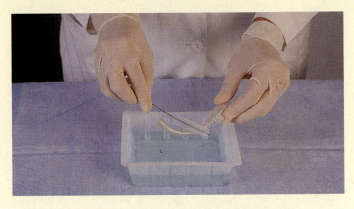

Figure 24-19. ■ Cleaning the inner cannula with a brush. (Photographer: Elena Dorfman.)

   - Clean the flange of the tube in the same manner.
   - Thoroughly dry the client's skin and tube flanges with dry gauze squares.

4. Clean the inner cannula.
   - Remove the inner cannula from the soaking solution.
   - Clean the lumen and entire inner cannula thoroughly, using the brush or pipe cleaners moistened with sterile normal saline (Figure 24-19 ■). Inspect the cannula for cleanliness by holding it at eye level and looking through it into the light.
   - Rinse the inner cannula thoroughly in sterile normal saline. *Thorough rinsing is important to remove the hydrogen peroxide from the inner cannula.*
   - After rinsing, use a pipe cleaner folded in half to dry only the inside of the cannula; do not dry the outside. *This removes excess liquid from the cannula and prevents possible aspiration by the client, while leaving a film of moisture on the outer surface to lubricate the cannula for reinsertion.*

5. Replace the inner cannula, securing it in place.
   - Insert the inner cannula by grasping the outer flange and inserting the cannula in the direction of its curvature.
   - Lock the cannula in place by turning the lock (if present) into position to secure the flange of the inner cannula to the outer cannula.
   - Replace disposable inner cannula. Secure both sides of the cannula firmly under lip of outer cannula.

6. Apply a sterile dressing.
   - Use a commercially prepared tracheostomy dressing of nonraveling material, or open and refold a 4 × 4 gauze dressing into a V shape as shown in Figure 24-20 ■. Avoid using cotton-filled gauze squares or cutting the 4 × 4 gauze. *Cotton lint or gauze fibers can be aspirated by the client, potentially creating a tracheal abscess.*
   - Place the dressing under the flange of the tracheostomy tube.

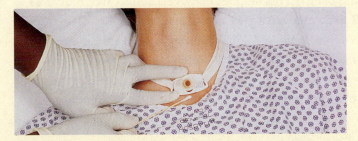

Figure 24-18. ■ Using an applicator stick to clean the tracheostomy site. (Photographer: Jenny Thomas.)

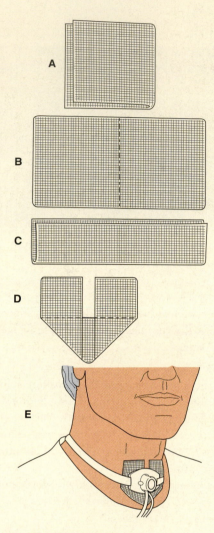

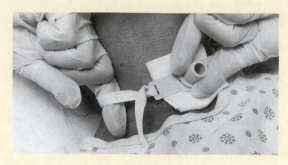

Figure 24-21. ■ Placing a finger underneath the tie tape before tying it. (Photographer: Jenny Thomas.)

7. Change the tracheostomy ties.

One-Strip Method
- Cut a length of twill tape 2.5 times the length needed to go around the client's neck from one tube flange to the other.
- Thread one end of the tape into the slot on one side of the flange.
- Bring both ends of the tape together, and take them around the client's neck, keeping them flat and untwisted.
- Thread the end of the tape next to the client's neck through the slot from the back to the front.
- Have the client flex the neck. Tie the loose ends with a square knot at the side of the client's neck, allowing for slack by placing one finger under the ties as shown in Figure 24-21 ■. Cut off long ends.

8. Check the tightness of the ties.
- Frequently check the tightness of the tracheostomy ties. *Neck movement may cause the ties to become too taut, interfering with coughing and circulation. Ties can loosen in restless clients, allowing the tracheostomy tube to extrude from the stoma.*

9. Document all relevant information.
- Record tracheostomy care and the dressing change, noting your assessments.

Figure 24-20. ■ Folding a 4 × 4 gauze to make a tracheostomy dressing.

- While applying the dressing, ensure that the tracheostomy tube is securely supported. *Excessive movement of the tracheostomy tube irritates the trachea.*

SAMPLE DOCUMENTATION: FOCUS CHARTING

Date	Time	Data Action Response
[date]	[time]	**D:** Encrustations noted around stoma; due for routine trach care. Breath sounds clear; no distress noted. **A:** Using aseptic technique, removed soiled trach dressing. Set up sterile field per P&P and removed inner cannula for cleaning. Cleansed stoma site & flange. Reinserted inner cannula & locked into place. Applied clean ties using the one-strip method; 2 fingers fit tightly under ties. Applied clean dressing around stoma and under flange. **R:** Patient tolerated procedure without SOB or distress noted. Tracheal stoma pink, free of encrustations and skin dry. Trach ties secure.

_____ N. Nurse, LVN

PROCEDURE 24-4   # Suctioning

Purposes

- To remove secretions that obstruct the airway
- To facilitate ventilation
- To obtain secretions for diagnostic purposes
- To prevent infection that may result from accumulated secretions

Equipment

- Towel or moisture-resistant pad (sterile towel for tracheal or endotracheal suctioning)
- Portable or wall suction machine with tubing and collection receptacle
- Sterile disposable container for fluids
- Sterile normal saline or water
- Sterile gloves
- Sterile suction catheter kit (#12 to #18 Fr. for adults; #8 to #10 Fr. for children, and #5 to #8 Fr. for infants); if both the oropharynx and the nasopharynx are to be suctioned, one sterile catheter is required for each
- Water-soluble lubricant (for nasopharyngeal suctioning)
- Y-connector
- Sterile gauzes
- Moisture-resistant disposal bag
- Sputum trap, if specimen is to be collected
- Resuscitation bag connected to 100% oxygen for tracheal or endotracheal care
- Goggles and mask if necessary
- Gown (if necessary)

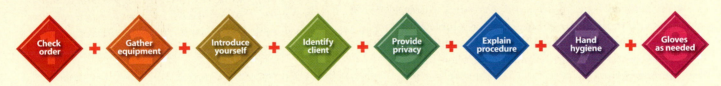

Check order + Gather equipment + Introduce yourself + Identify client + Provide privacy + Explain procedure + Hand hygiene + Gloves as needed

Part A: Oropharyngeal and Nasopharyngeal Cavities

Interventions

1. Prepare the client.
   - Explain to the client that suctioning will relieve breathing difficulty and that the procedure is painless but may be uncomfortable and stimulate the cough, gag, or sneeze reflex. *Knowing that the procedure will relieve breathing problems is often reassuring and enlists the client's cooperation.*
   - Position a conscious person who has a functional gag reflex in the semi-Fowler's position with the head turned to one side for oral suctioning or with the neck hyperextended for nasal suctioning. *These positions facilitate the insertion of the catheter and help prevent aspiration of secretions.*
   - Position an unconscious client in the lateral position, facing you. *This position allows the tongue to fall forward, so that it will not obstruct the catheter on insertion. Lateral position also facilitates drainage of secretions from the pharynx and prevents the possibility of aspiration.*
   - Place the towel or moisture-resistant pad over the pillow or under the chin.

2. Prepare the equipment.
   - Set the pressure on the suction gauge, and turn on the suction. Many suction devices are calibrated to three pressure ranges:

   Wall Unit

   Adult: 100 to 120 mm Hg

   Child: 95 to 110 mm Hg

   Infant: 50 to 95 mm Hg

   Portable Unit

   Adult: 10 to 15 mm Hg

   Child: 5 to 10 mm Hg

   Infant: 2 to 5 mm Hg
   - Open the lubricant if performing nasopharyngeal suctioning
   - Open the sterile suction package.
     a. Set up the cup or container, touching only its outside.
     b. Pour sterile water or saline into the container.
     c. Don sterile gloves and attach the catheter to the suction unit (Figure 24-22 ■). (The hand that touched the suction unit is no longer sterile.) *The sterile gloved hand maintains the sterility of the suction catheter, and the unsterile glove prevents the transmission of the microorganisms to the nurse.*

3. Make an approximate measure of the depth for the insertion of the catheter and test the equipment.
   - Measure the distance between the tip of the client's nose and the earlobe (about 13 cm [5 in.] for an adult).
   - Mark the position on the tube with the fingers of the sterile gloved hand.
   - Test the pressure of the suction and the patency of the catheter by applying your sterile gloved thumb to the

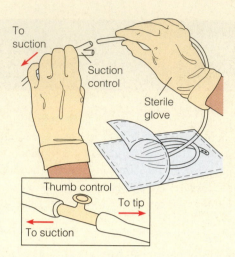

Figure 24-22. ■ Attaching the catheter to the suction unit.

port or open branch of the Y-connector (the suction control) to create suction.

4. Lubricate and introduce the catheter.
   ■ For nasopharyngeal suction, lubricate the catheter tip with sterile water, saline, or water-soluble lubricant; for oropharyngeal suction, moisten the tip with sterile water or saline. *This reduces friction and eases insertion.*

For an Oropharyngeal Suction
   ■ Pull the tongue forward, if necessary, using gauze.
   ■ Do not apply suction (that is, leave your thumb off the port) during insertion. *Applying suction during insertion causes trauma to the mucous membrane.*
   ■ Advance the catheter about 10 to 15 cm (4 to 6 in.) along one side of the mouth into the oropharynx. *Directing the catheter along the side prevents gagging.*

For a Nasopharyngeal Suction
   ■ Without applying suction, insert the catheter the premeasured or recommended distance into either nares, and advance it along the floor of the nasal cavity. *This avoids the nasal turbinates.*
   ■ Never force the catheter against an obstruction. If one nostril is obstructed, try the other.

5. Perform suctioning.
   ■ Apply your thumb to the suction control port to start suction, and gently rotate the catheter. *Gentle rotation of the catheter ensures that all surfaces are reached and prevents trauma to any one area of the respiratory mucosa due to prolonged suction.*
   ■ Apply suction for 5 to 10 seconds while slowly withdrawing the catheter, then remove your finger from the control, and remove the catheter.
   ■ A suction attempt should last only 10 to 15 seconds. During this time, the catheter is inserted, the suction is applied and discontinued, and the catheter removed.

(Keep in mind that the client is deprived of oxygen during the suction procedure.)
   ■ It may be necessary during oropharyngeal suctioning to apply suction to secretions that collect in the vestibule of the mouth and beneath the tongue.

6. Clean the catheter, and repeat suctioning as above.
   ■ Wipe off the catheter with sterile gauze if it is thickly coated with secretions. Dispose of the used gauze in a moisture-resistant bag.
   ■ Flush the catheter with sterile water or saline.
   ■ Relubricate the catheter, and repeat suctioning until the air passage is clear.
   ■ Allow 20- to 30-second intervals between each suction, and limit suction to 5 minutes total. *Applying suction for too long may cause secretion to increase or decrease the client's oxygen supply.*
   ■ Alternate nares for repeat suctionings. *This will decrease irritation to mucosal lining.*

7. Encourage the client to breathe deeply and to cough between suctionings. *Coughing and deep breathing help carry secretions from the trachea and bronchi into the pharynx, where they can be reached with the suction catheter.*

8. Promote client comfort.
   ■ Offer to assist the client with oral or nasal hygiene.
   ■ Assist the client to a position that facilitates breathing.

9. Dispose of equipment and ensure availability for the next suction.
   ■ Dispose of the catheter, gloves, water, and waste container. Wrap the catheter around your sterile gloved hand, holding it as the glove is removed over it for disposal.
   ■ Rinse the suction tubing as needed by inserting the end of the tubing into the used water container. Empty and rinse the suction collection container as needed or indicated by protocol. Change the suction tubing and container daily. *This provides good infection control.*
   ■ Ensure that supplies are available for the next suctioning (suction kit, gloves, water, or normal saline).

10. Assess the effectiveness of suctioning.
   ■ Auscultate the client's breath sounds to ensure they are clear of secretions. Observe skin color, dyspnea, and level of anxiety.

11. Document relevant data.
   ■ Record the procedure: the amount, consistency, color, and odor of sputum (e.g., foamy, white mucus; thick, green-tinged mucus; or blood-flecked mucus) and the client's breathing status before and after the procedure.
   ■ If the technique is carried out frequently, for example every hour, it may be appropriate to record only once, at the end of the shift; however, the frequency of the suctioning must be recorded.

Part B: Tracheostomy or Endotracheal Tube

Interventions

1. Prepare the client.
   - Inform the client that suctioning usually causes some intermittent coughing and that this assists in removing the secretions.
   - If not contraindicated because of health, place the client in semi-Fowler's position to promote deep breathing, maximum lung expansion, and productive coughing. *Deep breathing oxygenates the lungs, counteracts the hypoxic effects of suctioning, and may induce coughing. Coughing helps to loosen and move secretions.*
   - If necessary, provide analgesia prior to suctioning. *Endotracheal suctioning stimulates the cough reflex, which can cause pain for clients who have had thoracic or abdominal surgery or who have experienced traumatic injury. Premedication can increase the client's comfort during the suctioning procedure.*

2. Prepare the equipment.
   - Open the sterile supplies in readiness for use.
   - Place the sterile towel, if used, across the client's chest below the tracheostomy.
   - Turn on the suction, and set the pressure in accordance with agency policy. For a wall unit, pressure of about 100 to 120 mm Hg is normally used for adults, 50 to 95 mm Hg for infants and children.
   - Put on goggles, mask, and gown if necessary.
   - Put on sterile gloves. Some agencies recommend putting a sterile glove on the dominant hand and a nonsterile glove on the nondominant hand to protect the nurse.
   - Holding the catheter in the dominant hand and the connector in the nondominant hand, attach the suction catheter to the suction tubing (see Figure 24-22).

3. Flush and lubricate the catheter.
   - Using the dominant hand, place the catheter tip in the sterile saline solution.
   - Using the thumb of the nondominant hand, occlude the thumb control, and suction a small amount of the sterile solution through the catheter. *This determines that the suction equipment is working properly and lubricates the outside and the lumen of the catheter. Lubrication eases insertion and reduces tissue trauma during insertion. Lubricating the lumen also helps prevent secretions from sticking to the inside of the catheter.*

4. Quickly but gently insert the catheter without applying any suction.
   - With your nondominant thumb off the suction port, quickly but gently insert the catheter into the trachea through the tracheostomy tube (Figure 24-23 ■). *To prevent tissue trauma and oxygen loss, suction is not applied during insertion of the catheter.*
   - Insert the catheter about 13 cm (5 in.) for adults, less for children, or until the client coughs or you feel resistance. *Resistance usually means that the catheter tip has reached the carina (bifurcation of the trachea into the main bronchi). To prevent damaging the mucous membranes at the bifurcation, withdraw the catheter about 1 to 2 cm (0.4 to 0.8 in.) before applying suction.*

5. Perform suctioning.
   - Apply intermittent suction for 5 to 10 seconds by placing the nondominant thumb over the thumb port. *Suction time is restricted to 10 seconds or less to minimize oxygen loss.*
   - Rotate the catheter by rolling it between your thumb and forefinger while slowly withdrawing it. *This prevents tissue trauma by minimizing the suction time against any part of the trachea.*
   - Withdraw the catheter completely, and release the suction.
   - Ventilate the patient.
   - Then suction again.

6. Reassess the client's oxygenation status, and repeat suctioning.
   - Observe the client's respirations and skin color. Check the client's pulse if necessary, using your nondominant hand.
   - Encourage the client to breathe deeply and to cough between suctions.
   - Allow 2 to 3 minutes between suctions when possible. *This provides an opportunity for reoxygenation of the lungs.*
   - Flush the catheter, and repeat suctioning until the air passage is clear and the breathing is relatively effortless and quiet.
   - After each suction, pick up the resuscitation bag with your nondominant hand and ventilate the client with five breaths.

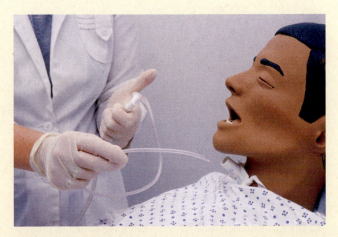

Figure 24-23. ■ Inserting the catheter into the trachea through the tracheostomy tube. (Photographer: Jenny Thomas.)

7. Dispose of equipment and ensure availability for the next suction.
   - Flush the catheter and suction tubing.
   - Turn off the suction, and disconnect the catheter from the suction tubing.
   - Wrap the catheter around your sterile hand, and peel the glove off so that it turns inside out over the catheter.
   - Discard the glove and the catheter in the moisture-resistant bag.
   - Replenish the sterile fluid and supplies so that the suction is ready to be used again. *Clients who require suction-ing often require it quickly, so it is essential to leave the equipment at the bedside ready for use.*

8. Provide for client comfort and safety.
   - Assist the client to a comfortable, safe position that aids breathing. *If the person is conscious, a semi-Fowler's position is frequently indicated. If the person is unconscious, the Sims' position aids in the drainage of secretions from the mouth.*

9. Document relevant data.
   - Record the suctioning, including the amount and description of suction returns, the amount of sterile saline instilled, and any other relevant assessments.

SAMPLE DOCUMENTATION: FOCUS CHARTING

Date	Time	Data Action Response
[date]	[time]	**D:** Client w/audibly moist breath sounds; RR 30 and labored. Weak, ineffective cough. Rhonchi and coarse crackles auscultated A&P. **A:** Positioned client in semi-Fowler's position. Maintaining sterile technique & following P&P, performed nasopharyngeal suctioning. **R:** Copious amounts of thick, yellow secretions removed. RR 26 and less labored. Breath sounds with minimal coarse crackles @ bases bilaterally.

_____ N. Nurse, LVN

PROCEDURE 24-5 Caring for and Maintaining Chest Tubes

Purpose
- To restore negative pressure and drain collected fluids or blood in the pleural cavity

Equipment
- Water-seal chest drainage system
- Padded hemostat at bedside

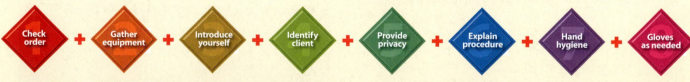
Check order + Gather equipment + Introduce yourself + Identify client + Provide privacy + Explain procedure + Hand hygiene + Gloves as needed

Interventions

Once the chest tube is in place and the water-seal chest drainage system is attached and functioning properly, the LPN/LVN may be responsible for maintaining the drainage system and caring for the tube.

The following procedural steps should be carried out at least once per shift.

1. Coil tubing loosely on the bed, checking to see that there is a straight line of tubing from the bed to the collection system. *Straight line tubing prevents pooling of fluids.*

2. Make sure tubing is free and not kinked. Do not use pins or restrain tubing. *Pins could puncture tubing, causing an air leak.*

3. Monitor water level daily in both water-seal chamber and suction control chamber.

4. Maintain pressure.
   - Keep drainage system below the level of the bed.
   - Maintain suction control negative pressure to create gentle bubbling.

- Maintain water-seal level (2 cm). *The water seal prevents room air from entering the pleural space.*

5. Maintain chest tube patency. Only if physician orders, milk chest tube to maintain drainage and tube patency.
   - Milk tube away from client toward the drainage receptacle.
   - If ordered, milk tube by alternately folding or squeezing and then releasing drainage tubing. *This provides intermittent suction to the chest tube but generates extreme negative pressure in the intrapleural space.*

6. Strip chest tube only if physician orders.
   - To strip chest tubes, pinch tubing close to the chest with one hand and using a lubricated thumb and forefinger, compress and slide fingers down the tube toward the receptacle. (Lubricant material is usually petrolatum or alcohol swab.)
   - Release pressure on the tube and repeat stripping action until the receptacle is reached. Note that increased negative pressure can occur. *Excessive negative pressure created by stripping and milking leads to increased negative pressure in the intrapleural space.*

clinical **ALERT**

Strip and milk chest tubes only with physician's orders. Also check your state's scope of practice and facility policy to determine if you are permitted to carry out these procedures.

7. Keep rubber-tipped hemostat at the client's bedside. *In an emergency, the tube can be clamped off nearest to the chest insertion site.*
8. Keep collection system below client's level. *This enables fluid to flow by gravity.*
9. Mark drainage on disposable system collection chamber every shift. Drainage should be measured at eye level. Report drainage exceeding 100 mL/h.
10. Assess client's status.
    - Instruct the client to deep breathe and cough at frequent intervals. *Frequent deep breathing helps to expand the lungs.*
    - Encourage the client to change positions frequently. Chest tube drainage does not limit client activity.
    - Observe and report any unusual respiratory signs or symptoms.

SAMPLE DOCUMENTATION: FOCUS CHARTING

Date	Time	Focus	Data Action Response
[date]	[time]	Chest tube	**D:** Chest tube in place; breath sounds diminished on left, VS: T 99.0, P 100, R 26, BP 134/90. Drainage 120 mL/8 h, pink tinged. Water-seal level 2 cm; suction control chamber water level 20 cm.
			A: Tube milked per physician's orders.
			R: Tube patent.
			_____ M. Stevens, LPN

PROCEDURE 24-6 # Applying a Sequential Compression Device

Purposes
- To facilitate venous return in immobilized clients
- To prevent thrombus formation

Equipment
- Measuring tape
- Antiemboli stockings
- Sequential compression device including disposable sleeves, air pump, and tubing

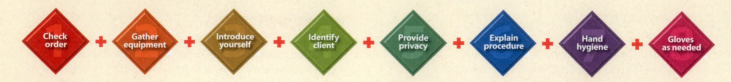

Interventions

1. Prepare the client.
   - Place the client in a dorsal recumbent or semi-Fowler's position. Provide for privacy, and drape the client appropriately.
   - Measure the client's legs as recommended by the manufacturer if a thigh-length sleeve is required. *Knee-length sleeves come in just one size; the thigh circumference determines the size needed for a thigh-length sleeve.*
   - Apply antiemboli stockings. *Antiemboli stockings provide added support and reduce skin irritation from the compression sleeve.*

2. Apply the sequential compression sleeves.
   - Place a sleeve under each leg with the opening at the knee.
   - Wrap the sleeve securely around the leg, securing the Velcro tabs (Figure 24-24 ■). Allow two fingers to fit between the leg and the sleeve. *This amount of space ensures that the sleeve does not impair circulation when inflated.*

3. Connect the sleeves to the control unit and adjust the pressure as needed.
   - Connect the tubing to the sleeves and control unit, ensuring that arrows on the plug and the connector are in alignment and that the tubing is not kinked or twisted. *Improper alignment or obstruction of the tubing by kinks or twists will interfere with operation of the SCD.*

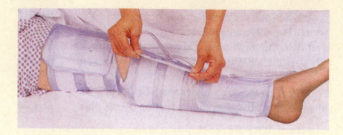

Figure 24-24. ■ Applying a sequential compression device to the leg. (Photographer: Jenny Thomas.)

   - Turn on the control unit and adjust the alarms and pressures as needed. The sleeve cooling control and alarm should be "on"; ankle pressure is usually set at 35 to 55 mm Hg. *It is important to have the sleeve cooling control on for comfort and to reduce the risk of skin irritation from moisture under the sleeve. Alarms warn of possible control unit malfunctions.*

4. Document the procedure.
   - Record baseline assessment data and application of the SCD. Note control unit settings.
   - Assess and document skin integrity and neurovascular status at least every 8 hours while the SCD is in place. Remove the unit and notify the physician if the client complains of numbness and tingling or leg pain. *These may be symptoms of nerve compression.*

SAMPLE DOCUMENTATION: FOCUS CHARTING

Date	Time	Data Action Response
[date]	[time]	**D**: Client is 1 day post Rt. THR. Antiemboli stockings & SCDs removed for bath. **A**: Assessed pedal and popliteal pulses. Assessed CMS status. Assessed skin integrity before replacing thigh-high antiemboli stockings and SCDs. Instructed client to report any numbness, tingling, or leg pain. **R**: CMS intact. The sleeve cooling control & alarm are "on" with sleeve pressure at 45 mm Hg. _____ N. Nurse, LPN

Chapter Review

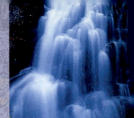

 ## KEY TERMS by Topic

Use the audio glossary feature of either the CD-ROM or the Companion Website to hear the correct pronunciation of the following key terms.

Introduction
respiration, ventilation

Structure and Function of the Respiratory System
epiglottis, inspiration, expiration, chronic obstructive pulmonary disease (COPD), pneumothorax, hemothorax, pleural effusion, diffusion, hemoglobin, erythrocytes, cardiac output, hematocrit, hypoxia, hypercarbia, hypercapnia, cyanosis, eupnea, tachypnea, bradypnea, apnea, hyperventilation, Kussmaul's breathing, dyspnea, shortness of breath (SOB), stridor

Structure and Function of the Cardiovascular System
atherosclerotic plaque, angina pectoris, myocardial infarction, anemia, dysrhythmias, ischemia, atherosclerosis, thrombus, embolus, exacerbations, hypovolemia, hypervolemia

Treatment of Oxygenation Problems
sputum, hemoptysis, electrocardiography, pulmonary function tests, tracheostomy, suctioning, cardiopulmonary resuscitation (CPR)

KEY Points

- The respiratory system includes pulmonary ventilation (the movement of air between the atmosphere and the lungs) and the diffusion of oxygen and carbon dioxide across the pulmonary membrane.

- The cardiovascular system transports these gases in the blood to the tissues, facilitates the diffusion of gases between the capillaries and body tissues, and carries away waste products from the tissues.

- Ninety-seven percent of oxygen is carried to the tissues loosely combined with hemoglobin in RBCs. Anemia, which is too few RBCs or low hemoglobin levels, impairs oxygen transportation.

- In most people, respirations are triggered by high carbon dioxide levels. However, some people with COPD have chronically high carbon dioxide levels, and their respirations are triggered by low oxygen (hypoxia). If they are given high levels of oxygen, they may stop breathing.

- Normal respirations are quiet and unlabored; altered respiratory patterns include tachypnea, bradypnea, hyperventilation, hypoventilation, and dyspnea. Shortness of breath is a subjective sensation of not getting enough air.

- A low-pitched snoring sound, stridor, and abnormal breath sounds may accompany partial airway obstruction.

- Diseases of the cardiovascular and/or respiratory systems, medications, stress, anger, and gender can affect O_2 delivery.

- Clients who have difficulty in ventilation, impaired gas exchange, or heart failure will require O_2 therapy to prevent hypoxia.

- Venous stasis must be prevented when the client has limited mobility. Antiemboli stockings and sequential compression devices are used for this purpose.

 ## EXPLORE MediaLink

Additional interactive resources for this chapter can be found on the Companion Website at www.prenhall.com/ramont. Click on Chapter 24 and "Begin" to select the activities for this chapter.

For chapter-related NCLEX®-style questions and an audio glossary, access the accompanying CD-ROM in this book.

Animations/Videos
- Carbon Dioxide Transport
- Incentive Spirometry

FOR FURTHER Study

For information about performing CPR, see Box 8-5.

For additional information about assessment of the respiratory system, see Chapter 19.

For more information about respiratory patterns and measuring blood pressure, see Boxes 20-6 and 20-7 respectively.

For additional information about preventing venous stasis, see Chapter 32.

Critical Thinking Care Map

Caring for a Client with Pneumonia

NCLEX-PN® Focus Area: Physiological Adaptation

Case Study: Johti Singh is a 39-year-old secretary who was admitted to the hospital with an elevated temperature, fatigue, and rapid labored respirations. Nursing history reveals that Ms. Singh has had a "bad cold" for several weeks that just wouldn't go away. She has been dieting for several months and skipping meals. In addition to her full-time job, she is attending college. She has smoked one pack of cigarettes per day since she was 18 years old. Chest x-ray confirms pneumonia.

Nursing Diagnosis: Ineffective Airway Clearance

COLLECT DATA

Subjective	Objective
_____	_____
_____	_____
_____	_____
_____	_____
_____	_____
_____	_____
_____	_____

Would you report this data? Yes/No

If yes, to: _____

What would you report? _____

Nursing Care

_____
_____
_____
_____
_____
_____
_____
_____
_____
_____
_____
_____

How would you document this?_____
_____
_____
_____

Compare your documentation to the sample provided in Appendix I.

Data Collected
(use those that apply)

- Height: 66"
- Weight: 120 lbs
- VS: T 103, P 82, R 24, BP 118/70
- Skin pale; cheeks flushed; chills; nasal flaring; use of accessory muscles; inspiratory crackles with diminished breath sounds right base; thick, yellow sputum.
- Chest x-ray: right lobar infiltration
- WBC 14,000
- pH 7.48
- HCO_3: 20 mEq/L
- Pa_{CO_2}: 80 mm Hg

Nursing Interventions
(use those that apply; list in priority order)

- Assist Ms. Singh to a sitting position with head slightly flexed.
- Determine healthy body weight for age and height.
- Encourage her to take a deep breath, hold for 2 seconds, and cough two or three times in succession.
- Arrange for dietary consult to determine calorie needs.
- Monitor rate, rhythm, depth, and effort of respirations.
- Administer antipyretic medication for patient comfort.
- Assess pain at least every 2 to 3 hours and administer analgesics as ordered.
- Ensure that shoulders are relaxed and knees are flexed.
- Provide written information as requested.
- Auscultate breath sounds, noting area of decreased or absent ventilations and presence of adventitious sounds.
- Encourage her to take several deep breaths.
- Monitor intake, output, and daily weight.
- Monitor respiratory secretions.
- Encourage use of incentive spirometry, as appropriate.
- Monitor increased restlessness, anxiety, and air hunger.

TEST-TAKING TIP When are you most awake? Some of us are morning people, and some of us are night or afternoon people. Keep this in mind when making your appointment to take the NCLEX® test. If you are an early morning riser, don't set your test time for late in the afternoon. Alternately, if you don't "wake up" until noon, don't take your exam first thing in the morning.

1 Your client is on strict bed rest. Which position facilitates the greatest expansion of the lungs?

1. Trendelenburg
2. low-Fowler's
3. Sims'
4. high-Fowler's

2 A breathing pattern in which respirations increase in rate and depth is known as:

1. Kussmaul's.
2. tachypnea.
3. dyspnea.
4. eupnea.

3 Which of the following data will receive highest priority when assessing your 33-year-old client with pneumonia?

1. size of pupils, presence of sneezing, location of pain
2. presence of hiccups, amount of sweating, BP
3. capillary refill, amount of sputum, trembling
4. restlessness, chest wall movement, color of nails

4 A client is experiencing an asthma attack. Which of the following outcomes will receive the highest priority in the care of this client:

1. The client will report a decrease in his anxiety level.
2. The client will maintain an open airway with adequate gas exchange.
3. The client will talk about how he feels about his disease.
4. The client will maintain adequate fluid balance.

5 A client with emphysema has severe difficulty breathing and orthopnea. Orthopnea means that the client:

1. is in respiratory distress.
2. has blood gases that indicate respiratory acidosis.
3. has periods of apnea.
4. has difficulty breathing unless he is sitting upright.

6 Uses of a tracheostomy tube include:

1. promotion of nutrition.
2. relief of flatus.
3. achievement of an artificial airway.
4. increasing dead space.

7 An 87-year-old client with pneumonia has just been admitted. Which of the following assessments takes first priority?

1. rapid, irregular respiration of 32/min
2. skin warm, flushed, and dry
3. temperature of 99.4°F (37.4°C)
4. dry, nonproductive cough

8 Your client with pneumonia presents with dyspnea. This means:

1. respirations are shallow.
2. the client is breathing very rapidly.
3. the client cannot breathe in a supine position.
4. breathing has become difficult and labored.

9 The physician has ordered O_2 via nasal cannula at 3 L/min. Safety precautions when oxygen is in use include:

1. making sure the room is well ventilated.
2. placing "No Smoking" signs in prominent places in the client's room.
3. keeping the flow rate <4 L/min to prevent toxicity.
4. avoiding use of any lotion for skin care.

10 With early signs of hypoxia, the nurse would expect to assess a client with emphysema for:

1. dyspnea, neurologic changes, hypertension, diminished breath sounds.
2. increased rate and depth of respirations, restlessness, decreased judgment, drowsiness.
3. orthopnea, use of accessory muscles to breathe, cyanosis of nail beds.
4. labored breathing, crowing respirations, inspiratory wheezing.

Answers and Rationales for Review Questions, as well as discussion of Care Plan and Critical Thinking Care Map questions, appear in Appendix I.

Chapter 25

Nutrition and Diet Therapy

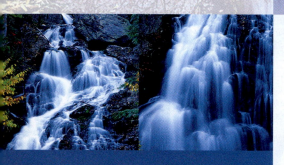

HISTORICAL Perspectives

Prior to rigorous academic study of individual nutrients in the early 1900s, many generations and populations were affected by malnutrition. Numerous accounts of diseases caused by nutritional deficiencies can be found throughout history. Some commonly recognized ones include scurvy, beriberi, and rickets. Although these conditions can still be found today, their causes have been identified, and they can be avoided through adequate intake of nutrients.

BRIEF Outline

NUTRITION
Nutrients
Standards for a Healthy Diet

LEARNING Outcomes

After completing this chapter, you will be able to:
1. Identify essential nutrients and the dietary sources of each.
2. Describe normal digestion, absorption, and metabolism of carbohydrates, proteins, and fats.
3. Explain essential aspects of energy balance.
4. Discuss body weight and body mass standards.
5. Identify developmental nutritional considerations.
6. Describe nursing interventions to promote good nutrition.

As healthcare providers, we work toward the goal that all people want to feel well, to enjoy good health. An essential part of this feeling of good health is to obtain the optimum nutrient supply for the body that is available. This chapter will introduce you to principles of nutrition and diet therapy, so that you can assist others in experiencing adequate nutrition.

NUTRITION

Nutrients

Nutrients are the organic, inorganic, and energy-producing substances found in foods. These nutrients are required for body functioning. The result of this interaction between nutrients and the human body is **nutrition**. Specific nutrients in food allow growth, maintenance of all body tissues, and normal functioning of all body processes.

Nutrients have three major functions. They provide energy for body processes and movement. They provide structural material for body tissues. They regulate body processes. When a person's food intake is adequate, there is a balance of these essential nutrients:

- Water
- Macronutrients: carbohydrates, proteins, and fats (lipids)
- Micronutrients: vitamins and minerals.

WATER

The body's most basic nutrient need is water. Water is vital to health and normal cellular function, serving as:

- A medium for metabolic reactions within cells
- A transporter for nutrients, waste products, and other substances
- A lubricant
- An insulator and shock absorber
- A means of regulating and maintaining body temperature.

Age, body fat, and gender affect total body water. Infants have 70% to 80% of their body weight in water. The proportion of body water decreases with aging; in people over age 60, it is less than half of body weight. Fat tissue is essentially free of water; lean tissue contains a significant amount of water. So, water makes up a greater percentage of a lean person's body weight than an obese person's. Women have proportionally more body fat than men, and so have a lower percentage of body water.

MACRONUTRIENTS

Macronutrients provide fuel that converts to energy. These nutrients are found in carbohydrates, proteins, and fats (lipids).

Carbohydrates

Carbohydrates are composed of the elements carbon (C), hydrogen (H), and oxygen (O). There are two basic kinds: simple carbohydrates (sugars) and complex carbohydrates (starches and fiber).

Sugars, the simplest of all carbohydrates, are water soluble. Both plants and animals produce sugars. (Lactose is a sugar formed by combining glucose and galactose and is found in milk.) However, sugars are mostly produced naturally by plants, especially fruits, sugar cane, and sugar beets. Processed or refined sugars (e.g., table sugar, molasses, and corn syrup) are those that have been extracted and concentrated from natural sources. Processed sugars are added to foods such as soft drinks, cookies, candy, ice cream, and some cereals.

Starches are *insoluble* (they do not dissolve in water). Starches are nonsweet forms of carbohydrate. Like sugars, nearly all starches exist naturally in plants, such as grains, legumes, and potatoes. Starches are in foods such as cereals, breads, flour, and puddings.

Fiber is a complex carbohydrate derived from plants. It cannot be digested by humans but supplies roughage, or bulk, to the diet. This bulk satisfies the appetite and also helps the digestive tract to eliminate wastes.

It is important that carbohydrate intake include natural as well as processed foods. Natural sources of carbohydrates supply protein, vitamins, minerals, and dietary fiber; these are often missing in processed foods. Because processed carbohydrate foods are relatively low in nutrients and high in calories, they are often referred to as "empty calories."

The end products of carbohydrate digestion are monosaccharides (glucose, fructose, and galactose). Some simple sugars, therefore, require no digestion. After the body breaks carbohydrates down into glucose, some glucose continues to circulate in the blood to maintain blood glucose levels and to provide a readily available source of energy. The remainder is either used as energy or stored. In healthy persons, essentially all digested carbohydrate is absorbed by the small intestine (see Figure 18-13 ⭕).

Insulin, a hormone secreted by the pancreas, is needed for glucose to be transported into the cells. So, the body's use of glucose is controlled by the pancreas's ability to produce insulin. When the pancreas is unable to produce insulin, or to produce enough insulin, the resulting condition is diabetes mellitus. Diabetes can negatively affect almost every body system.

Digested carbohydrates are maintained either as **glycogen** (the stored form of glucose) or as fat. The process of glycogen formation is called *glycogenesis*. All body cells are capable of storing glycogen; however, most glycogen is stored in the liver and skeletal muscles. Glycogen can be converted back to glucose when needed to maintain blood levels or to provide energy. Glucose that cannot be stored as glycogen is converted to fat.

Proteins

Proteins are organic substances composed of amino acids. Like carbohydrates, proteins contain carbon, hydrogen, and oxygen, but proteins also contain nitrogen. **Amino acids**, the building blocks of proteins, are categorized as essential or nonessential. *Essential amino acids* are those that cannot be manufactured in the body and must be supplied by ingesting protein. *Nonessential amino acids* are those that the body can manufacture. The body takes apart amino acids from food and reconstructs new ones from their basic elements (carbohydrates and nitrogen). See also Chapter 23 .

Proteins may be complete or incomplete. *Complete proteins* contain all of the essential amino acids plus many nonessential ones. Most animal proteins, including meats, poultry, fish, dairy products, and eggs, are complete proteins. *Incomplete proteins* lack one or more essential amino acids and are usually derived from vegetables. When an appropriate mixture of plant proteins is provided in the diet, a balance of essential amino acids can be achieved. For example, a combination of corn and beans is a complete protein. Specific combinations of two or more vegetables are called *complementary proteins.* Most protein is digested in the small intestine, where enzymes break it down into the end products of protein digestion, amino acids.

Amino acids are transported to the liver, where some are used to synthesize specific proteins such as albumin, globulin, and fibrinogen. Amino acids are also used to make protein for cell structures. In a sense, protein is "stored" as body tissue. The body cannot actually store excess amino acids for future use. However, a limited amount is available in the "metabolic pool" that exists as a result of the constant breakdown and buildup of the protein in body tissues.

Protein metabolism includes three activities: **anabolism** (building tissue), **catabolism** (breaking down tissue), and **nitrogen balance**. Because nitrogen is the element that distinguishes protein from lipids and carbohydrates, nitrogen balance reflects the status of protein nutrition in the body. Nitrogen balance is a measure of the intake and loss of nitrogen. When nitrogen intake equals nitrogen output, a state of nitrogen balance exists.

Lipids

Lipids are organic substances that are greasy and insoluble in water but soluble in alcohol or ether. *Fats* are lipids that are solid at room temperature; *oils* are lipids that are liquid at room temperature. In common use, the terms *fats* and *lipids* are used interchangeably. Lipids have the same elements (carbon, hydrogen, and oxygen) as carbohydrates, but they contain a higher proportion of hydrogen. Fatty acids, made up of carbon chains and hydrogen, are the basic structural units of most lipids. Based on their chemical structure, lipids are classified as simple or compound.

Glycerides, the simple lipids, are the most common form of lipids. **Triglycerides** (which have three fatty acids) account for over 90% of the lipids in food and in the body. Triglycerides may be saturated or unsaturated. *Saturated triglycerides* are found in animal products, such as butter, and are usually solid at room temperature. The hardness of the fat at room temperature indicates the amount of saturated fats present, harder fats such as beef tallow are more saturated than chicken fat, a softer fat. These saturated fats contribute to elevated blood cholesterol in humans and are considered detrimental to health. *Unsaturated triglycerides* are usually liquid at room temperature and are found in plant products, such as olive oil and corn oil. The unsaturated fats do not elevate but lower the blood cholesterol. Fish and low-fat foods would be included in selecting a diet with unsaturated fats. Knowing how to select fats that are less saturated can reduce the risk of heart disease.

Cholesterol is a fatlike substance that is both produced by the body and found in foods of animal origin. Most of the body's cholesterol is synthesized in the liver. However, some is absorbed from animal fats in the diet (e.g., from milk, egg yolk, and organ meats). Cholesterol is needed by the body to form bile acids and for the synthesis of steroid hormones. Cholesterol is also the primary lipid connected to heart disease. Testing for cholesterol levels is done to identify people at risk for developing coronary vessel disease. Lipids are digested mainly in the small intestine, where they are broken down to glycerol, fatty acids, and cholesterol. These are immediately reassembled inside the intestinal cells into triglycerides and cholesterol esters (cholesterol with a fatty acid attached to it), which are not water soluble. For these reassembled products to be transported and used, the small intestine and the liver must convert them into soluble compounds called lipoproteins. Lipoproteins are made up of various lipids and a protein. One of the roles of lipoproteins is to carry the cholesterol throughout the body. Cholesterol testing is ordered through *lipid profiles,* which test for lipoproteins and triglycerides. It is desirable to have a higher HDL (high-density lipoprotein) level and a lower LDL (low-density lipoprotein) level, because the risk of heart disease is greater when LDL is elevated. The LDL can be increased by the amount of saturated fats a person consumes.

MICRONUTRIENTS

Vitamins

A **vitamin** is an organic compound that cannot be manufactured by the body and is needed in small quantities to *catalyze* (or trigger) metabolic processes. Thus, when vitamins are lacking in the diet, metabolic deficits result. Vitamins are generally classified as fat soluble or water soluble. *Water-soluble vitamins* include C (ascorbic acid) and the B-complex vitamins: B_1 (thiamine), B_2 (riboflavin), B_3 (niacin or nicotinic acid), B_6 (pyridoxine), B_9 (folic acid), B_{12} (cobalamin), pantothenic acid, and biotin. The body cannot store water-soluble vitamins, so people must get a daily supply in the diet. Water-soluble vitamins can be affected by food processing, storage, and preparation. Vitamin content is highest in fresh foods that are consumed as soon as possible after harvest.

Fat-soluble vitamins include A, D, E, and K. The body can store these vitamins, though vitamins E and K can be stored only in limited amounts. Therefore, a daily supply of fat-soluble vitamins is not absolutely necessary.

Minerals

There are two categories of minerals. *Macrominerals* are those that people require daily in amounts over 100 mg. They include calcium, phosphorus, sodium, potassium, magnesium, chloride, and sulfur. *Microminerals* are those that people require daily in amounts less than 100 mg. They include iron, zinc, manganese, iodine, fluoride, copper, cobalt, chromium, and selenium. Both microminerals and macrominerals are found in vegetables, fruits, whole grains, and meats.

Nutritional needs are greatly affected by a person's age. Specific needs for macro- and micronutrients vary throughout the life span. Calorie requirements also rise and fall depending on the stage of life.

Standards for a Healthy Diet

Various daily food guides have been developed to help healthy people meet the daily requirements of essential nutrients and to facilitate meal planning. Food group plans emphasize the general types or groups of foods rather than the specific foods, because related foods are similar in composition and often have similar nutrient values. For example, all grains, whether wheat or oats, are significant sources of carbohydrates, iron, and the B vitamin thiamine. The Food Guide Pyramid (Figure 25-1 ■) was developed by the U.S. Department of Agriculture (USDA) as a graphic aid in making daily food choices. It divides foods into five groups of different sizes. Foods needed in the largest amounts (i.e., whole grains, cereal, rice, and pasta) appear in the largest block. Beside each block is the recommended number of daily servings. These are listed as ranges for meeting nutrient needs because individuals differ in size and activity level and therefore need different amounts of food. The USDA suggests that people eat a variety of whole foods to obtain the nutrients they need.

ENERGY BALANCE

Energy balance is the relationship between the energy obtained from food and the energy used by the body. The body gets energy in the form of **calories** (units of heat energy) from carbohydrates, protein, fat, and alcohol. The body uses energy for voluntary activities (like walking) and involuntary activities (like breathing and growing). A person's energy balance is determined by comparing energy intake with energy output. See also Chapter 32 ♾.

Metabolism is the term for all the biochemical and physiological processes by which the body grows and maintains itself. The basal metabolic rate (BMR) is the rate at which the body metabolizes food to maintain the energy requirements of a person who is awake and at rest. Lean, active people have a higher BMR than overweight and inactive people. In other words, they burn calories faster even when at rest.

NURSING CARE

ASSESSING

Size and weight are factors we notice almost without thinking. If a client is very thin or very heavy, this will be one of the first things the nurse observes. The nurse collects data about the client's height and weight. The nurse selects the appropriate type of scale to be used (Figures 25-2 ■ and 25-3 ■). Box 25-1 ■ provides guidelines about how to obtain a client's weight.

BOX 25-1	NURSING CARE CHECKLIST

Obtaining a Client's Weight

Adult Client

If client is able to stand

☑ Take measurement at the same time each day.

☑ Have the client wear the same kind and amount of clothing each day, and no shoes.

☑ Have client stand on the weighing platform while the nurse reads and records the weight (see Figure 25-3A).

If client cannot stand

☑ Weigh the client on a chair scale, *or*

☑ Weigh the client with a bed scale (canvas straps lift the client, and weight is recorded on a digital display or balance arm [see Figure 25-3B]).

Pediatric Client

☑ Lay neonates flat on the balance (see Figure 25-2D).

☑ Weigh infants without any clothing.

☑ Weigh young children in their underwear.

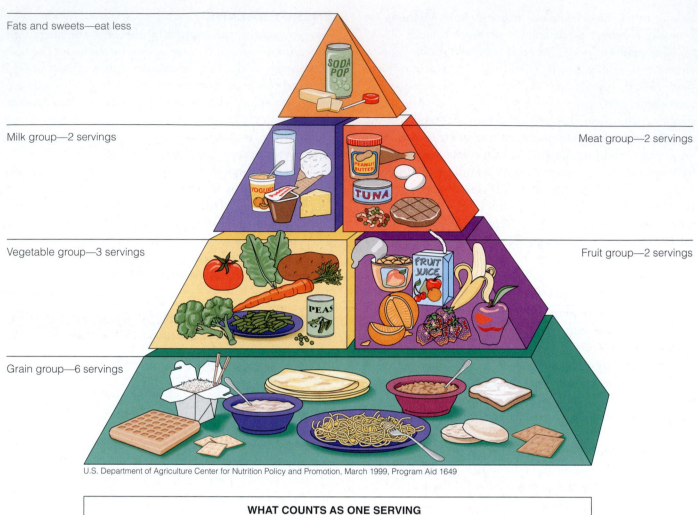

Fats and sweets—eat less

Milk group—2 servings

Meat group—2 servings

Vegetable group—3 servings

Fruit group—2 servings

Grain group—6 servings

U.S. Department of Agriculture Center for Nutrition Policy and Promotion, March 1999, Program Aid 1649

WHAT COUNTS AS ONE SERVING

GRAIN GROUP
1 slice of bread
1/2 cup of cooked rice or pasta
1/2 cup of cooked cereal
1 ounce of ready-to-eat cereal

VEGETABLE GROUP
1/2 cup of chopped raw
   or cooked vegetables
1 cup of raw leafy vegetables

FRUIT GROUP
1 piece of fruit or melon wedge
3/4 cup of juice
1/2 cup of canned fruit
1/4 cup of dried fruit

MILK GROUP
1 cup of milk or yogurt
2 ounces of cheese

MEAT GROUP
2 to 3 ounces of cooked lean
   meat, poultry, or fish

1/2 cup of cooked dry beans, or
1 egg counts as 1 ounce of lean
meat. 2 tablespoons of peanut
butter count as 1 ounce of
meat.

FATS AND SWEETS
Limit calories from these.

Four- to 6-year-olds can eat these serving sizes. Offer 2- to 3-year-olds less, except for milk.
Two- to 6 year-old children need a total of 2 servings from the milk group each day.

Figure 25-1. ■ The Food Guide Pyramid. (*Source:* U.S. Department of Agriculture. http://www.nal.usda.gov. Accessed October 12, 2006.)

Ideal body weight (IBW) is the weight recommended for optimal health. A person is said to be overweight when body weight exceeds IBW by up to 20%. A person whose body weight exceeds IBW by more than 20% is said to have **obesity**. Standardized tables can provide approximate ideal weights, but they are not precise.

For people over 18 years old, the body mass index (BMI) may be a better indicator of whether a person's weight is appropriate for height. The BMI also may provide a useful estimate of malnutrition. However, the results must be used with caution in people who have fluid retention (e.g., ascites or edema).

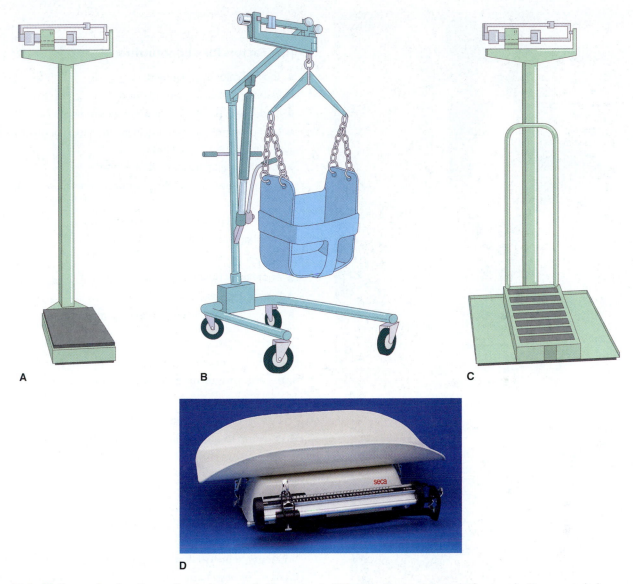

Figure 25-2. ■ Types of scales: **A.** standing balance scale; **B.** mechanical lift scale; **C.** wheelchair platform scale; **D.** neonate balance scale.

To calculate an individual's BMI, use this formula:

1. Measure the person's height in meters (1 meter = 3.3 ft, or 39.6 in.). Divide number of inches by 39.6 to find height in meters.
2. Measure the weight in kilograms (1 kg = 2.2 pounds). Divide number of pounds by 2.2 to find the weight in kilograms.
3. Calculate the BMI using the following formula:

$$\text{BMI} = \frac{\text{Weight in kilograms}}{(\text{Height in meters})^2}$$

4. Use the BMI number as follows: <16, malnourished; 16–19, underweight; 20–25, normal; 26–30, overweight; 31–40, moderately to severely obese; and >40, morbidly obese.

Problems of weight are among the most common health problems of adults. Excess body weight causes stress on body organs and contributes to chronic health problems such as hypertension and diabetes mellitus. Morbid obesity is obesity that interferes with mobility or breathing. Obese people may lack important nutrients even though they are eating excess calories.

Undernutrition means that nutrient intake is insufficient to meet daily energy requirements. It can occur because the person does not eat enough food, or because he or she cannot digest or absorb food. Risk factors for undernutrition are listed in Box 25-2 ■.

Protein–calorie malnutrition (PCM), once associated mostly with the starving children of third world countries, is now recognized as a significant problem of clients with

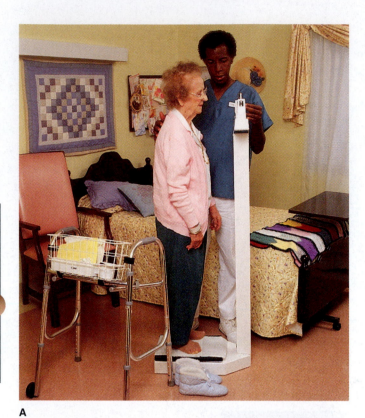

A

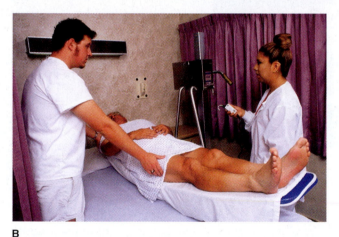

B

Figure 25-3. ■ Weighing the client: **A.** client on standing balance scale; **B.** client on bed scale.

cancer and chronic disease. Characteristics of PCM are weight loss and visible muscle and fat wasting.

DIAGNOSING, PLANNING, AND IMPLEMENTING

The most frequent nursing diagnoses related to nutrition are *Imbalanced Nutrition: More than Body Requirements, Imbalanced Nutrition: Less than Body Requirements,* and *Risk for Imbalanced Nutrition.* Nursing care of clients with imbalanced nutrition includes assisting with changes in diet, monitor-

---

BOX 25-2

Risk Factors for Undernutrition

- Too few calories consumed
- Inability to digest or absorb food
- Inadequate production of hormones or enzymes
- Medical condition resulting in inflammation or obstruction of the gastrointestinal tract
- Inability to acquire and prepare food
- Lack of knowledge about essential nutrients and a balanced diet
- Discomfort during or after eating
- Dysphagia (difficulty swallowing)
- Nausea or vomiting
- Anorexia or bulimia
- Severe depression
- Elderly living alone and/or on fixed incomes

---

ing blood glucose, stimulating appetite, assisting with meals, and providing enteral nutrition.

Providing Therapeutic Diets

Alterations in the client's diet are often needed to treat a disease process such as diabetes mellitus, to prepare for a special examination or surgery, to increase or decrease weight, to restore nutritional deficits, or to allow an organ to rest and promote healing. Diets may be modified in texture, calories, specific nutrients, seasonings, or consistency (Box 25-3 ■).

Clients who do not have special needs eat the *regular* (*standard* or *house*) *diet.* The house diet is a balanced diet that supplies the metabolic requirements of a sedentary person (about 2,000 kcal). Most agencies offer clients a daily menu from which to select their meals for the next day. Others provide standard meals to each client on the general diet. A

BOX 25-3   **CULTURAL PULSE POINTS**

Culture and Food Choices

Individual cultural practices often play a large role in the choice of food and diets. One's ethnic, national, and religious backgrounds have strong influences on food choices and eating patterns. Many immigrants from another country may show preferences for their native foods. For example, Southeast Asians enjoy a diet high in fish, duck, chicken, eggs, pork and soybean products, rice, noodles, and tea, and they prepare foods by stir frying and steaming. It is helpful to be aware of cultural food preferences and demonstrate appreciation and respect for clients' choices. It is also helpful to incorporate these dietary preferences when helping a client to adjust to a dietary restriction.

variation of the regular diet is the *light diet,* designed for postoperative and other clients who are not ready for the regular diet. Foods in the light diet are plainly cooked; fat, bran, and high-fiber foods are usually omitted. Not all agencies provide a light diet.

Diets that are modified in consistency are often given to clients before and after surgery or to promote healing in clients with gastrointestinal distress. These diets include nothing by mouth (NPO, from the Latin *nil per os*), clear liquid, full liquid, soft, and diet as tolerated.

NPO or Nothing by Mouth

On this diet, food and fluid are prohibited. This may be ordered before anesthesia or after surgery until bowel sounds return. IV fluids are often provided while a client is NPO to prevent dehydration. If a prolonged NPO diet is required, IV nutrition is usually ordered.

Clear Liquid Diet

This diet is limited to water, tea, coffee, clear broths, ginger ale or other carbonated beverages, strained and clear juices, and plain gelatin. This diet provides the client with fluid and carbohydrate (in the form of sugar) but does not supply adequate protein, fat, vitamins, minerals, or calories (no more than 600 kcal/day). It is a short-term diet (24 to 36 hours) provided for clients after certain types of surgery or when infection occurs in the gastrointestinal system. The major objectives of this diet are to relieve thirst, prevent dehydration, and minimize stimulation of the gastrointestinal tract.

Full Liquid Diet

This diet contains only liquids or foods that turn to liquid at body temperature, such as ice cream. Full liquid diets are often eaten by clients who have gastrointestinal disturbances or are otherwise unable to tolerate solid or semisolid foods. This diet is not recommended for long-term use because it is low in iron, protein, and calories. In addition, its cholesterol content is high because of the amount of milk offered. If a client is on this diet for long periods, a nutritionally balanced oral supplement, such as Ensure, is usually ordered. Six or more feedings per day may work best for the client who must stay on this diet for a long period.

Soft Diet

The soft diet is easily chewed and digested. It is often ordered for clients who have difficulty chewing and swallowing. It is a *low-residue* (low-fiber) diet with very few uncooked foods. The pureed diet is a modification of the soft diet. Liquid may be added to the food, which is then blended to a semisolid consistency.

Diet as Tolerated

Diet as tolerated is ordered when the client's appetite, ability to eat, and tolerance for certain foods change. For example, on the first postoperative day, a client may be given a clear liquid diet. If no nausea occurs, normal intestinal motility has returned, and the client feels like eating, the diet may be advanced to a full liquid, light, or regular diet.

Modifications for Disease

Many special diets may be prescribed to meet requirements for disease processes or altered metabolism. For example, a client with diabetes mellitus may need a diabetic diet recommended by the National Diabetic Association. An obese client may need a calorie-restricted diet. A cardiac client may need sodium and cholesterol restrictions. A client with allergies would need a nonallergenic diet. Some clients must follow certain diets (e.g., the diabetic diet) for a lifetime. If the diet is long term, the client must not only understand the diet but also develop a healthy, positive attitude toward it. All dietary instructions must be individually designed to meet the client's intellectual ability, motivation level, lifestyle, culture, and economic status.

Monitoring Blood Glucose

Clients who have diabetes may need to monitor random blood glucose levels throughout the day. This can be accomplished in the home setting by the client or family member, as well as by persons formally trained in medical care. By testing a single drop of blood, the client can receive a reading of the blood glucose present at the moment. Clients who understand the significance of this reading will be more likely to participate successfully in their therapeutic diet for an optimum management of their diabetes. Procedure 25-1 ■ on page 541 describes the procedure for monitoring blood glucose.

Stimulating the Appetite

Physical illness, unfamiliar or unpalatable food, environmental and psychological factors, and physical discomfort or pain may depress a client's appetite. A short-term decrease in food intake usually is not a problem for adults. However, over time, it leads to weight loss, decreased strength and stamina, and other nutritional problems. A decreased food intake is often accompanied by a decrease in fluid intake, which may cause dehydration. The nurse must determine the reason for a client's lack of appetite and then take steps to intervene. Reducing unpleasant odors, positioning the client comfortably, and sometimes cooling the room slightly are interventions that may help stimulate appetite.

Assisting Clients with Meals

Certain groups of people frequently require help with their meals. These groups include older adults who are infirm;

people with physical impairments, such as clients who are blind; those who must remain in a back-lying position; and those who cannot use their hands.

When feeding a client, ask in which order the client would like to eat the food. If the client cannot see, tell the client which food is being given. Always allow ample time for the client to chew and swallow the food before offering more. Also, provide fluids as requested. When the client is unable to communicate, offer fluids after every three or four mouthfuls of solid food. It is important to make the time a pleasant one, choosing topics of conversation that are of interest to clients who want to talk.

Although normal utensils should be used whenever possible, special utensils may be needed to assist a client to eat. Many adaptive feeding aids are available to help clients maintain independence. A standard eating utensil with a built-up or widened handle helps clients who cannot grasp objects easily. Plates with rims and plastic or metal plate guards enable the client to pick up the food by first pushing it against this raised edge. A suction cup or damp sponge or cloth may be placed under the dish to keep it from moving while the client is eating. No-spill mugs and two-handled drinking cups are especially useful for persons with impaired hand coordination. Stretch terry cloth and knitted or crocheted glass covers enable the client to keep a secure grasp on a glass. Lidded tip-proof glasses are also available. Clients are more likely to participate in mealtime if their meal is set up for them as needed. The nursing staff may need to open packages and cartons to make the food accessible. Meat may need to be cut, a sugar packet opened, or tea bags placed in the hot water. These simple preparations encourage the client to begin eating. They also give a few moments for the nurse and client to engage in pleasant conversation, another stimulant for eating.

Providing Enteral Nutrition

Two types of alternative feeding methods are **enteral nutrition** (through the gastrointestinal system) and parenteral (intravenous) nutrition. **Parenteral nutrition**, also referred to as total parenteral nutrition (TPN), is provided when the client is unable to ingest or absorb foods.

Enteral Access Devices

Enteral access is achieved by nasogastric or nasointestinal tubes, or gastrostomy or jejunostomy tubes.

A nasogastric tube is inserted through one of the nostrils, down the nasopharynx, and into the stomach or small intestine. Traditional *nasogastric tubes* are firm and larger than 12 Fr. in diameter. They are passed through the nose and pharynx to the stomach. An example is the Levin tube, a flexible rubber or plastic, single-lumen tube

with holes near the tip. The commonly used Salem sump tube has two lumens, the smaller of the two for air entry to reduce the risk of a vacuum forming should the tube affix itself to the mucosal lining of the stomach. Softer tubes that are more flexible and smaller than 12 Fr in diameter are frequently used for total enteral nutrition (TEN).

Nasogastric tubes are used for clients who have intact gag and cough reflexes, who have adequate gastric emptying, and who require short-term feedings. Procedure 25-2 ■ on page 541 provides guidelines for inserting and removing a nasogastric tube.

Nasogastric tubes may be inserted for reasons other than providing a route for feeding the client. These include:

- To prevent nausea, vomiting, and gastric distention following surgery. In this case, the tube is attached to a suction source.
- To remove stomach contents for laboratory analysis.
- To *lavage* (wash) the stomach in cases of poisoning or overdose of medications.

A *nasoenteric tube* is a longer tube than the nasogastric tube (at least 40 inches for an adult). It is inserted into one nostril and through the pharynx, esophagus, and stomach into the upper small intestine. Some agencies may require that specially trained nurses or physicians do this procedure. Nasoenteric tubes are used when risk for aspiration is high. Clients are at risk for aspiration if any of the following exist:

- Decreased level of consciousness
- Poor cough or gag reflexes
- Endotracheal intubation
- Recent extubation
- Inability to cooperate with the procedure
- Restlessness or agitation.

Gastrostomy and *jejunostomy devices* are used for long-term nutritional support, generally more than 6 to 8 weeks. Conventional tubes may be placed surgically or by laparoscopy through the abdominal wall into the stomach (**gastrostomy**) or into the jejunum (**jejunostomy**). More commonly, though, the percutaneous endoscopic gastrostomy (PEG) is used.

Testing Feeding Tube Placement

Before feedings are introduced, tube placement is confirmed by radiography, particularly when a small-bore tube has been inserted or when the client is at risk for aspiration. After placement is confirmed, the nurse marks the tube with indelible ink or tape at its exit point from the nose and documents the length of visible tubing for baseline data. Box 25-4 ■ lists items for the nurse to check prior to tube feeding.

<table>
<tr><td colspan="2">

BOX 25-4 | **NURSING CARE CHECKLIST**

</td></tr>
</table>

Verifying Tube Placement for Enteral Feedings

☑ Aspirate 20 to 30 mL of gastrointestinal secretions. *Note:* Small-bore tubes offer more resistance during aspirations than large-bore tubes and are more likely to collapse when negative pressure is applied.

☑ Measure the pH of aspirated fluid. This is the recommended method to determine tube placement. The pH of gastric fluid is normally 6 or lower, different from the pH of respiratory or intestinal fluids.

☑ Auscultate the epigastrium while injecting 5 to 20 mL of air. Air injected into the stomach produces whooshing, gurgling, or bubbling sounds over the epigastrium and the upper left quadrant. This method is less reliable than pH testing.

☑ Ensure initial radiographic verification of small-bore tubes.

☑ Closely observe the client for signs of obvious distress, and suspect tube dislodgment after episodes of coughing, sneezing, and vomiting.

Enteral Feedings

The frequency of feedings and amounts to be administered are ordered by the physician. Liquid feeding mixtures are available commercially, for example, Ensure, Osmolite, or Jevity. Enteral feedings may be ordered as intermittent or continuous. An **intermittent feeding** is the administration of 300 to 500 mL of enteral formula several times per day. These feedings are usually administered through the tube into the stomach over at least 30 minutes. **Continuous feedings** are generally administered over a 24-hour period using an infusion pump that guarantees a constant flow. Continuous feedings are essential when feedings are administered in the small bowel. *Cyclic feedings* are continuous feedings that are administered in less than 24 hours (e.g., 12 to 16 hours). These feedings, often administered at night and referred to as nocturnal feedings, allow the client to attempt to eat regular meals through the day. Because nocturnal feedings may use higher nutrient densities and higher infusion rates than the standard continuous feeding, the client should be assessed for fluid volume excess.

clinical ALERT

If a feeding tube accidentally becomes dislodged, formula could go into the lungs, causing aspiration or even death. Therefore, the nurse must verify that the tube is in the stomach before each intermittent feeding. In the case of continuous feedings, the nurse checks placement at least once per shift and before administering any medications through the tube.

Procedure 25-3 ■ on page 545 provides the essential steps for administering a tube feeding, and for administering and evaluating a gastrostomy or jejunostomy tube feeding.

Before administering a tube feeding, the nurse must check for any food allergies and assess tolerance to previous feedings. The nurse must also check the expiration date on a commercially prepared formula or the preparation date and time of agency-prepared solution. Any formula that has passed the expiration date or solution that has been at room temperature for more than 8 hours must be discarded.

Parenteral Nutrition

Feedings must sometimes be given intravenously when a client is unable to tolerate foods or formula through the gastrointestinal tract. Feeding is indicated when the patient has a need for intensive nutritional support, as seen with burns, sepsis, and multiple trauma, or at times when the intestinal tract and/or accessory organs are not functioning or need to be rested, as occurs with inflammatory bowel disorders such as Crohn's disease and pancreatitis. There are two forms of parenteral nutrition:

- *Peripheral vein infusions.* Various solutions containing dextrose, amino acids, vitamins, and minerals can be infused into peripheral veins. However, hypertonic solutions are irritating to peripheral veins and the concentrations of such solutions must be less than 10% dextrose. This limits the concentrations and amount of fluids and nutrients that can be safely administered. This method of feeding is only used when the need for nutritional support is short term, usually less than 2 weeks.
- *Central vein infusions.* When the nutritional needs are great, the use of a large central vein is desirable. TPN is infused through a catheter that is surgically inserted into a central vein, such as the subclavian or femoral vein, or through a peripherally inserted central catheter, which is inserted into a peripheral vein and is threaded forward into a large central vein. The central catheter allows for infusion of larger volumes of nutrients and for longer periods of time. They carry an added risk of infection and must be closely monitored.

EVALUATING

To evaluate the client with imbalanced nutrition, the nurse would compare baseline weight with current data and determine the client's compliance with the recommended diet. Goals for activity would be assessed. The client's support system and sense of satisfaction with changes in weight would be reviewed. If necessary, plans and goals would be adjusted.

CONTINUING CARE

The nurse must be an educator in helping clients with nutritional imbalances. Positive effects of changes in diet must be emphasized. Negative effects of continued imbalances must also be addressed. Every effort must be made to have the client participate in the planned changes, because food choice is a central part of people's lifestyles. Discuss with the client what goals they have in mind, and point out how their therapeutic diet will help them reach those goals. If clients are involved and empowered, believing that they can make a difference, their chances for success are much improved. It is important to assess the support of family and friends available to the client.

NURSING PROCESS CARE PLAN
Client with Altered Nutrition

Andrea Brown is a 20-year-old single woman who has been diagnosed as having anorexia. She is underweight, weighs 22% less than IBW, and weak. Despite her declining weight, she continues to make comments about being overweight such as "I am still too fat for my body build. I have no control over my life no matter what I do." Her hair appears to be thinning, and there are dark circles under her eyes. Upon collecting the meal tray one afternoon, the nurse notices that no food has been touched, and the client has requested soda crackers to go with her diet soda. Upon questioning, Ms. Brown states that she has had plenty to eat and is not hungry.

Assessment. VS: T 98, P 110, R 16, BP 110/74. Documentation of meals shows a poor intake, less than 25% at each meal since admission. Skin turgor is poor and mucous membranes dry. Lab tests indicate protein is below normal levels.

Nursing Diagnosis. The following important nursing diagnoses (among others) are established for this client:

- *Imbalanced Nutrition: Less than Body Requirements* related to anorexia
- *Adult Failure to Thrive* related to inadequate nutritive intake
- *Risk for Impaired Skin Integrity* related to alterations in nutritional state.

Expected Outcomes. The expected outcomes for the plan of care are that Ms. Brown will:

- Establish and maintain protein lab levels of normal value.
- Participate in psychiatric counseling program on a regular basis.
- Demonstrate stable weight without further losses in immediate future.

Planning and Implementation. The following nursing interventions are implemented for Ms. Brown. Assessments are done frequently to monitor her condition.

- Monitor weight daily.
- Record oral intake each meal.
- Dietitian consult to identify daily caloric intake necessary to stabilize weight loss and reach target weight.
- If client refuses to eat, notify physician.
- Work with healthcare team members and client to establish goals for weight gain and increased food intake.
- Establish an atmosphere of trust with the client.
- Request psychiatric consult order. Follow recommendations offered by mental health practitioner.
- Monitor skin for redness and breakdown daily during bath.

Evaluation. Although the client agrees to participate in the plan recommended by the healthcare team, progress is made slowly. Her weight loss is slowed, but continued monitoring and support of the healthcare team are necessary.

Critical Thinking in the Nursing Process

1. What possible interventions may need to be implemented to address a nutritional and fluid balance for Ms. Brown?
2. What would be the role of the psychiatric clinician when anorexia is demonstrated with physical characteristics?
3. Why would the diagnosis *Disturbed Body Image* be appropriate for Ms. Brown?

Note: Discussion of Critical Thinking questions appears in Appendix I.

Note: The references and resources for this and all chapters have been complied at the back of the book.

Monitoring Blood Glucose

Purposes

- To determine the client's blood glucose level
- To provide data for administering insulin in clients with diabetes mellitus

Equipment

- Chemical strips for reading glucose measurement
- Glucose monitor
- Lancet mechanism for obtaining blood
- Gloves
- Insulin sliding scale

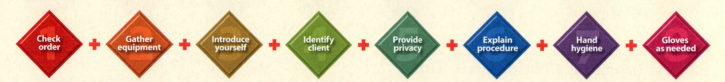

Check order + Gather equipment + Introduce yourself + Identify client + Provide privacy + Explain procedure + Hand hygiene + Gloves as needed

Interventions

1. Prepare the client. Explain that a drop of blood is needed to determine the client's blood glucose level. *This promotes cooperation.*
2. Confirm the correct chemical strips with the machine code. *Matching the codes prevents a misreading.*
3. Remove chemical strip from container and place it in the machine.
4. Prepare the lancet for puncture.
5. Don gloves. *This supports infection control.*
6. Hold chosen finger downward and squeeze gently from base to fingertip. *This helps bring blood to the puncture site.*
7. Wipe intended puncture site (lateral pads of fingers) per hospital protocol.
8. Place lancet against side of finger and release spring or stick finger with darting motion.
9. Allow drop of blood to accumulate onto chemical strip.
10. Activate timing device if monitor is not equipped with automatic timer.

11. Apply pressure to puncture site.
12. Allow the appropriate time for a digital readout.
13. Obtain results from the digital reading.
14. Discard soiled materials and gloves in proper containers.
15. Position client for comfort with the call bell within reach.
16. Document appropriate dose of regular insulin from sliding scale if provided.

SAMPLE DOCUMENTATION

[date]	BG: 250; Reg. Insulin 5 U given
[time]	SC per sliding scale.
	_____ N. Agarwal, LPN

Inserting and Removing Nasogastric Tubes

Purposes

- To administer tube feedings and medications directly into the GI tract for clients unable to eat by mouth or swallow a sufficient diet
- To establish a means for suctioning stomach contents to prevent gastric distention, nausea, and vomiting
- To remove stomach contents for laboratory analysis
- To *lavage* (wash) the stomach in case of poisoning, overdose of medications, or gastric bleeding

Equipment

- Nasogastric tube—Levine (single-lumen) or Salem sump (double-lumen)

- Towels, tissue, and an emesis basis
- Nonallergenic adhesive tape, 4 inches long and 1 inch wide or a NG tube clip
- Disposable gloves
- Water-soluble lubricant
- Glass of water and drinking straw
- Irrigating set with 20-mL syringe or 30-mL syringe with catheter tip
- pH test strip

- Stethoscope
- Clamp or plug for tubing
- Suction equipment if required
- Tincture of benzoin
- Tongue blade and penlight
- Rubber band and safety pin
- Plastic disposable bag
- Oral care supplies

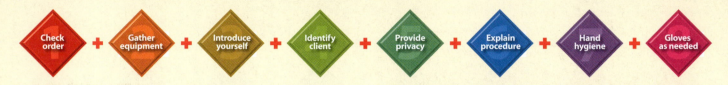

Check order + Gather equipment + Introduce yourself + Identify client + Provide privacy + Explain procedure + Hand hygiene + Gloves as needed

Part A: Inserting a Nasogastric Tube

Interventions

1. Prepare the client.
   - Explain to the client what you plan to do. *The passage of a gastric tube is not painful, but it is unpleasant because the gag reflex is activated during insertion.* Tell the client how to breathe and swallow upon your direction to facilitate insertion of the tube. Establish with the client what sign he or she could use (such as raising hand) to indicate for you to pause due to discomfort or gagging. *This form of communication gives client reassurance.*
   - Assist the client to a high-Fowler's position if health condition permits, and support the head on a pillow. *This facilitates passage of the tube into the esophagus.* Place a towel across the chest.
   - Remove the client's dentures so they do not become loose and interfere with insertion of the tube. Place tissues and emesis basin near client.

2. Assess the client's nares.
   - Ask the client if he or she has had nasal surgery, trauma, or a bleeding disorder. *A NG may be contraindicated in clients with such a history.*
   - Examine the nares for any obstructions or deformities by asking the client to breathe through one nostril while occluding the other.
   - Select the nostril that has the greater airflow.
   - Have client blow nose to clear.

3. Prepare the tube.
   - If needed, chill the tube for less flexibility, or warm the tube for increased flexibility. *A tube that is firm but not rigid will pass most easily and with the least amount of trauma.*

4. Determine how far to insert the tube.
   - Use the tube to mark off the distance from the tip of the client's nose to the tip of the earlobe and then from the tip of the earlobe to the tip of the sternum (Figure 25-4 ■). This length approximates the distance from

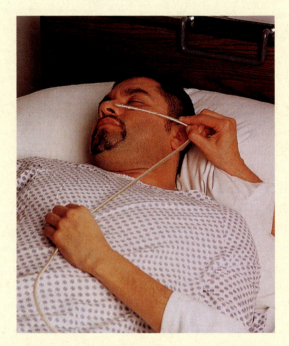

Figure 25-4. ■ Measuring the appropriate length of NG tube. (Photographer: Elena Dorfman.)

the nares to the stomach and may vary among individuals. Measuring the tube in this manner is more reliable than relying on tube markings and customizes the placement for this client. Mark the measured length with adhesive tape.

5. Insert the tube.
   - Lubricate the tip of the tube well with water-soluble lubricant or water to ease insertion, avoiding covering the holes on the tube with lubricant. *The lubricant reduces friction, thus reducing trauma. A water-soluble lubricant dissolves if the tube accidentally enters the lungs. An oil-based lubricant, such as petroleum jelly, will not dissolve and could cause respiratory complications if it enters the lungs.*

- Coil the tube's first 7 to 10 inches around your fingers to facilitate passage. Gently tip the client's head back and insert the tube, with its natural curve toward the client, into the selected nostril. Slowly advance the tube toward the nasopharynx by directing the tube toward the ear.
- If the tube meets resistance, withdraw it, relubricate it, and insert it in the other nostril. *The tube should never be forced against resistance, because of the possibility of trauma.*
- Once the tube reaches the pharynx the client will feel the tube in the throat and may gag and retch. You may need to pause and have the client rest for a few moments. Have the client take sips of water to calm the gag reflex.
- Ask the client to tilt the head forward, and encourage the client to drink sips of water and swallow. *Tilting the head forward facilitates passage of the tube into the posterior pharynx and esophagus rather than into the larynx; swallowing moves the epiglottis over the opening to the larynx* (Figure 25-5 ■).
- In cooperation with the client, pass the tube 5 to 10 cm (2 to 4 in.) with each swallow, until the indicated length is inserted.
- Stop the procedure and immediately remove tube if the client shows signs of coughing or cyanosis. *This could indicate that the tube has slipped into the trachea.*
- If the client continues to gag and the tube does not advance with each swallow, withdraw it slightly, and in-

spect the throat by looking through the mouth. *The tube may be coiled in the throat.* If so, withdraw it until it is straight, and try again to insert it.

6. Ascertain correct placement of the tube.
   - Ask the client to speak or hum. *If unable to do so, the tube may be passed through the vocal cords or coiled in the back of the throat.*
   - Auscultate air insufflation. This is done by attaching a syringe with 10 to 20 mL of air in it to the end of the tube. Place your stethoscope over the left upper quadrant of the abdomen, and listen while the air is injected. *You will hear the movement of air if the placement is in the stomach. If the client belches, the tube may be in the esophagus.*
   - With the syringe in place, withdraw stomach contents to determine placement of the tube in the stomach. If unable to withdraw contents, turn client on left side, advance the tube 1 to 2 inches, and attempt again.
   - If the signs do not indicate placement in the stomach, advance the tube 5 cm (2 in.), and repeat the tests.
   - Placement may be verified by x-ray. *It is unsafe to place the end of the tube in water to check placement, because it places the client at risk for aspiration.*

7. Connect the tube to suction or plug the tube end.

8. Apply tincture of benzoin to the bridge of the nose where tape will be placed. *Taping will improve the security of the tube.*

9. Prepare the tape by tearing it lengthwise halfway. Tape the unsplit end of tape to the nose and cross the split ends around the tubing (Figure 25-6 ■). *Do not tape tube to forehead because this may cause trauma to the nostril.*

10. To allow for client movement, make a slip knot with a rubber band around the tube. Secure the tube by pinning the rubber band to the client's gown.

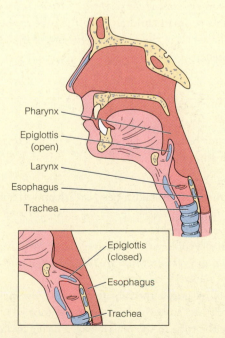

Pharynx
Epiglottis (open)
Larynx
Esophagus
Trachea

Epiglottis (closed)
Esophagus
Trachea

Figure 25-5. ■ Swallowing closes the epiglottis and allows passage of the nasogastric tube.

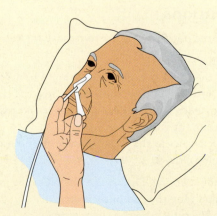

Figure 25-6. ■ Taping a NG tube to the bridge of the nose.

11. To connect to suction, attach the larger lumen of the Salem sump. This begins intermittent or continuous suction (as ordered).

12. Document the insertion of the tube, including time, type of tube, size of tube, and client response.

13. Ensure the client's comfort.

14. Irrigate the tube every 2 hours or as ordered.

15. Specific care of the Salem sump:
    - Inject 10 to 20 mL of air into the smaller lumen, the blue port. *This will clear the air vent, preventing gastric mucosal trauma if the tube adheres to the stomach lining. You can test for proper functioning of the air vent by putting the port near your ear. You will hear a hissing sound if patency exists.* Do not let the port hang downward or stomach contents may drain from it.

16. Clean the nares and provide oral care every shift and as needed to prevent infection and promote comfort. Assess nares for skin irritation.
    - Apply water-soluble lubricant to the nostril if it appears dry or encrusted.
    - Change the adhesive tape as required.
    - Position client in Semi-Fowler's position. *Head of bed must be elevated at least 30 degrees to minimize gastric reflux.*

17. Document placement checks and drainage amount, consistency, and color.

18. If suction is applied, ensure that the patency of both the nasogastric and suction tubes is maintained.
    - Irrigations of the tube with 30 mL of normal saline may be required at regular intervals. In some agencies, irrigations must be ordered by the physician.
    - Keep accurate records of the client's fluid intake and output, and record the amount and characteristics of the drainage. *This supports continuity of care.*

VARIATION: SMALL-BORE FEEDING TUBE

1. Prepare the tube for insertion.

2. Do not ice the tube or it will be too stiff.

3. Insert the stylet (guidewire) into the tube. Lubricate tube with water to activate lubricant.

4. After tube is in the stomach, have the client lean forward or to the right to help in advancing the tube. Leave the stylet in.

5. X-ray must confirm proper placement before any feeding is introduced. The stylet is removed after placement is confirmed.

PEDIATRIC CONSIDERATIONS

- For infants and young children, restraints may be necessary during tube insertion and throughout therapy. Restraints will prevent accidental dislodging of the tube.
- Place the infant in an infant seat, or position the infant with a rolled towel or pillow under the head and shoulders.
- When assessing the nares, obstruct one of the infant's nares, and feel for air passage from the other. If the nasal passageway is very small or is obstructed, an orogastric tube may be more appropriate.
- For infants and young children, measure appropriate NG tube length from the nose to the tip of the earlobe and then to the point midway between the umbilicus and the xiphoid process.
- If an orogastric tube is used, measure from the tip of the earlobe to the corner of the mouth to the xiphoid process.
- Do not hyperextend or hyperflex an infant's neck. *Hyperextension or hyperflexion of the neck could occlude the airway.*
- For infants or small children, tape the tube to the area between the end of the nares and the upper lip, as well as to the cheek.

Part B: Removing a Nasogastric Tube

Interventions

1. Confirm the physician's order to remove the tube.

2. Prepare the client.
   - Assist the client to a sitting position if health permits.
   - Place the towel or disposable pad across the client's chest to collect any spillage of mucous and gastric secretions from the tube.
   - Provide tissues to the client to wipe the nose and mouth after tube removal.

3. Discontinue suction. Disconnect the NG tube from the suction and plug the end of the tube.
   - Unpin the tube from the client's gown.
   - Remove the adhesive tape securing the tube to the nose.

4. Wash your hands and don disposable gloves to protect yourself from body fluids.

5. Remove the tube.
   - Ask the client to take a deep breath and to hold it. *This closes the glottis, thereby preventing accidental aspiration of any gastric contents.*
   - Pinch the tube with the gloved hand. *Pinching the tube prevents any contents inside the tube from draining into the client's throat.*
   - Slowly withdraw the tube for the first few inches, then quickly and smoothly withdraw the tube.
   - Place the tube in the plastic bag. *Placing the tube immediately into the bag prevents the transference of microorganisms from the tube to other articles or people.*

6. Ensure client comfort.
   - Provide oral care.
   - Assist the client as required to blow the nose. *Excessive secretions may have accumulated in the nasal passages.*

7. Dispose of the equipment appropriately.
   - Place the pad, bag with tube, and gloves in the receptacle designated by the agency. *Correct disposal prevents the transmission of microorganisms.*

8. Assess the nasogastric drainage if suction was used.
   - Measure the amount of gastric drainage, and record it on the client's fluid output record.
   - Inspect the drainage for appearance and consistency.

9. Document all relevant information.
   - Record the removal of the tube, the amount and appearance of any drainage if connected to suction, and any relevant assessments of the client.

SAMPLE DOCUMENTATION

[date] [time]	20-gauge Salem sump inserted through L nostril without difficulty. Low intermittent suction attached with immediate return of 200 mL green viscous fluid. Client tolerated procedure with minor discomfort. _____ J. Norris, LPN
[date] [time]	NG tube, Salem sump, draining 50 mL of clear fluid during past 4 hours. Patency verified through irrigation with 20 mL. NS. Placement confirmed. Oral care every 2 hours and upon request. Nares are free from irritation, with KY jelly applied. _____ J. Norris, LPN
[date] [time]	Bowel sounds present, passed flatus. NG tube removed without difficulty. Client tolerated procedure well, relieved to have tube removed. No n/v or abdominal discomfort present. _____ D. Hernandez, LPN

PROCEDURE 25-3 — Administering a Tube Feeding

Purpose

- To restore or maintain nutritional status

Equipment

- Tube feeding formula
- 20- to 50-mL syringe with an adapter
- Emesis basin
- Large catheter-tip syringe with plunger
  or
  Calibrated plastic feeding bag with tubing that can be attached to the feeding tube
  or
  Prefilled bottle with a drip chamber, tubing, and a flow-regulator clamp
- pH test strip
- Measuring container from which to pour the feeding (if using open system)
- Water (60 mL unless otherwise specified) at room temperature
- Feeding pump as required
- Correct amount of feeding solution
- Graduated container to hold the feeding
- Graduated container with 60 mL of water to flush the tubing
- Graduated container to measure residual formula
- Four 3- × 4-in. gauze squares to cover the end of the tube
- Elastic band
- Mild soap and water

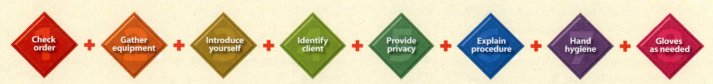
Check order → Gather equipment → Introduce yourself → Identify client → Provide privacy → Explain procedure → Hand hygiene → Gloves as needed

Part A: Nasogastric or Orogastric Feeding

Interventions

1. Confirm physician order for specific type and amount of feeding.

2. Prepare the client.
   - Assist the client to a Fowler's position in bed or a sitting position in a chair, the normal position for eating. If a sitting position is contraindicated, a slightly elevated right side-lying position is acceptable. The head of the bed should be raised 30 to 45 degrees. *These positions enhance the gravitational flow of the solution and prevent aspiration of fluid into the lungs.*

3. Assess tube placement.
   - Auscultate placement of 20 to 30 mL of air into the tube with your stethoscope positioned over the epigastric area.
   - Attach the syringe to the open end of the tube; aspirate alimentary secretions. Check the pH at least an hour after medications have been given. *Gastric content normal pH is 6 or below.*

4. Assess residual feeding contents.
   - Aspirate all the stomach contents, and measure the amount prior to administering the feeding, the residual. *This is done to evaluate whether undigested formula from a previous feeding remains or the stomach is emptying properly.*
   - If 75 to 150 mL (or more than half the last feeding) is withdrawn, check with the nurse in charge or refer to agency policy before proceeding. The precise amount to infuse is usually determined by the physician's order or by agency policy. *At some agencies, a feeding is withheld when the specified amount or more of formula remains in the stomach. In other agencies, the amount withdrawn is subtracted from the total feeding and that volume (less the undigested portion) is administered slowly.*
     or
     Reinstill the gastric contents into the stomach (to reduce fluid and electrolyte imbalance). Remove the syringe plunger, and pour the gastric contents via the syringe into the nasogastric tube. *Removal of the contents could disturb the client's electrolyte balance.*
   - If the client is on a continuous feeding, check the gastric residual every 4 hours or according to agency protocol.

5. Administer the feeding.
   - Before administering feeding:
     a. Check the expiration date of the feeding.
     b. Warm the feeding to room temperature. *An excessively cold feeding may cause cramps.*
   - When an open system is used, clean the top of the feeding container before opening it. *This minimizes the risk of contaminants entering the feeding syringe or feeding bag.*

FEEDING BAG (OPEN SYSTEM)
- Hang the bag from an infusion pole about 30 cm (12 in.) above the tube's point of insertion into the client.
- Clamp the tubing, and add the formula to the bag.
- Open the clamp, run the formula through the tubing, and reclamp the tube. *The formula will displace the air in the tubing, thus preventing the instillation of excess air into the client's stomach or intestine.*
- Attach the bag to the nasogastric tube (Figure 25-7 ■). Regulate the drip by adjusting the clamp, or secure the tubing in the feeding pump for regulated administration.

SYRINGE (OPEN SYSTEM)
- Remove the plunger from the syringe, and connect the syringe to a pinched or clamped nasogastric tube. *Pinching or clamping the tube prevents excess air from entering the stomach and causing distention.*
- Pour a small amount of feeding into the syringe barrel.
- Permit the feeding to flow in slowly at the prescribed rate. Raise or lower the syringe to adjust the flow as needed. Pinch or clamp the tubing to stop the flow for a minute if the client experiences discomfort. *If feeding is administered too quickly, flatus, crampy pain, and/or vomiting can occur.*

PREFILLED BOTTLE WITH DRIP CHAMBER (CLOSED SYSTEM)
- Remove the screw-on cap from the container, and attach the administration set with the drip chamber and tubing.
- Close the clamp on the tubing.

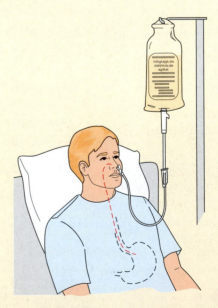

Figure 25-7. ■ Using a calibrated plastic bag to administer tube feeding.

- Hang the container on an intravenous pole about 30 cm (12 in.) above the tube's insertion point into the client. *At this height the formula should run at a safe rate into the stomach or intestine.*
- Squeeze the drip chamber to fill it to one-third to one-half of its capacity.
- Open the tubing clamp, run the formula through the tubing, and reclamp the tube. *The formula will displace the air in the tubing, thus preventing the instillation of excess air.*
- Attach the feeding set tubing to the feeding tube, and regulate the drip rate to deliver the feeding over the desired length of time. *Prefilled tube-feeding sets can be attached to a feeding pump to regulate the flow.*

6. Rinse the feeding tube immediately before all of the formula has run through the tubing.
   - Instill 50 to 100 mL of water through the feeding tube. *Water flushes the lumen of the tube, preventing future blockage by sticky formula.*
   - Be sure to add the water before the feeding solution has drained from the neck of a syringe or from the tubing of an administration set. Before adding water to a feeding bag or prefilled tubing set, first clamp and disconnect both feeding and administration tubes. *Adding the water before the syringe or tubing is empty prevents the instillation of air into the stomach or intestine and thus prevents unnecessary distention.*

7. Clamp and cover the feeding tube.
   - Clamp the feeding tube before all of the water is instilled. *Clamping prevents leakage of feeding or air from entering the tube.*
   - Cover the end of the feeding tube with gauze held by an elastic band. *Covering the tube end prevents leakage from it.*

8. Ensure client comfort and safety.
   - Pin the tubing to the client's gown by slip knotting a rubber band over the tube. *This minimizes pulling of the tube, thus preventing discomfort and dislodgment.*
   - Ask the client to remain sitting upright in Fowler's position or in a slightly elevated right lateral position for at least 30 minutes. *These positions facilitate digestion and movement of the feeding from the stomach along the alimentary tract, and prevent potential aspiration of the feeding into the lungs. The head of the bed must remain elevated 30 to 45 degrees when a continuous feeding is taking place.*

9. Dispose of equipment appropriately.
   - If the open system bag and connected tube are to be reused, wash them thoroughly with soap and water so that they are ready for reuse. Hang to air dry.

- Change the open system bag and connected tube every 24 hours or according to agency policy, as well as any syringes or irrigation fluid/set being used.

10. Monitor the client for possible problems.
    - Carefully assess clients receiving tube feedings for problems, particularly changes in lung sounds.
    - To prevent dehydration, give the client supplemental water in addition to the prescribed tube feeding as ordered.

11. Document all relevant information.
    - Document the feeding, including amount and kind of solution, duration of the feeding, and assessments of the client.
    - Record the volume of the feeding and water administered on the client's intake and output record.

VARIATION: CONTINUOUS-DRIP FEEDING

- If the feeding is a continuous-drip tube feeding, place a label on the container. *The label should indicate when the new feeding bag was hung.*
- Check residual as ordered or indicated by agency protocol. Then flush the tubing with 30 to 50 mL of water. *This verifies correct placement of the tube. If placement of a small-bore tube is questionable, a repeat x-ray should be done.*
- Determine agency protocol regarding withholding a feeding based on residual obtained. *Many agencies withhold the feeding for more than 75 to 150 mL of residual feeding.*
- To prevent spoilage or bacterial contamination, do not allow the feeding solution to hang longer than 8 hours. Check agency policy or manufacturer's recommendations regarding time limits.
- Follow agency policy regarding how frequently to change the feeding bag and tubing. *Changing the feeding bag and tubing every 24 hours reduces the risk of contamination.*

PEDIATRIC CONSIDERATIONS

- Feeding tubes may be reinserted at each feeding to prevent irritation of the mucous membrane, nasal airway obstruction, and stomach perforation that may occur if the tube is left in place continuously. Check agency practice.
- Position a small child or infant in your lap, provide a pacifier, and hold and cuddle the child during feedings. *This promotes comfort, supports the normal sucking reflex of the infant, and facilitates digestion.*
- Check agency policy or physician's orders for acceptable amounts of stomach aspirates and reinstillation of residual feedings.

Part B: Gastrostomy or Jejunostomy Feeding

1. Follow steps for NG feeding, including the following: Check placement, pour 15 to 30 mL of water into the syringe, remove the tube clamp, and allow the water to flow into the tube. *This determines the patency of the tube. If water flows freely, the tube is patent.* If the water does not flow freely, notify the nurse in charge and/or physician.

2. Administer the feeding.
   - Hold the syringe 7 to 15 cm (3 to 6 in.) above the os-tomy opening.
   - Slowly pour the solution into the syringe and allow it to flow through the tube by gravity.
   - Just before all the formula has run through and the sy-ringe is empty, add 30 mL of water. *Water flushes the tube and preserves its patency.*
   - If the tube is sutured in place, hold it upright, remove the syringe, and then clamp or plug the tube to prevent leakage. Cover the end of the tube with a 4 × 4 gauze, and secure the gauze with a rubber band.

3. Ensure client comfort and safety.
   - Assess status of peristomal skin. *Gastric or jejunal drainage contains digestive enzymes that can irritate the skin.* Document any redness and broken skin areas. Check or-ders about cleaning the peristomal skin, applying a skin protectant, and applying appropriate dressings. *Generally, the peristomal skin is washed with mild soap and water every shift and as needed.* Skin protectant may be ap-plied around the stoma.
   - Observe for common complications of enteral feedings: aspiration, hyperglycemia, abdominal distention, diar-rhea, and fecal impaction. Report findings to physician. *Often, a change in formula or rate of administration can cor-rect problems.*

VARIATION: PERCUTANEOUS ENDOSCOPIC GASTROSTOMY

- A percutaneous endoscopic gastrostomy (PEG) is kept in place with a short crosspiece or bolster near the skin level at the stoma.
- Clean the stoma daily with soap and water using a cot-ton swab or small piece of gauze in a circular motion.
- Rotate the bolster and clean the skin under it. Rotate the tube in a full circle between the thumb and forefin-ger daily.
- After cleaning, allow the skin to air dry.
- Report any signs of redness, pain, soreness, swelling, or drainage to the healthcare provider.
- Do not apply a dressing over the PEG. *A dressing and tape may result in skin excoriation and breakdown.*

4. Document all assessments and interventions.

SAMPLE DOCUMENTATION

[date] PEG-tube site assessed and cleaned.
[time] Client denies pain or soreness. No skin irritation present. Skin barrier cream applied.

_____ R. Diaz, LPN

Part C: Administering Medications via an Enteral Tube

Purpose
- To administer oral medications safely

Equipment
- 50- to 60-mL syringe
- Graduate conainer
- Medications to be administered
- Warm tap water (if needed to dissolve medications)
- Water for flushing tube
- Tongue blade or spoon to stir dissolved medications
- Disposable gloves
- pH test strip

1. Prepare the medications.
   - Determine if client is allergic to any of the prescribed medications.
   - Obtain any necessary client data, such as pulse, blood pressure, and lab values.
   - Determine if the medication can be safely given through a tube. Liquid medications are the best choice. If only a pill form is available, it helps to dissolve the pill in a small amount of warm water before administering, so as not to clog the tube. Some pills will need to be crushed and than dissolved.

Note: Enteric-coated and time-release pills should *NEVER* be crushed; if in a capsule form, do not open them. Crushing the pills or capsules alters their absorp-tion and metabolism, resulting in unpredictable drug effects and sometimes producing a bolus dosing of the drug. When unsure if a drug can be crushed, check with the pharmacy.

2. Administer the medications.
   - Don clean gloves.
   - Ensure proper placement of tube.
   - Check for residual when indicated. This is usually done when client is receiving a continuous feeding and per agency policy. Feedings may need to be held before or after certain medications (see step 4).
   - Attach 50- to 60- mL syringe to feeding tube. An adap-tor may be necessary for small-bore tubes.
   - Holding syringe upright at a 90-degree angle, adminis-ter 30 to 60 mL of tap water by pouring into syringe and allowing fluid to flow by gravity.
   - Administer medications, being sure to add sufficient water.
   - Administer another 30 to 60 mL of tap water after the medications have been administered. This helps to maintain tube patency.

3. Document medications.
   - Document fluid intake, being sure to include amount of fluid added to the medication.
4. Avoid drug–feeding interactions.
   - Never mix medications with the enteral feeding. The protein and mineral content of the feeding sometimes binds with the drug, thereby reducing drug absorption and availability.
   - Some medications that are known to interact with enteral feedings include:

   - *Antibiotics:* The mineral content reduces absorption of tetracycline, penicillin, and fluoroquinolones.
   - *Anticoagulants and antiepileptics:* The protein reduces absorption of warfarin (Coumadin) and phenytoin (Dilantin). Always check for specific interactions.
- The interactions can be minimized by holding feedings for 1 hour before or for 2 hours after administration of meds.

SAMPLE DOCUMENTATION

[date]   G tube client. 2.5 mL of residual noted.
[time]   Medications administered with 15 mL of H_2O. See MAR.
           G tube flushed with 30 mL of H_2O to maintain patency. Feeding continued, no c/o abdominal discomfort noted.
           _____ J. Norris, LPN

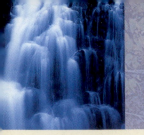

Chapter Review

 KEY TERMS by Topic

Use the audio glossary feature of either the CD-ROM or the Companion Website to hear the correct pronunciation of the following key terms.

Nutrients
nutrients, nutrition, glycogen, amino acids, anabolism, catabolism, nitrogen balance, lipids, triglycerides, vitamin

Standards of a Healthy Diet
calories, obesity, undernutrition, protein–calorie malnutrition, enteral nutrition, parenteral nutrition, gastrostomy, jejunostomy, intermittent feeding, continuous feedings

KEY Points

- For the body to grow, maintain body tissue, and perform all body functions normally, specific nutrients must be supplied. When a person is undernourished, carbohydrate reserves (stored as liver and muscle glycogen) meet energy requirements for a short time; then body protein is used. Over time, this may result in protein–calorie malnutrition.

- Homeostasis depends on many physiological processes. These processes regulate fluid intake and output. They also regulate the movement of water and dissolved substances between the body compartments.

- If diet therapy is long term, a client must not only understand the diet but also develop a healthy, positive attitude toward it. The client's belief that the diet will make a change is key to its success.

- After a feeding tube is inserted, and before feedings are introduced, tube placement is confirmed by radiography. Tube placement must be confirmed whenever possible dislodgment may have occurred, before administering medication or feeding through the tube, and at least daily for continuous feedings.

 EXPLORE MediaLink

Additional interactive resources for this chapter can be found on the Companion Website at www.prenhall.com/ramont. Click on Chapter 25 and "Begin" to select the activities for this chapter.

For chapter-related NCLEX®-style questions and an audio glossary, access the accompanying CD-ROM in this book.

Animations/Videos
- Carbohydrates
- Eating Disorders
- Lipids
- NG Tube

FOR FURTHER Study

To visualize the digestive track, see Figure 18-13.

For information on assessing vital signs, see Chapter 20.

For more about the role of nutrition in healing, see Chapter 23.

For more about nutrition's role in maintaining homeostasis, see Chapter 32.

Caring for a Client with Nasogastric Tube Feeding
NCLEX-PN® Focus Area: Physiological Adaptation

Case Study: Angelica Del Monico an 86-year-old female was admitted from long term care last evening for possible aspiration pneumonia. She has a history of CVA, with dysphagia, left side weakness. She has macular degeneration, which has severely compromised her vision; her hearing is assisted with bilateral hearing aids. Mrs. Del Monico is diabetic.

Nursing Diagnosis: Imbalanced Nutrition: Less than Body Requirements

COLLECT DATA

Subjective	Objective
_____	_____
_____	_____
_____	_____
_____	_____
_____	_____
_____	_____
_____	_____

Would you report this data? Yes/No

If yes, to: _____

What would you report? _____

Nursing Care

_____
_____
_____
_____
_____
_____
_____
_____
_____
_____
_____

How would you document this? _____
_____
_____

Data Collected
(use those that apply)

- Height: 150 cm (4'11")
- Weight: 39.55 kg (87 lbs)
- Temperature: 39°C (102.6°F)
- Pulse: 86 bpm
- Respirations: 30/min labored
- Blood Pressure: 130/82 mm Hg
- Skin pale and moist
- NPO, nasogastric tube 150 mL/hour Glucerna
- Blood glucose 236 at 7 A.M.
- Foley catheter in place draining dark amber urine
- Complaint of being thirsty
- Chest x-ray and urinalysis done—result pending
- WBC 28,000
- Client states "My chest hurts when I breathe"

Nursing Interventions
(use those that apply; list in priority order)

- VS q 4 hr. Tylenol gr. X for temp <101.6
- Cooling measures for temp <102
- Teach client to use incentive spirometer
- Blood glucose monitoring a.c. and h.s.
- Insulin per sliding scale
- Check tube placement and residual each shift and PRN
- Flush tube with 100 mL following medication administration
- Hold tube feeding for residual <150 mL
- Encourage coughing and deep breathing
- Instruct client to request prn pain medication before the pain is severe
- Create a quiet, nondisruptive environment with dim lights and comfortable temperature when possible.
- Offer oral fluids to increase urinary output
- Encourage self-feeding
- Encourage ambulation
- Elevate head of bed 30 degrees

Compare your documentation to the sample provided in Appendix I.

NCLEX-PN® Exam Preparation

1 A client who prefers vegetarian menus states that he has a greater need for carbohydrates and has not given thought to the amount of protein to consume. You would explain that the importance of eating at least the minimum daily requirements of protein is to allow the body to have:

1. adequate structural material for body tissues.
2. a limited amount of fat.
3. adequate calories for maintaining blood glucose.
4. adequate calcium for bone density.

2 You are teaching a client about limiting fat intake to reduce undesirable cholesterol and triglyceride levels. Which statement by the client would indicate that he or she would be most likely to succeed in keeping with the dietary changes?

1. "I think that if my spouse were here I would be sure to have the correct foods prepared for my meals."
2. "I think that a person only lives once, and what one eats will not really make that much difference in the long run."
3. "I think that I will be able to eat less fatty foods if I look at the food labels before I buy."
4. "I think that my spouse will be upset if I don't eat the same foods along with him/her."

3 When checking for proper placement of a nasogastric tube, gastric secretions are aspirated and the pH checked. Normal gastric pH should be _____.

4 A client's spouse who has coronary vessel disease (heart disease) asks you how best to prepare meals that would keep from promoting the disease. What should you say?

1. Cream sauces can be used to enhance the flavor of this diet.
2. Serve fish for the meat choice often, instead of other meats.
3. Seek assistance by shopping at health food stores.
4. Substitute onion salt and celery salt for table salt to enhance flavor.

5 A client visiting the clinic has heard about the dangers of obesity and wants to know if she is considered to be obese. You could accurately answer that:

1. anyone who is 10% or more above IBW is considered obese and at risk for health.
2. anyone who is 20% or less than IBW is considered to be obese and at risk for health.
3. anyone who is 20% or more above IBW is considered to be obese and at risk for health.
4. Anyone who is 20% or more above IBW but is physically active is not considered to be obese.

6 A client is receiving tube feeding and has inadvertently pulled out the tube. The nurse has replaced the tube and is ready to restart the feeding. What step must be taken before starting the feeding?

1. The client needs to be reweighed.
2. The client needs to have tube placement verified, perhaps even by x-ray.
3. The client should be tested on semisolid foods before returning to tube feeding.
4. The client should receive bolus feedings until tube placement is confirmed by x-ray.

7 A client has been diagnosed recently as having diabetes mellitus. You will assist the client in learning how to adjust to her newly prescribed diet, instructing her that the primary function of carbohydrates is to:

1. furnish the body with energy.
2. insulate the client to avoid loss of heat.
3. provide building blocks to repair new tissue.
4. supply client with adequate amounts of fiber.

8 A client has undergone colon surgery today and will be receiving a clear liquid diet. Which of the following foods would you expect to be on the client's meal tray?

1. milkshake
2. cranberry juice
3. apricot nectar
4. creamed soups

9 When giving medications through a Salem sump to a client, the proper procedure would be to:

1. administer the medications into the smaller blue port on the tube.
2. administer the medications orally if they are liquid or crushed.
3. administer the medications into the larger port on the tube.
4. administer the medications only after the tube was removed.

10 The nurse is preparing to insert a nasogastric tube. Which of the following supplies will it be necessary to collect? (Select all that apply.)

1. water-soluble lubricant
2. sterile gloves
3. emesis basin
4. stethoscope
5. measuring tape
6. scissors

Answers and Rationales for Review Questions, as well as discussion of Care Plan and Critical Thinking Care Map questions, appear in Appendix I.

Chapter 26

Fluids, Electrolytes, and Acid–Base Balance

BRIEF Outline

Body Fluids and Electrolyte Balance
Acid–Base Balance
Acid–Base Imbalances

LEARNING Outcomes

After completing this chapter, you will be able to:

1. Discuss the function, distribution, and regulation of fluids and electrolytes.
2. Identify factors affecting normal body fluids, electrolytes, and acid–base balance.
3. Identify nursing interventions for clients with acid–base disorders.
4. Teach clients measures to maintain fluid and electrolyte balances.
5. Identify nursing responsibilities in IV therapy.

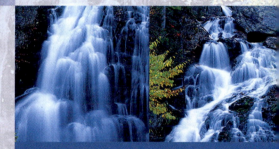

HISTORICAL Perspectives

The human body constantly strives to maintain homeostasis. Throughout the ages, man has achieved this through self-regulatory mechanisms. However, diseases often alter the body's ability to self-regulate, resulting in imbalances in fluids, electrolytes, and acid–base balance. Nurses play a vital role in assisting clients to maintain these balances. As the knowledge of disease and illness increased during the 19th century, the need for adequate fluid and electrolytes requirements became clear. Clients are now tested and treated in order to maintain the proper fluid and electrolyte levels.

In good health, homeostasis is maintained. Homeostasis is a delicate balance between fluids, electrolytes, and acids and bases in the body. Constant internal conditions such as chemistry, temperature, and blood pressure are maintained through homeostasis. Almost every illness has the potential to threaten this balance. Even in normal daily living, high temperatures or vigorous exercise without adequate water and salt intake can disturb homeostasis. Medical interventions such as diuretics or nasogastric suction without replacement of water and electrolytes can also cause fluid and electrolyte imbalances.

Body Fluids and Electrolyte Balance

The body's **fluid** is divided into two major compartments, intracellular and extracellular. **Intracellular fluid (ICF)** is found within the cells of the body. It accounts for approximately two-thirds of the total body fluid in adults and is vital to normal cell functioning. ICF contains oxygen, electrolytes, and glucose. **Extracellular fluid (ECF)** is found outside the cells and accounts for about one-third of total body fluid. The ECF is subdivided into three compartments: intravascular, interstitial, and transcellular (Figure 26-1 ■). ECF is the transport system that carries nutrients

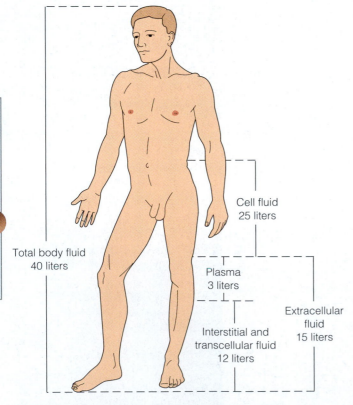

Figure 26-1. ■ Total body fluid represents 40 L in adult males weighing 70 kg. Fluid amounts are indicated for different body compartments.

Total body fluid 40 liters

Cell fluid 25 liters

Plasma 3 liters

Interstitial and transcellular fluid 12 liters

Extracellular fluid 15 liters

to, and waste products from, the cells. **Interstitial fluid** (three-quarters of the ECF) surrounds the cells and includes lymph. Interstitial fluid transports wastes from the cells by way of the lymph system, as well as directly into the blood plasma through capillaries. Intravascular fluid (or *plasma*) is found within the blood. Transcellular fluid, which some consider to be distinct from intracellular and extracellular fluids, includes cerebrospinal, pleural, peritoneal, and synovial fluids in the body.

COMPOSITION OF BODY FLUIDS

Extracellular and intracellular fluids contain oxygen, nutrients, carbon dioxide, and charged particles (called *ions*). Many salts break up into electrically charged ions when dissolved in water. These charged ions are called **electrolytes** because they are capable of conducting electricity. Ions that carry a positive charge are called *cations,* and ions carrying a negative charge are called *anions*. Examples of cations are sodium, potassium, calcium, and magnesium. Anions include chloride, bicarbonate, phosphate, and sulfate. The composition of fluids varies from one body compartment to another.

In extracellular fluid, the principal electrolytes are sodium, chloride, and bicarbonate. Other electrolytes such as potassium, calcium, and magnesium are present, but in much smaller quantities. Plasma and interstitial fluid, the two primary components of ECF, contain essentially the same electrolytes and solutes, except for protein. Plasma is rich in protein, containing large amounts of albumin; interstitial fluid contains little or no protein.

Intracellular fluid has a very different composition from ECF. Potassium and magnesium are the primary cations present in ICF; phosphate and sulfate are the major anions. Other electrolytes are present, but in much smaller concentrations. A balance of fluid volumes and electrolyte compositions in the fluid compartments of the body is essential to health. Normal and unusual fluid and electrolyte losses must be replaced if homeostasis is to be maintained.

Other body fluids, such as gastric and intestinal secretions, also contain electrolytes. When these fluids are lost from the body during severe vomiting, diarrhea, or gastric suctioning, electrolyte imbalance can result.

REGULATING BODY FLUIDS

In a healthy person, the volumes and chemical composition of the fluid compartments stay within narrow safe limits. Normally, fluid intake and fluid loss are balanced. Illness can upset this balance so that the body has too little or too much fluid.

Fluid Intake

During periods of moderate activity at moderate temperature, the average adult drinks about 1,500 mL per day but needs 2,500 mL per day, an additional 1,000 mL. This added volume is acquired from foods and as a by-product of food metabolism.

Fluid Output

Fluid losses from the body counterbalance the adult's 2,500-mL average daily intake of fluid. Fluid output occurs through several routes: urine, "insensible losses," and feces.

Urine formed by the kidneys and excreted from the urinary bladder is the major avenue of fluid output. Normal urine output for an adult is 1,400 to 1,500 mL per 24 hours, or at least 30 to 50 mL per hour. In healthy people, urine output may vary noticeably from day to day. Urine volume automatically increases as fluid intake increases. If fluid loss through perspiration is large, however, urine volume decreases to maintain fluid balance in the body.

Insensible losses occur through the skin and through the lungs. They are usually not noticeable and cannot be measured. Insensible fluid loss through the skin occurs in two ways: through diffusion and through perspiration. Water losses through diffusion are not noticeable but normally account for 350 to 400 mL per day. This loss can be significantly increased if the protective layer of the skin is damaged, as with burns or large abrasions. Perspiration varies depending on factors such as environmental temperature and metabolic activity. Fever and exercise increase metabolic activity and heat production, thereby increasing fluid losses through the skin.

Another type of insensible loss is the water in exhaled air. In an adult, this is normally 350 to 400 mL per day. When respiratory rate accelerates (as with exercise or an elevated body temperature), water loss can increase.

Loss through the intestines in feces usually amounts to 100 to 200 mL per day. The digested food that passes from the small intestine into the large intestine contains water and electrolytes. However, most fluid is reabsorbed in the proximal half of the large intestine.

REGULATING ELECTROLYTES

Electrolytes are present in all body fluids and fluid compartments. Just as maintaining the fluid balance is vital to normal body function, so is maintaining electrolyte balance (Box 26-1 ■). The concentration of specific electrolytes differs between fluid compartments, but a balance of *cations* (positively charged ions) and *anions* (negatively charged ions) should exist. Electrolytes are important for:

- Maintaining fluid balance
- Contributing to acid–base regulation
- Facilitating enzyme reactions
- Assisting neuromuscular reactions.

Most electrolytes enter the body through dietary intake and are excreted in the urine. Some electrolytes, like sodium and

chloride, are not stored and must be consumed daily to maintain normal levels. Table 26-1 ■ lists electrolytes of the body, their location, sources, and function, and Table 26-2 ■ lists major electrolytes and their signs and symptoms of hyper or hypo conditions.

Acid–Base Balance

Body fluids are maintained within a narrow range that is *alkaline* (slightly above 7 on a scale from 0 to 14). The normal pH of arterial blood is between 7.35 and 7.45.

Acids are continually produced during metabolism. Buffers in the digestive tract, the respiratory system, and the renal system work constantly to maintain the narrow pH range necessary for optimal function.

ACID–BASE REGULATORS

Buffer Regulation

Buffers neutralize excess acids or bases. They are the body's first line of defense against acid–base balance changes in the body. The major buffer systems in extracellular fluids are bicarbonate and carbonic acid. As long as a ratio of 20 parts of bicarbonate to 1 part of carbonic acid is maintained, the pH remains within its normal range of 7.35 to 7.45. If bicarbonate is depleted while neutralizing a strong acid, the pH may drop below 7.35, resulting in a condition called *acidosis*. Likewise, if a strong base is added to ECF and depletes carbonic acid, the pH may rise over 7.45, resulting in a condition called *alkalosis*.

Bicarbonate is present in both intracellular and extracellular fluids. Extracellular bicarbonate levels are regulated by the kidneys. The kidneys excrete bicarbonate when too much is present. They regenerate and reabsorb bicarbonate ions if more is needed. Unlike other electrolytes that must be consumed in the diet, adequate amounts of bicarbonate are produced by the body to meet the body's needs.

In addition to the bicarbonate–carbonic acid buffer system, plasma proteins, hemoglobin, and phosphates also function as buffers in body fluids.

TABLE 26-1

Location, Sources, and Function of Selected Electrolytes

ELECTROLYTE	LOCATION	SOURCES	FUNCTION
Sodium	Extracellular fluid (most abundant cation)	Bacon, ham, processed cheese, table salt	Controls and regulates water balance
Potassium	Intracellular fluid (most abundant cation)	Dark yellow and orange fruits, dark green leafy vegetables, meat, fish, and avocados	Helps maintain ECF and ICF water balance and acid–base balance; vital for skeletal, cardiac, and smooth muscle activity; supports ICF enzyme reactions
Calcium	Mostly in skeletal system, small amount in ECF	Milk and milk products very high; dark green leafy vegetables, canned salmon	1% of total calcium outside bones and teeth regulates muscle contraction/relaxation and neuromuscular and cardiac function. With aging, less calcium is absorbed in intestines and more is excreted via kidneys; weight-bearing exercise and vitamin D protect against osteoporosis and fractures
Magnesium	Primarily in skeleton and ICF; only about 1% in ECF	Cereal grains, nuts, dried fruit, legumes, green leafy vegetables, dairy products, meat, and fish	Aids intracellular metabolism, especially adenosine triphosphate (ATP) production; necessary for protein and DNA synthesis within cells. In ECF, helps regulate neuromuscular and cardiac function
Chloride	Major anion of ECF; major component of gastric juice as hydrochloric acid (HCl)	Found in the same foods as sodium	Functions with sodium to regulate serum osmolality and blood volume; concentration in ECF is regulated by sodium; is usually reabsorbed with sodium in the kidney; helps regulate acid–base balance; acts as buffer in the exchange of oxygen and carbon dioxide in red blood cells
Phosphate	Major anion of ICF; also is found in ECF, bone, skeletal muscle, and nerve tissue. Much higher levels in children, probably due to higher growth hormone	Found in many foods such as meat, fish, poultry, milk products, and legumes	Involved in many chemical actions of the cell; essential for functioning of muscles, nerves, and red blood cells; also involved in protein, fat, and carbohydrate metabolism; absorbed from the intestine
Bicarbonate	ICF and ECF; excreted and reabsorbed by kidneys	Produced in metabolic process, so dietary source unnecessary	Major body buffer involved in acid–base regulation

Respiratory System Regulation

The lungs help regulate acid–base balance by eliminating or retaining carbon dioxide, a potential acid. When carbon dioxide combines with water, it forms carbonic acid. This chemical reaction is reversible; carbonic acid breaks down into carbon dioxide and water. Working together with the buffer system, the lungs regulate acid–base balance and pH by altering the rate and depth of respirations. The response of the respiratory system to changes in pH is rapid, occurring within minutes.

Carbon dioxide is a powerful stimulator of the respiratory center. When blood levels of carbonic acid and carbon dioxide rise, respiratory center stimulation causes the rate and depth of respirations to increase. By contrast, when bicarbonate levels are excessive, the rate and depth of respirations are reduced.

Renal System Regulation

Although buffers and the respiratory system can compensate for changes in pH, the kidneys provide the primary long-term regulation of acid–base balance. However, their response is slower and more permanent and selective than that of the other systems. The kidneys maintain acid–base balance by selectively excreting or conserving bicarbonate and hydrogen ions. When excess hydrogen ion is present

TABLE 26-2	
Major Electrolytes	
ELECTROLYTE	**SIGNS AND SYMPTOMS**
Sodium (Na^+) ■ Major cation in ECF ■ Normal serum level: 135–147 mEq/L	*Hyponatremia:* muscle weakness, decreased skin turgor, headache, tremor, seizures *Hypernatremia:* thirst, fever, flushed skin, oliguria, and dry, sticky membranes
Potassium (K^+) ■ Major cation in ICF ■ Normal serum level: 3.5–5.0 mEq/L	*Hypokalemia:* decreased GI, skeletal muscle, and cardiac muscle function; decreased reflexes, rapid, weak, irregular pulse, muscle weakness, or irritability; decreased blood pressure; nausea and vomiting ileus *Hyperkalemia:* muscle weakness, nausea, diarrhea, oliguria
Calcium (Ca^{2+}) ■ Major cation in teeth and bones ■ Normal serum level: 8.5–10.5 mg/dL	*Hypocalcemia:* muscle tremor, muscle cramps, tetany, tonic-clonic seizures, paresthesia, bleeding, arrhythmias, hypotension *Hypercalcemia:* lethargy, headache, muscle flaccidity, nausea, vomiting, anorexia, constipation, polydipsia, hypertension, polyuria
Chloride (Cl^-) ■ Major anion in ECF ■ Normal serum level: 95–105 mEq/L	*Hypochloremia:* increased muscle excitability, tetany, decreased respirations *Hyperchloremia:* stupor, rapid deep breathing, muscle weakness
Phosphorus (P^{2-}) ■ Major anion in ICF ■ Normal serum level 3.5–4.5 mEq/dL	*Hypophosphatemia:* paresthesia (circumoral and peripheral), numbness, tingling, heightened sensitivity, lethargy, speech defects (such as stuttering or stammering) *Hyperphosphatemia:* renal failure, vague neuroexcitability to tetany and convulsions, arrhythmias and muscle twitching with sudden rise in phosphate levels
Magnesium (Mg^{2+}) ■ Major cation in ICF ■ Normal serum level: 1.3–2.1 mEq/L	*Hypomagnesemia:* dizziness, confusion, convulsions, tremor, leg and foot cramps, hyperirritability, arrhythmias, vasomotor changes, anorexia, nausea *Hypermagnesemia:* drowsiness, lethargy, coma, arrhythmias, hypotension, vague neuromuscular changes (tremor), vague GI symptoms (nausea), slow weak pulse

and the pH falls (*acidosis*), the kidneys reabsorb and regenerate bicarbonate and excrete hydrogen ion. When there is excess bicarbonate and a high pH (*alkalosis*), the kidneys excrete bicarbonate and retain hydrogen ions.

Acid–Base Imbalances

When a deficiency occurs in the respiratory process, the acid–base balance is disturbed: The alveoli of the lungs are unable to reduce the carbon dioxide levels. Such a condition can be acute, as in excessive sedation, or chronic, as in chronic pulmonary disease.

RESPIRATORY ACIDOSIS

As carbon dioxide is retained, it creates carbonic acid that builds up in the blood; the pH drops, creating **respiratory acidosis**. The changes in pH can be confirmed by an arterial blood gas (ABG) test showing a $PaCO_2$ (carbon dioxide measured in arterial blood) level above 45 mm Hg and a pH below 7.35 (Table 26-3 ■). When the pH falls, hemoglobin is altered to make it give up its oxygen. This altered hemoglobin is alkaline and begins mopping up the excess carbonic acid. Oxygen saturation will drop. The increase in

carbonic acid also causes changes in the respiratory center of the brain. Respirations become shallow and may even be ineffective. The client may exhibit headache, nausea and vomiting, and a change in mental status. If respiratory efforts

TABLE 26-3			
Interpretation of ABG Test			
1. Look at pH	⇑ = alkalosis		
	⇓ = acidosis		
2. Look at $PaCO_2$	= respiratory parameter		
3. Look at HCO_3	= metabolic parameter		
DISORDER	**pH**	**$PaCO_2$**	**HCO_3**
Respiratory acidosis	⇓	⇑	—
Respiratory alkalosis	⇑	⇓	—
Metabolic acidosis	⇓	—	⇓
Metabolic alkalosis	⇑	—	⇑

pH normal = fully compensated
All values abnormal = partially compensated
Two abnormal values = uncompensated

fail to correct the imbalance, the $PaCO_2$ continues to rise. This triggers the kidneys to hold onto bicarbonate and sodium, which combine to form sodium bicarbonate, another buffer to mop up carbonic acid. If these compensatory mechanisms fail to right the imbalance, hydrogen ions move into the cells and force the potassium out. With the potassium now unchecked, the client develops resultant hyperkalemia, heart arrhythmias, and a decreasing level of consciousness. The heart may experience such insult as to result in shock and even cardiac arrest. Treatment for respiratory acidosis is aimed at improving respiratory effort, including administration of oxygen.

RESPIRATORY ALKALOSIS

Respiratory alkalosis may develop when the opposite situation, hyperventilation, occurs. By breathing too rapidly, CO_2 (an acid) is blown off, causing a decrease in $PaCO_2$ and an elevated pH. This can occur when pain, anxiety reactions, or fever cause a client to hyperventilate. Arterial blood gases confirm this situation by showing a pH above 7.45 and $PaCO_2$ below 35 mm Hg. As the body defends itself, hydrogen ions leave the cells in exchange for potassium with resulting hypokalemia. The hydrogen ions join with the bicarbonate ions and lower the pH. As the $PaCO_2$ falls, the carotid and aortic bodies in the medulla are stimulated so the heart rate increases, but no change in the blood pressure occurs. There may be electrocardiographic (ECG) changes or chest pain, or the client may become restless and anxious. The blood vessels in the brain respond to the dropping $PaCO_2$ by constricting, reducing blood flow to the brain. The autonomic nervous system becomes overstimulated, and the client may exhibit dizziness and numbness or tingling in the fingers or toes. The client could be encouraged to breathe into a paper bag, which increases the level of CO_2 in the blood. After about 6 hours of uncompensated alkalosis, the kidneys pour off the bicarbonate and hold back hydrogen ions. The client may show a decreased respiratory rate and hypoventilation. Eventually, the central nervous system (CNS) and the heart are overcome by the alkalosis, resulting in a change in level of consciousness, hyper-reflexes, tetany, heart arrhythmias, seizures, and coma.

METABOLIC ACIDOSIS

Metabolic acidosis occurs when the bicarbonate is lost or acid is increased within the plasma. When fatty acids change to ketone bodies, perhaps from diabetes mellitus, starvation, or severe infection, metabolic acidosis may occur. Excessive loss of GI fluids may cause metabolic acidosis, as could renal insufficiency or failure. Arterial blood gases will confirm the imbalance with a pH below 7.35, a low bicarbonate level, and a low $PaCO_2$ level. The first clue

is hyperventilation as the respiratory system tries to blow off the acid. Although this will correct the imbalance initially, it will not be enough compensation to correct the metabolic imbalance. Deep and rapid respirations (*Kussmaul's respirations*) may eventually develop. The CNS and the heart become depressed. Decreased cardiac function and hypotension may develop. The client develops weakness and headache as the blood vessels in the brain dilate. The client will show a change in the level of consciousness. Diminished muscle tone and deep tendon reflexes may be present. Nausea and vomiting are likely to occur. The kidneys try to correct the imbalance by secreting hydrogen, which combines with ammonia or phosphate and is excreted in the urine. Sodium and bicarbonate are held back by the kidneys to correct the acidosis. Hydrogen goes into the blood, forcing potassium out.

Signs of hyperkalemia may be seen, such as diarrhea, numbness and tingling of fingers or toes, weak or flaccid extremities, slowed heart rate, and ECG changes. The excess hydrogen ions cause further imbalance in the electrolytes, thereby reducing nervous system responses, resulting in CNS depression, lethargy, headache, confusion or stupor, and coma. To treat the acidosis, the underlying cause must be found. Insulin needs to be given for the diabetic client. Insulin forces the potassium back into the cells, treating the hyperkalemia. A patent IV is necessary for effective reversal of this condition. Position the client to promote ventilation, record intake and output, and check oxygen saturation. Assess the level of consciousness frequently and make adaptations in the environment to promote the client's safety should confusion occur. In clients who fail to respond, the nurse should anticipate ventilatory support and possibly dialysis.

METABOLIC ALKALOSIS

Metabolic alkalosis occurs when the plasma loses hydrogen ions (acid) and gains bicarbonate. Arterial blood gases confirm this condition with a $PaCO_2$ greater than 45 mm Hg. The metabolic alkalosis often occurs from diuretics that fail to conserve potassium. Loss of gastric fluids, as in vomiting or NG tube suction, is another primary cause for alkalosis. The excessive bicarbonate ions that do not bind with the chemical buffers depress the vital sign center of the brain, and the client develops a decreased respiratory rate with slow and shallow respirations, thus increasing the $PaCO_2$. The kidneys let go of excess bicarbonate and hold on to the hydrogen ions to correct the imbalance. Sodium is thrown out by the kidneys, and the client shows polyuria followed by hypovolemia and thirst. To compensate for the hydrogen being thrown out by the kidneys, the potassium moves into the cells and the client shows signs of hypokalemia such as anorexia, weakness, and diminished reflexes. Also in response to hydrogen being thrown out, sodium moves into the nerve cells and overstimulates them. The client shows tetany, irritability, disorientation, and seizures. The underlying condition must be treated to reverse the imbalance. Untreated, the client may develop arrhythmias, and death may occur. A patent IV is required to treat this condition. Supplemental oxygen needs to be given when respiratory effort changes or oxygen saturations drop. NG suctioning should be discontinued, and nausea and vomiting treated with antiemetics. Seizure precautions need to be taken for client protection. As a precaution against metabolic alkalosis, NG tubes should be irrigated with normal saline instead of tap water.

NURSING CARE

ASSESSING

In assessing the client's fluid balance, it is important to consider unusual factors that may affect intake and output. If a client is extremely diaphoretic or has rapid, deep respirations, fluid loss is occurring even if it cannot be measured.

clinical ALERT

Report

When there is a significant discrepancy between intake and output or when fluid intake or output is inadequate, report this information to the charge nurse, physician, or other care provider.

Fluid imbalances may be difficult to detect. Poor skin turgor, or a rapid weak pulse with low blood pressure, may indicate dehydration. Noisy, wet respirations and edema may indicate fluid excess.

Acid–base imbalances may be detected initially by changes in respiratory effort or rate. Other vital signs may also be changing. The client may demonstrate a change in level of consciousness such as irritability/restlessness or lethargy, a change in muscle movement or reflexes, headache, nausea and vomiting, and a change in intake and output.

DIAGNOSING, PLANNING, AND IMPLEMENTING

Some common nursing diagnoses for clients with fluid and electrolyte or acid–base problems are *Deficient Fluid Volume*, *Excess Fluid Volume*, and *Impaired Gas Exchange* (see

Chapter 24 ⚭ for information on monitoring oxygenation status). Nursing interventions center on helping the client achieve and maintain homeostasis. Nurses assist clients by monitoring intake and output, monitoring intravenous infusions, and assisting with tubings, drains, and dressing changes.

Monitoring Intake and Output

Intake and output (I&O) is the measurement and recording of all fluid taken in and excreted during a 24-hour period. It provides important data about the client's fluid and electrolyte balance. Generally, I&O are measured for hospitalized at-risk clients. The decision to place a client on intake and output can be an independent nursing measure.

Most agencies have a form for recording I&O, usually a bedside record on which the nurse lists all items measured and their quantities per shift (Figure 26-2 ■). It is important to inform clients, family members, and all caregivers that accurate measurements of the client's fluid intake and output are required. Nursing staff should explain why the I&O is necessary and should emphasize the need to use a bedpan, urinal, commode, or in-toilet collection device. Clients who wish to be involved in recording fluid intake measurements need to be taught how to compute the values and what foods are considered fluids.

			PATIENT LABEL
	Intake and Output Record		
INTAKE	0600-1800	1800-0600	TOTAL
Oral			
Tube feeding			
IV (primary)			
IV Meds			
TPN			
Blood			
TOTAL			24-Hour Total
OUTPUT	0600-1800	1800-0600	TOTAL
Urine			
Emesis			
G.I. Suction			
Stool			
TOTAL			24-Hour Total

Figure 26-2. ■ Sample intake and output record. (Courtesy of El Camino Hospital, Mountain View, California.)

To measure fluid intake, the nurse records each item of fluid intake, specifying the time and type of fluid. All of the following fluids need to be recorded:

- *Oral fluids.* Include water, milk, juice, soft drinks, coffee, tea, cream, soup, and any other beverages. Include water taken with medications. To assess the amount of water taken from a water pitcher, measure what remains and subtract this amount from the volume of the full pitcher. Then refill the pitcher.
- *Ice chips.* Measure ice chips and record the amount of fluid intake as one-half the amount of the ice chips.
- Foods that are or become liquid at room temperature. These include ice cream, sherbet, custard, and gelatin. Do not measure foods that are pureed, because purees are simply solid foods prepared in a different form.
- *Tube feedings.* Record the amount of formula infused during the shift. Remember to include the 30- to 60-mL water rinse at the end of intermittent feedings or during continuous feedings.
- *Parenteral fluids.* The exact amount of intravenous fluid administered is to be recorded, since some fluid containers may be overfilled. Blood transfusions are included.
- *Intravenous medications.* Intravenous medications that are prepared with solutions such as normal saline (NS) and are administered as an intermittent or continuous infusion must also be included.
- *Catheter or tube irrigants.* Fluid used to irrigate urinary catheters, NG tubes, and intestinal tubes must be measured and recorded if not immediately withdrawn.

To measure fluid output, measure the following fluids (remember to observe appropriate infection control precautions):

- *Urinary output.* After the client voids, pour the urine into a measuring container. Measure the amount, then record the time and amount on the I&O form. For clients with retention catheters, empty the drainage bag into a measuring container at the end of the shift (or at prescribed times if output is to be measured more often). Note and record the amount of urine output. In intensive care areas, urine output often is measured hourly.
- *Vomitus and liquid feces.* Measure in a graduated cylinder. Record the amount and type of fluid and the time.
- *Tube drainage.* Record the amount of drainage from gastric or intestinal drainage tubes.
- *Wound drainage and draining fistulas.* Wound drainage may be documented by the type and number of dressings saturated with drainage or by measuring the exact amount of drainage collected in a vacuum drainage or gravity drainage system.

When the nurse compares total intake and total output for a 24-hour period, fluid imbalance will be evident. If intake is greater than output, fluid volume excess is the problem. If intake is less than output, fluid volume deficit is the problem.

Assisting with IV Therapy

When a client is unable to drink fluids, IV therapy is ordered to prevent fluid volume deficit and to provide necessary electrolytes.

Rules and regulations regarding the role of LPNs and LVNs in IV therapy vary from state to state. They are available from the Board of Nursing in each state. It is your responsibility to know what is legal for you to do; *always* perform duties within your scope of practice.

Intravenous Solutions

Intravenous solutions can be classified as isotonic, hypotonic, or hypertonic. Most IV solutions are isotonic, such as 0.9% sodium chloride (has the same concentration of solutes as blood plasma). **Isotonic** solutions are often used to restore vascular volume. **Hypertonic** solutions, such as 0.9% sodium chloride with 5% dextrose, have a greater concentration of solutes than plasma. **Hypotonic** solutions, such as 0.45% sodium chloride, have a lesser concentration of solutes.

IV solutions can also be categorized according to their purpose. *Nutrient solutions* contain carbohydrate in the form of dextrose. IV dextrose solution provide 3.4 calories per gram. For example, 1 L of 5% dextrose provides 170 calories. This amount of calories and fluid helps prevent dehydration and ketosis, but does not provide enough nutrients for body functions such as wound healing.

Electrolyte solutions contain varying amounts of cations and anions. Commonly used solutions are normal saline (0.9% sodium chloride solution), Ringer's solution (which contains sodium, chloride, potassium, and calcium), and lactated Ringer's solution (which contains sodium, chloride, potassium, calcium, and lactate). Saline and balanced electrolyte solutions commonly are used to restore vascular volume, particularly after trauma or surgery. They also may be used to replace fluid and electrolytes for clients with continuing losses, for example, because of gastric suction or wound drainage.

Volume expanders are used to increase the blood volume following severe loss of blood (e.g., from hemorrhage) or loss of plasma (e.g., from severe burns, which draw large amounts of plasma from the bloodstream to the burn site). Common volume expanders are dextran, plasma, and human serum albumin.

Assessing and Monitoring IV Infusion Sites

Monitoring IV infusion sites is a frequent responsibility of the LPN/LVN. Be aware of and assess visually for redness and swelling at the infusion site. Make sure bedding is not crushing the tubing or slowing flow and that blood is not backing up in the tubing. Notify the team leader if problems are noted. Be aware of IV bags that are near empty. Report them to the team leader so that they can be changed by trained personnel. Many facilities have IV infusion pumps equipped with alarms. If the pump alarm sounds, notify the team leader. Do not just turn it off.

Discontinuing an IV

The physician may order an IV to be discontinued when it is no longer necessary or to be converted to a saline or heparin lock to provide a route for medication administration.

Monitoring for Acid–Base Disorders

It may be impossible to determine the exact imbalance through signs and symptoms. Nurses work in collaboration with the physician and laboratory personnel to identify the problem. Laboratory results—ABGs—will be the determinant of the client's imbalance. The LPN/LVN needs to be aware of normal values and should routinely check lab results to confirm clinical signs. The client should be monitored for changes in vital signs, especially in respiratory effort or rate. Lung sounds may be diminished or absent. The pulse oximeter recordings should be monitored for decreasing oxygen levels. (See Chapter 24 🔗 for more information about supporting oxygenation.) Level of consciousness and presence of seizures need to be followed to determine the extent of the imbalance. Reflexes may be hyperreflexive or absent, depending on the particular imbalance. The client may complain of numbness or tingling in fingers or toes, lethargy, or headache. A change in urinary output or NG output would be significant to report. The nurse performs regular assessment of mental status and vital signs. Any client who has an intake and output imbalance is at risk for acid–base imbalance, and should be monitored closely until balance is achieved.

EVALUATING

The client with fluid and electrolyte or acid–base disorders must be monitored regularly and carefully. Data on vital signs and I&O should be collected. IV and respiratory therapy must be monitored as ordered. Changes in level of consciousness, abnormal or worsening vital signs, and fluid imbalances should be reported to the charge nurse or physician.

CONTINUING CARE

Teaching needs to take place addressing the underlying cause of imbalances. How the client should take his or her medications, especially new prescriptions, should be reviewed, and the client's questions should be answered. The client needs to know what signs might indicate that a respiratory compensation is beginning and what to report. Therapeutic dietary changes need to be reviewed.

NURSING PROCESS CARE PLAN
Client with Electrolyte Imbalance

Marcus Smith is a 69-year-old male who has been diagnosed with intrarenal renal failure. He has experienced damage to his nephrons and kidney tissue, resulting from an allergic reaction to contrasts dye administered during an IVP to r/o renal calculi. He has been on a sodium-restricted diet in an attempt to regulate fluid balance. His weight has increased 11 lbs. in one week's time, due to fluid retention. He has expressed concern that he will need to begin dialysis if his condition does not improve.

Assessment. VS: T 99, P 110, R 28, BP 188/94. Weight today 196, c/o nausea, and unable to eat. Urine output 200 mL/24 hours. Lab tests indicate elevated BUN and serum creatinine levels. Mr. Smith's daughter is concerned because he seems to her to be confused.

Nursing Diagnosis. The following nursing diagnoses (among others) are established for Mr. Smith:

- *Impaired Urinary Elimination*
- *Ineffective Renal Tissue Perfusion*
- *Fluid Volume Excess*
- *Acute Confusion*

Expected Outcomes. The expected outcomes for the plan of care are that Mr. Smith will:

- Decrease in weight of 1–2 lbs per day
- Participate in psychiatric counseling program on a regular basis
- Demonstrate stable weight without further losses in immediate future
- Serum electrolytes within normal limits.

Planning and Implementation. The following nursing interventions are implemented for Mr. Smith. Assessments are done frequently to monitor his condition.

- Monitor weight daily.
- Monitor for electrolyte imbalance.
- Monitor fluid intake and urine output.
- Administer antihypertensive and diuretics per physician's orders.

- Offer several small meals of sodium-restricted, low protein diet.
- Administer vitamin supplements as ordered.
- Reorient client as needed.
- Provide opportunity for client and family to express feelings concerning possibility of dialysis treatment.

Evaluation. Appetite improved, able to eat small amounts without nausea. Weight decreased to 190 lbs. Sodium, calcium, and potassium levels within normal limits. Urinary output 800 mL/24 hours. Mr. Smith and his daughter are asking questions about the dialysis.

Critical Thinking in the Nursing Process

1. Why would Mr. Smith be placed on a sodium-restricted diet when his sodium levels appear normal?
2. What is the probably cause of Mr. Smith's confusion and disorientation?
3. Mr. Smith's daughter asks how long he will need dialysis. What would be an appropriate answer to her question?

Note: Discussion of Critical Thinking questions appears in Appendix I.

Note: The references and resources for this and all chapters have been compiled at the back of the book.

Chapter Review

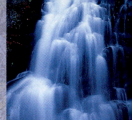

 ## KEY TERMS by Topic

Use the audio glossary feature of either the CD-ROM or the Companion Website to hear the correct pronunciation of the following key terms.

Body Fluids and Electrolyte Balance
fluid, intracellular fluid (ICF), extracellular fluid (ECF), interstitial fluid, electrolytes

Acid–Base Balance
buffers

Acid–Base Imbalances
respiratory acidosis, respiratory alkalosis, metabolic acidosis, metabolic alkalosis, intake and output (I&O), isotonic, hypertonic, hypotonic

KEY Points

- Homeostasis depends on many physiological processes. These processes regulate fluid intake and output. They also regulate the movement of water and dissolved substances between the body compartments.

- Fluid imbalances may signal the development of disease. Imbalances between fluid intake and fluid output need to be addressed without delay.

- Most electrolytes enter the body through dietary intake and are excreted in the urine. Some electrolytes, such as sodium and chloride, are not stored by the body and must be consumed daily to maintain normal levels.

- Changes in electrolyte levels and in acid–base balance can be life threatening. Clients with electrolyte or acid–base imbalances must be monitored often.

- If the flow of IV fluids is incorrect, problems such as hypervolemia, hypovolemia, or inadequate medication administration can result. The role of the LPN/LVN includes safe administration of such fluids. The LPN/LVN must consult a baseline assessment of the client's fluid status in order to evaluate fluid balance.

- The role of the LPN/LVN includes collecting data on the IV site at each assessment and before delivering medicated infusions.

 ## EXPLORE MediaLink

Additional interactive resources for this chapter can be found on the Companion Website at www.prenhall.com/ramont. Click on Chapter 26 and "Begin" to select the activities for this chapter.

For chapter-related NCLEX®-style questions and an audio glossary, access the accompanying CD-ROM in this book.

Animations/Videos
- Acid–Base Balance
- Fluids
- Membrane Transport

FOR FURTHER Study

See Chapter 24 for information on monitoring oxygenation status.

See Chapter 30 for more information on IV therapy.

Critical Thinking Care Map

Caring for a Client with Risk for Deficient Fluid Volume
NCLEX-PN® Focus Area: Physiological Integrity

Case Study: Patti Glove, a 40-year-old female, was admitted to an acute care hospital for treatment of intractable nausea/vomiting and diarrhea. Patti states that she has been experiencing the nausea and vomiting for the past 3 days, with the diarrhea beginning yesterday. She has not taken any medications at home for this condition. No fluids have been "kept down" for the 3 days. Patti states that she has been very weak and feels faint when she stands up.

Nursing Diagnosis: Deficient Fluid Volume

COLLECT DATA

Subjective	Objective
_____	_____
_____	_____
_____	_____
_____	_____
_____	_____
_____	_____
_____	_____

Would you report this? Yes/No

If yes, to: _____

What would you report? _____

Nursing Care

_____
_____
_____
_____
_____
_____
_____
_____
_____
_____
_____

How would you document this? _____
_____
_____

Compare your documentation to the sample provided in Appendix I.

Data Collected
(use those that apply)

- Weight: 145 lbs
- Blood pressure 98/62
- Pulse 110, regular
- Respirations, 16
- Mood: irritable, anxious
- States she is very thirsty
- Oxygen saturation: 93% on room air
- Nausea and vomiting present
- Mucous membranes dry
- Skin turgor poor
- Urine dark amber, 50 mL in last voiding

Nursing Interventions
(use those that apply; list in priority order)

- Monitor and report abnormal lab results.
- Monitor and document intake and output.
- Encourage fluid intake.
- Regularly monitor abdominal girth.
- Teach client to stand slowly.
- Monitor color, amount, and frequency of fluid loss.
- Assess for vertigo and hypotension.
- Take daily weights.
- Give and monitor effectiveness of antinausea medication as ordered.
- Give and monitor effectiveness of antidiarrheal medications as ordered.
- Monitor orthostatic blood pressure every 4 hours.
- Administer IV therapy as ordered.
- Provide frequent oral care.
- Teach client about intake/output measurement.

TEST-TAKING TIP Read all the choices for answers and eliminate those that you know are incorrect. If you narrow your choices down to two options, reread the stem (question) and decide which of the two choices *BEST* answers the question.

1 A client is in a lot of pain and breathing rapidly. The nurse recognizes this will cause CO_2 (carbon dioxide) to be exhaled and the client may develop which acid–base imbalance? _____.

2 The nurse is calculating the intake and output on a client. Which of the following client conditions would be considered an insensible fluid loss? The client:

1. has been perspiring heavily.
2. had a large emesis.
3. has a temperature of 36.8°C.
4. had a blood pressure reading of 92/50.

3 You are totaling the intake and output record for your shift. The client's IV fluid intake for the shift is 1,200 mL, and the output is 2,200 mL from a Foley catheter drainage bag. The client received 1,000 mL PO, and had emesis of 75 mL. What was the client's total output for your shift?

1. 3,125 mL
2. 2,275 mL
3. 2,200 mL
4. 2,125 mL

4 A client is receiving an intravenous solution of 0.45% sodium chloride. This is an example of which type of fluid replacement solution?

1. isotonic
2. hypotonic
3. hypertonic
4. osmotic

5 When assessing an intravenous site, the LPN/LVN observes redness and swelling. Which action should be taken by the LPN/LVN?

1. Elevate the affected extremity.
2. Apply a cool washcloth to the site.
3. Notify the primary nurse.
4. Reduce the flow rate of the intravenous solution.

6 The nurse is calculating the fluid intake of a client. Which of the following would not be included in the calculation?

1. ice chips
2. pureed foods
3. intravenous medications
4. nasogastric tube irrigation

7 When an isotonic solution is administered, fluid moves from an area of low concentration to an area of high concentration to achieve fluid balance. This occurs because the administered fluid:

1. has a lower concentration than the blood.
2. has a higher concentration than the blood.
3. will cause a shift in fluids to expand intravascular compartments.
4. has the same concentration as blood.

8 A client is admitted with diabetic ketoacidosis (DKA). Due to the ketone bodies formed, the client is most likely experiencing which of the following acid–base imbalances?

1. metabolic acidosis
2. metabolic alkalosis
3. respiratory acidosis
4. respiratory alkalosis

9 A client is experiencing a potassium deficiency secondary to diuretic therapy. The nurse recognizes this electrolyte deficiency could lead to:

1. osteoporosis.
2. abnormal cardiac function.
3. stress fractures.
4. excessive mucous production.

10 You are instructing a client on sodium restrictions about the purpose for the low-salt diet recently prescribed. You explain the importance of this diet, including the fact that the primary electrolyte for control and regulation of fluid balance in the body is

1. sodium.
2. potassium.
3. calcium.
4. magnesium.

Answers and Rationales for Review Questions, as well as discussion of Care Plan and Critical Thinking Care Map questions, appear in Appendix I.

Chapter 27

Urinary Elimination

BRIEF Outline

Physiology of Urinary Elimination
Factors Affecting Urinary Excretion
Altered Urine Production
Altered Urinary Elimination
Collaborative Care

HISTORICAL Perspectives

The yellow color of urine was previously thought to come from gold. Alchemists spent much time trying to extract gold from urine, and this led to some interesting discoveries such as white phosphorus by the German alchemist Hennig Brand in 1669 when he was distilling fermented urine. In 1773, the French chemist Hilaire Rouelle discovered the organic compound urea by boiling urine dry. The ancient Romans used urine as a bleaching agent for cleaning clothes, and as a teeth whitener.

Urine has also been historically used as an antiseptic. In times when other antiseptics were unavailable, urine, the darker the better, was utilized on open wounds to kill bacteria. Urine is known to be good against jellyfish stings because it neutralizes the pH of the venom. Urine from males is recommended because it is stronger.

LEARNING Outcomes

After completing this chapter, you will be able to:

1. Describe the process of urination.
2. Identify factors that influence urinary elimination.
3. Describe common alterations in urine production and elimination.
4. Describe nursing assessment of urinary function.
5. Identify normal and abnormal characteristics and constituents of urine.
6. List and describe basic urine tests, measure urinary output, and collect urine specimens.
7. Describe interventions to maintain normal urinary elimination.
8. Identify methods of preventing urinary infection.
9. Identify interventions for clients with retention catheters or urinary diversions.

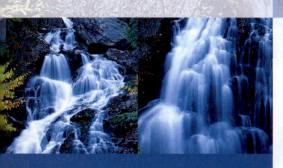

Urinary elimination is essential to health, and voiding can be postponed for only so long before the urge normally becomes too great to control. Urinary elimination depends on effective functioning of four urinary tract organs: kidneys, ureters, bladder, and urethra (Figure 27-1 ■).

Physiology of Urinary Elimination

KIDNEYS

The paired kidneys are situated on either side of the spinal column, behind the peritoneal cavity. They are the primary regulators of fluid and acid–base balance in the body. The functional units of the kidneys, the nephrons, filter the blood and remove metabolic wastes. In the average adult, 1,200 mL of blood pass through the kidneys every minute. Each kidney contains about 1 million nephrons. Each nephron has a glomerulus and a tuft of capillaries surrounded by Bowman's capsule (Figure 27-2 ■). The glomerular capillaries are porous, allowing fluid and solutes to move across this membrane into the capsule.

From the Bowman's capsule, the filtrate moves into the tubule of the nephron. In the proximal convoluted tubule, most of the water and electrolytes are reabsorbed. Solutes are reabsorbed in the loop of Henle, but in the same area

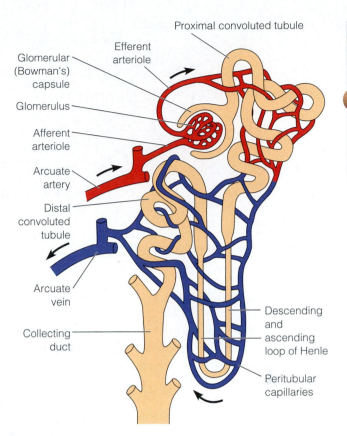

Figure 27-2. ■ The nephrons of the kidney are composed of six parts: the glomerulus, Bowman's capsule, proximal convoluted tubule, loop of Henle, distal convoluted tubule, and collecting duct.

other substances are secreted into the filtrate, concentrating the urine. In the distal convoluted tubule, additional water and sodium are reabsorbed under the control of hormones such as antidiuretic hormone (ADH) and aldosterone. When fluid intake is low or the concentration of solutes in the blood is high, more water is reabsorbed in the distal tubule, and less urine is excreted. The processes of controlled reabsorption specifically regulate fluid and electrolyte balance in the body.

URETERS

Once the urine is formed in the kidneys, it moves into the renal pelvis and from there into the ureters. The ureters are 10 to 12 in. long and about 0.5 in. wide in adults. The ureter is funnel shaped as it enters the kidney. The lower ends of the ureters enter the bladder at the posterior corners of the floor of the bladder (see Figure 27-1). At the junction between the ureter and the bladder, a valve prevents reflux (backflow) of urine up the ureters.

BLADDER

The urinary bladder is a hollow, muscular organ that serves as a reservoir for urine and as the organ of excretion. In males the bladder lies in front of the rectum and above the prostate

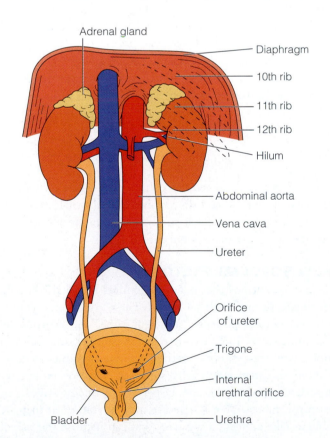

Figure 27-1. ■ Anatomic structures of the urinary tract.

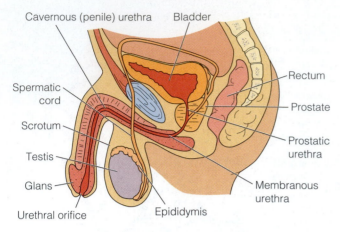

Figure 27-3. ■ The male urogenital system.

gland (Figure 27-3 ■). In females it lies in front of the uterus and vagina (Figure 27-4 ■). The base of the bladder is a triangular area marked by the ureter openings at the posterior corners and the opening of the urethra at the anterior inferior corner. Urine exits the bladder through the urethra.

The bladder is able to stretch because of rugae (folds) in the mucous membrane lining and because of the elasticity of its walls. When full, the bladder may extend above the symphysis pubis. In extreme situations it may extend as high as the umbilicus.

URETHRA

The urethra extends from the bladder to the urinary meatus (opening) external body and serves only as a passageway for the elimination of urine. The female's urinary meatus is located between the labia minora, in front of the vagina and below the clitoris. The female urethra is 1 to 1.5 in. long. The male urethra is about 8 in. long and serves as a passageway for semen as well as urine (see Figure 27-3). The male's urinary meatus is located at the distal end of the penis.

The internal sphincter muscle situated at the base of the urinary bladder is under involuntary control. The external

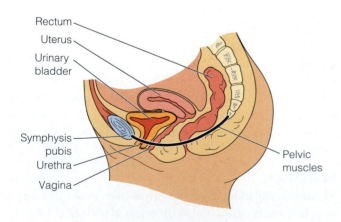

Figure 27-4. ■ The female urogenital system.

sphincter muscle is under voluntary control, allowing the individual to choose when urine is eliminated.

In both males and females, the urethra has a mucous membrane lining that is continuous with the bladder and the ureters. This structure facilities the spread of an infection of the urethra throughout the urinary tract to the kidneys. Women are particularly prone to urinary tract infections because of their short urethra and the proximity of the urinary **meatus** to the vagina and anus.

URINATION

Micturition, **voiding**, and *urination* all refer to the process of emptying the urinary bladder. Urine collects in the bladder until pressure stimulates special sensory nerve endings in the bladder wall called stretch receptors. These receptors respond when the adult bladder contains between 250 and 450 mL of urine by transmitting impulses to the spinal cord, causing the internal sphincter to relax and stimulating the urge to void. The conscious portion of the brain relaxes the external urethral sphincter muscle and urination takes place. If the time and place are inappropriate, voluntary controls allow the micturition reflex to subside until the bladder becomes more filled and the reflex is involuntarily stimulated again.

Voluntary control of urination is possible only if the nerves supplying the bladder and urethra, the neural tracts of the cord and brain, and the motor area of the cerebrum are intact. An individual must be able to sense that the bladder is full. Injury to any part of the nervous system above the level of the sacral region results in intermittent involuntary emptying of the bladder. Older people whose cognition is impaired may not be aware of the need to urinate or be able to respond appropriately to nervous system stimulus.

Factors Affecting Urinary Excretion

Numerous factors affect the volume and characteristics of the urine produced and the manner in which it is excreted.

See Table 27-1 ■ for a summary of the developmental changes affecting urinary output.

PSYCHOSOCIAL FACTORS

Certain conditions that relate to comfort or relaxation help stimulate the micturition reflex. These conditions include privacy, normal position, sufficient time, and occasionally running water. Inability to relax abdominal and perineal muscles and the external urethral sphincter inhibits voiding. People also may voluntarily suppress urination (voluntary **urinary retention**) because of perceived time pressures. For example, nurses often ignore the urge to void until they are able to take a break, a behavior that can increase the risk of urinary tract infections (UTIs).

TABLE 27-1	
Changes in Urinary Elimination through the Life Span	
STAGE	**VARIATIONS**
Fetus	The fetal kidney begins to excrete urine between the 11th and 12th week of development.
Infant	Ability to concentrate urine is minimal; therefore, urine appears light yellow.
	Because of neuromuscular immaturity, voluntary urinary control is absent.
Child	Kidney function reaches maturity between the first and second year of life; urine is concentrated effectively and appears a normal amber color.
	Between 18 and 24 months of age, the child starts to recognize bladder fullness and is able to hold urine beyond the urge to void.
	At approximately $2^1/_2$ to 3 years of age, the child can perceive bladder fullness, hold urine after the urge to void, and communicate the need to urinate.
	Full urinary control usually occurs at age 4 or 5 years; daytime control is usually achieved by age 3 years.
	The kidneys grow in proportion to overall body growth.
Adult	The kidneys reach maximum size between 35 and 40 years of age.
	After 50 years the kidneys begin to diminish in size and function. Most shrinkage occurs in the cortex of the kidney as individual nephrons are lost.
Older adult	An estimated 30% of nephrons are lost by age 80.
	Renal blood flow decreases because of vascular changes and a decrease in cardiac output.
	The ability to concentrate urine declines.
	Bladder muscle tone diminishes, causing increased frequency of urination and nocturia (awakening to urinate at night).
	Diminished bladder muscle tone and contractibility may lead to residual urine in the bladder after voiding, increasing the risk of bacterial growth and infection.
	Urinary incontinence may occur due to mobility problems or urologic impairments.

FLUID AND FOOD INTAKE

The healthy body maintains a balance between the amount of fluid ingested and the amount of fluid eliminated. When the amount of fluid intake increases, the output normally increases. Certain fluids, such as alcohol, increase fluid output by inhibiting the production of ADH. Fluids that contain caffeine (e.g., coffee, tea, and cola drinks) also increase urine production. By contrast, food and fluids high in sodium can cause fluid retention.

Some foods and fluids can change the color of urine. For example, beets and blackberries can cause urine to appear red; foods containing carotene can cause the urine to appear more yellow.

MEDICATION

Many medications, particularly those affecting the autonomic nervous system, interfere with the normal urination process and may cause retention. Included among the medications that may cause urinary retention are antispasmodics, antidepressants, antihypertensives, and antihistamines. **Diuretics** increase urine formation by preventing the reabsorption of water and electrolytes from the tubules of the kidney into the bloodstream. Diuretics are commonly prescribed for hypertension and cardiac disease to decrease fluid volume. Some medications also affect the color of urine.

MUSCLE TONE AND ACTIVITY

Regular exercise increases the muscle tone of the bladder and sphincters and also increases the metabolic rate. Clients who require a retention catheter for a long period may have poor bladder muscle tone because continuous drainage of urine prevents the bladder from filling and emptying normally. Abdominal muscle contraction assists in bladder emptying. Pelvic muscle tone is a factor in being able to retain urine voluntarily once the urge to urinate is perceived.

PATHOLOGIC CONDITIONS

Some diseases and pathologies can affect the formation and excretion of urine. Diseases of the kidneys may affect the ability of the nephrons to produce urine. Abnormal amounts of protein or blood cells may be present in the urine, or the kidneys may virtually stop producing urine altogether, a condition known as renal failure. Heart and circulatory disorders such as heart failure, shock, or hyperten-

Urinary or Male Reproductive System Disorders

African American males have a higher incidence of prostate cancer than any other race. They are also more likely to die from prostate cancer. Their mortality rate is more than double that of any other racial or ethnic group. Education about prevention and screening procedures is particularly important in the African American community, especially with young adult males. This age group does not routinely see a healthcare provider unless ill or injured.

Because of the high incidence of prostate cancer, it is recommended that all African American males have a yearly digital rectal examination and a prostate-specific antigen screening after the age of 40.

sion can affect blood flow to the kidneys, interfering with urine production. If abnormal amounts of fluid are lost through another route (e.g., vomiting or high fever), water is retained by the kidneys and urinary output falls.

A urinary stone (**calculus**) may obstruct a ureter, blocking urine flow from the kidney to the bladder. Hypertrophy of the prostate gland, a common condition affecting older men, may partially obstruct the urethra, impairing urination and bladder emptying. (Box 27-1 ■ discusses cultural aspects of prostate cancer.) Painful or difficult urination is termed **dysuria** and may be caused by multiple conditions.

Altered Urine Production

Although patterns of urination are highly individual, most people void about five to seven times a day: usually upon awakening, before going to bed, and around mealtimes. Evidence of blood in the urine is known as **hematuria**.

POLYURIA

Polyuria refers to the production of abnormally large amounts of urine by the kidneys. Polyuria can follow excessive fluid intake (*polydipsia*). It may be associated with diseases such as diabetes mellitus, diabetes insipidus, or chronic nephritis. **Diuresis** is another term for the production and excretion of large amounts of urine. This term is often used when medications are given to promote urine output. Polyuria or diuresis can cause excessive fluid loss, leading to intense thirst, dehydration, and weight loss. **Enuresis** is urinary incontinence usually occurring at night in children, commonly known as bedwetting. The causes may be stress, UTI, trauma, or disease.

OLIGURIA AND ANURIA

The terms *oliguria* and *anuria* are used to describe decreased urinary output. **Oliguria** is low urine output, usually less than 500 mL a day or 30 mL an hour. **Anuria** refers to a lack of urine production, with no effective urinary output. Although oliguria may occur as a result of abnormal fluid losses or a lack of fluid intake, it often indicates impaired blood flow to the kidneys or impending renal failure.

Altered Urinary Elimination

Despite normal urine production, a number of factors or conditions can affect urinary elimination. Selected factors associated with altered patterns of urine elimination are identified in Table 27-2 ■.

Collaborative Care

DIAGNOSTIC TESTS

Blood levels of urea and creatinine are routinely used to evaluate renal function. Both are normally eliminated by the kidneys through filtration. Urea, the end product of protein metabolism, is measured as blood urea nitrogen (BUN). Creatinine is produced in relatively constant quantities by the muscles. The creatinine clearance test uses 24-hour urine and serum creatinine levels to determine the glomerular filtration rate, a sensitive indicator of renal function.

Visualization procedures also may be used to evaluate urinary function. The KUB is an x-ray of the kidneys, ureters, and bladder. Intravenous pyelography (IVP) is a radiographic study used to evaluate the urinary tract. In IVP, contrast medium is injected intravenously. Following injection of the contrast medium, x-rays are taken to evaluate urinary tract structures. A computed axial tomography (CAT) scan is a painless, noninvasive x-ray procedure that distinguishes minor differences in the density of tissues. Renal ultrasonography is a noninvasive test that uses reflected sound waves to visualize the kidneys. During a cystoscopy, the bladder, ureteral orifices, and urethra can be visualized using a cystoscope, a lighted instrument inserted through the urethra.

Nurses are responsible for preparing clients for these studies and for follow-up care. Nurses also perform several tests on the unit. These are discussed later in the Diagnosing, Planning, and Implementing section that follows.

NURSING CARE

ASSESSING

The LPN/LVN is responsible for assessing the client's urinary function by collecting data and collaborating with the RN on findings related to the following factors: The nurse determines the client's normal voiding pattern and frequency, appearance of the urine and any recent changes, any past or current problems with urination, the presence of an ostomy, and factors influencing the elimination pattern.

TABLE 27-2

Selected Factors Associated with Altered Urinary Elimination

PATTERNS	SELECTED ASSOCIATED FACTORS
Polyuria (diuresis) (eliminating abnormally large amounts of urine)	Ingestion of fluids containing caffeine or alcohol Prescribed diuretic Presence of thirst, dehydration, and weight loss History of diabetes mellitus, diabetes insipidus, or kidney disease
Oliguria, anuria (low amounts of urine or no urine)	Decrease in fluid intake Signs of dehydration Presence of hypotension, shock, or heart failure History of kidney disease Signs of renal failure such as elevated blood urea nitrogen and serum creatinine, edema, hypertension
Frequency or nocturia (voiding more than usual; nocturia is voiding two or more times at night)	Pregnancy Increase in fluid intake Urinary tract infection Any known contributing or initiating causes, such as stress (small quantities voided 50–100 mL)
Urgency (feeling that voiding must occur immediately)	Presence of psychological stress Urinary tract infection
Dysuria (painful of difficult urination)	Urinary tract inflammation, infection, or injury Presence of other signs that may accompany dysuria, such as hesitancy, hematuria, pyuria (pus in the urine) and frequency. Burning may accompany or follow voiding
Enuresis (involuntary discharge of urine after voluntary control has normally been reached)	Family history of enuresis Difficult access to toilet facilities Home stresses
Incontinence (inability to control excretion)	Bladder inflammation or other disease Difficulties in independent toileting (mobility impairment) Leakage when coughing, laughing, sneezing Cognitive impairment
Retention	Distended bladder on palpation and percussion Associated signs, such as pubic discomfort, restlessness, frequency, and small urine volume Recent anesthesia Recent perineal surgery Presence of perineal swelling Prescribed medications Lack of privacy or other factors inhibiting micturition
Neurogenic bladder (dysfunction of nerves supplying the bladder	Lesions of the central nervous system or of nerves supplying the bladder

BOX 27-2

Assessment Interview: Urinary Elimination

Voiding Pattern

- How many times do you void during a 24-hour period?
- Has this pattern changed recently?
- Do you need to get out of bed to void at night? How often?

Description of Urine and Any Changes

- How would you describe your urine in terms of color, clarity (clear, transparent, or cloudy), and odor (faint or strong)?

Urinary Elimination Problems

- What problems have you had or do you now have with passing your urine?
- Passage of small amounts of urine?
- Voiding at more frequent intervals?
- Painful voiding?
- Difficulty starting urine stream?
- Frequent dribbling of urine or feeling of bladder fullness associated with voiding small amounts of urine?
- Accidental leakage of urine? If so, when does this occur?
- Past urinary tract illness such as infection of the kidney, bladder, or urethra; urinary calculi; surgery of kidney, ureters, or bladder?

Presence and Management of Urinary Diversion Ostomy

- What is your usual routine with your ostomy?
- What problems, if any, do you have with it?
- How can the nurse help you manage it?

Factors Influencing Urinary Elimination

- *Medications.* Do you take any medications that could increase urinary output (e.g., diuretic) or cause retention of urine (e.g., anticholinergic-antispasmodic, antidepressant-antipsychotic, anti-parkinsonism, antihistamines, antihypertensives)? Note specific medication and dosage.
- *Fluid intake.* What amount and kind of fluid do you take each day?
- *Environmental factors.* Do you have any problems with toileting?
- *Presence of long-term catheter.* How do you care for your catheter?
- *Stress.* Are you experiencing any long-term or short-term stress?
- *Disease.* Have you had or do you have any illnesses that may affect urinary function, such as hypertension, heart disease, neurologic disease (e.g., multiple sclerosis), cancer, prostatic enlargement, diabetes mellitus, or diabetes insipidus?

Examples of interview questions to elicit this information are presented in Box 27-2 ■.

Complete physical assessment of the urinary tract will be completed by the RN and usually includes palpation of the kidneys to detect areas of tenderness. Palpation of the bladder is also performed. The urethral meatus of both male and female clients may be inspected for swelling, discharge, and inflammation.

Because problems with urination can affect the elimination of wastes from the body, it is important for the LPN/LVN to observe the skin for color, texture, and tissue turgor as well as for the presence of edema. If incontinence, dribbling, or dysuria is noted in the history, the skin of the perineum should be inspected for irritation because contact with urine can excoriate the skin.

Urine Characteristics

Normal urine consists of 96% water and 4% solutes. Organic solutes include urea, ammonia, creatinine, and uric acid. Inorganic solutes include sodium, chloride, potassium, sulfate, magnesium, and phosphorus. Characteristics of normal and abnormal urine are shown in Table 27-3 ■.

DIAGNOSING, PLANNING, AND IMPLEMENTING

The North American Nursing Diagnosis Association (NANDA) includes one general diagnostic label for urinary elimination problems and subcategories that are more specific.

The goals established will vary according to the diagnosis and related defining characteristics. Examples of overall goals for clients with urinary elimination problems may include:

- Maintaining or restoring normal voiding pattern
- Regaining normal urine output
- Preventing associated risks such as infection, skin breakdown, fluid and electrolyte imbalance, and lowered self-esteem.

Examples of desired outcomes for these goals and others are listed in Table 27-4 ■.

Measuring Urinary Output

Normally, the kidneys produce urine at a rate of approximately 60 mL per hour or about 1,500 mL per day. Urine output is affected by many factors, including fluid intake, body fluid losses through other routes such as perspiration and breathing, and the cardiovascular and renal status of the individual.

Urine outputs below 30 mL per hour may indicate low blood volume or kidney malfunction and must be reported.

To measure fluid output, the nurse follows these steps:

1. Wear clean gloves to prevent contact with microorganisms or blood in urine.
2. Ask the client to void in a clean urinal, bedpan, commode, or toilet collection device ("hat").
3. Instruct the client to keep urine separate from feces and to avoid putting toilet paper in the urine collection container.
4. Pour the voided urine into a calibrated container.

TABLE 27-3

Characteristics of Normal and Abnormal Urine

CHARACTERISTIC	NORMAL	ABNORMAL	NURSING CONSIDERATIONS
Amount in 24 hours (adult)	1,200–1,500 mL	Under 1,200 mL Over 1,500 mL	Urinary output normally is approximately equal to fluid intake. Output of less than 30 mL/h may indicate decreased blood flow to the kidneys and should be immediately reported.
Color, clarity	Straw, amber Transparent	Dark amber Cloudy Dark orange Red or dark brown Mucous plugs, viscid, thick	Concentrated urine is darker in color. Dilute urine may appear almost clear, or very pale yellow. Some foods and drugs may color urine (e.g., beets, phenazopyridine, phenytoin). Red blood cells in the urine (hematuria) may be evident as pink, bright red, or rusty brown urine. Menstrual bleeding can also color urine but should not be confused with hematuria. White blood cells, bacteria, pus, or contaminants such as prostatic fluid, sperm, or vaginal drainage may cause cloudy urine.
Odor	Faint aromatic	Offensive	Some foods (e.g., asparagus) cause a musty odor; infected urine can have a fetid odor; urine high in glucose has a sweet odor.
Sterility	No microorganisms present	Microorganisms present	Urine specimens may be contaminated by bacteria from the perineum during collection.
pH	4.5–8	Under 4.5 Over 8	Freshly voided urine is normally somewhat acidic. Alkaline urine may indicate a state of alkalosis, urinary tract infection, or a diet high in fruits and vegetables. More acidic urine (low pH) is found in acidosis, starvation, diarrhea, or with a diet high in protein foods or cranberries.
Specific gravity	1.010–1.025	Under 1.010 Over 1.025	Concentrated urine has a higher specific gravity; diluted urine has a lower specific gravity.
Glucose	Not present	Present	Glucose in the urine indicates high blood glucose levels (>180 mg/dL), and may be indicative of undiagnosed or uncontrolled diabetes mellitus.
Ketone bodies (acetone)	Not present	Present	Ketones, the end product of the breakdown of fatty acids, are not normally present in the urine. They may be present in the urine of clients who have uncontrolled diabetes mellitus, are in a state of starvation, or who have ingested excessive amounts of aspirin.
Blood	Not present	Occult (microscopic) Bright red	Blood may be present in the urine of clients who have urinary tract infection, kidney disease, or bleeding from the urinary tract.

5. Holding the container at eye level, read the amount in the container.
6. If a specimen is required, pour some urine into the specimen container and discard the remainder, unless all urine is to be saved.
7. Record the amount on the fluid intake and output sheet, which may be at the client's bedside or in the bathroom.
8. Rinse the urine collection and measuring containers with cool water and store.
9. Remove gloves and wash hands.
10. Calculate and document the total output at the end of each shift and at the end of 24 hours on the client's chart.

Many clients can measure and record their own urine output when the procedure is explained to them.

When measuring urine from a client who has an indwelling catheter, the nurse follows these steps:

1. Wear clean gloves.
2. Take the calibrated container to the bedside.
3. Place the container under the urine collection bag so that the spout of the bag is above the container but not touching it. The calibrated container *is not* sterile; the inside of the collection bag *is* sterile.
4. Open the spout and permit the urine to flow into the container.
5. Close the spout, then proceed as described in the previous list.

Measuring Residual Urine

Residual urine (urine remaining in the bladder following the voiding) is normally not present or consists of only a few

---

TABLE 27-4

Evaluation Goals and Outcomes: Urinary Elimination

GOALS	EXAMPLES OF DESIRED OUTCOMES
Restore normal voiding pattern	Absence of pain, burning, hesitancy, or urgency with urination
	Voids at 3- to 4-hour intervals with no more than one voiding during the night
	Remains dry between voidings and at night
	Performs pelvic floor muscle exercises correctly at specified frequency
Perform toilet activities independently with or without assistive devices	Able to access toilet facilities or appropriate receptacle (urinal, commode) for voiding
	Able to manipulate clothing for voiding
	Able to get on and off toilet unassisted
	Cleans perineal area with tissue (and as necessary with soap and water) appropriately after voiding and defecating
Regain normal urine output	Quantity of urine at each voiding is within expected range (e.g., greater than 150 mL)
	Bladder empties completely with each voiding (e.g., bladder is nonpalpable and postvoid residual is less than 100 mL)
	Urinalysis values are within expected ranges (specific gravity, pH, protein, glucose, and ketones)
	Absence of manifestations of UTI such as dysuria, frequency, urgency, hematuria, or pyuria
	Identifies symptoms of and measures to prevent UTI
	Drinks at least 1,500 to 2,000 mL of fluid daily
	Fluid intake and output are balanced
	Serum electrolytes remain within expected values
Avoid complications associated with altered urinary elimination (urinary tract infection, skin breakdown, fluid and electrolyte imbalance, body image disturbance, social isolation)	Urine color, clarity, and odor are within normal limits
	Skin of perineal area and over bony prominences (sacrum, hips), or around urinary stoma if client has one, remains intact
	Cares for urinary stoma and drainage collection devices as instructed
	States or demonstrates acceptance of urinary diversion and ability to adjust to change in lifestyle
	Maintains or returns to previous social involvement

---

milliliters. A bladder outlet obstruction or loss of bladder muscle tone may interfere with complete emptying of the bladder during urination. Manifestations of urine retention may include frequent voiding of small amounts (e.g., less than 100 mL in an adult). Urinary stasis and UTI are possible consequences of incomplete bladder emptying. Residual urine is measured to assess the amount of retained urine after voiding and determine the need for interventions.

To measure residual urine, the nurse catheterizes the client immediately after voiding. The amount of urine voided and the amount obtained by catheterization are measured and recorded. An indwelling catheter may be inserted if the residual urine exceeds a specified amount.

Collecting Urine Specimens

The nurse is responsible for collecting urine specimens for a number of tests: clean voided specimens (for routine urinalysis), clean-catch or midstream urine specimens (for urine culture), timed urine specimens (for a variety of tests depending on the client's specific health problem), and indwelling catheter specimens.

Clean Voided Specimen

Many clients are able to collect a clean voided specimen and provide the specimen independently with minimal instruction. Male clients generally are able to void directly into the specimen container. Female clients usually sit or squat over the toilet, holding the container between their legs during voiding. About 120 mL (4 oz) of urine is generally required for this specimen. Clients who are seriously ill, physically incapacitated, or disoriented may need to use a bedpan or urinal in bed; others may require supervision or assistance in the bathroom. Whatever the situation, explicit directions are required:

- Keep the specimen free of fecal contamination.
- Female clients should discard the toilet tissue in the toilet or in a waste bag rather than in the bedpan.
- Tighten the lid on the container to prevent spillage and contamination of other objects.

The nurse must make certain that the specimen label and the laboratory requisition contain the correct information and are securely attached to the specimen. Incorrect identification of the specimen can lead to errors in diagnosis or treatment.

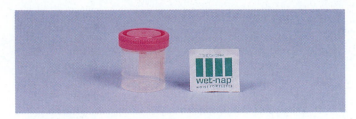

Figure 27-5. ■ Disposable clean-catch specimen equipment. (Photographer: Jenny Thomas.)

Clean-Catch or Midstream Specimen

Clean-catch or **midstream voided** specimens are collected when urine culture is ordered to identify microorganisms causing UTI. Although some contamination by skin bacteria may occur with a clean-catch specimen, the risk of introducing microorganisms into the urinary tract through catheterization is more significant. Care is taken to ensure that the specimen is as free as possible from contamination by microorganisms around the urinary meatus. Clean-catch specimens are collected in a sterile specimen container with a lid. Disposable clean-catch kits are available (Figure 27-5 ■). Procedure 27-1 ■ on page 585 explains how to collect a clean-catch urine specimen.

Timed Urine Specimen

Some urine examinations require collection of all urine produced and voided over a specific period of time, ranging from 1 to 2 hours to 24 hours. Timed specimens are generally refrigerated or contain a preservative to prevent bacterial growth or decomposition of urine components. To collect a timed urine specimen, follow these steps:

- Obtain a specimen container with preservative (if indicated) from the laboratory. Label the container with identifying information for the client, the test to be performed, time started, and time of completion.
- Provide a clean receptacle to collect urine (bedpan, commode, or toilet collection device).
- Post signs in the client's chart, Kardex, room, and bathroom alerting personnel to save all urine during the specified time.
- At the start of the collection period, have the client void and discard this urine. The time starts now.
- Save all urine produced during the timed collection period in the container, refrigerating or placing the container on ice as indicated. Avoid contaminating the urine with toilet paper or feces.
- At the end of the collection period, instruct the client to completely empty the bladder and save this voiding as part of the specimen. Take the entire amount of urine collected to the laboratory with the completed requisition.

- Record collection of the specimen, time started and completed, and any pertinent observations of the urine on appropriate records.

Indwelling Catheter Specimen

Sterile urine specimens can be obtained from closed drainage systems by inserting a sterile needle attached to a syringe through a drainage port in the tubing. Aspiration of urine from catheters can be done only with self-sealing rubber catheters. When self-sealing rubber catheters are used, the needle is inserted just above the place where the catheter is attached to the drainage tubing. To collect a specimen from a Foley (retention) catheter or a drainage tube, follow these steps:

- Wash hands.
- Wear disposable gloves.
- If there is no urine in the catheter, clamp the drainage tubing for about 30 minutes. This allows fresh urine to collect in the catheter.
- Wipe the area where the needle will be inserted with a disinfectant swab. The site should be distal to the tube leading to the balloon to avoid puncturing this tube. Disinfecting the needle insertion site removes any microorganisms on the surface of the catheter.
- Insert the needle at a 30- to 45-degree angle (Figure 27-6 ■). This angle of entrance facilitates self-sealing of the rubber.
- Unclamp the catheter.
- Withdraw the required amount of urine, for example, 3 mL for a urine culture or 30 mL for a routine urinalysis.
- Transfer the urine to the specimen container. Make sure the needle does not touch the outside of the container, if a sterile culture tube is used.
- Without recapping the needle, discard the syringe and needle in an appropriate sharps container.
- Cap the container.

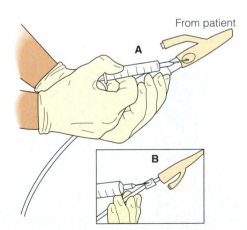

Figure 27-6. ■ Obtaining a urine specimen from a retention catheter: **A.** from a specific area near the end of the catheter; **B.** from an access port in the tubing.

- Remove gloves and discard appropriately and wash hands.
- Label the container, and send the urine to the laboratory immediately for analysis or refrigeration.
- Record collection of the specimen and any pertinent observations of the urine on the appropriate records.

Urine Testing

Several basic urine tests are often performed by nurses on the nursing units. These include tests for specific gravity, pH, and the presence of abnormal constituents such as glucose, ketones, protein, and occult blood.

Specific Gravity

The **specific gravity** of urine is a measure of its concentration, or the amount of solutes present in the urine. A urinometer, a hydrometer in a cylinder of urine (Figure 27-7 ■), a spectrometer, or a refractometer may be used to measure the specific gravity. The specific gravity of distilled water is 1.000. The specific gravity of urine normally ranges from 1.010 to 1.025. As urine becomes more concentrated, its specific gravity increases. Excess fluid intake or diseases affecting the ability of the kidneys to concentrate urine can result in low specific gravity readings. A high specific gravity may indicate fluid deficit or dehydration. Steps to measure specific gravity are outlined in Box 27-3 ■.

Urinary pH

Urinary pH is measured to determine the relative acidity or alkalinity of urine and to assess the client's acid–base status.

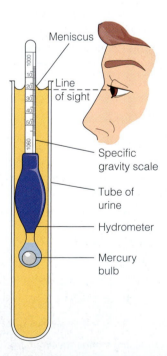

Figure 27-7. ■ A urinometer measurement of the specific gravity of the urine is taken at the base of the meniscus.

Meniscus
Line of sight
Specific gravity scale
Tube of urine
Hydrometer
Mercury bulb

BOX 27-3	NURSING CARE CHECKLIST

Measuring Specific Gravity of Urine

To Measure with a Urinometer

☑ Wear gloves and pour at least 20 mL of a fresh urine sample in the glass cylinder, or fill the cylinder three-quarters full.

☑ Place the urinometer into the cylinder and give it a gentle spin to prevent it from adhering to the sides of the cylinder.

☑ Hold the urinometer at eye level and read the measurement at the base of the meniscus at the surface of the urine (see Figure 27-7). The depth to which it sinks indicates the specific gravity.

To Measure with a Spectrometer or Refractometer

☑ Be sure to follow the manufacturer's directions.

☑ Don gloves, and place one or two drops of urine on the slide.

☑ Turn on the instrument light, and look into the instrument. The specific gravity will appear on a scope.

☑ Write down the number, then turn off the instrument.

☑ Remove the urine with a damp towel or gauze.

Following the Test

☑ Discard the urine. Clean the equipment with soap and water. Remove gloves.

☑ Document the results of the test on the client's record.

Quantitative measurements of urine pH are performed in the laboratory, but dipsticks or litmus paper often are used on nursing units or in clinics to obtain less precise pH measurements. Urine normally is slightly acidic, with an average pH of 6 (7 is neutral, less than 7 is acidic, greater than 7 is alkaline).

Glucose

Urine is tested for glucose to screen clients for diabetes mellitus and to assess clients for abnormal glucose tolerance during pregnancy. The amount of glucose in the urine is negligible in all healthy individuals.

Ketones

Ketone bodies, products of the breakdown of fatty acids, normally are not present in the urine, but are found in the urine of clients with poorly controlled diabetes. Urine ketone testing with reagent tablets or a dipstick also is used to evaluate ketoacidosis in clients who are alcoholic, fasting, starving, or consuming high-protein diets.

Protein

Protein molecules normally are too large to escape from glomerular capillaries into the filtrate. If the glomerular membrane has been damaged, however, proteins are able to escape into the renal filtrate and are removed in the urine. Urine testing for the presence of protein generally is done with a reagent strip (dipstick).

BOX 27-4	NURSING CARE CHECKLIST

Maintaining Normal Voiding Habits

Positioning

☑ Assist the client to a normal position for voiding: standing for males; for females, squatting or leaning slightly forward when sitting. These positions enhance movement of urine through the tract by gravity.

☑ If the client is unable to ambulate to the lavatory, use a bedside commode for females and a urinal for males standing at the bedside.

☑ If necessary, encourage the client to push over the pubic area with the hands or to lean forward to increase intra-abdominal pressure and external pressure on the bladder.

Relaxation

☑ Provide privacy for the client. Many people cannot void in the presence of another person.

☑ Allow the client sufficient time to void.

☑ Suggest the client read or listen to music.

☑ Provide sensory stimuli that may help the client relax. Pour warm water over the perineum of a female or have the client sit in a warm bath to promote muscle relaxation. Applying a hot water bottle to the lower abdomen of both men and women may also foster muscle relaxation.

☑ Turn on running water within hearing distance of the client to stimulate the voiding reflex and to mask the sound of voiding for people who find this embarrassing.

☑ Provide ordered analgesics and emotional support to relieve physical and emotional discomfort to decrease muscle tension.

Timing

☑ Assist clients who have the urge to void immediately. Delays only increase the difficulty in starting to void, and the desire to void may pass.

☑ Offer toileting assistance to the client at usual times of voiding, for example, on awakening, before or after meals, and at bedtime.

For Bed-Confined Clients

☑ Warm the bedpan. A cold bedpan may prompt contraction of the perineal muscles and inhibit voiding.

☑ Elevate the head of the client's bed to Fowler's position, place a small pillow or rolled towel at the small of the back to increase physical support and comfort, and have the client flex the hips and knees. This position simulates the normal voiding position as closely as possible.

Occult Blood

Normal urine is free from blood. When blood is present, it may be clearly visible or not visible (occult). Commercial reagent strips are used to test for occult blood in the urine.

Maintaining Normal Urinary Elimination

Most interventions to maintain normal urinary elimination are independent nursing functions. These include promoting adequate fluid intake, maintaining normal voiding habits, and assisting with toileting.

Promoting Fluid Intake

Increasing fluid intake increases urine production, which in turn stimulates the micturition reflex. A normal daily intake averaging 1,500 mL of measurable fluids is adequate for most adult clients.

Many clients have increased fluid requirements, necessitating a higher daily fluid intake. For example, clients who are perspiring excessively (have diaphoresis) or who are experiencing abnormal fluid losses through vomiting, gastric suction, diarrhea, or wound drainage require fluid to replace these losses in addition to their normal daily intake requirements.

Clients who are at risk for UTI or urinary calculi (stones) should consume 2,000 to 3,000 mL of fluid daily. Dilute urine and frequent urination reduce the risk of urinary tract infection as well as stone formation.

Increased fluid intake may be contraindicated for some clients such as people with kidney failure or heart failure. For these clients, a fluid restriction may be necessary to prevent fluid overload and edema.

Maintaining Normal Voiding Habits

Medical therapies often interfere with a client's normal voiding habits. When a client's urinary elimination pattern is adequate, the nurse helps the client adhere to normal voiding habits as much as possible. A nursing care checklist is provided in Box 27-4 ■.

Assisting with Toileting

Clients who are weakened by a disease process or impaired physically require assistance to toilet. The nurse should assist these clients to the bathroom and remain with them if they are at risk for falling. The bathroom should contain an easily accessible call signal to summon help if needed. Clients also need to be encouraged to use handrails placed near the toilet.

For clients unable to use bathroom facilities, the nurse positions urinary equipment close to the bedside (e.g., urinal, bedpan, commode) and provides the necessary assistance.

Preventing Urinary Tract Infections

The rate of UTI in women is about 20% yearly compared with a rate of 0.1% in men. UTI accounts for 40% of all nosocomial infections. Most UTIs are caused by bacteria common to the intestinal environment (e.g., *Escherichia coli*). Women are particularly at risk because of their short urethra and its proximity to the anal and vaginal areas.

For women who have experienced a UTI, nurses need to provide instructions about ways to prevent a recurrence. The following guidelines are useful for anyone:

- Drink eight 8-ounce glasses of water per day.
- Practice frequent voiding (every 2 to 4 hours) to flush bacteria out and prevent organisms from ascending into the bladder. Void immediately after intercourse.
- Avoid use of harsh soaps, bubble bath, powder, or sprays in the perineal area.
- Avoid tight-fitting pants or other clothing that creates irritation to the urethra and prevents ventilation of the perineal area.
- Wear cotton rather than nylon underclothes. Accumulation of perineal moisture facilitates bacterial growth and cotton enhances ventilation of the perineal area.
- Girls and women should always wipe the perineal area from front to back following urination or defecation.
- If recurrent urinary infections are a problem, take showers rather than baths.
- Increase the acidity of urine through regular intake of vitamin C and drinking two to three glasses of cranberry juice daily or take cranberry tablets.

Managing Urinary Incontinence

It is important to remember that urinary **incontinence** is not a normal part of aging and often is treatable. Independent nursing interventions for clients with urinary incontinence (UI) include a behavior-oriented continence training program, prompted voiding, pelvic muscle exercises, positive reinforcement, meticulous skin care, and for males, application of an external drainage device (condom).

Continence (Bladder) Training

A continence training program requires the involvement of the nurse, the client, and support people. Clients must be alert and physically able to follow a program. The goal of training is to decrease the frequency of UI. A bladder training program may include the following:

- Education of the client and support staff
- Bladder training, which requires that the client postpone voiding, resist or inhibit the sensation of urgency, and void according to a timetable rather than according to the urge to void
- Delayed voiding provides larger voided volumes and longer intervals between voiding. See Box 27-5 ■.

Pelvic Muscle Exercises

Pelvic muscle exercises, referred to as Kegel exercises, strengthen pelvic floor muscles in women and can reduce episodes of incontinence. The client can identify perineal

---

BOX 27-5	NURSING CARE CHECKLIST

Bladder Training

☑ Determine the client's voiding pattern and encourage voiding at those times, or establish a regular voiding schedule and help the client to maintain it, whether the client feels the urge or not. The stretching–relaxing sequence of such a schedule tends to increase bladder muscle tone and promote more voluntary control.

☑ Encourage the client to inhibit the urge-to-void sensation when a premature urge to void is experienced.

☑ Instruct the client to practice slow, deep breathing until the urge diminishes or disappears.

☑ When the client finds that voiding can be controlled, the intervals between voiding can be lengthened slightly without loss of continence.

☑ Regulate fluid intake, particularly during evening hours, to help reduce the need to void during the night.

☑ Encourage fluids about half an hour before the voiding time between the hours of 0600 and 1800.

☑ Avoid excessive consumption of citrus juices, carbonated beverages (especially those containing artificial sweeteners), alcohol, and drinks containing caffeine because these irritate the bladder, increasing the risk of incontinence.

☑ Schedule diuretics early in the morning.

☑ Explain to clients that adequate fluid intake is required to ensure adequate urine production to stimulate the micturition reflex.

☑ Apply protector pads to keep the bed linen dry, and provide specially made waterproof underwear to contain the urine and decrease the client's embarrassment.

☑ Assist the client with an exercise program to increase the tone of abdominal and pelvic muscles.

☑ Provide positive reinforcements to encourage continence.

---

muscles by stopping urination midstream or by tightening the anal sphincter as if to hold a bowel movement. Kegel exercises can be performed anytime, anywhere, sitting or standing—even when voiding.

Maintaining Skin Integrity

Skin that is continually moist becomes macerated. Urine that accumulates on the skin is converted to ammonia, which is very irritating to the skin. Because both skin irritation and maceration predispose the client to skin breakdown and ulceration, the incontinent person requires meticulous skin care. To maintain skin integrity, the nurse washes the client's perineal area with a mild soap and water, rinses it thoroughly, dries it, and provides clean, dry clothing or bed linen. If the skin is irritated, the nurse applies a barrier cream. If it is necessary to pad the client's clothes for protection, the nurse should use products that absorb wetness and leave a dry surface in contact with the skin.

Applying External Urinary Drainage Devices

The application of a condom or external catheter connected to a urinary drainage system is commonly prescribed for incontinent males. Use of a condom appliance is preferable to insertion of a retention catheter because the risk of UTI is minimal.

Methods of applying condoms vary according to how long the condom is worn. Condoms that are worn for a short period are generally applied with elastic tape only. If, however, the condom is to be worn for a longer period (e.g., a few days), additional measures are required to protect the foreskin and to ensure secure attachment. Procedure 27-2 ■ on page 586 describes how to apply and remove a drainage condom.

Managing Urinary Retention

Signs and symptoms of urinary retention are urgency, frequency, and bladder distention. The client is unable to empty the bladder fully. This may lead to incontinence, UTI, and other urinary complications. Interventions that assist the client to maintain a normal voiding pattern, discussed earlier, also apply to urinary retention. If these actions are unsuccessful, the physician may order a cholinergic drug such as bethanechol chloride (Urecholine) to stimulate bladder contraction and facilitate voiding. When all measures fail to initiate voiding, urinary catheterization may be necessary to empty the bladder completely. An indwelling Foley catheter may be inserted until the underlying cause is treated. Intermittent straight catheterization (every 3 to 4 hours) may be performed as an alternative because the risk of UTI is believed by some to be less than with an indwelling catheter.

Urinary Catheterization

Urinary **catheterization** is the introduction of a catheter through the urethra into the urinary bladder, usually performed only when absolutely necessary. The urinary structures are normally sterile except at the end of the urethra, so the danger exists of introducing microorganisms into the bladder when a catheter is used. Once an infection is introduced into the bladder, it can ascend the ureters and eventually involve the kidneys. Thus, strict sterile technique is used for catheterization.

Another hazard is trauma, particularly in the male client, whose urethra is longer and more tortuous. It is important to insert a catheter along the normal contour of the urethra. Damage to the urethra can occur if the catheter is forced through strictures or at an incorrect angle.

Catheters are commonly made of rubber or plastics, although they may also be made from latex or silicone. They are sized by the diameter of the lumen using the French (Fr.) scale: the larger the number, the larger the lumen. Either straight catheters, inserted to drain the bladder and

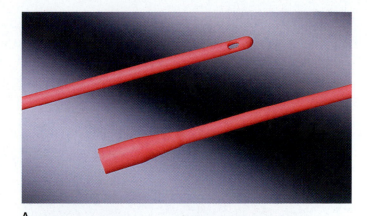

A

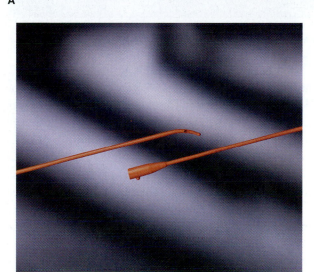

B

Figure 27-8. ■ Two types of straight catheters: **A.** a red-rubber catheter; **B.** a Coudé catheter. (Courtesy of Bard Medical Division.)

then immediately removed, or retention catheters, which remain in the bladder to drain urine, may be used.

The straight catheter is a single-lumen tube with a small eye or opening about 1/2 in. from the insertion tip (Figure 27-8A ■). The Coudé catheter is a variation of the straight catheter. It is more rigid than other straight catheters and has a tapered, curved tip (Figure 27-8B). This catheter may be used for men with prostatic hypertrophy because it is more easily controlled and less traumatic on insertion.

The retention, or Foley, catheter is a double-lumen catheter. The larger lumen drains urine from the bladder. A second, smaller lumen is used to inflate a balloon near the tip of the catheter to hold the catheter in place within the bladder (Figure 27-9 ■). Clients who require continuous or intermittent bladder irrigation may have a three-way Foley catheter. The three-way catheter has a third lumen through which sterile irrigating fluid can flow into the bladder. The fluid then exits the bladder through the drainage lumen, along with the urine.

MediaLink
Catheterization

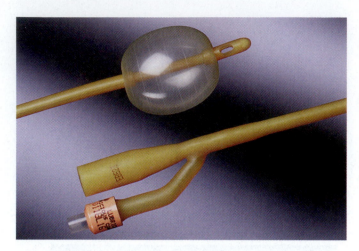

Figure 27-9. ◼ A retention (Foley) catheter with the balloon inflated. (Courtesy of Bard Medical Division.)

The balloons of retention catheters are sized by the volume of fluid used to inflate them. The two commonly used sizes are 5- and 30-mL balloons. The size of the balloon is indicated on the catheter along with the diameter, for example, "#18 Fr.—5 mL." Box 27-6 ◼ provides a checklist for catheter selection.

Retention catheters usually are connected to a closed gravity drainage system. This system consists of the catheter, drainage tubing, and a collecting bag for the urine. A closed system cannot be opened anywhere along the system, from catheter to collecting bag. Closed systems reduce the risk of microorganisms entering the system and infecting the urinary tract. Urinary drainage systems typically depend on the force of gravity to drain urine from the bladder to the collecting bag.

BOX 27-6	NURSING CARE CHECKLIST

Selecting an Appropriate Catheter

☑ Select the type of material in accordance with the estimated length of the catheterization period:
   a. Use plastic catheters for short periods only (e.g., 1 week or less), because they are inflexible.
   b. Use a latex or rubber catheter for periods of 2 or 3 weeks.
   c. Use silicone catheters for long-term use (e.g., 2 to 3 months) because they create less encrustation at the urethral meatus. However, they are expensive.

☑ Determine appropriate catheter length by the client's gender. For adult females, use a 22-cm catheter; for adult males, a 40-cm catheter.

☑ Determine appropriate catheter size by the size of the urethral canal. Use sizes such as #8 or #10 Fr. for children, #14 or #16 Fr. for adults. Men frequently require a larger size than women, for example, #18 Fr.

☑ Select the appropriate balloon size. For adults, use a 5-mL balloon to facilitate optimal urine drainage. A 30-mL balloon or larger is commonly used to achieve hemostasis of the prostatic area following a prostatectomy. Use 3-mL balloons for children.

Catheterization of females and males, using straight catheters, is described in Procedures 27-3 ◼ and 27-4 ◼ (starting on page 588), respectively. Procedure 27-5 ◼ outlines how to insert a retention catheter.

Helping Clients with Retention Catheters

Nursing care is largely directed toward preventing infection of the urinary tract and encouraging patent urinary flow. It includes encouraging large amounts of fluid intake, accurately recording the fluid intake and output, changing the retention catheter and tubing, maintaining the patency of the drainage system, preventing urinary backflow into the bladder, and teaching these measures to the client.

Fluids

The client with a retention catheter should drink up to 3,000 mL per day if permitted. Large amounts of fluid increase urine output, keeping the bladder flushed out and decreasing urinary stasis and subsequent infection. Large volumes of urine also minimize the risk of sediment or other particles obstructing the drainage tubing. Accurate recording of fluid intake and output is discussed in Chapter 26 ◯◯.

Dietary Measures

Acidifying the urine of clients with a retention catheter may reduce the risk of urinary tract infection and calculus formation. Foods such as eggs, meat, poultry, whole grains, cranberries, plums, and tomatoes tend to increase the acidity of urine.

Perineal Care

No special cleaning other than routine hygienic care is necessary for clients with retention catheters, nor is special meatal care recommended. The nurse should check agency practice in this regard.

Changing the Catheter and Tubing

Indwelling catheters are used only when necessary, and removed as soon as possible. However, some clients require long-term catheterization. Whenever possible, the closed catheter drainage system should be maintained, and the tubing not disconnected from the catheter for any reason. Routine changing of catheter and tubing is not recommended. Collection of sediment in the catheter or tubing or impaired urine drainage are indicators for changing the catheter and drainage system. When this occurs, a new sterile catheter with a closed drainage system is inserted.

A checklist on how to prevent catheter-associated UTIs is given in Box 27-7 ◼. Ongoing assessment of clients with retention catheters is a high priority. Box 27-8 ◼ provides guidelines.

Client Teaching

Usually nurses need to teach the client some principles about the gravity drainage system and the importance of a

BOX 27-7   NURSING CARE CHECKLIST

Preventing Catheter-Associated Urinary Infections

☑ Have an established infection control program in place.

☑ Catheterize clients only when necessary, by using aseptic technique, sterile equipment, and trained personnel.

☑ Maintain a sterile closed drainage system.

☑ Do not disconnect the catheter and drainage tubing unless absolutely necessary.

☑ Remove the catheter as soon as possible.

☑ Follow and reinforce good hand hygiene techniques.

☑ Provide routine perineal hygiene, including cleansing with soap and water after defecation.

☑ Prevent contamination of the catheter with feces in the incontinent client.

closed system. The client has to understand that the drainage tubing and bag need to be kept lower than the bladder at all times. Client instruction on methods to prevent tension on the catheter tubing, preventing kinks in the drainage tubing, and avoiding lying on the tubing can alleviate potential problems. Some clients also benefit from instruction about fluid intake measurement and perineal care.

Removing Retention Catheters

Retention catheters are removed after their purpose has been achieved, usually on the order of the physician. If the catheter has been in place for a short time (e.g., a few days), the client usually has little difficulty regaining normal urinary elimination patterns. Swelling of the urethra, however, may initially interfere with voiding, so the nurse should regularly assess the client for urinary retention until voiding is reestablished.

BOX 27-8   ASSESSING

Ongoing Assessment of Clients with Retention Catheters

■ Ensure that there are no obstructions in the drainage.

■ Check that there is no tension on the catheter or tubing, that the catheter is securely taped to the thigh or abdomen, and that the tubing is fastened appropriately to the bedclothes.

■ Ensure that gravity drainage is maintained and that the drainage receptacle is below the level of the client's bladder.

■ Ensure that the drainage system is well sealed or closed. Check that there are no leaks at the connection sites in open systems.

■ Observe the flow of the urine every 2 or 3 hours, and note color, odor, and any abnormal constituents. If blood clots are present, check the catheter more frequently to ascertain whether it is plugged.

Clients who have had a retention catheter for a prolonged period may require bladder retraining to regain bladder muscle tone. With an indwelling catheter in place, the bladder muscle does not stretch and contract regularly as it does when the bladder fills and empties by voiding. A few days prior to removal, the catheter may be clamped for specified periods of time (e.g., 2 to 4 hours), then released to allow the bladder to empty. This allows the bladder to distend and stimulates its musculature.

To remove a retention catheter, the nurse follows these steps:

■ Obtain a receptacle for the catheter (e.g., a disposable basin); a clean, disposable towel; disposable gloves; and a sterile syringe to deflate the balloon. The size of the balloon is indicated on the label at the end of the catheter.

■ Ask the client to assume a supine position as for a catheterization.

■ *Optional:* Obtain a sterile specimen before removing the catheter. Check agency protocol.

■ Remove the tape attaching the catheter to the client, don gloves, and then place the towel between the legs of the female client or over the thighs of the male.

■ Insert the syringe into the injection port of the catheter, and withdraw the fluid from the balloon. If not all the fluid can be removed, report this fact to the nurse in charge before proceeding.

■ Do not pull the catheter while the balloon is inflated; doing so may injure the urethra.

■ After all the fluid is withdrawn from the balloon, gently withdraw the catheter, and place it in the waste receptacle.

■ Dry the perineal area with a towel.

■ Remove gloves.

■ Measure the urine in the drainage bag, and record the removal of the catheter. Include in the recording (1) the time the catheter was removed; (2) the amount, color, and clarity of the urine; (3) the intactness of the catheter; and (4) instructions given to the client.

■ Following removal of the catheter, determine the time of the first voiding and the amount voided during the first 8 hours. Compare this output to the client's intake.

Urinary Irrigations

An **irrigation** is a flushing or washing-out with a specified solution. A bladder irrigation is carried out on a physician's order, usually to wash out the bladder and sometimes to apply a medication to the bladder lining, usually the RN's responsibility. Catheter irrigations may be performed to maintain or restore the patency of a catheter, for example, to remove blood clots blocking the catheter.

The closed method is the preferred technique for catheter or bladder irrigation because of the lower risk of UTI. Closed catheter irrigations may be either continuous

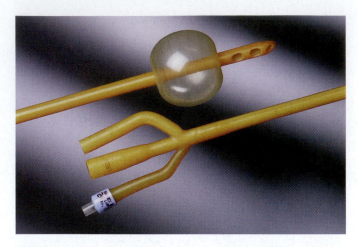

Figure 27-10. ■ A closed catheter or bladder irrigation system. (Courtesy of Bard Medical Division.)

or intermittent. A three-way, or triple lumen, catheter generally is used for closed irrigations. See Figures 27-10 ■ and 27-11 ■. Techniques for setting up and maintaining a continuous or intermittent closed catheter irrigation are outlined in Procedure 27-6 ■ on page 594.

Occasionally an open irrigation may be necessary to restore catheter patency. The risk of injecting microorganisms into the urinary tract is greater with open irrigations, because the connection between the indwelling catheter and the drainage tubing is broken. Strict precautions to maintain the sterility of the drainage tubing connector and interior of the indwelling catheter must be taken to minimize this risk.

The open method of catheter or bladder irrigation is performed with double-lumen indwelling catheters. It may be used for clients who develop blood clots and mucous fragments that occlude the catheter. It may also be used when it is undesirable to change the catheter. The steps involved in performing an open method of irrigation are shown in the Box 27-9 ■.

Urinary Diversions

A **urinary diversion** is the surgical rerouting of urine from the kidneys to a site other than the bladder. Urinary diversions are usually created when the bladder must be removed, for example, because of cancer or trauma. The ureters may be brought directly to the surface of the skin to form small stomas (*cutaneous ureterostomy*). The most common urinary diversion is the ileal conduit or ileal loop (Figure 27-12 ■). In this procedure, a segment of the ileum is removed, and the intestinal ends are reattached. One end of the portion removed is closed with sutures to create a pouch, and the other end is brought out through the abdominal wall to create a stoma. The ureters are implanted into the ileal pouch. The mucous membrane lining of the ileum also provides some protection from ascending infection. Urine drains continuously from the ileal pouch.

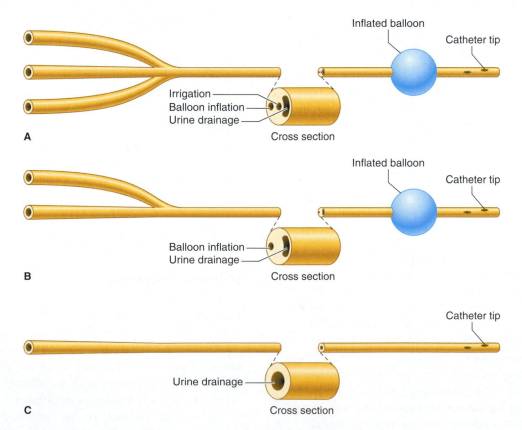

Figure 27-11. ■ **A.** A three-way Foley catheter. **B.** A normal retention catheter. **C.** A straight catheter.

BOX 27-9	NURSING CARE CHECKLIST

Open Method of Catheter Irrigation

☑ Obtain a sterile Asepto or piston syringe, sterile basin, and sterile irrigating solution at room temperature; sterile collection basin; sterile protective tubing cap; sterile waterproof drape; sterile gloves; and antiseptic swabs.

☑ Establish a sterile field close to the client's thigh. Place the sterile waterproof drape under the catheter and apply sterile gloves.

☑ Clean the junction between the catheter and the drainage tubing with antiseptic swabs.

☑ Disconnect the catheter and drainage tubing. Hold the catheter and tubing about 1 in. from their ends and place them on a sterile surface to avoid contaminating them.

☑ Cover the open end of the drainage tubing with the sterile protection cap.

☑ Draw irrigation fluid into the syringe and instill it slowly into the catheter.

☑ Remove the syringe and allow the irrigating solution to drain by gravity from the catheter into the collection basin.

☑ Repeat irrigations depending on the amount of solution to be instilled or until urine runs freely through the catheter and drainage is clear.

☑ Reconnect the catheter and drainage tubing, maintaining the sterility of the ends of the tubing and the inside of the catheter.

☑ Remove gloves.

☑ Assess and document the irrigation returns.

Highly motivated clients may be candidates for a continent urinary diversion. The Kock pouch, or continent ileal bladder conduit, also uses a portion of the ileum to form a reservoir for urine (Figure 27-13 ■). The client empties the pouch by inserting a clean catheter approximately every 4 hours. A small dressing is worn to protect the stoma and clothing.

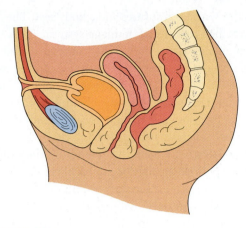

Figure 27-13. ■ A continent vesicostomy (Kock pouch).

When caring for clients with a urinary diversion, the nurse must accurately assess intake and output, note any changes in urine color, odor, or clarity (mucous shreds are commonly seen in the urine of clients with an ileal diversion), and frequently assess the condition of the stoma and surrounding skin. Clients who must wear a urine collection appliance are at risk for impaired skin integrity because of irritation by urine. The nurse should consult with an enterostomal therapist to identify the most appropriate appliance for the client's needs.

Suprapubic Catheter Care

A suprapubic catheter is inserted through the abdominal wall above the symphysis pubis into the urinary bladder (Figure 27-14 ■). The purpose of the suprapubic catheter is to divert the urinary output from the urethra to allow for healing or treatment. The physician inserts the catheter using local anesthesia or during bladder or vaginal surgery. The catheter may be secured in place with sutures, with a

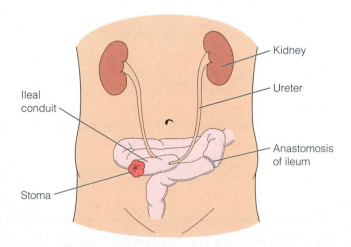

Figure 27-12. ■ An ileal conduit.

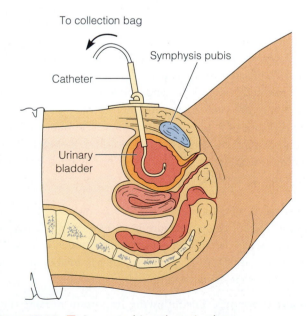

Figure 27-14. ■ A suprapubic catheter in place.

body seal, or with both sutures and a body seal. The catheter is then attached to a closed drainage system.

Care of clients with a suprapubic catheter includes regular assessments of the client's urine, fluid intake, and comfort; maintenance of a patent drainage system; skin care around the insertion site; periodic clamping of the catheter preparatory to removing it; and measurement of residual urine. Orders generally include leaving the catheter open to drainage for 48 to 72 hours, then clamping the catheter for 3- to 4-hour periods during the day until the client can void satisfactorily amounts. Satisfactory voiding is determined by measuring the client's residual urine after voiding.

Care of the catheter insertion site involves sterile technique. Dressings around the suprapubic catheter are changed whenever they are soiled with drainage to prevent bacterial growth and reduce the potential for infection. Procedures for cleaning wounds and changing dressings are discussed in Chapter 23 ∞. Any redness or discharge at the skin around the insertion site must be reported.

EVALUATING

Using the overall goals and desired outcomes identified in the planning stage (see Table 27-4), the nurse collects data to evaluate the effectiveness of nursing activities.

NURSING PROCESS CARE PLAN
Client with Impaired Urinary Elimination

Mrs. Kennedy, age 48, is recovering from a motor vehicle crash in which she sustained blunt trauma to her abdomen. She has a mild concussion. An indwelling urinary catheter is in place until she is able to communicate her need to urinate. Upon entering Mrs. Kennedy's room to collect a urine specimen ordered for culture and sensitivity, you note that Mrs. Kennedy is restless and moaning. Her abdominal dressing is dry and intact and her urinary bag contains about 200 mL of golden-colored urine. Her abdomen is tender and distended. When questioned, Mrs. Kennedy is able to communicate that she is in pain but is unable to communicate the specifics of her pain.

Assessment. VS: Temperature is 99.6, radial pulse is 86, respirations 24. Blood pressure is 130/90. WBC is 15,000. Her catheter is patent and urine is clear golden colored. IV is infusing with D_5W at 75 mL/h. She has an abdominal incision that is clean and dry, no redness noted.

Nursing Diagnosis. The following important nursing diagnoses (among others) are established for this client:

- *Pain*
- *Impaired Skin Integrity*
- *Impaired Urinary Elimination*
- *Anxiety*
- *Impaired Verbal Communication*
- *Risk for Infection*

Expected Outcomes. The expected outcomes for the plan of care are that:

- Pain will be controlled.
- Skin integrity will be effectively managed.
- Urinary output will be within normal limits.
- Client will be informed about procedures.
- Body language will be assessed for communication.
- Wound and catheter will be maintained without evidence of infection.

Planning and Implementation. The following nursing interventions are implemented for Mrs. Kennedy:

- Implement pain control measures.
- Monitor and document wound healing.
- Maintain and measure urinary output.
- Instruct client regarding procedures.
- Observe for body language communication.
- Monitor for signs and symptoms of infection.
- Maintain catheter care.

Evaluation. Mrs. Kennedy will remain in the hospital to determine the status of her concussion and results of tests. Her abdominal incision is approximated and healing without signs of infection. She is able to communicate her level of pain on a pain scale. Urinary output is adequate and is a clear straw color. The urinary C&S was positive for organisms and treated with antibiotics. She is ambulating with assistance.

Critical Thinking in the Nursing Process

1. What precautions should be taken when collecting a urine sample from a person with an indwelling urinary catheter and why?
2. What measures can be taken to prevent Mrs. Kennedy from developing a UTI if one is not already present?
3. Mrs. Kennedy's catheter was removed at 8 A.M. and at 12 noon. She voided 100 mL of clear yellow urine. The physician ordered a straight catheter for residual following first voiding. What is the reason for this order?

Note: Discussion of Critical Thinking questions appears in Appendix I.

Note: The references and resources for this and all chapters have been compiled at the back of the book.

Collecting a Urine Specimen for Culture and Sensitivity by the Clean-Catch Method

Purpose

- To determine the presence of microorganisms, the type of organism(s), and the antibiotics to which the organisms are sensitive

Equipment

Equipment used varies greatly from agency to agency. Some agencies use commercially prepared disposable clean-catch kits. Others use agency-prepared sterile trays. Both prepared trays and kits generally contain the following items:

- Disposable or sterile gloves
- Antiseptic towelette, such as povidone-iodine
- Sterile cotton balls or 2 × 2 gauze pads
- Sterile specimen container
- Specimen identification label

In addition, the nurse needs to obtain:

- Completed laboratory requisition form
- Urine receptacle, if the client is not ambulatory
- Basin of warm water, soap, washcloth, and towel for the nonambulatory client

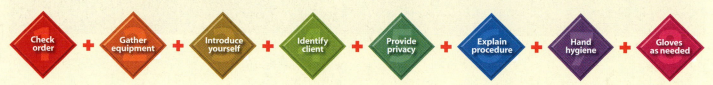

Check order ✛ Gather equipment ✛ Introduce yourself ✛ Identify client ✛ Provide privacy ✛ Explain procedure ✛ Hand hygiene ✛ Gloves as needed

Interventions

1. Instruct and assist the client appropriately.
   - Inform the client that a urine specimen is required. Give the reason and explain the method to be used to collect it.

2. For an ambulatory client who is able to follow directions, instruct the client how to collect the specimen.
   - Direct or assist the client to the bathroom.
   - Ask the client to wash and dry the genital and perineal area with soap and water. *This removes microorganisms that could contaminate the specimen.*
   - Instruct the client how to clean the urinary meatus with antiseptic towelettes.

For Female Clients

- Use each towelette only once. Clean the perineal area from front to back, and discard the towelette. Use all towelettes provided (usually two or three). *Cleaning from front to back cleans the area of least contamination to the area of greatest contamination.*

For Male Clients

- If uncircumcised, retract the foreskin slightly to expose the urinary meatus.
- Using a circular motion, clean the urinary meatus and the distal portion of the penis. Use each towelette only once, then discard. Clean several inches down the shaft of the penis. *This cleans from the area of least contamination to the area of greatest contamination.*

3. For a client who requires assistance, prepare the client and equipment.

- Wash the perineal area with soap and water; rinse and dry. Assist the client onto a clean commode or bedpan. If using a bedpan or urinal, position the client as upright as allowed or tolerated.
- Open the clean-catch kit, taking care not to contaminate the inside of the specimen container or lid.
- Wear clean gloves.
- Clean the urinary meatus and perineal area as described in step 2.

4. Collect the specimen from a nonambulatory client or instruct an ambulatory client how to collect it.
   - Instruct the client to start voiding. *Bacteria in the distal urethra and at the urinary meatus are cleared by the first few milliliters of urine expelled.*
   - Place the specimen container into the stream of urine and collect the specimen, taking care not to touch the container to the perineum or penis. Avoid contaminating the interior of the specimen container and the specimen itself.
   - Collect 30 to 60 mL of urine in the container.
   - Cap the container tightly, touching only the outside of the container and the cap.
   - If necessary, clean the outside of the specimen container with disinfectant.
   - Remove gloves if handling another person's urine. Wash hands.

5. Label the specimen and transport it to the laboratory.
   - Ensure that the specimen label and the laboratory requisition carry the correct information. Attach them securely to the specimen.

■ Arrange for the specimen to be sent to the laboratory immediately. *Bacterial cultures must be started immediately, before any contaminating organisms can grow, multiply, and produce false results.*

6. Document pertinent data.
   ■ Record collection of the specimen, any pertinent observations of the urine in terms of color, odor, and consistency, and any difficulty in voiding that the client experienced.

SAMPLE DOCUMENTATION

[date]   Urine C&S to lab. Urine straw
[time]   colored, clear and free from odor.
          No abnormal constituents noted.
          Client voided freely without
          complaints of difficulty.
          _____ D. Haus, LVN

PROCEDURE 27-2   # Applying a Condom Catheter

Purposes

■ To collect urine and control urinary incontinence
■ To permit the client physical activity without fear of embarrassment because of leaking urine
■ To prevent skin irritation as a result of urine incontinence

Equipment

■ Leg drainage bag with tubing or urinary drainage bag with tubing

■ Condom sheath
■ Bath blanket
■ Disposable gloves
■ Basin of warm water and soap
■ Washcloth and towel
■ Elastic tape or Velcro strap

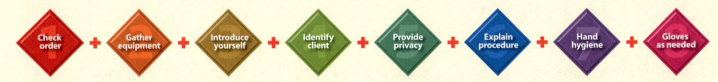

Check order + Gather equipment + Introduce yourself + Identify client + Provide privacy + Explain procedure + Hand hygiene + Gloves as needed

Interventions

1. Prepare the equipment.
   ■ Assemble the leg drainage bag or urinary drainage bag for attachment to the condom sheath.
   ■ Roll the condom outward onto itself to facilitate easier application. *On some models an inner flap will be exposed. This flap is applied around the urinary meatus to prevent the reflux of urine (Figure 27-15 ■).*

2. Position and drape the client.
   ■ Position the client in either a supine or a bed-sitting position.
   ■ Drape the client appropriately with the bath blanket, exposing only the penis.

3. Inspect and clean the penis.
   ■ Don gloves.
   ■ Inspect the penis for skin irritation (contact dermatitis), excoriation, swelling, or discoloration. *The nurse needs to obtain baseline data.*

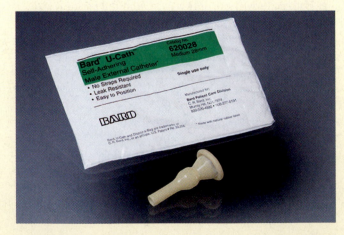

Figure 27-15. ■ Before application, roll the condom outward onto itself. (Courtesy of Bard Medical Division.)

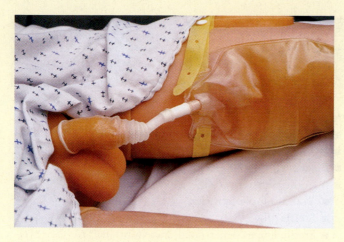

Figure 27-16. ■ The condom rolled over the penis.

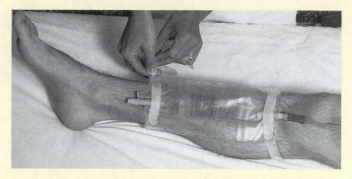

Figure 27-17. ■ Attaching the urinary drainage bag to the leg.

- Clean the genital area, and dry it thoroughly. *This minimizes skin irritation and excoriation after the condom is applied.*

4. Apply and secure the condom.
   - Roll the condom smoothly over the penis, leaving 1 in. between the end of the penis and the rubber or plastic connecting tube (Figure 27-16 ■). *This space prevents irritation of the tip of the penis and provides for full drainage of urine.*
   - Secure the condom firmly, but not too tightly, to the penis by wrapping a strip of elastic tape or Velcro around the base of the penis over the condom. *The elastic or Velcro strip should not come in contact with the skin and should hold the condom in place without impeding blood circulation to the penis.*

5. Securely attach the urinary drainage system.
   - Make sure that the tip of the penis is not touching the condom and that the condom is not twisted. *A twisted condom could obstruct the flow of urine.*
   - Attach the urinary drainage system to the condom.
   - Remove gloves.
   - If the client is to remain in bed, attach the urinary drainage bag to the bed frame.
   - If the client is ambulatory, attach the bag to the client's leg (Figure 27-17 ■). *Attaching the drainage bag to the leg helps control the movement of the tubing and prevents twisting of the thin material of the condom appliance at the tip of the penis.*

6. Teach the client about the drainage system.
   - Instruct the client to keep the drainage bag below the level of the condom and to avoid loops or kinks in the tubing.

7. Document pertinent data.
   - Record the application of the condom, the time, and pertinent observations, such as irritated areas on the penis.

8. Inspect the penis 30 minutes following the condom application, and check urine flow.
   - Assess the penis for swelling and discoloration, which indicates that the condom is too tight.

9. Change the condom daily, and provide skin care.
   - Remove the elastic or Velcro strip and roll off the condom.
   - Wash the penis with soapy water, rinse, and dry it thoroughly.
   - Assess the foreskin for signs of irritation, swelling, and discoloration.

SAMPLE DOCUMENTATION

[date]	Condom catheter applied and at-
[time]	tached to gravity drainage. Client

tolerated procedure well, no complaints of pain. Urine clear, straw colored.

_____ D. Haus, LVN

PROCEDURE 27-3

Female Urinary Catheterization Using a Straight Catheter

Before inserting a urinary catheter, check (1) the order authorizing the catheterization, (2) whether the order or policy specifies a maximum amount of urine to be removed during the catheterization (if the client is retaining urine), and (3) the client's chart for any direction about the type or size of catheter to use.

Purposes

- To relieve discomfort due to bladder distention or to provide gradual decompression of a distended bladder
- To assess the amount of residual urine if the bladder empties incompletely
- To obtain a urine specimen
- To empty the bladder completely prior to surgery

Equipment

- Flashlight or lamp
- Mask, if required by agency policy
- Bath blanket or drape
- Soap, a basin of warm water, a washcloth, and a towel
- Disposable gloves
- Bladder ultrasound device (optional)
- A sterile catheterization kit containing
  - Water-soluble lubricant
  - Sterile gloves
  - Sterile drapes, fenestrated drape (optional) to place over the perineum
  - Antiseptic solution
  - Cotton balls or gauze squares
  - Forceps
  - Basin for urine (base of kit can be used)
- Sterile catheter of appropriate size (e.g., for an adult #14 or #16 Fr. is often used)
- Specimen container as required
- Bag or receptacle for disposal of the cotton balls

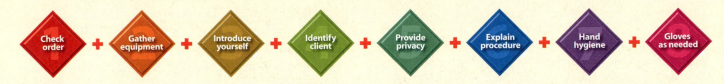

Check order + Gather equipment + Introduce yourself + Identify client + Provide privacy + Explain procedure + Hand hygiene + Gloves as needed

Interventions

1. Assess for urinary retention.
   - To palpate the bladder, indent the skin more than 1.3 cm (0.5 in.) just above the pubic symphysis by pressing the fingers of one hand on the fingers of the other. *This increases the pressure for palpation.*

2. Prepare the client.
   - Explain the catheterization to the client, and provide privacy. *Exposure of the genitals is embarrassing to most clients. Some people fear that the procedure will be painful; explain that normally a catheterization is painless and that there may be a sensation of pressure.*
   - Assist the client to a supine position, with knees flexed and thighs externally rotated. Pillows can be used to support the knees and to elevate the buttocks. *Raising the client's pelvis gives the nurse a better view of the urinary meatus and reduces the risk of contaminating the catheter.*
   - Drape the client. *This maintains comfort and prevents unnecessary exposure.* Cover the client's chest and abdomen with a bath blanket. Pull the client's gown up over her hips. Cover her legs and feet as for perineal care.
   - Wear disposable gloves.
   - Wash the perineal–genital area with warm water and soap. *Cleaning reduces the number of microorganisms around*

the urinary meatus and the possibility of introducing microorganisms with the catheter.
   - Rinse and dry the area well. *Rinsing removes soap that could inhibit the action of an antiseptic, if used later.*
   - Remove disposable gloves.
   - Obtain assistance if the client requires help in maintaining the required position. *The client must remain still throughout the procedure to maintain a clear view of the urinary meatus and prevent contamination of the sterile field.*

3. Prepare the equipment.
   - Adjust the light to view the urinary meatus. It may be necessary to use a flashlight or to place a gooseneck lamp at the foot of the bed.
   - Put on a mask, gown, and cap if required by agency policy.

4. Create a sterile field.
   - At the client's bedside, open a sterile kit and the catheter, if it is packaged separately, and put on the sterile gloves.
   - Drape the client with the sterile drape, being careful to protect its sterility and the sterility of your gloves. Place the drape under the buttocks while keeping the

edges cuffed over your gloves. *This prevents contamination of the gloves against the client's buttocks.* If a fenestrated drape is provided, place it over the perineal area, exposing only the labia.

- Place the sterile kit on the drape between the client's thighs. *This facilitates access to supplies.*
- Pour the antiseptic solution over the cotton balls, if they are not already prepared and if meatal cleansing with an antiseptic is agency practice (see step 5).
- Lubricate the insertion tip of the catheter liberally, and place it in the sterile container ready for use. *Water-soluble lubricant facilitates insertion of the catheter by reducing friction. Lubrication is done at this point because the nurse will subsequently have only one sterile hand available.*
- Open the urine specimen container, and keep the top sterile. This prepares the container for specimen collection.

5. Clean the meatus with antiseptic (if recommended by the agency).
   - Check agency protocol about cleaning the meatus. *There is controversy regarding the value of meatal cleansing using antiseptics before catheterization.*
   - Using the nondominant hand, separate the labia minora with your thumb and one finger or another two fingers.
   - Expose the urinary meatus adequately by retracting the tissue of the labia minora in an upward (anterior) direction (Figure 27-18 ■). Clean first from the meatus downward and then on either side, using a new swab for each stroke (Figure 27-19 ■). Once the meatus is cleaned, do not allow the labia to close over it. *Keeping the labia apart prevents the risk of contaminating the urinary meatus. Note: Your hand that touches the client becomes unsterile. It remains in position exposing the urinary meatus,*

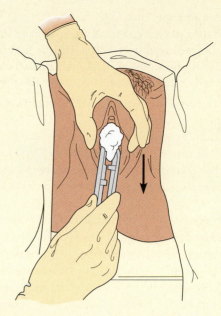

Figure 27-19. ■ When cleaning the urinary meatus, move the swab downward.

while your other hand remains sterile holding the sterile forceps.

6. Inspect the meatus.
   - With the urinary meatus exposed, assess any signs, such as excoriation of the tissues surrounding the urinary meatus, swelling of the urinary meatus, or the presence of discharge around the urinary meatus. *This assessment provides baseline data.* If any discharge is present, obtain a culture swab.

7. Insert the catheter until urine flows.
   - Place the drainage end of the catheter in the urine receptacle. Pick up the insertion end of the catheter with your uncontaminated, sterile, gloved hand, holding it about 2 in. from the insertion tip. *Because the adult female urethra is approximately 1.5 in. long, the catheter is held far enough from the end to allow full insertion into the bladder and to maintain control of the tip of the catheter so it will not accidentally become contaminated.*
   - Gently insert the catheter into the urinary meatus until urine flows. Insert the catheter in the direction of the urethra. If the catheter meets resistance during insertion, do not force it. *Forceful pressure against the urethra can produce trauma.* Ask the client to take deep breaths. *This helps relax the external sphincter.* If this does not relieve the resistance, discontinue the procedure and report the problem to the nurse in charge. Exercise caution to prevent the catheter tip from becoming contaminated. If it becomes contaminated, discard it.
   - When the urine flows, transfer your hand from the labia to the catheter to hold it in place. *This prevents its expulsion by a possible bladder contraction.*

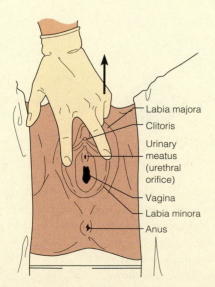

Labia majora
Clitoris
Urinary meatus (urethral orifice)
Vagina
Labia minora
Anus

Figure 27-18. ■ To expose the urinary meatus, separate the labia minora and retract the tissue upward.

8. Collect a urine specimen.
   - Pinch the catheter, and transfer the drainage end of it into the sterile specimen bottle. Usually 30 mL of urine is sufficient for a specimen. Securely place the top on the specimen container, and set it aside for labeling later.
9. Empty or partially drain the bladder, and then remove the catheter.
   - For adults experiencing urinary retention, some orders limit the amount of urine drained to 1,000 mL. Limiting the amount of urine drained has been a controversial issue. Rapid removal of large amounts of urine was once thought to induce engorgement of the pelvic blood vessels and hypovolemic shock. However, retained urine may serve as a reservoir for microorganisms to multiply. Usually agency policy or the physician indicates the amount to be removed and times at which the remaining urine is to be withdrawn. Research findings support the premise that complete drainage of a distended bladder is likely to be more comfortable and certainly seems as safe as threshold clamping.
   - Pinch the catheter. *This prevents leakage of urine.* Remove the catheter slowly.
10. Promote client comfort.
    - Dry the client's perineum with a towel or drape. *Excess lubricant and solution in the area can irritate the skin.*

11. Assess the urine.
    - Inspect the urine for color, clarity, odor, and the presence of any abnormal constituents, such as blood.
    - Measure the amount of urine.
12. Document the catheterization.
    - Include assessments before and after the procedure; type and size of catheter inserted; time; characteristics and amount of urine obtained; whether a specimen was sent to the laboratory; and client response to the procedure.

SAMPLE DOCUMENTATION

[date]
[time]
Urinary straight catheter inserted, urine spontaneous 300 mL, clear and straw colored. Urinalysis and C&S to lab. Catheter removed. Client tolerated procedure well.
_____ D. Haus, LVN

PROCEDURE 27-4

Male Urinary Catheterization Using a Straight Catheter

Purposes
- See Procedure 27-3, page 588

Equipment
- See Procedure 27-3. A #16 or #18 Fr. catheter is often used for an adult male.

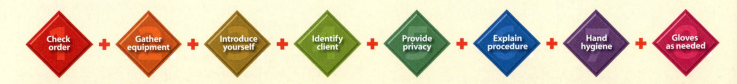

Check order + Gather equipment + Introduce yourself + Identify client + Provide privacy + Explain procedure + Hand hygiene + Gloves as needed

Interventions

1. Assess for urinary retention.
   - Palpate the bladder
2. Prepare the client.
   - Explain the catheterization, as in Procedure 27-3. Assist the client to a supine position, with the knees slightly flexed and the thighs slightly apart. *This allows greater relaxation of the abdominal and perineal muscles and permits easier insertion of the catheter.*

- Drape the client by folding the top bedclothes down so that the penis is exposed and the thighs are covered. Use a bath blanket to cover the client's chest and abdomen.
- Wear disposable gloves.
- Wash the penis and dry it well.
- Remove disposable gloves.
3. Create a sterile field.
   - Open the sterile tray, and don the sterile gloves.

- Place a drape under the penis and a second drape above the penis over the pubic area. If a fenestrated drape is available, place it over the penis and pubic area, exposing only the penis.
- Place the sterile kit on the sterile drape over the client's thighs or next to the thigh.
- Pour the antiseptic solution over the cotton balls, if they are not already prepared.
- Lubricate the insertion tip of the catheter liberally for about 2 to 6 in. Place it in the sterile container ready for insertion. *Water-soluble lubricant facilitates insertion of the catheter by reducing friction. This step is done before cleaning because the nurse will subsequently have only one sterile hand available.*

4. Clean the urinary meatus with antiseptic (if recommended by the agency).
- Grasp the penis firmly behind the glans with the nondominant hand, and spread the meatus between the thumb and forefinger. Retract the foreskin of an uncircumcised male. The hand holding the penis is now considered contaminated. Grasp the penis firmly to avoid stimulating an erection.
- With the dominant hand, use sterile forceps to pick up a swab. Clean the meatus first, and then wipe the tissue surrounding the meatus in a circular motion. Discard each swab after only one wipe. *Using forceps maintains the sterility of your gloves.*

5. Insert the catheter.
- Place the drainage end of the catheter in the urine receptacle. Then pick up the insertion end of the catheter with your uncontaminated, sterile, gloved hand, holding it about 3 to 4 in. from the insertion tip for an adult or about 1 in. for a baby or small boy. *In some agencies, the catheter is picked up with forceps.* The male urethra is approximately 8 in. long. Holding the catheter far enough from the end to maintain control of the tip of the catheter avoids accidental contamination.
- Lift the penis to a position perpendicular to the body (90-degree angle), and exert slight traction (pulling or tension upward). Insert the catheter steadily about 8 in. or until

urine begins to flow. *Lifting the penis so that it is perpendicular to the body straightens the downward curvature of the urethra.*
- To bypass slight resistance at the sphincters, twist the catheter, or wait until the sphincter relaxes. Ask the client to take deep breaths or try to void. If difficult resistance is met, discontinue the procedure and report the problem to the nurse in charge. *Slight resistance is normally encountered at the external and internal urethral sphincters. Deep breathing can help to relax the external sphincter. Forceful pressure exerted against a major resistance can traumatize the urethra.*
- While the urine flows, lower the penis, and transfer your hand to hold the catheter in place at the meatus.

6. Drain the urine from the bladder.
- Collect a urine specimen (if required) after the urine has flowed for a few seconds. Pinch the catheter, and transfer the drainage end of the catheter into the sterile specimen bottle, taking care not to contaminate the specimen container. Usually 30 mL of urine is sufficient for a specimen.
- Empty the bladder, or drain the amount of urine specified in the order. See Procedure 27-3, step 9.

7. Make the client comfortable.
- Dry the penis with a towel or drape.
- Replace the foreskin. *This prevents a mechanical phimosis (constriction), which may compromise circulation to the glans.*

8. Assess the client and the urine, as in Procedure 27-3, and document the procedure and the assessments.

SAMPLE DOCUMENTATION

[date]
[time]   Straight catheter inserted without difficulty. Urine C&S sent to the lab. Urine cloudy, with occasional mucous threads. Client tolerated procedure well.

_____ D. Haus, LVN

| PROCEDURE 27-5 | **Inserting a Retention (Indwelling) Catheter** |

Purposes

- To facilitate accurate measurement of urinary output for critically ill clients whose output needs to be monitored hourly
- To provide for intermittent or continuous bladder drainage and irrigation
- To prevent urine from contacting an incision after perineal surgery
- To manage incontinence when other measures have failed

Equipment

In addition to the equipment used for a straight catheterization, the following equipment is needed:

- Sterile retention catheter (#14 or #16 Fr. for adults, #8 or #10 Fr. for children are often used)
- Prefilled syringe (sterile water is often used)

- Nonallergenic tape or a catheter stabilizing or strapping device (e.g., urologic cath-strap)
- Safety pin or clip
- Urine collection bag and tubing (the tubing may be attached to the retention catheter if a closed drainage system is used)

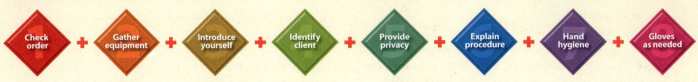

Interventions

1. Prepare the client and the equipment.
   - Explain to the client why the retention catheter is to be inserted, how long it will be in place, and how the urinary drainage equipment needs to be handled to maintain and facilitate the drainage of urine. Reassure the client that the procedure is painless. *Some clients experience the urge to void during insertion of the catheter and for a short time after the catheter is in place. Reassure these clients that the catheter drains the urine and that the urge to void will disappear.*
   - Follow the procedure for straight catheterization up to and including creating a sterile field.

2. Test the catheter balloon.
   - Attach the prefilled syringe to the balloon valve, and inject the fluid. *Sterile water rather than sterile saline should be used because the saline can crystallize and prevent complete deflation of the balloon.* The balloon should inflate appropriately and not leak. Withdraw the fluid and set aside the catheter with the syringe attached for later use. If the balloon leaks or does not inflate adequately, replace the catheter. In such a case, withdraw the fluid, and detach the syringe for later use. Ask another nurse to obtain a second catheter and open the package for you, then test the new balloon, or remove the equipment and obtain another catheter; then start again with the new sterile equipment.

3. Follow the steps as for straight catheterization.
   - Lubricate the insertion tip of the catheter.
   - Remove the sterile cap from the specimen container.
   - Expose and clean the urinary meatus and surrounding tissues with antiseptic if recommended.
   - Insert the catheter and inflate the balloon.
   - Collect a urine specimen as required.

4. Move the catheter farther into the bladder, and inflate the balloon.
   - Insert the catheter an additional 1 to 2 in. beyond the point at which urine began to flow. *The balloon of the catheter is located behind the opening at the insertion tip, and sufficient space needs to be provided to inflate the balloon. This ensures that the balloon is inflated inside the bladder and not in the urethra, where it could produce trauma.*

- Inflate the balloon by injecting the contents of the prefilled syringe into the valve of the catheter (Figure 27-20A ■). Placement of the catheter and balloon in a male client is shown in Figure 27-20B. If the client complains of discomfort or pain during the balloon inflation, withdraw the fluid, insert the catheter a little farther, and inflate the balloon again. Insert no more fluid than the balloon size indicates (e.g., 5 or 30 mL), and remove the syringe. A special valve prevents backflow of the fluid out of the

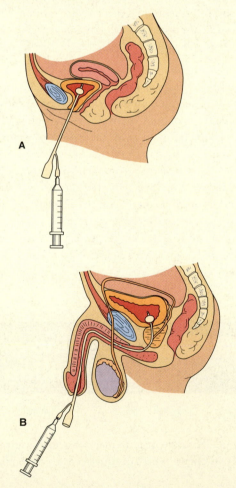

Figure 27-20. ■ Placement of retention catheter and inflated balloon: **A.** in female client; **B.** in male client.

catheter. Follow agency policy when using a 30-mL balloon. Some agency policies state that only 15 mL of fluid is injected for inflation.

5. Ensure effective balloon inflation.
   - When the balloon is safely inflated, apply slight tension on the catheter until you feel resistance. *Resistance indicates that the catheter balloon is inflated appropriately, and that the catheter is well anchored in the bladder.*
   - Then move the catheter slightly back into the bladder. *This keeps the balloon from exerting undue pressure on the neck of the bladder.*

6. Anchor the catheter.
   - Tape the catheter with nonallergenic tape to the inside of a female's thigh (Figure 27-21 ■) or to the thigh or abdomen of a male client (Figure 27-22 ■). Some nurses prefer taping the male catheter to the abdomen whenever there is increased risk of excoriation at the penile–scrotal junction. *Taping restricts the movement of the catheter, thus reducing friction and irritation in the urethra when the client moves. It also prevents skin excoriation at the penile–scrotal junction in the male.*

7. Establish effective drainage.
   - Ensure that the emptying base of the drainage bag is closed.
   - Secure the drainage bag to the bed frame, using the hook or strap provided. Suspend the bag off the floor, but keep it below the level of the client's bladder (see Figure 27-21). *Urine flows by gravity from the bladder to*

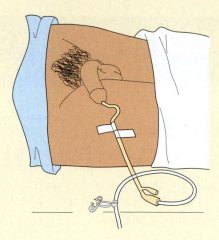

Figure 27-22. ■ Tape the catheter to the thigh or abdomen of a male client.

the drainage bag. The bag should be off the floor so that the emptying spout does not become grossly contaminated.
   - Coil the drainage tubing loosely beside the client so that the remaining tubing runs in a straight line down to the drainage bag. Fasten the vertical tubing to the bedclothes with tape, a tubing clamp, or a safety pin and elastic band (see Figures 27-21 and 27-22). *The drainage tubing should not loop below its entry into the drainage bag, which would impede the flow of urine by gravity.*

8. Document pertinent data.
   - Record the time and date of the catheterization; the type and size of catheter; the reason for catheterization; how much fluid was used to inflate the balloon; assessments before and after the procedure, including amount, color, and clarity of urine obtained; whether a specimen was taken and sent to the laboratory; whether all urine was emptied from the bladder; and the client's response.

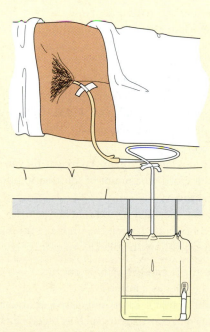

Figure 27-21. ■ Tape the catheter to the inside of a female's thigh.

SAMPLE DOCUMENTATION

[date]	Retention catheter #16 Fr inserted.
[time]	Urine spontaneous 300 mL, yellow straw colored. Client tolerated procedure well.
	_____ D. Haus, LVN

<table>
<tr><td>PROCEDURE 27-6</td><td># Irrigating a Catheter or Bladder (Closed System)</td></tr>
</table>

Before irrigating a catheter or bladder, check (1) the reason for the irrigation; (2) the order authorizing the continuous or intermittent irrigation (in most agencies, a physician's order is required); (3) the type of sterile solution, the amount and strength to be used, and the rate (if continuous); and (4) the type of catheter in place. If these are not specified on the client's chart, check agency protocol.

Purposes

■ To maintain the patency of a urinary catheter and tubing (continuous irrigation)
■ To free a blockage in a urinary catheter or tubing (intermittent irrigation)

Equipment

■ Disposable gloves
■ Disposable water-resistant sterile towel
■ Three-way retention catheter in place
■ Sterile drainage tubing and bag (if not in place)
■ Sterile antiseptic swabs
■ Sterile receptacle
■ Sterile irrigating solution warmed or at room temperature
■ Infusion tubing
■ IV pole

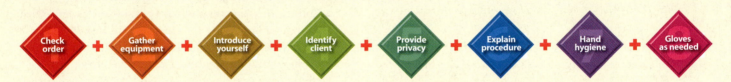

Check order + Gather equipment + Introduce yourself + Identify client + Provide privacy + Explain procedure + Hand hygiene + Gloves as needed

Interventions

1. Prepare the client.
   ■ Explain the procedure and its purpose to the client.
   ■ Provide for privacy and drape the client as needed to allow access to the retention catheter.
   ■ Don gloves.
   ■ Empty, measure, and record the amount and appearance of urine present in the drainage bag. Discard urine and gloves. *Emptying the drainage bag allows more accurate measurement of urinary output after the irrigation is in place or completed. Assessing the character of the urine provides baseline data for later comparison.*

2. Prepare the equipment.
   ■ Connect the irrigation infusion tubing to the irrigating solution and flush the tubing with solution.
   ■ Connect the irrigation tubing to the input port of the three-way catheter. Connect the drainage bag and tubing to the urinary drainage port if not already in place.

3. Irrigate the bladder.
   ■ For continuous irrigation, open the flow clamp on the urinary drainage tubing (if present). *This allows the irrigating solution to flow out of the bladder continuously.*
   a. Open the regulating clamp on the irrigating tubing and adjust the flow rate as prescribed by the physician or to 40 to 60 drops per minute if not specified.
   b. Assess the drainage for amount, color, and clarity. The amount of drainage should equal the amount of irrigant entering the bladder plus expected urine output.

■ For intermittent irrigation, determine whether the solution is to remain in the bladder for a specified time.
   a. If the solution is to remain in the bladder (a bladder irrigation or instillation), close the flow clamp on the urinary drainage tubing. *Closing the flow clamp allows the solution to be retained in the bladder and in contact with bladder walls.*
   b. If the solution is being instilled to irrigate the catheter, open the flow clamp on the urinary drainage tubing. Irrigating solution will flow through the urinary drainage port and tubing, removing mucous shreds or clots.
   c. Open the flow clamp on the irrigating tubing, allowing the specified amount of solution to infuse. Clamp the tubing.
   d. After the specified period that the solution is to be retained has passed, open the drainage tubing flow clamp and allow the bladder to empty.

4. Assess the client and the urinary output.
   ■ Assess the client's comfort.
   ■ Assess the amount, color, and clarity of drainage; note any abnormal constituents such as blood clots, pus, or mucous shreds.
   ■ To document urine output, empty the drainage bag and measure the contents. Subtract the amount of irrigant instilled from the total volume of drainage to obtain urine output.

5. Document the irrigation.
   - Include all assessments obtained before and after performing the irrigation.

VARIATION: CLOSED IRRIGATION USING A TWO-WAY INDWELLING CATHETER

1. Assemble the equipment, including:
   - Clean disposable gloves
   - Disposable water-resistant towel
   - Sterile irrigating solution
   - Sterile basin
   - Sterile 30- to 50-mL syringe with a #18- or #19-gauge needle
   - Sterile antiseptic swabs

2. Prepare the client (see step 1 of main procedure for catheter irrigation).

3. Prepare the equipment.
   - Perform hand hygiene and don gloves.
   - Place the disposable water-resistant towel under the catheter.
   - For a bladder irrigation or instillation, clamp the drainage tubing distal to the injection port on the tubing or catheter. *Clamping prevents the urine and solution from draining into the drainage bag.* For a catheter irrigation, leave the tubing unclamped.
   - Using aseptic technique, open supplies and pour the irrigating solution into the sterile basin or receptacle. *Aseptic technique is vital to reduce the risk of instilling microorganisms into the urinary tract during the irrigation.*
   - Remove the cap from the needle and draw the prescribed amount of irrigating solution into the syringe, maintaining the sterility of the syringe and solution.
   - Using the antiseptic swab, clean the port on the catheter or drainage tubing through which the solution will be instilled.

4. Irrigate the bladder.
   - Insert the needle into the port.
   - Gently inject the solution into the catheter. In adults, about 30 to 40 mL generally is instilled for catheter irrigations; 100 to 200 mL may be instilled for bladder irrigation or instillation. Smaller amounts are used for children.
   - When the total amount to be instilled has been injected (or for catheter irrigation, when urine is flowing freely), remove the needle from the port and discard the syringe and uncapped needle in an appropriate receptacle (sharps container).
   - After the prescribed dwelling time for a bladder irrigation, remove the clamp from the drainage tubing and allow the urine and irrigating solution to drain into the drainage bag.
   - Assess the drainage for amount, color, and clarity. *The amount of drainage should equal the amount of irrigant entering the bladder plus expected urine output.*

5. Assess the client and the urinary output and document the procedure as previously noted.

SAMPLE DOCUMENTATION

[date]
[time]
Continuous bladder irrigation maintained. Occasional clots noted, urine output at 700 mL this shift. Bladder nondistended and no complaints of discomfort.
_____ D. Haus, LVN

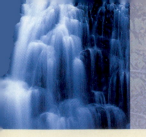

Chapter Review

KEY TERMS by Topic

Use the audio glossary feature of either the CD-ROM or the Companion Website to hear the correct pronunciation of the following key terms.

Physiology of Urinary Elimination
meatus, micturition, voiding

Factors Affecting Urinary Excretion
urinary retention, diuretics, calculus, dysuria

Altered Urine Production
hematuria, polyuria, diuresis, enuresis, oliguria, anuria

Collaborative Care
residual urine, midstream voided, specific gravity, incontinence, catheterization, irrigation, urinary diversion

KEY Points

- Urinary elimination depends on normal functioning of the urinary, cardiovascular, and nervous systems.

- Urine is formed in the nephron, the functional unit of the kidney, through a process of filtration, reabsorption, and secretion. Hormones such as ADH and aldosterone affect the reabsorption of sodium and water, thus affecting the amount of urine formed.

- The normal process of urination is stimulated when sufficient urine collects in the bladder to stimulate stretch receptors.

- In the adult, urination generally occurs after 250 to 450 mL of urine has collected in the bladder.

- Many factors influence a person's urinary elimination including growth and development, fluid intake, stress, activity, medications, and various diseases.

- Alterations in urine production and elimination include polyuria, oliguria, anuria, frequency, nocturia, urgency, dysuria, enuresis, hematuria, incontinence, and retention.

- Assessment of a client's urinary function includes (1) normal voiding patterns, recent changes, past and current problems with urination, and factors influencing the elimination pattern; (2) a physical assessment of the genitourinary system; (3) inspection of the urine for amount, color, clarity, and odor; and, if indicated, (4) testing of urine for specific gravity, pH, and the presence of glucose, ketone bodies, protein, and occult blood.

- Many NANDA-approved nursing diagnoses may apply to clients with altered urinary elimination patterns, for example, *Urinary Retention*, and related diagnoses such as *Risk for Infection*.

- Bladder training can often reduce episodes of incontinence.

- Clients with urinary retention are at risk of UTI.

- The most common cause of UTI is invasive procedures such as catheterization and cystoscopic examination. Females in particular are prone to ascending UTIs because of their short urethras.

- Nursing interventions for urinary elimination problems include (1) assisting the client to maintain an appropriate fluid intake, (2) assisting the client to maintain normal voiding patterns, (3) monitoring the client's daily fluid intake and output, and (4) maintaining cleanliness of the genital area.

- Urinary catheterization is frequently required for clients with urinary retention.

- Care of clients with indwelling catheters is directed toward preventing infection of the urinary tract and encouraging urinary flow through the drainage system.

- Bladder or catheter irrigations may be used to apply medication to bladder walls or maintain catheter patency.

- When the urinary bladder is removed, a urinary diversion is formed to allow urine to be eliminated from the body. The ileal conduit or ileal loop is the most common diversion and requires that the client wear a urine collection device continually over the stoma.

EXPLORE MediaLink

Additional interactive resources for this chapter can be found on the Companion Website at www.prenhall.com/ramont. Click on Chapter 27 and "Begin" to select the activities for this chapter.

For chapter-related NCLEX®-style questions and an audio glossary, access the accompanying CD-ROM in this book.

Animations/Videos
- Catheterization
- The Kidney

FOR FURTHER Study

For more information about wound care, see Chapter 23.
For more on recording fluid intake and output, see Chapter 26.

Caring for a Client with Impaired Urinary Elimination

NCLEX-PN® Focus Area: Physiological Integrity

Case Study: Mr. Lee Jay, a 54-year-old client, is being treated for out-of-control type 1 diabetes. He is incontinent of foul-smelling urine. He complains of thirst and frequent urination. He is 6′3″, weighs 200 lbs, and states, "I try to maintain my diabetic diet, but I'm on a fixed income." Mr. Jay is alert and oriented to person, place, and time. He monitors his glucose about once a week and gives himself insulin injections. He has diminished pedal pulses, and his feet are cool to the touch. The physician has ordered lab tests and an indwelling catheter.

Nursing Diagnosis: Impaired Urinary Elimination

COLLECT DATA

Subjective	Objective
_____	_____
_____	_____
_____	_____
_____	_____
_____	_____
_____	_____
_____	_____

Would you report this data? Yes/No

If yes, to: _____

What would you report? _____

Nursing Care

_____
_____
_____
_____
_____
_____
_____
_____
_____
_____
_____

How would you document this? _____
_____
_____

Compare your documentation to the sample provided in Appendix I.

Data collected
(use those that apply)

- Diabetes out of control
- Incontinent
- Foul-smelling urine
- Cloudy urine
- Mucous threads in urine
- Alert and oriented
- Weakened
- Diminished pedal pulses
- Glucose 440
- Temp. 99
- BP 140/80
- Tired
- Catheter to gravity drainage
- Thirst
- Diabetic care compliance

Nursing Interventions
(use those that apply; list in priority order)

- Take vital signs every 4 hours.
- Maintain catheter asepsis.
- Ambulate client tid.
- Monitor lab tests.
- Observe urine for output.
- Assess pedal pulses.
- OB stool. Stool for occult blood.
- Assess urine for abnormal constituents.
- Take daily weights.

NCLEX-PN® Exam Preparation

1 The fact that females are more prone to urinary tract infections (UTIs) is attributed to the length of the:

1. ureters.
2. urethra.
3. renal pelvis.
4. glomeruli.

2 The production of abnormally large amounts of urine by the kidneys is known as:

1. oliguria.
2. anuria.
3. polydipsia.
4. diuresis.

3 The normal adult amount of urine excreted per day is approximately:

1. 5,000 mL.
2. 3,500 mL.
3. 1,500 mL.
4. 500 mL.

4 The purpose of a urine culture is to determine:

1. whether pathogenic bacteria are present.
2. glucose level.
3. urine concentration.
4. occult blood.

5 The physician has ordered a 24-hour urine specimen. After instructing the client, the nurse will:

1. determine the specific gravity.
2. discard the first void and time the specimen.
3. test the urine for glucose.
4. begin timing the 24-hour specimen.

6 When obtaining a urine sample from a catheter, the nurse can clamp the catheter for:

1. 10 minutes.
2. 20 minutes.
3. 30 minutes.
4. 60 minutes.

7 The specific gravity of normal urine is between

1. 1.000 and 1.005.
2. 1.010 and 1.025.
3. 1.025 and 1.030.
4. 1.030 and 1.050.

8 Fluid restriction may be initiated for a client with:

1. diabetes.
2. renal calculi.
3. kidney failure.
4. UTI.

9 Identify a measure to prevent UTI recurrence:

1. Limit water intake.
2. Encourage the use of nylon underclothes.
3. Bathe frequently.
4. Drink cranberry juices and take vitamin C.

10 Your client has returned from surgery with a suprapubic catheter in place. This catheter is introduced through the client's:

1. ureter.
2. kidney.
3. urethra.
4. abdomen.

Answers and Rationales for Review Questions, as well as discussion of Care Plan and Critical Thinking Care Map questions, appear in Appendix I.

Chapter 28

Gastrointestinal Elimination

BRIEF Outline

Physiology of Defecation
Factors That Affect Defecation
Common Fecal Elimination Problems
Fecal Diversion Ostomies

LEARNING Outcomes

After completing this chapter, you will be able to:

1. Describe the functions of the lower intestinal tract.
2. Identify factors that influence fecal elimination and patterns of defecation.
3. Distinguish normal from abnormal characteristics and constituents of feces.
4. Describe methods used to assess the intestinal tract.
5. Differentiate five common fecal elimination problems.
6. Describe how to collect stool specimens and test for occult blood.
7. Discuss ways to assist the development of healthy defecation patterns.
8. Identify care and management for an ileostomy and colostomy.
9. Describe types of enemas and describe the procedure for administering an enema.

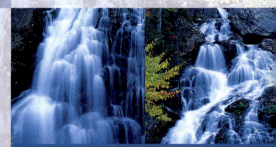

HISTORICAL Perspectives

Gastroenterology is a relatively new specialty but has roots dating back to 1868. Gabriella and Rudolph Schindler pioneered humane methods of performing gastroscopies with a semiflexible gastroscope that is still used today. Their method included numbing of the throat, instruction about the examination to encourage cooperation, and spoken guidance and encouragement during the procedure. This history demonstrates the creativity and dedication of the founders of gastroenterology.

Nurses frequently are involved in assisting clients with elimination problems. These problems can be embarrassing to clients and can cause considerable discomfort.

Physiology of Defecation

Elimination of the waste products of digestion from the body is essential to health. The excreted waste products are referred to as **feces** or *stool*.

LARGE INTESTINE

The large intestine extends from the ileocecal (ileocolic) valve, which lies between the small and large intestines, to the anus. The colon (large intestine) in the adult is generally about 125 to 150 cm (50 to 60 in.) long. It has seven parts: the cecum; ascending, transverse, and descending colons; sigmoid colon; rectum; and anus or external orifice (Figure 28-1 ■).

The large intestine is a muscular tube lined with mucous membrane. The muscle fibers are both circular and longitudinal, permitting the intestine to enlarge and contract in both width and length. This expansion and contraction enables **peristalsis**, a wavelike motion that propels intestinal contents forward.

The colon's main functions are the absorption of water and electrolytes, the mucal protection of the intestinal wall, and fecal elimination. The colon produces bacteria necessary for the synthesis of vitamin K. Vitamin K is necessary for coagulation of the blood. The waste products that leave the stomach through the small intestine and then pass through the ileocecal valve are called **chyme**. As much as 1,500 mL of chyme passes into the large intestine daily. Most of it is absorbed in the proximal colon; approximately 100 mL of fluid is excreted in the feces.

The colon also serves a protective function through mucous secretion. Mucus protects the intestinal wall from bacterial activity and helps hold fecal material together. Products of elimination include flatus and feces. **Flatus** is largely air and the by-products of the digestion of carbohydrates.

RECTUM AND ANAL CANAL

The rectum in the adult is usually 10 to 15 cm (4 to 6 in.) long; the most distal portion, 2.5 to 5 cm (1 to 2 in.) long, is the anal canal. When the veins in this area become distended, a condition known as hemorrhoids occurs.

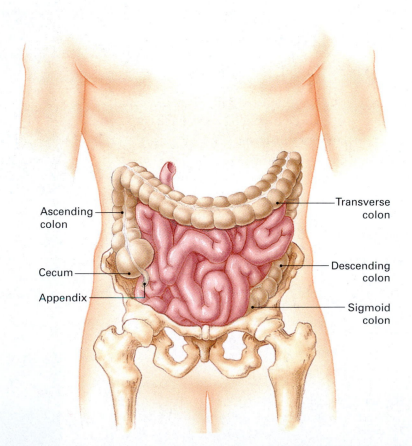

Ascending colon

Transverse colon

Cecum

Descending colon

Appendix

Sigmoid colon

Figure 28-1. ■ The large intestine. (*Source:* Fremgen, Bonnie F., Frucht, Suzanne S., Medical Terminology: A Living Language, 3rd ed. © 2005. Electronically reproduced with permission of Pearson Education, Inc., Upper Saddle River, New Jersey.)

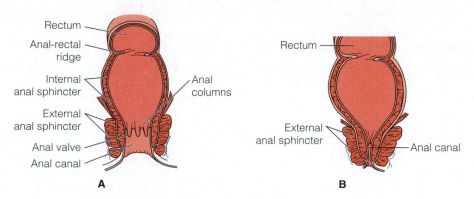

Figure 28-2. ■ The rectum, anal canal, and anal sphincters: **A.** open; **B.** closed.

The anal canal is bounded by an internal and an external sphincter muscle (Figure 28-2 ■). The internal sphincter is under involuntary control, and the external sphincter normally is voluntarily controlled.

Defecation

Defecation or *bowel movement* is the expulsion of feces from the anus and rectum. The frequency of defecation is highly individual, varying from several times per day to two or three times per week. The amount defecated also varies from person to person. When peristalsis moves the feces into the sigmoid colon and the rectum, the sensory nerves in the rectum are stimulated and the individual becomes aware of the need to defecate.

Expulsion of the feces is assisted by contraction of the abdominal muscles and the diaphragm. This maneuver causes an increase in abdominal pressure, which moves the feces through the anal canal. People who ignore the defecation reflex or who consciously inhibit it may eventually lose sensitivity to the defecation response. Constipation can be the end result.

Feces

Normal feces are made of about 75% water and 25% solid materials. They are soft but formed. If the feces are propelled very quickly along the large intestine, there is not time for most of the water to be reabsorbed and the feces will be more fluid. Normal feces require a normal fluid intake; feces that contain less water may be hard and difficult to expel.

Feces are normally brown, chiefly due to the presence of *bilirubin* (a red pigment in bile). Another factor that affects fecal color is the action of bacteria such as *Escherichia coli* or staphylococci, normally present in the large intestine. The action of microorganisms on the chyme contributes to the odor of feces. Table 28-1 ■ describes normal and abnormal characteristics of feces.

An adult usually forms 7 to 10 L of flatus (gas) in the large intestine every 24 hours. Air can be swallowed with food and fluids taken by mouth. Other gases are formed through the action of bacteria on the chyme in the large intestine.

Factors That Affect Defecation

AGE AND DEVELOPMENT

Defecation material and patterns change dramatically from birth to 2½ years. Bowel patterns are established at an early age and are maintained through most of life.

DIET

Sufficient bulk (cellulose, fiber) in the diet is necessary to provide fecal volume. Fiber stimulates peristalsis to maintain regularity. Low-residue foods, such as rice, eggs, and lean meats, move more slowly through the intestinal tract. Increasing fluid intake with such foods increases their rate of movement.

Certain foods and irregular eating can result in digestive upsets and, in some instances, the passage of watery stools. Individuals who eat at the same times every day usually have a regularly timed, physiological response to the food intake and a regular pattern of peristaltic activity in the colon.

Spicy foods can produce diarrhea and flatus in some individuals. Other foods that may influence bowel elimination include the following:

- Gas-producing foods, such as cabbage, onions, cauliflower, bananas, and apples
- Laxative-producing foods, such as bran, prunes, figs, chocolate, and alcohol
- Constipation-producing foods, such as cheese, pasta, eggs, and lean meat.

FLUIDS

Daily fluid intake of 2,000 to 3,000 mL is necessary to promote a normal soft formed stool. When fluid intake is inadequate or output is excessive, the body continues to reabsorb

TABLE 28-1

Characteristics of Normal and Abnormal Feces

CHARACTERISTIC	NORMAL	ABNORMAL	POSSIBLE CAUSE
Color	Adult: brown Infant: yellow	Clay or white	Absence of bile pigment (bile obstruction): diagnostic study using barium
		Black or tarry	Drug (e.g., iron); bleeding from upper gastrointestinal tract (e.g., stomach, small intestine); diet high in red meat and dark green vegetables (e.g., spinach)
		Red	Bleeding from lower gastrointestinal tract (e.g., rectum); some foods (e.g., beets)
		Pale	Malabsorption of fats; diet high in milk and milk products and low in meat
		Orange or green	Intestinal infection
Consistency	Formed, soft, semisolid, moist	Hard, dry	Dehydration; decreased intestinal motility resulting from lack of fiber in diet, lack of exercise, emotional upset, laxative abuse
		Diarrhea	Increased intestinal motility (e.g., due to irritation of the colon by bacteria)
Shape	Cylindrical (contour of rectum) about 2.5 cm (1 in.) in diameter in adults	Narrow, pencil-shaped, or stringlike stool	Obstructive condition of the rectum
Amount	Varies with diet (about 100–400 g/day)		
Odor	Aromatic: affected by ingested food and person's own bacterial flora	Pungent	Infection, blood
Constituents	Small amounts of undigested roughage, sloughed dead bacteria and epithelial cells, fat, protein, dried constituents of digestive juices (e.g., bile pigments), inorganic matter (calcium, phosphates)	Pus	Bacterial infection
		Mucus	Inflammatory condition
		Parasites	
		Blood	Gastrointestinal bleeding
		Large quantities of fat	Malabsorption
		Foreign objects	Accidental ingestion

fluid. As a result, the feces become hardened and drier than normal. If chyme moves abnormally quickly through the large intestine, however, there is less time for fluid to be absorbed into the blood; as a result, the feces are soft or even watery.

ACTIVITY

Activity stimulates peristalsis, thus facilitating the movement of chyme along the colon. Weak abdominal and pelvic muscles are often ineffective in increasing the intra-abdominal pressure during defecation or in controlling defecation. Weak muscles can result from lack of exercise, immobility, or impaired neurologic functioning. Clients confined to bed are often constipated.

PSYCHOLOGICAL FACTORS

Some people who are anxious or angry experience increased peristaltic activity and subsequent diarrhea. In contrast, people who are depressed may experience slower intestinal motility, resulting in constipation.

DEFECATION HABITS

Hospitalized clients may suppress the urge because of embarrassment about using a bedpan, lack of privacy, or because defecation is too uncomfortable.

MEDICATIONS

Some drugs have side effects that can interfere with normal elimination. Some cause diarrhea; others, such as tranquilizers, morphine, and codeine, cause constipation because they decrease gastrointestinal activity. Iron tablets act more locally on the bowel mucosa to cause constipation.

Some medications are intended to directly affect elimination. Laxatives and cathartics are medications that stimulate bowel activity and assist fecal elimination. Other medications soften stool, facilitating defecation. Certain medications, such as dicyclomine hydrochloride (Bentyl), suppress peristaltic activity and sometimes are used to treat diarrhea.

Some medications affect the appearance of the feces. Any drug that causes gastrointestinal bleeding as a side effect (e.g., aspirin products) can cause the stool to be red or black (**tarry**). Iron preparations may cause the stool to be black. Antibiotics may cause a gray-green discoloration because of effects on digestion; and antacids may cause a whitish discoloration or white specks in the stool.

DIAGNOSTIC PROCEDURES

Common diagnostic procedures for the gastrointestinal system include a barium swallow (upper gastrointestinal series) in which the client swallows a radiopaque substance that provides an outline of the alimentary canal. Films are obtained to identify abnormalities and diagnosis. A barium enema (lower gastrointestinal series) is given to the client as a contrast barium enema and x-rays are taken. This procedures identifies disorders of the colon. Before certain diagnostic procedures, such as visualization of the sigmoid colon (**sigmoidoscopy**), the client is often restricted from ingesting food or fluid. The client may also be given a cleansing enema prior to the examination.

ANESTHESIA AND SURGERY

General anesthetics cause the normal colon movements to cease or slow down by blocking parasympathetic stimulation. Clients who have regional or spinal anesthesia are less likely to experience this problem.

Surgery that involves direct handling of the intestines can cause intestinal movement to cease temporarily. This condition, called **paralytic ileus**, usually lasts 24 to 48 hours. Listening for bowel sounds that reflect intestinal motility is an important nursing assessment following surgery.

PATHOLOGICAL CONDITIONS

Spinal cord injuries and head injuries can decrease the sensory stimulation for defecation. Impaired mobility may limit the client's ability to respond to the urge to defecate, resulting in constipation. Poorly functioning anal sphincters may cause the client to experience fecal incontinence.

PAIN

Clients who experience discomfort when defecating often suppress the urge to defecate to avoid the pain. They experience constipation as a result.

Common Fecal Elimination Problems

Five common problems are related to fecal elimination: constipation, fecal impaction, diarrhea, bowel incontinence, and flatulence.

CONSTIPATION

Constipation is defined as fewer than three bowel movements per week. The client has small, dry, hard stool, or

---

BOX 28-1

Manifestations of Constipation

- Decreased frequency of defecation
- Hard, dry, formed stools
- Straining at stool; painful defecation
- Reports of rectal fullness or pressure or incomplete bowel evacuation
- Abdominal pain, cramps, or distention
- Use of laxatives
- Decreased appetite
- Headache

---

passes no stool for a period of time. Constipation occurs when the movement of feces through the large intestine is slow, allowing time for additional reabsorption of fluid from the large intestine. Constipation is associated with difficult evacuation of stool and increased effort or straining of the voluntary muscles of defecation. It is not associated with a specific number of bowel movements in a set time, because the range of normal varies. Assessment of the person's habits is necessary before a diagnosis of constipation is made. See Box 28-1 ■ for defining characteristics of constipation.

Constipation can be hazardous to some clients. Straining associated with constipation often is accompanied by holding the breath (**Valsalva maneuver**). This maneuver can present serious problems to people with heart disease, brain injuries, or respiratory disease. Holding the breath increases the intrathoracic and intracranial pressures. To some degree, this pressure can be reduced if the person exhales through the mouth while straining. However, avoiding straining altogether is the best precaution.

FECAL IMPACTION

Fecal **impaction** is a mass or collection of hardened, putty-like feces in the folds of the rectum. Impaction results from prolonged retention and accumulation of fecal material. Fecal impaction is recognized by the passage of liquid fecal seepage and no normal stool. The liquid portion of the feces seeps out around the impacted mass (Figure 28-3 ■).

The client may experience symptoms that include a frequent but nonproductive urge to defecate, as well as rectal pain. A generalized feeling of illness results. The client becomes anorexic, the abdomen becomes distended, and nausea and vomiting may occur.

The causes of fecal impaction are usually poor defecation habits and constipation. As mentioned, certain medications affect elimination and can contribute to impactions. Substances such as the barium used in radiologic examinations

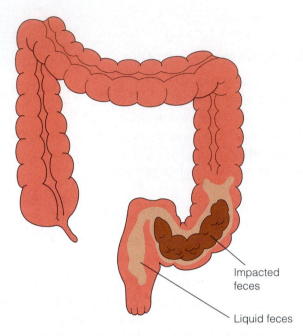

Impacted feces

Liquid feces

Figure 28-3. ■ A fecal impaction with liquid feces passing around the impaction.

of the upper and lower gastrointestinal tracts can also be a causative factor. After examinations of the lower gastrointestinal tract, measures are usually taken to ensure removal of the barium and prevent complications.

Impaction can be assessed by digital examination of the rectum, during which the hardened mass can often be palpated. Digital examination of the impaction through the rectum should be done gently and carefully, because stimu-

lation of the **vagus nerve** in the rectal wall can slow the client's heart.

Although fecal impaction can generally be prevented, digital removal of impacted feces is sometimes necessary. When fecal impaction is suspected, the client is often given an oil retention enema, a cleansing enema 2 to 4 hours later, and daily additional cleansing enemas, suppositories, or stool softeners. If these measures fail, manual removal is often necessary.

DIARRHEA

Diarrhea refers to the passage of liquid feces and increased frequency of defecation. Rapid passage of chyme reduces the time available for the large intestine to reabsorb water and electrolytes. The person with diarrhea finds it difficult or impossible to control the urge to defecate. Bowel sounds are increased, and spasmodic cramps occur. Sometimes the client passes blood and excessive mucus; nausea and vomiting may also occur. With persistent diarrhea, irritation of the anal area, the perineum, and buttocks generally results. Fatigue, weakness, and dehydration with possible electrolyte imbalance are the results of prolonged diarrhea.

When the cause of diarrhea is irritants in the intestinal tract, diarrhea is thought to be a protective mechanism. However, it can create serious fluid and electrolyte losses in the body. Table 28-2 ■ lists some of the major causes of diarrhea and the physiological responses of the body.

BOWEL INCONTINENCE

Bowel **incontinence**, also called fecal incontinence, refers to the loss of voluntary fecal control and gaseous elimina-

TABLE 28-2
Major Causes of Diarrhea

CAUSE	PHYSIOLOGICAL EFFECT
Psychological stress (e.g., anxiety)	Increased intestinal motility and mucous secretion
Medications	
Antibiotics	Inflammation and infection of mucosa due to overgrowth of pathogenic intestinal microorganisms
Iron	Irritation of intestinal mucosa
Cathartics	Irritation of intestinal mucosa
Allergy to food, fluid, drugs	Incomplete digestion of food or fluid
Intolerance of food or fluid	Increased intestinal motility and mucous secretion
Diseases of the colon	
Malabsorption syndrome	Reduced absorption of fluids
Crohn's disease	Inflammation of the mucosa often leading to ulcer formation
Others	
Surgical operations	Variable

tion through the anus. The incontinence may occur at specific times, such as after meals, or it may occur irregularly.

Fecal incontinence is generally associated with impaired functioning of the anal sphincter or its nerve supply, such as in some neuromuscular diseases, spinal cord trauma, and tumors of the external anal sphincter muscle.

Fecal incontinence is an emotionally distressing problem that can lead to embarrassment and social isolation. Incontinent feces are acidic and contain digestive enzymes that are highly irritating to skin. Therefore, the area around the anal region should be kept clean and dry and protected with a moisture barrier ointment.

FLATULENCE

There are three primary causes of flatus: (1) action of bacteria on the chyme in the large intestine, (2) swallowed air, and (3) gas that diffuses from the bloodstream into the intestine.

Flatulence is the presence of excessive *flatus* (gas) in the intestines. It leads to stretching and inflation of the intestines (intestinal distention). Large amounts of air and other gases can accumulate in the stomach, resulting in gastric distention.

Most gases that are swallowed are expelled through the mouth by **eructation** (belching or burping). Flatulence can occur in the colon, from a variety of causes, such as foods (e.g., cabbage, onions), abdominal surgery, or narcotics. If the gas is propelled by increased colon activity, it may be expelled through the anus. If excessive gas cannot be expelled through the anus, it may be necessary to insert a rectal tube or to provide a return flow enema (also called a Harris flush) to remove it. Procedure 28-1 ■ on page 614 explains how to insert a rectal tube.

Fecal Diversion Ostomies

An **ostomy** is an opening in the abdominal wall for the elimination of feces or urine. There are many types of ostomies. An **ileostomy** is an opening into the *ileum* (small bowel). A **colostomy** is an opening into the *colon* (large bowel). The purpose of bowel and urinary ostomies is to divert and drain waste material. Bowel diversion ostomies are often classified according to (1) status (permanent or temporary), (2) their location, and (3) the construction of the stoma.

PERMANENCE

Temporary colostomies are generally performed for traumatic injuries or inflammatory conditions of the bowel. They allow the distal diseased portion of the bowel to rest and heal. Permanent colostomies are performed to provide a means of elimination when the rectum or anus is nonfunctional as a result of a birth defect or a disease such as cancer of the bowel. The diseased portion may or may not be removed.

ANATOMIC LOCATION

An ileostomy generally empties from the distal end of the small intestine. An *ascending colostomy* empties from the as-

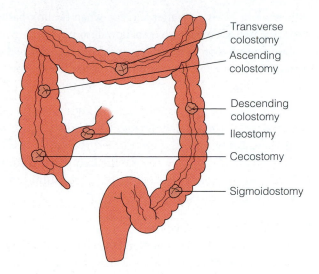

Figure 28-4. ■ The locations of bowel diversion ostomies.

cending colon. A *transverse colostomy* empties from the transverse colon. A *descending colostomy* empties from the descending colon. A *sigmoidostomy* empties from the sigmoid colon. A cecostomy empties from the cecum (Figure 28-4 ■).

STOMA CONSTRUCTION

Ostomy construction can be classified in the following ways.

End Colostomy or Single-Barrel

The functioning end of the intestine (the section of bowel that remains connected to the upper gastrointestinal tract) is brought out onto the surface of the abdomen, forming the stoma by cuffing the intestine back on itself and suturing the end to the skin. A stoma is an artificial opening created to the surface of the body. The distal portion of bowel (now connected only to the rectum) may be removed, or sutured closed and left in the abdomen. An end colostomy is usually a permanent ostomy, resulting from trauma, cancer, or another pathological condition.

Double-Barrel Colostomy

This colostomy involves the creation of two separate stomas on the abdominal wall. The proximal (nearest) stoma is the functional end that is connected to the upper gastrointestinal tract and will drain stool. The distal stoma, connected to the rectum and also called a mucous fistula, drains small amounts of mucus material. This is most often a temporary colostomy performed to rest an area of bowel, and to be later closed.

Loop Colostomy

This colostomy is created by bringing a loop of bowel through an incision in the abdominal wall. The loop is held in place outside the abdomen by a plastic rod slipped beneath it. An incision is made in the bowel to allow the passage of stool through the loop colostomy. The supporting rod is removed approximately 7–10 days after surgery, when healing has occurred that will prevent the loop of bowel from retracting into the abdomen. A loop colostomy is most often performed for creation of a temporary stoma to divert stool away from an area of intestine that has been blocked or ruptured.

The location of the ostomy affects the character and management of the fecal drainage. The farther along the bowel the ostomy is, the more formed the stool, because the large bowel reabsorbs water. So the frequency of stomal discharge can be controlled better by establishing an ostomy in the large intestine.

OSTOMY MANAGEMENT

Clients with **fecal diversions** need considerable psychological support, instruction, and physical care. Many agencies contract with enterostomal therapy nurses to assist these clients.

STOMA AND SKIN CARE

Fecal material (**effluent**) from a colostomy or ileostomy is irritating to the peristomal skin. Ileal effluent (products of elimination) is especially irritating, because it contains digestive enzymes. The nurse assesses the peristomal skin for irritation each time the appliance is changed. See Box 28-2 ■ for assessing a stoma. Any skin irritation or breakdown needs to be treated immediately.

The skin is kept clean by washing off any excretion and drying the skin thoroughly. An **appliance** (pouch or bag) is then fitted securely to the stoma. Drying the skin before attaching the appliance is crucial, because pouches do not adhere to moist skin, and effluent will leak out. All appliances have three features in common: a pouch to collect the effluent, an outlet at the bottom for easy emptying, and a faceplate. The faceplate is an adhesive ring placed on the client's skin; the pouch attaches to the faceplate.

Odor control is essential to clients' self-esteem. Selecting the appropriate kind of appliance promotes odor control. An intact appliance contains odors. The appliance should be rinsed thoroughly when it is emptied. Deodorizers can be placed in the pouch of the appliance. Oral intake of bismuth subcarbonate can be prescribed by the physician to help control odor.

Disposable ostomy appliances can be used for up to 5 to 7 days. They need to be changed whenever the effluent leaks onto the **peristomal** skin or when effluent cannot be rinsed completely away. The bag should be monitored for drainage and emptied when it is one-third full. This prevents pulling on the appliance and accidental soiling. If the skin is erythematous (red), eroded, denuded, or ulcerated, it should be changed every 24 to 48 hours to allow appropriate treatment of the skin. If the client complains of pain or discomfort, the area should be carefully inspected. Procedure 28-2 ■ on page 614 explains how to change a bowel diversion ostomy appliance, and Procedure 28-3 ■ on page 617 lists the steps for irrigating a colostomy.

Procedure 28-2 ■ on page 614 ... Procedure 28-3 ■ on page 617

BOX 28-2

Assessing a Stoma

- *Stoma color.* The stoma should appear red, similar in color to the mucosal lining of the inner cheek. Very pale or darker-colored stomas with a bluish or purplish hue indicate impaired blood circulation to the area.

- *Stoma size and shape.* Most stomas protrude slightly from the abdomen. New stomas normally appear swollen, but swelling generally decreases over 2 or 3 weeks or may take as long as 6 weeks. Failure of swelling to recede may indicate a problem, such as blockage.

- *Slight bleeding.* Initially the stoma bleeds slightly when it is touched, but other bleeding should be reported.

- *Status of peristomal skin.* Any redness and irritation of the peristomal skin—the 5 to 13 cm (2 to 5 in.) of skin surrounding the stoma—should be noted.

- *Amount and type of feces.* For ileal effluent and feces (effluent from a colostomy), assess amount, color, odor, and consistency. Inspect for abnormalities, such as pus or blood.

- *Complaints.* Complaints of a burning sensation under the faceplate may indicate skin breakdown. The presence of abdominal discomfort or distention also needs to be determined.

COLLABORATIVE CARE

Diagnostic and Laboratory Studies

Diagnostic studies of the gastrointestinal tract include direct visualization techniques, indirect visualization techniques, and laboratory tests for abnormal constituents.

Visualization Techniques

Direct visualization techniques include:

- *Anoscopy,* the viewing of the anal canal
- *Proctoscopy,* the viewing of the rectum
- *Proctosigmoidoscopy,* the viewing of the rectum and sigmoid
- *Colonoscopy,* the viewing of the large intestine.

Indirect visualization of the gastrointestinal tract is achieved by *roentgenography (x-ray films).* X-rays of the gastrointestinal (GI) tract can detect strictures, obstructions, tumors, ulcers, inflammatory disease, or other structural changes such as hiatal hernias. Introduction of a radiopaque substance such as barium enhances visualization of the GI tract. For examination of the upper GI tract or small bowel, the client drinks the barium sulfate (barium swallow). For examination of the lower GI tract, the client is given an enema containing the barium, commonly referred to as a barium enema. These x-rays usually include fluoroscopic examination. That is, the x-ray films are projected onto a screen, which permits continuous observation of the flow of barium. The LPN/LVN prepares the patient for the test, maintains NPO status prior to the test if necessary, and follows a physician-established protocol.

BOX 28-3 **NURSING CARE CHECKLIST**

Obtaining Stool Specimens

When obtaining stool samples:

☑ Follow medical aseptic technique.

☑ Wear disposable gloves to prevent contamination of the hands or of the outside of the specimen container.

☑ Use clean tongue blades to transfer the specimen to the container and then dispose of them in the waste container.

☑ Collect the amount of stool required. Usually about 1 in. of formed stool or 15 to 30 mL of liquid stool is adequate. For some timed specimens, the entire stool passed may need to be sent.

☑ Include visible pus, mucus, or blood in sample specimens.

☑ For a stool culture, dip a sterile swab into the specimen, preferably where purulent fecal matter is present. Using sterile technique, place the swab in a sterile test tube.

☑ Send the specimens to the laboratory immediately (fresh specimens provide the most accurate results). In some instances refrigeration is indicated, because bacteriologic changes take place in stool specimens left at room temperature.

Stool Specimens

The nurse is responsible for collecting stool specimens for testing. Before obtaining a specimen, the nurse needs to determine the correct method of obtaining and handling it. In many situations, only a single specimen is required. In others, timed specimens are necessary, which require that every stool passed be collected within a designated time period and sent to the laboratory immediately (if ordered).

Nurses need to give clients the following instructions:

■ Defecate in a clean **bedpan** (receptacle for urine or feces) or bedside commode.

■ Empty the bladder before specimen collection. If possible, do not contaminate the specimen with urine or menstrual discharge.

■ Do not place toilet tissue in the bedpan after defecation. Contents of the paper can affect the results.

■ Notify the nurse as soon as possible after defecation.

Box 28-3 ■ provides guidelines for obtaining a stool specimen.

NURSING CARE

ASSESSING

The LPN/LVN gathers data by performing a physical examination of the abdomen, rectum, and anus; inspecting the feces; and reviewing any data obtained from relevant diagnos-

tic tests. Collected data are used in collaboration with the RN when planning care.

Physical examination of the abdomen includes inspection, auscultation, and light palpation. Auscultation is done before palpation, because palpation can alter peristalsis. Examination of the rectum and anus includes inspection and palpation.

Inspecting the Feces

The client's stool is inspected for color, consistency, shape, amount, odor, and the presence of abnormalities. See Table 28-1 for a summary of normal and abnormal characteristics of stool and possible causes.

Testing Feces for Occult Blood

Stool is tested for **occult** (hidden) **blood** to detect gastrointestinal bleeding that is not visible to the eye. Bleeding can occur as a result of ulcers, inflammatory disease, or tumors. The test for occult blood, often referred to as the **guaiac test** (which uses blood-sensitive guaiac paper), can be readily performed by the nurse in the clinical area or by the client at home. Refer to Box 28-4 ■ for client instructions in testing the stool for occult blood.

Certain foods, medications, and vitamin C can produce inaccurate test results. False-positive results can occur if the client has recently ingested (1) red meat; (2) raw vegetables

BOX 28-4 **CLIENT TEACHING**

Assessing Stool for Occult Blood

■ Avoid restricted foods, medications, and vitamin C for the period recommended by the manufacturer and during the test.

■ Label the specimens with your name, address, age, and date of specimen. Three specimens are collected from consecutive and different bowel movements, to confirm negative results and avoid false-positive results.

■ Avoid collecting specimens during your menstrual period and for 3 days afterward, or if you have bleeding hemorrhoids or blood in your urine.

■ Avoid contaminating the specimen with urine or toilet tissue. Empty your bladder before the test. To facilitate specimen collection, transfer the stool to a clean, dry container. Wear disposable gloves.

■ Use the tongue blade provided to transfer the specimen to the test folder or tape. Only a small amount of stool is required. Take the sample from the center of a formed stool to ensure a uniform sample.

■ For a Hemoccult test, a thin layer of feces is smeared over the boxes inside the envelope, and a drop of developing solution is applied on the opposite side of the specimen paper. For the Hematest, a thin layer of feces is smeared onto guaiac filter paper, a tablet is placed in the middle of the specimen, and two or three drops of water are added to the tablet.

or fruits, particularly radishes, turnips, horseradish, and melons; or (3) certain medications that irritate the gastric mucosa and cause bleeding, such as aspirin, iron preparations, and anticoagulants.

DIAGNOSING, PLANNING, AND IMPLEMENTING

The LPN/LVN should be aware of appropriate nursing diagnoses related to bowel elimination. Some common NANDA diagnoses for fecal elimination problems are *Constipation, Diarrhea,* and *Risk for Imbalanced Fluid Volume.*

The major goals for clients with fecal elimination problems are to:

- Maintain or restore normal bowel elimination pattern.
- Maintain or regain normal stool consistency.
- Prevent associated risks such as fluid and electrolyte imbalance, skin breakdown (see hygiene discussions in Chapter 22 ⊘), abdominal distention, and pain. Refer to Box 28-5 ■ for discharge instructions regarding healthy defecation.

Promoting Regular Defecation

The nurse can help clients in the clinical setting to achieve regular defecation by providing (1) privacy, (2) a regular time for defecation, (3) nutrition and fluids, (4) exercise, and (5) correct positioning.

Privacy

Privacy during defecation is extremely important, but the nurse may need to stay with clients who are too weak to be left alone.

Timing

A client should be encouraged to defecate when the urge to defecate is recognized. Many people have well-established times and routines for defecation that should be part of the client's schedule. Clients should not be hurried but given adequate time to defecate.

BOX 28-5

Discharge Teaching for Healthy Defecation

- Establish a regular exercise regimen.
- Include high-fiber foods, such as vegetables, fruits, and whole grains, in the diet.
- Maintain fluid intake of 2,000 to 3,000 mL a day.
- Do not ignore the urge to defecate.
- Allow time to defecate, preferably at the same time each day.
- Avoid over-the-counter medications to treat constipation and diarrhea.

Nutrition and Fluids

The diet a client needs for regular normal elimination varies, depending on the kind of feces the client currently has, the frequency of defecation, and the types of foods that the client finds assist normal defecation.

- *For constipation:* Increase daily fluid intake, and instruct the client to drink hot liquids and fruit juices, especially prune juice. Include fiber-rich foods in the diet, such as prunes, raw fruit, bran products, and whole-grain cereals and bread.
- *For diarrhea:* Encourage oral intake of fluids and bland food. Eating small amounts of bland foods can be helpful because they are more easily absorbed. Diarrhea can lead to potassium losses. Highly spiced foods and high-fiber foods can aggravate diarrhea. See Box 28-6 ■ for details about managing diarrhea in the clinical setting and at home.
- *For flatulence:* Limit carbonated beverages, the use of drinking straws, and chewing gum. These increase the ingestion of air. Gas-forming foods, such as cabbage, beans, onions, and cauliflower, should also be avoided.

Exercise

Regular exercise helps clients develop a regular defecation pattern. Weak abdominal and pelvic muscles impede

---

BOX 28-6   **CLIENT TEACHING**

Managing Diarrhea

- Drink at least eight glasses of water per day to prevent dehydration.
- Avoid alcohol, beverages with caffeine, and excessively cold fluids, which aggravate the problem.
- Ingest foods with sodium and potassium. Most foods contain sodium. Potassium is found in dairy products, meats, and many vegetables and fruits, especially tomatoes, potatoes, bananas, peaches, and apricots.
- Limit foods containing insoluble fiber, such as whole-wheat and whole-grain breads and cereals, and raw fruits and vegetables.
- Increase foods containing soluble fiber, such as oatmeal and skinless fruits and potatoes.
- Limit fatty foods (e.g., dairy products and packaged processed meats).
- Thoroughly clean and dry the perianal area after passing stool to prevent skin irritation and breakdown. Use soft toilet tissue to clean and dry the area. Apply a moisture-barrier cream or ointment, such as zinc oxide or petrolatum, as needed.
- Discontinue medications or foods that cause diarrhea.
- When diarrhea has stopped, reestablish normal bowel flora by eating fermented dairy products, such as yogurt or buttermilk.

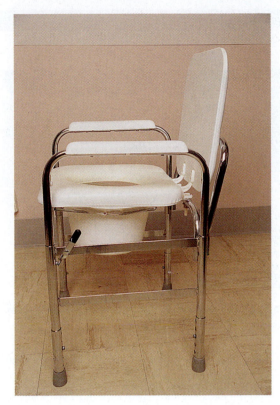

Figure 28-5. ■ Commode with overlying seat. (Photographer: Elena Dorfman.)

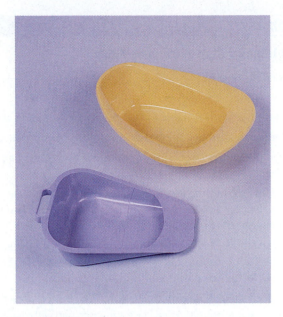

Figure 28-6. ■ The high-back or regular bedpan and the fracture or slipper pan. (Photographer: Jenny Thomas.)

normal defecation. In the clinical setting, encourage ambulatory clients to walk frequently in the room or the hallway.

Positioning

To aid defecation, the best position on a toilet seat for most people seems to be leaning forward. For clients who have difficulty moving themselves to and from the toilet, an elevated toilet seat can be attached to a regular toilet. A bedside commode is often used for the adult client who can get out of bed but is unable to walk to the bathroom (Figure 28-5 ■).

Clients restricted to bed may need to use a bedpan. The two main types of bedpans are the regular high-back pan and the fracture (or slipper) pan (Figure 28-6 ■). The fracture pan has a low back and is used for clients who cannot raise their buttocks. Nursing guidelines for giving and removing a bedpan are presented in Box 28-7 ■. Female clients use a bedpan for both urine and feces. Male clients use a bedpan for feces and a urinal for urine.

Most male clients are able to use a urinal independently either in bed or when standing at the bedside. The nurse must remain with clients who need support to stand at the bedside. For clients who cannot stand at the bedside, place the urinal between the client's legs with the handle uppermost so that urine will flow into it.

Teaching about Medications

Antidiarrheal Medications

These medications are usually reserved for treatment of chronic diarrhea (more than 3 to 4 weeks). They slow the motility of the intestine or absorb excess fluid in the intestine.

Antiflatulent Medications

Antiflatulent agents such as simethicone do not decrease the formation of flatus. They do coalesce the gas bubbles and facilitate their passage by belching through the mouth or expulsion through the anus.

Cathartics and Laxatives

Cathartics are drugs that induce defecation. They can have a strong, purging effect. A **laxative** is mild when compared to a cathartic. Laxatives produce frequent soft or liquid stools that are sometimes accompanied by abdominal cramps. Table 28-3 ■ describes the different types of laxatives. Some laxatives are given in the form of suppositories. These act in various ways: by softening the feces, by releasing gases such as carbon dioxide to distend the rectum, or by stimulating the nerve endings in the rectal mucosa.

Laxative abuse is believed to be a common problem. Older adults in particular often use laxatives improperly. Continual use of laxatives weakens the bowel's natural responses to fecal distention and results in chronic constipation.

clinical ALERT

Laxatives are contraindicated in the client who has nausea, cramps, fever, vomiting, or undiagnosed abdominal pain.

BOX 28-7   **NURSING CARE CHECKLIST**

Giving and Removing a Bedpan

☑ Provide privacy.

☑ Wear disposable gloves.

☑ If the bedpan is metal, warm it by rinsing it with warm water.

☑ Adjust the bed to a height appropriate to prevent back strain.

☑ Elevate the side rail on the opposite side to prevent the client from falling out of bed.

☑ Ask the client to assist by flexing the knees, resting the weight on the back and heels, and raising the buttocks, or by using a trapeze bar, if present.

☑ Help lift the client as needed by placing one hand under the lower back, resting your elbow on the mattress, and using your forearm as a lever.

☑ Place a regular bedpan so that the client's buttocks rest on the smooth, rounded rim. Place a fracture pan with the flat, low end under the client's buttocks (Figure 28-7 ■).

☑ For the client who cannot assist, obtain the assistance of another nurse to help lift the client onto the bedpan. Or, place the client on his or her side, place the bedpan against the buttocks (Figure 28-8 ■), and roll the client back onto the bedpan.

☑ To provide a more normal position for the client's lower back, elevate the client's bed to a semi-Fowler's position, if permitted. If elevation is contraindicated, support the client's back with pillows as needed to prevent hyperextension of the back.

☑ Cover the client with bed linen to maintain comfort and self-dignity.

☑ Provide toilet tissue, place the call light within reach, lower the bed to the low position, elevate the side rail if indicated, and leave the client alone.

☑ Answer the call bell promptly.

☑ When removing the bedpan, return the bed to the position used when giving the bedpan. Hold the bedpan steady to

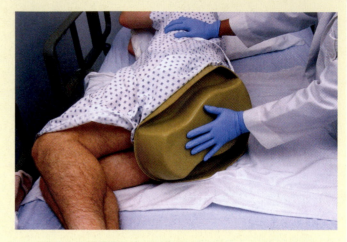

Figure 28-8. ■ Placing a bedpan against a client's buttocks.

prevent spillage of its contents. Cover the bedpan, and place it on the bedside chair.

☑ If the client needs assistance with cleaning, don gloves and wipe the client's perineal area with several layers of toilet tissue. If a specimen is to be collected, discard the soiled tissue into a moisture-proof receptacle other than the bedpan. For female clients, clean from the urethra toward the anus to prevent the transfer of rectal microorganisms into the urinary meatus.

☑ Wash the perineal area of dependent clients with soap and water as indicated, and dry the area thoroughly.

☑ For all clients, offer warm water, soap, a washcloth, and a towel to wash the hands.

☑ Assist the client to a comfortable position, empty and clean the bedpan, and return it to the bedside.

☑ Remove and discard your gloves and wash your hands.

☑ Document color, odor, amount, and consistency of urine and feces, and the condition of the perineal area.

Assessment Interview Fecal Elimination

Defecation Pattern

☑ What is the frequency and time of day of defecation?

☑ Has this pattern changed recently?

Description of Feces and Any Changes

☑ How would you describe your stool in terms of color, texture (hard, soft, watery), shape, odor?

☑ Have you noticed any changes in your stool recently?

Fecal Elimination Problems

☑ What problems have you had or do you now have with your bowel movements (constipation, diarrhea, excessive flatulence, seepage, or incontinence)?

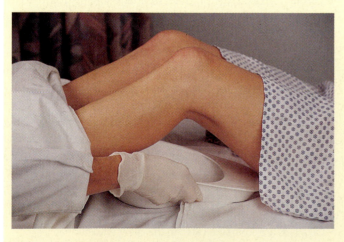

Figure 28-7. ■ Placing a fracture or slipper pan under the buttocks.

☑ When and how often does it occur?

☑ What causes it (food, fluids, exercise, emotions, medications, disease, surgery)?

☑ What methods have you used to remedy the problem, and how effective were they?

Factors Influencing Elimination

☑ *Use of elimination aids.* What routines do you follow to maintain your usual defecation pattern? Do you use natural aids, laxatives, or enemas to maintain elimination?

☑ *Diet.* What foods do you believe affect defecation? What foods do you typically eat? What foods do you always avoid? Do you take meals at regular times?

☑ *Fluid.* What amount and kind of fluid do you take each day?

☑ *Exercise.* What is your usual daily exercise pattern?

☑ *Medications.* Have you taken any medications that could affect the gastrointestinal tract (e.g., iron, antibiotics)?

☑ *Stress.* Are you experiencing any long-term or short-term stress?

The client's medication regimen should be examined by the physician and RN to see whether it could be the cause of constipation.

Administering Enemas

An **enema** is a solution introduced into the rectum and large intestine. The purpose of an enema is to distend the intestine and sometimes to irritate the intestinal mucosa, in order to increase peristalsis and excretion of feces and flatus.

Enemas are classified into three groups: cleansing, retention, and return-flow.

Cleansing Enemas

Cleansing enemas are intended to remove feces. They are given chiefly to:

■ Prevent the escape of feces during surgery.

■ Prepare the intestine for certain diagnostic tests such as x-ray or visualization tests (e.g., colonoscopy).

TABLE 28-3

Types of Laxatives

TYPE	ACTION	EXAMPLES	PERTINENT TEACHING INFORMATION
Bulk forming	Increases the fluid, gaseous, or solid bulk in the intestines.	Psyllium hydrophilic mucilloid (Metamucil)	May take 12 or more hours to act. Sufficient fluid must be taken.
Emollient/stool softener	Softens and delays the drying of the feces; permits fat and water to penetrate feces.	Docusate sodium (Colace)	Refrigerated oil has less odor. Mixing syrup with fruit juice decreases unpleasant taste.
Wetting agents	Lowers the surface tension of the feces, thus helping water to penetrate the feces.	Docusate sodium (Colace)	Slow acting; may take several days.
Stimulant/irritant	Irritates the intestinal mucosa or stimulates nerve endings in the wall of the intestine, causing rapid propulsion of the contents.	Bisacodyl (Dulcolax)	Acts more quickly than bulk-forming agents. Fluid is passed with the feces. May cause cramps. Prolonged use may cause fluid and electrolyte imbalance.
Lubricant	Lubricates the feces in the colon.	Mineral oil (Haley's M-O)	Prolonged use inhibits the absorption of some fat-soluble vitamins.
Saline/osmotic	Draws water into the intestine by osmosis, distends bowel, and stimulates peristalsis.	Epsom salts, magnesium hydroxide (milk of magnesia), magnesium citrate, sodium phosphate (Fleet enema)	May be rapid acting. Can cause fluid and electrolyte imbalance, particularly in elderly people and children with cardiac and renal disease. Should not be used by elderly clients. Prolonged use inhibits the absorption of some fat-soluble vitamins.

TABLE 28-4

Commonly Used Enema Solutions

SOLUTION	CONSTITUENTS	ACTION	TIME TO TAKE EFFECT	POTENTIAL ADVERSE EFFECTS
Hypertonic	90–120 mL of solution (e.g., sodium phosphate)	Draws water into the colon.	5–10 min	Retention of sodium
Hypotonic	500–1,000 mL of tap water	Distends colon, stimulates peristalsis, and softens feces.	15–20 min	Fluid and electrolyte imbalance; water intoxication
Isotonic	500–1,000 mL of normal saline (9 mL NaCl to 1,000 mL water)	Distends colon, stimulates peristalsis, and softens feces.	15–20 min	Possible sodium retention
Soapsuds	500–1,000 mL (3–5 mL soap to 1,000 mL water)	Irritates mucosa, distends colon.	10–15 min	Irritates and may damage mucosa
Oil (mineral, olive, cottonseed)	90–120 mL	Lubricates the feces and the colonic mucosa.	30–60 min	

- Remove feces when there is constipation or impaction.
- Establish regular bowel function as part of a bowel training program.

Cleansing enemas use a variety of solutions. Table 28-4 ■ lists commonly used solutions.

Cleansing enemas may also be described as high or low. A *high enema* is given to cleanse as much of the colon as possible. The *low enema* is used to clean the rectum and sigmoid colon only. The client maintains a left lateral position during administration.

The force of flow of the solution is governed by the (1) height of the solution container, (2) size of the tubing, (3) viscosity of the fluid, and (4) resistance of the rectum. The higher the solution container is held above the rectum, the faster the flow and the greater the force (pressure) in the rectum. During most adult enemas, the solution container should be no higher than 30 cm (12 in.) above the rectum. During a high cleansing enema, however, the solution container is usually held 30 to 45 cm (12 to 18 in.) above the rectum. This instills the fluid farther to clean the entire bowel.

Retention Enema

Retention enemas introduce oil into the rectum and sigmoid colon. The oil is retained for a relatively long period (e.g., 1 to 3 hours). It acts to soften the feces and to lubricate the rectum and anal canal, thus facilitating passage of the feces.

Return-Flow Enema

A return-flow enema (or Harris flush) is used occasionally to expel flatus. Alternating flow of 100 to 200 mL of fluid into and out of the rectum and sigmoid colon stimulates peristalsis. This process is repeated five or six times until the flatus is expelled and abdominal distention is relieved.

Commercially prepared, low-volume, disposable enema kits are commonly used today. The kit includes a flexible bottle of solution with a prelubricated, firm tip. Procedure 28-4 ■ on page 618 describes how to administer an enema.

Digital Removal of a Fecal Impaction

Digital removal involves breaking up the fecal mass with the finger and removing it in portions. Because the bowel mucosa can be injured during this procedure, some agencies limit who can perform digital disimpactions. Rectal stimulation is also contraindicated for some people, because it may result in cardiac arrhythmia.

Manual removal of an impaction can be painful. Use a well-lubricated, gloved finger and insert the finger into the anal canal as far as you can reach. Loosen and dislodge stool by gently massaging around it. Break up stool by working the finger into the hardened mass, taking care to avoid injury to the mucosa of the rectum. Carefully work stool downward to the end of the rectum and remove it in small pieces. Manual stimulation should be minimal.

Decreasing Flatulence

There are a number of ways to reduce or prevent flatus. They include avoiding gas-producing foods and using straws, increasing exercise, moving in bed, and ambulation. Movement stimulates peristalsis, escape of flatus, and reabsorption of gases in the intestinal capillaries. If these measures fail, flatulence may be treated by insertion of a rectal tube (see Procedure 28-1).

Bowel Training Programs

For clients who have chronic constipation, frequent impactions, or fecal incontinence, bowel training programs may be helpful. The program is based on factors within the client's control and is designed to help the client establish normal defecation. Such matters as food and fluid intake, exercise, and defecation habits are all considered. Before beginning such a program, clients must understand it and want to be involved.

EVALUATING

Data are collected to determine whether the client has achieved goals established during the planning phase. Steps toward achieving or maintaining normal bowel elimination patterns and stool consistency are assessed and documented. For clients with ostomies, steps toward self-care are reviewed. If outcomes are not achieved, the nurse should discuss the situation with the RN participating in the client's care.

CONTINUING CARE

The nurse plays an important role in educating clients about bowel elimination. Refer back to Box 28-5 for instructions the nurse can share with clients about maintaining healthy elimination patterns.

To make toileting easier in the home, teach clients and their families to:

- Ensure safe and easy access to the toilet. Make sure lighting is appropriate, scatter rugs are removed or securely fastened, and so on.
- Provide instruction as needed about transfer techniques.
- Suggest ways that garments can be adjusted to make disrobing easier for toileting.
- If appropriate, instruct the client to keep a record of time and frequency of stool passage, any associated pain, and color and consistency of the stool.
- Provide information about required food and fluid alterations to promote defecation or to manage diarrhea.
- Discuss problems associated with overuse of laxatives, if appropriate, and the use of alternatives (e.g., Metamucil) to laxatives, suppositories, and enemas.
- If the client is taking a constipating medication (e.g., narcotic analgesic), discuss the addition of a fiber supplement once a day and increasing oral fluids.
- Provide instructions associated with specific elimination problems and treatment, such as constipation, diarrhea, or ostomy care, as discussed earlier.

NURSING PROCESS CARE PLAN
Client with Constipation

Mrs. Emma Brown is a 78-year-old widow of 9 months. She lives alone in a low-income housing complex for older people. Her two children live with their families in a city 150 miles away. She has always enjoyed cooking; however, now that she is alone, she does not cook for herself. As a result, she has developed irregular eating patterns and tends to prepare soup-and-toast meals. She gets little exercise and has had bouts of insomnia since her husband's death. For the past month, Mrs. Brown has been having a problem with constipation. She states she has a bowel movement about every 3 to 4 days and her stools are hard and painful to excrete.

Assessment. VS: 98.6, P (radial) 78, R 22, BP 130/84. She complains of anorexia and her abdomen is bloated. Bowel sounds diminished.

Nursing Diagnosis. The following important nursing diagnoses (among others) are established for this client:

- *Constipation*
- *Risk for Loneliness*
- *Imbalanced Nutrition: Less than Body Requirements*
- *Pain*

Expected Outcomes

- Establishes an elimination pattern suitable to lifestyle.
- Examines possible community resources and seek referrals for coping with loneliness.
- Understands fluid importance in stool consistency.
- Participates in planning a routine diet regimen that includes high-fiber foods to decrease constipation.
- Controls pain associated with bowel movements.

Planning and Implementation

- Review bowel pattern and lifestyle.
- Provide resources to client for senior interaction and activity.
- Increase fluid intake and exercise.
- Provide information regarding intestinal physiology.
- Offer a variety of easy-to-prepare diet menus high in fiber.
- Discuss aids to soften stool.
- Identify pain level associated with bowel movements.

Evaluation. Mrs. Brown has joined a senior center and signed up for an exercise class. She is drinking more fluids. Her diet has more fiber and bran. Mrs. Brown has established a morning routine that provides a relaxing unhurried time in the bathroom. She heeds the urge to defecate rather than delaying the process. She is preparing more varied foods at scheduled times.

Critical Thinking in the Nursing Process

1. Describe the process of defecation.
2. Teach Mrs. Brown measures and the rationale that will assist her in preventing constipation.
3. Explain why it is not recommended for clients to use laxatives or enemas to encourage bowel movements on a long term basis.

Note: Discussion of Critical Thinking questions appears in Appendix I.

Note: The references and resources for this and all chapters have been compiled at the back of the book.

PROCEDURE 28-1   # Inserting a Rectal Tube

Purpose

- To promote removal of flatulence following abdominal surgery or for clients who have swallowed excessive air.

Equipment

- Rectal tube, 22–30 Fr. (12–18 Fr. for children)

- Plastic bag or stool specimen container
- Hypoallergenic tape
- Water-soluble lubricant
- Bed protector
- Clean gloves

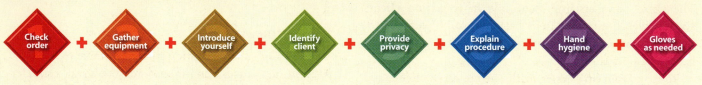

Check order + Gather equipment + Introduce yourself + Identify client + Provide privacy + Explain procedure + Hand hygiene + Gloves as needed

Interventions

1. Position the client on the left side in a recumbent position and drape. *This position facilitates insertion of the tube following normal curve of rectum and sigmoid colon.*

2. Tape a plastic bag around the distal end of the rectal tube or place it in the specimen container and vent the upper side of plastic bag. *Venting will prevent inflation of the plastic bag.*

3. Lubricate proximal end of rectal tube with water-soluble lubricant. *To ease the insertion of the tube into the rectum.*

4. Gently separate buttocks and ask client to take a deep breath. *Taking a deep breath relaxes the anal sphincter and prevents tissue trauma during tube insertion.*

5. Gently insert tube into client's rectum, past the external and internal sphincters (approximately 5 in.). *To allow tube to reach area where flatus is trapped.*

6. Gently tape tube in place with paper tape. *To maintain proper position of the tube.*

7. Leave tube in place no longer than 20 minutes. *Prolonged stimulation of the anal sphincter may result in loss of*

neuromuscular response. Prolonged presence of the catheter may cause pressure necrosis of mucosa.

8. Remove tube and provide perianal care as needed.

SAMPLE DOCUMENTATION

[date]	
[time]	**D**—P 68. Abdomen distended and hard. Client states "Unable to pass gas." **A**—30 French rectal tube inserted without difficulty.
1550	**R**—tube removed; abdomen soft, nondistended; client admits to feeling more comfortable. P 72. Tolerated procedure well.
	_____ C. Lasko, LVN

PROCEDURE 28-2   # Changing a One-Piece, Drainable Bowel Diversion Ostomy Appliance

Before changing a bowel diversion ostomy appliance, determine the kind of ostomy and its placement on the abdomen. It is important to confirm which is the functioning stoma and any orders about the care of the stomas.

Purposes

- To assess and care for the peristomal skin

- To collect effluent for assessment of the amount and type of output
- To minimize odors for the client's comfort and self-esteem

Equipment

- Disposable gloves
- Electric or safety razor

- Bedpan
- Solvent (presaturated sponges or liquid)
- Moisture-proof bag (for disposable pouches)
- Cleaning materials, including tissues, warm water, mild soap (optional), washcloth or cotton balls, towel
- Tissue or gauze pad
- Skin barrier (paste, powder, water, or liquid skin sealant)
- Stoma measuring guide

- Pen or pencil and scissors
- Clean ostomy appliance, with optional belt
- Tail closure clamp
- Special adhesive, if needed
- Stoma guide strip, if needed
- Deodorant (liquid or tablet) for a non–odor-proof colostomy bag

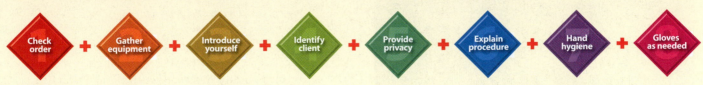

Interventions

1. Determine the need for an appliance change.
   - Assess the used appliance for leakage of effluent. *Effluent can irritate the peristomal skin.*
   - Ask the client about any discomfort at or around the stoma. *A burning sensation may indicate breakdown beneath the faceplate of the pouch.*
   - Assess the fullness of the pouch. *Pouches need to be emptied when they are one-third to one-half full. The weight of an overly full bag may loosen the faceplate and separate it from the skin, causing the effluent to leak and irritate the peristomal skin.*
   - If there is pouch leakage or discomfort at or around the stoma, change the appliance.

2. Select an appropriate time.
   - Avoid times close to meal or visiting hours. *Ostomy odor and effluent may reduce appetite or embarrass the client.*
   - Avoid times immediately after the administration of any medications that may stimulate bowel evacuation. *It is best to change the pouch when drainage is least likely to occur.*

3. Prepare the client and support people.
   - Explain the procedure to the client and support people. *Changing an ostomy appliance should not cause discomfort, but it may be distasteful to the client. Support persons are often more supportive if properly informed.*
   - Communicate acceptance and support to the client. *It is important to change the appliance competently and quickly.*
   - Provide privacy, preferably in the bathroom, where clients can learn to deal with the ostomy as they would at home.
   - Assist the client to a comfortable sitting or lying position in bed or preferably a sitting or standing position in the bathroom. *Lying or standing positions may facilitate smoother pouch application, that is, avoid wrinkles.*
   - Don gloves, and unfasten the belt if the client is wearing one.

4. Shave the peristomal skin of well-established ostomies as needed.
   - Use an electric or safety razor on a regular basis to remove excessive hair. *Hair follicles can become irritated or*

infected by repeated pulling out of hairs during removal of the appliance and skin barrier.

5. Empty and remove the ostomy appliance.
   - Empty the contents of the pouch through the bottom opening into a bedpan. *Emptying before removing the pouch prevents spillage of effluent onto the client's skin.*
   - Assess the consistency and the amount of effluent.
   - Peel the bag off slowly while holding the client's skin taut. *Holding the skin taut minimizes client discomfort and prevents abrasion of the skin.*
   - If the appliance is disposable, discard it in a moisture-proof bag.

6. Clean and dry the peristomal skin and stoma.
   - Use toilet tissue to remove excess stool.
   - Use warm water, mild soap (optional), and cotton balls or a washcloth and towel to clean the skin and stoma. Check agency practice on the use of soap. *Soap is sometimes not advised because it can be irritating to the skin.*
   - Use a special skin cleanser to remove dried, hard stool. *This emulsifies the stool, making removal less damaging to the skin.*
   - Dry the area thoroughly by patting with a towel or cotton balls. *Excess rubbing can abrade the skin.*

7. Assess the stoma and peristomal skin.
   - Inspect the stoma for color, size, shape, and bleeding.
   - Inspect the peristomal skin for any redness, ulceration, or irritation. *Transient redness after the removal of adhesive is normal.*
   - Place a piece of tissue or gauze pad over the stoma, and change it as needed. *This absorbs any seepage from the stoma.*

8. Apply paste-type skin barrier if needed.
   - Fill in abdominal creases or dimples with paste. *This establishes a smooth surface for application of the skin barrier and pouch.*
   - Allow the paste to dry for 1 to 2 minutes or as recommended by the manufacturer.

9. Prepare and apply the skin barrier (peristomal seal).

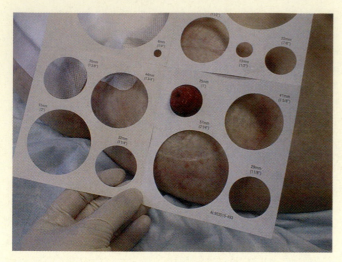

Figure 28-9. ■ A guide for measuring the stoma. (*Source:* Cory Patrick Hartley, San Ramon Regional Medical Center, San Ramon, CA. Reprinted with permission.)

For a Solid Wafer or Disk Skin Barrier

- Use the guide (Figure 28-9 ■) to measure the size of the stoma.
- On the backing of the skin barrier, trace a circle the same size as the stomal opening.
- Cut out the traced stoma pattern to make an opening in the skin barrier. Make the opening no more than 0.3 to 0.4 cm (1/8 to 1/6 in.) larger than the stoma. *This minimizes the risk of effluent contacting peristomal skin.*
- Remove the backing to expose the sticky adhesive side.
- Center the skin barrier over the stoma, and gently press it onto the client's skin, smoothing out any wrinkles or bubbles (Figure 28-10 ■).

For Liquid Skin Sealant

- Cover the stoma with a gauze pad. *This prevents contact with the skin sealant.*

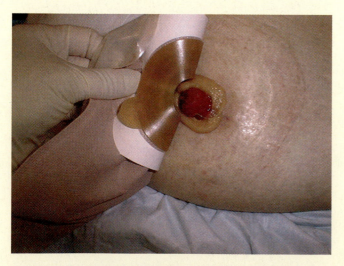

Figure 28-10. ■ Centering the skin barrier over the stoma. (*Source:* Cory Patrick Hartley, San Ramon Regional Medical Center, San Ramon, CA. Reprinted with permission.)

- Either wipe or apply the product evenly around the peristomal skin to form a thin layer of the liquid plastic coating to the same area.
- Allow the skin barrier to dry until it no longer feels tacky.

10. Fill in any exposed skin around an irregularly shaped stoma.
- Apply paste to any exposed skin areas. Use a non–alcohol-based product if the skin is excoriated. *Alcohol may cause stinging and burning.*
  or
  Sprinkle peristomal powder on the skin, wipe off the excess, and dab the powder with a slightly moist gauze or an applicator moistened with a liquid skin barrier. *This creates a barrier or seal.*

11. Prepare and apply the clean appliance.
- Remove the tissue over the stoma before applying the pouch.

For a Disposable Pouch with Adhesive Square

- If the appliance does not have a precut opening, trace a circle 0.3 to 0.4 cm (1/8 to 1/6 in.) larger than the stoma size on the appliance's adhesive square. The opening is made slightly larger than the stoma to prevent rubbing, cutting, or trauma to the stoma.
- Cut out a circle in the adhesive. Take care not to cut any portion of the pouch.
- Peel off the backing from the adhesive seal.
- Center the opening of the pouch over the client's stoma, and apply it directly onto the skin barrier (Figure 28-11 ■).
- Gently press the adhesive backing onto the skin and smooth out any wrinkles, working from the stoma outward. Wrinkles allow seepage of effluent, which can irritate the skin or soil clothing.
- Remove the air from the pouch. Removing the air helps the pouch lie flat against the abdomen.

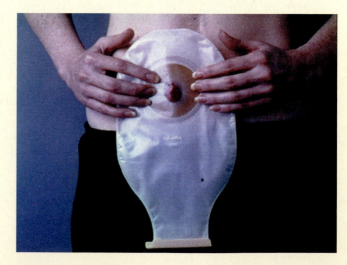

Figure 28-11. ■ Applying the disposable pouch. (*Source:* Courtesy of Convatec, a Bristol-Meyers Squibb Company.)

- Place a deodorant in the pouch (optional).
- Close the pouch by turning up the bottom a few times, fanfolding its end lengthwise, and securing it with a tail closure clamp.

Adjust the teaching plan and nursing care plan as needed. Include on the teaching plan the equipment and procedure used. *Client learning is facilitated by consistent nursing interventions.*

VARIATION: APPLYING THE SKIN BARRIER AND APPLIANCE AS ONE UNIT

If a disk- or wafer-type skin barrier is used, the skin barrier and appliance can be applied as one unit. Applying the skin barrier and the appliance together not only is quicker but also is thought to reduce the chance of wrinkles. It also is easier for the client to apply without help.

- Prepare the skin barrier by measuring the size of the stoma, tracing a circle on the backing of the skin barrier, and cutting out the traced stoma pattern to make an opening in the skin barrier.
- Prepare the appliance by cutting an opening 0.3 to 0.4 cm (1/8 to 1/6 in.) larger than the stoma size (if not already present) and peeling off the backing from the adhesive seal.
- Center the opening of the pouch over the skin barrier.
- Remove the skin barrier backing to expose the sticky adhesive side.
- Center the skin barrier and appliance over the stoma, and press it onto the client's skin.

SAMPLE DOCUMENTATION

[date] [time] Ostomy measured, appliance applied. Ostomy is brick red in color; no bleeding noted. Effluent dark brown, watery. Peristomal skin clean and dry. Bag secured with ostomy clasp. Client tolerated procedure well.

_____ D. Haus, LVN

PROCEDURE 28-3 Irrigating a Colostomy

Purpose
- To manage regular bowel elimination

Equipment
- Solution container
- 1,000 mL warm water
- Irrigating tube with cone
- Irrigating sleeve long enough to reach water level in the toilet
- Washcloths or gauze sponges to clean skin and stoma
- IV pole
- Water-soluble irrigant
- Plastic bag for disposing used pouch
- Clean gloves
- Replacement clean pouch and closure device
- Skin barrier

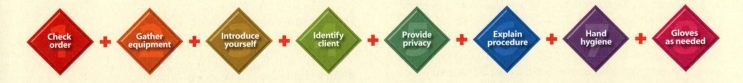

Interventions

1. Remove used pouch and dispose of it in the plastic bag. *Proper disposal of body waste if done for infection control.*

2. Assess pulse and blood pressure. *Assess pulse and BP for client susceptible to vagal response before procedure and monitor closely for early signs of hypotension, bradycardia, or loss of consciousness.*

3. Clean stoma and skin with warm water and soft cloth. *To remove any feces from the area around the stoma.*

4. Assess for signs of irritation or breakdown. *To prevent skin breakdown and to provide timely treatment for skin problems.*

5. Prepare irrigation solution: Fill the container with 750 to 1,000 mL of lukewarm water solution at 105° to 110°F.

(40.6° to 43.3°C) *Solutions that are too hot or cold can cause cramping.*

6. Hang the container on IV pole next to the toilet or commode. *Solution is positioned 18 in. (45.7 cm) above the insertion site to promote gravity flow.*

7. Allow solution to run through the tubing so that air is removed. Clamp tube. *If air is instilled during procedure, the client may experience discomfort as a result of distention of colon.*

8. Assist client to sit on the toilet/commode or on a chair in front of the toilet.

9. Place sleeve between client's thighs and direct end into toilet. *To prevent soiling the client or the floor.*

10. Lubricate cone tip with water-soluble lubricant. *Danger of perforation of the colon is greater when using a catheter for irrigation. Use of an irrigation cone is safer and results in better water flow.*

11. Position cone in sleeve by placing top through opening. If cone cannot be inserted easily, do not force. Hold cone snugly against the stoma. *This prevents solution backflow.*

12. Remove cone and close off or fold over top of sleeve after solution is instilled.

- Allow client to remain seated while majority of stool and solution return, usually 10 to 15 minutes.
- Clean client's skin and stoma with warm water. Dry thoroughly.
- Apply skin barriers and clean pouch.

SAMPLE DOCUMENTATION

[date]   750 mL of warm water instilled.
[time]   Large amount of soft brown, semi-
           soft stool returned with solution.
           Stoma and peristomal skin intact
           with no signs of bleeding or exco-
           riation. Skin barrier and pouch
           reapplied. Client assisted back to
           bed. Tolerated procedure well.
           P 72, BP 122/70.
           _____ S. Ceaders, LPN

PROCEDURE 28-4 Administering an Enema

Before administering an enema, determine whether a physician's order is required. At some agencies, a physician must order the kind of enema and the time to give it, for example, the morning of the examination. When the client has rectal disease, the physician may also specify the size of the rectal tube to use. At other agencies, enemas are given at the nurses' discretion (ie, as necessary on a prn order). In addition, determine the presence of kidney or cardiac disease that contraindicates the use of a hypotonic solution.

Purposes

- To stimulate a bowel movement.
- To remove accumulated stool from sigmoid colon in preparation for diagnostic test or surgery

Equipment

- Disposable underpad
- Bath blanket

- Bedpan or commode
- Disposable gloves
- Water-soluble lubricant if tubing not prelubricated

For a Large-Volume Enema

- Solution container with tubing of correct size and tubing clamp
- Correct solution, amount, and temperature (see Box 28-4 on page 612.)

For a Small-Volume Enema

- Prepackaged container of enema solution with lubricated tip

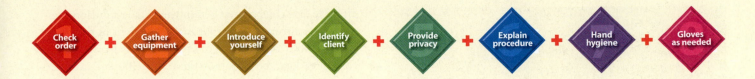

Interventions

1. Prepare the client.
   - Explain the procedure to the client. Indicate that the client may experience a feeling of fullness while the solution is being administered.
   - Assist the adult client to a left lateral position, with the right leg as acutely flexed as possible (Figure 28-12 ■). This position facilitates the flow of solution by gravity into the sigmoid and descending colon, which are on the left side. Having the right leg acutely flexed provides for adequate exposure of the anus.
   - Place the underpad under the client's buttocks to protect the bed linen, and drape the client with the bath blanket.

2. Prepare the equipment.
   - Lubricate about 5 cm (2 in.) of the rectal tube (some commercially prepared enema sets already have lubricated nozzles). *Lubrication facilitates insertion through the sphincters and minimizes trauma.*
   - Run some solution through the connecting tubing of a large-volume enema set and the rectal tube to expel any air in the tubing; then close the clamp. *Air instilled into the rectum, although not harmful, causes unnecessary distention.*

3. Wear gloves, and insert the rectal tube.
   - For clients in the left lateral position, lift the upper buttock to ensure good visualization of the anus.
   - Insert the tube smoothly and slowly into the rectum, directing it toward the umbilicus (Figure 28-13 ■). The angle follows the normal contour of the rectum. Slow insertion prevents spasm of the sphincter.
   - Insert the tube 7 to 10 cm (3 to 4 in.) in an adult. *Because the anal canal is about 2.5 to 5 cm (1 to 2 in.) long in the adult, insertion to this point places the tip of the tube beyond the anal sphincter into the rectum.*

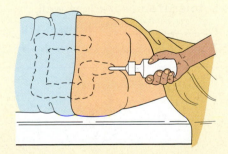

Figure 28-12. ■ Assuming a left lateral position for an enema. Note the commercially prepared enema.

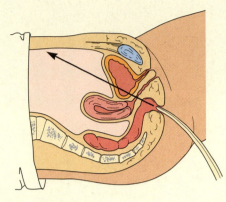

Figure 28-13. ■ Inserting the rectal tube following the direction of the rectum.

   - If resistance is encountered at the internal sphincter, ask the client to take a deep breath, then run a small amount of solution through the tube to relax the internal anal sphincter.
   - Never force tube entry. If resistance persists, withdraw the tube, and report the resistance to the nurse in charge.

4. Slowly administer the enema solution.
   - Raise the solution container, and open the clamp to allow fluid flow.
     or
     Compress a pliable container by hand.
   - During most adult low enemas, hold the solution container no higher than 30 cm (12 in.) above the rectum. The higher the solution container is held above the rectum, the faster the flow and the greater the force (pressure) in the rectum. During a high enema, hold the solution container a little higher (e.g., 45.7 cm [18 in.]). *The fluid must be instilled farther to clean the entire bowel.*
   - Administer the fluid slowly. If the client complains of fullness or pain, use the clamp to stop the flow for 30 seconds, and then restart the flow at a slower rate. *Administering the enema slowly and stopping the flow momentarily decrease the likelihood of intestinal spasm and premature ejection of the solution.*
   - If you are using a plastic commercial container, roll it up as the fluid is instilled. *This prevents subsequent suctioning of the solution.* See Figure 28-14 ■.
   - After all the solution has been instilled or when the client cannot hold any more and wants to defecate (the urge to defecate usually indicates that sufficient fluid has been administered), close the clamp, and remove the rectal tube from the anus.

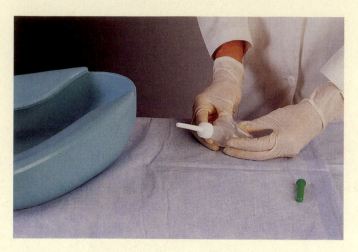

Figure 28-14. ■ Rolling up a commercial enema container.

■ Place the rectal tube in a disposable towel as you withdraw it.

5. Encourage the client to retain the enema.
   ■ Ask the client to remain lying down. *It is easier for the client to retain the enema when lying down than when sitting or standing, because gravity promotes drainage and peristalsis.*
   ■ Ensure that the client retains the solution for the appropriate amount of time, for example, 5 to 10 minutes for a cleansing enema or at least 30 minutes for a retention enema.

6. Assist the client to defecate.
   ■ Assist the client to a sitting position on the bedpan, commode, or toilet. *A sitting position facilitates the act of defecation.*
   ■ Ask the client who is using the toilet not to flush it. *The nurse needs to observe the feces.*
   ■ If a specimen of feces is required, ask the client to use a bedpan or commode.

7. Record and report relevant data.
   ■ Record administration of the enema; type of solution; length of time solution was retained; the amount, color, and consistency of the returns; and the relief of flatus and abdominal distention.

VARIATION: ADMINISTERING AN ENEMA TO AN INCONTINENT CLIENT

■ Occasionally a nurse needs to administer an enema to a client who is unable to control the external sphincter

muscle and thus cannot retain the enema solution for even a few minutes. In that case, the client assumes a supine position with knees flexed on a bedpan. The head of the bed can be elevated slightly, to 30 degrees if necessary for easier breathing, and the client's head and back are supported by pillows. Pressing the buttocks together may help the client to retain the solution. The nurse wears gloves to prevent direct contact with the solution and feces that are expelled over the hand into the bedpan during the administration of the enema.

VARIATION: ADMINISTERING A RETURN-FLOW ENEMA OR HARRIS FLUSH

■ For a return-flow enema, the solution (100 to 200 mL for an adult) is instilled into the client's rectum and sigmoid colon. Then the solution container is lowered so that the fluid flows back out through the rectal tube into the container. The inflow–outflow process is repeated five or six times (to stimulate peristalsis and the expulsion of flatus), and the solution is replaced several times during the procedure if it becomes thick with feces.

Large-Volume Enemas

Age	Volume (mL)
18 months	50–200
18 months–5 years	200–300
5–12 years	300–500
12 years and older	500–1,000

Temperature

For adult: 40°–43°C (105°–110°F)
For children: 37.7°C (100°F)

SAMPLE DOCUMENTATION

[date]	Cleansing enema given, Client toler-
[time]	ated 750 mL of tap water. Returned
	soft brn stool and water. Client
	tolerated procedure well.
	_____ D. Haus, LVN

Chapter Review

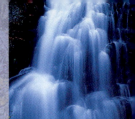

 ## KEY TERMS by Topic

Use the audio glossary feature of either the CD-ROM or the Companion Website to hear the correct pronunciation of the following key terms.

Physiology of Defecation
feces, peristalsis, chyme, flatus, defecation

Factors That Affect Defecation
tarry, sigmoidoscopy, paralytic ileus

Common Fecal Elimination Problems
constipation, Valsalva maneuver, impaction, vagus nerve, diarrhea, incontinence, flatulence, eructation

Fecal Diversion Ostomies
ostomy, ileostomy, colostomy, fecal diversions, effluent, appliance, peristomal, bedpan

Nursing Care
occult blood, guaiac test, cathartics, laxative, enema

KEY Points

- Primary functions of the large bowel are the excretion of digestive waste products and the maintenance of fluid balance.

- A regular pattern of fecal elimination with formed, soft stools is essential to health and a sense of well-being.

- Factors that affect defecation are developmental level, diet, fluid intake, activity and exercise, psychological factors, regular defecation, medications, diagnostic procedures, anesthesia, and pathological conditions.

- Common fecal elimination problems include constipation, fecal impaction, diarrhea, bowel incontinence, and flatulence.

- When inspecting the client's stool, the nurse must observe its color, consistency, shape, amount, odor, and the presence of abnormal constituents.

- An adverse effect of constipation is straining during defecation, during which the Valsalva maneuver may be used. Cardiac problems may ensue.

- An adverse effect of prolonged diarrhea is fluid and electrolyte imbalance.

- Digital removal of an impaction should be carried out gently because of vagal nerve stimulation and subsequent depressed cardiac rate. An order is often necessary.

- Normal defecation is often facilitated in both well and ill clients by providing privacy, teaching clients to attend to defecation urges promptly, assisting clients to normal sitting positions whenever possible, encouraging appropriate food and fluid intake, and scheduling regular exercise.

- Clients who have bowel diversion ostomies require special care, with attention to psychological adjustment, diet, and stoma and skin care.

 ## EXPLORE MediaLink

Additional interactive resources for this chapter can be found on the Companion Website at www.prenhall.com/ramont. Click on Chapter 28 and "Begin" to select the activities for this chapter.

For chapter-related NCLEX®-style questions and an audio glossary, access the accompanying CD-ROM in this book.

Animations/Videos
- Enema

FOR FURTHER Study

Assessment of abdomen is discussed in detail in Chapter 19.
Hygiene is discussed in detail in Chapter 22.
Perineal care is explained in Chapter 22 and Procedure 22-1.
Nutrition is discussed in Chapter 25.
Fluid balance is discussed in Chapter 26.

Critical Thinking Care Map

Caring for a Client with Ulcerative Colitis

NCLEX-PN® Focus Area: Physiological Adaptation

Case Study: Mrs. Dora Davis is a 60-year-old client being treated for ulcerative colitis. She was hospitalized for a colectomy and has a permanent ileostomy. Today marks her third postoperative day. She continues to have pain, and when you empty her ileostomy bag, she throws the cover over her head. She is due for discharge in 2 days. The enterostomal nurse has visited and initiated teaching care of the ostomy. Mrs. Davis worries that the bag will break when she gets up. She has confided that she is fearful that her husband will find her unattractive.

Nursing Diagnosis: Deficient Knowledge Related to Ostomy Management

COLLECT DATA

Subjective	Objective
_____	_____
_____	_____
_____	_____
_____	_____
_____	_____
_____	_____
_____	_____

Would you report this data? Yes/No

If yes, to: _____

What would you report? _____

Nursing Care

_____
_____
_____
_____
_____
_____
_____
_____
_____
_____
_____
_____

How would you document this? _____
_____
_____

Compare your documentation to the sample provided in Appendix I.

Data Collected
(use those that apply)

- Ileostomy rt. abdomen
- Stoma brick red
- Effluent watery, dark brown, flecks of blood
- Refuses to look at the ileostomy
- Pain
- Anxious
- Fearful
- Peristomal area reddened
- Weight: 110 lbs
- Hemoglobin 10
- WBC 12,000
- Gait steady
- UA shows 2+ bacteria
- BP 120/86
- Temperature 99.4
- Skin turgor slow

Nursing Interventions
(use those that apply; list in priority order)

- Monitor intake and output.
- Take daily weights.
- Increase fluid intake.
- Assess stoma.
- Inspect peristomal skin.
- Monitor lab values.
- Take VS every 4 hours.
- Assess skin turgor.
- Assess coping mechanisms.
- Provide referrals to ostomy association.
- Include family in teaching.

NCLEX-PN® Exam Preparation

TEST-TAKING TIP Do not spend a long time on one question; go on to the next question. On a written test, mark the question and return to it when you have time. When testing on a computer, look at the key words in the question, read all your possible answers, choose an answer, and move on.

1 When movement of the intestine ceases temporarily after abdominal surgery, it is known as:
1. constipation.
2. volvulus.
3. ulcerative colitis.
4. paralytic ileus.

2 Using digital removal of a fecal impaction causes rectal stimulation and is contraindicated for:
1. renal diseases.
2. cancer.
3. cardiac disease.
4. neurologic disorders.

3 Peristalsis is described as:
1. gas expulsion from the intestine.
2. stool formation.
3. fluid elimination from the intestine.
4. wavelike contractions of the intestinal muscles.

4 Which measure is most often used for the client with a fecal impaction?
1. rectal tube
2. Harris flush
3. oil retention enema
4. cathartic

5 Effluent from an ileostomy is irritating to the skin because it contains:
1. digestive enzymes.
2. electrolytes.
3. bile.
4. organic salts.

6 A stool specimen being tested for blood is called the:
1. C&S test.
2. guaiac test.
3. steatorrhea test.
4. albumin test.

7 A common complication of diarrhea is:
1. calculus.
2. potassium loss.
3. fluid overload.
4. hypoactive bowel sounds.

8 A major side effect of this drug will cause a decrease in gastrointestinal activity leading to constipation.
1. Colace
2. codeine
3. Catapres
4. clonidine

9 A postoperative client is complaining about gas pains. What initial intervention would you suggest?
1. bed rest
2. drinking with a straw
3. ambulation
4. Lomotil

10 The peristomal site of an ileostomy is reddened and ulcerated. How often would the appliance be changed?
1. every 5 days
2. every 4 hours
3. every 24 to 48 hours
4. once a week

Answers and Rationales for Review Questions, as well as discussion of Care Plan and Critical Thinking Care Map questions, appear in Appendix I.

Chapter 29

Medications

BRIEF Outline

Drug Standards

Effects of Drugs

Medication Orders

Systems of Measurement

Equipment

Routes of Administration

HISTORICAL Perspectives

Doctor Alexander Wood, of the Royal College of Physicians of Edinburgh in 1850, had been experimenting with a hollow needle for the administration of drugs. He published a short paper titled "A New Method of Treating Neuralgia by the direct application of Opiates to the Painful Points." In this paper, he showed that the method was not limited to the administration of opiates. In 1954, the first mass-produced disposable syringe and needle, produced in glass was developed for mass administration of the new Salk polio vaccine to 1 million American children. In 1955, Roehr Products introduced a plastic disposable hypodermic syringe called the Monoject, which has been developed into the type of syringe that nurses use every day.

LEARNING Outcomes

After completing this chapter, you will be able to:

1. Define selected terms related to the administration of medications.
2. Describe legal aspects of administering drugs.
3. Identify physiological factors and individual variables affecting medication action.
4. Describe physiological variables that alter medication administration and effectiveness.
5. Describe various routes of medication administration.
6. Identify essential parts of a medication order.
7. Recognize abbreviations commonly used in medication orders.
8. List six essential steps to follow when administering medication.
9. Demonstrate an understanding of the system of measurements used for medications and how to convert units of weight and measure.
10. Identify equipment required for parenteral medications.
11. Outline steps required to administer oral medications safely.
12. Outline steps required for nasogastric and gastrostomy tube medication administration.
13. Describe LPN's/LVN's responsibilities in monitoring IV drip rate.
14. Describe how to mix selected drugs from vials and ampules.
15. Identify sites used for intradermal, subcutaneous, and intramuscular injections.
16. Describe essential steps for safely administering parenteral medications by intradermal, subcutaneous, and intramuscular routes.
17. Describe essential steps in safely administering topical medications: dermatologic, ophthalmic, otic, nasal, vaginal, rectal, and respirator inhalation preparations.

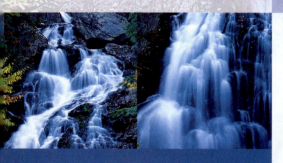

A **medication** is a substance administered for the diagnosis, cure, treatment, relief, or prevention of disease. In the health-care context, the words *medication* and *drug* are used interchangeably.

In the United States and Canada, medications are usually dispensed by the order of physicians and dentists. The written direction for the preparation and administration of a drug is called a **prescription**.

A drug may have four different names:

1. The **generic** (family) name, given before a drug becomes official.

2. The *official* name, the name under which it is listed in one of the official publications (e.g., the *United States Pharmacopeia*).

3. The *chemical* name, which describes the drug constituents precisely.

4. The *trademark,* or *brand name,* which is the name used by the drug manufacturer. Because a drug may be manufactured by several companies, it can have several trade names. Medications are often available in a variety of forms. Examples are given in Table 29-1 ■.

TABLE 29-1	
Types of Drug Preparations	
TYPE	**DESCRIPTION**
Aerosol spray or foam	A liquid, powder, or foam deposited in a thin layer on the skin by air pressure
Aqueous solution	One or more drugs dissolved in water
Aqueous suspension	One or more drugs finely divided in a liquid such as water
Caplet	A solid form, shaped like a capsule, coated and easily swallowed
Capsule	A gelatinous container that holds a drug in powder, liquid, or oil form
Cream	A nongreasy, semisolid preparation used on the skin
Elixir	A sweetened and aromatic solution of alcohol used as a vehicle for medicinal agents
Extract	A concentrated form of a drug made from vegetables or animals
Gel or jelly	A clear or translucent semisolid that liquefies when applied to the skin
Liniment	A medication mixed with alcohol, oil, or soapy emollient and applied to the skin
Lotion	A medication in a liquid suspension applied to the skin
Lozenge (troche)	A flat, round, or oval preparation that dissolves and releases a drug when held in the mouth
Ointment (salve, unction)	A semisolid preparation of one or more drugs used for application to the skin and mucous membrane
Paste	A preparation like an ointment, but thicker and stiff, that penetrates the skin less than an ointment
Pill	One or more drugs mixed with a cohesive material, in oval, round, or flattened shapes
Powder	A finely ground drug or drugs; some are used internally, others externally
Suppository	One or several drugs mixed with a firm base such as gelatin and shaped for insertion into the body (e.g., the rectum); the base dissolves gradually at body temperature, releasing the drug
Syrup	An aqueous solution of sugar often used to disguise unpleasant-tasting drugs
Tablet	A powdered drug compressed into a hard, small disk; some are readily broken along a scored line; others are enteric coated to prevent them from dissolving in the stomach
Tincture	An alcohol or water-and-alcohol solution prepared from drugs derived from plants
Transdermal patch	A semipermeable membrane shaped in the form of a disk or patch that contains a drug to be absorbed through the skin over a long period of time

Drug Standards

Drugs may have natural (e.g., plant, mineral, and animal) sources, or they may be synthesized in the laboratory. For example, digitalis is plant derived, sodium chloride is a mineral, insulin has animal or human sources, and propoxyphene hydrochloride (the analgesic Darvon) is synthesized in a laboratory.

Drugs vary in strength and activity. Drugs must be pure and of uniform strength if drug dosages are to be predictable in their effect. Therefore, drug standards have been developed to ensure uniform quality. In the United States, official drugs are those designated by the Federal Food, Drug, and Cosmetic Act. These drugs are officially listed in the *United States Pharmacopeia* (USP) and described according to their source, physical and chemical properties, tests for purity and identity, method of storage, assay, category, and normal dosages. In Canada, the *British Pharmacopoeia* is used for the same purpose, although some drugs used in Canada conform to the USP because they are obtained from the United States.

LEGAL ASPECTS OF DRUG ADMINISTRATION

The administration of drugs is controlled by law. Table 29-2 ■ summarizes drug legislation for the United States and Canada.

Nurses must:

1. Know how nursing practice acts in their areas define and limit their functions. *Note:* The LPN/LVN must never function outside his or her scope of practice. He or she should be in constant communication with the RN. Knowing one's scope and reporting to the RN whenever necessary will ensure that the LPN/LVN is operating within the legal limits of the license as it relates to drug administration.
2. Be able to recognize the limits of their own knowledge and skill.

Under the law, nurses are responsible for their own actions whether or not a written order exists. Nurses administer thousands of medications and are responsible for assessing drug effects, including recognizing unfavorable reactions. Since it is impossible to memorize pertinent information about every drug, nurses must rely on references, such as the *Physician's Desk Reference* (PDR) or *Nurse's Drug Guide.* If a physician writes an incorrect order (e.g., Demerol 500 mg instead of Demerol 50 mg), the nurse who administers the incorrect dosage is responsible for the error. Therefore, nurses should question any order that appears unreasonable and refuse to give the medication until the order is clarified.

TABLE 29-2	
Important Drug Legislation for United States and Canada	
LEGISLATION	**CONTENT**
Pure Food and Drug Act (U.S. 1906)	First government intervention that established consumer protection in the manufacture of drugs and foods. It requires all drugs to meet minimal standards of strength, purity, and quality. Drug preparations containing morphine must be labeled as such. Established written resources for officially approved drugs, which became the *United States Pharmacopeia*/National Formulary (USP/NF).
Proprietary or Patent Medicine Act (Can. 1908)	Protects the public against unsafe and ineffective over-the-counter drugs.
Food, Drug, and Cosmetic Act (U.S. 1938)	Implemented by Food and Drug Administration (FDA); requires that labels be accurate and that all drugs be tested for harmful effects.
Durham-Humphrey Amendment (U.S. 1952)	Clearly differentiates drugs that can be sold only with a prescription, those that can be sold without a prescription, and those that should not be refilled without a new prescription.
Canada Food and Drugs Act (Can. 1953)	Prohibits advertising any food, drug, cosmetic, or device as a cure for certain specified diseases. Sets standards for manufacture, distribution, and sale of all drugs, with the exception of narcotics.
Canadian Narcotic Control Act (Can. 1961)	Allows only authorized people to possess narcotics. Specifies records about narcotics that must be kept.
Kefauver-Harris Amendment (U.S. 1962)	Requires proof of safety and efficacy of a drug for approval.
Comprehensive Drug Abuse Prevention and Control Act (U.S. 1970) (Controlled Substances Act)	Categorizes controlled substances and limits how often a prescription can be filled; established government-funded programs to prevent and treat drug dependence. (The Drug Enforcement Administration was established as a bureau of the Department of Justice to enforce provisions of the act. This act also established five schedules of drugs based on their degree of danger for abuse or addiction, beginning with C-I for most abuse potential to C-V for low abuse potential. [Woodrow, 2002].)

Another aspect of nursing practice governed by law is the use of controlled substances. In hospitals, controlled substances are kept in a locked drawer, cupboard, medication cart, or computer-controlled dispensing system. Agencies have special forms for recording the use of controlled substances. The information required usually includes the name of the client, drug name, the date and time of administration, the dosage, and the signature of the person who prepared and gave the drug. The name of the physician who ordered the drug may also be part of the record.

Included on this record are the controlled substances wasted during preparation. When a dose or portion of a dose is not used, it must be disposed of according to facility procedure. A second licensed nurse must witness and sign that the drug was wasted and disposed of properly. In most agencies, counts of controlled substances are taken at the end of each shift. The count total should tally with the total at the end of the last shift minus the number used. Discrepancies must be reported immediately.

Effects of Drugs

The **therapeutic effect** of a drug, also referred to as the *desired effect,* is the reason the drug is prescribed. See Table 29-3 ■ for kinds of therapeutic actions.

A drug side effect is an unintended drug action. Unfavorable **side effects** are called *untoward effects.* Untoward effects may be tolerated for the sake of therapeutic effect. More severe side effects, also called **adverse effects** or *drug reactions,* may justify discontinuing the drug.

Drug toxicity (deleterious effects of a drug on an organism or tissue) results from overdosage, ingestion of a drug intended for external use, and **cumulative effect** (buildup of the drug in the blood because of impaired metabolism or excretion). Some toxic effects become apparent immediately; some are not apparent for weeks or months. Drug toxicity may be avoided by close monitoring of the drug dose and client response.

A **drug allergy** is an immunologic reaction to a drug. When a person is first exposed to a foreign substance (antigen), such as a drug, the body may react by producing antibodies, triggering an allergic reaction called anaphylaxis. Check for allergies before giving medications. See Table 29-4 ■ for common mild allergic responses.

Drug tolerance occurs when a person requires increases in dosage to maintain the therapeutic effect. Habituating drugs such as opiates, barbiturates, ethyl alcohol, and nicotine produce tolerance. A cumulative effect is the increasing response to repeated doses of a drug, which occurs when the rate of administration exceeds the rate of metabolism or excretion. As a result, the drug builds up in the client's body unless the dosage is adjusted.

An **idiosyncratic effect** (unexpected unique bodily response) causes unpredictable abnormal symptoms in clients, including opposite drug actions and over- and underresponse to medications.

A **drug interaction** occurs when the administration of one drug alters the effect of another drug. The effect of each drug may increase (*potentiating* or *synergistic effect*) or decrease (*inhibiting effect*). Drug interactions may be beneficial or harmful. Foods and other natural substances, such as herbal supplements, may interact adversely with a medication. For example, tetracycline should not be given with milk or milk products because it will decrease the effectiveness of the medication.

TABLE 29-3		
Therapeutic Actions of Drugs		
DRUG TYPE	**DESCRIPTION**	**EXAMPLES**
Palliative	Relieves the symptoms of a disease but does not affect the disease itself.	Morphine sulfate, aspirin for pain
Curative	Cures a disease or condition.	Penicillin for infection
Supportive	Supports body function until other treatments or the body's response can take over.	Norepinephrine bitartrate for low blood pressure; aspirin for high body temperature
Substitutive	Replaces body fluids or substances.	Thyroxine for hypothyroidism, insulin for diabetes mellitus
Chemotherapeutic	Destroys malignant cells.	Busulfan for leukemia
Restorative	Returns the body to health.	Vitamin, mineral supplements, B_{12} injections for pernicious anemia

---

TABLE 29-4

Common Mild Allergic Responses

SYMPTOM	DESCRIPTION/RATIONALE
Skin rash	Either an intraepidermal vesicle rash or a rash typified by an urticarial wheal or macular eruption; rash is usually generalized over the body
Pruritus	Itching of the skin with or without a rash
Angioedema	Edema due to increased permeability of the blood capillaries
Rhinitis	Excessive watery discharge from the nose
Lacrimal tearing	Excessive tearing
Nausea, vomiting	Stimulation of these centers in the brain
Wheezing and dyspnea	Shortness of breath and wheezing upon inhalation and exhalation due to accumulated fluids and swelling of the respiratory tissues
Diarrhea	Irritation of the mucosa of the large intestine

Iatrogenic disease (disease caused unintentionally by medical therapy) can be due to drug administration.

ACTIONS OF DRUGS IN THE BODY

The action of a drug in the body can be described in terms of its half-life. **Half-life** is the time interval required for the body's elimination processes to reduce the concentration of the drug in the body by one-half. For example, if a drug's half-life is 8 hours, then the amount of drug in the body is as follows:

Initially: 100%
After 8 hours: 50%
After 16 hours: 25%
After 24 hours: 12.5%
After 32 hours: 6.25%

Because the purpose of most drug therapy is to maintain a constant drug level in the body, repeated doses are required to maintain that level. A person may not respond in the same manner to successive doses. See Box 29-1 ■ for an explanation of the four processes of drug actions (absorption, distribution, metabolism, and excretion).

FACTORS AFFECTING MEDICATION ACTION

Various factors affect the action of a medication, and they vary based on the individual. For instance, an idiosyncratic effect is unexpected and individual. The drug may have a completely different effect from the normal one or cause unpredictable and unexplained symptoms.

Ethnicity and culture may contribute to differences in responses to medications. It is thought that a toxic reaction may be due to a genetic defect that causes a person to be unable to eliminate a drug or to metabolize a drug too quickly.

Cultural practices can also affect a drug's actions. Herbal remedies may counteract prescribed medications. Age and development may also have an effect on medication. Box 29-2 ■ lists age-related considerations for medication administration.

Routes of Administration

The route of administration affects medication action. Pharmaceutical preparations are generally designed for

---

BOX 29-1

Key Terms Related to Drug Action

- *Onset of action:* The time after administration when the body initially responds to the drug
- *Peak plasma level:* The highest plasma level achieved by a single dose when the elimination rate of a drug equals the absorption rate
- *Drug half-life (elimination half-life):* The time required for the elimination process to reduce the concentration of the drug to one-half what it was at initial administration
- *Plateau:* A maintained concentration of a drug in the plasma during a series of scheduled doses
- **Absorption:** The process by which a drug passes into the bloodstream
- *Distribution:* The process by which the drug is sent to various body tissues
- *Metabolism:* The process by which some drugs are converted in the liver to inactive compounds
- *Excretion:* The process by which drugs are eliminated from the body, which most often occurs via the renal system

BOX 29-2

Age-Related Considerations for Medication Administration

Infants and Children

- Knowledge of human growth and development is essential for the nurse. Oral medications for children are usually prepared in sweetened liquid form to make them more palatable. Never disguise with a necessary food (like formula, milk, or juice), because the child may refuse that food in the future. Parents may provide suggestions.
- Infants usually require small dosages because of their body size and the immaturity of their organs, especially the liver and kidneys. They often do not have all of the enzymes required for drug metabolism and therefore may require different medications than adults. In adolescence or adulthood, allergic reactions may occur with drugs formerly tolerated.
- Children tend to fear any unfamiliar procedures, especially those in which needles are used. The nurse must acknowledge that the child will experience pain; denying this fact only fosters distrust. After an injection, the nurse (or parent) should cuddle and speak softly to the infant and/or give a toy to dispel the child's association of the nurse with pain.

Variation: Giving Oral Medications to Infants and Children

- Select an appropriate vehicle to measure and administer the medication, for example, a plastic disposable cup, plastic syringe without needle, or tuberculin syringe. Whenever possible, give children a choice about use of a spoon, dropper, or syringe.
- Dilute the oral medication, if indicated, with a small amount of water. Many oral medications are readily swallowed if they are diluted with a small amount of water. If large quantities of water are used, the child may refuse to drink the entire amount and receive only a portion of the medication.
- Unless contraindicated, crush medications that are not supplied in liquid form and mix them with substances available on most pediatric units, such as honey, flavored syrup, jam, or a fruit puree. *Note:* When selecting a substance to mix with a medication, avoid *essential* food items such as milk, cereal, and orange juice. If these foods are used, the child may refuse them in the future.
- Disguise disagreeable-tasting medications with sweet-tasting substances mentioned previously. However, present any altered medication to the child honestly and not as a food or treat.
- To prevent nausea, pour a carbonated beverage over finely crushed ice and give it before or immediately after the medication is administered.
- To prevent aspiration and choking, position infants in a semi-reclining position, and administer the medication slowly in divided doses by spoon or a plastic syringe.
- If using a spoon, retrieve and refeed medication that is thrust outward by the infant's tongue.
- If using a syringe, place it along the side of the infant's tongue. This position prevents gagging and expulsion of the medication.
- A child's parents or guardians may be able to provide valuable information on how best to give the child medications. However, a nurse may need to partially restrain a child who refuses to cooperate or consistently resists despite explanation, en-

couragement, and attempts to determine the reason for the behavior.
  a. Place the child in your lap with the right arm behind you.
  b. Grasp the child's left hand firmly with your left hand.
  c. Secure the head between your arm and body.
- Follow all medication with a drink of water, juice, a soft drink, or a Popsicle or frozen juice bar. This removes any unpleasant aftertaste.
- For children who take sweetened medications on a long-term basis, follow the medication administration with oral hygiene. These children are at high risk for dental caries.
- For a young child, use a doll to demonstrate the procedure. This facilitates cooperation and decreases anxiety.
- For a young child or infant, enlist assistance to immobilize the arms and head. The parent may hold the infant or young child. This prevents accidental injury during medication administration.

Adults

- Maternal health considerations: During pregnancy, women must be very careful about taking medications. Most drugs are contraindicated because of the possible adverse effects on the fetus.
- Older adult physiological changes that affect responses to medications include the following:
  - Decreases in liver and renal function can affect the excretion of drugs leading to an accumulation of the drug in the body, thereby increasing the risk for drug toxicity.
  - Decreased gastric mobility and decreased gastric acid production and blood flow can impair drug absorption.
  - Increased adipose tissue and decreased total body fluid proportionate to the body mass can increase the possibility of drug toxicity.
  - Decreased number of protein-binding sites and changes in the blood–brain barrier can occur. The latter permits fat-soluble drugs to move readily to the brain, often resulting in dizziness and confusion. This is particularly evident with beta blockers.
  - Impaired circulation delays the action of medications given intramuscularly or subcutaneously. Digitalis, which is frequently taken by older people, can accumulate to toxic levels and be lethal.
  - Older adults usually require smaller dosages of drugs, especially CNS depressants. Their reactions to medications, particularly sedatives, are unpredictable and often bizarre. Reactions to sedatives include irritability, confusion, disorientation, restlessness, and incontinence. Nurses therefore need to observe clients carefully for untoward reactions.
  - Because memory and visual acuity of older adults may be impaired, the nurse needs to develop simple, realistic plans for clients to follow at home. For example, clients are more likely to remember to take medications if they are scheduled to be taken with meals or at bedtime. If they are likely to forget whether they have taken their medications, a special container for medications can be employed. An empty container indicates that the person has already taken the pills. If the person has poor visual acuity, the nurse or a family

(continued)

member can be write out the plan in block letters large enough to be read.

■ Older adult psychosocial problems (related to physiological changes, past experiences, and established attitudes toward medications) include these:

■ Taking several different medications daily. The possibility of error increases with the number of medications taken.

■ The greater number of medications also compounds the problem of drug interactions. A general rule to follow is to take as few medications as possible.

■ Attitudes of older people toward medical care and medications vary. Older people tend to believe in the wisdom of the physician more readily than younger people. Some older people are bewildered by the prescription of several medications and may passively accept their medications

and "cheek" them, spitting out tablets or capsules after the nurse leaves the room. For this reason, the nurse is advised to stay with clients until they have swallowed the medications. Others may be suspicious of medications and actively refuse them.

■ Older people are mature adults capable of reasoning. Therefore, the nurse needs to explain the reasons for and the effects of medications. This education can prevent clients from continuing to take a medication long after there is a need for it or discontinuing a drug too quickly. For example, clients should know that diuretics will cause them to urinate more frequently and may reduce ankle edema. Instructions about medications need to be given to all clients. These instructions should include when to take the drugs, what effects to expect, and when to consult a physician.

one or two specific routes of administration. Table 29-5 ■ lists the advantages and disadvantages of various routes of administration. The route of administration should always be indicated when the drug is ordered. When administering a drug, the nurse needs to ensure that the pharmaceutical preparation is appropriate for the route specified.

Medication Orders

A physician determines the client's medication needs and orders medications. Usually, the order is written, although telephone and verbal orders are acceptable in a number of agencies. Nursing students need to know the agency policies about medication orders. In some hospitals, for example, only licensed nurses are permitted to accept telephone and verbal orders.

TABLE 29-5

Routes of Administration

ROUTE	ADVANTAGES	DISADVANTAGES
Oral	Most convenient Usually least expensive Safe, does not break skin barrier Administration usually does not cause stress	Inappropriate for clients with nausea or vomiting Drug may have unpleasant taste or odor Inappropriate when gastrointestinal tract has reduced motility Inappropriate if client cannot swallow or is unconscious Cannot be used before certain diagnostic tests or surgical procedures Drug may discolor teeth or harm tooth enamel Drug may irritate gastric mucosa Drug can be aspirated by seriously ill clients
Sublingua	Same as for oral, *plus* Drug can be administered for local effect Drug is rapidly absorbed into the bloodstream More potent than oral route because drug directly enters the blood and bypasses the liver	If swallowed, drug may be inactivated by gastric juice Drug must remain under tongue until dissolved and absorbed
Buccal	Same as for sublingual	Same as for sublingual
Rectal	Can be used when drug has objectionable taste or odor Drug released at slow, steady rate	Dose absorbed is unpredictable
Vaginal	Provides local therapeutic effect	Limited use
Topical	Provides a local effect Few side effects	May be messy and may soil clothes Drug can enter body through abrasions and cause systemic effects

TABLE 29-5

Routes of Administration (*continued*)

ROUTE	ADVANTAGES	DISADVANTAGES
Transdermal	Prolonged systemic effect Few side effects Avoids gastrointestinal absorption problems	Leaves residue on the skin that may soil clothes May cause skin irritation
Subcutaneous	Onset of drug action faster than oral	Must involve sterile technique because breaks skin barrier More expensive than oral Can administer only small volume Slower than intramuscular administration Some drugs can irritate tissues and cause pain Can be anxiety producing
Intramuscular	Pain from irritating drugs is minimized Can administer larger volume than subcutaneous Drug is rapidly absorbed	Breaks skin barrier Some drugs can irritate tissues and cause pain Can be anxiety producing
Intradermal	Absorption is slow (this is an advantage in testing for allergies)	Amount of drug administered must be small Breaks skin barrier
Intravenous	Rapid effect	Limited to highly soluble drugs Anxiety producing and causes pain
Inhalation	Introduces drug throughout respiratory tract Rapid localized relief Drug can be administered to unconscious client	Drug intended for localized effect can have systemic effect Of use only for the respiratory system

Four common medication orders are the stat order, the single order, the standing order, and the prn order.

1. A **stat order** indicates that the medication is to be given immediately and only once.
2. The **single order** or *one-time order* is for medication to be given once at a specified time.
3. The **standing order**, sometimes referred to as a *routine order,* may or may not have a termination date. A standing order may be carried out indefinitely (e.g., multiple vitamins daily) until an order is written to cancel it, or it may be carried out for a specified number of days.
4. A **prn order**, or *as-needed order,* permits the nurse to give a medication when, in the nurse's judgment, the client requires it. The nurse must use good judgment about when the medication is needed and when it can be safely administered.

ESSENTIAL PARTS OF A MEDICATION ORDER

The drug order has seven essential parts, as listed in Box 29-3 ■. Unless it is a standing, or routine order, the order should state the number of doses or the number of days the drug is to be administered.

BOX 29-3

Essential Parts of a Drug Order

- Full name of the client
- Date and time the order is written
- Name of the drug to be administered
- Dosage of the drug
- Route of administration
- Frequency of administration
- Signature of the person writing the order

COMMUNICATING A MEDICATION ORDER

A drug order is written on the client's chart by a physician or by a nurse who receives a telephone or verbal order from a physician. The medication order is then copied by a nurse or clerk to a medication administration record (MAR), often a Kardex. Increasingly, nurses are provided with daily computer-generated MARs. This method saves time and reduces errors caused by hand copying of the physician's order.

Medication administration records (Figure 29-1 ■) vary in form, but all include the client's name, room, and bed number; drug name and dose; and times and method of

☐ Seton Medical Center 100 Spurway Ave • Daly City ☐ Seton Medical Center Coastside 100 Marine Blvd • Moss Beach	**MEDICATION ADMINISTRATION RECORD**		**PAGE 1 OF 1** 5 0507-02

MEDICATION ADMINISTRATION RECORD

PRN#:

MRN#:   AGE:

ADM: 08-04-01   SEX:

VERIFIED BY: _____ DATE: _____

DOB: HT:

DR.   HT:

DIAGNOSIS: *#ALOC
                *#PNEUMONIA

GENERATED: 08-07-08   07:32am

ALLERGIES: NO KNOWN DRUG ALLERGIES

FOR PERIOD: 08-07-08   08:00
THROUGH: 08-08-08   07:59

START	STOP	MEDICATION/I.V./IVPB/IRRIGATION		0800-1559	1600-2359	0000-0759
08-06 17	09-05 16	FERROUS SULFATE 300MG=5ML TWICE A DAY PO (FESO4)	(973539)	09	17	
08-06 17	09-05 16	DOCUSATE SODIUM 100MG=1UDCUP TWICE A DAY PO (COLACE) 100MG/30ML UD HOLD FOR LOOSE STOOL	(973532)	09	17	
08-05 09	09-04 08	ASCORBIC ACID 500MG=1TAB TWICE A DAY PO (VITAMIN C) 500MG TAB	(972096)	09	17	
08-05 09	09-04 08	LEVOTHYROXINE 0.05MG=1TABDAILY PO (SYNTHROID) 0.05MG TAB	(972095)	09		
08-05 09	09-04 08	ASPIRIN 325MG=1 TAB DAILY PO (ASPIRIN) 325MG TAB *W/FOOD TO AVOID GI UPSET	(972094)	09		
08-04 23	08-14 22	CEFUROXIME ADDV. 1.500GM=1VIAL EVERY 8 HOUS IV (KEFUROX) 1.5GM ADDV *ATTACH TO D5W 50ML ADDV BAG *ACTIVATE BEFORE UNFUSION* * INFUSE OVER 30 MINS*	(971776)	14	22	06
		——— **PRN ORDERS** ———				
08-04 23	09-03 22	ACETAMINOPHEN 650MG=1SUPP EVERY 4 HOURS AS NEEDED PR (TYLENOL) 650MG SUPP	(971779)			

INITIALS	SIGNATURE	SHIFT	INITIALS	SIGNATURE	SHIFT	INITIALS	SIGNATURE	SHIFT

SITE CODES:	A. Right Upper Outer Gluteus B. Left Upper Outer Quadrant Gluteus	C. Right Outer Aspect Arm D. Left Outer Aspect Arm	E. Right Ventrogluteal F. Left Ventrogluteal	G. Abdomen H. Right Thigh	J. Left Thigh

Figure 29-1. ■ Medication administration record. (*Source:* Courtesy of Seton Medical Center, Daly City, CA. Reprinted with permission.)

administration. In some agencies, the date the order was prescribed and the date the order expires are also included.

The nurse should always question the physician about any order that is *ambiguous* (unclear or difficult to read), *unusual* (e.g., an abnormally high dosage of a medication), or contraindicated by the client's condition. When the LPN/LVN determines that a physician-ordered medication is inappropriate, the following actions are required:

1. Discuss the order with the RN and/or the nursing supervisor.
2. Contact the physician and discuss the rationale for believing the medication or dosage to be inappropriate.
3. Document in notes the following: time the physician was notified, by whom, information conveyed to the physician, and the physician's response (using the physician's words, if possible).
4. If the physician cannot be reached, document all attempts to contact the physician and the reason for withholding the medication.
5. If someone else gives the medication, document data about the client's condition before and after the medication.
6. If an incident report is indicated, clearly document factual information.

Systems of Measurement

Three systems of measurement are used for the administration of medication: the metric system, the apothecaries' system, and the household system.

METRIC SYSTEM

The **metric system** is a decimal system based on units of 10. Units can be multiplied or divided by 10 to form secondary units. Multiples are calculated by moving the decimal point to the right, and division is accomplished by moving the decimal point to the left.

Basic units of measurement are the meter, the liter, and the gram. Prefixes (from Latin) indicate subdivision of the basic unit: *deci-* (1/10 or 0.1), *centi* (1/100 or 0.01), and *milli-* (1/1,000 or 0.001). Multiples of the basic units (from Greek) are *deka-* (10), *hecto-* (100), and *kilo-* (1,000). See Figure 29-2 ■ for examples. In nursing practice, the kilogram (kg) is the only multiple of the gram used, and the milligram (mg) and microgram (mcg) are subdivisions. Fractional parts of the liter are usually expressed in milliliters (mL).

APOTHECARIES' SYSTEM

The **apothecaries' system** predates the metric system. The basic unit of weight in the apothecaries' system is the grain (gr), likened to a grain of wheat, and the basic unit of volume is the minim, a volume of water equal in weight to a grain of wheat. The word *minim* means "the least." Other units of weight are the dram, the ounce, and the pound. The

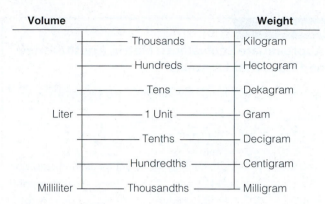

Figure 29-2. ■ Basic metric measurements of volume and weight.

units of volume are the fluid dram, the fluid ounce, the pint, the quart, and the gallon.

Quantities in the apothecaries' system are often expressed by lowercase Roman numerals (ii, iv, ix, etc.), particularly when the unit of measure is abbreviated. The Roman numeral follows the unit of measure. Although rarely used today, some medications are still being ordered in apothecary measurement.

HOUSEHOLD SYSTEM

Household system measures may be used when more accurate systems of measure are not required. Included in household measures are drops, teaspoons, tablespoons, cups, and glasses. Although pints and quarts are often found in the home, they are defined as apothecaries' measures.

Table 29-6 ■ lists measurement equivalents for the metric, apothecaries', and household systems.

clinical ALERT

A household teaspoon may hold 7.5 mL. This caution should be included in discharge instructions. It is advisable to use a medication cup or spoon with milliliter markings to prevent overdose of a drug.

CONVERTING UNITS OF WEIGHT AND MEASURE

Sometimes drugs are dispensed from the pharmacy in grams when the order specifies milligrams, or they are dispensed in milligrams though ordered in grains. For example, a physician orders morphine gr 1/4. The medication is available only in milligrams. The nurse knows that 1 mg equals 1/60 gr or 60 mg equals 1 grain. To convert the ordered dose to milligrams, the nurse calculates as follows:

$$\text{If } 60 \text{ mg} = 1 \text{ gr}$$
$$\text{Then } x \text{ mg} = 1/4 \text{ gr } (or\ 0.25 \text{ gr})$$
$$x = \frac{(60 \times 0.25)}{1}$$
$$x = 15 \text{ mg}$$

TABLE 29-6

Approximate Equivalents: Metric, Apothecaries', and Household Systems

METRIC	APOTHECARIES'	HOUSEHOLD
Volume		
1 mL	15 minims (min or m)	15 drops (gtt)
5 mL	75 min	1 measuring teaspoon
7.5 mL	112.5 min	1 household teaspoon
15 mL	4 fluid drams (dr)	1 tablespoon (Tbsp) (= 3 teaspoons)
30 mL	1 fluid ounce (oz)	1 fluid ounce
240 mL	8 oz	1 cup
500 mL	1 pint (pt)	1 pint
1,000 mL	1 quart (qt)	1 quart
4,000 mL	1 gallon (gal)	1 gallon
Weight		
1 milligram (mg)	1/60 grain	—
60 mg	1 grain (gr)	—
1 gram (g)	15 grains	—
4 g	1 dram	—
30 g	1 ounce	—
500 g	1.1 pound (lbs)	—
1,000 g (1 kilogram [kg])	2.2 lbs	—

Converting Weights within the Metric System

It is quite simple to find equivalent units of weight within the metric system, because the system is based on units of 10. Only three metric units of weight are used for drug dosages: the gram (g), milligram (mg), and microgram (mcg); 1,000 mg or 1,000,000 mcg equals 1 g. Equivalents are computed by dividing or multiplying. For example, to change milligrams to grams, the nurse divides the number of milligrams by 1,000. The simplest way to divide by 1,000 is to move the decimal point three places to the left:

$$500 \text{ mg} = ? \text{ g}$$

Move the decimal point three places to the left:

$$\text{Answer} = 0.5 \text{ g}$$

Conversely, to convert grams to milligrams, multiply the number of grams by 1,000, or move the decimal point three places to the right:

$$0.006 \text{ g} = ? \text{ mg}$$

Move the decimal point three places to the right:

$$\text{Answer} = 6 \text{ mg}$$

Converting Weights and Measures between Systems

When preparing client medications, a nurse may need to convert weights or volumes from one system to another.

The units of weight most commonly used in nursing practice are the gram, milligram, and kilogram; and the grain and the pound. Household units of weight are generally not applicable (see Table 29-6). Learning these equivalents helps the nurse make weight conversions easily.

CALCULATING DOSAGES

Several formulas can be used to calculate drug dosages. One formula uses ratios:

$$\frac{\text{Dose on hand}}{\text{Quantity on hand}} = \frac{\text{Desired dose}}{\text{Quantity desired } (n)}$$

For example, erythromycin 500 mg is ordered. It is supplied in a liquid form containing 250 mg in 5 mL. To calculate the dosage, the nurse uses the formula

$$\frac{\text{Dose on hand (250 mg)}}{\text{Quantity on hand (5 mL)}} = \frac{\text{Desired dose (500 mg)}}{\text{Quantity desired } (n)}$$

Then the nurse cross-multiplies:

$$250 \times n = 5 \times 500$$
$$250 \times n = 2,500$$
$$n = \frac{2,500}{250}$$
$$n = 10 \text{ mL}$$

Therefore, the dose ordered is 10 mL. The nurse can also use the following formula to calculate dosages:

$$\frac{\text{Desired dose}}{\text{Dose on hand}} \times \text{Quantity on hand}$$

For example, heparin is often distributed in large vials in prepared dilutions of 10,000 units per mL. If the order calls for 5,000 units, the nurse can use the formula above to calculate:

$$n = \frac{5,000}{10,000} \times 1 \text{ mL}$$
$$n = 1/2 \text{ mL} = 0.5 \text{ mL}$$

Therefore, the nurse injects 0.5 mL for a 5,000-unit dose.

Dosages for Children

Although dosage is stated in the medication order, nurses must understand something about the safe dosage for children. Unlike adult dosages, children's dosages are not always standard. Body size significantly affects dosage.

BODY SURFACE AREA. Body surface area is determined by using a **nomogram** and the child's height and weight. This is considered to be the most accurate method of calculating a child's dose. Standard nomograms give a child's body surface area according to weight and height (Figure 29-3 ■).

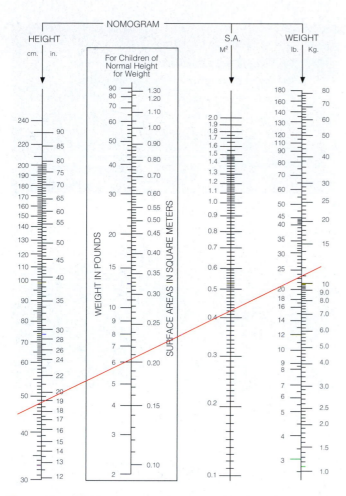

Figure 29-3. ■ Nomogram with estimated body surface area. A straight line is drawn between the child's height (on the left) and the child's weight (on the right). The point at which the line intersects the surface area column is the estimated body surface area.

The formula is the ratio of the child's body surface area to the surface area of an average adult (1.7 square meters, or 1.7 m^2), multiplied by the normal adult dose of the drug:

$$\text{Child's dose} = \frac{\text{Surface area of child (m}^2)}{1.7 \text{ m}^2} \times \text{Normal adult dose}$$

For example, a child who weighs 10 kg and is 50 cm tall has a body surface area of 0.4 m^2. Therefore, the child's dose of tetracycline corresponding to an adult dose of 250 mg would be as follows:

$$\text{Child's dose} = \frac{0.4 \text{ m}^2}{1.7 \text{ m}^2} \times 250 \text{ mg}$$
$$= 0.23 \times 250 = 58.82 \text{ mg}$$

Equipment

SYRINGES

To administer parenteral medications, nurses use injectable equipment. **Syringes** have three parts: the *tip,* which con-

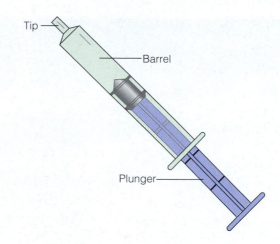

Figure 29-4. ■ The three parts of a syringe.

nects with the needle; the *barrel,* or fluid chamber, on which the scales are printed; and the *plunger,* which fits inside the barrel (Figure 29-4 ■).

To handle a syringe aseptically, the nurse may only touch the outside of the barrel and the plunger handle. The nurse must avoid letting any unsterile object contact the tip or inside of the barrel, the shaft of the plunger, or the shaft or tip of the needle.

Syringes differ in size, shape, and material. The three most commonly used types are the standard hypodermic syringe, the insulin syringe, and the tuberculin syringe (Figure 29-5 ■). Hypodermic syringes come in 2-, 2.5-, and 3-mL sizes. They usually have two scales marked on them: the minim and the milliliter. The milliliter scale is the one normally used.

Insulin syringes are similar to hypodermic syringes, but they have a specially calibrated scale for use with U-100 insulin. In North America, all insulin syringes are calibrated this way. Most insulin syringes are disposable and have a nonremovable needle. Low-dose insulin syringes are also available. The correct choice of syringe is based on the insulin dose.

The tuberculin syringe is a narrow-barrel syringe, calibrated in tenths and hundredths of a milliliter (up to 1 mL)

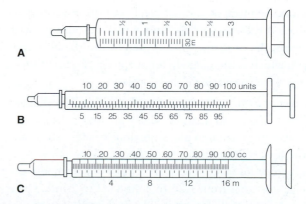

Figure 29-5. ■ Three kinds of syringes: **A.** hypodermic syringe marked in tenths (0.1) of milliliters and in minims; **B.** insulin syringe marked in 100 units; **C.** tuberculin syringe marked in tenths (0.1) and hundredths (0.01) of cubic millimeters and in minims.

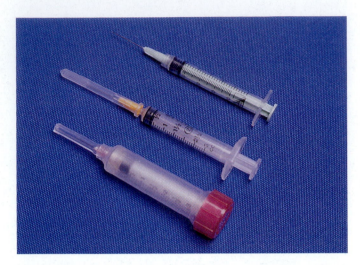

Figure 29-6. ■ Disposable plastic syringes and needles: top, with syringe and needle exposed; middle, with plastic cap over the needle; bottom, with plastic case over the needle and syringe. (Photographer: Elena Dorfman.)

on one scale and in sixteenths of a minim (up to 1 minim) on the other scale. Originally designed to administer tuberculin, this syringe is useful for administering other drugs, particularly when a small, precise measurement is necessary (e.g., pediatric doses).

Other syringes are manufactured in several sizes such as 5, 10, 20, and 50 mL. Most syringes used today are made of plastic and are individually packaged for sterility in a paper wrapper or a rigid plastic container (Figure 29-6 ■). The syringe and needle may be packaged together or separately.

Injectable medications are frequently supplied in disposable, prefilled unit-dose systems such as (1) ready-to-use syringes or (2) prefilled sterile cartridges and needles that require the attachment of a reusable holder (injection system) before use (Figure 29-7 ■). Examples of the latter system are the Tubex and Carpuject injection systems. The manufacturers provide specific directions for use.

NEEDLES

Needles are made of stainless steel, and most are disposable. A needle has three parts: the **hub**, which fits onto the syringe; the **cannula**, or shaft, which is attached to the hub; and the **bevel**, which is the slanted part of the tip (Figure 29-8 ■).

Needles have variable characteristics:

1. *Slant or length of the bevel.* Bevel length varies. Long-bevel needles are sharpest. They are best for subcutaneous and intramuscular injections because they cause the least discomfort.
2. *Length of the shaft.* The shaft length of commonly used needles varies from 1.25 to 5 cm (1/2 to 2 in.). The appropriate needle length is chosen according to the client's muscle development, the client's weight, and the type of injection.

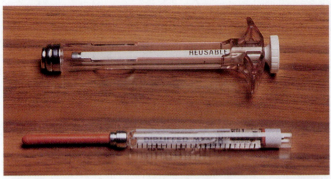

A

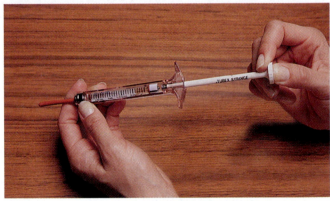

B

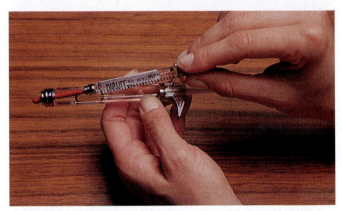

C

Figure 29-7. ■ **A.** Syringe and prefilled sterile cartridge with needle. **B.** Assembling the device. **C.** The cartridge slides into the syringe barrel, turns, and locks at the needle end. The plunger then screws into the cartridge end. (Photographer: Elena Dorfman.)

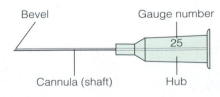

Figure 29-8. ■ The parts of a needle.

3. *Gauge (or diameter) of the shaft.* The gauge varies from 16 to 28. The larger the gauge number, the smaller the diameter of the shaft. Smaller gauges produce less tissue trauma, but larger gauges are necessary for viscous medications, such as penicillin.

Additional equipment is need for intravenous administration.

Routes of Administration

ORAL MEDICATIONS

The oral route is the most common medication route. As long as a client can swallow effectively and retain the drug in the stomach, this is the route of choice. Procedure 29-1 ■ on page 650 describes how to give oral medications. Oral medications are contraindicated when a client is vomiting, has gastric or intestinal suction, is unconscious, or has swallowing difficulty, such as after a stroke. Such clients in the hospital are usually on orders for "nothing by mouth" (**NPO**).

There are two variations on the oral medication transmucosal route: sublingual and buccal. In **sublingual** administration, the drug is placed under the tongue (Figure 29-9 ■). The drug is absorbed into the blood vessels on the underside of the tongue. Nitroglycerin is one example of a drug commonly given in this manner.

Buccal means "pertaining to the cheek." In buccal administration, the tablet is held in the mouth next to the mucous membranes of the cheek until it dissolves (Figure 29-10 ■). The medication acts locally on the mucous membrane or systemically when the drug is absorbed into the blood vessels of the cheek (the same as the sublingual medication route).

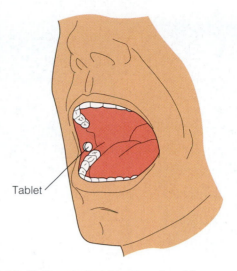

Figure 29-10. ■ Buccal administration of a tablet.

NASOGASTRIC AND GASTROSTOMY MEDICATIONS

For the client who is NPO and has a nasogastric (NG) or gastrostomy (G) tube in place, medication may be administered via the tube. Medication is absorbed enterally because the medication is delivered directly into the stomach or small intestine. See also Procedures 25-2 and 25-3 ⬤.

PARENTERAL MEDICATIONS

LPNs/LVNs give **parenteral** (injectable) medications. The routes are **intradermal** (ID or into the dermis or skin), **subcutaneous** (Sub-Q, subQ, or subcutaneously [per JCAHO standards], below the skin), **intramuscular** (IM or into the muscle), and, in some states, **intravenous** (IV or into the vein). Figure 29-11 ■ illustrates the different angles of these injections and different ways of holding the syringe to administer them. Administration of medications via the parenteral route is discussed in the Nursing Care section of this chapter.

Because parenteral medications are absorbed rapidly and are irretrievable once injected, the nurse must prepare and administer them carefully and accurately. Administering parenteral drugs requires the same nursing knowledge as for oral and topical drugs. However, because injections are invasive procedures, aseptic technique must be used to minimize the risk of infection.

TOPICAL MEDICATIONS

Topical medications are those that are applied locally to the skin or to mucous membranes in areas such as the eye, external ear canal, nose, vagina, and rectum. Traditionally, topical application to the skin was limited to medications intended to produce a local effect at the administration site. However, several medications (e.g., nitroglycerin and estrogen) have been "packaged" in special transdermal

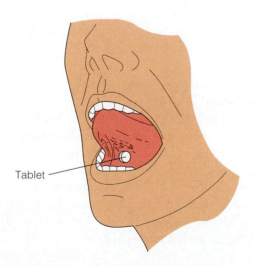

Figure 29-9. ■ Sublingual administration of a tablet.

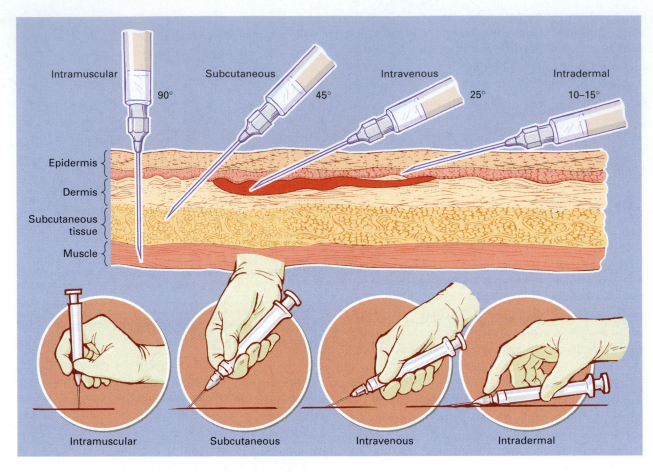

Figure 29-11. ■ Angles of needle insertion for four types of injection.

delivery systems that gradually release a predictable amount of active substance into the bloodstream for as long as a week.

NURSING CARE

ASSESSING

When LPNs/LVNs are assigned the responsibility of administering medication, they must review the client's chart, including the medication history and nursing notes for assessment data, and discuss any concerns with the RN or physician.

DIAGNOSING, PLANNING, AND IMPLEMENTING

Providing Safety in Medication Administration

When administering any drug, regardless of the route of administration, the nurse must follow certain procedures. For a description of these procedures, see Table 29-7 ■. Box 29-4 ■ lists the six "rights" and the three "checks" for accu-

rate drug administration. The nurse who prepares the medication must also administer it to the client. Medications must never be left unattended on the medication cart or at the client's bedside.

Clients may take cultural remedies when they are ill, or they may have prohibitions against certain medications based on cultural and religious beliefs (Box 29-5 ■). These practices must be considered in the care of and planning for the client.

Observing Client's Response to the Drug

The kinds of behavior that reflect the action or lack of action of a drug and its untoward effects (both minor and major) are as variable as the purposes of the drugs themselves. For example, the effectiveness of a sedative–hypnotic may be directly observed by how well the client sleeps. The effectiveness of an antispasmodic must be based on the client's report of pain relief. It is essential to chart the client's drug response, but written notes are only one facet of communication needed for continuity of care. The LPN/LVN should also verbally report the client's response to the team leader or physician.

TABLE 29-7

Rules for Medication Administration

THE NURSE MUST ALWAYS	DESCRIPTION
Identify the client	In hospitals, most clients wear some sort of identification (ID), such as a wristband with name and hospital ID number. Before giving the client any drug, check the ID band against the MAR. As a double check, ask the client to state his or her name and birth date. JCAHO requires the use of two identifiers—neither of which can be the client's room number.
Inform the client	If the client is unfamiliar with the medication, the nurse should explain the intended action as well as any side effects or adverse effects that might occur.
Administer the drug	Read medication orders and records carefully; check both the client and drug name against the names on the drug packaging. If the client's medication is kept in a medication cart or computerized dispensary, check against this also.
Provide adjunctive interventions as indicated	Clients may need physical assistance, such as positioning for an injection. They may need teaching about measures to enhance drug effectiveness, such as changes in diet and fluid intake. Clients may express fear of medication. The LPN/LVN can allay fear through active listening and by offering factual information and emotional support.
Record the drug	Documentation must be completed immediately following the administration of a medication; never prechart medications. The name of the drug, dosage, method of administration, specific relevant data such as pulse rate, and any other pertinent information (e.g., date to be discontinued) are recorded in the chart in ink or by computer printout after being transcribed from the physician's order sheet. The record should also include the exact time of administration and the signature of the nurse providing the medication. Many medication records are designed in flowchart style so that the nurse signs once on the page and initials each medication administered. Any prn or stat medications, as well as the client's response to the drug, are recorded separately and should be documented in the nursing/progress notes. Nurses must be aware of all the medications a client is taking, and be alert for drug–drug or drug–food interactions.
Evaluate the client's response to the drug	In all nursing activities, nurses need to be aware of the medications that a client is taking and record their effectiveness as assessed by the client and the nurse on the client's chart. The nurse may also report the client's response to the RN or the physician.

Administering Oral Medications

The nurse provides oral medications and water or other liquid as appropriate for the client. The nurse remains with the client while the client swallows the medicine and assists if necessary. (*Note:* The nurse should be aware that some clients "pouch" medications in the cheek instead of swallowing them.)

Sublingual and buccal medications are placed under the tongue or between the cheek and the gum. They are not swallowed but allowed to dissolve in the mouth.

BOX 29-4

Six "Rights" and Three "Checks" of Drug Administration

Right Client
Right Drug
Right Dose
Right Route
Right Time
Right Documentation

Compare drug to MAR when removed from drawer.
Compare drug to MAR when pouring into cup.
Compare drug to MAR when returning container to drawer.

Administering Nasogastric and Gastrostomy Medications

Clients may be NPO because of illness, surgery, or another procedure. Medication may then be administered via nasogastric or gastrostomy tube. Guidelines for administering medications by NG or G tubes are shown in Box 29-6 ■.

BOX 29-5   CULTURAL PULSE POINTS

Cultural Remedies and Prohibitions

Cultural practices may affect which medications are acceptable to clients. For example, clients who follow strict Jewish dietary laws are not permitted to use pork insulin to treat diabetes. Muslims also do not consume pork products, but they are allowed to use medications made from pork. Many cultures prescribe herbal remedies based on cultural views of the nature of the illness. Many Native Americans, Hispanics, and Asians employ native health treatments before, or along with, Western medicine. These groups may consult an herbalist or medicine man. There is much more acceptance of alternative remedies in society now than in the past, but there still is need for caution. The client's record should always include herbs, remedies, or alternate medical practices as an important part of the client's database.

BOX 29-6	NURSING CARE CHECKLIST

Administering Medications by Nasogastric or Gastrostomy Tube

☑ Always check with the pharmacist to see if the client's medications come in liquid form, because liquids are less likely to cause tube obstruction.

☑ If not available, determine if the drug may be safely crushed. Enteric-coated, sustained-action, buccal, and sublingual medications should never be crushed.

☑ Dissolve crushed tablets in warm water. Cold liquids may congeal or cause client discomfort.

☑ Read medication labels carefully before opening a capsule.

☑ Open capsules and mix the contents with water only with the pharmacist's advice.

☑ Do not administer whole or undissolved medications.

☑ If the tube is connected to suction, disconnect the suction and keep the tube clamped for 20 to 30 minutes after giving the medication to enhance absorption. Positioning the patient toward the right side may facilitate gastric emptying.

☑ Always check and confirm NG tube placement before administering medications by checking gastric pH or by auscultating air.

☑ Flush the tube with at least 15 to 30 mL (5 to 10 mL for children) of water before administering medications.

☑ If you are giving several medications, administer each one separately and flush with at least 5 mL (3 mL for children) of water between each.

☑ When you have finished administering all medications, flush with another 15 to 30 mL of water to clear the tube.

Sources: Data from Lehmann, S., & Barber, J. (1991, November). Giving medication by feeding tube: How to avoid problems. *Nursing 91*, p. 61; and Petrosino, B. M., Christian, B. J., Wolfe, J., et al. (1989, December). Implications of selected problems with nasoenteral tube feeding. *Critical Care Quarterly, 12*, 1.

Assisting with IV Medication Administration

LPNs/LVNs, once licensed and certified in IV therapy, may be responsible for starting and hanging IVs. Until then, the LPN/LVN is responsible for assessing the site and removing the delivery system, once an order has been given to discontinue. Box 29-7 ■ provides instructions for discontinuing an intravenous infusion. See also Procedure 30-11 ⚭.

Preparing Injectable Medications

Injectable medications can be prepared by withdrawing the medication from an ampule or vial into a sterile syringe, using prefilled syringes, or via a needleless injection system.

BOX 29-7	NURSING CARE CHECKLIST

Discontinuing an Intravenous Device

☑ Check physician's order.

☑ Gather appropriate equipment.

☑ Identify the client and explain the procedure.

☑ Wash hands and don gloves.

☑ Stabilize needle or catheter while removing tape.

☑ Remove needle or catheter carefully and smoothly, keeping it almost flush with skin.

☑ Do not press down on top of needle point while it is in the vein.

☑ Once the catheter is removed, quickly press sterile pad over venipuncture site, and hold firmly until bleeding stops.

☑ Hold pressure for several minutes if client's drug therapy prolongs bleeding.

☑ Apply clean pad and tape in place.

☑ Elevate arm to reduce venous pressure and help facilitate clot formation.

☑ Observe venipuncture site for redness, swelling, or hematoma.

☑ Dispose of equipment.

☑ Wash hands.

☑ Check site again in 15 minutes.

☑ Record volume infused on intake and output (I&O) sheet.

☑ Document.

Ampules and Vials

Ampules and vials (Figure 29-12 ■) are frequently used to package sterile parenteral medications. An **ampule** is a clear glass container with a distinctive shape usually designed to hold a single dose of a drug. Ampule capacity ranges from 1 mL to 10 mL or more. Most ampules have colored score markings for opening. Refer to Procedure 29-2 ■ on page 653 for steps in preparing medications from ampules and vials.

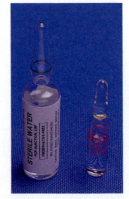
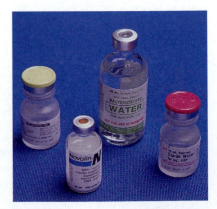

A **B**

Figure 29-12. ■ A. Ampules; **B.** vials.

A **vial** is a small glass bottle with a sealed rubber cap. Vials come in different sizes, from single to multidose, and have a metal or plastic cap that protects the rubber seal.

Mixing Medications in One Syringe

Frequently, clients need more than one drug injected at the same time. To spare the client the experience of being injected twice, two drugs (if compatible) can be mixed together in one syringe. (See Procedure 29-2C for how to mix medications in one syringe.)

Preventing Needle-Stick Injuries

One of the most potentially hazardous procedures that healthcare personnel face is using and disposing of needles and sharps.

clinical ALERT

Needle-stick injuries present a major risk for infection with hepatitis B virus, human immunodeficiency virus (HIV), and many other pathogens. Standards have been set by the Occupational Safety and Health Administration to prevent such injuries.

To prevent needle-stick injury, the nurse must follow these guidelines carefully and consistently:

- Always use the designated puncture-proof disposal container provided (Figure 29-13 ■). Never throw sharps in

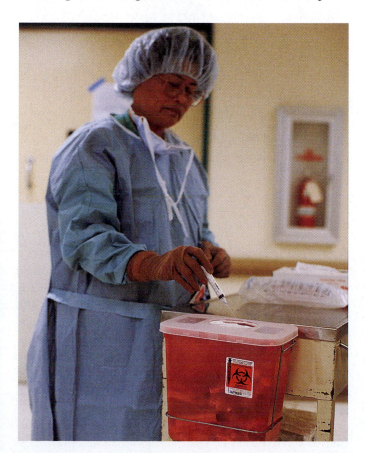

Figure 29-13. ■ Disposal container for contaminated needles and other sharps. (Photographer: Elena Dorfman.)

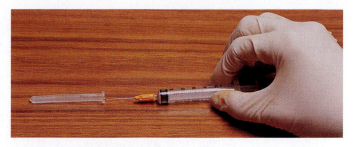

Figure 29-14. ■ Recapping a used needle using the scoop method. (Photographer: Elena Dorfman.)

wastebaskets. Never leave sharps unattended in public or client care areas.
- Handle all sharps with care, including any items that can cut or puncture skin, such as needles, surgical blades, lancets, razors, broken glass (including capillary pipettes and open ampules), exposed dental wires, reusable items (e.g., large-bore needles, hooks, rasps, drill points), or ANY SHARP INSTRUMENT!
- Never bend or break needles before disposal.
- Never recap used needles except under specified circumstances (e.g., when transporting a syringe to the laboratory for an arterial blood gas or blood culture).
- If you must recap a needle, use the one-handed "scoop" method. Set the needle cap and syringe horizontally on a flat surface. Insert the needle into the cap, using one hand (Figure 29-14 ■). Use your other hand to pick up the cap and tighten it to the needle hub.

If an accidental needle-stick injury occurs, follow specific steps outlined by the agency. A summary of these steps is provided in Box 29-8 ■. Safety syringes are now available to protect healthcare workers.

Administering Intradermal Injections

An intradermal injection is the administration of a drug into the dermal layer of the skin just beneath the epidermis (see

BOX 29-8

What to Do If Needle Stick Occurs

If you experience a needle-stick or sharp injury or are exposed to the blood or other body fluids of a client during the course of your work, immediately follow these steps or those prescribed by the facility:

- Wash needle sticks and cuts with soap and water.
- Flush splashes to nose, mouth, or skin with clean water.
- Irrigate eyes with clean water, saline, or sterile irrigants.
- Report the incident to your supervisor and complete an incident report.
- Immediately seek medical treatment.

Source: Recommendations courtesy of the National Institute for Occupational Health and Safety.

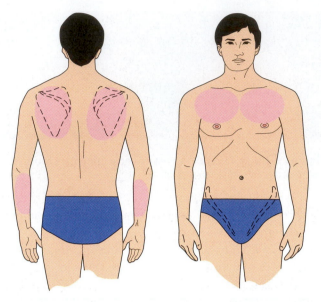

Figure 29-15. ■ Body sites commonly used for intradermal injections.

Figure 29-11). Intradermal injections generally use only a small amount of liquid, such as 0.1 mL. This method of administration is frequently indicated for allergy and tuberculin tests and for vaccinations. Common sites for intradermal injections are the inner lower arm, the upper chest, and the back beneath the scapulae (Figure 29-15 ■). Typically, the left arm is used for tuberculin tests and the right arm is used for all other tests.

The equipment normally used is a 1-mL syringe calibrated into hundredths of a milliliter. The needle is short and fine. After the site is cleaned, the skin is held tautly, and the syringe is held at about a 15-degree angle to the skin, with the bevel of the needle upward. The needle is then inserted through the epidermis into the dermis, and the fluid is injected. The drug produces a small bleb just under the skin (Figure 29-16 ■). The needle is then withdrawn quickly, and the site is very lightly wiped with an antiseptic swab. The area is not massaged because the medication may disperse into the tissue or out through the needle insertion site. Intradermal injections are absorbed slowly through blood capillaries in the area.

Administering Subcutaneous Injections

Many kinds of drugs (such as insulin and heparin) are administered *subcutaneously* (just beneath the skin). Common sites for subcutaneous injections are the outer aspect of the upper arms and the anterior aspect of the thighs. These areas are convenient and normally have good blood circulation. Other areas that can be used are the abdomen, the scapular areas of the upper back, and the upper ventrogluteal and dorsogluteal areas (Figure 29-17 ■). Only small doses (0.5 to 1 mL) of medication are usually injected via

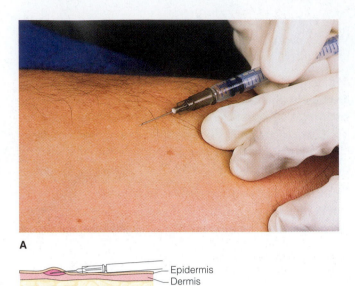

Figure 29-16. ■ For an intradermal injection: **A.** the needle enters the skin at a 15-degree angle; **B, C.** the medication forms a bleb under the epidermis.

the subcutaneous route. Refer to Procedure 29-3 ■ on page 657 for instructions about subcutaneous injections.

Administering Intramuscular Injections

Injections into muscle tissue (IM injections) are absorbed more quickly than subcutaneous injections because of the greater blood supply to the body muscles. Muscles can also take a larger volume of fluid without discomfort than subcutaneous tissues can, although the amount varies somewhat, depending on muscle size, muscle condition, and the site used. An adult with well-developed muscles can usually safely tolerate up to 4 mL of medication in the gluteus medius and gluteus maximus muscles.

A major consideration in the administration of IM injections is the selection of a safe site located away from large blood vessels, nerves, and bone. Several body sites can be

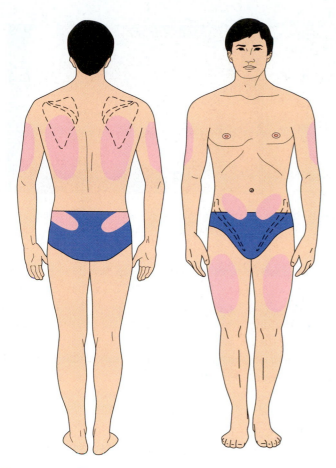

Figure 29-17. ■ Body sites commonly used for subcutaneous injections.

used for IM injections (Figure 29-18 ■). See Procedure 29-3A for administering IM injections.

Ventrogluteal Site

The ventrogluteal site is in the gluteus medius muscle, which lies over the gluteus minimus. The ventrogluteal site

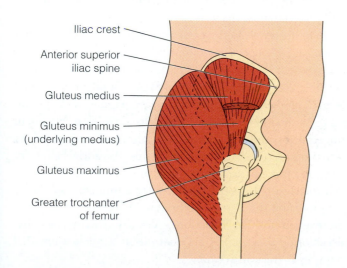

Figure 29-18. ■ Lateral view of the right buttock showing the three gluteal muscles used for intramuscular injections.

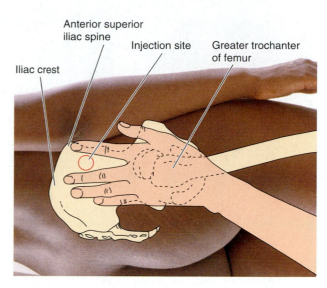

Figure 29-19. ■ The ventrogluteal site for an intramuscular injection.

is the preferred site for IM injections because the area (1) contains no large nerves or blood vessels, (2) provides the greatest thickness of gluteal muscle consisting of both the gluteus medius and gluteus minimus, (3) is sealed off by bone, and (4) contains consistently less fat than the buttock area, thus eliminating the need to determine the depth of subcutaneous fat.

The client position for the injection can be a supine, prone, or side-lying position. To establish the exact site, the nurse places the heel of the hand on the client's greater trochanter, with the fingers pointing toward the client's head. The right hand is used for the left hip, and the left hand for the right hip. With the index finger on the client's anterior superior iliac spine, the nurse stretches the middle finger dorsally, palpating the crest of the ilium and then pressing below it. The triangle formed by the index finger, the third finger, and the crest of the ilium is the injection site (Figure 29-19 ■).

Vastus Lateralis Site

The vastus lateralis muscle is usually thick and well developed in both adults and children. It is recommended as the site of choice for IM injections for infants. Because there are no major blood vessels or nerves in the area, it is desirable for infants whose gluteal muscles are poorly developed. It is located on the anterior lateral aspect of the thigh (Figure 29-20 ■). The middle third of the muscle is suggested as the site. This is established by dividing the area between the greater trochanter of the femur and the lateral femoral condyle into thirds and selecting the middle third (Figure 29-20B). The client can assume a back-lying or a sitting position for an injection into this site.

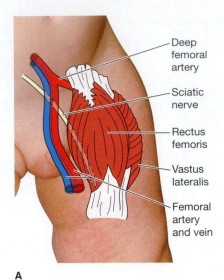

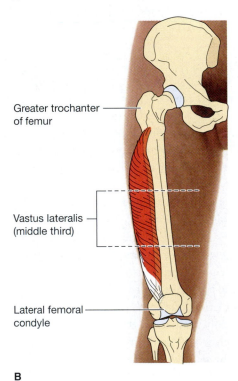

Figure 29-20. ■ **A.** The vastus lateralis muscle of the upper thigh, used for intramuscular injections. **B.** The vastus lateralis site of the right thigh, used for an intramuscular injection. (*Source:* Custom Medical Stock Photo, Inc.)

Dorsogluteal Site

The dorsogluteal site is composed of the thick gluteal muscles of the buttocks (Figure 29-21 ■). The dorsogluteal site can be used for adults and for children with well-developed gluteal muscles. Because these muscles are developed by walking, this site should not be used for children under 3 years unless the child has been walking for at least 1 year. The nurse must choose the injection site carefully to avoid striking the sciatic nerve, major blood vessels, or bone.

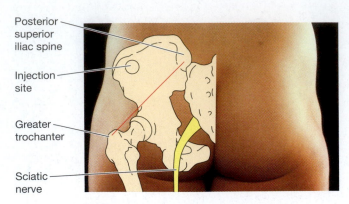

Figure 29-21. ■ The dorsogluteal site for an intramuscular injection. (*Source:* Custom Medical Stock Photo, Inc.)

The nurse palpates the posterior superior iliac spine, and then draws an imaginary line to the greater trochanter of the femur. This line is lateral to and parallel to the sciatic nerve. The injection site is lateral and superior to this line. Palpating the ilium and the trochanter is important. Visual calculations alone can result in an injection that is too low and that injures other structures.

The client needs to assume a prone position with the toes pointed inward, or a side-lying position with the upper knee flexed and in front of the lower leg. These positions promote muscle relaxation and minimize discomfort from the injection.

Deltoid Site

The deltoid muscle is found on the lateral aspect of the upper arm. It is not used often for IM injections, because it is a relatively small muscle and is very close to the radial nerve and radial artery. It is sometimes considered for use in adults because of rapid absorption from the deltoid area, but no more than 1 mL of solution can be administered. This site is recommended for the administration of hepatitis B vaccine in adults.

To locate the densest part of the muscle, the nurse palpates the lower edge of the acromion and the midpoint on the lateral aspect of the arm that is in line with the axilla. A triangle within these boundaries indicates the deltoid muscle about 5 cm (2 in.) below the acromion process (Figure 29-22 ■). Another method of establishing the deltoid site is to place four fingers across the deltoid muscle, with the first finger on the acromion process. The site is three fingerbreadths below the acromion process (see Figure 29-22B).

Procedure 29-3A describes how to administer an IM injection using the Z-track technique. This technique is recommended for IM injections. Vistaril (hydroxyzine hydrochloride solution) is an example of a medication that requires Z-track injection.

Although it is common practice to add 0.2 mL of air following the drawing up of medication, research has shown

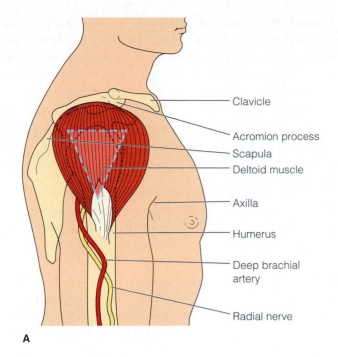

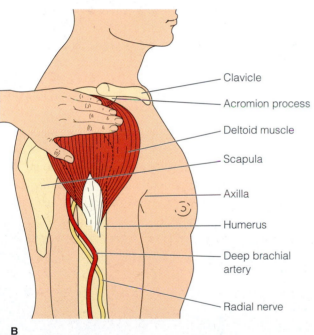

Figure 29-22. ■ **A.** The deltoid muscle of the upper arm, used for intramuscular injections. **B.** A method of establishing the deltoid muscle site for an intramuscular injection.

that use of an air bubble in the syringe is unnecessary with modern disposable syringes and can be potentially dangerous, causing overdoses (Beyea & Nicoll, 1996, pp. 34–35). Syringes are now calibrated to deliver correct dosages without the use of an air bubble. Some sources still advise the addition of 0.2 to 0.5 mL of air when administering medication Z-track to clear the needle in order to prevent tracking of medication when the needle is withdrawn.

Administering Topical Applications

Skin Applications

Topical skin or dermatologic preparations include ointments, pastes, creams, lotions, powders, sprays, and patches (see Table 29-1 earlier in this chapter). Before applying a dermatologic preparation, thoroughly clean the area with mild soap and water and pat it dry. Medication absorption is affected by the buildup of skin secretions and previous topical medication. Human skin harbors microorganisms, so nurses should wear gloves when administering skin applications and always use surgical asepsis when an open wound is present.

Ophthalmic Instillations

Preparations for the eye (**ophthalmics**) come as liquids or ointments. Procedure 29-4 ■ on page 662 illustrates how to administer ophthalmic medications.

Otic Instillations

Medical aseptic technique is used to instill **otics** (ear preparations) unless the tympanic membrane is damaged, in which case sterile technique is required. The position of the external auditory canal varies with age. In the child under 3 years of age, it is directed upward. In the adult, the external auditory canal is a short tube about 2.5 cm (1 in.) long. Procedure 29-5 ■ on page 664 explains how to administer otic instillations.

Nasal Instillations

Nasal instillations (nose drops and sprays) usually are instilled for their *astringent* effect (to shrink swollen mucous membranes), to loosen secretions and facilitate drainage, or to treat infections of the nasal cavity or sinuses. Nasal decongestants are the most common nasal instillations. Many of these products are available without a prescription. Clients need to be taught to use these agents with caution. Chronic use of nasal decongestants may lead to a *rebound effect* (an increase in nasal congestion after the decongestant action has ended). If excess decongestant solution is swallowed, serious systemic effects may also develop, especially in children. Saline drops are safer as a decongestant for children.

Usually, clients self-administer sprays. In the supine position with the head tilted back, the client holds the tip of the container just inside the nares and inhales as the spray enters the nasal passages. For clients who use nasal sprays repeatedly, the nares need to be assessed for irritation. In children, nasal sprays are given with the head in an upright position to prevent excess spray from being swallowed.

The client should also be instructed to (1) blow the nose prior to nasal instillation, (2) breathe through the mouth to prevent aspiration of medication into the trachea and bronchi, (3) remain in a back-lying position for at least 1 minute so that the solution will come into contact with all of the nasal surface, and (4) avoid blowing the nose for several minutes.

Vaginal Instillations

Vaginal medications, or instillations, are inserted as creams, jellies, foams, or suppositories to treat infection or to relieve vaginal discomfort, such as itching, dryness, or pain. See Procedure 29-6 ■ on page 665 for guidelines on administering vaginal instillations.

Rectal Instillations

Insertion of medications into the rectum in the form of suppositories is a frequent practice. Rectal administration is a convenient and safe method of giving certain medications.

When rectal medication is to be given for constipation, the nurse should check the chart for the last bowel movement (BM) recorded. If no BM is recorded, then a digital exam should be done before giving a suppository. To insert a rectal suppository:

- Assist the client to a left lateral position, with the upper leg flexed.
- Fold back the top bedclothes to expose the buttocks.
- Don a glove on the hand used to insert the suppository.
- Unwrap the suppository and lubricate the smooth rounded end, or see manufacturer's instructions. The rounded end is usually inserted first. The lubricant reduces irritation of the mucosa and facilitates insertion.
- Lubricate the gloved index finger.
- Encourage the client to relax by breathing through the mouth.
- Insert the suppository gently into the anal canal, rounded end first (or according to manufacturer's instructions), along the rectal wall using the gloved index finger (Figure 29-23 ■). For an adult, insert the suppository beyond the internal sphincter (i.e., 10 cm [4 in.]); for a child or infant, insert it 5 cm (2 in.) or less.

- Avoid embedding the suppository in feces.
- Press the client's buttocks together for a few minutes.
- Ask the client to remain in the left lateral or supine position for at least 5 minutes to help retain the suppository. The suppository should be retained for at least 30 to 40 minutes or according to manufacturer's instructions.

Medication is occasionally given by enema. An example of this would be Kayexalate (sodium polystyrene sulfonate) to treat hyperkalemia (excessive potassium).

Respiratory Inhalation Drugs

Medications administered by inhalation, such as bronchodilators, are frequently prescribed for clients with chronic respiratory disease such as asthma, emphysema, or bronchitis. Medications by inhalation are often administered by a respiratory therapist via *nebulizer* (a machine that aerosolizes liquid as a fine mist delivered by mouthpiece or facial mask). A nebulizer is a type of inhaler that sprays a fine, liquid mist of medication. This is done through a mask or mouthpiece, using oxygen, air under pressure, or an ultrasonic machine. An ultrasonic machine is often used by persons who cannot use a metered-dose inhaler, such as infants and young children, and persons with severe asthma. The nebulizer is connected to a machine via plastic tubing to deliver the medication. A *metered-dose inhaler* (MDI) can be used by clients to self administer measured doses of an aerosol medication. See Chapter 24 ⬗ for more information.

To ensure correct delivery of the prescribed medication, nurses need to instruct clients on correct MDI use. To release medication through the mouthpiece, the client compresses the canister by hand while inhaling, and medication is released (Figure 29-24 ■). An extender or spacer may be

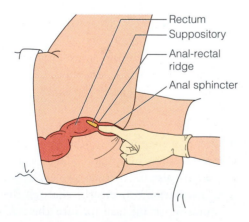

Figure 29-23. ■ Inserting a rectal suppository beyond the internal sphincter and along the rectal wall.

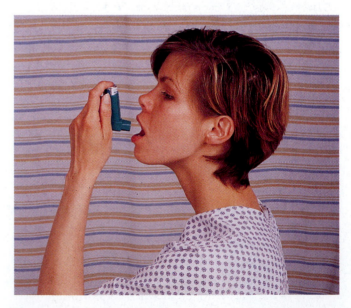

Figure 29-24. ■ The inhaler positioned away from the open mouth. (Photographer: Jenny Thomas.)

attached to the mouthpiece to facilitate medication absorption for better results. *Spacers* are holding chambers into which the medication is fired and from which the client inhales, so that the dose is not lost by exhalation. Box 29-9 ■ provides instructions for clients about using a MDI. Newer, breath-activated MDIs are being produced in which inhalation triggers the release of a premeasured dose of medication.

BOX 29-9	CLIENT TEACHING

Using a Metered-Dose Inhaler

- Make sure the canister is firmly and fully inserted into the inhaler.
- Remove the mouthpiece cap and, holding the inhaler upright, shake the inhaler for 3 to 5 seconds to mix the medication evenly.
- Tilt the head back slightly.
- Hold the canister upside down.
  a. Hold the MDI 1 to 2 cm (0.5 to 1 in.) from the open mouth (see Figure 29-24).
  b. If using a spacer, put the mouthpiece far enough into the mouth so that it extends beyond the teeth. Close the lips tightly around the mouthpiece. An MDI with a spacer or extender is always placed in the mouth.

Administering the Medication

- Inhale and exhale for several breaths, inhaling slowly and deeply through the nose.
- Then inhale slowly and deeply through the mouth while at the same time pressing down once on the medication canister. Continue to inhale for 2 to 3 seconds.
- Hold your breath for 5 to 10 seconds or longer, if possible.
- Remove the inhaler from or away from the mouth.
- Exhale slowly through pursed lips.
- If another puff is prescribed, wait for 1 to 3 minutes before the next inhalation. Remember to reshake the inhaler.
- After the inhalation is completed, rinse mouth with tap water and blow the nose to remove any remaining medication and reduce irritation and risk of infection.
- Clean the MDI mouthpiece after each use. Use mild soap and water, rinse it, and let it air dry before replacing it on the device.
- Disinfect the mouthpiece weekly by soaking it for 20 minutes in 1 pint of water and 2 ounces of vinegar.
- Store the canister at room temperature. Avoid extremes of temperature.
- Follow the physician's orders about frequency of use.
- Report adverse reactions such as restlessness, palpitations, nervousness, or rash to your physician.

Sources: Data from Weixler, D. (1994, July). Correcting metered dose inhaler misuse. *Nursing 94, 24,* 62–64; and Borkgren, M., & Gronkiewicz, C. (1995, January). Update your asthma care from hospital to home. *American Journal of Nursing, 95*(1), 28.

Irrigations

An irrigation (or *lavage*) is the washing out of a body cavity by a stream of water or other fluid, which may contain medication. Guidelines for administering eye and ear irrigations are shown in Box 29-10 ■.

EVALUATING

After administering medication, the nurse observes the client to determine the effectiveness of the medication. The nurse also monitors the client for possible adverse effects and reports these to the team leader and physician. The nurse must promptly document administration of medications to provide client safety and prevent accidental overdose of medications.

NURSING PROCESS CARE PLAN
Client with an Emergency Appendectomy

Kevin Ketron is a 20-year-old client who has just returned to the nursing unit from surgery after undergoing an emergency appendectomy.

Assessment. Client is awake and complaining of incisional pain at a level of 8/10. Dressing is dry and intact. Intravenous infusion of lactated Ringer's solution is running at 125 mL/h. Following surgery he received Kefzol (a cephalosporin antibiotic) 1 g intravenously every 4 hours until he was able to tolerate fluids. He now has been placed on oral Suprax (cefixime) 200 mg twice daily until discharged and for 1 week after returning home. He also has an order for morphine sulfate 10 mg to be given every 3 hours IM as necessary for pain.

Nursing Diagnosis. The following important nursing diagnoses (among others) are established for this client:

- *Risk for Deficient Fluid Volume* related to fluid restriction (although in the assessment it is stated that the client is receiving IV fluid until able to tolerate fluids).
- *Impaired Home Maintenance* related to deficient knowledge regarding self-care following appendectomy
- *Acute Pain* related to surgical incision
- *Risk for Infection* related to surgical incision

Expected Outcomes The expected outcomes for the plan of care are:

- Maintains fluid volume balance.
- Maintains normal blood pressure, pulse, and body temperature.
- Follows mutually agreed-on healthcare home maintenance plan.
- Uses pain rating scale to identify current level of pain intensity and determine a comfort level.
- Remains free from symptoms of infection.

Planning and Implementation

- Monitor intake and output, skin turgor, and vital signs every 4 hours; observe for decreased pulse volume and increase in body temperature.
- Provide fresh water and oral fluids preferred by the client; provide prescribed diet and snacks.
- Ensure that follow-up appointment is scheduled before discharge.
- Provide detailed instruction for self-care, medications, and wound care; evaluate understanding of discharge instructions.
- Tell client to report location, intensity (using pain scale), and quality when experiencing pain.
- Describe adverse effects of unrelieved pain.
- Discuss client's fear of undertreated pain, overdose, and addiction.
- When opioids are administered, assess pain intensity, sedation, and respiratory status.
- Use proper hand hygiene techniques before and after giving care to client.
- Follow Standard Precautions and wear gloves during any contact with blood and body fluids.
- Perform dressing changes using sterile technique.
- Ensure client's appropriate hygienic care with correct hand hygiene; bathing; and hair, nails, and perineal care performed by the nurse or client.

Evaluation. Vital signs on second postoperative day are T 98.8, P 76, R 18, BP 128/78. He is taking a clear liquid diet, tolerated well with no complaints of nausea or vomiting. Discharge planning was initiated. The client will check with his roommate on ability to drive him to his follow-up appointment. Mr. Ketron was able to identify signs and symptoms of infection and describe when a physician should be notified. He understands the need to request pain medication while pain is still manageable. His pain is being maintained at a 2 to 3 level with prn M/S every 4 hours. The incision site is clean and dry with no drainage. Edges are well approximated, staples removed and Steri-Strips applied. Client has taken a shower.

Critical Thinking in the Nursing Process

1. It is always possible that a person receiving antibiotic drugs may experience side effects or an allergic reaction to the drug. How does an allergic reaction differ from a drug side effect?
2. Mr. Ketron is complaining of pain, and you have prepared his IM injection of morphine. How will you select the best site to give the morphine injection?
3. Mr. Ketron has been placed on oral antibiotics now that he is able to tolerate food and oral fluids. What difference, if any, does it make if this drug is given before or after meals?

Note: Discussion of Critical Thinking questions appears in Appendix I.

Note: The references and resources for this and all chapters have been compiled at the back of the book.

BOX 29-10	NURSING CARE CHECKLIST

Administering Eye and Ear Irrigations

☑ Assess the site and surrounding structures for exudate, erythema, swelling, discharge, or other lesions before the irrigation. Determine the client's chief complaints (burning, pain, itching, etc.).

☑ Assemble required equipment: irrigating solution; appropriate irrigating syringe; receptacle to receive irrigation returns (e.g., kidney-shaped basin); moisture-proof drape; and cotton swabs as needed.

☑ Position the client appropriately in a sitting or lying position with the head tilted toward the affected eye or ear.

☑ Place the fluid-receiving receptacle below the affected area and a moisture-resistant pad beneath the receptacle.

☑ Put on disposable gloves.

☑ Clean the eyelids or ear meatus before the irrigation as necessary, using moistened cotton swabs.

Administering the Irrigation

Eye Irrigation

☑ Expose the lower conjunctival sac by separating the lids with the thumb and forefinger to prevent reflex blinking. Or, to irrigate in stages, first hold the lower lid down, then hold the upper lid up. Exert pressure on the bony prominences of the cheekbone and beneath the eyebrow when holding the eyelids to minimize the possibility of pressing the eyeball and causing discomfort.

☑ Fill and hold the eye irrigator about 2.5 cm (1 in.) above the eye to ensure an even, safe pressure of the solution.

☑ Irrigate the eye, directing the solution on the lower conjunctival sac and from the inner canthus to the outer canthus.

Directing the solution in this way prevents possible injury to the cornea and prevents fluid and contaminants from flowing down the nasolacrimal duct.

☑ Irrigate until the solution leaving the eye is clear (no discharge is present) or until all the solution has been used.

☑ Dry around the eye with tissue or gauze.

Ear Irrigation

☑ Straighten the ear canal up and back in the adult and down and back in the child under 3 years of age.

☑ Insert a rubber-tipped syringe into the auditory meatus, and direct the solution gently upward against the top of the canal. The solution is instilled gently because strong pressure from the fluid can cause discomfort and damage the tympanic membrane.

☑ Dry the outside of the ear with absorbent cotton balls. Place a cotton fluff in the auditory meatus to absorb the excess fluid.

☑ Assist the client to a side-lying position on the affected side. Lying with the affected side down helps drain the excess fluid by gravity.

For All Irrigations

☑ Assess the client for any discomfort and the appearance and odor of the fluid returns.

☑ Document all relevant information, including all nursing assessments and interventions relative to the procedure; the type, concentration, amount, and temperature of the solution used; the appearance of the returns; and the presence of any discomfort.

Purpose

- To provide a medication that has systemic effects or local effects on the gastrointestinal tract or both (see specific drug action for each medication administered)

Equipment

- Medication tray or cart
- Disposable medication cups: small paper or plastic cups for tablets and capsules, waxed or plastic calibrated medication cups for liquids
- Medication administration record (MAR) or computer printout
- Pill crusher

or

Syringe of appropriate size for child's mouth and medication amount
- Straws to administer medications that may discolor the teeth or to facilitate the ingestion of liquid medication for certain clients
- Water and water cups
- Applesauce or pudding may be needed to facilitate medication administration when pills must be crushed and for patients with swallowing difficulties

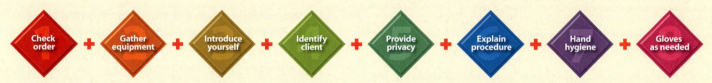

Interventions

1. Verify the client's ability to take medication orally.
   - Determine whether the client can swallow well, is NPO, nauseated or vomiting, has gastric suction, or has diminished or absent bowel sounds. Also, check for medication allergies.

2. Verify the order for accuracy.
   - Check the accuracy of the MAR or of the printout with the physician's written order. *It should contain the following information: client's name, drug name and dosage, time for administration, and route of administration.*
   - Check the expiration date.
   - Report any discrepancies in the order to the nurse in charge or the physician, as agency policy dictates.

3. Obtain appropriate medication.
   - Read the MAR and take the appropriate medication from the shelf, drawer, or refrigerator. The medication may be dispensed from the bottle, box, or unit-dose package.
   - Compare the label of the medication container or unit-dose package against the order on the MAR. If these are not identical, recheck the client's chart. If there is still a discrepancy, check with the nurse in charge or the pharmacist. *These checks are essential in providing the correct medication.*

4. Prepare the medication.
   - Prepare the correct amount of medication for the required dose, using aseptic technique.

- While preparing the medication, recheck the MAR with each prepared drug and container. *This second check reduces the chance of error.*

TABLETS OR CAPSULES

- Pour the required number into the bottle cap, and then transfer the medication to the disposable cup without touching the tablets (Figure 29-25 ■). Usually, all tablets or capsules to be given to the client are placed in the same cup.
- Keep narcotics and medications that require specific assessments, such as pulse measurements, respiratory rate or depth, or blood pressure, separate from the others. *This enables the nurse to withhold the medication if indicated.*
- Break scored tablets as needed to obtain the correct dosage. Use a file or cutting device if necessary

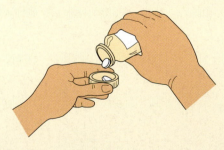

Figure 29-25. ■ Pouring a tablet into the container cap.

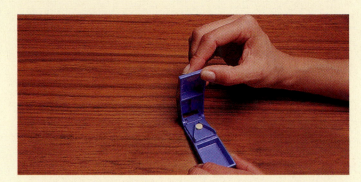

Figure 29-26. ■ A cutting device can be used to divide tablets. (Photographer: Elena Dorfman.)

(Figure 29-26 ■). Discard unused tablet pieces according to agency policy.

■ If the client has difficulty swallowing, crush the tablets to a fine powder with a pill crusher or between two medication cups or spoons. Mix the powder with a small amount of soft food (e.g., custard, applesauce). *Note:* Check with pharmacy before crushing tablets. *Sustained-action, enteric-coated, buccal, or sublingual tablets should not be crushed.*

■ Place packaged unit-dose capsules or tablets (Figure 29-27A ■) directly into the medicine cup. Do not remove the wrapper until at the bedside. *The wrapper keeps the medication clean and facilitates identification.*

LIQUID MEDICATION

■ Thoroughly mix the medication before pouring. Discard any mixed medication changed in appearance. *Changes in appearance may indicate contamination or expiration of the medication.*

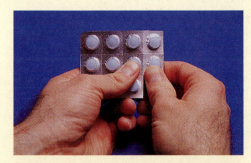

A

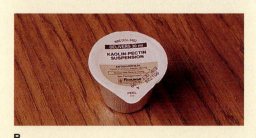

B

Figure 29-27. ■ Unit-dose packages: **A.** tablets; **B.** liquid medications. (Photographer: Elena Dorfman.)

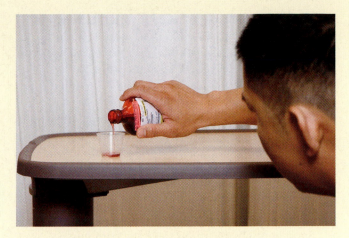

Figure 29-28. ■ Pouring a liquid medication from a bottle.

■ Remove the cap and place it upside down on the countertop. *This helps to avoid contaminating its inside.*

■ Hold the bottle so the label is next to your palm, and pour the medication away from the label (Figure 29-28 ■). *This prevents the label from becoming soiled and illegible as a result of spilled liquids.*

■ Hold the medication cup at eye level and fill it to the desired level, using the bottom of the meniscus (crescent-shaped upper surface of a column of liquid) to align with the container scale (Figure 29-29 ■). (Marking the level with an indelible marker or with one's finger helps to prevent overpouring of medication.) *This method ensures accuracy of measurement. Overage amounts may not be poured back into the bottle.*

■ Before capping the bottle, wipe the lip with a paper towel. *This prevents the cap from sticking.*

■ When giving small amounts of liquids (e.g., less than 5 mL), prepare the medication in a sterile syringe without the needle.

■ Keep unit-dose liquids in their package and open them at the bedside.

ORAL NARCOTICS

■ If an agency uses a manual recording system for controlled substances, check the narcotic record for the pre-

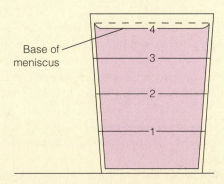

Base of meniscus

Figure 29-29. ■ The bottom of the meniscus is the measuring guide.

vious drug count and compare it with the current supply available. *Some medications, including narcotics, are kept in plastic containers that are sectioned and numbered. This allows the drugs to be controlled securely.*

- Remove the next available tablet and drop it in the medicine cup.
- After removing a tablet, record the necessary information on the appropriate narcotic control record and sign it. *Note: Computer-controlled dispensing systems allow access only to the selected drug and automatically record its use.*
- Any time a narcotic must be wasted, it should be disposed of per agency protocol. A second licensed nurse must observe the wastage and both nurses must sign on the appropriate space on the narcotic record.

ALL MEDICATIONS

- Place the prepared medication and MAR together on the tray or cart.
- Return the bottle, box, or envelope to its storage place and recheck the label on the container. *This third check further reduces the risk of error.*
- Avoid leaving prepared medications unattended. *This precaution prevents potential mishandling errors.*

5. Administer the medication at the correct time.
   - Identify the client by comparing the name and hospital number on the medication record or list with the name and number on the client's identification bracelet and by asking the client's name. *Accurate identification is essential to prevent error. Remember, JCAHO requires the use of two identifiers.*
   - Explain the purpose of the medication and how it will help, using language that the client can understand. Include relevant information about effects; for example, tell the client receiving a diuretic to expect an increase in urine. *Information facilitates acceptance of and compliance with the therapy.*
   - Assist the client to a sitting position or, if not possible, to a side-lying position. *These positions facilitate swallowing and prevent aspiration.*
   - Take the required assessment measures, such as pulse and respiratory rates or blood pressure. Take the apical pulse rate before administering digitalis preparations. Take blood pressure before giving hypotensive drugs. Take the respiratory rate prior to administering narcotics. *Narcotics depress the respiratory center.* If any of the findings are above or below the predetermined parameters, consult the physician before administering the medication.
   - Give the client sufficient water or preferred juice to swallow the medication. Before using juice, check for any food and medication incompatibilities. *(Grapefruit*

juice is contraindicated when administering most antihypertensive drugs.) Fluids ease swallowing and facilitate absorption from the gastrointestinal tract.

- If the client is unable to hold the pill cup, use the pill cup to introduce the medication into the client's mouth, and give only one tablet or capsule at a time. *Putting the cup to the client's mouth maintains the cleanliness of the nurse's hands. Giving one medication at a time eases swallowing.*
- If an older child or adult has difficulty swallowing, ask the client to place the medication on the back of the tongue before taking the water. *Stimulation of the back of the tongue produces the swallowing reflex.*
- If the medication has an objectionable taste, ask the client to suck a few ice chips beforehand, or give the medication with juice, applesauce, or bread if there are no contraindications. *The cold will desensitize the taste buds, and juices or bread can mask the taste of the medication.*
- If the client says that the medication you are about to give is different from what the client has been receiving, do not give the medication without checking the original order. *Most clients are familiar with the appearance of medications taken previously. Unfamiliar medications may signal a possible error.*
- Stay with the client until all medications have been swallowed. *The nurse must see the client swallow the medication before the drug administration can be recorded. This practice additionally allows the nurse to monitor the client for choking. A physician's order or agency policy is required for medications left at the bedside.*

6. Document each medication given.
   - Record the medication given, dosage, time, any complaints or assessments of the client, and your signature.
   - If medication was refused or omitted, record this fact on the appropriate record; document the reason, when possible, and the nurse's actions according to agency policy. *Recording the fact and the reason communicates the greatest amount of information, so that the charge nurse or physician can follow up.*

7. Dispose of all supplies appropriately.
   - Return the medication records to the appropriate file for the next administration time.
   - Replenish stock (e.g., medication cups) and return cart to medicine room.
   - Discard used disposable supplies.

8. Evaluate the effects of the medication.
   - Return to the client when the medication is expected to take effect (usually 30 minutes). *This allows you to evaluate the effects of the medication on the client.*

SAMPLE DOCUMENTATION

[date]	Digoxin 0.5 mg held. AP 54. Will reassess in 1 hour. (VS, i.e., BP 110/76, T 98.6, R 16).
[time]	No c/o chest pain or dyspnea.
	_____ M. Wirthwood, LVN

Or use the DAR method:

[time]	**D:** Apical pulse 54, BP 110/76, T 98.6, R 16. No c/o chest pain or dyspnea. Lungs clear to auscultation. No s/s of digoxin toxicity.
	A: Digoxin 0.5 mg held. Physician notified. Order for digoxin level received. Will re-assess apical pulse in 1 hour.
[time]	**R:** Apical pulse 62.
	_____ M. Wirthwood, LVN

PROCEDURE 29-2   # Preparing Medications

Purpose

- To prepare medication for administration to client using safety and infection control rules

Equipment

- MAR or computer printout
- Ampule of sterile medication, or two vials of medication, or one vial and one ampule, or two ampules, or one vial or ampule and one cartridge
- File (if ampule is not scored) and small gauze square, or ampule opener
- Antiseptic swabs
- Sterile needle and syringe
- Filter needle (optional) (now mandated by JCAHO for use with ampule)
- Additional sterile subcutaneous or intramuscular needle (optional)
- Sterile water or normal saline, if drug is in powdered form

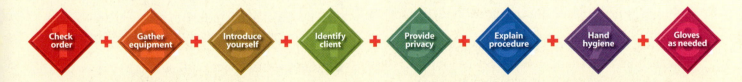

Check order + Gather equipment + Introduce yourself + Identify client + Provide privacy + Explain procedure + Hand hygiene + Gloves as needed

Part A: Preparing Medications from Ampules

Interventions

1. Check the medication order, including drug administration. *This ensures accuracy.*
   - Check the label on the ampule carefully against the MAR or client's chart to make sure that the correct medication is being prepared.
   - Follow the three checks for administering medications. Read the label on the medication (1) before it is taken off the shelf, (2) before withdrawing the medication, and (3) after placing it back on the shelf.

2. Prepare the medication ampule for drug withdrawal.
   - Flick the upper stem of the ampule several times with a fingernail or, holding the upper stem of the ampule, make a large circle with the arm extended. *This will bring all the medication down to the main portion of the ampule.*

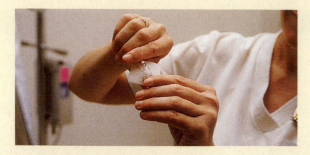

Figure 29-30. ■ Breaking the neck of an ampule. (Photographer: Jenny Thomas.)

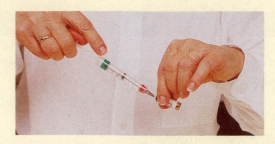

Figure 29-31. ■ Withdrawing a medication from an ampule. (Photographer: Jenny Thomas.)

- Partially file the neck of the ampule, if necessary, to start a clean break.
- Place a piece of sterile gauze between your thumb and the ampule neck or around the ampule neck, and break off the top by bending it toward you (Figure 29-30 ■). *The sterile gauze protects the fingers from the broken glass and any glass fragments will spray away from the nurse.*
  or
  Place the antiseptic wipe packet over the top of the ampule before breaking off the top. *This method ensures that all the glass fragments fall into the packet and reduces the risk of cuts.*
- Dispose of the top of the ampule in the sharps container.
3. Withdraw the medication.
  - Place the ampule on a flat surface.

- Obtain a filter needle to withdraw the medication. Disconnect the existing needle with cap on; attach the filter needle to the syringe. *Filter needles prevent glass particles from being drawn up with the medication.*
- Remove the cap from the filter needle and insert the needle into the center of the ampule. Do not touch the rim of the ampule with the needle to keep it sterile. Withdraw the required dosage.
- If necessary, tilt the ampule slightly to access all the medication (Figure 29-31 ■).
- If a filter needle was used to withdraw the medication, replace it with a regular needle; tighten the cap at the hub before injecting the client.
- If a filter needle was not used, recap the needle using a safety device. *This prevents needle-stick injury while transporting medication to client's room.*

Part B: Preparing Medications from Vials

Interventions

1. Check the medication order, including drug administration, to ensure accuracy.
  - Check the label on the vial carefully against the MAR or client's chart to make sure that the correct medication is being prepared.
  - Follow the three checks for administering medications. Read the label on the medication (1) before it is taken off the shelf, (2) before withdrawing the medication, and (3) after placing it back on the shelf.

2. Prepare the medication vial for drug withdrawal.
  - Mix the solution, if necessary, by rotating the vial between the palms of the hands, not by shaking. *Some vials contain aqueous suspensions, which settle when they stand. In some instances, shaking is contraindicated because it may cause the mixture to foam.*
  - Remove the protective metal or plastic cap, and clean the rubber cap of a previously opened vial with an antiseptic wipe by rubbing in a circular motion and allow it

to air dry. *The antiseptic cleans the cap of dust or grease and reduces the number of microorganisms.*

3. Withdraw the medication.
  - Attach a filter needle as agency practice dictates to draw up premixed liquid medications from multidose vials. *The filter prevents any solid particles from being drawn up through the needle.*
  - Ensure that the needle is firmly attached to the syringe.
  - Remove the cap from the needle; then draw up into the syringe the amount of air equal to the volume of the medication to be withdrawn. *This practice will help to equalize pressure within the closed system of the vial.*
  - Carefully insert the needle into the upright vial through the center of the rubber cap, maintaining the sterility of the needle.
  - Inject the air into the vial, keeping the bevel of the needle above the surface of the medication (Figure 29-32 ■). *The air will allow the medication to be drawn out easily*

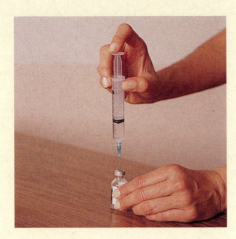

Figure 29-32. ■ Injecting air into a vial. (Photographer: Jenny Thomas.)

because negative pressure will not be created inside the vial. The bevel is kept above the medication to avoid creating bubbles in the medication.

■ Withdraw the prescribed amount of medication using either of the following methods:

a. Hold the vial down (i.e., with the base lower than the top); move the needle tip so that it is below the fluid level; and withdraw the medication (Figure 29-33 ■). Avoid drawing up the last drops of the vial. *Proponents of this method say that keeping the vial in the upright position while withdrawing the medication allows particulate matter to precipitate out of the solution. Leaving the last few drops reduces the chance of withdrawing foreign particles.*

or

b. Invert the vial; ensure the needle tip is below the fluid level; and gradually withdraw the medication (Figure 29-33B). *Keeping the tip of the needle below the fluid level prevents air from being drawn into the syringe.*

■ Hold the syringe and vial at eye level to determine that the correct dosage of drug is drawn into the syringe. Eject air remaining at the top of the syringe into the vial.

■ When the correct volume of medication is obtained, withdraw the needle from the vial, and replace the cap over the needle (using the scoop method), thus maintaining its sterility.

■ If necessary, tap the syringe barrel to dislodge any air bubbles present in the syringe. *The tapping motion will cause the air bubbles to rise to the top of the syringe where they can be ejected out of the syringe.*

■ Replace the filter needle, if used, with a regular needle of the correct gauge and length before injecting the client.

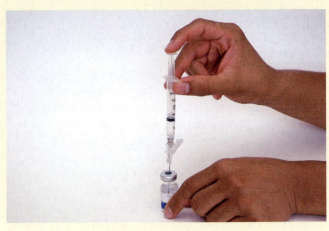

A

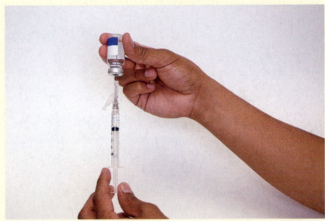

B

Figure 29-33. ■ **A.** Withdrawing a medication from a vial that is held with the base down. **B.** Withdrawing a medication from an inverted vial. (Photographer: Elena Dorfman.)

VARIATION: PREPARING AND USING VIALS FOR RECONSTITUTION

■ Read the manufacturer's directions to determine the amount and type of solution to be used for reconstitution. *Some solutions are unstable in solution and must be distributed in powder or crystalline form to be reconstituted at the time dosage is due.*

■ Add the amount of sterile water or saline indicated in the directions. An equivalent amount of air as the amount of solvent must be removed from the vial in order to equalize air pressure within the vial.

■ If a multidose vial is reconstituted, label the vial with the date and time it was prepared, the amount of drug contained in each milliliter of solution, and your initials. *Time is an important factor to consider in the expiration of these medications.*

■ Once the medication has been reconstituted, store it in a refrigerator or as recommended by the manufacturer.

Part C: Mixing Medications Using One Syringe

Interventions

1. Check the medication order for accuracy.
   - Check the label on the ampule or vial carefully against the MAR or client's chart. *This makes sure that the correct medication is being prepared.*
   - Follow the three checks for administering medications. Read the label on the medication (1) before it is taken off the shelf, (2) before withdrawing the medication, and (3) after placing it back on the shelf.
   - Before preparing and combining the medications, ensure that the total volume of the injection is appropriate for the injection site.

2. Prepare the medication ampule or vial for drug withdrawal.
   - See Part A of this procedure for an ampule and Part B for a vial.
   - Inspect the appearance of the medication for clarity. *Some medications are always cloudy. Preparations that have changed in appearance should be discarded.*
   - If using insulin, thoroughly mix the solution in each vial prior to administration. Rotate the vials between the palms of the hands and invert the vials. Do not shake the vials. *Mixing ensures an adequate concentration and thus an accurate dose. Shaking insulin vials can make the medication frothy, making precise measurement difficult.*
   - Clean the tops of the vials with antiseptic swabs.

3. Withdraw the medications.

MIXING MEDICATIONS FROM TWO VIALS

- Withdraw a volume of air equal to the total volume of medications to be withdrawn from vials A and B.
- Inject a volume of air equal to the volume of medication to be withdrawn into vial A.
- Withdraw the needle from vial A and inject the remaining air into vial B.
  or
  Draw up the volume of air equal to the amount of solution to be drawn from vial A and inject into vial A. Next, draw up the volume of air equal to the amount of solution to be drawn from vial B and inject into vial B. Leaving the needle in the vial, invert vial B and withdraw the prescribed amount of medication.
- Withdraw the required amount of medication from vial B. The same needle is used to inject air into and withdraw medication from the second vial. *It must not be contaminated with the medication in vial A.*
- Using a newly attached sterile needle, withdraw the required amount of medication from vial A. If using a syringe with a fused needle, withdraw the medication from vial A. The syringe now contains a mixture of medications from vials A and B. *With this method, neither vial is contaminated by microorganisms or by medication from the other vial.*
- See also the variation on mixing insulins later in this procedure.

MIXING MEDICATIONS FROM ONE VIAL AND ONE AMPULE

- First prepare and withdraw the medication from the vial. Ampules do not require the addition of air prior to withdrawal of the drug.
- Then withdraw the required amount of medication from the ampule.

MIXING MEDICATIONS FROM ONE CARTRIDGE AND ONE VIAL OR AMPULE

- First ensure that the correct dose of the medication is in the cartridge. Discard any excess medication and air.
- Draw up the required medication from a vial or ampule into the cartridge. Note that when withdrawing medication from a vial, an equal amount of air must first be injected into the vial.
- If the total volume to be injected exceeds the capacity of the cartridge, use a syringe with sufficient capacity to withdraw the desired amount of medication from the vial or ampule, and transfer the required amount from the cartridge to the syringe. When withdrawing medication from a cartridge, one must first withdraw medication from the vial or ampule. The needle from the cartridge must be removed, and the rubber stopper is pierced with the needle of the syringe in order to extract the contents. It is not necessary to first instill air into a cartridge.

VARIATION: MIXING INSULINS

The following is an example of mixing 10 units of regular insulin and 30 units of NPH insulin. *Regular, or clear insulin, must be drawn first and NPH, or cloudy insulin, is drawn second.*

- Inject 30 units of air into the NPH vial and withdraw the needle. (There should be no insulin in the needle.) The needle should not touch the insulin (Figure 29-34 ■, step 1).
- Inject 10 units of air into the regular insulin vial and immediately withdraw 10 units of regular insulin (Figure 29-34, steps 2 and 3).
- Reinsert the needle into the NPH insulin vial and withdraw 30 units of NPH insulin (Figure 29-34, step 4). (The air was previously injected into the vial.)
  By using this method, you avoid adding NPH insulin to the regular insulin.

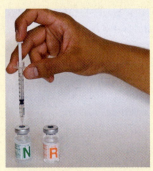

Step 1

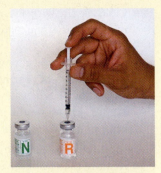

Step 2

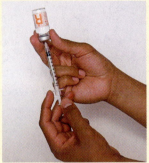

Step 3

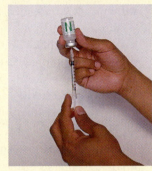

Step 4

Figure 29-34. ■ Mixing two types of insulin together.

PROCEDURE 29-3   **Administering Injections**

Purposes

- To provide a medication the client requires (see specific drug action)
- For subcutaneous: To allow slower absorption of a medication compared with either the intramuscular or intravenous route

Equipment

- Client's MAR or computer printout
- Sterile medication (usually provided in an ampule or vial)
- Syringe and needle of a size appropriate for the amount of solution to be administered
- Antiseptic swabs
- Dry sterile gauze for opening an ampule (optional)
- Disposable gloves

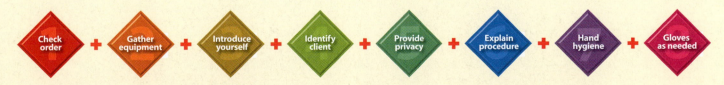

Check order + Gather equipment + Introduce yourself + Identify client + Provide privacy + Explain procedure + Hand hygiene + Gloves as needed

---

Part A: Intramuscular Injection

Interventions

1. Check the medication order for accuracy.
   - See Procedure 29-1, step 2.

2. Prepare the medication from the vial or ampule.
   - See Procedure 29-2 (ampule or vial).

- Whenever feasible, change the needle on the syringe before the injection. *Because the outside of a new needle is free of medication, it does not irritate subcutaneous tissues as it passes into the muscle.*

- Invert the syringe needle uppermost and expel all excess air. (Some institutions subscribe to the practice of drawing up 0.2 to 0.3 mL of air to expel contents of syringe to prevent tracking through tissue layers and/or to seal medication into the site of injection.)

3. Identify the client, and assist the client to a comfortable position.
   - Check the client's identification band, and ask the client to tell you his or her name and date of birth (as a second identifier). *This verifies identity.*
   - Assist the client to a supine, lateral, prone, or sitting position, depending on the chosen site. If the target muscle is the gluteus medius (ventrogluteal site), have the client in the supine position flex the knee(s); in the lateral position, flex the upper leg; and in the prone position, "toe in." *Appropriate positioning promotes relaxation of the target muscle.*
   - Obtain assistance to immobilize an infant or young child. The parent may hold the infant or young child. *This prevents accidental injury during the procedure.*

4. Select, locate, and clean the site.
   - Perform hand hygiene.
   - Select a site free of skin lesions, tenderness, swelling, hardness, or localized inflammation and one that has not been used frequently.
   - If injections are to be frequent, alternate sites. If necessary, discuss with the prescribing physician an alternative method of providing the medication.
   - Determine whether the size of the muscle is appropriate to the amount of medication to be injected. *An average adult's deltoid muscle can usually absorb 0.5 mL of medication, although some authorities believe 1 mL can be absorbed by a well-developed deltoid muscle. The gluteus medius muscle can often absorb 1 to 4 mL, although 4 mL may be very painful.*
   - Locate the exact site for the injection. (See the discussion of sites earlier in this chapter.)
   - Don gloves.

- Clean the site with an antiseptic swab. Using a circular motion, start at the center and move outward about 5 cm (2 in.).
- Transfer and hold the swab between the third and fourth fingers of your nondominant hand in readiness for needle withdrawal, or position the swab on the client's skin above the intended site. Allow skin to dry prior to injecting medication.

5. Prepare the syringe for injection.
   - Remove the needle cover without contaminating the needle.
   - Confirm that the medication and the dose are both correct.
   - If using a prefilled unit-dose medication, be careful to avoid dripping medication on the needle prior to injection. If this does occur, wipe the medication off the needle with a sterile gauze. *Medication left on the needle can cause pain when it is tracked through the subcutaneous tissue.*

6. Inject the medication using a Z-track technique.
   - Use the nondominant hand to pull the skin laterally and downward approximately 2.5 cm (1 in.) at the site (Figure 29-35 ■). Under some circumstances, such as for an emaciated client or an infant, the muscle may be pinched. *Pulling the skin and subcutaneous tissue or pinching the muscle makes it firmer and facilitates needle insertion.*
   - Holding the syringe between the thumb and forefinger (as if holding a pencil), pierce the skin quickly at a 90-degree angle (Figure 29-36 ■), and insert the needle into the muscle. *Using a quick motion lessens the client's discomfort.*
   - Aspirate by holding the barrel of the syringe steady with your nondominant hand and by pulling back on the plunger with your dominant hand. If blood appears in the syringe, withdraw the needle, discard the

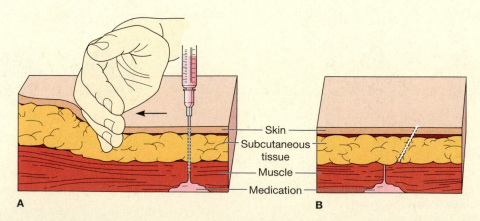

A   Skin
Subcutaneous tissue
Muscle
Medication   B

Figure 29-35. ■ Inserting an intramuscular needle at a 90-degree angle using the Z-track method: **A.** Skin pulled to the side; **B.** skin released. *Note:* When the skin returns to its normal position after the needle is withdrawn, a seal is formed over the intramuscular site. This prevents seepage of the medication into the subcutaneous tissues and subsequent discomfort.

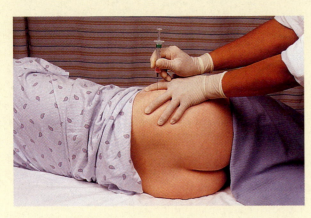

Figure 29-36. ■ Administering an intramuscular injection into the ventrogluteal site. (Photographer: Jenny Thomas.)

syringe, document the occurrence, and prepare a new injection. *This step determines whether the needle has been inserted into a blood vessel.*

■ If blood does not appear, inject the medication steadily and slowly, holding the syringe steady. *Injecting medication slowly permits it to disperse into the muscle tissue, thus decreasing the client's discomfort. Holding the syringe steady minimizes discomfort.*

7. Withdraw the needle and then release hand that has been holding skin laterally.
   ■ Withdraw the needle slowly and steadily. *This minimizes tissue injury.*
   ■ Apply gentle pressure at the site with a dry sponge. If contraindicated, do not massage the site. *Massaging the site can result in tissue irritation.*
   ■ If bleeding occurs, apply pressure with a dry sterile gauze until it stops.

8. Dispose of supplies appropriately.
   ■ Discard the uncapped needle and attached syringe into designated receptacles. *Proper disposal protects the nurse and others from injury and contamination. The CDC recommends not capping the needle before disposal to reduce the risk of needle-stick injuries.*
   ■ Remove gloves. Perform hand hygiene.

9. Document all relevant information.
   ■ Include the time of administration, drug name, dose, route, and the client's reactions.

10. Assess effectiveness of the medication at the time it is expected to act.

Part B: Subcutaneous Injection

Interventions

1. Check the medication order for accuracy.
   ■ See Procedure 29-1, step 2.

2. Prepare the medication from the vial or ampule.
   ■ See Procedure 29-2 (ampule or vial).

3. Identify the client, and assist the client to a comfortable position.
   ■ Check the client's identification band, and ask the client to tell you his or her name and date of birth (as a second identifier). *This verifies identity.*
   ■ Assist the client to a position in which the arm, leg, or abdomen can be relaxed, depending on the site to be used. *A relaxed position of the site minimizes discomfort.*
   ■ Obtain assistance in holding an uncooperative client or small child. *This prevents injury due to sudden movement after needle insertion.*

4. Select and clean the site.
   ■ Select a site free of tenderness, hardness, swelling, scarring, itching, burning, or localized inflammation. Select a site that has not been used frequently. *These conditions could hinder the absorption of the medication and also increase the likelihood of injury and discomfort at the injection site.*
   ■ Don gloves.
   ■ Cleanse the skin with antiseptic per agency protocol. Swab the center of the site in a widening circle to

about 5 cm (2 in.). Let the skin dry completely. *The mechanical action of swabbing removes skin secretions, which contain microorganisms.*
   ■ Hold the swab between the third and fourth fingers of the nondominant hand, or position the swab on the client's skin above the intended site. *This keeps the swab accessible when the needle is withdrawn.*

5. Prepare the syringe for injection.
   ■ Remove the needle cap while waiting for the antiseptic to dry. Pull the cap straight off to avoid contaminating the needle by the outside edge of the cap. *The needle will become contaminated if it touches anything but the inside of the cap, which is sterile.*
   ■ Confirm that the medication and the dosage are both correct. *This prevents medication error.*

6. Inject the medication.
   ■ Grasp the syringe in your dominant hand by holding it between your thumb and fingers. With palm facing to the side or upward for a 45-degree-angle insertion, or with the palm downward for a 90-degree-angle insertion, prepare to inject (Figure 29-37 ■; see also Figure 29-11).
   ■ Using the nondominant hand, pinch or spread the skin at the site, and insert the needle using the dominant hand and a firm steady push. *The nondominant hand can be used to immobilize the extremity of an infant or a young*

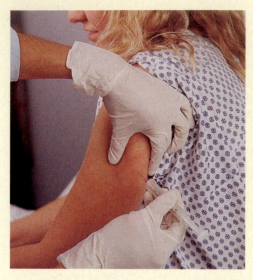

Figure 29-37. ■ Administering a subcutaneous injection into pinched tissue. (Photographer: Elena Dorfman.)

child as the needle is inserted. Recommendations vary about whether to pinch or spread the skin and at what angle to administer subcutaneous injections. The most important consideration is the depth of the subcutaneous tissue in the area to be injected. *If the client has more than 1/2 inch of adipose tissue in the injection site, it would be safe to administer the injection at a 90-degree angle with the skin spread. If the client is thin or lean and lacks adipose tissue, the subcutaneous injection should be given with the skin pinched and at a 45- to 60-degree angle.*

- When the needle is inserted, move your nondominant hand to the end of the plunger. Some nurses find it easier to move the nondominant hand to the barrel of the syringe and the dominant hand to the end of the plunger. If the nondominant hand is holding the extremity of an infant or small child, use the dominant hand to aspirate and inject the medication.

- Aspirate by pulling back on the plunger. If blood appears, withdraw the needle, discard the syringe, document the occurrence, and prepare a new injection. If no blood appears, inject the medication. *Subcutaneous medications can be very dangerous if injected directly into the bloodstream since these drugs require slow absorption.* See variation for administering a heparin injection.

- Inject the medication by holding the syringe steady and depressing the plunger with a slow, even pressure.

Holding the syringe steady and injecting the medication at an even pressure minimizes discomfort for the client.

7. Remove the needle.
   - Remove slowly and smoothly, pulling along the line of insertion while depressing the skin with your nondominant hand. *Depressing the skin places countertraction on it and minimizes the client's discomfort when the needle is withdrawn.*
   - If bleeding occurs, apply pressure to the site with dry sterile gauze until it stops. *Bleeding rarely occurs after subcutaneous injection.*

8. Dispose of supplies appropriately.
   - Discard the uncapped needle and attached syringe into designated receptacles. *Proper disposal protects the nurse and others from injury and contamination. The CDC recommends not capping the needle before disposal to reduce the risk of needle-stick injuries.*
   - Remove gloves. Perform hand hygiene.

9. Document all relevant information.
   - Document the medication given, dosage, time, route, any assessments, and add your signature.
   - Many agencies prefer that medication administration be recorded on the medication record. *The nurse's notes are used when prn medications are given or when there is a special problem.*

10. Assess the effectiveness of the medication at the time it is expected to act.

VARIATION: ADMINISTERING A HEPARIN INJECTION

The subcutaneous administration of heparin requires special precautions because of the drug's anticoagulant properties.

- Select a site on the abdomen away from the umbilicus and above the level of the iliac crests. *Some agencies support the practice of subcutaneous injection of heparin in the thighs or arms as alternate sites to the abdomen.*
- Use a 5/8-in., 25- or 26-gauge needle, and insert it at a 90-degree angle. If a client is very lean or wasted, insert it at a 45-degree angle.
- Do not aspirate when giving heparin by subcutaneous injection. *Aspiration can possibly damage the surrounding tissue and cause bleeding as well as bruising.*
- Do not massage the site after the injection. *Massaging could cause bleeding and ecchymosis and hasten drug absorption.*
- Alternate the sites of subsequent injections.

Part C: Intradermal Injection

Interventions

1. Check the medication order for accuracy.
   - See Procedure 29-1, step 2.

2. Prepare the medication from the vial or ampule.
   - See Procedure 29-2 (ampule or vial).

3. Identify the client, and assist the client to a comfortable position.
   - Check the client's identification band, and ask the client to tell you his or her name and date of birth (as a second identifier). *This verifies identity.*

■ Assist the client to a position in which the arm (or sometimes back) can be relaxed and easily available. *A relaxed position of the site minimizes discomfort.*

4. Select and clean the site.
   ■ Select a site on the forearm or upper back free of tenderness, hardness, swelling, scarring, itching, burning, or localized inflammation. *These conditions could hinder the absorption of the medication and increase the likelihood of injury and discomfort at the injection site. Since most intradermal injections are used to test for allergic reactions, any blemish may conceal a response.*
   ■ Don gloves.
   ■ Cleanse the skin with antiseptic per agency protocol. Swab the center of the site in a widening circle to about 5 cm (2 in.). Let the skin dry completely. *If you inject the skin before it dries, you might introduce antiseptic into the skin causing discomfort or an interference with test results.*

5. Prepare the syringe for injection. *Use a TB syringe or a 0.5- to 1-mL syringe, 26- or 27-gauge, 3/8-in. needle and do not draw up more than 0.1 mL of solution for injection for the intradermal route.*
   ■ Confirm that the medication and the dosage are both correct. *This prevents medication error.*
   ■ Remove the needle cap while waiting for the antiseptic to dry. Pull the cap straight off to avoid contaminating the needle by the outside edge of the cap. *The needle will become contaminated if it touches anything but the inside of the cap, which is sterile.*
   ■ Hold the client's arm in your nondominant hand and stretch the skin taut. *Stretching the skin tightly allows for ease of needle insertion.*

6. Inject the medication.
   ■ Hold the needle with the bevel side up at a 10- to 15-degree angle from the skin (almost parallel to the skin surface).
   ■ Slowly insert the needle into the first layer of skin so that the bevel is completely covered by the skin. The point of the needle should be slightly visible through the skin.
   ■ Inject the medication very slowly until a bleb or wheal (small white bubble) is formed just under the skin surface. *If no bubble forms, withdraw the needle slightly as it may be too deep. If solution leaks out as you inject, the needle is not deep enough. Do not aspirate when administering an intradermal injection because there are only small capillaries and no large vessels in the dermal layer of skin.*

7. Remove the needle.
   ■ Withdraw needle at same angle as insertion and lightly pat area with a sterile gauze pad. *Do not massage because this action may interfere with test results.*

8. Dispose of supplies appropriately.
   ■ Discard the uncapped needle and attached syringe into designated receptacles. *Proper disposal protects the nurse and others from injury and contamination. The CDC recommends not capping the needle before disposal to reduce the risk of needle-stick injuries.*
   ■ Remove gloves. Perform hand hygiene.

9. Document all relevant information.
   ■ Document the medication given, dosage, time, route, any assessments, injection site, and your signature.
   ■ Many agencies prefer that medication administration be recorded on the medication record. *The nurse's notes are used when prn medications are given or when there is a special problem.*
   ■ Clients undergoing allergy testing must be observed for a minimum of 30 minutes after the test for possible anaphylactic reaction. Emergency equipment and medication must be available before administering allergy testing.
   ■ Clients should be provided written instructions regarding when to return for reading. Clients should be instructed to avoid scrubbing, scratching, or rubbing the area of the injection and to report to an emergency facility if dyspnea, hives, or rash develops.

10. Assess the effectiveness of the medication at the time it is expected to act.
   ■ Since many intradermal injections are given for purposes of allergy sensitivity or tuberculosis testing, follow-up documentation may be required. *Tuberculosis testing, sometimes called a Mantoux or PPD skin test must be read 48 to 72 hours after the test has been administered. Each agency has a policy on how the patient reaction is to be evaluated and recorded.*

SAMPLE DOCUMENTATION

[date]	Pen VK 500,000 units IM rt.
[time]	thigh.
	Client tolerated well.
	_____ P. Bullock, LPN

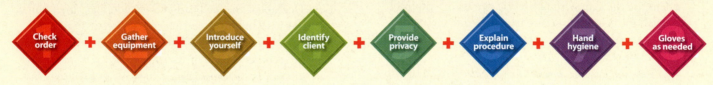

Administering Ophthalmic Instillations

Purpose

- To provide an eye medication the client requires (e.g., an antibiotic) to treat an infection or for other reasons (see specific drug action)

Equipment

- Disposable gloves
- Sterile absorbent sponges soaked in sterile normal saline
- Medication
- Dry sterile absorbent sponges
- Sterile eye dressing (pad) as needed and paper tape to secure it

Check order + Gather equipment + Introduce yourself + Identify client + Provide privacy + Explain procedure + Hand hygiene + Gloves as needed

Interventions

1. Check the medication order and the medication.
   - Carefully check the physician's order for the preparation, strength, and number of drops. Also, confirm the prescribed frequency of the instillation and which eye is to be treated. Abbreviations are frequently used to identify the eye: OD (right eye), OS (left eye), and OU (both eyes).

2. Prepare the client.
   - Check the client's identification band, and ask the client to tell you his or her name and date of birth (as a second identifier). *This verifies identity.*
   - Explain the technique to the client or to the parents of an infant or child. *The administration of an ophthalmic medication is not usually painful. Ointments are often soothing to the eye, but some liquid preparations may sting initially.*
   - Assist the client to a comfortable position, either sitting or lying.

3. Clean the eyelid and the eyelashes.
   - Don sterile gloves.
   - Use sterile cotton balls moistened with sterile irrigating solution or sterile normal saline, and wipe from the inner canthus to the outer canthus. *If not removed, material on the eyelid and lashes can be washed into the eye. Cleaning toward the outer canthus prevents contamination of the other eye and the lacrimal duct.*

4. Administer the eye medication.
   - Check the ophthalmic preparation for the name, strength, and number of drops if a liquid is used. Draw the correct number of drops into the shaft of the dropper if a dropper is used. If ointment is used, discard the first bead. *Checking medication data is essential to prevent a medication error. The first bead of ointment from a tube is considered to be contaminated.*
   - Instruct the client to look up to the ceiling. Give the client a dry sterile absorbent sponge. *The client is less likely*

to blink if looking up. While the client looks up, the cornea is partially protected by the top eyelid. A sponge is needed to press on the nasolacrimal duct after a liquid instillation or to wipe excess ointment from the eyelashes after an ointment is instilled.

   - Expose the lower conjunctival sac by placing the thumb or fingers of your nondominant hand on the client's cheekbone just below the eye and gently drawing down the skin on the cheek. If the tissues are edematous, handle the tissues carefully to avoid damaging them. *Placing the fingers on the cheekbone minimizes the possibility of touching the cornea, avoids putting any pressure on the eyeball, and prevents the person from blinking or squinting.*
   - Approach the eye from the side and instill the correct number of drops onto the outer third of the lower conjunctival sac. Hold the dropper 1 to 2 cm (0.4 to 0.8 in.) above the sac (Figure 29-38 ■). *The client is less likely to blink if a*

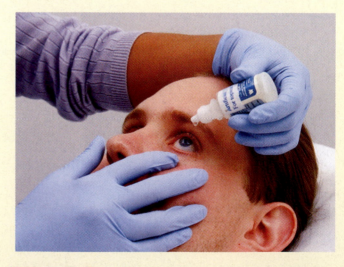

Figure 29-38. ■ Instilling an eyedrop into the lower conjunctival sac. (Photographer: Elena Dorfman.)

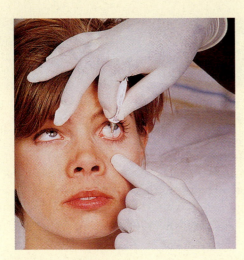

Figure 29-39. ■ Instilling eye ointment into the lower conjunctival sac. (Photographer: Jenny Thomas.)

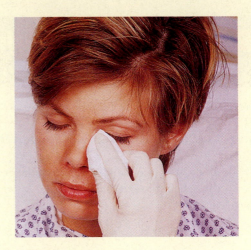

Figure 29-40. ■ Pressing on the nasolacrimal duct. (Photographer: Jenny Thomas.)

side approach is used. When instilled into the conjunctival sac, drops will not harm the cornea as they might if dropped directly on it. The dropper must not touch the sac or the cornea.

or

Holding the tube above the lower conjunctival sac, squeeze 2 cm (0.8 in.) (or amount prescribed) of ointment from the tube into the lower conjunctival sac from the inner canthus outward (Figure 29-39 ■).

■ Instruct the client to close the eyelids but not to squeeze them shut. Closing the eye spreads the medication over the eyeball. *Squeezing can injure the eye and push out the medication.*

■ For liquid medications, press firmly or have the client press firmly on the nasolacrimal duct for at least 30 seconds (Figure 29-40 ■). Check agency practice. *Pressing on the nasolacrimal duct prevents the medication from running out of the eye and down the duct.*

5. Clean the eyelids as needed. Wipe the eyelids gently from the inner to the outer canthus to collect excess medication.

6. Apply an eye pad if needed, and secure it with paper tape.

7. Assess the client's response.
   ■ Assess responses immediately after the instillation and again after the medication should have acted.

8. Document all relevant information.
   ■ Record nursing assessments and interventions. Include the name of the drug, the strength, the number of drops if a liquid, the time, and the response of the client.

SAMPLE DOCUMENTATION

[date]
[time]   Presented at ER following work-related injury. Experienced severed pain in rt. eye while using grinding wheel. Fluorescein NA 2 gtts instilled OD. Seen by Dr. Wilson 0.5-mm metal sliver removed. Eye irrigated with 25 mL NSS. Eye patch applied.

_____ R. Nelson, LPN

PROCEDURE 29-5 # Administering Otic Instillations

Purposes

- To soften earwax so that it can be readily removed at a later time
- To provide local therapy to reduce inflammation, destroy infective organisms in the external ear canal, or both
- To relieve pain

Equipment

- Disposable gloves (optional)
- Cotton-tipped applicator
- Correct medication bottle with a dropper
- Flexible rubber tip (optional) for the end of the dropper, which prevents injury from sudden motion, for example, by a child or disoriented client
- Cotton fluff

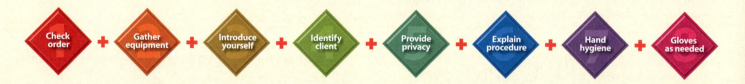

Check order + Gather equipment + Introduce yourself + Identify client + Provide privacy + Explain procedure + Hand hygiene + Gloves as needed

Interventions

1. Check the medication order.
   - Carefully check the physician's order for the kind of medication; the time, amount, and dosage; and which ear is to be treated.

2. Prepare the client.
   - Check the client's identification band, and ask the client to tell you his or her name and date of birth (as a second identifier). *This verifies identity.*
   - Explain the procedure to the client or to the parents of an infant or child. Client will need to remain in a side-lying position during and following procedure so that the medication will remain in ear canal.
   - Obtain assistance to immobilize an infant or young child. *This prevents accidental injury due to sudden movement during the procedure.*
   - Assist the client to a side-lying position with the ear being treated uppermost.

3. Clean the pinna of the ear and the meatus of the ear canal.
   - Don gloves if infection is suspected.
   - Use cotton-tipped applicators and solution to wipe the pinna and auditory meatus. Remove any discharge before the instillation so that it won't be washed into the ear canal.

4. Administer the ear medication.
   - Warm the medication container in your hand, or place it in warm water for a short time. *This promotes client comfort.*
   - Partially fill the ear dropper with medication.
   - Straighten the auditory canal. For an infant, gently pull the pinna down and back (Figure 29-41 ■). For an adult

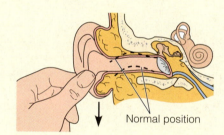

Normal position

Figure 29-41. ■ Straightening the ear canal of a child by pulling the pinna down and back.

or a child older than 3 years of age, pull the pinna upward and backward. *The auditory canal is straightened so that the solution can flow the entire length of the canal.*

- Instill the correct number of drops along the side of the ear canal (Figure 29-42 ■).

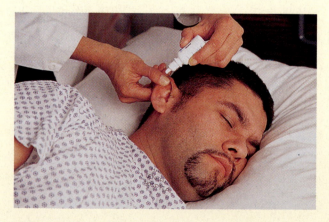

Figure 29-42. ■ Instilling eardrops.

- Press gently but firmly a few times on the tragus of the ear. Pressing on the tragus assists the flow of medication into the ear canal.
- Ask the client to remain in the side-lying position for about 5 minutes. *This prevents the drops from escaping and allows the medication to reach all sides of the canal cavity.*
- Insert a small piece of cotton fluff loosely at the meatus of the auditory canal for 15 to 20 minutes. Do not press it into the canal. *The cotton helps retain the medication when the client is up. If pressed tightly into the canal, the cotton would interfere with the action of the drug and the outward movement of normal secretions.*

5. Assess the client's response.
   - Assess the character and amount of discharge, appearance of the canal, discomfort, and so on, immediately after the instillation and again when the medication is expected to act. Inspect the cotton ball for any drainage.

6. Document all relevant information.
   - Document all nursing assessments and interventions relative to the procedure.

- Include the time, the dose, and any complaints of pain. *Many agencies use flow sheets; others may require that a notation be made on the nurse's notes.*

SAMPLE DOCUMENTATION

[date]	Impacted cerumen ×2 weeks.
[time]	Debrox gtts ii each ear daily ×5 days. Prepared for ear irrigation. 100 mL warm H_2O via Asepto syringe. Otoscopic exam revealed clear ear canal. Tolerated procedure well.

_____ O. Pearson, LVN

PROCEDURE 29-6 Administering Vaginal Instillations

Purposes

- To treat or prevent infection
- To reduce inflammation
- To relieve vaginal discomfort

Equipment

- Drape
- Correct vaginal suppository or cream
- Applicator for vaginal cream
- Disposable gloves
- Lubricant for a suppository
- Disposable towel
- Clean perineal pad

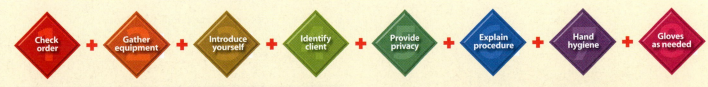

Check order + Gather equipment + Introduce yourself + Identify client + Provide privacy + Explain procedure + Hand hygiene + Gloves as needed

Interventions

1. Check the medication order.
   - Carefully check the physician's order for the specific medication ordered, its dosage, and the time of administration.

2. Prepare the client.
   - Check the client's identification band, and ask the client to tell you his or her name and date of birth (as a second identifier). *This verifies identity.*
   - Explain to the client that a vaginal instillation is normally a painless procedure, and in fact may bring relief from itching and burning if an infection is present. *Many clients feel embarrassed about this procedure, and some may prefer to perform the procedure themselves if instruction is provided.*
   - Provide privacy, and ask the client to void. *If the bladder is empty, the client will have less discomfort during the treatment, and the possibility of injuring the vaginal lining is decreased.*

3. Position and drape the client appropriately.
   - Assist the client to a back-lying position with the knees flexed and the hips rotated laterally.

■ Drape the client appropriately so that only the perineal area is exposed.

4. Prepare the equipment.
   ■ Unwrap the suppository, and put it on the opened wrapper.
   or
   Fill the applicator with the prescribed cream, jelly, or foam. Directions are provided with the manufacturer's applicator.

5. Assess and clean the perineal area.
   ■ Don gloves. *Gloves prevent contamination of the nurse's hands from vaginal and perineal microorganisms.*
   ■ Inspect the vaginal orifice; note any redness, edema, odor, or discharge from the vagina; and ask about any vaginal discomfort.
   ■ Provide perineal care to remove microorganisms. *This decreases the chance of moving microorganisms into the vagina.*

6. Administer the vaginal suppository, cream, foam, or jelly.

VAGINAL SUPPOSITORY
   ■ Lubricate the rounded (smooth) end of the suppository, which is inserted first. *Lubrication facilitates insertion.*
   ■ Lubricate your gloved index finger.
   ■ Expose the vaginal orifice by separating the labia with your nondominant hand.
   ■ Insert the suppository about 8 to 10 cm (3 to 4 in.) along the posterior wall of the vagina, or as far as it will go (Figure 29-43 ■). The posterior wall of the vagina is about 2.5 cm (1 in.) longer than the anterior wall because the cervix protrudes into the uppermost portion of the anterior wall. The anterior wall is usually about 6 to 7.5 cm (2.5 to 3 in.).
   ■ Withdraw the finger, and remove the gloves, turning them inside out. Discard appropriately. *Turning the gloves inside out prevents the spread of microorganisms.*
   ■ Ask the client to remain lying in the supine position for 5 to 10 minutes following insertion. The hips may also

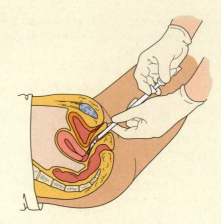

Figure 29-44. ■ Using an applicator to instill a vaginal cream.

be elevated on a pillow. *This position allows the medication to flow into the posterior fornix after it has melted.*

VAGINAL CREAM, JELLY, OR FOAM
   ■ Gently insert the applicator about 5 cm (2 in.).
   ■ Slowly push the plunger until the applicator is empty (Figure 29-44 ■).
   ■ Remove the applicator and place it on the towel. *The applicator is put on the towel to prevent the spread of microorganisms.*
   ■ Discard the applicator if disposable or clean it according to the manufacturer's directions.
   ■ Remove the gloves, turning them inside out. Discard appropriately.
   ■ Ask the client to remain lying in the supine position for 5 to 10 minutes following the insertion.

7. Ensure client comfort.
   ■ Dry the perineum with tissues as required.
   ■ Apply a clean perineal pad and a T-binder if there is excessive drainage.

8. Document all relevant information.
   ■ Record the instillation and assessments as for other medications and instillations.

9. Assess and document the client's response.

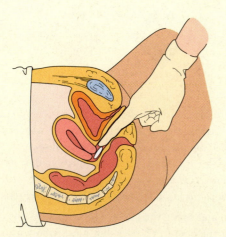

Figure 29-43. ■ Instilling a vaginal suppository.

SAMPLE DOCUMENTATION

[date]	C/o of vaginal itching, white
[time]	cheese-like discharge and burning on urination. Completed 10-day course of ABT. Terconazole via applicator intravaginally.
	_____ T. Mallesen, LPN

Chapter Review

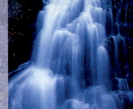

 KEY TERMS by Topic

Use the audio glossary feature of either the CD-ROM or the Companion Website to hear the correct pronunciation of the following key terms.

Introduction
medication, prescription, generic

Effects of Drugs
therapeutic effect, side effects, adverse effects, drug toxicity, cumulative effect, drug allergy, drug tolerance, idiosyncratic effect, drug interaction, iatrogenic disease, half-life, absorption

Medication Orders
stat order, single order, standing (routine) order, prn order

Systems of Measurement
metric system, apothecaries' system, household system, nomogram

Equipment
syringes, hub, cannula, bevel

Routes of Administration
NPO, sublingual, buccal, parenteral, intradermal, subcutaneous, intramuscular, intravenous, ampule, vial, ophthalmics, otics

KEY Points

- Nursing practice acts define limits on the nurse's responsibilities regarding medications.

- Medications have several names. Nurses need to know the generic and trade names of a medication and be aware of both its therapeutic and side effects.

- Adverse effects of medications include drug toxicity, drug allergy, drug tolerance, idiosyncratic effect, and drug interactions.

- Various routes are used to administer medications: oral, sublingual, buccal, rectal, vaginal, parenteral (IV, IM, SubQ, ID), topical, transdermal, inhalation, or via a nasogastric or gastrostomy tube.

- Medication orders must include the client name, date and time the order is written, name of the medication, dosage, route, frequency of administration, and signature of the person writing the order. Nurses must question any unclear orders before implementing the order.

- Three systems of measurement are used: the metric system, the apothecaries' system, and the household system. Weights and measures may need to be converted by the nurse within these three systems.

- When administering medications, the nurse observes the six "rights" to ensure accurate administration. When preparing medications, the nurse checks the medication container label against the medication card form or printout three times.

- The nurse who prepares the medication administers it and must never leave a prepared medication unattended.

- The nurse always identifies the client appropriately before administering a medication and stays with the client until the medication is taken.

- Medications, once given, are documented as soon as possible after administration.

- When mixing insulins in the same syringe, air should be injected into the cloudy (intermediate- or long-acting) insulin vial first, followed by air into the clear (short-acting) vial. The short-acting (clear) insulin should be drawn up first, followed by the cloudy (intermediate- or long-acting). There should never be contamination of the short-acting insulin.

- Proper site selection is essential for an intramuscular injection to prevent tissue, bone, and nerve damage. The nurse should always palpate anatomic landmarks when selecting a site.

- Clients receiving a series of injections should have the injection sites rotated.

- After use, needles should not be recapped but must be placed in puncture-resistant containers.

 EXPLORE MediaLink

Additional interactive resources for this chapter can be found on the Companion Website at www.prenhall.com/ramont. Click on Chapter 29 and "Begin" to select the activities for this chapter.

For chapter-related NCLEX®-style questions and an audio glossary, access the accompanying CD-ROM in this book.

Animations/Videos
- Drug Metabolization
- Injections
- Pharmacology and the Elderly

∞ FOR FURTHER Study

For more details on respiratory therapy, see Chapter 24.

For further information about inserting a nasogastric tube, see Procedure 25-2.

For information about administering tube feedings, see Procedure 25-3.

For information about discontinuing an intravenous device, see Procedure 30-11.

Critical Thinking Care Map

Caring for a Client with Insulin-Dependent Diabetes Mellitus

NCLEX-PN® Focus Area: Health Promotion and Maintenance

Case Study: Marissa Gonsalves is a 27-year-old elementary schoolteacher newly diagnosed with type 1 diabetes mellitus. She also attends school at night with plans to complete her master's degree in the spring. She lives with three roommates who have shared a house since their college days. She expresses concern over her diagnosis. "It will be hard to follow the diet at home. I don't eat on a regular schedule on my school nights and my roommates are big snackers."

Nursing Diagnosis: Ineffective Therapeutic Regimen Management

COLLECT DATA

Subjective	Objective
_____	_____
_____	_____
_____	_____
_____	_____
_____	_____
_____	_____
_____	_____

Would you report this data? Yes/No

If yes, to: _____

What would you report? _____

Nursing Care

_____
_____
_____
_____
_____
_____
_____
_____
_____
_____
_____
_____
_____

How would you document this? _____
_____
_____

Compare your documentation to the sample provided in Appendix I.

Data Collected
(use those that apply)

- Weight: 156 lbs
- Fasting blood sugar 164 mg/mL
- Urine shows presence of ketones
- VS: T 99, P 132, R 28, BP 100/54
- Complains of excessive thirst and frequent urination
- States, "I have been so tired, but it is probably because I am working and going to school."
- Started on insulin injection and blood glucose monitoring; client hesitant to perform monitoring and injections herself
- 1,800-calorie ADA diet

Nursing Interventions
(use those that apply, list in priority order)

- Review daily actions that are not therapeutic.
- Pay meticulous attention to foot care.
- Monitor skin condition at least once a day; determine whether client is experiencing loss of sensation.
- Demonstrate and allow client to perform monitoring and self-injection under supervision.
- Observe and report signs of infection such as redness, warmth, discharge, and increased body temperature.
- Provide information about the therapeutic regimen in various formats (video, brochures, written instructions).
- Deliberate with the client on changes that are possible to meet therapeutic goals.
- Assess client's locus of control related to her health.

1 Demerol 50 mg has been ordered for your client. On checking the narcotic cabinet, you find a Demerol 75-mg prefilled syringe on hand. Which of the following is the appropriate action?

1. Inform your client that he will have to wait until the pharmacy brings the correct dose of medication.
2. Call the physician and request a different order.
3. Waste 25 mg of Demerol in front of a licensed witness.
4. Give your client an injection of 50 mg and dispose of the syringe with the remainder in the sharps container.

2 The physician has written an order that is illegible. It appears to be to 5 mg of Ativan. The order in fact was 0.5 mg. Who is responsible for the error?

1. The nurse who administers the incorrect dosage is responsible for the error.
2. The physician who wrote the illegible order is responsible.
3. The unit secretary who transcribed the order is responsible.
4. The charge nurse who verified the order is responsible.

3 The reason the drug is prescribed is known as the:

1. side effect.
2. untoward effect.
3. therapeutic effect.
4. adverse effect.

4 Your client is experiencing unpredictable abnormal symptoms including opposite drug action. You know this to be a(n):

1. drug tolerance.
2. idiosyncratic effect.
3. iatrogenic disease.
4. drug interaction.

5 The physician has ordered Valium 5 mg "stat" for agitation. You understand the order to mean:

1. the drug is to be given as needed.
2. the medication is to be given immediately and only once.
3. the order may be carried out indefinitely until an order is written to cancel it.
4. the drug is to be given according to the facility policy.

6 A preop order is given for atropine 1/300 gr. On hand you have a multidose vial containing 1 mg/mL. What volume of the drug would you give?

1. 1/3 mL
2. 0.2 mL
3. 1 mL
4. 2 mL

7 You are providing discharge instructions for a mother of a 2-year-old. The physician has written a prescription for 1 teaspoon amoxicillin every 6 hours × 10 days. Which of the following statements would ensure that the mother understands the instructions?

1. "I will use his favorite spoon to measure his medication."
2. "I will disguise the medicine in his milk to be sure he will take it."
3. "I will give him the medication with meals and his last dose before he goes to bed."
4. "I will need to use a medicine cup to measure the correct dose."

8 You are preparing a subcutaneous injection of heparin for your client. You will be giving 4,000 units. On hand you have 5,000 unit/mL. Which of the following is the best syringe to use?

1. an insulin syringe because it is calibrated in units with a 5/8-inch needle
2. A tuberculin syringe because it is calibrated in tenths (0.1)
3. A 2-mL syringe with a 22-gauge 2.5-cm (1-in.) needle
4. A 3-mL syringe with a 23-gauge 3-cm (1.5-in.) needle

9 The primary reason why nurses should wear gloves when administering topical medications is:

1. human skin harbors microorganisms.
2. topical medication can cause skin irritation on the nurse.
3. topical medications on the nurse's hands can be transferred to another client.
4. skin preparations must be applied using sterile technique.

10 The dorsogluteal site should not be used for infants because:

1. it is difficult to restrain a child in the proper position to use this site.
2. this muscle is developed by walking so it should not be used until the child has been walking for 1 year.
3. medication is absorbed slowly from this location.
4. the area is very vascular so there is a tendency for extensive bruising.

Answers and Rationales for Review Questions, as well as discussion of Care Plan and Critical Thinking Care Map questions, appear in Appendix I.

Chapter 30

IV Therapy

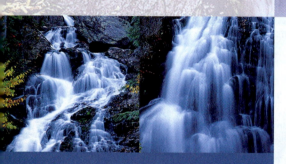

HISTORICAL Perspectives

Modern IV therapy is less than a century old. In Europe in the mid-1600s, medical researchers used a quilled bladder to inject opium into dogs. In 1667 lamb's blood was infused into a 15-year-old Parisian boy. The boy did not survive the infusion. In 1834, the medical community decided that only human blood was safe for transfusion. In 1930, intravenous infusions were done in the critically ill only, and only by doctors, with nurses assisting them. It was a major procedure done with sterile gowns, masks, surgical caps, etc. The nurses also used and reused sharpened and sterilized steel needles.

BRIEF Outline

Legal Implications
Fluids and Electrolytes
Equipment Overview
Preparing the Client for IV Therapy
Anatomy of Peripheral Veins
Factors Affecting IV Site Solution
Venipuncture Procedure
Peripheral IV Therapy Complications
Blood Transfusions
IV Rate Calculations

LEARNING Outcomes

After completing this chapter, you will be able to:

1. Discuss the objectives of IV therapy.
2. Identify the types of infusion devices used in parenteral therapy.
3. Identify peripheral veins appropriate for use in IV therapy.
4. Describe factors that influence needle selection.
5. Demonstrate proper venipuncture procedure.
6. Identify complications associated with infusion therapy.
7. Demonstrate accurate calculations for determining IV rates.
8. Demonstrate changing a sterile central line dressing.
9. Discuss the procedure for administering blood products.

The LPN/LVN must be knowledgeable and skillful when delivering IV therapy. You should first understand and review the practical/vocational nurse practice act for scope of practice for the state in which you reside. The LPN/LVN must be trained in IV therapy before they can start IVs. In some states LPN/LVN students must complete their nurse's training before they can take the IV course. Once the new graduate has taken boards and completed the IV therapy training, the term "IV Certified" will usually be added to his or her license upon the first renewal. Follow the policy and procedures set forth by the agency in which you perform nursing practice. It is the responsibility of the nurse to be the client advocate in observation of potential complications and early intervention. Preparing and educating the client about IV therapy will ensure client cooperation and promote a therapeutic relationship. It is essential for the nurse to be fully aware of the standards of practice involved in IV therapy. Managing IV therapy is one of the most important roles that an LPN/LVN undertakes.

Legal Implications

Laws differ from state to state, so you must be knowledgeable about the laws in your state. This section provides an overview of significant issues. There are four sources of law in the United States: constitutional law, statutory law, administrative law, and common law. Common law is court-made law and is most commonly found in the area of malpractice. Criminal law relates to a wrong against the public for which the government authority can prosecute criminal acts with imprisonment or fines. If carried out in an unlawful manner, IV therapy administration can be a criminal offense. Civil law applies to the legal rights of private persons/corporations. A private wrong or act of omission can result in a civil tort. Intentional torts that could be related to IV therapy are negligence, assault and battery, false imprisonment, slander, libel, and invasion of privacy. For example, to force a rational adult client to allow placement of an IV cannula could constitute assault and battery charges.

Negligence is the failure to do something that a reasonable prudent person would do. Malpractice is acting in a manner that departs from the accepted standards of practice that the average qualified healthcare provider would deliver. *Note:* If an act of malpractice does not create harm, legal action cannot be initiated. The rule of personal liability states that every person is liable for his or her own tortuous conduct; therefore, nurses are liable for their own wrongdoings in carrying out physician orders. If an LPN/LVN in his or her professional judgment does not feel confident performing a particular IV task, then he or she can properly refuse to do so.

BREACH OF DUTY

Breaches of duty are certain events that may foreseeably cause a specific harm, for example, delay in medication administration, unfamiliarity with the drug, inappropriate route of administration, failure to qualify orders, and negligence in client teaching. More specific litigation for nurses can result from infiltration and phlebitis, extravasations, broken central venous catheters, nerve injury, and poor or inaccurate documentation.

STANDARDS OF CARE

The client is the focus of standards of care. The Joint Commission on Accreditation of Healthcare Organizations (JCAHO) has indicated that standards of care must be developed within organizations to measure quality based on expectations of service. Sources of standards of care include federal regulators, the Occupational Safety and Health Administration (OSHA), the Food and Drug Administration (FDA), and the Centers for Disease Control and Prevention (CDC). State regulators include departments of health and human services, which enforce Health Insurance Portability and Accountability Act (HIPAA) regulations. Professional standards of care include those published by the American Nurse Association (ANA), the Infusion Nurses Society (INS), JCAHO, the American Association of Blood Banking (AABB), and the Environmental Protection Agency (EPA). Standards of care address nursing process, accountability, currency in practice and outcomes of care and focus for the client.

OCCURRENCE/INCIDENT REPORT

A report should be filed every time something unusual occurs or a deviation from the standard of care occurs. These reports are used for internal quality assurance purposes and as a record of an event. Incidents should be reported to the charge nurse/supervisor and objectively charted but not referenced in the client legal record. See Figure 36-1 ⚭ for an example of an Occurrence/Incident Report.

CDC/OSHA GUIDELINES

All nursing personnel must follow Standard Precautions. All body fluids (not including sweat) are treated as if known to be infectious with HIV, hepatitis B and C, and other bloodborne pathogens. The main barriers include gloves in combination with hand hygiene practices, eye protection, and mucous membrane protection (face shield or goggles and mask).

The Needlestick Safety and Prevention Act of November 2000 reinforced the need to use safe needles in order to reduce needle-stick injuries. Needleless systems and needle safety devices are being used to protect the safety of healthcare personnel. Built-in safety features such as syringes with a sliding sheath that shields the attached needle after use, needles that retract into a syringe after use, shielded or retracting catheters, and intravenous medical delivery systems that use a catheter port with a needle housed in a protective covering are currently being used.

If you are stuck by a needle or other sharp, or get blood or other potentially infectious materials in your eyes, nose, mouth, or on broken skin:

- Immediately flood the exposed area with water and clean any wound with soap and water or a skin disinfectant if available.
- Report this immediately to your employer.
- Seek immediate medical attention.

POSTEXPOSURE PROPHYLAXIS

Healthcare agencies are required to have a plan in place prior to an exposure occurring. The treating agency will evaluate the risk of exposure, evaluate the source client, evaluate the exposed person, and decide on postexposure prophylaxis (PEP) or therapy and follow-up care.

Contaminated sharps have to be placed in a puncture-resistant, leak-proof, and labeled container. They must be easily accessed, maintained upright, and replaced routinely. Hepatitis B vaccine must be offered at no charge to an employee "at a reasonable time and place" and "within ten days of initial assignment."

PHYSICAL HAZARDS

Additional hazards noted are abrasions, contusions, chemical exposure, and latex allergy. Small or undetected skin abrasions/contusions can be potential portals for microorganisms. Hand hygiene practice helps to prevent the invasion of microorganisms. The handling of cytotoxic drugs can be hazardous and associated with human cancers. Latex allergies develop with an exposure to natural rubber latex. Reactions range from asthma to anaphylaxis. There is no treatment for latex allergy other than avoidance of latex. Nonlatex personal protective equipment is provided to personnel with a latex sensitivity.

Fluid and Electrolytes

Water is the largest component of the body. The functions of body fluids are to:

- Maintain blood volume
- Transport nutrients to and from cells
- Regulate body temperature
- Assist in digestion

Body water found within cells is referred to as intracellular fluid (ICF). Fluid found outside the cells is known as extracellular fluid (ECF). ECF further consists of two compartments between interstitial (tissue) space and intravascular (plasma) space. An exchange of fluid occurs continuously between the ICF and ECF. These changes occur as a result of changes in the volume or concentration of the plasma. Homeostasis of the internal environment occurs with intake and output that is relatively equal as in healthy adults. (See Box 30-1 ■.)

BOX 30-1	
Fluid Imbalances	
FLUID IMBALANCE	**ASSESSMENT**
Fluid deficit	Low body temperature
	Weight loss
	Pulse rate can be increased or decreased
	Low blood pressure
	Sunken eyes
	Poor skin turgor
	Dry, cracked lips
	Cool extremities
	Diminished urine output
	Increased hematocrit
	Elevated electrolytes and BUN levels
	Increased serum osmolarity
Fluid excess	Weight gain
	High blood pressure
	Bounding pulse
	Jugular vein distention
	Increased respiratory rate
	Dyspnea
	Moist crackles or rhonchi
	Edema
	Puffy eyelids
	Periorbital edema
	Low hematocrit
	Decreased serum electrolytes and BUN levels
	Low serum osmolarity

FLUID TRANSPORT

Movement of particles occurs through transport mechanisms. Passive transport is the movement of solutes through membranes without energy expenditure. **Passive diffusion** is the movement of molecules randomly in all directions from a region of high concentration to an area of low concentration. There is no force to stop diffusion and particles distribute themselves evenly. An example is how ink spreads in water. **Osmosis** is the passage of water from an area of lower particle concentration toward an area of higher concentration of particles. An example is what happens to a hot dog when boiled in water; "it plumps when you cook it." **Osmotic pressure** develops as solute particles collide against each other. The concentration of solution with increased solute particles increases the collisions and creates increased osmotic pressure, causing the movement of fluid. The term **osmolarity** is the total number of osmotically active particles and refers to the concentration of a solute in a volume of solution. These two terms are similar and are used interchangeably. **Filtration** is the transfer of water and dissolved substances from a region of high pressure to a region of low pressure. Filtration moves in one direction due to hydrostatic pressure and results in water and electrolytes moving from capillaries to interstitial fluid. An example would be that of pouring a solution through a strainer in which the size of the opening determines the size of particles to be filtered.

Active transport occurs when it is necessary for electrolytes to move from an area of low concentration to an area of high concentration. Energy must be expended for movement to occur against a concentration gradient. Energy is released from the cell in the form of adenosine triphosphate (ATP) to enable substances to pass through the cell membrane.

ELECTROLYTES

Electrolytes separate in solution and become electrically charged particles called ions. They are either negatively charged anions "−" or positively charged cations "+". Ions are expressed in mEq (milliequivalents) per liter rather than mg (milligrams). Milliequivalents measure chemical activity rather than weight. The total cations and anions in a given compartment must be equal to have balance. A loss or gain upsets a delicate chemical balance. See Chapter 26 ⚭, Table 26-2 ⚭ in particular, for more about electrolytes.

DIAGNOSING AND PLANNING

Nursing diagnoses common to IV therapy are:

- *Deficient Fluid Volume*
- *Risk for Deficient Fluid Volume*
- *Excess Fluid Volume*
- *Risk for Imbalanced Fluid Volume*
- *Imbalanced Nutrition: Less than Body Requirements*
- *Deficient Knowledge*
- *Risk for Infection*

Desired outcomes for clients with IV therapy might include:

- Client will maintain fluid volume balance.
- Client's electrolytes will be maintained within normal limits.
- Client will maintain a balanced nutrition status.
- Client will understand the purpose and medical treatment plan for IV therapy.
- Client will remain free from infection related to IV therapy.

IV SOLUTIONS

Solutions used for IV therapy may be isotonic, hypotonic, or hypertonic. The type ordered is dependent on the need to change or maintain the client's body fluid status. The effect an IV solution has on the fluid compartments depends on how the solution's osmolarity compares with the client's serum osmolarity. Normally, serum has the same osmolarity as other body fluids. A lower serum osmolarity suggests fluid overload; a higher osmolarity suggests hemoconcentration and dehydration. See Table 30-1 ■.

TABLE 30-1		
IV Solutions		
SOLUTION	**IV EXAMPLE**	**NURSING IMPLICATIONS**
Isotonic	Lactated Ringer's (LR) 0.9% NS D_5W	■ These solutions expand the intravascular compartment. Monitor client for signs of fluid overload particularly if the client has hypertension or chronic heart failure (CHF). ■ Don't give LR if the client has liver disease because of the inability to metabolize lactate. ■ Avoid giving D_5W to a client at risk for increased intracranial pressure (ICP). It acts like a hypotonic solution after administration. D_5W is quickly metabolized, leaving only water—a hypotonic solution.
Hypotonic	0.45% NS (½NS) 0.33% NS $D_{2.5}W$	■ These solutions contain less sodium than ICF. They move water into cells, causing cells to swell and possibly burst. ■ These solutions can cause a sudden fluid shift from blood vessels into cells. This can cause cardiovascular collapse from intravascular fluid depletion and increased ICP from fluid shift into brain cells. ■ Avoid hypotonic solutions to clients at risk for ICP, CVA, stroke, head trauma, or neurosurgery. ■ Avoid hypotonic solutions for clients at risk for third spacing fluid shifts such as burns, trauma, or low serum protein levels.
Hypertonic	D 5% 0.45% NS (D_5½NS) D 5% 0.9% NS (D_5NS) D 5% LR (D_5LR)	■ These solutions greatly expand the intravascular compartment. Monitor your client for circulatory overload. ■ Hypertonic solutions pull fluid from the ICF compartment. Avoid these solutions in clients with a condition that causes cellular dehydration such as diabetic ketoacidosis. ■ Avoid these solutions in clients with impaired heart or kidney function because this client is unable to manage extra fluid.

ACID–BASE BALANCE

The key to **acid–base balance** is the regulation of hydrogen ion concentration of body fluids. The kidneys and the lungs are the major organs in regulating acid–base balance. There are two types of acid–base imbalances:

- Metabolic (base bicarbonate deficit and excess) acidosis and alkalosis
- Respiratory (carbonic acid deficit and excess) acidosis and alkalosis.

The pH of fluid refers to the hydrogen ion concentration of that fluid. Normal pH is 7.35 to 7.45. A pH of less than 7.35 reflects an increase of hydrogen ions, which can send the client into acidosis. A pH of greater than 7.45 reflects a decrease in hydrogen ions, which can send the client into alkalosis. A variation of 0.4 above or below can prove to be fatal. Three main regulators maintain the pH of the blood:

1. Chemical buffer systems act like sponges and combine with acid or alkali to prevent excessive changes in the hydrogen ion concentration. The body has a strong tendency toward acidity and needs a buffering system that is more base than acid. The main buffer pair is sodium bicarbonate ($NaHCO_3$) and carbonic acid (H_2CO_3); they are responsible for 45% of hydrogen ion buffering. The ratio of bicarbonate is 20 parts to 1 part carbonic acid (Figure 30-1 ■). Phosphate buffers react with acids and bases to form compounds that alter pH. Phosphate buffers are particularly effective in the renal tubules. Protein buffers are abundant in the body. Composed of hemoglobin and other proteins, they bind with acids and bases to cause neutralization.

2. The lungs effectively regulate the blood levels of CO_2. CO_2 combines with H_2O to form carbonic acid. Increased levels of CO_2 decrease pH level. Receptors in the brain identify pH changes and vary rate and depth of breathing to compensate. Faster, deeper respirations reduce the CO_2 level in the lungs. The decrease in CO_2 increases the pH level. Respiratory response is rapid but short lived.

3. The kidneys reabsorb or excrete acids and bases into the urine. They can produce bicarbonate to refill lost stores. The kidneys have a slower response, but long-term effects result.

Ranges for arterial blood gases are as follows: (Refer to Chapter 26 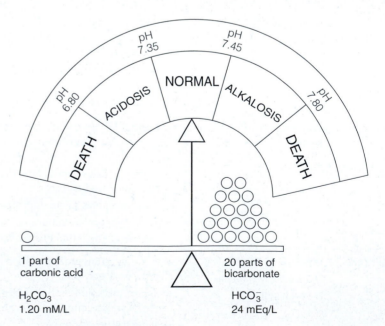 for complete coverage of arterial blood gases.)

- pH = 7.35–7.45
- Pa_{CO_2} = 35–45 mm Hg
- HCO_3 = 22–26 mEq/L

The ranges listed above are average values.

DETERMINING ACID–BASE IMBALANCE

1. Verify the pH level. A high level leads to alkalosis; a low one to acidosis.

2. Establish the primary cause of the disturbance. Ascertain the Pa_{CO_2} and HCO_3 in relationship to the pH.

   a. pH > 7.45, Pa_{CO_2} < 35 mm Hg: The major imbalance is respiratory alkalosis. *Pa_{CO_2} is usually opposite of the pH. If the pH is low and Pa_{CO_2} is high or if pH is high with low Pa_{CO_2}, then it is respiratory in origin.*

   b. pH > 7.45, HCO_3 > 26 mEq/L: The major imbalance is metabolic alkalosis. *HCO_3 levels usually follow the pH level. If the pH is high and HCO_3 is high or if the pH is low with low HCO_3, then it is metabolic in origin.*

   c. pH < 7.35, Pa_{CO_2} > 45 mm Hg: The primary imbalance is metabolic acidosis.

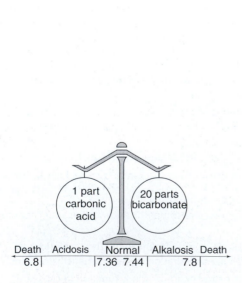

Death	Acidosis	Normal	Alkalosis	Death
6.8		7.36 7.44		7.8

Figure 30-1. ■ pH.

BOX 30-2

Acid–Base Imbalances

IMBALANCE	ETIOLOGY	SIGNS/SYMPTOMS	TREATMENT
Metabolic acidosis	Diarrhea Diabetic ketoacidosis Renal failure Acid ingestion Fistulas	Nausea and vomiting Kussmaul's breathing Headache Drowsiness Increased breathing	Reverse underlying cause. Administer sodium bicarbonate per physician order.
Metabolic alkalosis	Gastric suctioning Vomiting Hypokalemia Potassium-losing diuretics Excessive alkali ingestion	Dizziness Tingling of the fingers Carpopedal spasm Depressed respirations Circumoral paresthesia	Reverse underlying cause. Administer chloride for the kidneys to excrete bicarbonate. Restore normal fluid volume.
Respiratory acidosis	Aspiration Cardiac arrest Severe pneumonia Emphysema Pulmonary edema Pneumothorax	Dizziness Palpitations Convulsions Weakness Mental changes Ventricular fibrillation	Improve ventilation. Use bronchodilators. Administer oxygen and fluids.
Respiratory alkalosis	Hyperventilation Anxiety Hypoxemia High fever Pulmonary emboli	Light-headedness Numbness and tingling of extremities Tinnitus Palpitations Blurred vision Chest tightness	Treat source of anxiety. Ask client to breathe slowly into a paper bag. Administer sedatives as ordered.

d. pH < 7.35, HCO_3 < 22 mEq/L: The primary imbalance is metabolic acidosis.

3. The next step is to decide if compensation has started. Monitor the value other than the major source of the imbalance. The other value shows the body's attempt to compensate. Compensation involves opposites. *If the major imbalance is metabolic acidosis, compensation will be accomplished by respiratory alkalosis.*

4. Partial compensation occurs when the pH remains outside of the normal range.

See Box 30-2 ■.

Equipment Overview

The LPN's/LVN's knowledge about IV equipment is essential in the safe delivery of IV therapy. Identifying the appropriate equipment and understanding the purpose of IV therapy for the client will assist the nurse in the selection of the necessary equipment. Typically IV containers are changed every 24 hours or per facility policy, this is usually performed with tubing changes. An IV container that is at a "keep open" or slow rate could conceivably run as long as 24 hours and would need to be replaced in that time frame.

Two types of infusion systems are used: glass or plastic systems. Glass bottles have a partial vacuum and require air vents. The glass system has the advantages of being very clear, so the fluid level is more accurately read and it is inert. The disadvantages are breakage, storage difficulties, rigidity, and difficult disposal. Glass construction is made with mixed materials that could cause incompatibilities with fluids or additives. Additionally, the potential for coring exists due to the rubber bung (stopper) when the administration set is inserted. In an open glass system, air enters through a plastic tube in the container and collects in the air space in the bottle allowing for displacement of the solution. In a closed glass system, air is filtered into the container via vented tubing in order to allow air into the container.

Plastic containers are used 90% to 95% of the time. They create no vacuum and they are flexible and collapsible. Plastic IV bags do not need air to replace fluid flowing from the container. Plastic containers are completely closed systems, lightweight, easy to store, and are made of polyvinyl

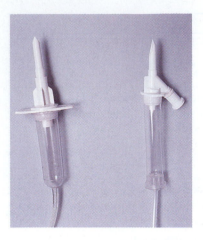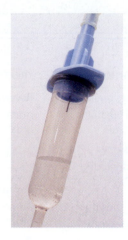

Figure 30-2. ■ Infusion spikes and drip chambers.

chloride (PVC). Bags can be spiked with either a vented or nonvented administration set (Figure 30-2 ■).

Disadvantages of plastic bags are that determining fluid level is more difficult and the bag can puncture easily. Plastic containers are made up of plasticizers and are not completely inert, so never use markers to write on the bag because the ink could be absorbed into the plastic.

All containers require some type of administration set to deliver fluid to the client. The most commonly used ones are the primary or *macrodrip* set and the pediatric or *microdrip* set. In the pediatric setting, buretrols and burettes are used to deliver a precise amount of fluid and prevent fluid overload.

The primary sets are the basic administration sets used for infusion of primary parenteral fluids. The drop factors of these commercial sets vary according to the manufacturer. Usually a macrodrip set ranges from 10 to 20 gtt/mL and the microdrip set is 60 gtt/mL. A secondary administration set, called a *piggyback* set or a volume (meter or burette) controlled set, can be added to the primary line. (See Procedure 30-1 ■ on page 694.)

Primary and secondary continuous administration sets must be changed every 72 hours and immediately upon suspected contamination or compromise of product or system. When an increased rate of cannula-related infections occurs, the organization should return to a 48-hour administration set change. Many hospitals adopt a 48-hour change rather than 72 hours; check your facility policy.

ADMINISTRATION SET COMPONENTS

■ *Spike/piercing pin:* Sharp plastic end designed to be inserted into the IV fluid container. Connected to the flange, drop orifice, and drip chamber.
■ *Flange:* Plastic guard that assists in protecting against contamination upon insertion of the spike.
■ *Drop orifice:* The size and shape of the opening that determines the drop factor.
■ *Drip chamber:* A flexible clear plastic tube that encloses the drop orifice and is connected to the tubing.

■ *Tubing:* It is long (66–100 in.) for primary and shorter (32–42 in.) for secondary tubing.

A mixture of clamps, ports, connectors, or filters may be built in to the system.

■ *Clamp:* A control device that compresses the tubing wall. The most common are a slide, roller or screw clamp. The slide clamp is less precise when determining fluid control.
■ *Injection ports:* A port is an access point into the tubing. Ports are used for medication administration; smaller gauge needles are recommended to ensure resealing.
■ *Check valve:* This valve allows the main IV solution to continue after a secondary solution (IVPB, intravenous piggyback) has infused.
■ *Hub:* An adaptor that connects the administration set to the IV catheter or needleless system. It is referred to as a male Luer lock.
■ *Filter:* The final filter removes foreign particulate from the solution (Figure 30-3 ■). Some are included in the administration set or can be added. A 0.22-micron filter is considered adequate for bacterial/particulate reduction.

Extension tubing may be utilized to allow the IV tubing to be changed away from the insertion site, decreasing the risk of contamination. An IV loop also enables the tubing to be changed away from the device and promotes stabilization of the device. A T-connector is useful for simultaneous administration of fluids and drugs. It eliminates the need for insertion of a second venipuncture device. (See Procedures 30-2 ■, 30-3 ■, and 30-4 ■.)

Blood administration sets come in a Y-shaped or straight single tubing. The Y tubing allows for infusion of 0.9% normal saline before and after each blood product infusion. Blood administration sets come with an inline filter; the minimum pore size is 170 to 260 microns. Microaggregate blood filters can be added or may be inline. These filters are recommended for blood that has been stored longer than

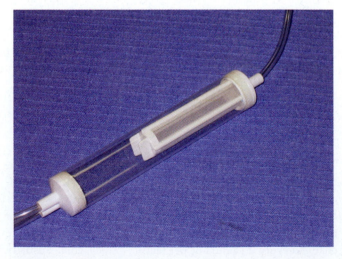

Figure 30-3. ■ Filter.

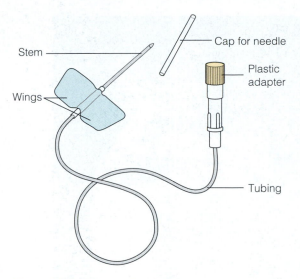

Figure 30-4. ■ Butterfly needle.

5 days and when administering multiple units; refer to your facility's policy on adding these filters.

PERIPHERAL INFUSION DEVICES

Several types of peripheral infusion devices are available. Scalp vein needles (butterfly needles) and over-the-needle catheters (ONCs) are commonly used. When selecting a cannula it should be of the smallest gauge and shortest length possible to accommodate the necessary therapy. Cannulas have radiopaque material in them so that they are visible to x-rays.

Scalp Vein (Butterfly) Needles

Scalp vein (butterfly) needles are used for short-term therapy (Figure 30-4 ■). Gauges range from 17, 19, 21, and 23 to 25 at the smallest, length is 0.5 to 1.0 in., and plastic tubing extends from the wings that is 3 to 12 in. long. Single-dose therapy, blood withdrawal, and clients who are allergic to nylon or Teflon would be good reasons to choose a butterfly needle. They are also used for infants, children, elderly, and adults with small veins. The wings assist with easy insertion and securing of the device. Butterfly needles, however, are stainless steel and not flexible, which may cause easy needle displacement. There is also increased risk of contamination with a stainless steel needle.

Guide to ONC Use

GAUGE	USE
14–16	Multiple trauma, heart surgery, and transplants
18	Major surgery or trauma and blood administration
20	Minor surgery or trauma and blood administration
22–24	Pediatric clients, clients with small veins, for platelets and plasma (Avoid this small gauge with packed RBCs, whole blood, and antibiotics).

Over-the-Needle Catheter

An ONC is used for long-term peripheral infusion therapy for the delivery of viscous fluids (i.e., blood) (Figure 30-5 ■). Gauges range from 14, 16, 18, 20, and 22 to 24 largest to smallest. Catheter length varies from 0.5 to 2.0 in. The point of the needle extends beyond the tip of the catheter, so that after the venipuncture, the needle is withdrawn and discarded, leaving the flexible catheter in the vein. These catheters are easy to insert and are patent longer than a steel needle. Infiltration rate is lower and they are radiopaque. Catheters with wings are easily taped. Some disadvantages are an increased risk of phlebitis; the stylet is long and inflexible, adding to the risk of puncture; and some hubs are more difficult to tape. See Box 30-3 ■.

CENTRAL LINE DEVICES

Central line devices were developed for long-term IV therapy access. These devices are designed for client comfort and to decrease complications associated with numerous therapy needs. A central venous catheter is inserted into the subclavian vein or the internal jugular vein. The catheter tip end may be positioned in the superior vena cava or in the right atrium. The LPN/LVN needs to be aware of three types of central line devices: centrally placed percutaneous catheters, central venous tunneled catheters, and implanted ports that must be inserted by a physician. The third

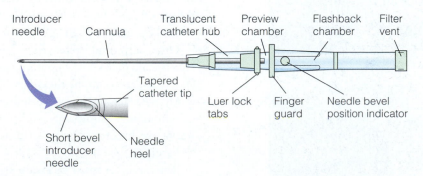

Figure 30-5. ■ Over-the-needle catheter (ONC).

catheter is a peripherally inserted central catheter (PICC), which can be inserted by a trained RN. Common catheter names are Groshong, Hickman, and Broviac. They are typically double or triple lumens, but can be a single lumen. The LPN/LVN who is certified in IV therapy can change the site dressing on a central line, PICC line, or midline catheter. Check for the LPN/LVN scope of practice with regard to IV therapy in your state. (See Procedure 30-5 ■ on page 700.)

ELECTRONIC INFUSION DEVICES

The two basic groups of electronic infusion devices are controllers and pumps. These devices will provide better control of the infusion flow rate. They are designed with alarms to signal a change in the normal flow of the IV solution. Electronic equipment has improved the accuracy of IV infusions but the responsibility and accuracy remain with the nurse monitoring the IV. Machines are not infallible and must be checked for accuracy of the IV rates. The nurse using these machines must understand their use, their mechanical operation, and how to troubleshoot problems.

A controller regulates IV flow rate by relying on gravity rather than exertion or pressure (Figure 30-6 ■). Use of a controller is appropriate for a large percentage of infusions not requiring the accuracy of the volumetric pump. The drop size may vary among administration sets, which requires a controller device to be more accurate. A controller is unable to detect an infiltration and the flow rate is affected

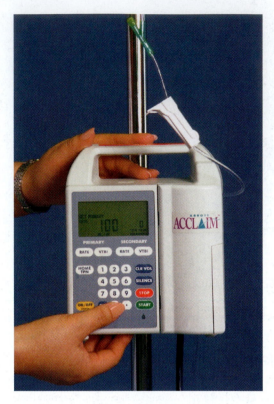

Figure 30-7. ■ Positive-pressure pump.

by the height of the IV bag in relation to the IV site. The LPN/LVN should frequently visually monitor the IV site for signs of infiltration.

An infusion pump is classified as a positive-pressure pump (Figure 30-7 ■). These pumps are programmed to deliver high volumes of fluid more accurately than the controller. They have more features such as keeping track of the fluid volume infused and more sensitive alarms. Volumetric pumps may require a type of cassette or cartridge to be used with the machine. Peristaltic pumps are used primarily to deliver enteral feedings; they use a rotary disk or rollers to compress the tubing, which propels the fluid forward. (See Procedure 30-6 ■ on page 702.)

Syringe pumps provide precise infusion by controlling the rate by means of the drive speed and syringe size. It is valuable for critical infusions and small doses of high-potency drugs. This technology is being used with patient-controlled analgesia (PCA).

Other advanced systems are also in use, such as multi-channel and dual-channel pumps that are computer generated and deliver several medications concurrently or intermittently with the infusion solution (Figure 30-8 ■). Portable or ambulatory pumps are compact and lightweight. The life of the battery system is limited and requires frequent recharging.

The caregiver must be aware of the functional characteristics of the selected device prior to its use. Always read the manufacturer's directions before using any infusion pump.

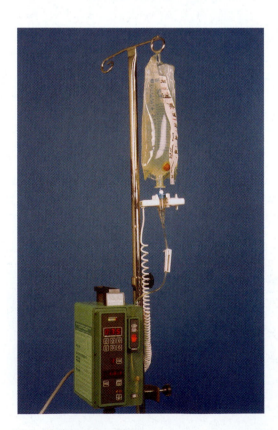

Figure 30-6. ■ Controller device.

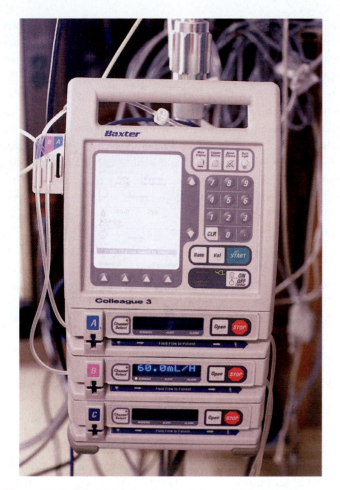

Figure 30-8. ■ Multichannel or dual channel infusion pump.

Typically the facility that employs you will provide you with in-services on the electronic devices used.

Nursing Considerations for Infusion Devices

- Peristaltic regulators are not appropriate for administration of blood due to their squeezing action.
- The administration set's drip chamber must be only half full to allow the sensor to monitor the drip sensor; most sensors are placed at the top of the chamber.
- Tubing cassettes should be inverted for priming.
- Rate regulation devices do not take the place of nursing assessment but rather verify accurate function of the machine at regular intervals.
- All solutions should be labeled with flow strip tubing.
- Piggyback administration sets increase the risk of introducing air bubbles. Place them above the air detector device.
- Always check the package instruction to determine if a filter is compatible with a pump or controller.
- If the electronic device's alarm is going off, check for the most obvious problems in a systematic way: Follow the IV tubing from the insertion site to the IV bag. Look for kinked tubing; for instance, the client may be sitting on it. Check that roller/slide clamps are released. If the

problem is the result of an infiltrate, remove and restart the IV in another location either above the previous site or in the other arm.

ACCESSORY EQUIPMENT

Fluid/blood warmers are available and may be indicated when a rapid or massive transfusion or a neonatal transfusion exchange is necessary or for a client with potent cold agglutinins. Most transfusions do not need to be warmed.

INTERMITTENT INFUSION DEVICE (PERIPHERAL SALINE LOCK/HEPARIN LOCK, PRN DEVICE)

An intermittent infusion device maintains venous access in the client who must receive IV medications regularly or intermittently but who doesn't require a continuous flow of fluids. The advantages of this device are that it:

- Minimizes the risk of fluid overload and electrolyte imbalance.
- Reduces cost.
- Increases client comfort and mobility.
- Reduces client anxiety.
- Allows for collection of blood samples.
- Allows access for emergency administration of medication.

The CDC recommends that heparin be used only when intermittent infusion devices are used for blood sampling. Studies indicate that 0.9% sodium chloride (normal saline) is just as effective as heparin in maintaining catheter patency and reducing phlebitis at IV site. Routine flushing is necessary to ensure and maintain patency of the cannula. It also prevents mixing of medications and solutions that are incompatible. LPNs/LVNs who hold an IV therapy certificate can instill a minute amount of heparin or normal saline into an intermittent infusion lock for the purpose of patency. Licensees must demonstrate competence prior to the performance of the procedure. (See Procedure 30-7 ■ on page 704.)

Preparing the Client for IV Therapy

Fear and anxieties are minimized through teaching. The LPN/LVN should instruct the client on the purpose of the IV, the mechanics of the insertion process, and the degree of discomfort expected. If the client is agitated or in pain, delaying the procedure might be advisable. Distraction techniques are encouraged. Taking deep breaths and releasing them slowly during insertion is a strong technique. Alternately, tensing and relaxing muscle groups tend to focus the client on the action rather than the IV insertion. Should the client be prescribed pain medication, doing the procedure during the drug's peak effectiveness is recommended.

An infant's response is reflexive with body movements, pulling back extremity, and crying. Use distractions such as shaking a rattle, singing a song, or providing a toy. After the procedure cuddle and rock the baby using soothing tones. The toddler response is physical—hitting, biting, or kicking and screaming. The child may use the entire body to resist the nurse. Allow the toddler to explore equipment such as the armboard or to hold the tape. Use a treatment room to insert the IV instead of the child's room, so that it remains a "safe" place.

The child 3 to 7 years old should be prepared for IV therapy right before the procedure is performed. Allow the child as much control as possible. Tell the child that crying is permitted but that it is important to hold still. An assistant should help manage the child. Suggest the child take a deep breath and blow air as if blowing bubbles. Another technique is to have the child push hands together thereby concentrating on the motion rather than the IV injection.

Anatomy of Peripheral Veins

To perform IV therapy, it is the responsibility of the LPN/LVN to accurately understand the integumentary and venous systems. It is important to develop the ability to assess veins and determine suitability for venous access. Review the integumentary system in Chapter 23 ◯◯ and Figure 30-9 ■.

Veins are thin walled and less muscular than arteries (Box 30-4 ■). They can be easily distended under minimal pressure. Vein walls have three layers: The outermost layer, the tunica adventitia, surrounds and supports the vessel. It is made up of connective tissue and its appearance is likened to that of tree bark. This is the part of the vein that allows movement with the skin; you will hear this referred to as a rolling vein. When the vein is accessed with a venous catheter, the nurse can feel a pop upon entering the vein. The middle layer is labeled the tunica media. This layer is composed of the muscle and

elastic tissues that constrict and distend the vein. This venous layer can go into venospasm, causing pain and partially occluding the vessel. This layer is less rigid than the outermost layer and can have a tendency to collapse veins, which are often referred to as disappearing veins. The innermost layer is the tunica intima, referred to as the endothelial lining. This layer is thin and supports the valves pointing toward the heart that prevent blood backflow. When a tourniquet is applied, the valves can be identified as a visible bulge along the distended vein. Inaccurate venipuncture may traumatize the tunica intima, producing roughened endothelial edges. Platelets can adhere to the roughened area and lead to clot formation. (See Procedure 30-8 ■ on page 705.)

The most common sites for venipuncture are the veins of the hands and arms. When assessing suitability of a vein, the nurse palpates for a round, stable, elastic vein (Table 30-2 ■). The vein should feel bouncy, spongy, rubbery—similar to the feel of a water balloon.

Factors Affecting IV Site Selection

When selecting an IV site, these factors must first be considered:

- *Duration of IV therapy:* Select a vein that can support IV therapy for at least 72 hours. Begin therapy at the most distal area for long-term therapy avoiding fingers. Follow routine site rotation and alternate arms.
- *Cannula size:* Hemodilution is important to prevent vein irritation. The gauge of the cannula should be as small as possible. The appropriate size for most situations is a 20- to 22-gauge cannula.

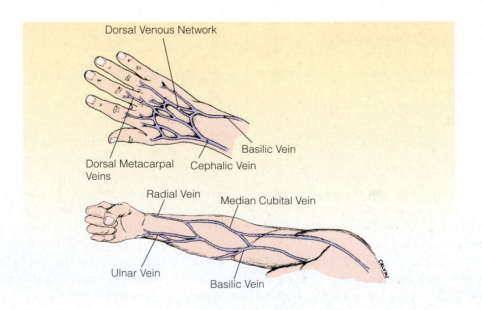

Figure 30-9. ■ Sites for venipuncture.

BOX 30-4

Differences Between Veins and Arteries

	VEINS	ARTERIES
Blood color	Dark red, unoxygenated blood	Bright red, oxygenated blood
Pulse	No pulse	Pulsation with ventricle contraction
Valves	Presents as a bulge along the vein. Keeps the blood flowing toward the heart.	Does not occur in arteries. Blood flows away from the heart.
Location	Superficial veins are found just under the skin.	Arteries are found deeper in the skin and surrounded by muscle to protect them. One to 10 arteries are superficially located and identified as aberrant arteries.
Tissue supplied	Veins are multiple and appear in a network formation. An injury to one usually isn't serious because another will perform its function.	An artery supplies one area. An injury or occlusion can endanger the tissue supplied.

TABLE 30-2

Superficial Veins of the Arm and Their Suitability for IV Therapy

VEINS	LOCATION	IV SUITABILITY
Digital vein	Found along lateral and dorsal areas of the fingers	Used when other sites are unavailable, for short-term therapy. Isotonic solutions and small-gauge (22-gauge) needles are appropriate for these veins. Use armboard or tongue blade to securely place.
Metacarpal vein	Found on the dorsum of the hand, and formed by union of the digital veins between the knuckles	The hand veins are the best place to begin IV therapy because they are the most distal, allowing the veins above to be used as they are needed. Venous cannulas of 22 to 20 gauge with a short needle are easily inserted. Wrist mobility limited.
Cephalic vein	Formed by the metacarpal veins and function in the radial part of the forearm and upper arm	These veins can handle large-gauge needles (16 to 22 gauge). Veins may have a tendency to roll. Larger veins can be used for rapid fluid infusion. Hypertonic fluids and fluids that irritate the veins can be infused more easily.
Antecubital cephalic vein	Found in the antecubital fossa, in front of the elbow	Antecubital site should be avoided unless warranted by an emergency. This area is difficult to splint and may be uncomfortable. Change site within 24 hours.
Accessory cephalic vein	Found along the radial bone following the metacarpal veins of the thumb	Veins may be shorter in length than cephalic veins. These are medium to large veins accommodating 18- to 20-gauge cannulas. May be more difficult to palpate than other veins.
Basilic vein	Follows along the ulnar side of the forearm	This area is a more difficult access than veins on the radial side of forearm but can be approached by bending the arm upward at the elbow. Eighteen- to 22-gauge cannulas can be easily inserted. Veins have a tendency to roll.
Median vein	Forms from veins on the palm of the hand and extends up the front of the forearm on the ulnar side	Veins are easily accessible for IV therapy. Various cannula sizes can be inserted. Median antebrachial areas have many nerve endings and should be avoided. Infiltration occurs easily.
Great saphenous vein	Found at the internal malleolus of the foot	Used as a last resort. Excellent for short-term IV therapy when other sites are unavailable. Large veins can accommodate larger cannulas. Can impair circulation of the lower leg and there is an increased risk of deep venous thrombosis. Avoid in the diabetic client.
Dorsal venous network	Found on the dorsal area of the foot	Suitable for infants and toddlers and can be used for adults as a last resort. Veins are difficult to see. Increased risk of deep venous thrombosis. Avoid in the diabetic client.

- *Type of solution:* Hypertonic solutions, potassium chloride, and antibiotics are irritating to the vein walls. Select a large vein to accommodate these solutions.
- *Condition of the vein:* Choose a soft, straight vein for venipuncture. Palpate the vein and move your finger down the vein observing how it refills. A sluggish refill indicates that the vein is prone to collapsing. Avoid veins that are bruised, red, swollen, or found near a previously infected site. Restart IV infusion above a previous site.
- *Client's level of consciousness:* A combative client may cause a challenge to securing the IV site. Use an armboard to protect the site. Avoid the wrist area if restraints are being used.
- *Client activity:* If the client is using crutches or a walker or uses hands to steady movement and to get up and around, avoid the wrist and hands.
- *Client's age:* Veins in the elderly are more fragile; approach their veins cautiously and gently. Determine the need for a tourniquet. Infants have fewer available IV sites. Children under age 4 have increased body fat, so veins in the hands and feet may be the only accessible sites.
- *Dominant hand:* The dominant hand usually has the most identifiable veins; avoid if possible. Active movement of the extremity can displace the cannula. Take into account the preference of the client.
- *Presence of preexisting disease:* Clients with dehydration or vascular disease can have limited available veins. Avoid sites affected by cerebrovascular accident, mastectomy, amputation, and orthopedic surgery or plastic surgery of the hand or arm. Clients on chemotherapy may have poor venous access. An extremity that has a shunt or graft access for dialysis should not be used for IV insertion. Clients on anticoagulants have a tendency to bleed.

The nurse is responsible for taking necessary precautions when choosing an IV site. Some guidelines include limiting tourniquet pressure for venous distention and use of the smallest cannula necessary to accomplish the necessary infusion.

Venipuncture Procedure

Prior to inserting an IV catheter, the LPN/LVN will check the physician's order, perform hand hygiene, collect and prepare the equipment, prepare and assess the client, and select the appropriate site. (See Procedure 30-2.) In preparing the IV site, the nurse may need to remove excess hair to facilitate catheter insertion, taping, and dressing adherence. Infusion Nurse Society (INS) suggests the use of scissors for this. A razor can cause impairment of the skin integrity. Ensure that the client does not have an iodine allergy prior to prepping the skin. Prep with alcohol using a circular motion from the inside out and allow drying for 1 minute. Alcohol is an antimicrobial agent, removes oils from the skin, and can be used alone if the client has an allergy to Betadine. Betadine is the next step, a germicidal solution that is effective for up to 6 hours after drying for 1 minute.

Successful first sticks depend on proper preparation. Feeling rushed or nervous may lead to failure of the insertion. Put the client at ease by engaging in conversation. When the client is extremely nervous and has a needle phobia, a vasovagal response can ensue. The client can present with tachycardia and hypertension prior to insertion. Post-cannulation the client can experience bradycardia and a drop in blood pressure, pallor, diaphoresis, and syncope. The onset is usually immediate. Keep the needle out of sight until the last minute, this may decrease the severity of the symptoms.

Here are some options for tourniquets (Figure 30-10 ■):

- A *flat rubberized band* can be used, but be careful not to pull hair. Avoid twisting the band and keep the tails of the band away from the insertion site.

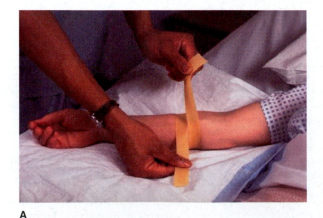

A

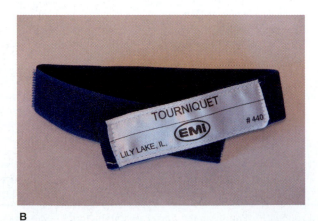

B

Figure 30-10. ■ **A.** Rubber tourniquet; **B.** Velcro tourniquet.

- A *Velcro-closure band* is more comfortable and easier to handle than the traditional rubberized band.
- A *blood pressure cuff* at 30 mm Hg is preferred by some clinicians, especially with elderly clients or those with fragile veins. It prevents excessive engorgement.

(See Procedure 30-8.)

LOCAL ANESTHETIC

Lidocaine 1% without epinephrine can be used to numb the skin prior to a needle stick. There is controversy regarding this practice. The INS has stated that local anesthesia, including lidocaine, should not be routinely used for the insertion of a cannula. The IV nurse must receive instruction in the proper procedure and demonstrate knowledge, skill, and ability. Finally, have a physician order. The client feels touch and pressure, but not pain, and will have muscle control. The effect is felt within 15 to 30 seconds and last 30 to 45 minutes. The nurse checks for history of allergies. The dose used is 0.1 mL of 1% lidocaine. The use of lidocaine may expose the client to complications, including:

- Allergic reaction
- Anaphylaxis
- Inadvertent injection of drug into the vascular system
- Obliteration of the vein.

TECHNIQUES IN VENIPUNCTURE

Two methods are used for vein entry. Gloves should be applied before venipuncture is initiated.

- *Direct method or one-step entry:* The cannula enters the skin directly over the vein in one quick motion.
- *Indirect method:* Two steps are required; the cannula is inserted through the skin, and then the vein is relocated and entered.

Approaching the vein with the bevel up and to the side of the vein allows the nurse to feel the pop upon entering the vein. Hold the skin taut and pull down on the vein slightly; this will make the vein wall easier to penetrate.

Several methods are used to advance the cannula. Smooth cannula insertion and advancement of the catheter prevents the cannula from being displaced.

1. Floating the cannula into the vein, advance the cannula one-third to one-half its length into the vein or until you see a backflow of blood. Attach the tubing and start the IV solution at a slow rate. Use one hand to maintain vein stretch while advancing the cannula with one hand.
2. For a two-handed method, insert the cannula into the vein half the length of the cannula or until you see a backflow of blood. With one hand hold the hub of the cannula while retracting the stylet with the other hand. Maintain the vein stretch and advance the cannula until it is inserted completely.

3. The one-step technique is used by the more experienced nurse. In a one-step insertion, the cannula enters the skin and is advanced in one step.
4. When using catheters with a raised lip on the hub. Push the cannula off the stylet, advancing the cannula halfway into the vein and pressing your forefinger or thumb against the hub's lip, sliding the cannula forward. It will move off the stylet and into the vein.
5. Do not spend too much time probing for a vein; gently feel for the tip of the cannula. This gives you an idea of whether the cannula is above, below, to the right or left of the vein. If you are unable to locate the vein remove the cannula and attempt venipuncture in another site.

Stabilize the catheter by one of three methods:

- U method
- H method
- Chevron method.

Determine whether an armboard is necessary to stabilize the catheter. Implement dressing management, with either a gauze dressing or transparent semipermeable membrane (TSM). (See also Procedures 30-9 ■ and 30-10 ■ starting on page 706.)

Documentation of IV therapy includes date of insertion, location, gauge and length of cannula, type of solution administered, client's response, and signature of the nurse inserting the IV.

Placing IV cannulas in infants requires expertise and specialized training. Scalp veins in infants are suitable for use until about 12 to 18 months of age. When scalp veins are used, always point the cannula downward in the direction of the infant's heart. Lower extremity veins are suitable for infants and toddlers, but are used as a last resort in adults.

Peripheral IV Therapy Complications

Complications that occur from IV therapy are classified by location. The nurse must take contributing factors into consideration:

- Age of the client
- Client's medical condition
- Skin integrity
- Site of infusion
- Duration of infusion
- Method of infusion
- Site and line maintenance
- Client activity
- Insertion technique.

Careful and frequent observation of the IV site will lead to early intervention of local complications. (Tables 30-3 ■ and 30-4 ■). (See also Procedure 30-11 ■ on page 712.)

TABLE 30-3

Local IV Complications

COMPLICATION	CAUSE	NURSING INTERVENTIONS AND PREVENTIONS

Phlebitis
Tenderness at the tip of the catheter
Redness at the tip of the catheter and along the vein
Edema
Febrile
Vein is hardened on palpation
Types of phlebitis
   Mechanical
   Chemical
   Bacterial
	Friction related to cannula movement
	Cannula left in the vein for an extended period of time
	Clotting at the tip of the catheter
	High pH, low pH, or high osmolarity solutions causing vein irritation
	Rapid infusion
	Infection
	Increased risk with total parenteral nutrition (TPN), burns, multiple sticks, and immunosuppression
		Remove cannula.
		Warm compress.
		Notify physician.
		Document signs and symptoms, phlebitis scale (Table 30-4), and interventions.
		Prevention Techniques:
		Tape cannula securely.
		Use filter.
		Review insertion technique.

Infiltration Edema above the IV site Uncomfortable, painful burning Coolness at the site No backflow when IV bag lowered Tightness and blanching at the site IV rate decreased	Cannula dislodged or has perforated through the vein	Discontinue cannula. Apply cold pack and then warm compress. Elevate extremity. Assess circulation and capillary refill. Reinsert cannula above infiltration site or use other extremity. Document. *Prevention Techniques:* Observe site frequently. Avoid obscuring the site. Teach client to observe and report changes. Do not use tape that encircles the arm, causing constriction and obscuring the site.
Hematoma Tenderness at IV site Bruising around the site Inability to advance or flush IV site	Vein has perforated through other vein wall at the time of insertion Leakage of blood from needle displacement	Remove venipuncture device. Apply pressure and warm compresses. Check for continued bleeding. Document. *Prevention Techniques:* Select a vein that accommodates the catheter needing to be inserted. Use a blood pressure cuff for a tourniquet. Release tourniquet once insertion is achieved.
Venospasm First symptom is pain along the vein Slow flow rate Blanched skin over the site	Common with blood transfusion or cold fluids Severe vein irritation from drugs or fluids Rapid IV flow rate	Apply warm compress over the vein. Slow the IV flow rate. *Prevention Techniques:* Use a blood warmer device. Use fluids at room temperature when possible.
Vasovagal Response Vein collapse during venipuncture Pallor	Anxiety or pain	Lower the head of the bed. Ask client to take deep breaths. Check vital signs. *Prevention Techniques:*

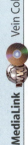

MediaLink Vein Collapse

TABLE 30-3		
Local IV Complications (*continued*)		
COMPLICATION	**CAUSE**	**NURSING INTERVENTIONS AND PREVENTIONS**
Sweating, faintness, dizziness, and nausea Low blood pressure		Prepare and reassure the client. Use a local anesthetic if nurse has been authorized to do so.
Thrombosis Painful, reddened, and edematous vein Sluggish IV rate Febrile Malaise Unable to flush medication lock	Injury to the endothelial cells of the vein; platelets adhere and development of thrombus ensues Multiple sticks Through and through perforations of the vein	Remove venipuncture device. Reinsert IV in other extremity. Apply warm compresses. Be observant of potential infection process. Document. *Prevention Techniques:* Review venipuncture techniques. Use infusion devices to avoid blood from backing up. Use filters.
Thrombophlebitis Severe pain Reddened; edema; and vein is hardened Visible red line above the insertion site	Thrombosis and inflammation Use of lower extremity for infusion High pH, low pH, or high osmolarity solutions, causing vein irritation Insertion technique Client's condition	Remove venipuncture device. Reinsert IV in other extremity. Apply warm compresses. Document. *Prevention Techniques:* Observe site frequently. Secure catheter to prevent movement. Use proper IV insertion technique.
Nerve, Tendon, or Ligament Damage Severe pain similar to an electrical shock Numbness Muscle contraction May suffer delayed reaction Paralysis Deformity	Venipuncture technique Improper splinting or taping is too tight	Stop procedure. Document. *Prevention Techniques:* Review venipuncture technique. Avoid repeated attempts to insert venipuncture device into the same tissues. Tape securely without being too constricting. Pad armboards.
Extravasation (severe infiltration of a vesicant solution into the surrounding tissue) Severe pain or burning Skin sloughing Tissue necrosis Edema Skin tightness Coolness over the site Blanching Slow infusion rate Dressing may be moist	Venipuncture device dislodged Perforation of the vein wall Mechanical friction	Stop infusion and aspirate any fluid. Administer antidote per facility policy immediately. Apply cold packs unless vinca alkaloids are being infused. Cold application would be contraindicated. Photograph site per facility policy. Elevate arm per facility policy. Notify physician. Document. *Prevention Techniques:* Be skilled at IV insertion technique. Have knowledge of vesicant solutions. Access blood return of IV prior to infusion. Assess the condition of client's vein. Assess visibility of IV site.

TABLE 30-4

Phlebitis Scale

STAGE	INDICATORS	NURSING INTERVENTIONS
0	No pain, redness, or edema at site	None
1+	Redness may extend above the IV site up to 1½ in.; may or may not be painful	Remove cannula.
2+	Redness may extend above the IV site up to 1½ in.; painful, edema	Remove cannula. Elevate extremity. Apply cool pack first and then warm compresses.
3+	Redness, edema, painful, and palpable cord less than 3 in. above the IV site	Remove cannula. Elevate extremity. Apply cool pack first and then warm compresses. Notify physician.
4+	Redness, edema, painful, induration, palpable cord less than 3 in. above the IV site	Remove cannula and culture tip. Elevate extremity. Apply cool pack first and then warm compresses. Notify physician.
5+	Purulent drainage, redness, edema, painful, induration, palpable cord less than 3 in. above the IV site	Remove cannula. Culture drainage, tip of the cannula. Elevate extremity. Apply cool pack first and then warm compresses. Notify physician.

SYSTEMIC COMPLICATIONS

Systemic complications can develop quickly or insidiously. They can be life threatening and must be recognized early to initiate prompt treatment. See Table 30-5 ■ Systemic Complications.

Blood Transfusions

To provide safe therapeutic transfusion therapy, the nurse must be knowledgeable about the circulatory system and the management of blood products. The LPN/LVN is responsible for understanding and carrying out the facility criteria, policies, and procedures in transfusion therapy. Careful observation of the client for signs and symptoms of transfusion reactions and condition changes can avert potential life-threatening problems. The use of 0.9% sodium chloride (NS) is used with transfusion therapy and is established in policies and procedures. (Box 30-5 ■ discusses cultural considerations surrounding blood transfusions.)

Clients receiving transfusions are tested for ABO and Rh grouping. Antibody screening and compatibility testing are performed prior to infusion of blood or blood products. The purpose is to prevent antigen–antibody reactions and identify antibodies that the recipient may have.

There are three types of blood donor collection methods. **Homologous** collection is a blood donation by someone other than the person receiving the blood. Strict guidelines have been in place to make sure the blood is safe for use. **Autologous** blood donation is when the client provides his or her own blood. This option is for a person who is likely to need blood for an elective surgery and donates prior to

---

BOX 30-5   **CULTURAL PULSE POINTS**

Blood Transfusions

Jehovah's Witnesses believe that the Bible prohibits the consumption, storage, and transfusion of blood even in cases of emergency. In the last 20 years there has been a strong interest in bloodless surgery. This surgery may involve the use of techniques such as cell salvage, in which a device recycles and cleans blood from a client during an operation and redirects it back to the client's body. Other options include the use of blood substitutes that expand blood volume to prevent shock. Laser or sonic scalpels can be used to minimize bleeding during an operation.

TABLE 30-5

Systemic Complications

COMPLICATION	CAUSE	NURSING INTERVENTIONS AND PREVENTION
Circulatory Overload		
Uncomfortable	Flow rate too rapid	Raise the head of bed.
Neck vein engorgement	Error in fluid requirements	Administer oxygen.
Respiratory distress (pulmonary edema)	Client with renal or cardiac conditions	Notify physician.
Crackles		Administer medications per physician order.
Changes in I&O		Document.
		Prevention Techniques:
		Use infusion devices appropriately.
		Monitor infusions frequently.
		Make accurate fluid calculations.
Septicemia/Bacteremia		
Fluctuating febrile state	Nosocomial infection	Notify physician.
Chills	Primarily staphylococci and enterococci infections	Check vital signs.
Elevated WBC		Monitor condition changes.
Malaise	Lack of consistent hand hygiene	Start antimicrobial therapy per physician order.
IV site contaminated; no signs of infection at site	Client risk factors: age, immunity, other infections	Reinsert IV catheter in opposite extremity.
Hypotension	Infusion factors: catheter, solutions, insertion site, length of infusion	Obtain cultures of equipment and client's blood.
Tachycardia and tachypnea	Inadequately maintained insertion site	Document.
Mental status changes		*Prevention Techniques:*
Diarrhea		Practice consistent hand hygiene.
Vascular collapse, shock, and death		Inspect equipment and solutions for malfunctions.
		Use Betadine for antimicrobial action.
		Ensure sterile dressing to insertion site.
		Monitor insertion site routinely.
		Change site per facility/INS protocol.
Air Embolism		
Respiratory distress (dyspnea, cyanosis, tachypnea, wheezes, cough, and pulmonary edema)	Solution runs dry	Place in Trendelenburg position.
	Hanging a new IV bag and not clearing the line of air from a bag that ran dry	Call for assistance.
Inconsistent breath sounds	Air in administration tubing cassettes	Administer oxygen.
Weakened pulse	Improper technique for tubing changes	Check vital signs.
Palpitations, chest pain, and tachycardia	Loose connections	Notify physician.
Confusion, anxiousness, seizures		Keep emergency equipment on hand.
Mental status changes		Document.
Hemiplegia, aphasia, coma, and death		*Prevention Techniques:*
		Remove air from administration sets.
		Vent air from ports using a syringe.
		Use filters.
		Follow routine changes for tubing and dressings.
		Hang IV solutions prior to the bag running dry.
		Use infusion devices to monitor fluid infusion.

(continued)

TABLE 30-5

Systemic Complications (*continued*)

COMPLICATION	CAUSE	NURSING INTERVENTIONS AND PREVENTION
Allergic Reactions		
Itching	Allergens, medications	Stop infusion immediately.
Runny nose		Ensure patent airway.
Bronchospasm		Notify physician.
Wheezing		Administer antihistamine, steroid, anti-inflammatory, and antipyretic per physician order.
Rash		
Edema at site		Epinephrine is usually administered and can be repeated.
Anaphylactic reaction (within minutes up to an hour after exposure)		Document.
Flushing, chills, anxiety, itching, agitation, ear throbbing, wheezing, coughing, convulsions, and death		*Prevention Techniques:*
		Check client's allergy history.
		Test dose of, e.g., antibiotics.
		Monitor clients in the first 15 minutes of the infusion of a new drug.
Speed Shock		
(Foreign substance-medication is introduced into the vascular system rapidly)	IV administration of medications or fluids at a rapid rate	Ask for assistance.
Dizziness		Notify the physician.
Headache		Administer antidote.
Chest tightness		Administer emergency medications.
Hypotension		Document.
Irregular pulse		*Prevention Techniques:*
Shock		Use microdrop administration sets (60 gtt/mL).
		Use infusion control flow devices.
		Avoid movement of the catheter.
		Monitor piggyback infusion.

the operation. **Designated** blood is blood that is donated by friends and relatives of the client.

The main functions of the cardiovascular system are to deliver oxygenated blood and nutrients to the tissues. This transport system then removes waste substances from the tissues. Objectives for administering a blood transfusion are to:

- Restore and maintain blood volume.
- Improve the oxygen-carrying capacity of the circulatory system.
- Restore and maintain coagulation factors.
- Treat blood deficiencies such as anemia and other hematologic disorders.
- Permit neonatal blood exchange.

Various types of blood or blood components may be transfused (Table 30-6 ■). The client's condition and lab values determine the type of blood required. (See Procedure 30-12 ■.)

TRANSFUSION REACTIONS

Blood transfusions create a significant risk to clients for transfusion reactions (Tables 30-7 ■ and 30-8 ■). The nurse infusing blood products is charged with recognizing adverse signs and symptoms of a transfusion reaction. Implementing immediate action to stop or reverse transfusion reaction effects can be lifesaving. Treat all reactions seriously until proven otherwise. Upon suspicion of a transfusion reaction, stop the transfusion, change the IV tubing, and start a saline solution infusion at a keep-open rate. Do not discard the blood container or administration set; they will be returned to the blood bank. Notify the physician.

TABLE 30-6

Blood/Blood Components

COMPONENT	INDICATOR	NURSING INTERVENTIONS
Whole blood (500 mL) Composed of RBCs, plasma, WBCs, and platelets	To restore blood volume, most whole blood is broken down into three components.	Rarely transfused today Use 20-gauge catheter or larger for infusion Rate is 2–4 hours Whole blood requires type and crossmatching and must be ABO identical
Red Blood Cells (250–300 mL)	Improve oxygen-carrying capacity in symptomatic anemia Increase RBC mass Hemoglobin/hemocrit (H/H) values Client symptoms Blood loss Surgical procedures with blood loss of >1200 mL	Determine severity of anemia and whether diet or vitamins could be an alternative Assess client's age, presence of cardiopulmonary or vascular problems Administer over 1–3 hours; never exceed 4 hours Use 16- to 20-gauge catheter Check vital signs
Leukocyte-reduced RBCs (Poor RBCs) (200 mL)	Prevention of febrile, nonhemolytic transfusion reactions Client with multiple transfusions (e.g., with leukemia or hemophilia)	Use Pall filter Infuse over 1½ to 4 hours Administer same as whole blood and PRBCs Watch for hypotension
Platelets (50–500 mL) Responsible for hemostasis Lives up to 12 days in blood Fragmented cells without nuclei, hemoglobin and are unable to reproduce. Normal platelet value: 150,000–300,000/μL	Prevent or control bleeding from platelet deficiencies Platelet counts <10,000/μL Thrombocytopenia Acute leukemia Control active bleeding with platelet counts of <50,000 μL Prophylactic with massive blood transfusions Prophylactic with cardiopulmonary bypass	Transfusions can be repeated every 1–3 days Rapid transfusion Usual rate 5–10 min Effectiveness can be altered if fever, infection, or active bleeding present Use filter Pooled platelets should be transfused within 4 hours
Plasma and fresh frozen plasma (FFP) (200–250 mL)	*Plasma:* Replace plasma proteins *FFP:* Provide replacement coagulation factors (V, XI) Client with multiple coagulation factor deficiencies secondary to liver disease, DIC Coumarin drug reversal Thrombotic thrombocytopenia purpura	*Plasma:* Infusion rate: 220 mL/h Medications/diluents never added to plasma *FFP:* Infusion rate: 1–2 hours PT > 19 or PTT > 53 Must be thawed prior to infusion, about 30 min ABO compatibility
Cryoprecipitate (5–20 mL/unit volumes) Factor VIII Made from insoluble portion of plasma	Factor I, VIII, XIII, and von Willebrand factor deficiency Hypofibrinogenemia Uremic clients to control bleeding	Rate 1–2 mL/min ABO compatible Use 170 micron filter Rapid transfusion Must be thawed prior to transfusion Units are usually pooled
Recombinant Factor VIII Recombinant DNA technology	Hemophilia Factor VIII or IX deficiency	Bolus infusion Store in refrigerator Allergic reactions
Albumin 5%–25% (50–250 mL) Colloid volume expander Heat treated to prevent viral activation and hepatitis free Equal volume to plasma	Increase plasma volume Hypovolemic shock from trauma or surgery Support blood pressure Induce diuresis	Supplied in glass bottles Use within 4 hours of opening No filters not required Rapid infusion Watch for fluid overload

TABLE 30-7

Transfusion Reactions

REACTIONS	CAUSE	SIGNS AND SYMPTOMS/NURSING INTERVENTIONS
Acute hemolytic transfusion reaction	Hemolysis occurs when antibodies in plasma attach to antigens on the donors RBCs.	Tachycardia, tachypnea, burning sensations along the vein, flushing, bleeding, low back, flank pain. Vascular collapse, shock, death *Nursing Interventions:* Stop transfusion. Treat shock. Maintain blood pressure. Administer diuretics as ordered. Monitor urine output. Prepare for potential dialysis. Obtain urine/blood samples required with a transfusion reaction. Document.
Delayed hemolytic reaction	Occurs as a consequence to RBC destruction by alloantibodies. Immunogenicity. Previous immunization through pregnancy.	Lowered H/H, low-grade fever, jaundice, malaise *Nursing Interventions:* Treatment is nonspecific. Monitor H/H. Monitor renal function.
Allergy reaction	Recipient has sensitivity to donor's plasma proteins.	Rash, hives, itching, facial flushing, runny eyes and nose, anxiety, dyspnea, and wheezing *Nursing Interventions:* Stop transfusion. Treat with antihistamine per order. Restart transfusion slowly if a mild reaction. Monitor vital signs. Mild reactions can precede major allergic reactions.
Circulatory overload	Rapid blood administration; the body is unable to make adjustment to fluid load.	Cough, dyspnea, hypertension, pulmonary congestion/edema, hypervolemia, neck vein distention, and chest constriction *Nursing Interventions:* Stop transfusion. Elevate head of bed. Administer diuretics. Administer oxygen. Notify physician. Collect blood and urine specimens.
Febrile nonhemolytic reaction	Client has sensitivities to leukocyte, platelet, or protein antigens; bacterial contamination.	Fever, chills, headache, nausea and vomiting, chest pain, cough, and malaise *Nursing Interventions:* Stop transfusion. Monitor vital signs. Administer antipyretic per order. Notify physician. Restart transfusion slowly.
Anaphylactic transfusion reaction	Occurs when donor blood with IgA proteins is transfused into an IgA-deficient recipient who has developed an IgA antibody.	Anxiety, urticaria, wheezing, hypotension, shock, cardiac arrest or death *Nursing Interventions:* Stop transfusion. Resuscitate with CPR. Maintain blood pressure. Monitor vital signs. Administer steroids per order. Administer IV fluids.

TABLE 30-8		
Transfusion Complications		
COMPLICATIONS	**CAUSE**	**SIGNS AND SYMPTOMS/NURSING INTERVENTIONS**
Hepatitis B/C	Viral infection; is spread by blood and serum. Incubation is 90 days.	Anorexia, dark urine, increased liver enzymes, jaundice, pharyngitis *Nursing Interventions:* Treat symptomatically. Encourage client to rest. Prevent transmission to others.
Graft versus host disease	Recipient reacts to donor lymphocytes; T lymphocytes are activated and proliferate, attacking the host tissue cells. Client is immunocompromised.	Fever, diarrhea, rash, and hepatitis *Nursing Interventions:* Treat symptomatically. Realize that morbidity is high. Use leukocyte reducing filter. Use irradiated blood.
HIV-1	Viral infection is transmitted by bodily secretions from HIV-positive individual.	Flulike symptoms, six stages of Walter Reed classification system, chronic fungal and viral infections *Nursing Interventions:* Realize there is no cure. Treat symptomatically. Follow CDC Standard Precautions.
Hyperkalemia (potassium toxicity)	Occurs most often in multiple transfusions. Potassium is released into blood during RBC destruction.	EKG changes, bradycardia, muscle twitching, asystole, diarrhea, oliguria to anuria to renal failure *Nursing Interventions:* Stop or slow transfusion. Notify physician. Monitor EKG and potassium levels. Remove excess potassium.
Sepsis	Occurs when blood is contaminated.	Febrile, chills, nausea and vomiting, diarrhea, hypotension, shock *Nursing Interventions:* Stop transfusion. Return blood container and tubing to the blood bank. Obtain blood culture. Administer antibiotics, fluid, steroids, and vasopressors as ordered.

Monitor vital signs and remain with the client. Notify the blood bank and laboratory because urine and blood samples will need to be obtained. Verify labels on blood containers with corresponding client identifications. Document time of the reaction, data, nursing interventions, including vital signs, specimens sent, treatment, and the client's response. Many facilities require a transfusion reaction report form.

IV Rate Calculations

IV rates can be calculated in a variety of ways. The infusion rate of the IV solution passes through the drip chamber and is regulated by the drip chamber. Drip factors vary by manufacturer and are found on the administration set box (Box 30-6 ■). When the physician writes an IV therapy order it includes type of solution, quantity of infusate, the time frame for administration, and, depending on the facility, the milliliters per hour. The flow rate is regulated by the nurse manually or by an electronic infusion device.

The nurse is responsible for the regulation of flow rates by determining the infusion time or the total hours to be infused. Calculating milliliters per hour, and drops per minute. The nurse adjusts the rate by using the roller clamp on the tubing and counting the drops per minute. Hold the watch up to the drip chamber at eye level to count the drops manually for 1 minute. The nurse may also set the infusion

BOX 30-6

Drop Factors

INFUSION ADMINISTRATION SETS	gtt/mL
Standard sets (macrodrip)	10
	15
	20
Minidrip (microdrip; pediatric drip)	60
Buretrol set	60
Blood administration set	10
	6

rate on an electronic infusion device; see the following standard formula:

$$\frac{\text{Amount of fluid (in mL)} \times \text{drop factor}}{\text{Time to infuse in minutes}} = \text{drops per minute}$$

Problem: 1,000 mL of D₅W is to run over 8 hours with a drip factor of 10. What are the drops per minute?

$$\frac{\text{Amount of fluid } (\mathbf{1,000\ mL}) \times \text{drop factor } (\mathbf{10})}{\text{Time to infuse in minutes } (\mathbf{8\ hours})}$$
$$= \text{drops per minute}$$

Determine the fluid per hour: **1,000 mL** divided by **8 hours** = **125 mL**. Time to infuse is now 60 minutes or 1 hour.

$$\frac{\text{Amount of fluid } (\mathbf{125\ mL}) \times \text{drop factor } (\mathbf{10})}{\text{Time to infuse in minutes } (\mathbf{60\ min})}$$
$$= \text{drops per minute}$$

$$\frac{125 \times 10}{60} = \text{gtt/mL}$$

$$\frac{125 \times 1}{6} = 21\ \text{gtt/mL}$$

Here is a shorter, more practical method:

$$\frac{60\ (\text{minutes})}{\text{Drop factor}}$$

The drop factor divided into 60 will give a number to be divided into the milliliters per hour. If the milliliters per hour rate is known, it is easy to find the drops per minute. The infusion time in hours divided into the amount to be infused gives milliliters per hour.

Problem: IV infusion of D₅LR 1,000 mL to run at 125 mL/h. The drop factor is 20 gtt/mL. What is the rate in gtt/min?

$$60 \div 20 = 3$$
$$125 \div 3 = 41.6 \text{ or } 42\ \text{gtt/minute (round off to the nearest whole number)}$$

Intravenous medications are not typically given by the LPN/LVN by secondary lines, push, or bolus. Check your state's nurse practice act for scope of practice.

NURSING PROCESS CARE PLAN
Client with Dehydration

Margaret Greene is an 80-year-old woman living in an assisted living facility, but being for the most part self-sufficient. Her nurse's aide found her in her apartment very confused, still in her pajamas at 2:00 P.M. She told the aide that she had been throwing up and not able to keep anything down since last night. The aide tried to get some fluids down her but she refused. When the aide attempted to get some vital signs she became combative, which was unusual for this very gentle woman.

Assessment. VS: T 100.6, P 58 weak, R 24, BP 88/50. Client's skin is dry, skin turgor is tented. UA and C&S specimen were obtained and sent to the lab; urine was dark and concentrated. A serum blood BUN and H/H were also obtained. Ms. Greene continues to be confused but is taking sips of water. IV of D₅W at 100 mL/h placed per paramedics on transfer to the hospital.

Nursing Diagnosis. The following important nursing diagnoses (among others) are established for this client:

- *Deficient Fluid Volume* related to fluid loss related to vomiting
- *Confusion* related to dehydration

Expected Outcomes

- Adequate hydration will be achieved.
- Confusion will dissipate with adequate hydration.
- Skin turgor will be improved.
- Electrolytes will return to balanced state.

Planning and Implementation

- Orient client to time, place, and surroundings.
- Monitor IV fluids and oral intake.
- Monitor electrolyte, BUN, and hematocrit lab values.
- Avoid fluid overload.
- Keep accurate intake and output records.
- Weigh client every day.
- Assess for skin turgor in the elderly over the sternum or forehead. (Skin elasticity is retained in this area in the elderly.)
- Monitor temperature. (Temperature may not appear elevated as the elderly client's normal body temperature is often degrees lower than that of a younger person.)

Evaluation. Ms. Greene is less disoriented and confused. IV infusion replaced lost fluids; I&O is balanced. Client is taking clear liquids at least 50%. Urine is yellow, straw colored.

Critical Thinking in the Nursing Process

1. Describe the difference between isotonic solutions and hypotonic solutions. Which solutions are used in the treatment of dehydration?
2. What symptoms might Ms. Greene exhibit if she is becoming overhydrated? What nursing implications are indicated?

3. Calculate drops per minute for an IV of D_5W to run at 100 mL/h with a drop factor of 15.

Note: Discussion of Critical Thinking questions appears in Appendix I.

Note: The references and resources for this and all chapters have been compiled at the back of the book.

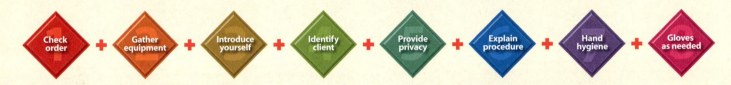

| PROCEDURE 30-1 | **Using a Volume Control Set** |

Purposes

- To deliver limited amounts of medications or solution
- To monitor fluids for pediatric and critically ill clients
- To deliver intermittent administration of measured volumes of fluid with a calibrated chamber

Equipment

- IV solution
- Volume control administration set
- Extension tubing if desired
- Medication syringe (for RN's use)
- Antimicrobial swab
- Label

Check order + Gather equipment + Introduce yourself + Identify client + Provide privacy + Explain procedure + Hand hygiene + Gloves as needed

Interventions

1. Add extension tubing to the volume control unit if necessary.
2. Close slide/roller clamps.
3. Open the air vent located on the top of the volume chamber.
4. Hang the IV solution and remove the plastic cap for insertion.
5. Remove the plastic covering from the spike. *Keep fingers below the flange to avoid contamination of the spike.*
6. Insert the spike into the IV bag.
7. Open the upper roller clamp that is between the IV bag and volume control set. Fill the chamber to about one-third full (Figure 30-11 ■).
8. Close the upper roller clamp.
9. Open the lower clamp and squeeze the drip chamber under the volume control set to about one-half full.
10. Prime the rest of the tubing and close the clamp.
11. Attach the tubing to the IV catheter site and begin infusion.
12. Medication infusion (**RN responsibility and scope**)
    a. Swab injection port located on top of the volume control chamber with an antimicrobial solution. *The applicable INS standard indicates that injection access ports should be aseptically cleansed with an approved antimicrobial solution immediately before use.*
    b. Instill previously prepared medication into chamber and gently mix medication with IV solution.
    c. If further dilution is needed, add more IV solution to the chamber.
    d. Open the clamp below the IV chamber and adjust the prescribed drip rate.

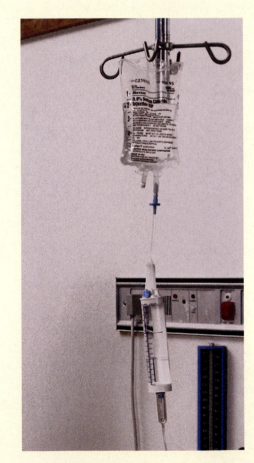

Figure 30-11. ■ Buretrol.

    e. Label the volume control chamber and include the client's name, medication, dose, and the time the medication was started.

Note: A volume control set may also be referred to as a metered-volume chamber or buretrol.

SAMPLE DOCUMENTATION

[date]   Initiated first dose Kefzol 1 g in 50 mL of D$_5$ NS per physician order. Client tolerated
[time]   well no complaints noted.
_____ M. Dedio, LVN

Note: This may be documented in the medication administration record (MAR) or IV therapy record rather than in the nurse narrative note.

PROCEDURE 30-2 | # Preparing an Intravenous Solution

Purposes

- To maintain fluid and electrolyte balance
- To maintain daily nutritional requirements
- To restore and replace fluid losses

Equipment

- Infusate/IV solution in a bag (*Some glass bottles are used today for infusing certain medications.*)

- Primary administration tubing set
- Add-on particulate filter (*used according to facility policy*)
- Electronic infusion device or free-standing IV pole for gravity infusion
- Needleless Luer lock cannula
- Tubing date sticker
- Time strip

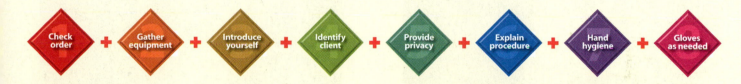

Check order + Gather equipment + Introduce yourself + Identify client + Provide privacy + Explain procedure + Hand hygiene + Gloves as needed

Interventions

1. Remove outer plastic wrap by tearing at the precut tab. *There may be condensation on the bag and it may be wet.*

2. Examine bag carefully for any tears or leaks. Inspect the bag for discoloration, cloudiness, or particulate matter. *Evidence of change may indicate contamination. If contaminated, the bag must be discarded per facility policy.*

3. Hang the bag on the IV pole and affix the time strip (Figure 30-12 ■). *Avoid using a felt pen to write on the IV bag, the ink may leak through to the solution.*

4. Close the roller/slider clamp on the administration set (Figure 30-13 ■).

5. Remove the plastic cover on the tubing spike and the plastic protector on the bag port (Figure 30-14 ■).

6. While squeezing the drip chamber, insert the spike into the bag port (Figure 30-15 ■). *Squeezing the drip chamber prevents air from entering the bag. Keep fingers below the flange to avoid contamination of the spike.*

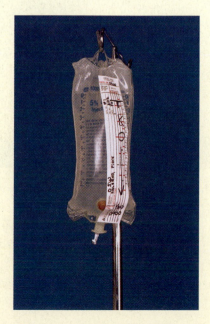

Figure 30-12. ■ IV time strip/bag suspended.

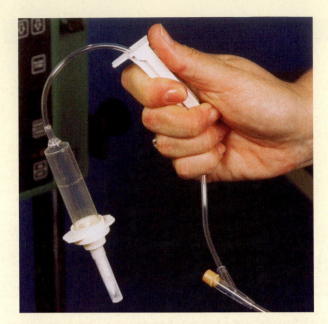

Figure 30-13. ■ Close to clamp.

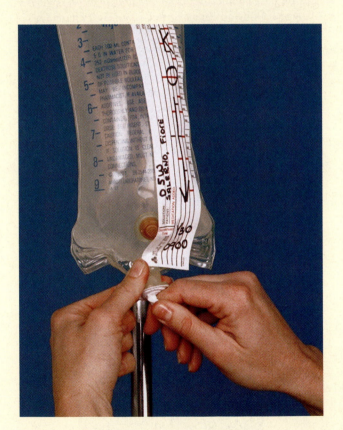

Figure 30-14. ■ Remove plastic protector on the IV tubing spike.

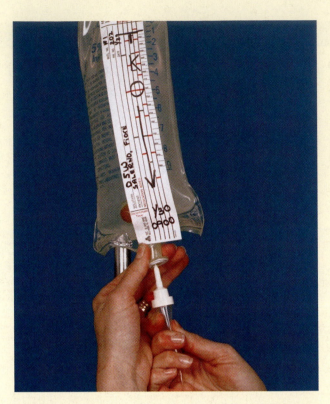

Figure 30-15. ■ Insert tubing spike while squeezing the drip chamber.

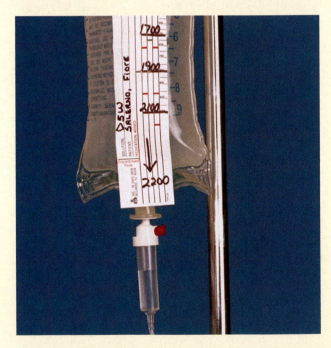

Figure 30-16. ■ Drip chamber partially full.

7. Release pressure to the drip chamber until it is half full of fluid (Figure 30-16 ■). *The drip chamber allows the monitoring of solution delivery.*

8. Attach add on terminal filter when indicated (Figure 30-17 ■). *Filters reduce risk of infection or particulate contamination.*

9. Remove the protective cover at the end of tubing. Open the roller/slider clamp and prime/purge the tubing and filter of air. Hold the tubing tip at a higher level than the tubing loop while priming (Figure 30-18 ■). *Air rises and will pass out of the tubing as the fluid purges the tubing.*

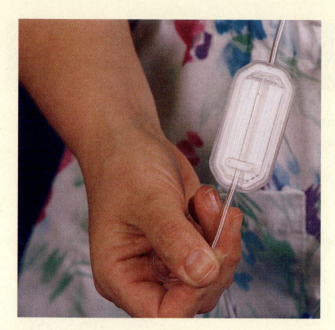

Figure 30-17. ■ Filter.

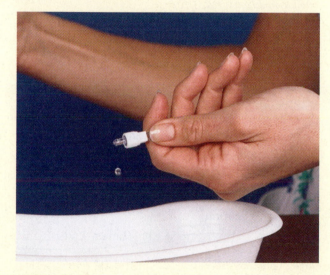

Figure 30-18. ■ Priming tubing.

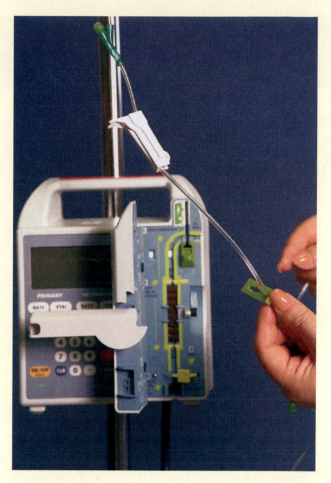

Figure 30-19. ■ Close tubing clamp when priming complete.

13. Attach sticker with date of tubing use. *To maintain consistency of tubing changes according to the facility's policy. INS standards recommend that primary tubing be changed every 72 hours or upon suspicion of contamination or compromise.*

14. Load administration set into the electronic device according to the manufacturer's directions. *Most devices require their tubing be used with detailed loading instructions.*

SAMPLE DOCUMENTATION

[date]
[time]
IV infusion of D₅W 1,000 mL at 125 mL per hour initiated with #22 ONC to the left hand. IV site is clean and dry without evidence of erythema or edema. Client tolerated procedure well; no complaints of pain at the site.
_____ C. Porter, LVN

---

10. Invert and tap Y injection ports to remove air bubbles as the tubing is primed. *Follow directions included in the administration set for priming pump cassettes. Careful air removal from the tubing prevents air embolism and supports administration set function.*

11. Hold filter (if attached) downward, allowing it to fill halfway and then invert the filter to complete the priming process. Tap the filter to remove air out of the filter as it primes.

12. Close the roller clamp when priming is complete. Attach the needleless cannula on the end of the tubing (Figure 30-19 ■). *Maintain sterility before infusion is initiated. Needleless connections protect against needle sticks.*

Changing IV Solution Containers

Purposes

- To follow physician orders for a change in IV solution
- To continue the prescribed regimen for IV therapy with the next solution

Equipment

- IV solution

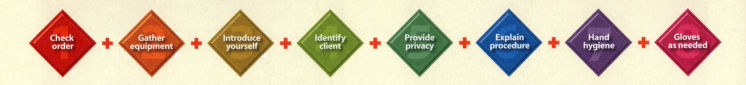

Check order + Gather equipment + Introduce yourself + Identify client + Provide privacy + Explain procedure + Hand hygiene + Gloves as needed

Interventions

1. Remove outer plastic wrap by tearing at the precut tab. *There may be condensation on the bag and it may be wet.*

2. Examine bag carefully for any tears or leaks. Inspect the bag for discoloration, cloudiness, or particulate matter. *Evidence of change may indicate contamination. If contaminated, the bag must be discarded per facility policy.*

3. Hang the new IV container on the IV pole.

4. Remove the protective cap or tear the tab from the tubing insertion port. *Follow the manufacturer's direction to expose the insertion site of the IV bag.*

5. Slide the flow clamp closed on the administration set or close the roller clamp proximal to the IV bag.

6. Remove the current IV solution from the IV pole.

7. With one hand on the bag and one hand on the spike under the flange, loosen the spike from the IV solution. *Keep fingers below the flange to avoid contamination of the spike.*

8. While squeezing the drip chamber, insert the spike into the new bag port. *Squeezing the drip chamber prevents air from entering the bag.* Release pressure to the drip chamber until it is half full of fluid. *The drip chamber allows the monitoring of solution delivery.*

9. Open the slide/roller clamp and regulate the fluid rate as prescribed by physician order.

SAMPLE DOCUMENTATION

[date]
[time]   IV container changed from D$_5$W to LR 1,000 mL at 125 mL per hour per physician order. IV is infusing with no evidence of redness or edema.

_____ K. James, LVN

Note: This may be recorded on the IV therapy flow sheet or I&O form in the client's chart rather than in narrative form in the nurse's notes.

PROCEDURE 30-4 | # Changing IV Tubing

Purposes

- To change IV tubing every 72 hours as recommended by INS
- To maintain asepsis and Standard Precautions at all times

Equipment

- Gloves
- Administration set
- 2 × 2 sterile gauze
- Time strip
- IV tubing label
- Infusate/IV solution in a bag

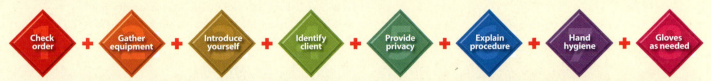

Check order ✚ Gather equipment ✚ Introduce yourself ✚ Identify client ✚ Provide privacy ✚ Explain procedure ✚ Hand hygiene ✚ Gloves as needed

Interventions

1. Follow directions in Procedure 30-2, steps 1 through 13. *Changing IV tubing is normally done when the next IV solution is due.*

2. Determine the condition of the IV site. Observe for signs of redness, phlebitis, or infiltration. *The INS standard indicates that a peripheral short catheter should be removed every 72 hours and immediately when phlebitis, infiltration, or contamination to the site is suspected.*

3. Explain to the client the reason for changing the IV tubing. *Explaining the procedure to the client gives him or her information to enlist compliance and cooperation.*

4. Apply clean gloves.

5. Loosen tape that is securing the existing tubing to the catheter.

6. Clamp off the existing IV and remove it from the electronic monitoring device.

7. Open the 2 × 2 package, maintaining sterility.

8. Tear off tape strips to be used to secure tubing.

9. Detach the IV tubing. *Make sure the IV catheter is stabilized by gently twisting the tubing to loosen it. Put the 2 × 2 gauze under the IV site to contain any drops from the IV disconnection.*

10. Attach the new IV tubing to the catheter. *Twist the end of the new IV tubing into the catheter to lock into place.*

11. Retape the tubing securely.

12. Attach sticker with date of tubing change (Figure 30-20 ■). *To maintain consistency of tubing changes according to the facility's policy. INS standards recommend that primary tubing be changed every 72 hours or upon suspicion of contamination or compromise.*

13. Load administration set into the electronic device according to the manufacturer's directions. *Most devices require their tubing be used with detailed loading instructions.*

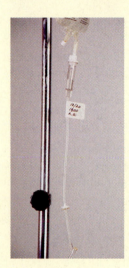

Figure 30-20. ■ IV bag with label.

SAMPLE DOCUMENTATION

[date]
[time]
IV tubing changed with #3 bag of D₅ 1/2NS at 100 mL per hour. IV site is clean and dry, no evidence of redness or edema.

_____ B. Jones, L.V.N.

Note: Tubing change can be noted on the IV therapy flow sheet or I&O form in the client's chart rather than in narrative form in the nurse's notes.

PROCEDURE 30-5   Changing a Central Line Dressing

Purposes

- To protect the central line catheter from contamination
- To prevent the central line catheter from becoming displaced
- To provide a visual means to observe the central line site

Equipment

- Betadine (povidone-iodine) swabs (3)
- Alcohol swabs (3)
- Central line dressing kit (optional)

- Transparent semipermeable dressing
- Precut sterile drain gauze (optional)
- Tape
- Receptacle for soiled dressing
- Clean gloves
- Sterile gloves
- Face mask (2)
- Sterile long-sleeved gown (check facility policy)
- Skin preparation/tincture of benzoin (check facility policy)

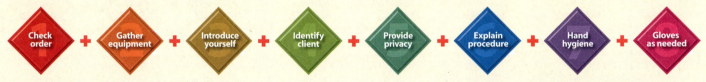

Check order ✚ Gather equipment ✚ Introduce yourself ✚ Identify client ✚ Provide privacy ✚ Explain procedure ✚ Hand hygiene ✚ Gloves as needed

Interventions

1. Explain the procedure to the client. *Giving instructions to the client prior to the procedure will prepare the client and encourage his or her cooperation during the procedure.*

2. Assist the client to a comfortable position while providing the client with privacy.

3. Expose the central line site. Apply a face mask. Assist the client to apply a mask if tolerated or ask the client to turn the head away from the central line dressing site. *This decreases the airborne risk of infection.*

4. Prepare the equipment needed. Open sterile supplies (Figure 30-21 ■).

5. Apply clean gloves and gently remove the soiled dressing and adhesive from the skin. Start at the edges of the dressing and work toward the insertion site (Figure 30-22 ■). Do not touch catheter insertion site. *Careful removal will prevent the central line catheter from being tugged or displaced.*

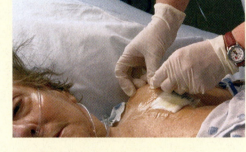

Figure 30-22. ■ Remove old dressing.

6. Discard the soiled dressing in the proper disposal receptacle. Remove clean gloves (Figure 30-23 ■).

7. Observe the site for signs and symptoms of infection, inflammation, and infiltration (Figure 30-24 ■). Examine the site for loose sutures, drainage, and odor. Inspect the skin for changes and assess the length of the catheter.

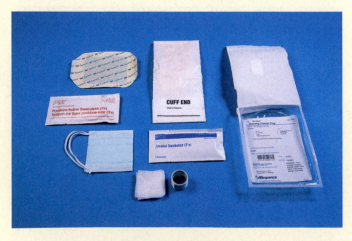

Figure 30-21. ■ Central dressing equipment.

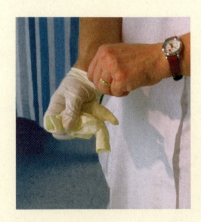

Figure 30-23. ■ Remove gloves.

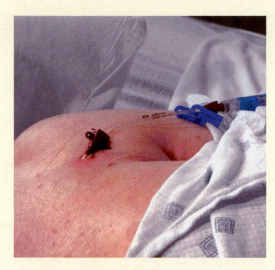

Figure 30-24. ■ Inspect insertion site.

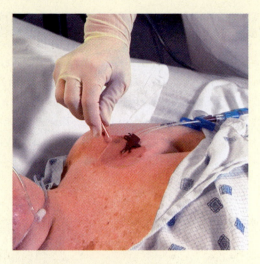

Figure 30-26. ■ Cleanse insertion site.

Abnormal findings must be documented and the physician notified. A culture of the drainage may be necessary.

8. Apply sterile gloves (Figure 30-25 ■). Cleanse the insertion site with three alcohol swabs in a circular motion working from the catheter insertion site outward 4 to 6 in. and allow the skin to dry (Figure 30-26 ■). Discard the swabs after each wipe. Repeat this same procedure with the three Betadine (povidone-iodine) swabs and allow the skin to dry. *Cleaning from the insertion site outward prevents contamination.*

9. Apply the precut sterile gauze dressing around the catheter. *The gauze is used to absorb exudate in the first 24 hours following the insertion of the catheter. Check facility policy with regards to using gauze dressing.*

10. Tincture of Benzoin or a skin preparation can be applied to the skin and allowed to dry. *The skin preparation protects the skin and promotes adhesion of the dressing.*

11. Apply a transparent semipermeable dressing (Figure 30-27 ■). *This type of dressing allows easy visualization of the site and skin. It allows gas exchange but is impermeable to fluids and*

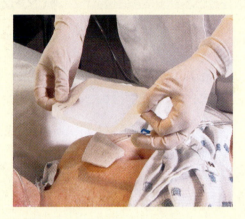

Figure 30-27. ■ Sterile transparent dressing.

microorganisms. Dressing changes may vary according to the facility. The INS recommends dressing changes at routine intervals. Most facilities require central line changes every 72 to 96 hours and immediately if the dressing becomes wet or is leaking.

12. Secure the catheter tubing. *Looping the tubing and taping it securely prevents pulling on the catheter and potential dislodgement of the catheter.*

13. Label the dressing with the date, time and the initials of the nurse performing the dressing change (Figure 30-28 ■).

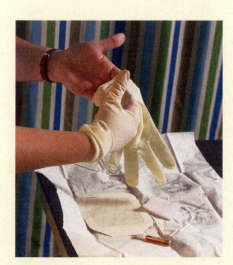

Figure 30-25. ■ Apply sterile gloves.

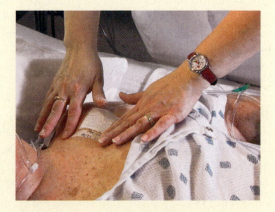

Figure 30-28. ■ Label dressing with date and initial.

SAMPLE DOCUMENTATION

[date]   The central line dressing to the left upper chest area was changed using sterile
[time]   technique. The insertion site is reddened at the suture area. Nursing will monitor for
increased redness to the suture site. No drainage, edema, or odor noted. TSM applied
and secured in place. The client tolerated the procedure without pain or complaints.
_____ Nellie Nguyen, LVN

PROCEDURE 30-6   # Setting the IV Flow Rate

Purposes

- To accurately set the prescribed IV rate
- To maintain fluid and electrolyte balance
- To maintain and restore fluid losses

Equipment

- Infusion device or pump
- IV administration set (compatible with device)
- Gloves
- Needleless cannula
- Tubing label

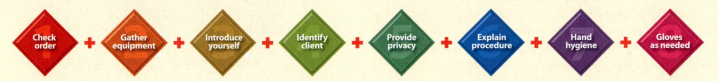

Check order + Gather equipment + Introduce yourself + Identify client + Provide privacy + Explain procedure + Hand hygiene + Gloves as needed

Interventions

1. Follow the steps found in Procedure 30-2 for preparing intravenous solution. *Use the correct administrative set for the infusion device being utilized. Most pumps have dedicated tubing and require a specific method to load the machine. If using tubing with a cassette follow the manufacturer's instructions for priming the line.*

2. Explain to the client about the purpose of the infusion controller/pump, the various sounds and sensitivity of the machine. Include when to notify the nurse if the alarm sounds. Inform the client that it runs on batteries when unplugged allowing for the client to be mobile. *Providing instruction regarding the equipment will promote client cooperation.*

   Continue for controller infusion. For pump infusion, go to page 703 and continue at #3.

CONTROLLER INFUSION

3. Affix the controller to the IV pole and connect to the electrical outlet. *This device is less commonly used today. The function depends on gravity flow.*

4. Attach the eye sensor to the drip chamber above the level of fluid but below the drop opening. Make sure

the photoelectric eye sensor is connected firmly into the controller. *The eye must be able to sense the fluid drop in order to give an accurate rate.*

5. Open the door of the device and insert the IV tubing into the controller. *Follow the manufacturer's instruction.* Close the door to the device and latch the handle.

6. Perform venipuncture or affix tubing to the existing IV catheter. (Follow the steps found in Procedure 30-9 for performing a venipuncture.

7. Open all slide/roller clamps and turn on the power to the controller to initiate infusion.

8. Set the controls on the front of the controller to the appropriate infusion rate and volume. *Setting the volume to 50 to 100 mL less than the total volume gives the nurse time to attach a new bag before the previous bag is depleted.*

9. Count the drops for 15 seconds and multiply by 4 (Figure 30-29 ■). *Verifying the drops per minute ensures the device is working correctly.*

10. Ensure that the volume on the alarm is turned on. *The purpose of the alarm is to alert the nurse that the infusion is not proceeding as scheduled.*

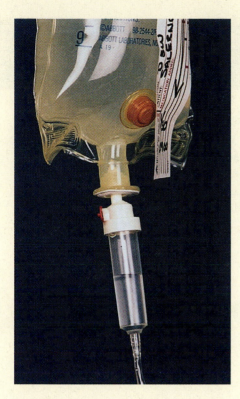

Figure 30-29. ■ Count drips per minute.

11. Monitor the infusion every hour. Assess the volume that has been infused and compare to the time label on the bag. *This intervention will verify that the machine is functioning properly and the client is receiving the correct amount of fluid per hour.*

12. Troubleshoot if the machine alarms. Check:
    a. For kinks in the line
    b. The fluid level in the drip chamber; ensure it is half full allowing the electronic eye to sense the drop
    c. The placement of the electronic eye on the drip chamber
    d. The position of the extremity with IV site can cause the machine to alarm
    e. The rate and volume; verify accuracy
    f. That the IV site is patent and free flowing
    g. That IV tubing slide/roller clamps are open
    h. Fluid in the IV container.

PUMP INFUSION

3. Affix the pump to the IV pole at eye level and connect to the electrical outlet. *This is a positive-pressure infusion, so the solution is delivered by applying pressure to the infusion to maintain the prescribed flow rate. It is extremely beneficial when administering viscous solutions, when the client's activity increases venous back pressure, or when the venipuncture catheter is a small gauge. The device can be placed at any level because it does not rely on gravity to function.*

4. Open the door of the device and insert the IV tubing into the controller. *Follow the manufacturer's instruction. If the tubing has a cassette attached, make sure that the cassette has been completely filled with fluid. It may need to be tilted and tapped to eliminate air bubbles. If air bubbles remain, it may cause the alarm to sound.* Close the door to the device and latch the handle.

5. Perform venipuncture or affix tubing to the existing IV catheter. Follow the steps found in Procedure 30-9 for performing a venipuncture.

6. Open all slide/roller clamps and turn on the power to the controller to initiate infusion.

7. Press the number pad for the prescribed drops per minute or milliliters per hour and push the start button.

8. Ensure that the volume on the alarm is turned on. *The purpose of the alarm is to alert the nurse that the infusion is not proceeding as scheduled.*

9. Monitor the infusion every hour. Assess the volume that has been infused and compare to the time label on the bag. *This intervention will verify that the machine is functioning properly and the client is receiving the correct amount of fluid per hour.*

10. Troubleshoot if the machine alarms. Check:
    a. For kinks in the line
    b. The fluid level in the drip chamber; ensure it is half full allowing the electronic eye to sense the drop
    c. The placement of the electronic eye on the drip chamber
    d. The position of the extremity with an IV, can cause the machine to alarm
    e. The rate and volume; verify accuracy
    f. That the IV site is patent and free flowing
    g. That IV tubing slide/roller clamps are open
    h. Fluid in the IV container.

SAMPLE DOCUMENTATION

[date] [time]	IV initiated with D$_5$W infusing at 125 mL per hour using infusion pump. Venipuncture performed to the right hand with 20-gauge ONC. IV site is clean and dry. Client tolerated procedure well without complaints.
	_____ Y. Yanez, LVN

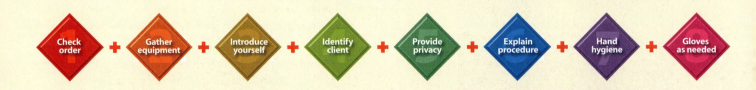

Inserting a Medication Lock

Purposes

- To maintain a venous access for intermittent IV medication infusion
- To increase client's mobility and comfort
- To allow blood collection without repeated venipunctures
- To provide venous access for emergency medication delivery

Equipment

- Medication lock, prn device, or intermittent IV lock
- Needleless syringe
- Normal saline solution vial
- 2 × 2 sterile gauze
- Clean gloves

Check order + Gather equipment + Introduce yourself + Identify client + Provide privacy + Explain procedure + Hand hygiene + Gloves as needed

Interventions

1. Determine the patency of the IV. Observe for signs of redness, phlebitis, or infiltration. *The INS standard indicates that a peripheral short catheter should be removed every 72 hours and immediately when phlebitis, infiltration, or contamination to the site is suspected.* Establish a new line (following the steps in Procedure 30-9 for performing a venipuncture using the ONC procedure) or use the existing line if patent.

2. Explain to the client the reason for an intermittent IV lock.

3. Apply clean gloves.

4. Loosen tape that may be obstructing the insertion of the intermittent device.

5. Clamp off the IV. It may be necessary to disconnect the IV from the electronic monitoring device when converting the existing IV line to an intermittent lock.

6. Open the 2 × 2 gauze package maintaining sterility.

7. Open the intermittent lock package and maintain sterility (Figure 30-30 ■).

8. Detach the IV tubing. *Make sure to stabilize the IV catheter, gently twist the tubing to loosen it. Put the 2 × 2 gauze under the IV site to contain any drops from the IV disconnection.*

9. Attach the lock to the hub of the cannula. *Remove the protective cap. Twist the intermittent lock into place.*

10. Clean the needleless injection port with an antimicrobial swab (Figure 30-31 ■). *The INS standard indicates*

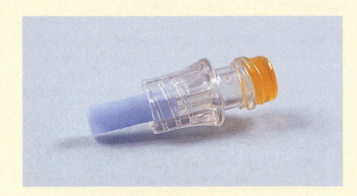

Figure 30-30. ■ Intermittent lock.

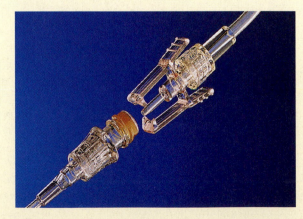

Figure 30-31. ■ Needle-free device. (Photograph reprinted courtesy of (BD) Becton, Dickinson and Company and courtesy of Baxter Healthcare Corporation. All rights reserved.)

that injection access ports should be aseptically cleansed with an approved antimicrobial solution immediately before use.

11. Infuse the saline solution as directed in the facility's procedures.

12. Retape the catheter and intermittent device into place. The chevron or U method is recommended. A protective gauze bandage can be applied such as a stretch netting or a Kerlix dressing.

SAMPLE DOCUMENTATION

[date]
[time]

IV was converted to an intermittent lock. The client was given information as to the purpose of the intermittent lock. The client tolerated the procedure well. The IV site is clean and dry without evidence of redness or edema.

_____ M. Della, LVN

PROCEDURE 30-8   # Applying a Tourniquet

Purposes

- To dilate a vein
- To perform intravenous venipuncture
- To perform phlebotomy

Equipment

- Alcohol swabs
- Blood pressure cuff (optional)

- Clean gloves when inserting IV needle/cannula
- IV insertion kit (optional)
- Tourniquet (flat, soft, 5 cm [2 in.] wide)
- Towel or disposable waterproof pad
- Velcro tourniquet (optional)
- Warm moist towel

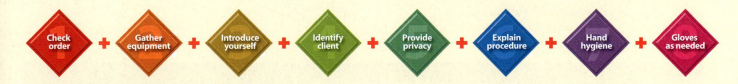

Check order + Gather equipment + Introduce yourself + Identify client + Provide privacy + Explain procedure + Hand hygiene + Gloves as needed

Interventions

1. Assess the condition of the veins. Use a straight, soft, bouncy vein. Avoid previously used veins or area that has been infected or is reddened (graft, fistula, mastectomy, IV site, paralysis). Avoid valves in the veins. *A straight, soft, bouncy vein is easiest to access. Previously used veins and areas of potential infection or compromise all could be difficult to access and may lead to complications. Entering the vein at a valve could cause injury to the valve.*

2. Check that the cannula gauge is appropriate for the client's age and size. *A gauge that is too large may cause unnecessary discomfort and possible damage.*

3. Check the length of therapy and the client's activities. *The length and type of therapy may determine the type of gauge used as well as the client's extremity use.* Determine whether the client is using antithrombotics or anticoagulants. *Clotting time will be delayed in clients using these drugs.*

4. Select the nondominant hand first, unless one of the diseases/conditions listed in step 1 is present. Client preference is accommodated if possible. The most used veins are cephalic and basilic veins. The least used are feet and legs veins. *Use of the nondominant hand usually means the extremity is used less often than the dominant extremity when performing routine ADLs, diminishing movement and pressure to the extremity.*

5. Apply the tourniquet. Avoid rolling of the tourniquet. If it becomes twisted, reapply the tourniquet. Place the

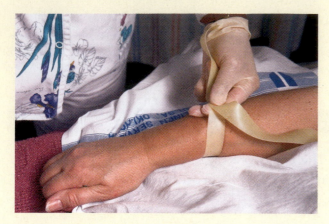

Figure 30-32. ■ Tourniquet applied.

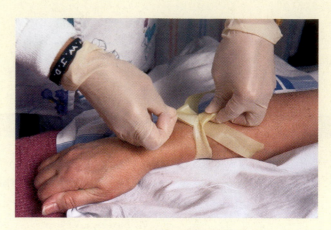

Figure 30-33. ■ Overlap with ends away from the site.

tourniquet flat 15 cm (6 in.) above the planned puncture site. Apply the two ends together; put one end on top of the other. Lift and stretch the tourniquet, then tuck the end on top underneath the tourniquet (Figure 30-32 ■). The tails should be out of the way of the planned site insertion or above the tourniquet (Figure 30-33 ■). Avoid pinching hair or skin. *This distends the vein.*

6. The tourniquet should be snug but avoid occluding the radial pulse. Leave the tourniquet in place for approximately 2 minutes. Observe for color changes or client complaints of a tingling sensation. *Marked darkening of the skin and complaints by the client can signal that tissue is not adequately perfused. Check the radial pulse. If it is absent, reapply the tourniquet.*

7. Have the client open and close his or her fist four to six times. *Opening and closing the fist dilates the vein.*

8. You can gently flick/tap the site or rub alcohol swabs on the skin. Avoid slapping the site. *Alcohol swabs and tapping distend the vein. Slapping will redden the skin and cause discomfort but will not increase the likelihood of finding a vein.*

9. Use your index finger to feel for an insertion site. *The index finger is the most sensitive for palpation.*

10. If you are unable to find an adequate site for insertion, you can place the hand in a dependent position and/or use a warm compress then reapply the tourniquet. *These measures increase blood to the extremity.*

11. Repeat steps 7 through 10.

SAMPLE DOCUMENTATION

See Procedure 30-9.

PROCEDURE 30-9 **Performing Venipuncture**

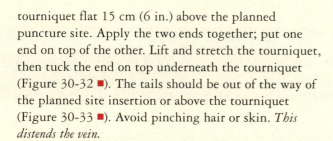

Purposes

- To initiate vascular access for intravenous therapy
- To administer fluids and electrolytes
- To maintain parenteral nutrition
- To administer blood or blood components
- To provide vascular access for intravenous medications

Equipment

- Alcohol swabs
- Blood pressure cuff (optional)
- Clean gloves when inserting IV needle/cannula
- IV insertion kit (optional)

- Tourniquet (flat, soft, 5 cm [2 in.] wide)
- Towel or disposable waterproof pad
- Velcro tourniquet (optional)
- Warm moist towel
- Povidone-iodine wipes
- Scalp vein (butterfly or winged) needle *or* over-the-needle catheter (ONC)
- Prepared IV administration setup (see Procedure 30-2)
- Transparent semipermeable dressing
- Tape
- Armboard (optional)

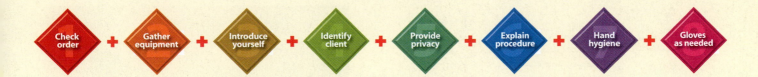

Interventions

1. See applying a tourniquet (Procedure 30-8).

2. Prepare the site with povidone-iodine wipe, use alcohol prep (70%) if the client is allergic to iodine. Allow the preparation to dry completely. *Germicidal action occurs when the skin preparation dries. An antibacterial barrier can decrease risk for infection at the puncture site.*

3. Select appropriate scalp vein/butterfly/winged needle or an ONC device. *A winged needle is used primarily for short-term therapy, usually less than 24 hours. The butterfly needle has low rates of inflammation and phlebitis. The steel needle is not flexible and therefore has a tendency to dislodge or puncture the vein, increasing the risk of infiltration. The ONC is easy to insert and floats in the vein. It is used for long-term therapy; the material used in its manufacture is designed to minimize local reactions.*

   Continue for scalp vein/butterfly/winged needle. For over-the-needle catheter, go to page 709 and continue at #4.

SCALP VEIN/BUTTERFLY/WINGED NEEDLE

4. Attach the end of the IV tubing to end of the scalp vein/butterfly/winged needle tubing.

5. Remove the plastic cover from the butterfly/winged needle and prime the fluid through the needle (Figure 30-34 ■). Clamp the tubing and replace the needle protector.

6. Anchor the vein by pulling the skin taut with the thumb of the nondominant hand beneath the selected site. *Controlling the vein prevents rolling and facilitates needle insertion.*

7. Holding the butterfly/winged needle by the wings with the bevel up, enter the client's skin at a 30-degree

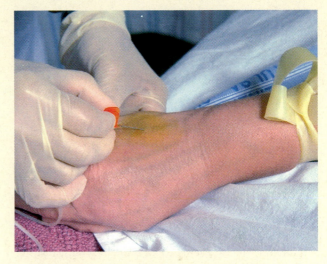

Figure 30-35. ■ Anchor vein and insert at 30-degree angle.

angle (Figure 30-35 ■). Two methods used to enter the vein:

   a. Enter the skin next to or along the vein. Drop the needle to a 15-degree angle and when the needle is under the skin enter the vein.

   b. Insert the needle into the skin below the intended site and directly into the vein. *Using the one-thrust method can result in hematoma formation.*

8. A pop is felt when the vein is entered. Observe for a flashback of blood in the tubing. Follow the course of the vein and advance the needle to the wings.

9. Release the tourniquet.

10. Attach sterile resealable injection cap. Inject normal saline for peripheral saline lock (PSL) (Figure 30-36 ■), or connect to IV tubing. *The injection cap is used to flush the lock or when connecting to the infusion.* Open the roller clamp and monitor

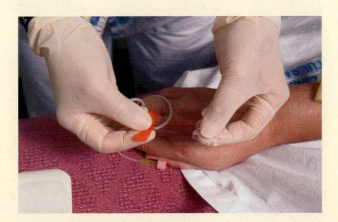

Figure 30-34. ■ Remove winged needle cap.

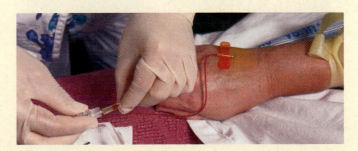

Figure 30-36. ■ Lock attached to butterfly.

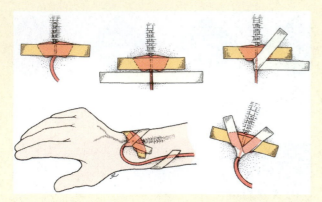

Figure 30-37. ■ Chevron method.

the drip chamber. *The fluid should be free flowing: observe for swelling at the insertion site.*

11. Slow the infusion to a keep-open rate, and secure the needle and tubing to avoid the needle from becoming dislodged. Using ½-inch-wide tape with the adhesive side up under the tubing, cross the tape over the wings (Chevron method) (Figure 30-37 ■). Another taping method is to fold the tape end over the wings, making a U shape securing the needle (Figure 30-38 ■). Place another piece of tape across the wings of the chevron. Avoid adhering tape over the insertion site. *This allows for assessment and access.* Gloves can be removed here or after all taping is completed. *Wash hands if gloves have been removed.*

12. Loop the butterfly/winged needle tubing to the side of the insertion site (Figure 30-39 ■). *Leave enough of a loop so as to avoid kinking the tubing at the wings.*

13. Apply the occlusive semipermeable transparent dressing (Figure 30-40 ■) over the insertion site. A 2 × 2 gauze square, taped occlusively can also be used.

14. Label the dressing with date, time, and initials; include the size of needle used.

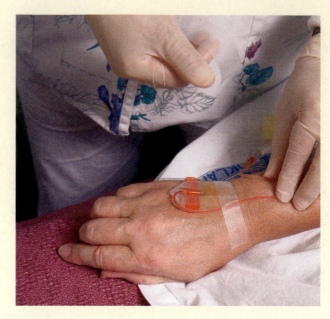

Figure 30-39. ■ Loop tubing and secure.

15. Regulate the infusion rate by pump or calculate the drip rate by gravity flow per minute.

16. Affix armboard to immobilize the hand in a flexion position. *This reduces risk of cannula displacement.*

17. Change IV every 48 to 72 hours. *INS recommends that a peripheral catheter be removed every 72 hours or immediately with suspected contamination or complications. An increased risk of phlebitis and bacteria colonization occuring after 72 hours has been documented.*

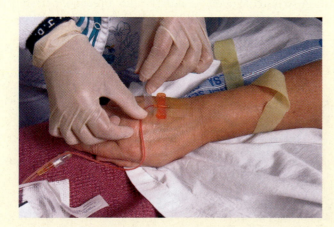

Figure 30-38. ■ Using U shape to tape.

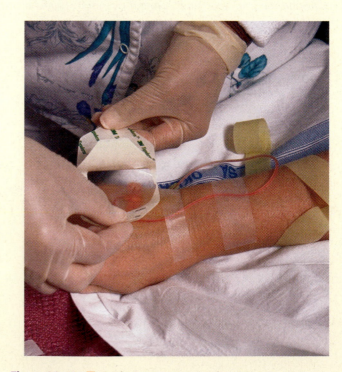

Figure 30-40. ■ Occlusive transparent dressing.

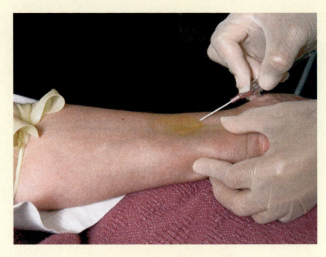

Figure 30-41. ■ Over the ONC, stabilize device.

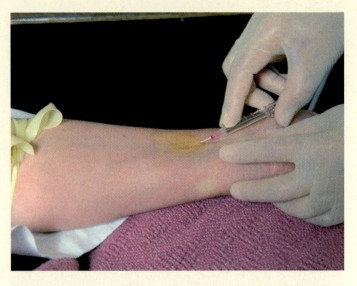

Figure 30-43. ■ After skin insertion, reduce angle and advance.

OVER-THE-NEEDLE CATHETER

4. Position the client's arm or hand. Select the appropriate size ONC for the purpose of the infusion. Open the catheter package and inspect for any product compromise.

5. Anchor the vein by pulling the skin taut with the nondominant thumb.

6. Stabilize the catheter with the needle bevel up and insert into the skin at a 45-degree angle (Figure 30-41 ■). As with the winged needle, the catheter can be inserted along the vein or distal to the site and directly into the vein.

7. Lower the cannula angle to 30 degrees and enter the vein. A pop sensation is usually felt. A backflash of blood will be seen in the plastic hub (Figure 30-42 ■). *A backflash of blood indicates the cannula is in the vein. If no blood is seen and you did not feel the catheter enter the vein, assess the vein's position. You can pull back slightly without exiting the vein and reattempt venipuncture. After two attempts at venipuncture without success, the nurse should notify the charge nurse or team leader for assistance.*

8. Holding onto the needle/stylet, advance only the catheter into the lumen of the vein (Figure 30-43 ■). *By holding onto the needle/stylet there is a decreased risk of puncturing the vein. The catheter slides over the needle/stylet.*

9. Release the tourniquet. Leave the needle/stylet in place while taping the catheter in place. Tape the catheter wings in place and across the body of the catheter. Avoid touching the insertion site and the hub catheter junction to maintain aseptic technique.

10. Apply pressure to the distal end of the catheter and then remove the needle/stylet. *This action prevents blood loss.* If using a needleless catheter, use the button to retract the needle (Figure 30-44 ■).

11. Connect the end of the catheter to the primed administration set or needleless cap.

12. Open the roller clamp and observe the fluid flow in the drip chamber. Monitor the insertion site for signs of infiltration.

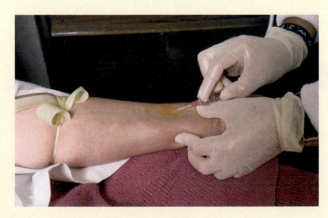

Figure 30-42. ■ Bevel up, blood flash.

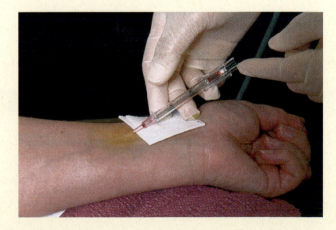

Figure 30-44. ■ Release tourniquet, gauze pad under hub, withdraw stylet, leaving catheter in place.

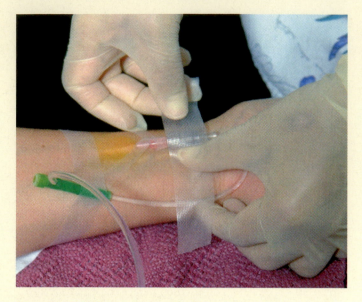

Figure 30-45. ■ Secure cannula with tape using the chevron method.

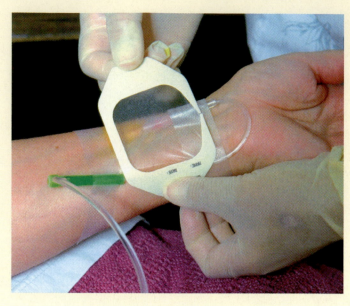

Figure 30-46. ■ Apply transparent dressing over site.

13. Decrease fluid flow and continue taping the catheter using the chevron method (Figure 30-45 ■).

14. Apply the occlusive semipermeable transparent dressing over the insertion site (Figure 30-46 ■). A 2 × 2 gauze square, taped occlusively can also be used.

15. Loop the administration set tubing to the side of the insertion site and secure by taping.

16. Label the dressing with date, time, and initials (Figure 30-47 ■); include the size of needle used.

17. Regulate the infusion rate by pump or calculate the drip rate by gravity flow per minute.

18. Remove gloves and wash hands.

19. Change IV every 48 to 72 hours. *INS recommends that a peripheral catheter be removed every 72 hours or immediately with suspected contamination or complications. An increased risk of phlebitis and bacteria colonization occuring after 72 hours has been documented.*

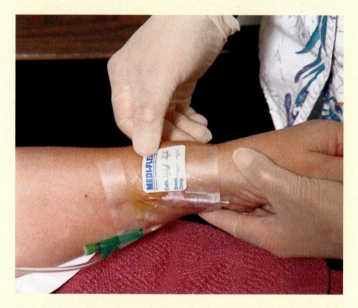

Figure 30-47. ■ Label with initials and date.

SAMPLE DOCUMENTATION

[date]   IV infusion of D$_5$W 1,000 mL at 125 mL per hour initiated with #22 ONC to the left
[time]   hand. IV site is clean and dry without evidence of erythema or edema. Client tolerated
procedure well; no complaints of pain at the site.
_____ C. Porter, LVN

PROCEDURE 30-10 # Assessing and Maintaining an IV Insertion Site

Purposes

- To assess the IV site regularly
- To evaluate for changes in the patency of the system
- To maintain the prescribed infusion rate
- To assess for complications and report to the physician

Equipment

- Clean gloves
- Tape

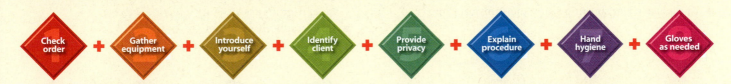

Check order + Gather equipment + Introduce yourself + Identify client + Provide privacy + Explain procedure + Hand hygiene + Gloves as needed

Interventions

1. Explain the procedure to the client and enlist his or her co-operation. *The IV site should be evaluated every 8 hours for complications or more frequently if the client's condition warrants it.*

2. Provide the client with privacy.

3. Check the physician order and the sequence of the IV bags. Compare the IV label name and the client's identification band. *This confirms that the infusion is being given to the right client. If the IV bag and the ID band do not match, slow the IV container to a keep-open rate until corrective action can be implemented. Follow agency policy requiring incident reporting.*

4. Monitor the rate of flow and the volume infused hourly. Check the time strip as to the fluid remaining in the IV bag. *Although electronic devices used to monitor the volume and rate have improved IV therapy, they are not infallible and sometime need adjustment. Ultimately the responsibility lies with the nurse caring for the client. To read the volume remaining in the bag stretch the upper edges of the bag. If the rate is too slow, make adjustments to the predetermined rate. If the rate is too fast, the physician may need to be notified; follow agency policy. Infusing fluid too quickly can lead to fluid overload.*

5. Observe for the patency of the IV tubing and catheter. *Check that the drip chamber is half full and make adjustments if needed. Examine the tubing for kinks and obstructions. The client laying on the tubing can be an impediment to the flow.* If the flow is less than prescribed, lower the IV bag and look for a blood return at the IV site. *A blood return indicates that the needle is intact and properly placed in the vein. Venous pressure is stronger than the fluid pressure in the IV tubing giving a blood return. If no blood is returned, it may indicate that the catheter is no longer placed in the vein or is partially obstructed. Be aware that a soft catheter may not demonstrate a blood return and still be placed properly.*

6. Apply gloves. Palpate the site gently through the transparent dressing. *Note any redness or infiltration at the site. Observe for leakage and determine the cause. It could be a loosening at the catheter hub, in which case, tighten the connection. If that does not stop the leakage, change the tubing. If the flow continues to be less than ordered, adjust the level of the catheter bevel slowly. If by raising the catheter the fluid flow improves place a 2 × 2 gauze under the hub and tape securely. The catheter bevel can be up against the wall of the vein, causing a partial obstruction of the infusate solution or a tendency to be positional.*

7. Check the date on the peripheral IV label. Change the IV to a new proximal site every 72 hours according to facility policy. *INS standards indicate that a peripheral short catheter should be removed every 72 hours and immediately upon suspected contamination.* See Procedure 30-9.

8. Check the date on the administration set and extension tubing. Change every 72 hours according to facility policy. This preventive measure can be routinely done with a new IV bag infusion. *INS standards indicate that primary and secondary administration sets should be changed every 72 hours and immediately upon suspected contamination.*

SAMPLE DOCUMENTATION

[date]	IV of D5LR #2 bag infusing at
[time]	80 mL per hour. IV seems to be
	positional, will monitor for changes.
	IV site to the right hand is clean
	and dry; there is no evidence of
	pain, redness or edema.
	_____ A. Parra, LVN

PROCEDURE 30-11 | **Discontinuing or Terminating IV Therapy**

Purposes

- To replace a compromised cannula
- To change an IV site after 72 to 96 hours (following hospital policy)
- To discontinue or terminate an IV per physician order
- To change an IV infiltration site
- To replace a site showing signs and symptoms of infection
- To discontinue an IV upon discharge of the client
- To discontinue an IV upon placement of a central line that takes over the peripheral function

Equipment

- Clean gloves
- Sterile (2 × 2 or 4 × 4) gauze pads (Avoid use of an alcohol wipe, it promotes stinging and bleeding.)
- Tape or adhesive bandage
- Disposable hazardous waste container

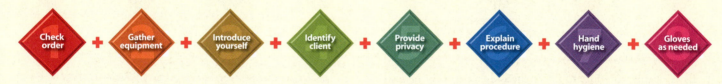

Check order + Gather equipment + Introduce yourself + Identify client + Provide privacy + Explain procedure + Hand hygiene + Gloves as needed

Interventions

1. Turn off the infusate with the slide/roller clamp (Figure 30-48 ■). Gloves optional. *This prevents the fluid from flowing out of the catheter onto the bed or client.*

2. Apply clean gloves. Loosen tape and dressing toward the cannula, while holding the needle or cannula firmly in place (Figure 30-49 ■). Apply countertraction to the skin. Adhesive remover can be used for the client who is particularly sensitive. *Movement of the catheter or cannula can injure the vein and cause the client discomfort. Countertraction prevents pulling the skin and causing discomfort or trauma.*

3. Stabilize the cannula. *Stabilizing the cannula avoids movement that can traumatize the site, causing increased bleeding and pain.*

4. Hold folded gauze over site while removing cannula/needle. Avoid pressure to site until cannula/needle is removed smoothly (Figure 30-50 ■). *Pressure applied prior to cannula removal causes the client discomfort.*

5. Apply gauze pressure to insertion site (Figure 30-51 ■). *Pressure stops bleeding. Avoid the use of an alcohol wipe, it promotes bleeding and causes stinging to the site.* Hold pressure for a few minutes, longer if client is taking antithrombotics/anticoagulants. Do not walk away until bleeding has ceased. *Clotting time will be prolonged in clients using these drugs.* Hold the client's limb above the level of the heart if bleeding persists. *Raising the limb decreases blood flow to the area.*

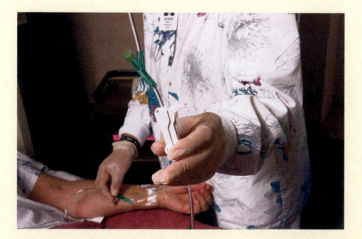

Figure 30-48. ■ Turn off infusion, discontinue IV.

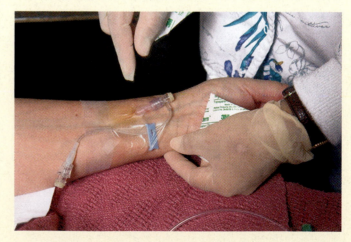

Figure 30-49. ■ Loosen dressing and tape.

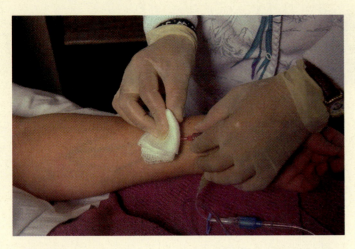

Figure 30-50. ■ Remove needle carefully and smoothly.

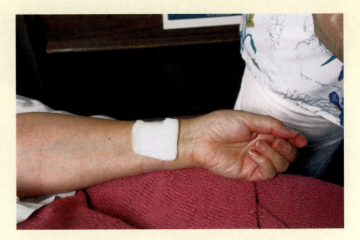

Figure 30-52. ■ Tape gauze into place.

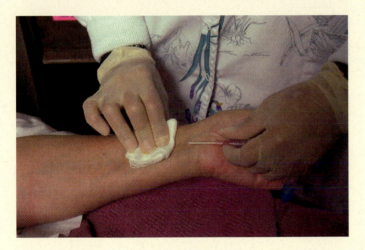

Figure 30-51. ■ Apply pressure to puncture site.

6. Observe for signs of hematoma, redness or swelling. Examine the catheter to make certain that it is intact. *These signs are potential complications of IV insertion. If a piece of the catheter or tubing remains in the client's vein, it could move toward the heart or lungs, causing serious problems. Immediately apply a tourniquet above the insertion site and report it to the physician and charge nurse.*

7. Tape gauze into place or use adhesive bandage (Figure 30-52 ■). *The dressing inhibits microorganisms from entering the open site.*

8. Dispose of equipment and gloves in the appropriate container. *Proper disposal inhibits transmission of microorganisms.*

9. Document pertinent relevant information. Record the cannula size that was removed and document the fluid infused on the intake and output form according to the agency practice. Include the container number, type of solution, time of the IV discontinuance, and the client's response.

SAMPLE DOCUMENTATION

[date]   NS bag #2 and IV discontinued as
[time]   per physician order, cannula
         22 gauge fully intact. Site clean
         and dry; no evidence of further
         bleeding. Pressure dressing ap-
         plied. Client tolerated the proce-
         dure well; no complaints of pain,
         edema, or ecchymosis at the site.
         _____ J. Ian, LVN

Transfusing Blood or Blood Components

Purposes

- To restore or expand blood volume
- To treat blood deficiencies such as anemia and other hematologic disorders
- To improve the oxygen-carrying capacity of the circulatory system

Equipment

- Normal saline solution (NSS), 500 mL
- Blood or component unit
- Y-set blood tubing with filter (170- to 240-micron filter)
- Venipuncture set (if site not established)
- Over-the-needle cannula (ONC), recommended 18–20 gauge or larger (22 gauge for limited transfusions)
- Needleless cannula
- Antimicrobial swabs
- Tape
- Electronic monitoring device designed for blood administration or free-standing IV pole
- Blood warming device (not required for routine transfusions)

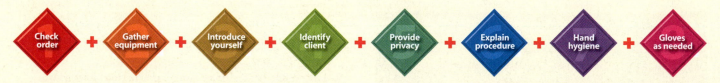

Check order + Gather equipment + Introduce yourself + Identify client + Provide privacy + Explain procedure + Hand hygiene + Gloves as needed

Interventions

1. Verify physician's order. *The physician's order should be specific to the blood/blood components and the duration of transfusion.* Follow the facility's policies and procedures for transfusion therapy.

2. Check client's identification band, and ask client to state his or her name. *INS standards indicate that nurses are responsible for verification of patient identification.*

3. Obtain or check the client's signed transfusion consent form. *INS standards indicate that the nurse is responsible for confirmation of an informed patient consent.*

4. Assess the client's understanding of the purpose of blood transfusion and associated risks. *INS standards specify that nurses are responsible for client education.* Gather information regarding the client's previous blood transfusion response or allergic reactions.

5. Determine that the type and crossmatch has been processed and the blood/blood component is available in the blood bank.

6. Assess the patency of the client's current intravenous therapy. Initiate infusion with NSS 0.9%, using the Y-set blood tubing with filter (Figure 30-53 ■). *Normal saline is an isotonic solution that has an osmolarity equal to that of serum. Hypotonic solutions cause blood cells to burst, resulting in hemolysis, and hypertonic solutions cause blood cells to dilute and shrink. Blood and blood components should be filtered; the minimum pore size of a blood filter is between 170 and 260 microns.* Establish an intravenous line for the transfusion if IV is not available. Follow the steps in Procedure 30-9 for performing a venipuncture using the

ONC procedure with a cannula gauge of 18 to 20. *A cannula size of 18 to 20 gauge is necessary to provide adequate transfusion flow. A 22 gauge can be used for plasma products.*

7. Check the client's pretransfusion vital signs for baseline information. *An existing temperature elevation must be reported to the physician before proceeding.*

8. Obtain the blood or blood component from the blood bank (Figure 30-54 ■). The nurse verifies the blood/blood component bag with the laboratory technician, by checking component type, ABO and Rh, unit number, expiration date, and client identification number. The nurse's and laboratory technician's signatures/initials are required to validate and document that proper procedure has been followed. *Blood/blood component cannot be returned to the blood bank after it has been checked out for 20 minutes. Blood transfusion should be initiated within 30 minutes after being checked out of the blood bank. Blood is refrigerated at 33.6 to 42.8°F (1–6°C) in the blood bank; do not refrigerate blood on the nursing unit. Blood bank refrigerators are carefully monitored for constant control.* Check the blood unit for bubbles, cloudiness, color, and sediment. *These signs indicate bacterial contamination. If these signs are present, return the blood unit immediately and document your observations.*

9. The nurse returns to the unit and will again double check the blood/blood component with another licensed nurse before proceeding (Figure 30-55 ■). The nurse verifies the blood/blood component bag by checking component type, ABO and Rh, unit number, expiration date, and client identification number.

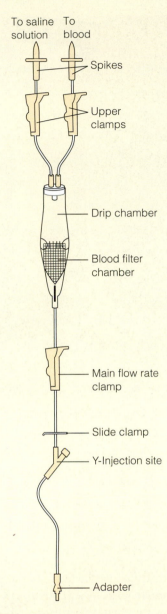

To saline   To
solution   blood

Spikes

Upper
clamps

Drip chamber

Blood filter
chamber

Main flow rate
clamp

Slide clamp

Y-Injection site

Adapter

Figure 30-53. ■ Blood Tubing.

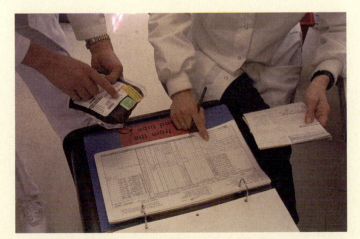

Figure 30-54. ■ Obtain ordered typed and matched blood or blood component bag from blood bank.

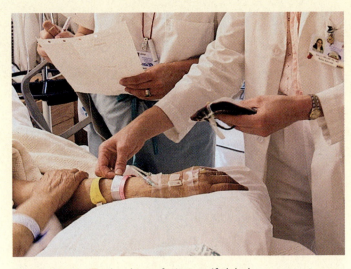

Figure 30-55. ■ Blood transfusion, verify label.

10. Record and document VS 5 minutes prior to initiating blood/blood component bag transfusion. The nurse verifies the client's name, identification number, checking component type, ABO and Rh, unit number, and expiration date at the bedside.

11. Perform hand hygiene and apply clean gloves.

12. Prime tubing with NSS then close all clamps on the Y-set tubing (Figure 30-56 ■). Once the tubing has been primed attach the needleless cannula.

13. Remove the protective covering on the bag port and spike the blood bag with the Y-set. Open the clamps to the blood. Prime the tubing with blood/blood component. Agitate the blood/blood component bag. *This facilitates the mixing of blood with the anticoagulant additive in the bag.*

14. Initiate the blood transfusion slowly, it is recommended to start with 5 mL/min for the first 15 minutes of the transfusion. *Slowing the administration allows the nurse time to observe for adverse blood transfusion reactions (Figure 30-57 ■). Blood/blood component should be infused within 4 hours. Packed cells are routinely infused within 1½ to 2 hours. Do not mix medications with blood/blood components. Stop the infusion immediately if an adverse transfusion reaction is apparent and notify the physician. Keep the vein open with a NSS. Follow agency policy for transfusion reactions, which may include sending the first voided urine specimen to the laboratory, documenting vital signs, and returning the blood container and tubing to the laboratory for further testing.*

15. Ensure that the electronic monitoring device being used is designed for use with blood/blood components. *Other types of infusion devices can cause hemolysis. Infusion devices control and regulate transfusion rate.*

16. Blood warming devices are not used for most transfusions but may be indicated for rapid transfusions

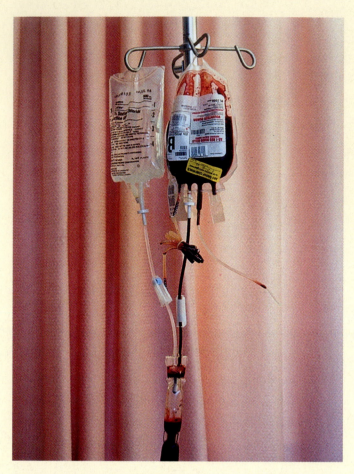

Figure 30-56. ■ Prime blood administration with normal saline before starting infusion with Y-set tubing.

or neonatal transfusion exchanges and clients receiving cold agglutinins. Follow manufacturer's instructions. *Do not attempt to warm blood in a microwave or hot water.*

17. Vital signs are taken 15 minutes after the transfusion begins followed by 30 minutes and 60 minutes thereafter until transfusion is completed. Follow your agency policy for routine vital signs for blood transfusions.

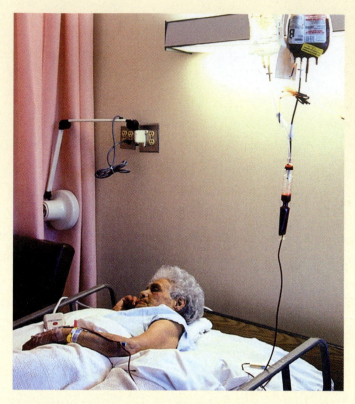

Figure 30-57. ■ Observe client for adverse signs.

18. When the transfusion has been completed, close the clamps leading to the blood and open the clamp from the NSS flushing the tubing.

19. Vital signs are taken post-transfusion.

20. Discard the blood bag in an appropriate biohazard waste container.

21. Document the type, unit, and amount of blood/blood component that was administered. Be clear about the time the infusion began and was terminated. Note vital signs and how the client tolerated the procedure. Detail any reactions and include nursing interventions initiated. Record physician notification.

SAMPLE DOCUMENTATION

[date]	Pretransfusion VS: T 98.7, P 76, R 16, BP 110/72. IV patent with NSS infusing at keep-
0825	open rate. Transfusion of 1 unit of 250 mL of packed red blood cells initiated at 0830.
0845	VS: T 98.5, P 78, R 18, BP 108/70.
0915	VS: T 98.6, P 78, R 16, BP 110/78.

Transfusion completed at 1,000. Post-transfusion VS: T 98.6, P 76, R 16, BP 112/78. Client tolerated the procedure well. 100 mL of NSS infused. No adverse reactions noted. IV site is clean and dry.

_____ J. French, LVN

Chapter Review

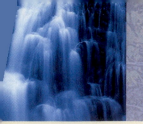

 KEY TERMS by Topic

Use the audio glossary feature of either the CD-ROM or the Companion Website to hear the correct pronunciation of the following key terms.

Fluids and Electrolytes
passive diffusion, osmosis, osmotic pressure, osmolarity, filtration, active transport, acid–base balance

Blood Transfusions
homologous, autologous, designated

KEY Points

- The LPN/LVN must be knowledgeable and skillful when delivering IV therapy.
- Intentional torts related to IV therapy are negligence, assault and battery, false imprisonment, slander, libel, and invasion of privacy.
- A departure from the accepted standards of practice related to IV therapy is considered malpractice.
- Standards of care must be developed within organizations to measure quality based on expectations of service. Organizations involved in IV therapy are OSHA, FDA, CDC, DHS, HIPAA, ANA, INS, JCAHO, AABB, and EPA.
- Water is the largest component of the body. Its functions include maintenance of blood volume, transportation of nutrients to and from cells, regulation of body temperature, and assistance with digestion.
- The kidneys and lungs are the major organs in regulating acid–base imbalances.
- Understanding equipment and administration of IV therapy will promote safety in the delivery process.

- Knowledge of the integumentary and venous systems assists the nurse to determine vein suitability for IV therapy.
- Three types of blood donation collection methods include homologous, autologous, and designated.

 EXPLORE Media Link

Additional interactive resources for this chapter can be found on the Companion Website at www.prenhall.com/ramont. Click on Chapter 30 and "Begin" to select the activities for this chapter.

For chapter-related NCLEX®-style questions and an audio glossary, access the accompanying CD-ROM in this book.

☋ FOR FURTHER Study

Chapter 23 covers the integumentary system.
See Chapter 26, Table 26-2 in particular, for more about electrolytes.

Caring for a Client Requiring a Blood Transfusion

NCLEX-PN® Focus Area: Physiological Adaptation

Case Study: Margaret Woods is a 50-year-old woman who underwent a surgical procedure for a right hip replacement. Prior to admission for her surgery she participated in an autologous blood donation for two units of blood. Postoperatively, she returned to the hospital unit with a dressing to the right hip with some drainage and a Hemovac drain to suction that drained 150 mL of serosanguineous drainage.

Nursing Diagnosis: Deficient Fluid Volume

COLLECT DATA

Subjective	Objective
_____	_____
_____	_____
_____	_____
_____	_____
_____	_____
_____	_____
_____	_____

Would you report this data? Yes/No

If yes, to: _____

What would you report? _____

Nursing Care

_____
_____
_____
_____
_____
_____
_____
_____
_____
_____
_____
_____
_____

How would you document this? _____
_____
_____

Compare your documentation to the sample provided in Appendix I.

Data Collected
(use those that apply)

- 50-year-old female
- Surgery: right hip replacement
- Height: 5 ft 4 in.
- Weight: 200 lbs
- VS: T 99, P 110, R 22, BP 90/55
- Hemoglobin 6 g/dL, hematocrit 22%
- Hemovac 150 mL, serosanguineous drainage
- CXR clear
- Blood sugar 120
- Abductor pillow placed
- Pain level 8
- Ferrous sulfate 325 mg
- Demerol 75 mg every 4 hours prn for pain
- D_5W at 125 mL
- Soft diet
- Lethargic

Nursing Interventions
(use those that apply; list in priority order)

- Arrange PT consult.
- Reinforce surgical dressing.
- Monitor I&O.
- Drain Hemovac and record drainage.
- Increase diet to Reg.
- Monitor H/H.
- Transfuse client with 1 unit PRBCs if H/H is <7 g/dL or 22%.
- Monitor VS every 4 hours.
- Elevate legs.

NCLEX-PN® Exam Preparation

1 When preparing to start an IV in a client who will be receiving blood, which of the following is the best choice of catheter sizes?

1. 18-gauge
2. 10-gauge
3. 25-gauge
4. 22-gauge

2 Which of the following solutions would you hang with or add to blood or blood components?

1. D_5W
2. $D_5\frac{1}{2}NS$
3. LR
4. NS

3 What is the purpose of an intermittent infusion device?

1. Prevent phlebitis.
2. Provide vascular access.
3. Prevent infiltration.
4. Administer solutions at a rapid rate.

4 A client has the following signs and symptoms: moist rales, increased respiratory rate, dyspnea, and 3+ edema of the ankles. Which of the following nursing diagnoses might you suspect?

1. *Deficient Fluid Volume*
2. *Excess Fluid Volume*
3. *Impaired Tissue Integrity*
4. *Ineffective Tissue Perfusion*

5 Which peripheral vein is most appropriate for antibiotic therapy or blood administration?

1. cephalic
2. dorsal metacarpal vein
3. digital vein
4. median antecubital vein

6 Which of the following organs are considered the regulatory organs in acid–base balance?

1. lungs and liver
2. lungs and the kidneys
3. kidneys and hypothalamus
4. pituitary and pineal glands

7 The nurse noted that a client exhibited irritability, fatigued muscles, nausea, and anorexia. She reviewed his serum electrolytes and found the following: chloride 92, potassium 3.1. The nurse would anticipate the following electrolyte imbalance:

1. hyponatremia
2. hyperchloremia
3. hypokalemia
4. hypernatremia

8 Minidrip administration sets, which deliver 60 gtt/mL, are primarily used for:

1. any hospitalized client.
2. diabetic clients.
3. pediatric clients.
4. cardiac clients.

9 Which of the following signs and symptoms would indicate metabolic alkalosis (bicarbonate excess)?

1. Kussmaul's breathing, confusion, increased respiratory rate
2. tetany, soft tissue calcification, low pH
3. poor skin turgor, sunken eyeballs, rapid pulse
4. dizziness, tingling of fingers and toes, decreased respirations, and cardiac dysrhythmias

10 A client receiving IV therapy via a central line is exhibiting fluctuating fever, profuse sweating, nausea, and a blood pressure that is lower than normal. You would suspect:

1. local infection.
2. septicemia.
3. venous spasm.
4. circulatory overload.

Answers and Rationales for Review Questions, as well as discussion of Care Plan and Critical Thinking Care Map questions, appear in Appendix I.

Chapter 31

Perioperative Nursing

BRIEF Outline

Preoperative Phase
Intraoperative Phase
Postoperative Phase

LEARNING Outcomes

After completing this chapter, you will be able to:

1. Describe the phases of the perioperative period.
2. Discuss various types of surgery according to degree of urgency, degree of risk, and purpose.
3. Identify nursing responsibilities in planning perioperative nursing care.
4. Describe essential preoperative teaching, including pain control, moving, leg exercises, and coughing and deep-breathing exercises.
5. Describe essential aspects of preparing a client for surgery, including skin preparation.
6. Identify potential postoperative complications and describe nursing interventions to prevent them.
7. Describe appropriate wound care for a postoperative client.

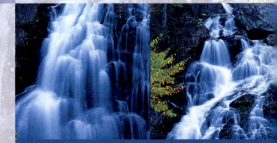

HISTORICAL Perspectives

Historically, the term operating room (OR) nursing *was used to characterize nursing care activities circumscribed to the geographic limits of the surgical suite. The current view of perioperative nursing denotes the delivery of client care in the preoperative, intraoperative, and postoperative phases of the client's surgical experience through the framework of the nursing process. The perioperative nurse engages in client assessment and in collecting, organizing, and prioritizing client data; establishes nursing diagnoses; identifies optimal client outcomes; develops and implements a plan of nursing care; and evaluates that care in terms of desired outcomes to be achieved by the client. This is all performed in a collaborative practice with other healthcare practitioners.*

BOX 31-1

Purpose of Surgical Procedures

Diagnostic procedures confirm or establish a diagnosis (e.g., biopsy of a mass in a breast).

Palliative procedures relieve or reduce pain or symptoms of a disease; do not cure (e.g., resection of nerve roots).

Ablative procedures remove a diseased body part (e.g., removal of a gallbladder [cholecystectomy]).

Reconstructive procedures restore function or appearance that has been lost or reduced (e.g., breast implant).

Transplant procedures replace malfunctioning structures (e.g., liver transplant).

Surgery is a unique experience of a planned physical alteration encompassing three phases: preoperative, intraoperative, and postoperative. The *preoperative phase* occurs prior to surgery; the *intraoperative phase* occurs during surgery; and the *postoperative phase* occurs following surgery. These three phases are together referred to as the **perioperative period**. The LPN's/LVN's responsibilities are usually confined to client care in the postoperative period, although preoperative preparation is within the scope of the LPN/LVN.

Surgical procedures are commonly grouped in one of three ways:

1. *Purpose.* Surgical procedures may be categorized according to their purpose (Box 31-1 ■).
2. *Degree of urgency.* Surgery is classified by its urgency and necessity to preserve the client's life, body part, or body function. **Emergency surgery** is performed immediately to preserve function or the life of the client. **Elective surgery** is performed when a condition is not immediately life threatening or to improve the client's life.
3. *Degree of risk.* Surgery is also classified as major or minor according to the degree of risk to the client. *Major surgery* involves a high degree of risk. In contrast, *minor surgery* normally involves little risk, produces few complications, and is often performed on an outpatient basis as "day surgery." The degree of risk involved in a surgical procedure is affected by the client's age, general health, nutritional status, use of medications, and mental status. Box 31-2 ■ lists health problems that increase surgical risk.

Preoperative Phase

PREOPERATIVE CONSENT

Prior to any surgical procedure and before receiving any sedative medication, clients must sign a surgical consent form, which is supplied by the medical facility. The consent form lists the surgical procedure and any risks that might

BOX 31-2

RISK FACTORS FOR CLIENTS NEEDING SURGERY

- Malnutrition can lead to delayed wound healing, infection, and reduced energy. Protein and vitamins are needed for wound healing; vitamin K is essential for blood clotting.
- Obesity leads to hypertension, impaired cardiac function, and impaired respiratory ventilation. Obese clients are also more likely to have delayed wound healing and wound infection because adipose tissue impedes blood circulation and its delivery of nutrients, antibodies, and enzymes required for wound healing.
- Cardiac conditions such as angina pectoris, recent myocardial infarction, hypertension, and congestive heart failure weaken the heart. Well-controlled cardiac problems generally pose minimal operative risk.
- Blood coagulation disorders may lead to severe bleeding, hemorrhage, and subsequent shock.
- Upper respiratory tract infections or chronic obstructive lung diseases such as emphysema adversely affect pulmonary function, especially when exacerbated by the effects of general anesthesia. They also predispose the client to postoperative lung infections.
- Renal disease or insufficiency impairs regulation of the body's fluids and electrolytes and excretion of drugs and other toxins.
- Diabetes mellitus predisposes the client to wound infection and delayed healing.
- Liver disease (e.g., cirrhosis) impairs the liver's abilities to detoxify medications used during surgery, produce the prothrombin necessary for blood clotting, and metabolize nutrients essential for healing.
- Uncontrolled neurologic disease such as epilepsy may result in seizures during surgery or recovery.
- Aspirin and some herbal medications and supplements increase blood coagulation time and risk of hemorrhage; they need to be discontinued several days prior to surgery.

be involved from the surgery or anesthesia and protects clients from having an undesired surgical procedure. It also protects the medical facility and the health personnel from a claim by the client or family that permission was not granted for the procedure. The consent form becomes a part of the client's record and goes to the operating room with the client.

SCREENING TESTS

The physician orders preoperative diagnostic screening tests and examinations to determine abnormalities. Abnormalities may delay the surgical procedure or warrant treatment prior to surgery. Table 31-1 ■ lists routine preoperative screening tests.

TABLE 31-1

Routine Preoperative Screening Tests

TEST	RATIONALE
Complete blood count (CBC)	RBCs, hemoglobin (Hgb), and hematocrit (Hct) are important to the oxygen-carrying capacity of the blood; WBCs are an indicator of immune function or infection
Blood grouping and cross-matching	Determined in case blood transfusion is required during or after surgery
Serum electrolytes (Na^+, K^+, Ca^{2+}, Mg^{2+}, Cl^-, HCO_3^-)	To evaluate fluid and electrolyte status
Fasting blood glucose	High levels may indicate undiagnosed diabetes mellitus
Blood urea nitrogen (BUN) and creatinine	To evaluate renal function
ALT, AST, LDH, and bilirubin	To evaluate liver function
Serum albumin and total protein	To evaluate nutritional status
Urinalysis	To determine urine composition and possible abnormal components (e.g., protein or glucose) or infection
Chest x-ray	To evaluate respiratory status and heart size
Electrocardiogram (ECG)	To identify preexisting cardiac problems or disease

NURSING CARE

ASSESSING

Preoperative assessment includes collecting and reviewing specific client data to determine the client's needs both pre- and postoperatively. Physical, psychological, and social needs are determined during assessment.

Preoperatively, the nurse performs a brief but complete physical assessment, paying particular attention to systems that could affect the client's response to anesthesia or surgery. Respiratory and cardiovascular assessments provide baseline data for evaluating the client's postoperative status. They also may alert care providers to a problem (e.g., a respiratory infection or irregular pulse rate) that may affect the client's response to surgery and anesthesia.

DIAGNOSING, PLANNING, AND IMPLEMENTING

A number of NANDA nursing diagnoses may be appropriate for the preoperative client. The LPN/LVN will help implement many of the interventions. Two common nursing diagnoses for perioperative clients are *Anxiety* and *Deficient Knowledge.*

Planning should involve the client and support persons. The length of the preoperative period affects preoperative care and planning. Today, unlike the past, the preoperative period is usually a couple of hours before surgery. Because of the lack of time, a nursing care plan and teaching plan have to be developed quickly. The nurse has to be familiar with nursing diagnoses and surgical procedure prerequisites. Goals for preoperative clients are to be physically, mentally, and emotionally prepared for surgery.

Preoperative Teaching

Preoperative teaching is a vital part of nursing care. Studies have shown that preoperative teaching reduces clients' anxiety and postoperative complications. It also increases their satisfaction with the surgical experience. Good preoperative teaching aids the client's return to work and other activities of daily living (ADLs).

Preoperative instructions for all clients are summarized in Box 31-3 ■. Procedure 31-1 ■ on page 735 provides guidelines for teaching clients preoperatively about the moving, leg exercises, deep breathing, and coughing they will be doing during their postoperative period.

Providing Physical Preparation

Preoperative physical preparation of the client includes the following areas: nutrition and fluids, elimination, hygiene, rest, care of valuables and prostheses, medications, and special orders. A preoperative checklist is used on the day of surgery. The nurse checks the medical facility's forms and

BOX 31-3	CLIENT TEACHING

Preoperative Instructions

- Explain the need for preoperative tests (e.g., laboratory, x-ray, ECG).
- Discuss bowel preparation, if required.
- Discuss skin preparation, including operative area and pre-operative bath or shower.
- Discuss preoperative medications, if ordered.
- Explain individual therapies ordered by the physician, such as intravenous therapy, the insertion of a urinary catheter or nasogastric tube, or use of a spirometer or antiembolism stockings.
- Discuss the visit by the anesthesia provider.
- Explain the need to restrict food and oral fluids at least 8 hours before surgery.
- Provide a general timetable for perioperative events, including the time of surgery.
- Discuss the need to remove jewelry, makeup, and all prostheses (e.g., eyeglasses, hearing aids, complete or partial dentures, wig) immediately before surgery. Discuss the disposition of these articles.
- Inform client about the preoperative holding area, and give the location of the waiting room for support persons.
- Teach deep-breathing and coughing exercises, leg exercises, ways to turn and move (see Procedure 31-1), and splinting techniques.

follows appropriate recording procedures. Two things are essential:

1. All pertinent records (laboratory records, x-ray films, consents) must be assembled and completed so that operating and recovery room personnel can refer to them for the client's baseline data.
2. All physical preparation must be completed to ensure client safety.

Nutrition and Fluids

Proper hydration and nutrition promote healing. Nurses record any signs of malnutrition or fluid imbalance.

Many preoperative clients are listed as NPO (nothing by mouth). Because anesthetics depress gastrointestinal functioning and create a danger that the client may vomit and aspirate vomitus during administration of a general anesthetic, the client is told to fast at least 6 to 8 hours before surgery. However, some studies have indicated that a shorter fasting period for clear liquids may be acceptable. Facility policy and anesthesia provider preference should be followed.

Elimination

Enemas before surgery are no longer routine, but cleansing enemas may be ordered if bowel surgery is planned. After surgery involving the intestines, peristalsis often does not return for 24 to 48 hours. Stool softeners may be ordered to prevent the client from experiencing constipation.

Prior to surgery, a urinary catheter may be ordered to ensure that the bladder remains empty. This helps prevent inadvertent injury to the bladder, particularly during pelvic surgery. If the client does not have a catheter, it is important for the client to empty the bladder prior to receiving preoperative medications.

Hygiene

In some settings, clients are asked to bathe or shower and shampoo their hair the evening or morning of surgery (or both depending on the type of surgery scheduled). The purpose of hygienic measures is to reduce the risk of wound infection.

The surgical skin preparation is carried out during the intraoperative phase. The purpose of surgical skin prep is to prepare the surgical site and reduce the risk of postoperative infection. Shave preps are often performed in the labor and delivery unit in the client's room prior to a cesarean section. Surgeons usually prefer a minimal shave prep to the pubic area instead of a full prep as was a former practice. See Procedure 31-2 ■ on page 737.

The client is encouraged to remove all cosmetics and nail polish so that the nail beds, skin, and lips are visible for assessing circulation during and after surgery. It is also important for the nails to be clear so that the pulse oximeter can be used on the fingers during and after surgery to measure the client's oxygen concentration.

The client may be required to wear a surgical hat/cap for surgery. The surgical cap contains the client's hair and traps microorganisms on the hair and scalp from escaping into the air during surgery and possibly contaminating the surgical site.

Immediately before surgery, the nurse removes, or asks the client to remove, all hair pins and clips. Clips can cause pressure or accidental damage to the scalp when the client is unconscious. In most medical facilities, the client also removes personal clothing and puts on a client gown.

Valuables

Client valuables such as jewelry and money should be given to a support person by the client. If this is impossible, the valuables are labeled and placed in safekeeping (see discussion in Chapter 10 ⬤⬤ and Figure 10-2 ⬤⬤). If the client does not want to remove a wedding band, the nurse can tape it in place. However, wedding bands must be removed for surgery on the left hand or if there is danger of the fingers swelling after surgery. Among situations requiring removal of rings are cast application to an arm and mastectomy with removal of the lymph nodes, because these procedures may cause edema of the arm and hand.

Prostheses

All **prostheses** (artificial body parts, partial or complete dentures, contact lenses, artificial eyes, and artificial limbs) and eyeglasses, wigs, and false eyelashes must be removed before surgery. These items are considered client valuables and are handled in the same way as all valuables.

Medications

Preoperative medications may be given on the hospital unit or after the client goes to the operating room. Commonly used preoperative medications include:

- Sedatives and tranquilizers, such as secobarbital and midazolam (Versed), to reduce anxiety, produce an amnesic effect, and ease anesthetic induction
- Narcotic analgesics, such as morphine and meperidine (Demerol), to provide client sedation if the client is experiencing discomfort or pain preoperatively or if discomfort is anticipated during invasive procedures or during the administration of a regional anesthetic
- Anticholinergics, such as atropine, scopolamine, and glycopyrrolate (Robinul), to reduce oral and pulmonary secretions and prevent laryngospasm
- Histamine-receptor antihistamines, such as cimetidine (Tagamet) and ranitidine (Zantac), to reduce gastric fluid volume and gastric acidity, or Reglan may be given to reduce the incidence of nausea and vomiting
- Neuroleptanalgesic agents, such as Innovar, to induce general calmness and sleepiness.

Preoperative medications are given at a scheduled time or "on call," when the operating room notifies the client's nurse to give the medication.

Vital Signs

The nurse assesses and records physical measurements or vital signs for baseline data. Abnormal findings, such as elevated blood pressure or elevated temperature, must be reported.

Antiemboli Stockings

Antiemboli stockings are firm elastic hose that compress the veins of the legs and facilitate the return of venous blood to the heart. They are intended to prevent the formation of blood clots in the legs and edema of the legs and feet. These stockings can be applied preoperatively or postoperatively. For shorter procedures, unless ordered because of the client's venous status, these stockings are not ordered. See Procedure 31-3 ■ on page 738 for steps in applying antiembolism stockings.

Sequential Compression Devices

It is common for a **sequential compression device (SCD)** to be ordered for the surgical client to promote venous return from the legs. SCDs inflate and deflate plastic sleeves that the nurse applies to the client's legs to promote venous flow. See Procedure 24-6 ⬭ for steps in applying sequential compression sleeves and hooking up the sleeves to the SCD device.

EVALUATING

The nurse evaluates specific desired client outcomes. For example, the nurse assesses whether the client's vital signs are stable, if the client understands and is ready for surgery, and if the client has learned about and can perform postoperative exercises.

Intraoperative Phase

RNs work intraoperatively as members of the surgical team. The RN functions as the client's advocate, maintains the client's safety, and continually assesses the needs of the client and the surgical team.

TYPES OF ANESTHESIA

Anesthesia, the alteration in the level of sensation and consciousness, is classified as *general* (comprehensive) or *regional* (specific). **Conscious sedation**, in which a client is conscious and has an increased pain threshold during surgery, is another form of anesthesia. Anesthetic agents usually are administered by an anesthesiologist or nurse anesthetist. Box 31-4 ■ provides a detailed explanation of the types of anesthesia.

Postoperative Phase

Nursing care during the postoperative phase is especially important for the client's recovery. Anesthesia impairs the ability of clients to respond to environmental stimuli and to help themselves, although the degree of consciousness of clients will vary. Moreover, surgery traumatizes the body by disrupting protective mechanisms and homeostasis.

IMMEDIATE POSTANESTHETIC PHASE

In the recovery room (postanesthesia care unit or PACU), the unconscious client is usually cared for by an RN. The nurse stabilizes the client and ensures the client's vital signs are stable. The nurse also assesses if the client has a normal gag reflex before ice chips or sips of water can be given. After the client has been stabilized, he or she will be transferred to a nursing unit where an LPN/LVN may be assigned to continue postoperative care.

PREPARING FOR ONGOING CARE OF THE POSTOPERATIVE CLIENT

While the client is in the operating room, the client's bed and room are prepared for the postoperative phase. The nurse must obtain and set up any special equipment, such as

---

BOX 31-4

Types of Anesthesia

General anesthesia is the loss of all sensation and consciousness.

- Protective reflexes such as cough and gag reflexes are lost.
- Blocks awareness centers in the brain so that amnesia (loss of memory), analgesia (insensibility to pain), hypnosis (artificial sleep), and relaxation (rendering a part of the body less tense) occur.
- Administered by intravenous infusion or by inhalation of gases through a mask or an endotracheal tube.

Regional anesthesia is the temporary interruption of the transmission of nerve impulses to and from a specific area or region of the body.

- *Topical* (surface) *anesthesia* is applied directly to the skin and mucous membranes, open skin surfaces, wounds, and burns.
- *Local anesthesia* (infiltration) is injected into a specific area and is used for minor surgical procedures such as suturing a small wound or performing a biopsy. *Nerve block* is a technique in which the anesthetic agent is injected into and around a nerve or small nerve group that supplies sensation to a small area of the body.
- *Spinal anesthesia* is injected, by way of a lumbar puncture, into the subarachnoid space surrounding the spinal cord. Spinal anesthesia is often categorized as a low, mid, or high spinal. Spinal anesthesia may evoke several physiological responses that can result in major problems if not properly monitored. The nurse must be aware of these potential problems following spinal anesthesia which include:
  - Hypotension
  - Possible paralysis of the respiratory muscles (when total spinal anesthesia is used), which requires immediate intubation
  - Postdural puncture headache (postspinal headache), which is one of the most frequent client complaints following spinal anesthesia.
  - *Epidural anesthesia* is an injection of an anesthetic agent (usually lidocaine, bupivacaine, and chloroprocaine) into the epidural space, which is the area inside the spinal column but outside the dura mater.

Conscious sedation produces minimal depression of the client's level of consciousness.

- It can be used alone or in conjunction with regional anesthesia for diagnostic tests and surgical procedures.
- It gives the client the ability to consciously maintain a patent airway and verbally and physically respond.
- It increases the client's pain threshold.
- Conscious sedation induces a degree of amnesia but allows for prompt reversal of its effects.
- It allows the client to return to normal activities of daily living quickly.

---

an intravenous pole, suction, oxygen equipment, and orthopedic appliances (e.g., traction) if applicable. If these items are not requested on the client's record, the nurse consults with the perioperative nurse or surgeon about verifying if these items are needed for the optimal care of the client.

NURSING CARE

ASSESSING

As soon as the client returns to the nursing unit, the RN conducts an initial assessment. The sequence of these activities varies with the situation. The surgeon's postoperative orders are consulted to obtain the following information:

- Food and fluids permitted by mouth
- Type of intravenous solutions and intravenous medications
- Position in bed
- Medications ordered (e.g., analgesics, antibiotics)
- Laboratory tests
- Intake and output, which in some facilities are monitored for all postoperative clients
- Activity permitted, including ambulation.

The nurse assesses the client and also checks the PACU record for the following data:

- Operation performed
- Presence and location of any drains
- Anesthetic used
- Postoperative diagnosis
- Estimated blood loss
- Medications administered in the PACU.

Assessments are usually made every 15 minutes until vital signs stabilize. Today, clients can go home the same day as their surgery due to the less invasive nature of most surgeries. Clients who have undergone more intensive surgery (e.g., open heart surgery, extensive bowel surgery) are admitted to the medical facility from the PACU. The nurse takes the client's vital signs every hour for the next 4 hours, then every 4 hours for the next 2 days. *Note:* Assessments *must* be made as often as the client's condition requires. The nurse performs the assessments described next.

Level of Consciousness

Assess the client's orientation to time, place, and person. Most clients are fully conscious but drowsy when returned to their unit. Assess reaction to verbal stimuli and ability to move extremities.

Vital Signs

Take the client's vital signs (pulse, respiration, blood pressure, and oxygen saturation level) every 15 minutes until stable or in accordance with the medical facility's protocol. Compare initial findings with PACU recorded data. In addition, assess the client's lung sounds and assess for signs of common circulatory problems, such as postoperative hypotension, hemorrhage, or shock. (See Procedures in Chapter 24 ⬭ for more about oxygenation.) Potential postoperative problems, with related manifestations and preventive measures, are listed in Table 31-2 ∎.

TABLE 31-2

Potential Postoperative Problems

PROBLEM/DESCRIPTION	CAUSE	CLINICAL SIGNS	PREVENTIVE INTERVENTIONS
Respiratory			
Pneumonia—inflammation of the alveoli	Infection, toxins, or irritants causing inflammatory process	Elevated temperature, cough, expectoration of blood-tinged or purulent sputum, dyspnea, chest pain	Deep-breathing exercises and coughing, moving in bed, early ambulation
Infectious pneumonia—may be limited to one or more lobes (*lobar*) or occur as scattered patches throughout the lungs (*bronchial*); also can involve interstitial tissues of lungs	Common organisms include *Streptococcus pneumoniae*, *Haemophilus influenzae*, and *Staphylococcus aureus*		
Hypostatic pneumonia	Immobility and impaired ventilation result in atelectasis and promote growth of pathogens		
Aspiration pneumonia—inflammatory process caused by irritation of lung tissue by aspirated material, particularly hydrochloric acid (HCl) from the stomach	Aspiration of gastric contents, food, or other substances; often related to loss of gag reflex		
Atelectasis—a condition in which alveoli collapse and are not ventilated	Mucous plugs blocking bronchial passageways, inadequate lung expansion, analgesics, immobility	Dyspnea, tachypnea, tachycardia; diaphoresis, anxiety; pleural pain, decreased chest wall movement; dull or absent breath sounds; decreased oxygen saturation (SpO_2)	Deep-breathing exercises and coughing, moving in bed, early ambulation
Pulmonary embolism—blood clot that has moved to the lungs and blocks a pulmonary artery, thus obstructing blood flow to a portion of the lung	Stasis of venous blood from immobility, venous injury from fractures or during surgery, use of oral contraceptives high in estrogen, preexisting coagulation or circulatory disorder	Sudden chest pain, shortness of breath, cyanosis, shock (tachycardia, low blood pressure)	Turning, ambulation, antiemboli stockings, SCDs
Circulatory			
Hypovolemia—inadequate circulating blood volume	Fluid deficit, hemorrhage	Tachycardia, decreased urine output, decreased blood pressure	Early detection of signs; fluid and/or blood replacement
Hemorrhage—internal or external bleeding	Disruption of sutures, insecure ligation of blood vessels	Overt bleeding (dressings saturated with bright blood; bright, free-flowing blood in drains or chest tubes), increased pain, increasing abdominal girth, swelling or bruising around incision	Early detection of signs
Hypovolemic shock—inadequate tissue perfusion resulting from markedly reduced circulating blood volume	Severe hypovolemia from fluid deficit or hemorrhage	Rapid weak pulse, dyspnea, tachypnea; restlessness and anxiety; urine output less than 30 mL/h; decreased blood pressure; cool, clammy skin, thirst, pallor	Maintain blood volume through adequate fluid replacement, prevent hemorrhage; early detection of signs

(continued)

TABLE 31-2

Potential Postoperative Problems (*continued*)

PROBLEM/DESCRIPTION	CAUSE	CLINICAL SIGNS	PREVENTIVE INTERVENTIONS
Thrombophlebitis—inflammation of the veins, usually of the legs and associated with a blood clot	Slowed venous blood flow due to immobility or prolonged sitting; trauma to vein, resulting in inflammation and increased blood coagulability	Aching, cramping pain; affected area is swollen, red, and hot to touch; vein feels hard; discomfort in calf when foot is dorsiflexed or when client walks (Homans' sign)	Early ambulation, leg exercises, antiemboli stockings, SCDs, adequate fluid intake
Thrombus—blood clot attached to wall of vein or artery (most commonly the leg veins)	As for thrombophlebitis for venous thrombi; disruption or inflammation of arterial wall for arterial thrombi	*Venous:* same as thrombophlebitis *Arterial:* pain and pallor of affected extremity; decreased or absent peripheral pulses	*Venous:* same as thrombophlebitis *Arterial:* maintaining prescribed position; early detection of signs
Embolus—foreign body or clot that has moved from its site of formation to another area of the body (e.g., lungs, heart, or brain)	Venous or arterial thrombus; broken intravenous catheter, fat, or amniotic fluid	In venous system, usually becomes a pulmonary embolus (see pulmonary embolism); signs of arterial emboli may depend on the location	As for thrombophlebitis or thrombus; careful maintenance of IV catheters
Urinary Urinary retention—inability to empty the bladder, with excessive accumulation of urine in the bladder	Depressed bladder muscle tone from narcotics and anesthetics; handling of tissues during surgery on adjacent organs (rectum, vagina)	Fluid intake larger than output; inability to void or frequent voiding of small amounts, bladder distention, suprapubic discomfort, restlessness	Monitoring of fluid intake and output, interventions to facilitate voiding, urinary catheterization as needed
Urinary tract infection (UTI)—inflammation of the bladder, ureters, or urethra	Immobilization and limited fluid intake, instrumentation of the urinary tract	Burning sensation when voiding, urgency, cloudy urine, lower abdominal pain	Adequate fluid intake, early ambulation, aseptic straight catheterization only as necessary, good perineal hygiene
Gastrointestinal Nausea and vomiting	Pain, abdominal distention, ingesting food or fluids before return of peristalsis, certain medications, anxiety	Complaints of feeling sick to the stomach; retching or gagging	IV fluids until peristalsis returns; then clear fluids, full fluids, and regular diet; antiemetic drugs if ordered; analgesics for pain
Constipation—infrequent or no stool passage for abnormal length of time (e.g., within 48 hours after solid diet started)	Lack of dietary roughage, analgesics (decreased intestinal motility), immobility	Absence of stool elimination, abdominal distention, and discomfort	Adequate fluid intake, high-fiber diet, early ambulation
Tympanites—retention of gases	Slowed motility of the intestines due to handling of the bowel during surgery and the effects of anesthesia	Hollow drumlike sound produced when the abdomen is tapped, obvious abdominal distention, abdominal discomfort (gas pains), absence of bowel sounds	Early ambulation; avoid using a straw; provide ice chips or water at room temperature
Paralytic ileus—intestinal obstruction characterized by lack of peristaltic activity	Anesthesia, handling the bowel during surgery, electrolyte imbalance, wound infection	Abdominal pain and distention; constipation; absent bowel sounds; vomiting	IV fluids until peristalsis returns; gradual reintroduction of oral feeding; early ambulation

TABLE 31-2

Potential Postoperative Problems (*continued*)

PROBLEM/DESCRIPTION	CAUSE	CLINICAL SIGNS	PREVENTIVE INTERVENTIONS
Wound			
Wound infection—inflammation and infection of incision or drain site	Poor aseptic technique; laboratory analysis of wound swab identifies causative microorganism	Purulent exudate, redness, tenderness, elevated body temperature, wound odor	Keeping wound clean and dry, surgical aseptic technique when changing dressings
Wound dehiscence—separation of a suture line before the incision heals	Malnutrition (emaciation, obesity), poor circulation, excessive strain on suture line	Increased incision drainage, tissues underlying skin become visible along parts of the incision	Adequate nutrition, appropriate incisional support, and avoidance of strain
Wound evisceration—extrusion of internal organs and tissues through the incision	Same as for wound dehiscence	Opening of incision and visible protrusion of organs	Same as for wound dehiscence
Psychological			
Postoperative depression—mental disorder characterized by altered mood	Weakness, surprise nature of emergency surgery, news of malignancy, severely altered body image, or other personal matter; may be a physiological response to some surgeries	Anorexia, tearfulness, loss of ambition, withdrawal, rejection of others, feelings of dejection, sleep disturbances (insomnia, excessive sleeping)	Adequate rest, physical activity, opportunity to express anger and other negative feelings

Skin Color and Temperature

Skin color and temperature, particularly of the lips and nail beds, are indicators of **tissue perfusion** (passage of blood through the vessels). Pale, cyanotic, cool, and moist skin may indicate circulatory problems.

Comfort

Assess the client's comfort level when taking vital signs and as needed between vital sign measurements. Assess the location and intensity of the pain. Do not assume that reported pain is incisional. Other causes may include muscle strains, flatus, and angina. Ask the client to rate the pain on a scale of 0 to 10, with 0 being no pain and 10 the worst pain imaginable. Evaluate the client for objective indicators of pain: pallor, perspiration, muscle tension, and reluctance to cough, move, or ambulate. Determine when and what analgesics were last administered, and assess the client for any side effects of medication such as nausea and vomiting. (See Chapter 21 ∞ for an in-depth discussion of pain.)

Fluid Balance

Assess the type and amount of intravenous fluids that have been ordered, the flow rate, and infusion site. LPN/LVN responsibilities related to IV therapy are defined in the scope of practice in each individual state. Monitor the client's fluid intake and output. In addition to assessing the client for shock, assess for signs of circulatory overload, and monitor serum electrolytes.

Dressing and Bedclothes

Inspect the client's dressings and sheets for drainage underneath the client. Excessive bloody drainage on dressings or on the sheets under the client can indicate hemorrhage. Record amount of drainage on dressings by describing the diameter of the stains or by noting the number and type of dressings saturated with the drainage.

Drains and Tubes

Determine color, consistency, and amount of drainage from all tubes and drains. All tubes should be *patent* (open), and tubes and suction equipment should be functioning. Drainage bags must be hanging properly and not dragging on the floor. See Chapter 23 ∞ for more information about wound care.

Document the client's time of arrival and all assessments. Most medical facilities have progress flow records the nurse uses for documentation either on hardcopy or electronically. Customize the frequency, parameters, and priorities necessary to meet the individual needs of the client.

DIAGNOSING, PLANNING, AND IMPLEMENTING

Surgery can involve many body systems both directly and indirectly and is a complex experience for the client. Nursing diagnoses focus on a wide variety of actual, potential, and collaborative problems. See Appendix II ∞ for a list of NANDA diagnoses for the postoperative client. Some of the most common nursing diagnoses for postoperative clients are *Impaired Skin Integrity* and *Risk for Infection.* Potential problems that may be experienced by the postoperative client are summarized in Table 31-2.

Postoperative care planning and discharge planning begin in the preoperative phase when preoperative teaching is implemented.

Major client outcomes/goals after surgery include maintaining comfort, healing, achieving wellness, and avoiding complications of surgery.

Pain Management

The client will start to experience pain after the effects of the anesthesia wear off. As prescribed diet and activity increases, the client's pain usually decreases. (See Chapter 21 ⊂⊃ for a more in-depth discussion of pain and pain management.) During the initial postoperative period, the physician may prescribe one of the following:

1. Patient-controlled analgesia (PCA) (self-administration of opioid and other potent pain medications by a programmed infusion pump).
2. Continuous analgesic administration through an intravenous or epidural catheter. PRN parenteral or oral analgesics are administered on a routine basis (usually every 2 to 6 hours, depending on the drug, route, and dose) for the first 24 to 36 hours. When routine analgesic administration is no longer necessary, the prescribed analgesic is generally given before scheduled activities and rest periods. Clients need to be reminded that analgesics are most effective when taken on a regular basis or before pain becomes severe. An anti-inflammatory agent is often administered in conjunction with a narcotic analgesic to enhance pain relief.

Nurses can provide nonpharmacologic measures in addition to prescribed analgesia. These include ensuring that the client is warm, providing back rubs, position changes, diversional activities, and adjunctive measures such as use of imagery.

Positioning

Position the client as ordered. Clients who have had spinal anesthetics are usually ordered to lie flat for 8 to 12 hours after the procedure until the anesthetic has left their system. Activity after a spinal anesthetic can cause the client to have a severe headache. An unconscious or semiconscious client is placed on the side with the head slightly elevated, if possible, or in a position that allows fluids to drain from the mouth to prevent aspiration. Unless contraindicated, elevation of affected extremities (e.g., following foot surgery) with the distal extremity higher than the heart promotes venous drainage and reduces swelling.

Deep-Breathing and Coughing Exercises

Deep-breathing exercises help remove mucus, which can form and remain in the lungs due to the effects of general anesthetic and analgesics. These anesthetic drugs depress the action of both the cilia of the mucous membranes lining the respiratory tract and the respiratory center in the brain. Deep breathing increases lung expansion and prevents the accumulation of secretions. It helps prevent pneumonia and **atelectasis** (collapse of the alveoli), which may result from stagnation of fluid in the lungs (see Procedure 31-1).

An incentive spirometer is often ordered for the postoperative client to encourage deep breathing. This device measures the flow of air inhaled through a mouthpiece. See Chapter 24 ⊂⊃ for information about how to use an incentive spirometer. The client is instructed to breathe in through the mouthpiece until a certain level on the meter is achieved (usually measured by a ball within an enclosed chamber). Inhalation and ventilation are enhanced using the incentive spirometer.

Deep breathing frequently initiates the coughing reflex. Voluntary coughing in conjunction with deep breathing helps the client move and expel accumulated respiratory tract secretions (see Procedure 31-1).

Encourage the client to do deep-breathing and coughing exercises hourly, or at least every 2 hours, during waking hours for the first few days. Assist the client to a sitting position in bed or on the side of the bed. The client can splint the incision (exert light to medium pressure against the incisional area) with a pillow when coughing, or the nurse can splint the incision for the client to reduce discomfort. Splinting the incision provides stability to the incisional site so the client does not experience as much pain when coughing or walking.

Leg Exercises

Encourage the client to perform leg exercises taught in the preoperative period every 1 to 2 hours during waking hours. Muscle contractions compress the veins, preventing the stasis of blood in the veins, which is a cause of thrombus formation and subsequent thrombophlebitis and emboli. Contractions also promote arterial blood flow (see Procedure 31-1).

Moving and Ambulation

Encourage the client to turn from side to side at least every 2 hours. This allows alternate lungs to expand fully (the uppermost lung will have full expansion). Clients who practice turning before surgery usually find it easier to do after surgery. Avoid placing pillows or rolls under the client's knees because pressure on the popliteal blood vessels can reduce blood circulation to and from the lower extremities.

The client should ambulate as soon as possible after surgery in accordance with the surgeon's orders. Generally, clients begin ambulation the evening of the day of surgery or the first day after surgery, unless contraindicated. Early ambulation prevents respiratory, circulatory, urinary, and gastrointestinal complications. It also prevents general muscle weakness. Schedule ambulation for periods after the client has taken an analgesic or when the client is comfortable. Ambulation should be gradual, starting with the client sitting on the bed and dangling the feet over the side.

A client who cannot ambulate is periodically assisted to a sitting position in bed, if allowed, and turned frequently. The sitting position permits the greatest lung expansion.

Hydration

Intravenous infusions replace body fluids lost either before or during surgery. When oral intake is permitted, initially offer only ice chips or small sips of water. Large amounts of water can induce vomiting because of the affects of anesthetics and narcotic analgesics on stomach motility. The client who cannot take fluids by mouth may be allowed by the surgeon's orders to take ice chips. Provide mouth care and place mouthwash at the client's bedside. Postoperative clients often complain of thirst and a dry, sticky mouth. These discomforts are a result of the preoperative fasting period, preoperative medications (such as atropine), and loss of body fluid.

Measure the client's fluid intake and output for at least 2 days or until fluid balance is stable without an intravenous infusion. Ensuring adequate fluid balance is important. Sufficient fluids keep the respiratory mucous membranes and secretions moist, thus facilitating the expectoration of mucus during coughing. Also, an adequate fluid balance is important to maintain renal and cardiovascular function.

Diet

The surgeon orders the client's postoperative diet. Depending on the extent of surgery and the organs involved, the client may be allowed nothing by mouth (NPO) for several days or may be able to resume oral intake when nausea is no longer present. When "diet as tolerated" is ordered, offer the client clear liquids first. If the client tolerates clear liquids without nausea, the diet can often progress to full liquids and then to a regular diet, provided gastrointestinal functioning has returned to normal. Assess the return of peristalsis by auscultating the abdomen (see Chapter 19 ⭕). Gurgling and rumbling sounds indicate peristalsis. Bowel sounds should be carefully assessed every 4 to 6 hours. Oral fluids and food are usually started after the return of peristalsis. Very weak clients will need assistance to eat.

Observe the client's tolerance of the food and fluids ingested. Note and report the passage of flatus, abdominal distention, and bowel movements.

Urinary Elimination

Provide measures that promote urinary elimination. For example, help male clients stand at the bedside, or female clients to a bedside commode to urinate if allowed. Ensure that fluid intake is adequate and recorded. Report to the

surgeon if a client does not void within 8 hours following surgery, unless another time frame is specified. Most facilities have parameters for the nurse to follow.

Generally, I&O is recorded (see Figure 26-2 ⭕) for at least 2 days or until the client reestablishes fluid balance without an IV or catheter in place.

Suction

Some clients return from surgery with a nasogastric (NG) tube in place with orders to connect the tube to suction. For more information about NG tubes, see Chapter 25 ⭕. The suction ordered can be continuous or intermittent. Intermittent suction is applied when a single-lumen gastric tube is used to reduce the risk of damaging the mucous membrane near the distal port of the tube. Continuous suction may be applied if a double-lumen tube is in place. Fluids and electrolytes must be replaced intravenously when gastric suction or continuous drainage is ordered due to the loss of fluids through suctioning. NG tubes may be irrigated if the lumen becomes clogged, and they are generally irrigated before and after tube feedings or the instillation of medications. Nasogastric irrigation may require a physician's order, particularly following gastrointestinal surgery. Procedure 31-4 ■ on page 740 describes the management of NG suction. See also Procedure 25-3 ⭕.

Suction may also be applied to other drainage tubes such as chest tubes or a wound drain. The type and amount of suction is ordered by the physician. A suction regulator with a drainage receptacle connects to a wall outlet that provides negative pressure. Check the receptacle frequently to prevent excess drainage from interfering with the suction apparatus. Empty or change the receptacle according to facility policy. Portable electric suction units or pumps (e.g., the Gomco pump) may be used in the home or when wall suction is not available in the facility.

Wound Care

Most clients return from surgery with a sutured wound covered by a dressing, although in some cases the wound may be left unsutured. Dressings are inspected regularly to ensure that they are clean, dry, and intact. Excessive drainage may indicate hemorrhage, infection, or a wound that has **dehisced** (opened on the suture line). Any abnormal, excessive drainage must be reported to the physician.

See Chapter 23 ⭕ for information about wound drainage, cleaning wounds, wound irrigation, hot and cold applications, and supporting and immobilizing wounds.

When dressings are changed, the nurse assesses the wound for appearance, size, drainage, swelling, pain, and the status of a drain or tubes. Details about these assessments are outlined in Box 31-5 ■.

Not all surgical dressings require changing. Sometimes surgeons in the operating room apply a dressing that remains in place until the sutures are removed, and no further

| BOX 31-5 | NURSING CARE CHECKLIST |

Assessing Surgical Wounds

☑ *Appearance.* Inspect color of wound and surrounding area and approximation of wound edges.

☑ *Size.* Note size and location of the wound. Note if there is a dehiscence (partial or total rupturing of a sutured wound). If internal organs are visible (evisceration), notify physician immediately!

☑ *Drainage.* Observe location, color, consistency, odor, and degree of saturation of dressings. Note number of dressings saturated or diameter of drainage on dressing.

☑ *Swelling.* Observe the amount of swelling; minimal to moderate swelling is normal in early stages of wound healing.

☑ *Pain.* Expect severe to moderate postoperative pain for 3 to 5 days; persistent severe pain or sudden onset of severe pain may indicate internal hemorrhaging or infection.

☑ *Drains or tubes.* Inspect drain security and placement, amount and character of drainage, and functioning of collecting apparatus, if present.

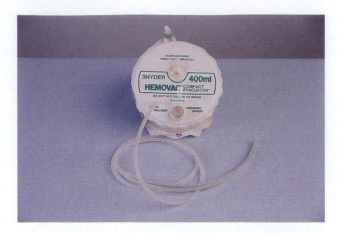

Figure 31-1. ■ Closed wound drainage system (Hemovac).

drainage tubes are sutured in place and connected to a reservoir. These portable wound suctions also provide for accurate measurement of the drainage. Generally, the suction is discontinued from 3 to 5 days postoperatively or when the drainage is minimal. Nurses are responsible for maintaining the wound suction, which hastens the healing process by draining excess exudate that might otherwise interfere with the formation of granulation tissue and healing.

When emptying the container, the nurse wears gloves and avoids touching the drainage port.

dressings are required. In many situations, however, surgical dressings are changed regularly, using sterile technique to prevent the growth of microorganisms.

In some instances, a client may have a Penrose drain inserted directly into the incision or adjacent to the incision. In this situation, the main surgical incision is considered cleaner than the surgical stab wound made for the drain insertion, because there is usually considerable drainage from the drainage site. The main incision is therefore cleaned first. Cleaning a wound and applying a sterile dressing are detailed in Procedure 31-5 ■ on page 742

clinical ALERT

Materials that were used to clean a stab wound are never used again to clean the main incision. The main incision must be kept free of the microorganisms around the stab wound.

Wound Drains and Suction

Surgical drains, such as a Penrose drain, are inserted to permit the drainage of excess serosanguineous fluid and purulent material and to promote healing of underlying tissues. These drains may be inserted and sutured through the incision line, but they are most commonly inserted through stab wounds a few centimeters away from the incision line so that the incision itself may be kept dry. Without a drain, some wounds would heal on the surface but trap the discharge inside. When this happens an abscess can form.

A **closed wound drainage system** consists of a drain connected to either an electric suction or a portable mechanical drainage suction, such as a Hemovac (Figure 31-1 ■) or Jackson-Pratt. The closed system reduces the possible entry of microorganisms into the wound through the drain. The

Sutures

Sutures are threads used to sew body tissues together. Sutures used to attach tissues beneath the skin are often made of an absorbable material that disappears in several days. Skin sutures, by contrast, are made of a variety of nonabsorbable materials. Silver wire clips or staples are also used for wound closures. Usually, skin sutures and clips are removed 7 to 10 days after surgery. Many surgeons prefer to use surgical adhesives on the wound that are a gluelike substance. This material takes the place of sutures and **approximates** (brings together the two skin sides) the wound very well.

The surgeon orders the removal of sutures, clips, or staples. In some facilities, only the surgeon removes the sutures; in others, registered nurses and nursing students with appropriate supervision may do so. The LPN/LVN should review the LPN/LVN scope of practice regarding suture and staple removal. Many states permit LPN/LVNs to remove these on well-approximated, uncomplicated surgical wounds. Usually the client is home before the time of the suture or staple removal and these are removed in the surgeon's office. (For a review of wound healing, see Chapter 23 ⬤.)

Sterile technique and special suture scissors are used in suture removal. The scissors have a short, curved cutting tip that readily slides under the suture (Figure 31-2 ■). Wire clips or staples are removed with a special instrument that squeezes the center of the clip to remove it from the skin (Figure 31-2B). Nursing care guidelines for removing sutures are provided in Box 31-6 ■.

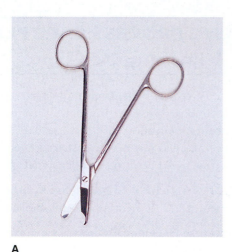

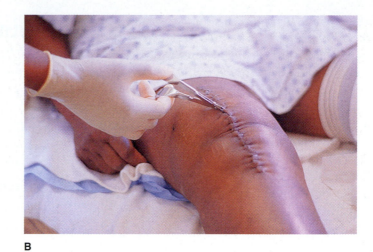

A   **B**

Figure 31-2. ■ **A.** Suture scissors. **B.** Removing surgical clips.

BOX 31-6	NURSING CARE CHECKLIST

Removing Skin Sutures, Clips, or Staples

☑ Before removing skin sutures, clips, or staples, verify the orders for removal and whether a dressing is to be applied following the removal.

☑ Inform the client that the removal may produce slight discomfort, such as a pulling or stinging sensation, but should not be painful.

☑ Put on gloves to remove dressings and dispose of gloves and dressing in appropriate container.

☑ Put on sterile gloves. Clean the incision in accordance with medical facility protocol.

Removing Plain Interrupted Sutures (vs. Running Sutures)

☑ Grasp the suture at the knot with a pair of forceps.

☑ Place the curved tip of the suture scissors under the suture as close to the skin as possible, either on the side opposite the knot (Figure 31-3 ■) or directly under the knot. Cut the suture. *Sutures are cut as close to the skin as possible on one side of the visible suture line because the suture material that is visible to the eye is in contact with resident bacteria on the skin and must not be pulled beneath the skin during removal. Suture material that is beneath the skin is considered free from bacteria.*

☑ With the forceps, pull the suture out in one piece. Inspect the suture carefully to make sure that all suture material is removed. *Suture material left beneath the skin acts as a foreign body and causes inflammation.*

☑ Discard the suture onto a piece of sterile gauze or into a moisture-proof bag. Be careful not to contaminate the tips of the forceps.

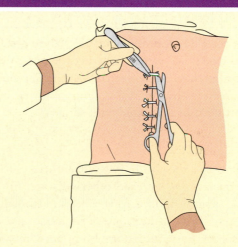

Figure 31-3. ■ Removing a plain interrupted skin suture.

☑ Remove alternate sutures so that remaining sutures keep the skin edges in close approximation and prevent dehiscence. If no dehiscence occurs, remove the remaining sutures. If dehiscence does occur, do not remove the remaining sutures and report the dehiscence to the nurse in charge.

☑ Some surgeons prefer to use running sutures, which are not visible and are absorbable. Many times the surgeon will use Steri-Strips over these incisions to maintain the suture line integrity. If Steri-Strips are ordered by the physician, apply them to the wound after removing the sutures or clips. Reapply a sterile dressing, if indicated.

☑ Instruct the client about follow-up wound care, such as contacting the physician if wound discharge, pain or swelling appears.

Orthopedic Wound Care: Care for Clients with Skeletal Traction

Clients with serious orthopedic fractures will have to have the fractures stabilized in surgery with skeletal traction. This kind of traction includes an external fixation device (pins or other orthopedic apparatus) that is passed through the skin through the bone to be stabilized and exits to the opposite side of the initial entry. These appliances or devices require special care by the nurse. Often the term *pin care* is ordered for the client with these appliances. The "pin" is a stainless steel or titanium fixation device used to immobilize the involved area. See Procedure 31-6 ■ on page 744.

Caring for Clients with an Extremity Amputation

Postoperative care of the client with an amputation can be challenging. The client has body disturbance issues and must relearn ADLs.

The nurse follows facility and surgeon protocol when caring for the postoperative client with an amputation. Generally, the nurse provides care for these clients following the protocol listed in Procedure 31-7 ■ on page 745.

EVALUATING

Using the goals developed during the planning stage, the nurse collects data to evaluate whether the identified goals and desired outcomes have been achieved. The nurse collects data about client comfort, healing, restoring wellness, and preventing risks associated with surgery.

CONTINUING CARE

The nurse reviews the client's self-care abilities, such as the ability to manage hygiene and other self-care, to perform wound care as needed, to manage tubes and stomas, and to manage prescribed medications. The nurse teaches the client and/or family about required supplies (dressings, hypoallergenic tape, etc.) or assistive devices (cane, raised toilet seat, grab bars in the shower). The client must know what occurrences might indicate a complication, and when to call the nurse or physician. Referrals and support systems are reviewed before discharge (Box 31-7 ■).

BOX 31-7	**CULTURAL PULSE POINTS**

Surgical Clients and Cultural Practices

The perioperative nurse must be familiar with the different cultural practices of clients undergoing surgery and attempt to honor these cultural practices as closely as possible but within the confines of the sterile OR environment. The nurse must ensure that clients understand the rationale for OR procedures with the ultimate goal of client safety and return to optimal functioning.

NURSING PROCESS CARE PLAN
A Postsurgical Client

Mr. Teng is a 77-year-old client with a history of chronic obstructive pulmonary disease. Currently, his respiratory condition is being controlled with medications, and he is free of infection. He has just been transferred to the PACU following a hernia repair performed under spinal anesthesia.

Assessment. Mr. Teng's BP is 132/88, P 84, R 28, and tympanic temperature 97.8° F. He is awake and stable.

Nursing Diagnosis. The following important nursing diagnosis (among others) is established for this client:

- *Ineffective Breathing Pattern*

Expected Outcomes

- Performs deep breathing, coughing, and incentive spirometry as instructed.
- Has normal breath sounds on auscultation.
- Has adequate respiratory excursion (depth).

Planning and Implementation

- Monitor respiratory rate, depth, and ease of respiration.
- Monitor client's oxygen saturation and blood gases.
- Encourage client to take deep breaths at prescribed intervals and do controlled coughing.
- Assist client to splint abdomen with pillow while coughing.
- Teach client to use incentive spirometer.

Evaluation. Client demonstrates ability to use incentive spirometer, cough, and deep breathe every 2 h while awake. Mr. Teng splints abdomen while coughing to decrease discomfort. Lungs clear; no signs and symptoms of respiratory infection. Client remains flat due to spinal anesthesia until all sensation has returned to the extremities or as ordered by the surgeon.

Critical Thinking in the Nursing Process

1. What factors place Mr. Teng at increased risk for the development of complications during and after surgery?
2. Speculate about why Mr. Teng's surgeon and anesthesiologist decided to perform Mr. Teng's surgery under regional anesthesia as opposed to general anesthesia?
3. What postoperative precautions are especially important for Mr. Teng in view of his chronic lung condition?

Note: Discussion of Critical Thinking questions appears in Appendix I.

Note: The references and resources for this and all chapters have been compiled at the back of the book.

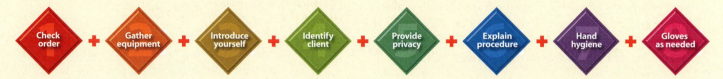

PROCEDURE 31-1

Teaching Moving, Leg Exercises, Splinting, Deep Breathing, and Coughing and Use of a Continuous Passive Motion Machine

Purposes

- To maintain blood circulation
- To stimulate respiratory function and lung aeration, preventing atelectasis and pneumonia
- To decrease stasis of gas in the intestines
- To facilitate early ambulation

- To stimulate blood circulation, thereby preventing thrombophlebitis and thrombus formation

Equipment

- Pillow or towel roll
- Continuous passive motion machine

Check order + Gather equipment + Introduce yourself + Identify client + Provide privacy + Explain procedure + Hand hygiene + Gloves as needed

Interventions

1. Demonstrate to the client ways to turn in bed and to get out of bed in a manner to decrease discomfort.
   - Instruct the client who has a right abdominal incision or a right-sided chest incision to turn to the left side of the bed and sit up as follows:
     a. Flex the knees.
     b. Splint the wound by holding the left arm and hand or a small pillow against the incision. *This minimizes pressure against the incision and reduces pain.*
     c. Turn to the left while pushing with the right foot and grasping a partial side rail on the left side of the bed with the right hand. *This puts the least amount of pressure on the operative side.*
     d. Bring self to a sitting position on the side of the bed by using the right arm and hand to push down against the mattress and swing the feet over the edge of the bed.
   - Teach the client with left abdominal or left-sided chest incision to perform the same procedure but splint with the right arm and turn to the right.
   - For clients with orthopedic surgery (e.g., hip surgery), use special aids, such as a trapeze, to assist with movement.

2. Teach the client the following three leg exercises to increase circulation to the lower extremities and maintain muscle tone.
   - Alternate dorsiflexion and plantar flexion of the feet (Figure 31-4 ■). This exercise is sometimes referred to as calf pumping, because it alternately contracts and relaxes the calf muscles, including the gastrocnemius muscles (see also Figures 32-12 ⬭ and 32-28 ⬭).
   - Flex and extend the knees, and press the backs of the knees into the bed while dorsiflexing the feet. Instruct

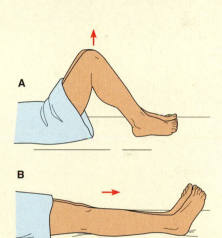

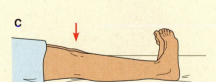

Figure 31-4. ■ Flexing and extending the knees.

clients who cannot raise their legs to do isometric exercises that contract and relax the muscles.
   - Raise and lower the legs alternately from the surface of the bed. Flex the knee of the stable leg and extend the knee of the moving leg (Figure 31-5 ■). This exercise contracts and relaxes the quadriceps muscles.

3. Show the client how to hold pressure with a pillow or towel roll against the incisional site. This maneuver is called *splinting* the incisional site because it adds support

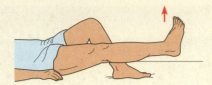

Figure 31-5. ■ Raising and lowering the legs.

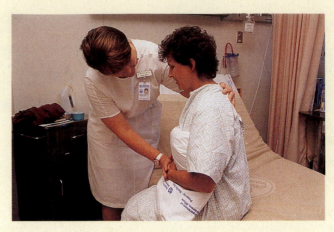

Figure 31-7. ■ Splinting an incision with a pillow while coughing. (Photographer: Elena Dorfman.)

to muscles weakened by surgery and is helpful when moving or coughing. *By exerting pressure against the incision, the client can have a sense of control over the incisional pain. The pressure decreases the strain against the incision.*

4. Show the client how to support the incision by placing the palms of the hands on either side of the incisional site or directly over the incisional site, holding the palm of one hand over the other. *Coughing uses the abdominal and other accessory respiratory muscles. Splinting the incision may reduce pain while coughing if the incision is near any of these muscles.*

5. Show the client how to splint the abdomen with clasped hands and a firmly rolled pillow or towel roll held against the client's abdomen.

6. Demonstrate deep-breathing (diaphragmatic) exercises as follows:
   - Place hands palms down on the border of the rib cage, and inhale slowly and evenly through the nose until the greatest chest expansion is achieved (Figure 31-6 ■).
   - Hold the breath for 2 to 3 seconds.
   - Exhale slowly through the mouth.
   - Continue exhalation until maximum chest contraction has been achieved.

7. Help the client perform deep-breathing exercises.
   - Ask the client to assume a sitting position.
   - Place the palms of your hands on the border of the client's rib cage to assess respiratory depth. Explain this to the client because some clients may be uncomfortable with anyone touching their rib cage.
   - Ask the client to perform deep breathing, as described in step 6.

8. Instruct the client to cough voluntarily, splinting the incisional site (Figure 31-7 ■) after a few deep inhalations.
   - Ask the client to inhale deeply, hold the breath for a few seconds, and then cough once or twice.
   - Ensure that the client coughs deeply and does not just clear the throat.

9. Inform the client about the expected frequency of these exercises. *This prepares the client mentally to perform them in the recovery period.*
   - Instruct the client to start the exercises as soon as possible after surgery. This promotes good oxygenation.
   - Encourage clients with abdominal or chest surgery to carry out deep breathing and coughing at least every 2 hours, taking a minimum of five breaths at each session. Note, however, that the number of breaths and frequency of deep breathing varies with the client's condition. *Clients who are susceptible to pulmonary problems may need deep-breathing exercises every hour. Clients with chronic respiratory disease may need special breathing exercises (e.g., pursed-lip breathing), abdominal breathing, exercises using various kinds of incentive spirometers.* See Chapter 24 ∞.

10. Document the teaching and all assessments.

CONTINUOUS PASSIVE MOTION MACHINE USE FOR POSTOPERATIVE CLIENTS

The continuous passive motion (CPM) machine (Figure 31-8 ■) is a postoperative treatment method that is designed to assist in recovery after joint surgery. In most clients, after extensive

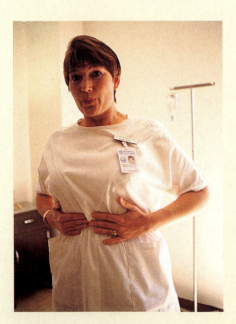

Figure 31-6. ■ Demonstrating deep breathing. (Photographer: Elena Dorfman.)

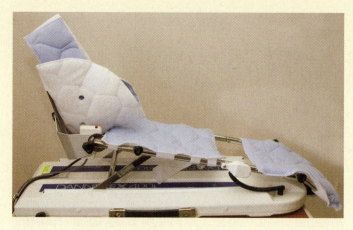

Figure 31-8. ■ CPM machine.

joint surgery, attempts at joint motion cause pain and, as a result, the client guards against joint movement. When this happens, the tissue around the joint becomes stiff and scar tissue forms, resulting in a joint that has limited range of motion.

Passive range of motion means that the joint is moved without the client's muscles being used. Applied postopera-

tively, often in the PACU, a CPM device may be used on an inpatient or outpatient basis. By using a motorized device to gradually move the joint, it is possible to significantly accelerate recovery time by increasing range of motion, decreasing soft tissue stiffness, promoting healing of joint surfaces and soft tissue, and preventing the development of motion-limiting adhesions (scar tissue).

CPM devices are available for the knee, ankle, shoulder, elbow, wrist, and hand. The surgeon prescribes how the CPM unit should be used by the client (speed, duration of usage, amount of motion, rate of increase of motion, etc.)

SAMPLE DOCUMENTATION

[date]	Client coughing and deep breathing
[time]	every 2 hours. Splinting abdomen
	while coughing. Lungs clear.
	_____ T. Thompson, LPN

PROCEDURE 31-2   # Performing a Presurgical Skin Prep

Purpose

■ To remove hair from skin and surface microorganisms prior to surgical procedures

Equipment

■ Gloves-sterile and non-sterile
■ Surgical prep tray or disposable razor

■ Soap or shaving cream
■ Gauze pads
■ Surgical prep solution

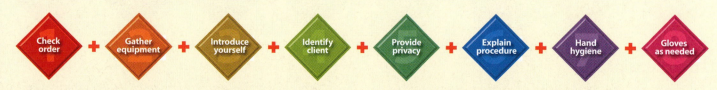

Check order + Gather equipment + Introduce yourself + Identify client + Provide privacy + Explain procedure + Hand hygiene + Gloves as needed

Interventions

1. Perform hand hygiene and gather supplies.

2. Identify client and explain procedure. *To assure procedure is performed on correct client.*
   ■ Identify the body part that requires the surgical prep (read chart, ask client, read operative consent form). *For conformation of proper site to avoid wrong site surgery.*

3. Don nonsterile gloves.

4. Trim any long hair with bandage scissors. *To prevent tugging and pulling when shaving.*
   ■ Use of a disposable electric razor is preferred. *To prevent small cuts, which would be a port of entry for microorganisms.* If using a standard disposable razor, wet the gauze with prep solution/shaving cream and apply to the hair/skin in the area to be prepared for surgery.

- Remove the prescribed amount of hair per surgeon preference.
- Use dry gauze or tape to pick up loose hair.
- Clean the area so it is free of loose hair. Hair can be a source of microorganisms

5. Perform the surgical prep in the preoperative area or in the surgical suite.
   - Supplies and equipment
   - Open the prep kit and follow directions for use of the items inside. Most will have sponges on a handle, surgical skin prep solution, and the sterile barriers required). Open the prep kit or all packages using sterile technique. To maintain sterility.

6. Apply sterile gloves

7. Using sterile technique, place a sterile barrier under the site to be prepped.

8. The skin prep is performed from the center of the surgical site to the outside. *The center needs to be the cleanest part.* Scrub in a circular motion outward. If the site is a digit on a hand or foot, then scrub all the way around the toes

and the foot from clean to contaminated as efficiently as possible
   - Use all of the sponges/gauze with the surgical prep solution and let the prep solution remain on the skin. *This will allow the solution to continue to inhibit or kill microorganisms on the skin.*
   - Cover the surgically prepped site with sterile drapes. *To ensure the site remains free of microorganisms.*

9. Document area prepped for surgery as an additional precaution against incorrect surgical intervention.

SAMPLE DOCUMENTATION

[date] Left great toe shaved and prepped
[time] for surgical removal per sterile
        technique. Site covered with sterile
        drapes.

_____ L. Cruz, LPN

PROCEDURE 31-3 ## Applying Antiemboli Stockings

Purposes

- To facilitate venous return from the lower extremities
- To prevent venous stasis and venous thrombosis
- To reduce peripheral edema

Equipment

- Tape measure
- Clean antiemboli stockings of appropriate size and of the type ordered

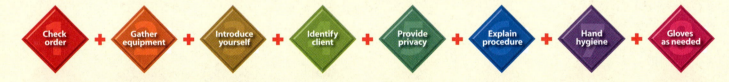

Check order + Gather equipment + Introduce yourself + Identify client + Provide privacy + Explain procedure + Hand hygiene + Gloves as needed

Interventions

1. Take measurements as needed to obtain the appropriate size stockings.
   - Measure the length of both legs from the heel to the gluteal fold (for thigh-length stockings) or from the heel to the popliteal space (for knee-length stockings).
   - Measure the circumference of each calf and each thigh at the widest point.
   - Compare the measurements to the size chart to obtain stockings of correct size. Obtain two sizes if there is a significant difference. *Stockings that are too large for the*

client do not place adequate pressure on the legs to facilitate venous return and may bunch, increasing the risk of pressure and skin irritation. Stockings that are too small may impede blood flow to the feet and cause discomfort.

2. Select an appropriate time to apply the stockings.
   - Apply stockings in the morning, if possible, before the client arises. *In sitting and standing positions, the veins can become distended so that edema occurs; the stockings should be applied before this happens.*

- Assist the client who has been ambulating to lie down and elevate the legs for 15 to 30 minutes before applying the stockings. *This facilitates venous return and reduces swelling.*

3. Prepare the client.
   - Assist the client to a lying position in bed.
   - Wash and dry the legs as needed.

4. Apply the stockings.
   - Reach inside the stocking from the top, and grasping the heel, turn the upper portion of the stocking inside out over the foot portion. *Firm elastic stockings are easier to fit over the foot and calf when inverted in this manner rather than bunching the stocking up.*
   - Ask the client to point the toes, and position the stocking on the client's foot, taking care to place the toe and heel portions of the stocking appropriately (Figure 31-9A ■). *Pointing the toes makes application easier.*
   - Grasp the upper edge of the stocking and gently pull the stocking over the leg, turning it right side out in the process (Figure 31-9B).

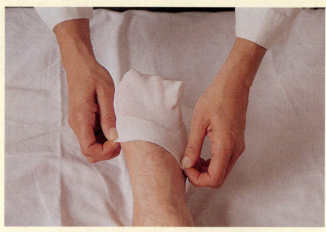

A

clinical ALERT

If you are having trouble adjusting stockings over a client's foot, this technique may help. Place the foot in a small plastic bag. (A clean bedside trash bag works well.) Adjust the stocking over the bag-covered foot and up the leg. Once the stocking has been adjusted, pull the plastic bag out through the open toe of the stocking. The elastic stocking will be smooth and wrinkle free without discomfort to the client.

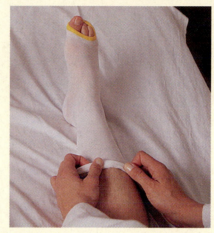

B

Figure 31-9. ■ A. Applying the inverted stocking over the toes. **B.** Pulling the stocking snugly over the leg. (Photographer: Elena Dorfman.)

- Inspect the client's leg and stocking, smoothing any folds or creases. Ensure that the stocking is not rolled down or bunched at the top or ankle. *Folds and creases can cause skin irritation under the stocking; bunching of the stocking can further impair venous return.*
- Remove the hose for 30 minutes every 8 hours, inspecting the legs and skin while the hose are off. *This allows early detection of problems.*
- Soiled hose may be laundered by hand with warm water and mild soap. Hang to dry.

5. Document the procedure.
   - Record the procedure, your assessment data, and when the stockings are removed and reapplied.

SAMPLE DOCUMENTATION

[date]
[time]
Antiemboli stockings removed for bathing. Bilateral pedal pulses strong and regular. Skin warm, dry, and pink. No evidence of edema. Homans' sign negative. Stockings replaced, client ambulated from bed to chair.
_____ K. Turner, LVN

PROCEDURE 31-4 **Managing Nasogastric Suctioning**

Purposes

- To relieve abdominal distention
- To maintain gastric decompression after surgery
- To remove blood and secretions from the gastrointestinal tract
- To relieve discomfort (e.g., when a client has a bowel obstruction)
- To maintain the patency of the NG tube

Equipment

- NG tube in place in the client
- Basin
- 50-mL syringe with an adapter
- Stethoscope
- Suction device for either continuous or intermittent suction
- Connector and connecting tubing
- Disposable gloves
- Graduated container as required to measure gastric drainage
- Cotton-tipped applicators
- Ointment or lubricant
- Disposable irrigating set containing a sterile 50-mL syringe, moisture-resistant pad, basin, and graduated container
- Sterile normal saline (500 mL) or the ordered solution

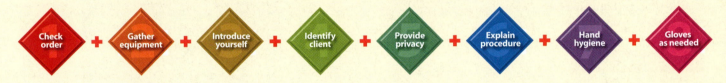

Interventions

INITIATING SUCTION

1. Position the client appropriately.
   - Assist the client to a semi-Fowler's position if it is not contraindicated. *In semi-Fowler's position, the NG tube is not as likely to lie against the wall of the stomach and will therefore suction most efficiently. Semi-Fowler's position also prevents reflux of gastric contents, which could lead to aspiration.*

2. Confirm that the NG tube is in the stomach.
   - Aspirate stomach contents and check their acidity using a pH test strip.
   - Insert air into the NG tube with the syringe and listen with a stethoscope over the stomach (just below the xiphoid process) for a swish of air or gurgling.
   - Use other methods in accordance with facility protocol.

3. Set and check the suction.
   - Connect the appropriate suction regulator to the wall suction outlet and the collection device to the regulator. Intermittent suction regulators generally are used with single-lumen tubes. Apply suction for a set interval (15 to 60 seconds), followed by an interval of no suction. Intermittent suction is set at 80 to 100 mm Hg or as ordered by the physician. Check the suction level by occluding the drainage tube and observing the regulator dial during a suction cycle. Continuous suction regulators are used with double-lumen (e.g., Salem sump) nasogastric tubes. Set continuous suction as ordered by the physician, or at 60 to 120 mm Hg.

   - If using a portable suction machine, turn on the machine and regulate the suction as above. The Gomco pump has two settings: low intermittent for single-lumen tubes, and high for double-lumen tubes.
   - Test for proper suctioning by holding the open end of the suction tube to the ear and listening for a swishing noise or by occluding the end of the tube with a thumb.

4. Establish gastric suction.
   - Connect the NG tube to the tubing from the suction by using the connector.
   - If a Salem sump tube is in place, connect the larger lumen to the suction equipment. This double-lumen tube has a smaller tube running inside the primary suction tube. *The smaller tube provides a continuous flow of atmospheric air through the drainage tube at its distal end and prevents excessive suction force on the gastric mucosa at the drainage outlets. Damage to the gastric mucosa is thus avoided.*
   - Always keep the air vent tube of a Salem sump tube open and above the level of the stomach when suction is applied. *Closing the vent can stop the sump action and cause mucosal damage. Keeping the end of the air vent tube higher than the stomach prevents reflux of gastric contents into the air lumen of the tube.*
   - After suction is applied, monitor the tubing for a few minutes until the gastric contents appear to be running through the tubing into the receptacle. A Salem sump tube makes a soft, hissing sound when it is

hooked up to the suction apparatus and is functioning correctly.

- If the suction apparatus is not working properly, check that all connections are tight and that the tubing is not kinked.
- Coil and secure the tubing on the bed so that it does not loop below the suction bottle. *If the tubing falls below the suction bottle, the suction may be obstructed because of the pressure required to push the fluid against gravity.*

5. Assess the drainage.
   - Observe the amount, color, odor, and consistency of the drainage. *Normal gastric drainage has a thick consistency and is either colorless or yellow-green because of the presence of bile. A coffee-grounds color and consistency may indicate bleeding.*
   - Test the gastric drainage for pH and blood (by using Hematest) when indicated. *A person who has had gastrointestinal surgery can be expected to have some blood in the drainage.*

MAINTAINING SUCTION

6. Assess the client and the suction system regularly.
   - Assess the client every 30 minutes until the system is running effectively and then every 2 hours, or as the client's health indicates, to ensure that the suction is functioning properly. *If the client complains of fullness, nausea, or epigastric pain or if the flow of gastric secretions is absent in the tubing or in the collection receptacle, ineffective suctioning or blockage of the nasogastric tube is likely.*
   - Inspect the suction system for patency of the system (e.g., kinks or blockages in the tubing) and tightness of the connections. *Loose connections can permit air to enter and decrease the effectiveness of the suction by decreasing the negative pressure.*

7. Relieve blockages if present.
   - Don gloves.
   - Check the suction equipment. To do this, disconnect the NG tube from the suction holding the tubing over a collecting basin (to collect gastric drainage). With the suction turned on, place the end of the suction tubing in a basin of water. *If water is drawn into the drainage receptacle, the suction equipment is functioning properly and the nasogastric tube is either blocked or positioned incorrectly.*
   - Reposition the client (e.g., to the other side) if permitted. *This may facilitate drainage.*
   - If the nasogastric tube is taped in place, caution must be used when untaping the tube from the nares. Rotate the NG tube, and reposition it and tape back in place. Taping the NG tube to the nares secures the tube and prevents dislodging. Rotating the NG tube is contraindicated in clients who have had gastrointestinal surgery. *Moving the tube may interfere with gastric sutures.*
   - Irrigate the nasogastric tube as agency protocol states or by the order of the physician. See steps 11 to 13.

8. Prevent reflux into the vent lumen of a Salem sump tube. *Reflux of gastric contents into the vent lumen may occur when*

stomach pressure exceeds atmospheric pressure. In this situation, gastric contents follow the path of least resistance and flow out the vent lumen rather than the drainage lumen. To prevent reflux:
   - Place the NG tubing higher than the client's stomach.
   - Keep the drainage collection container below the level of the client's stomach and do not allow it to become overfull. *A collection device placed above the level of fluid in the stomach or that is too full may interfere with drainage, allowing reflux of gastric contents into the air lumen.*
   - Keep the drainage lumen free of particulate matter that may obstruct the lumen. See steps 11 to 13 for irrigating a NG tube.

9. Ensure the client's comfort.
   - Clean the client's nostrils as needed, using the cotton-tipped applicators and water. Apply a water-soluble lubricant or ointment.
   - Provide mouth care every 2 to 4 hours and as needed. *Some postoperative clients with an NG tube are permitted to suck ice chips or a moist cloth to maintain the moisture of the oral mucous membranes.*

10. Empty the drainage receptacle according to agency policy or physician's order.
    - Clamp the NG tube, and turn off the suction.
    - Don gloves.
    - If the receptacle is graduated, determine the amount of drainage.
    - Disconnect the receptacle.
    - If the receptacle is not graduated, empty the contents into a graduated container and measure.
    - Inspect the drainage carefully for color, consistency, and presence of substances (e.g., blood clots).
    - Discard and replace a full receptacle and reattach it to the suction apparatus. Check the facility policy.
    - Turn on the suction and unclamp the NG tube.
    - Observe the system for several minutes to make sure function is reestablished.
    - Go to step 14.

IRRIGATING A NG TUBE

11. Prepare the client and the equipment.
    - Place the moisture-resistant pad under the end of the NG tube.
    - Turn off the suction.
    - Don gloves.
    - Disconnect the NG tube from the connector.
    - Determine that the tube is in the stomach. See step 2 above and Chapter 25 ∞. *This ensures that the irrigating solution enters the client's stomach.*

12. Irrigate the tube.
    - Draw up the ordered volume of irrigating solution in the syringe; 30 mL of solution per instillation is usual, but up to 60 mL may be given per instillation if ordered.

- Attach the syringe to the NG tube, and slowly inject the solution.
- Gently aspirate the solution. *Forceful withdrawal could damage the gastric mucosa.*
- If you encounter difficulty in withdrawing the solution, inject 20 mL of air and aspirate again, and/or reposition the client or the NG tube. *Air and repositioning may move the end of the tube away from the stomach wall.* If aspirating difficulty continues, reattach the tube in intermittent low suction, and notify the nurse in charge or physician.
- Repeat the preceding steps until the ordered amount of solution is used.
- *Note:* A Salem sump tube can also be irrigated through the vent lumen without interrupting suction. However, only small quantities of irrigant can be injected through this lumen compared to the drainage lumen.
- After irrigating the NG tube, inject 10 to 20 mL of air into the vent lumen while applying suction to the drainage lumen. *This tests the patency of the vent and ensures sump functioning.*

13. Reestablish suction.
   - Reconnect the NG tube to suction.
   - If a Salem sump tube is used, inject the air vent lumen with 10 mL of air after reconnecting the tube to suction.
   - Observe the system for several minutes to make sure it is functioning.

14. Document all relevant information.
   - Record the time suction was started. Also record the pressure established, the color and consistency of the drainage, and nursing assessments.
   - During maintenance, record assessments, supportive nursing measures, and data about the suction system.
   - When irrigating the tube, record verification of tube placement; the time of the irrigation; the amount and type of irrigating solution used; the amount, color and consistency of the returns; the patency of the system following the irrigation; and nursing assessments. *Remember the saying, "If it isn't documented, it wasn't done."*

SAMPLE DOCUMENTATION

[date]	Abdominal distention decreased;
[time]	bowel sounds present in all 4 quadrants; 450 mL of dark coffee-grounds gastric drainage; oral mucous membrane pink and moist.
	_____ D. Wilson, LPN

PROCEDURE 31-5

Cleaning a Sutured Wound and Applying a Sterile Dressing

Purposes

- To promote wound healing by primary intention
- To prevent infection
- To assess the healing process
- To protect the wound from mechanical trauma

Equipment

- Bath blanket (if necessary)
- Moisture-proof bag
- Mask (optional)
- Acetone or another solution (if necessary to loosen adhesive tape)
- Disposable gloves
- Sterile gloves
- Sterile dressing set; if not available, gather the following sterile items from a central supply cart:
  - Drape or towel
  - Gauze squares or available dressing
  - Container for the cleaning solution
  - Cleaning solution (e.g., normal saline)
  - Two pairs of forceps
  - Gauze dressings and Surgipads
  - Applicators or tongue blades to apply ointments
  - Additional supplies required for the particular dressing (e.g., extra gauze dressings and ointment, if ordered)
- Tape, tie tapes, or binder

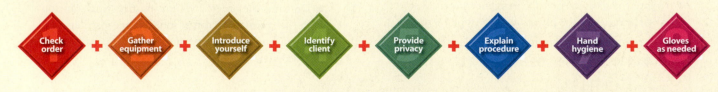

Interventions

1. Prepare the client and assemble the equipment.
   - Acquire assistance for changing a dressing on a restless or confused adult. *The restless or confused client might move and contaminate the sterile field or the wound.*
   - Assist the client to a comfortable position in which the wound can be readily exposed. Expose only the wound area, using a bath blanket to cover the client, if necessary. *Unnecessary exposure is physically and psychologically distressing to most people.*
   - Make a cuff on the moisture-proof bag for disposal of the soiled dressings, and place the bag within reach. It can be taped to the bed side rails or bedside table. *Making a cuff helps keep the outside of the bag free from contamination by the soiled dressings and prevents subsequent contamination of the nurse's hands or of sterile instrument tips when discarding dressing or sponges. Placement of the bag within reach prevents the nurse from reaching across the sterile field and the wound and potentially contaminating these areas.*
   - Put on a face mask, if required. *Some agencies require that a mask be worn for surgical dressing changes to prevent contamination of the wound by droplet spray from the nurse's respiratory tract.*

2. Remove binders (if used) and tape.
   - Remove binders, if used, and place them aside. Untie tie tapes, if used.
   - Remove the tape by holding down the skin and pulling the tape gently but firmly toward the wound. *Pressing down on the skin provides countertraction against the pulling motion. Tape is pulled toward the incision to prevent strain on the sutures or wound.*
   - Use a solvent to loosen tape, if required. *Moistening the tape with acetone or a similar solvent lessens the discomfort of removal, particularly from hairy surfaces.*

3. Remove and dispose of soiled dressings appropriately.
   - Put on clean disposable gloves, and remove the outer dressing or Surgipad.

   - Lift the outer dressing so that the underside is away from the client's face. *The appearance and odor of the drainage may be upsetting to the client.*
   - Place the soiled dressing in the moisture-proof bag without touching the outside of the bag. *Contamination of the outside of the bag is avoided to prevent the spread of microorganisms to the nurse and others.*
   - Remove the dressings, taking care not to dislodge any drains. If the gauze sticks to the drain, support the drain with one hand and remove the gauze with the other.
   - Assess the location, type (color, consistency), and odor of wound drainage, and the number of gauzes saturated or the diameter of drainage collected on the dressings.
   - Discard the soiled dressings in the bag as before.
   - Remove gloves, dispose of them in the moisture-proof bag, and wash hands.

4. Set up the sterile supplies.
   - Open the sterile dressing set, using surgical aseptic technique.
   - Place the sterile drape beside the wound.
   - Open the sterile cleaning solution, and pour it over the gauze sponges in the plastic container.
   - Put on sterile gloves.

5. Clean the wound, if indicated.
   - Clean the wound, using your sterile gloved hands or forceps and gauze swabs moistened with cleaning solution.
   - If using forceps, keep the forceps tips lower than the handles at all times. *This prevents their contamination by fluid traveling up to the handle and nurse's wrist and back to the tips.*
   - Use the cleaning methods illustrated and described in Figure 31-10 ■ or one recommended by facility protocol.

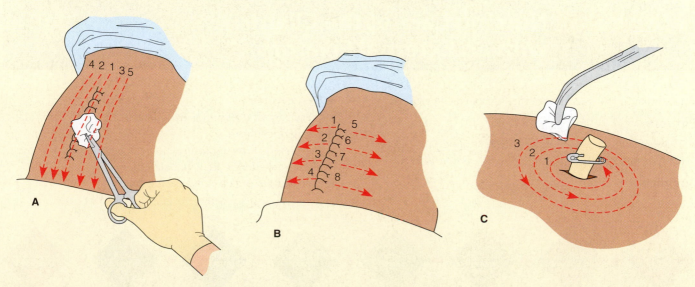

Figure 31-10. ■ Methods of cleaning surgical wounds: **A.** Cleaning the wound from top to bottom, starting at the center. **B.** Cleaning a wound outward from the incision. **C.** Cleaning around a drain site. For all methods, a clean sterile swab is used for each stroke.

- Use a separate swab for each stroke, and discard each swab after use. *This prevents the introduction of microorganisms to other wound areas.*
- If a drain is present, clean it next, taking care to avoid reaching across the cleaned incision. Clean the skin around the drain site by swabbing in half or full circles from around the drain site outward, using separate swabs for each wipe (Figure 31-10C). *This ensures that clean areas are not contaminated.*
- Support and hold the drain erect while cleaning around it. Clean as many times as necessary to remove the drainage.
- Dry the surrounding skin with dry gauze swabs as required. Do not dry the incision or wound itself. *Moisture facilitates wound healing.*

6. Apply dressings to the drain site and the incision.
   - Place a precut 4 × 4 gauze snugly around the drain (Figure 31-11 ■), or open a 4 × 4 gauze to 4 × 8, fold it lengthwise to 2 × 8, and place the 2 × 8 around the drain so that the ends overlap. *This dressing absorbs the*

drainage and helps prevent the drainage from excoriating the skin. Using precut gauze or folding it as described, instead of cutting the gauze, prevents any threads from coming loose and getting into the wound, where they could cause inflammation and provide a site for infection.

- Apply the sterile dressings one at a time over the drain and the incision. Place the bulk of the dressings over the drain area and below the drain, depending on the client's usual position. *Layers of dressings are placed for best absorption of drainage, which flows by gravity.*
- Apply the final Surgipad, remove gloves, and dispose of them. Secure the dressing with tape or ties.

7. Document the procedure and all nursing assessments.

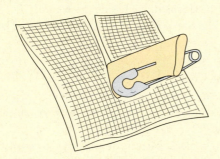

Figure 31-11. ■ Precut gauze in place around a drain.

SAMPLE DOCUMENTATION

[date]   Incision clean and dry, edges pink,
[time]   well approximated, sutures in place.
         Moderate amount of serosan-
         guineous drainage on dressing, no
         evidence of inflammation or odor.
         Incisional pain 4/10. Incision
         cleaned with normal saline. Covered
         with sterile dressing and secured
         with tape.

                    _____ B. Harvey, LVN

PROCEDURE 31-6 Nursing Care of the Client with an External Fixator

An external fixator is a pin or other orthopedic device.

Purpose

- To remove drainage and exudate from around pin sites and prevent infection

Equipment

- Sterile gloves
- Sterile barrier
- Sterile applicators and gauze sponges
- Kling or conform
- Prescribed cleansing solution (check for allergies as some clients are allergic to povidone/iodine)
- Sterile basin or cup for cleansing solution

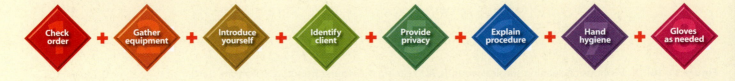

Interventions

1. Check the physician's orders regarding pin site care.
2. Perform hand hygiene.
3. Identify client and explain procedure.
4. Medicate client for pain as needed before cleaning procedure.
5. Ensure the client is in the correct position for maintaining proper alignment. If traction is used, make sure the proper weight is used. Assess the distal extremity for color and edema.
6. Remove dressings.
   - Don nonsterile gloves and remove and discard pin site dressings, observing dressing for drainage amount, color, and odor. *To assess for signs of infection.*
   - Visually assess pin site, noting any redness, swelling, or drainage and make a mental note for later documentation. *To assess for signs of infection.*
   - Remove and dispose of gloves.
7. Set up sterile field.
   - Open applicator and gauze packages and drop onto sterile field.
   - Open prescribed cleansing solution into sterile basin or cup.
   - Don sterile gloves. *To maintain sterility.*
8. Apply cleansing solution to applicators and, maintaining sterile technique, clean area around pin site using the following technique:
   - Clean starting at the pin insertion site and work outward (away from pin site), removing any crust or exudate that has accumulated. Using a new applicator, clean several times around each insertion site using gentle pressure to ease tissue down on pin. *This prevents cross contamination of site.* Once the pin insertion site has been cleaned, work from the clean to dirty area. Never go back to the pin site with the applicator once you have used it away from the site.
   - Loosely dress each pin site by wrapping sterile gauze around the base of the pin. *To prevent microorganisms from entering the wound.*
   - Use the Kling or conform to cover the rest of the surgical wound area by starting the wrapping procedure at the distal end of the extremity and wrapping proximally. *To protect area and keep dressing in place.*
9. Discard materials and remove gloves. Perform hand hygiene.
10. Document pin site assessment and site care given.

SAMPLE DOCUMENTATION

[date] [time]	Pin care performed using sterile procedure on left arm. No drainage or odor apparent. Pin sites free of redness, powder ointment applied to skin surrounding each pin and covered with sterile gauze. Arm wrapped c̄ conforming gauze. Procedure tolerated. _____ B. Schmidt, LPN

PROCEDURE 31-7 Postoperative Stump Care for Extremities

Purposes
- Observation and assessment of surgical site
- Shrinking and molding of residual limb

Equipment
- Two elastic bandages: 4-in. size for below the knee and 6-in. size for above the knee
- Dressings as ordered
- Cleansing solution
- Sterile basin
- Tape
- Sterile and nonsterile gloves

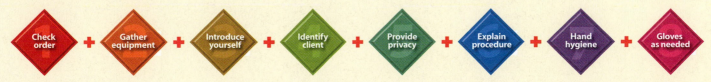

Check order ✚ Gather equipment ✚ Introduce yourself ✚ Identify client ✚ Provide privacy ✚ Explain procedure ✚ Hand hygiene ✚ Gloves as needed

Interventions

1. Check provider's order.

2. Perform hand hygiene.

3. Identify client and explain procedure.

4. Prepare any sterile supplies needed for wound care.
   - Position impervious barrier under the area.
   - Don nonsterile gloves.

5. Remove elastic bandages and dressings observing wound and dressing for drainage, amount, and color. Dispose of dressings and gloves properly. *To assure that standard precautions are carried out.*

6. Don sterile gloves.

7. Wash stump with prescribed cleansing solution and rinse with normal saline starting from the wound and working to the perimeter.
   - Allow area to dry.

8. Inspect wound for signs of infection (redness, swelling, drainage). *To recognize early signs of infection.*

9. Teach client how to assess wound and stump for neuro and circulatory status. *To begin early client teaching of self care.*

10. Dress the wound per provider's order.
    - Explain to client the purpose of the elastic wrap. The wrap is used to form a conical stump for a future prosthetic.
    - Begin by placing the start of the elastic wrap across the bottom of the stump from anterior to posterior. Continue with diagonal spiral turns upward covering the beginning end to secure it. Wrap using a figure-eight fashion stretching the elastic bandage to one- to two-thirds of the bandage limits. *Do not wrap stump in a circular fashion. Doing so will constrict the stump circulation.* Continue to wrap upward toward the groin area, avoiding any creases in the bandage. (Pressure should be directed upward and outward from the end of the stump as you wrap.) *To promote proper shrinking and molding of stumps.*
    - Continue as needed with a new elastic wrap attached to the wrap in place (either by sewing or some other method).

- The bandage should be wrapped from the inside of the thigh, upward and outward across the front of the hip joint.
- Continue the wrap behind the hips at the level of the hip bones.
- Return the elastic wrap to the stump and finish wrapping with figure-eight turns.
- Secure the end of the wrap using the Velcro closure or tape. (Avoid using safety pins or clips to prevent injury to the skin. Tape should not be used on the skin directly to prevent any loss of skin integrity.) *Clips and pins can pierce the skin.*
- Repeat every 4 to 6 hours or as prescribed by the physician or when the bandages become loose. *To assure that equal and constant compression will be applied to stump.*
- Some facilities have stump "shrinker sheaths" for the purpose of readying the stump for the prosthesis. If this is available, stretch and roll down the sheath using the plastic ring. Fit onto the end of the stump and follow directions for application assuring there are no wrinkles.

11. Document.

SAMPLE DOCUMENTATION

[date]
[time]

Incision well approximated, clean, no redness, swelling or drainage. Stump wash and dried and dressed per physicians orders by client. Instruction for wrapping provided as procedure performed. Questions encouraged. Client stated "I would like a try to do wrapping next time."

_____ M. Lee, LPN

Chapter Review

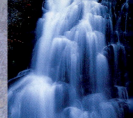

KEY TERMS by Topic

Use the audio glossary feature of either the CD-ROM or the Companion Website to hear the correct pronunciation of the following key terms.

Introduction
surgery, perioperative period, emergency surgery, elective surgery, diagnostic, palliative, ablative, reconstructive, transplant

Preoperative Phase
prostheses, antiemboli stockings, sequential compression device (SCD)

Intraoperative Phase
anesthesia, conscious sedation

Postoperative Phase
tissue perfusion, atelectasis, dehisced, closed wound drainage system, sutures, approximates

KEY Points

- Surgery is a unique experience that creates stress and necessitates physical and psychological changes. Factors such as age, general health, nutritional status, medication use, and mental status affect a client's risk during surgery.

- Clients must agree to surgery and sign a surgical consent before they are sedated for surgery.

- Preoperative teaching should include moving, leg exercises, and coughing and deep-breathing exercises. Good postoperative teaching helps prevent postoperative complications.

- Physical preparation includes the following areas: nutrition and fluids, elimination, hygiene, rest, medications, care of valuables and prostheses, special orders, and surgical skin preparation.

- A preoperative checklist provides a guide to and documentation of a client's preparation before surgery.

- Initial and ongoing assessment of the postoperative client includes level of consciousness, vital signs, oxygen saturation, skin color and temperature, comfort levels, fluid balance, dressings, drains, and tubes.

- The overall goals of nursing care during the postoperative period are to promote comfort and healing, restore the highest possible level of wellness, and prevent associated risks such as infection or respiratory and cardiovascular complications.

- Surgical aseptic technique (sterile technique) is used when changing dressings on surgical wounds to promote healing and reduce the risk of infection. Sutures, wire clips, or staples are generally removed 7 to 10 days after surgery.

EXPLORE MediaLink

Additional interactive resources for this chapter can be found on the Companion Website at www.prenhall.com/ramont. Click on Chapter 31 and "Begin" to select the activities for this chapter.

For chapter-related NCLEX®-style questions and an audio glossary, access the accompanying CD-ROM in this book.

Animations/Videos
- Preoperative and Postoperative Care

FOR FURTHER Study

For handling of client valuables prior to surgery, see discussion in Chapter 10 and Figure 10-2.

For information about auscultating the abdomen to assess for the return of peristalsis, see Chapter 19.

For a more in-depth discussion of pain and pain management, see Chapter 21.

For in-depth discussion of stages of wound healing, information about wound drainage, cleaning wounds, wound irrigation, hot and cold applications, and supporting and immobilizing wounds, see Chapter 23.

For more about oxygenation and client instructions on using an incentive spirometer, see Chapter 24.

For more information on use of sequential compression devices, see Chapter 24 and Procedure 24-6.

For more information about gastrointestinal tubes, see Chapter 25 and Procedure 25-3.

For an illustration of an intake and output record, see Figure 26-2.

For an illustration of leg exercises, see Figures 32-12 and 32-28.

Critical Thinking Care Map

Caring for a Client with an Amputated Arm
NCLEX-PN® Focus Area: Psychosocial Integrity: Coping and Adaptation

Case Study: Tim Broughton is a 22-year-old college student. Six days ago, he was involved in a motorcycle crash resulting in a severe injury to his right arm. After every attempt to save his right arm, amputation to his right arm below the right shoulder was performed 2 days ago.

Nursing Diagnosis: Disturbed Body Image

COLLECT DATA

Subjective	Objective
_____	_____
_____	_____
_____	_____
_____	_____
_____	_____
_____	_____
_____	_____

Would you report this data? Yes/No

If yes, to: _____

What would you report? _____

Nursing Care

_____
_____
_____
_____
_____
_____
_____
_____
_____
_____
_____

How would you document this?_____
_____
_____

Compare your documentation to the sample provided in Appendix I.

Data Collected
(use those that apply)

- Vital signs stable
- Complains of pain
- Refuses to respond to nurse's questions about pain level
- Will not look at limb during dressing change
- States, "I wish I had died in the accident; life will never be the same."
- Dressing dry and intact
- Wound healing without signs of infection

Nursing Interventions
(use those that apply; list in priority order)

- Contact physician for social worker or psychologist referral.
- Acknowledge denial, anger, or depression as normal.
- Teach the importance of range-of-motion exercises.
- Ask client to describe past experiences with pain and effectiveness of methods used to manage pain.
- Encourage client to make own decisions, participate in plan of care, and accept both inadequacies and strengths.
- Obtain assistive devices needed for activity.
- Allow client gradual exposure to body change.
- Help client to accept help from others.
- Teach family appropriate care of surgical site.

1 Preoperative teaching is a vital part of nursing care of the client scheduled for surgery. Good preoperative teaching by the nurse has the following goals:

1. It can lengthen the client's hospitalization.
2. It facilitates the client's return to jogging and exercise.
3. It can reduce postoperative pain and teaches the client coping mechanisms to deal with postoperative discomfort.
4. It increases anxiety in the client and the client's support persons.

2 You are preparing clients for surgery. Several clients have requested to be allowed to wear their wedding rings. Of the following, which client must remove his or her wedding ring, rather than leaving it on the left hand and secured with tape?

1. a 65-year-old male scheduled for a TURP (transurethral resection of the prostate)
2. a 31-year-old female having a repeat c-section
3. a 72-year-old female having a total hip replacement
4. a 49-year-old female scheduled for a left modified radical mastectomy

3 Postoperative assessments are usually made every 15 minutes until vital signs stabilize. Of the following, which client requires vital signs every hour?

1. a client with stable vital signs on the day of discharge
2. a client with stable vital signs within 3 hours after surgery
3. a client with hypotension and depressed respirations 2 hours after surgery
4. a client with a temperature of 99.8°F on the second postoperative day

4 A client returns to the unit following surgery in which spinal anesthesia was administered. You need to give instructions to the nursing assistant about positioning the client. Of the following positions, which is the most appropriate for this client?

1. reverse Trendelenburg
2. positioned on his or her left side with head slightly elevated
3. flat for 8 to 12 hours
4. semi-Fowler's position

5 You are teaching deep breathing and coughing to your client who is having surgery later today. Which of the following statements indicates the need for further teaching?

1. "I will lie prone and flat while coughing to control pain."
2. "I will hold a pillow against my abdomen during coughing."
3. "After taking a deep breath, I will cough forcefully."
4. "I will take a deep breath through my nose prior to coughing."

6 A postoperative client is complaining of pain. Of the following, which is the most accurate way to assess the severity of pain?

1. Assess the client's vital signs.
2. Ask the client if the pain is mild, moderate, or severe.
3. Observe physiological signs such as grimace or sweating.
4. Ask the client to rate the pain using a scale of 0 to 10.

7 One day following surgery your client is to start ambulating. He asks, "Why can't I just stay in bed until I feel better?" Of the following, which would be the best response?

1. "Your doctor has written an order for you to walk, and I must follow the doctor's orders."
2. "If you walk to the chair, it will be easier to change the bed while you are up."
3. "Walking is one of the best ways to prevent respiratory and circulatory complications."
4. "You will never feel better if you just lie in bed."

8 You are preparing your client for surgery. Of the following assessment information, what needs to be reported to the physician immediately?

1. His vital signs are: temperature 98.8, pulse 84, respirations 20, BP 132/80.
2. The client reports he took his pills with sips of water as instructed before coming to the hospital.
3. The client tells you he doesn't understand what they are going to do, and he is not sure he wants to go through with the surgery.
4. The client is allergic to morphine sulfate.

9 Reflux of gastric contents into the NG tube vent lumen may occur when stomach pressure exceeds atmospheric pressure. To prevent this, you would:

1. clamp the NG tube vent lumen and turn up the suction.
2. place the NG tubing higher than the client's stomach.
3. place the NG tube lower than the stomach.
4. irrigate the NG tubing.

10 You are removing staples on a client with an abdominal surgical incision. The wound opens and a portion of the intestine protrudes from the opening. You know this occurrence to be:

1. secondary intention.
2. dehiscence.
3. evisceration.
4. granulation.

Answers and Rationales for Review Questions, as well as discussion of Care Plan and Critical Thinking Care Map questions, appear in Appendix I.

Chapter 32

Activity, Rest, and Sleep

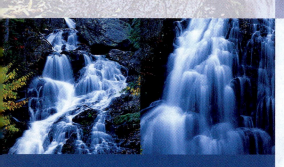

BRIEF Outline

ACTIVITY

Normal Movement

Factors Affecting Body Alignment and Activity

Effects of Immobility

REST AND SLEEP

Physiology of Sleep

Functions of Sleep

Factors Affecting Sleep

Common Sleep Disorders

HISTORICAL Perspectives

History has shown that simple animals became inactive whenever possible in order to restore and maintain their nervous system. As humans have evolved, the nervous system has become increasingly important as a maintenance system to promote health through rest and restoration. A daily cycle of activity, rest, and sleep is essential in restoring the nervous system. Sleep is probably devoted to the removal of waste products from the nervous system especially the buildup of neurotransmitters and hormones between cells. Sleep occurs in cycles for most humans; they quickly move into restorative sleep, then back up toward wakefulness, then down again. It is daylight that awakes us and the release of a hormone called melatonin that tells us to sleep.

LEARNING Outcomes

After completing this chapter, you will be able to:

1. Describe basic elements of normal movement.
2. Compare effects of exercise and immobility on body systems.
3. Identify and assess factors influencing human mobility including body alignment, activity–exercise patterns, and activity tolerance.
4. Use proper body mechanics when positioning, moving, lifting, and ambulating clients.
5. Explain the dynamics of sleep.
6. Describe variations in sleep patterns throughout the life span.
7. Identify factors that affect normal sleep.
8. Describe common sleep disorders.
9. Describe interventions to promote normal sleep.

Balanced activity, rest, and sleep are essential to health. Most people equate physical well-being with freedom of mobility. Mobility is vital to independence. Inability to perform routine activities of daily living (ADLs) such as bathing, cooking, shopping, and engaging in recreational sports or work can adversely effect a client's self-esteem and mental health.

ACTIVITY

Normal Movement

Body movement is dependent on the integrated and interdependent activity of the musculoskeletal, nervous, and *vestibular* (inner ear) systems. Normal movement involves four bodily aspects: *alignment* (posture), joint mobility, *balance* (stability), and coordination. Alignment and joint mobility are discussed briefly here.

ALIGNMENT AND POSTURE

When the body is aligned, organs are properly supported. This allows them to function at their best, while also maintaining balance.

The **line of gravity** is an imaginary vertical line drawn through the body's center of gravity (Figure 32-1 ■). The **center of gravity** is the point at which all of the body's mass is centered and the base of support (the foundation on which the body rests) achieves balance. In humans, the usual line of gravity is drawn from the top of the head, down between the shoulders, through the trunk slightly anterior to the sacrum, and between the weight-bearing joints (hips, knees) and base of support (feet). In the upright position, the center of gravity occurs in the pelvis approximately midway between the umbilicus and the symphysis pubis. When standing, an adult must center body weight symmetrically along the line of gravity to maintain stability. Greater stability and balance are achieved in the sitting or supine position because a chair or bed provides a wider base of support with a lower center of gravity. When the body is well aligned, there is little strain on the joints, muscles, tendons, or ligaments.

The musculoskeletal system continuously works to maintain erect posture and to offset the constant pull of gravity. The sustained muscle contraction required to maintain the upright position is called **postural tonus**. Posture is one criterion for assessing general health, physical fitness, and beauty. Posture reflects the mood, self-esteem, and personality of an individual.

JOINT MOBILITY

Most skeletal muscles are attached to two bones at the joint. These muscles are defined by the movement they produce and are therefore called flexors, extensors, internal rotators, and so on. Types of synovial joint movement are shown in Table 32-1 ■.

Flexors are stronger than extensors, so when a person is inactive, joints become pulled into the *flexed* (bent) position. Constant immobility causes muscles to shorten permanently and become fixed in the "flexed" position (see later section on immobility). The **range of motion (ROM)** of a joint is the maximum movement possible for that joint. Range of motion varies by individual and is determined by heredity, age, injury or disease, and level of physical activity. Many mechanisms are responsible for maintaining human balance.

Equilibrium (the sense of balance) depends on the integration of stimuli from several organs: the muscles and tendons of the head and neck (vestibulospinal input), the eyes (vestibulo-ocular input), and the inner ear. The inner ear or **labyrinth** consists of the cochlea, vestibule, and semicircular canals. The semicircular canals and vestibule govern equilibrium.

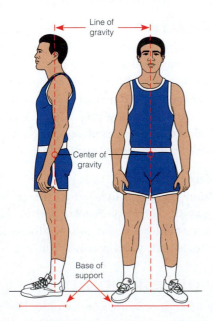

Figure 32-1. ■ Center of gravity and the line of gravity influence standing alignment.

TABLE 32-1

Synovial Joint Movements and Their Actions

MOVEMENT	ACTION	MOVEMENT	ACTION
Flexion	Decreasing the angle of the joint (e.g., bending the elbow)	Eversion	Turning the sole of the foot outward by moving the ankle joint
Inversion	Increasing the angle of the joint (e.g., straightening the arm at the elbow)	Inversion	Turning the sole of the foot inward by moving the ankle joint
Hyperextension	Further extension or straightening of a joint (e.g., bending the head backward)	Pronation	Moving the bones of the forearm so that the palm of the hand faces downward when held in front of the body
Abduction	Movement of the bone away from the midline of the body	Supination	Moving the bones of the forearm so that the palm of the hand faces upward when held in front of the body
Adduction	Movement of the bone toward the midline of the body	Protraction	Moving a part of the body forward in the same plane parallel to the ground
Rotation	Movement of the bone around its central axis	Retraction	Moving a part of the body backward in the same plane parallel to the ground
Circumduction	Movement of the distal part of the bone in a circle while the proximal end remains fixed		

Factors Affecting Body Alignment and Activity

Numerous factors affect an individual's body alignment, mobility, and daily activity level. These include growth and development, physical health, mental health, nutrition, personal values and attitudes, and other external factors.

GROWTH AND DEVELOPMENT

A person's age and musculoskeletal and nervous system development affect posture, body proportions, body mass, body movements, and reflexes. Refer to Chapter 11 ⚭ for age-related considerations.

PHYSICAL HEALTH

Mobility is directly affected by any disorder of the musculoskeletal or nervous systems, or by any vestibular (inner ear) disorders. Congenital anomalies, such as hip dysplasia and spina bifida, affect motor function. Musculoskeletal trauma limiting mobility includes strains, sprains, fractures, joint dislocations, amputations, and joint replacement. Nervous system disorders such as cerebral palsy, Parkinson's disease, multiple sclerosis, tumors, infections (e.g., meningitis), and injuries to the spinal cord or brain such as cerebrovascular accidents (strokes) may leave muscles weakened, paralyzed, spastic (with too much muscle tone), or flaccid (without muscle tone). Disorders of the vestibular apparatus, such as an ear infection or Ménière's disease, cause **vertigo**, a strong sensation of spinning around in space, which impairs balance.

Illnesses that limit the supply of oxygen to vital organs affect activity tolerance. Examples include chronic obstructive pulmonary disease (COPD), emphysema, anemia, angina, and congestive heart failure (CHF).

MENTAL HEALTH

Mental or *affective* (emotional) disorders affect personal motivation. Anxiety may produce an increase in physical activity. Chronic stress, however, depletes the body's energy reserves, producing fatigue. Slumped posture may indicate lassitude or depression. A depressed client may lack the physical energy required for daily hygiene. Exercise is necessary to mental health. Movement energizes the client and facilitates coping.

NUTRITION

Undernutrition and overnutrition influence body alignment and mobility. Obesity distorts posture and balance, causing strain on muscles and joints. More energy is expended on movement, which produces fatigue.

Effects of Immobility

A sedentary lifestyle or history of inactivity due to injury or illness increases the risk of major disease. The level of risk depends on the duration of inactivity, the client's general health, and sensory awareness. Nurses must understand these risks and encourage client mobility. Early ambulation after illness or surgery is an essential preventive measure.

MUSCULOSKELETAL SYSTEM

Signs of prolonged immobility are most often manifested in the musculoskeletal system. Muscular strength decreases in the absence of physical activity. Common musculoskeletal problems resulting from prolonged immobility include:

- *Disuse osteoporosis.* Without the stress of weight-bearing activity, bones demineralize. Calcium, which gives bones density and strength, becomes depleted. Despite adequate calcium in the diet, this demineralization process, known as **osteoporosis**, continues during immobility. Bones become spongy and deformed, and they fracture easily.
- *Disuse atrophy.* Unused muscles **atrophy** (decrease in size), losing most of their normal strength and function.
- *Contractures.* When muscle fibers are not able to shorten and lengthen for a prolonged time, a contracture (permanent shortening of the muscle) develops. This process involves the tendons, ligaments, and joint capsules, causing permanent fixation of the joint—irreversible except by surgical intervention. Joint deformities such as foot drop (Figure 32-2 ■) and external hip rotation occur when a stronger muscle dominates the opposite muscle.
- *Joint pain and stiffness.* Without movement, *collagen* (connective tissue) at the joint becomes **ankylosed** (permanently immobile). In addition, as the bones demineralize, excess calcium may deposit in the joints, contributing to stiffness and pain.

CARDIOVASCULAR SYSTEM

Diminished Cardiac Reserve

Decreased mobility creates an imbalance in the autonomic nervous system, resulting in increased heart rate. During immobility a rapid heart rate reduces diastolic pressure, coronary blood flow, and heart capacity available to respond to metabolic demands. Because of this diminished reserve, an immobilized person may experience tachycardia and angina with minimal exertion.

Increased Use of the Valsalva Maneuver

The Valsalva maneuver occurs when forceful exhalation against the closed glottis increases intrathoracic pressure, which in turn reduces venous blood return to the heart. This is the kind of breath holding that is done when straining to make a bowel movement or attempting to move up in bed. As the glottis opens and breath is released, blood suddenly surges to the heart. Tachycardia or cardiac arrhythmia may result.

Orthostatic Hypotension

Orthostatic hypotension (postural hypotension) is common with prolonged bed rest. It is marked by a sudden drop in blood pressure when a client stands and blood pools in the lower extremities. Cerebral perfusion is compromised, creating dizziness or fainting. This sequence is usually accompanied by a sudden and marked increase in heart rate, the body's effort to protect the brain from an inadequate blood supply.

Venous Vasodilation and Stasis

The skeletal muscles of an active person contract with each movement. They compress the blood vessels to pump the blood back to the heart against gravity. Valves in the leg veins, which remain constricted, aid in venous return to the heart by preventing backflow. Atrophied muscles cannot assist in pumping blood back to the heart against gravity. Blood pools in the leg veins, causing vasodilation and engorgement (Figure 32-3 ■).

Dependent Edema

When venous pressure is great, serum is forced from the blood vessels into the surrounding interstitial space, causing

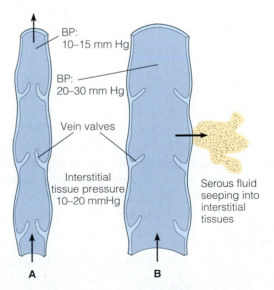

Figure 32-3. ■ Leg veins: **A.** in a mobile person; **B.** in an immobile person.

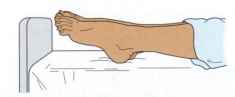

Figure 32-2. ■ Plantar flexion contracture (foot drop).

edema (swelling). Edema occurs most commonly in the lower body, below the level of the heart. Prolonged bed rest is likely to cause edema at the sacrum. Prolonged sitting generally causes edema in the lower legs.

Thrombophlebitis and Emboli

Venous vasodilation and stasis predispose the client to **thrombus** (blood clot) formation. Impaired venous return to the heart, blood hypercoagulability, and injury to a vessel wall may result in **thrombophlebitis** (one or more clots loosely attached to an inflamed vessel wall). Thrombi become very dangerous when they break loose. **Emboli** (clots moved from their place of origin, causing circulatory obstruction elsewhere) may lodge in vessels supplying vital organs. Large pulmonary (lung) emboli may cause **infarction** (death of tissue) and sudden death. Emboli in the coronary or cerebral vessels are equally life threatening.

RESPIRATORY SYSTEM

Decreased Respiratory Movement

In a recumbent, immobile client, ventilation of the lungs is passively altered. The rigid bed presses against the body and curtails chest movement. Abdominal organs push against the diaphragm, further restricting chest movement and lung expansion. An immobile recumbent person rarely sighs, because muscle atrophy affects the respiratory muscles. Without periodic stretching movements, the cartilaginous intercostal joints become fixed in an *expiratory* (sunken chest) position, further restricting the potential for maximum ventilation. These changes produce shallow respirations and reduced **vital capacity** (the maximum volume of air that can be exhaled after maximum inhalation). Up to 25% to 50% of normal vital capacity may be compromised in an immobile, paralyzed client. For more information about oxygenation, see Chapter 24 ⚭.

Pooling of Respiratory Secretions

Secretions are normally expelled by coughing and posture changes. Inactivity allows respiratory secretions to pool by gravity (Figure 32-4 ■), interfering with the normal exchange of oxygen and carbon dioxide in the alveoli. Cough may be diminished due to loss of respiratory muscle tone, dehydration (which thickens mucus), or sedatives, which depress the cough reflex. Poor oxygenation and buildup of carbon dioxide in the blood can result in respiratory acidosis, a potentially lethal imbalance of body pH.

Atelectasis

As a result of changes in pulmonary blood flow, bed rest decreases surfactant production. *Surfactant* enables the alveoli to remain open. Decreased surfactant combined with mucous blockage of a bronchiole may cause **atelectasis** (the collapse of

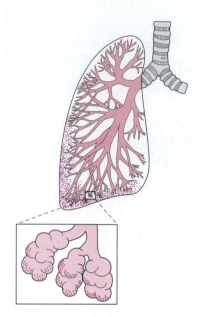

Figure 32-4. ■ Pooling of secretions in the lungs of an immobile person.

a lobe or of an entire lung) distal to the blockage. Immobile, elderly, postoperative clients are at greatest risk of atelectasis.

Hypostatic Pneumonia

Pneumonia (inflammation of the lung) caused by static secretions in the alveoli is a common cause of death among weakened immobile persons, especially heavy smokers.

METABOLIC SYSTEM

Anorexia

Loss of appetite (*anorexia*) occurs as a result of decreased metabolic rate and increased catabolism. Reduced caloric intake is usually a response to decreased energy requirements. Reduced dietary protein intake increases the risk of negative nitrogen balance and malnutrition.

Negative Calcium Balance

Negative calcium balance occurs as a result of calcium loss from bone.

URINARY SYSTEM

Urinary Stasis

Gravity plays an important role in the emptying of the kidneys and bladder. The client in a supine (back-lying) position must push upward against gravity (Figure 32-5 ■) to urinate. **Urinary stasis** occurs when urine *stagnates* in (does not move out of) the urinary tract.

Renal Calculi

Negative calcium balance causes increased excretion of calcium salts in the urine, which precipitate as crystals or

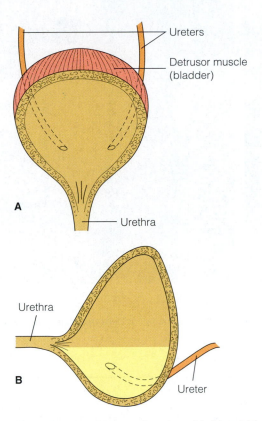

A

Ureters

Detrusor muscle (bladder)

Urethra

B

Urethra

Ureter

Figure 32-5. ■ Pooling of urine in the urinary bladder: **A.** The client is in an upright position. **B.** The client is in a back-lying position.

calculi (kidney stones). Prolonged horizontal positioning causes the renal pelvis to become filled with stagnant alkaline urine, creating an ideal environment for calculi formation.

Urinary Retention

Static urine is an excellent medium for bacterial growth. Urinary tract infections (UTIs) are most commonly caused by *Escherichia coli,* the colon bacillus. The normally sterile urinary tract may be contaminated by improper perineal care, an indwelling urinary catheter, or urinary *reflux* (backward flow). See Chapter 27 ◐ for conditions related to the urinary tract.

GASTROINTESTINAL SYSTEM

Decreased peristalsis, colon motility, and strength of the abdominal and perineal muscles used in defecation cause constipation. Disruption of normal bowel habits, caused by the embarrassment or discomfort of using a bedpan, may cause the client to postpone or ignore the urge for elimination. Repeated postponement suppresses the urge and weakens the defecation reflex. A bedfast person may lack the strength required to expel hardened stool. See Chapter 28 ◐ for discussion of concerns related to bowel elimination.

INTEGUMENTARY SYSTEM

Reduced Skin Turgor

Skin can atrophy as a result of prolonged immobility. Shifts in body fluids between fluid compartments can affect the consistency and health of the dermis and subcutaneous tissues, eventually causing a gradual loss in skin *turgor* (elasticity). See Chapter 23 ◐ for a full discussion of the skin.

Skin Breakdown

Normal blood circulation relies on muscle activity. Immobility impedes circulation and diminishes the supply of nutrients. As a result, skin breakdown and formation of pressure ulcers can occur (see Chapter 23 ◐).

PSYCHONEUROLOGICAL SYSTEM

People who are unable to carry out usual activities related to their roles (e.g., breadwinner, spouse, parent, or athlete) become dependent on others. Loss of independence damages self-esteem, and may in turn provoke exaggerated emotional response. Reactions vary considerably. Some individuals become apathetic or withdrawn; others become angry or aggressive.

COLLABORATIVE CARE

Hospitalized clients with limited mobility due to surgery, trauma, or a disease process may need assistive devices in order to regain mobility (Figure 32-6 ■). In most facilities, selection, fitting, and training in use of these devices is the responsibility of the physical therapy department. It is the LPN's or LVN's responsibility to reinforce the teaching and ensure that the client can use them safely both in the hospital and at home after discharge. See Box 32-1 ■ for teaching clients to use walking aids.

Mobility Devices

CANES.   Three types of canes are used today: the standard straight-legged cane; the tripod or crab cane, which has three feet; and the quad cane, which has four feet and provides the most support.

WALKERS.   Walkers are mechanical devices for ambulatory clients who need more support than a cane provides. Walkers come in many shapes and sizes, with devices suited to individual needs. The standard type of walker is made of polished aluminum. It has four legs with rubber tips and plastic hand grips (Figure 32-6B). Many walkers have adjustable legs.

Two- or four-wheeled walkers do not need to be picked up to be moved. However, they are less stable than the standard walkers. Wheeled walkers are used by clients who are too weak or unstable to pick up and move the walker with each step.

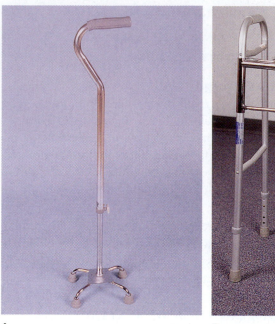
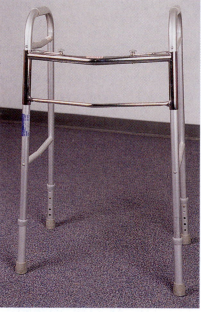
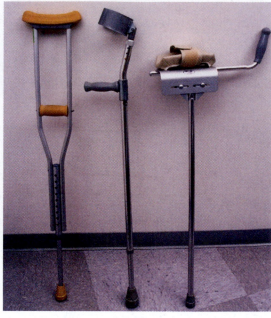

A   B   C

Figure 32-6. ■ Walking aids: **A.** Quad cane. (Photographer: Jenny Thomas.) **B.** Standard walker. (Photographer: Elena Dorfman.) **C.** Three types of crutches: C1, axillary crutch; C2, Lofstrand crutch; C3, Canadian, or elbow extensor, crutch.

BOX 32-1	CLIENT TEACHING

Using Walking Aids

Canes

- Hold the cane with the hand on the stronger side of the body to provide maximum support and appropriate body alignment when walking.
- Position the tip of a standard cane (and the nearest tip of other canes) about 15 cm (6 in.) to the side and 15 cm (6 in.) in front of the near foot, so that the elbow is slightly flexed.

When Maximum Support Is Required

- Move the cane forward about 30 cm (1 ft), or a distance that is comfortable while the body weight is borne by both legs.
- Then move the affected (weak) leg forward to the cane while the weight is borne by the cane and stronger leg.
- Next, move the unaffected (stronger) leg forward ahead of the cane and weak leg while the weight is borne by the cane and weak leg.
- Repeat the steps. This pattern of moving provides at least two points of support on the floor at all times.

As You Become Stronger and Require Less Support

- Move the cane and weak leg forward at the same time, while the weight is borne by the stronger leg.
- Move the stronger leg forward, while the weight is borne by the cane and the weak leg.

Walkers

When Maximum Support Is Required

- Move the walker ahead about 15 cm (6 in.) while your body weight is borne by both legs.

- Then move the right foot up to the walker while your body weight is borne by the left leg and both arms.
- Next, move the left foot up to the right foot while your body weight is borne by the right leg and both arms.

If One Leg Is Weaker than the Other

- Move the walker and the weak leg ahead together about 15 cm (6 in.) while your weight is borne by the stronger leg.
- Then move the stronger leg ahead while your weight is borne by the affected leg and both arms.

Crutches

- Follow the plan of exercises developed for you to strengthen your arm muscles before beginning crutch walking.
- Have a healthcare professional establish the correct length for your crutches and the correct placement of the handpieces. Crutches that are too long force your shoulders upward and make it difficult for you to push your body off the ground. Crutches that are too short will make you hunch over and develop an improper body stance.
- The weight of your body should be borne by the arms rather than the axillae (armpits). Continual pressure on the axillae can injure the radial nerve and eventually cause crutch palsy, a weakness of the muscles of the forearm, wrist, and hand.
- Maintain an erect posture as much as possible to prevent strain on muscles and joints and to maintain balance.
- Each step taken with crutches should be a comfortable distance for you. It is wise to start with a small rather than large step.
- Inspect the crutch tips regularly, and replace them if worn.
- Keep the crutch tips dry and clean to maintain their surface friction. If the tips become wet, dry them well before use.
- Wear a tie shoe with a low heel that grips the floor.

CRUTCHES. Crutches may be a temporary need for some people and a permanent one for others. Crutches should enable a person to ambulate independently, so it is important to learn to use them properly. There are several kinds of crutches (Figure 32-6C). The most frequently used are the underarm crutch or axillary crutch with hand bars, and the Lofstrand or forearm crutch, which extends to the forearm. The Lofstrand crutch is a single adjustable tube of aluminum to which a curved piece of steel, a rubber-covered hand bar, and a metal forearm cuff are attached. The Canadian or elbow extensor crutch, like the Lofstrand, is made of a single tube of aluminum with lateral attachments, a hand bar, and a cuff for the forearm, but it also has a cuff for the upper arm. This crutch is usually used by clients who require support for weak extensor muscles of the arm (e.g., weak triceps brachii).

All crutches require suction tips, usually made of rubber, which help to prevent the crutches from slipping on a floor surface. Proper measurement for and fitting of crutches is essential to ensure client safety.

NURSING CARE

The LVN/LPN collects information from the client, from other nurses, and from the client's records. The examination and history are important sources of information about disabilities affecting the client's mobility and activity status, such as contractures, edema, pain in the extremities, or generalized fatigue.

An activity and exercise history is usually part of the comprehensive nursing history form and includes daily activity level, activity tolerance, type and frequency of exercise, and factors affecting mobility. If the client indicates a recent pattern change or difficulties with mobility, a more detailed history is required. This detailed history should include the specific nature of the problem; when it first began and its frequency; its causes, if known; how the problem affects daily living; client coping strategies; and whether these methods have been effective.

ASSESSING

Body Alignment

Assessment of body alignment includes an inspection of the client while the client stands. To assess alignment the nurse views the client from lateral, anterior, and posterior perspectives.

The "slumped" posture (Figure 32-7 ■) is the most common problem that occurs when people stand. The neck is flexed far forward, the abdomen protrudes, the pelvis is thrust forward to create *lordosis* (an exaggerated curvature of

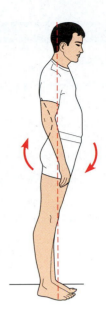

Figure 32-7. ■ Poor trunk alignment. The arrows indicate the direction in which the pelvis is tilted.

the lumbar spine), and the knees are markedly hyperextended. Lower back pain and fatigue occur quickly in people with poor posture. Refer to Figure 32-1 for correct posture.

Gait

The characteristic pattern of a person's *gait* (walk) is assessed to determine the client's mobility and risk for injury due to falling. The nurse assesses gait as the client walks into the room or asks the client to walk a distance of 10 feet down a hallway and observes for the following:

- Head is erect, gaze is straight ahead, and vertebral column is upright.
- Heel strikes the ground before the toe.
- Feet are dorsiflexed in the swing phase.
- Arm opposite the swing-through foot moves forward at the same time.
- Gait is smooth, coordinated, and rhythmic, with even weight borne on each foot; it produces minimal body swing from side to side and directs movement straight ahead; and it starts and stops with ease.

The nurse should also note the client's need for a prosthesis or assistive device, such as a cane or walker. For a client who uses assistive aids, the nurse assesses gait without the device and compares the assisted and unassisted gaits.

Appearance and Movement of Joints

Physical examination of the joints involves inspection; palpation; assessment of range of active motion; and, if active motion is not possible, assessment of range of passive motion. The following joints may be given special attention: neck,

---

BOX 32-2   NURSING CARE CHECKLIST

Active ROM Exercises

☑ Perform each ROM exercise as taught to the point of slight resistance, but not beyond, and never to the point of discomfort.

☑ Perform the movements systematically, using the same sequence during each session.

☑ Perform each exercise three times.

☑ Perform each series of exercises twice daily.

For Older Adults

☑ For older adults, it is not essential to achieve full range of motion in all joints. Instead, emphasize achieving a sufficient range of motion to carry out activities of daily living (ADLs), such as walking, dressing, combing hair, showering, and preparing a meal.

---

shoulder, elbow, wrist, hip, knee, and ankle. Box 32-2 ■ gives points for the nurse to remember in teaching clients to do active ROM exercises. Assessment of range of motion should not be unduly fatiguing, and the joint movements need to be performed smoothly, slowly, and rhythmically. No joint should be forced. Uneven, jerky movement and forcing can injure the joint and its surrounding muscles and ligaments.

The nurse also assesses the amount of assistance the client requires for the following:

■ Moving in the bed. In particular, observe for the amount of assistance the client requires for turning:
  ■ From a supine position to a lateral position
  ■ From a lateral position on one side to a lateral position on the other
  ■ From a supine position to a sitting position in bed.
■ Rising from a lying position to a sitting position on the edge of the bed. Healthy people can normally rise without support from the arms.
■ Rising from a chair to a standing position. Normally this can be done without pushing with the arms.
■ Range of motion of joints needed to complete transfer movements (see previous section).
■ Coordination and balance. Determine the client's abilities to hold the body erect, to bear weight and keep balance in a standing position on both legs or only one, to take steps, and to push off from a chair or bed.

See Procedure 32-1 ■ on page 772 for instruction in providing passive ROM exercises.

Activity Tolerance

By observation of certain activities, the nurse can predict whether the client has the strength and endurance to participate in activities that require similar expenditures of energy. The most useful measures in predicting activity tolerance are heart rate, strength, and rhythm; respiratory rate, depth, and rhythm; and blood pressure. If the client tolerates an activity well, and if the client's heart rate returns to baseline within 5 minutes after activity, the activity is considered safe. This activity, then, can serve as a standard for predicting the client's tolerance for similar activities.

When collecting data pertaining to the problems of immobility, the nurse uses inspection, palpation, and auscultation; monitors results of laboratory tests; and takes measurements, including body weight, fluid intake, and fluid output.

DIAGNOSING, PLANNING, AND IMPLEMENTING

The LVN/LPN in collaboration with the RN develops a nursing care plan using a NANDA list. Examples of NANDA diagnoses that relate to activity are *Activity Intolerance, Impaired Physical Mobility,* and *Risk for Injury.* See Appendix II ∞ for a complete NANDA list. Positioning, transferring, and ambulating clients are almost always independent nursing functions. The physician usually orders specific body positions only after surgery, anesthesia, or trauma involving the nervous and musculoskeletal systems. All clients should have an activity order written by a physician on admission.

As part of planning, the nurse is responsible for identifying clients who need assistance with body alignment and determining the degree of assistance required. The nurse must be sensitive to the client's need for independence, yet must provide assistance when warranted.

Most clients require specific knowledge to achieve and maintain proper body mechanics. The nurse is responsible for teaching such skills. For example, a client with a back injury must learn how to get out of bed safely and comfortably; a client with an injured leg needs to know how to transfer from bed to wheelchair safely; and a client with a newly acquired walker needs to learn how to use it safely. Nurses often teach family members or caregivers safe moving, lifting, and transfer techniques in the home setting.

The goals established for clients vary according to the nursing diagnosis and anticipated outcome for each individual. Examples of overall goals for clients with actual or potential problems related to mobility or activity follow:

■ Increase tolerance for physical activity.
■ Avoid injury from falling or improper use of body mechanics.
■ Avoid any complications associated with immobility.

Nursing strategies to maintain or promote body alignment and mobility involve positioning clients appropriately, moving and turning clients in bed, transferring clients, providing ROM exercises, ambulating clients with or without mechanical aids, and preventing the complications of immobility. Whenever positioning, moving, lifting, and ambulating clients, nurses must use proper body mechanics to avoid personal injury. Refer to Chapter 8 ∞ for more information related to body mechanics and the nurse.

Positioning Clients

Positioning a client in good body alignment and changing position regularly and systematically are essential aspects of nursing practice. Clients who move easily automatically reposition for comfort. These people generally require minimal assistance from nurses, other than guidance about ways to maintain body alignment and exercise their joints. However, those who are weak, frail, in pain, paralyzed, or unconscious rely on nurses to provide or assist with position changes. For all clients, it is important to assess the skin and provide skin care before and after a position change.

Any position, if unchanged for a prolonged period, becomes detrimental. Frequent changes of position prevent muscle discomfort, pressure damage to superficial nerves and blood vessels, decubiti, and contractures. Position changes maintain muscle tone and stimulate postural reflexes.

When the client is not able to move independently or assist with moving, the preferred method is to have two or more people move or turn the client. Appropriate assistance reduces the risk of muscle strain and body injury to both the client and nurse. See Procedure 32-2 ■ on page 776 for moving a client in bed.

Sometimes a person who appears well aligned may be experiencing discomfort. To promote the client's proper body alignment, comfort and safety, the nurse should:

- *Make sure the mattress is firm and level* yet yields enough to fill in and support natural body curvatures. Mattress inspection in the home setting is particularly important. A sagging or too soft mattress or an underfilled water bed may contribute to development of hip flexion contractures or low back strain and pain. A plywood bedboard may be placed beneath a sagging mattress to add support. Some bedboards are hinged to allow the head of the bed to be raised. Bedboards are strongly recommended for clients who are at risk for back problems.
- *Ensure that the bed is clean and dry.* Wrinkled or damp sheets increase the risk of pressure ulcer formation (see Chapter 22). Make sure extremities can move freely whenever possible. For example, top sheets need to be loose for the client to move the feet.
- *Place support devices in specified areas* according to the client's position. See Box 32-3 ■ for commonly used support devices. Use only those devices needed to maintain alignment (such as a trochanter roll, Figure 32-8 ■) and prevent stress on muscles and joint. If the person is mobile, too many devices limit movement and increase the potential for injury.
- *Avoid placing one body part, particularly one with bony prominences, directly on top of another body part.* Excessive pressure can damage veins and predispose the client to thrombus formation. Pressure against the popliteal space can damage nerves and blood vessels in this area.

BOX 32-3

Support Devices

- *Pillows.* Different sizes are available. Used for support or elevation of a body part (e.g., an arm). Specially designed dense pillows can be used to elevate the upper body.
- *Mattresses.* There are two types of mattresses: ones that fit on the bed frame (e.g., standard bed mattress) and mattresses that fit on the standard bed mattress (e.g., egg-crate mattress). Mattresses should be evenly supportive. See Chapter 22 for additional information and Table 23-5 for devices that reduce pressure on body parts.
- *Bedboards.* Bedboards are usually made of wood and are placed under the mattress to provide support.
- *Chair beds.* These beds can be placed into the position of a chair for clients who cannot move from the bed but require a sitting position.
- *Foot boot.* These are made of a variety of substances. They usually have a firm exterior and padding of foam to protect the skin. They provide support to the feet in a natural position and keep the weight of covers off the toes. Without support, an immobilized client's feet assume a plantar flexion position (foot drop). Prolonged assumption of this position results in permanent contracture of the gastrocnemius muscle and tendon.
- *Footboard.* A flat panel often made of plastic or wood. It keeps the feet in dorsiflexion to prevent plantar flexion.

- *Plan a systematic 24-hour schedule for position changes.* See Chapter 22 .

Positioning the Bed

Fowler's Position

Fowler's position, or a semisitting position, is a bed position in which the head and trunk are raised 45 to 60 degrees. In low-Fowler's or semi-Fowler's position, the head and trunk are raised 15 to 45 degrees. In high-Fowler's position, the head and trunk are raised 60–90 degrees. See illustrations of positions in Table 32-2 ■ (Figures 32-9A–E ■). In this position, the knees may or may not be flexed.

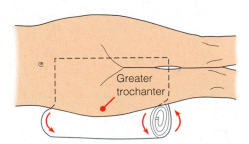

Figure 32-8. ■ Making a trochanter roll: (1) Fold the towel in half lengthwise. (2) Roll the towel tightly, starting at one narrow edge and rolling within approximately 30 cm (1 ft) of the other edge. (3) Invert the roll. Then palpate the greater trochanter of the femur and place the roll with the center at the level of the greater trochanter; place the flat part of towel under the client; then roll the towel snugly against the hip.

TABLE 32-2

Positions

POSITIONS	UNSUPPORTED POSITION
Fowler's position (Figure 32-9A) Low-Fowler's (semi-Fowler's) position (supported). Note that arm support is omitted in this instance. The amount of support depends on the needs of the individual client. 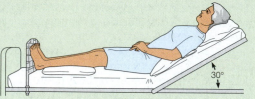 **Figure 32-9A.** ■ Low-Fowler's (semi-Fowler's) position (supported).	Bed-sitting position with upper part of body elevated 15–90° commencing at hips Head rests on bed surface Arms fall at sides Legs lie flat and straight on lower bed surface Legs are externally rotated Heels rest on bed surface Feet are in plantar flexion Posterior flexion of lumbar curvature
Dorsal Recumbent position (supported) (Figure 32-9B) 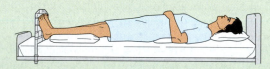 **Figure 32-9B.** ■ Dorsal recumbent position (supported).	Head is flat on bed surface Lumbar curvature of spine is apparent Legs may be externally rotated Legs are extended Feet assume plantar flexion position Heels on bed surface Pillow at lower back (lumbar region) to support lumbar region
Prone position (supported) (Figure 32-9C) 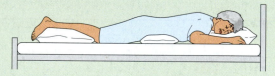 **Figure 32-9C.** ■ Prone position (supported).	Head is turned to side and neck is slightly flexed Body lies flat on abdomen accentuating lumbar curvature Toes rest on bed surface; feet are in plantar flexion Hyperextension of lumbar curvature; difficulty breathing; pressure Small pillow or roll under abdomen just below diaphragm on breasts (women); pressure on genitals (men) Plantar flexion of feet (foot drop)
Lateral position (supported) (Figure 32-9D) 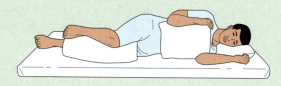 **Figure 32-9D.** ■ Lateral (supported).	Body is turned to side, both arms in front of body, weight resting primarily on lateral aspects of scapula and ilium Upper arm and shoulder are rotated internally and adducted Upper thigh and leg are rotated internally and adducted Internal rotation and adduction of femur; twisting of the spine Pillow under head and neck to provide good alignment Pillow under leg and thigh to place them in good alignment Internal rotation and adduction of femur; twisting of the spine
Sims' (semiprone) position (unsupported) Sims' position (supported) (Figure 32-9E) 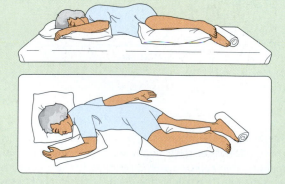 **Figure 32-9E.** ■ Sims' position (unsupported and supported).	Head rests on bed surface; weight is borne by lateral aspects of cranial and facial bones Upper shoulder and arm are internally rotated Upper leg and thigh are adducted and internally rotated Feet assume plantar flexion

PROBLEM TO BE PREVENTED	CORRECTIVE MEASURE
Posterior flexion of lumbar curvature	Pillow at lower back (lumbar region) to support lumbar region
Hyperextension of neck	Pillows to support head, neck, and upper back
Shoulder muscle strain, possible dislocation of shoulders, edema of hands and arms with flaccid paralysis, flexion contracture of the wrist	Pillow under forearms to eliminate pull on shoulder and assist venous blood flow from hands and lower arms
Hyperextension of knees	Small pillow under thighs to flex knees
External rotation of hips	Trochanter roll lateral to femur (Figure 32-8)
Pressure on heels	Pillow under lower legs
Plantar flexion of feet (foot drop)	Footboard to provide support for dorsal flexion
Hyperextension of neck in thick-chested person	Pillow of suitable thickness under head and shoulders if necessary for alignment
Posterior flexion of lumbar curvature	Roll or small pillow under lumbar curvature
External rotation of legs	Roll or sandbag placed laterally to trochanter of femur (optional)
Hyperextension of knees	Small pillow under thigh to flex knee slightly
Plantar flexion (foot drop)	Footboard or rolled pillow to support feet in dorsal flexion
Pressure on heels	Pillow under lower legs
Flexion or hyperextension of neck	Small pillow under head unless contraindicated because of promotion of mucous drainage from mouth
Hyperextension of lumbar curvature; difficulty breathing; pressure on breasts (women); pressure on genitals (men)	Small pillow or roll under abdomen just below diaphragm
Plantar flexion of feet (foot drop)	Allow feet to fall naturally over end of mattress, or support lower legs on a pillow so that toes do not touch the bed
Lateral flexion and fatigue of sternocleidomastoid muscles	Pillow under head and neck to provide good alignment
Internal rotation and adduction of shoulder and subsequent limited function; impaired chest expansion	Pillow under upper arm to place it in good alignment; lower arm should be flexed comfortably
Internal rotation and adduction of femur; twisting of the spine	Pillow under leg and thigh to place them in good alignment; shoulders and hips should be aligned
Lateral flexion of neck	Pillow supports head, maintaining it in good alignment unless drainage from the mouth is required
Internal rotation of shoulder and arm; pressure on chest, restricting expansion during breathing	Pillow under upper arm to prevent internal rotation
Internal rotation and adduction of hip and leg	Pillow under upper leg to support it in alignment
Foot drop	Sandbags to support feet in dorsal flexion

Nurses need to clarify the meaning of the term *Fowler's position* in a particular agency. Fowler's position may refer to elevation of the upper part of the body without knee flexion, and the term *semi-Fowler's* may refer to the sitting position with knee flexion.

Fowler's position is the position of choice for people who have difficulty breathing and for clients with heart problems. When the client is in this position, gravity pulls the diaphragm downward, allowing greater chest expansion and lung ventilation.

A common error nurses make when aligning clients in Fowler's position involves pillow usage. Overly plump or multiple pillows placed behind the client's head promote the development of neck flexion contractures. The nurse should encourage the client to rest without a pillow for several hours each day to extend the neck fully and counteract the effects of poor neck alignment.

Orthopneic Position

The orthopneic position is an adaptation of high-Fowler's position in which the client sits in bed or at bedside with an overbed table across the lap (Figure 32-10 ■). This position allows maximum chest expansion, eases breathing, and is especially helpful to clients with COPD. In this position, the client can press the lower chest against the edge of the overbed table to assist with exhalation.

Dorsal Recumbent Position

In the *dorsal recumbent* (back-lying) position, the client's head and shoulders are slightly elevated on a small pillow. In some agencies, the terms *dorsal recumbent* and *supine* are used interchangeably. However, in the supine or dorsal position, the head and shoulders are not elevated (see Figure 32-9B). In both positions, the client's forearms may be elevated on pillows or placed at the client's sides. Supports are similar in both positions, except for the head pillow (see Table 32-2). The dorsal recumbent position is used to provide comfort and to facilitate healing after certain surgeries or anesthetics (e.g., spinal).

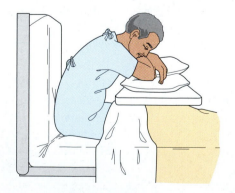

Figure 32-10. ■ Orthopneic position.

Prone Position

In the *prone* position (see Figure 32-9C), the client lies on the abdomen with the head turned to one side. The hips are not flexed. Both children and adults often sleep in this position, at times with one or both arms flexed over their heads. This position has several advantages. Prone is the only bed position that allows full extension of the hip and knee joints. When used periodically, the prone position helps to prevent flexion contractures of the hips and knees, thereby counteracting a problem caused by all other bed positions. Prone position promotes drainage from the mouth and is especially useful for unconscious clients or those clients recovering from surgery of the mouth or throat.

The prone position also has distinct disadvantages. The pull of gravity on the trunk produces a marked lordosis in most people, so that the neck is rotated laterally to a significant degree. For this reason, the prone position must be avoided by clients with spinal abnormalities and employed only when the client's back is properly aligned and maintained only for a brief time. This position also causes plantar flexion. Clients with cardiac or respiratory problems can find the prone position confining or suffocating because chest expansion is inhibited. Infants should not be placed in the prone position to sleep; sleeping prone is considered a risk for the occurrence of sudden infant death syndrome (SIDS).

Lateral Position

In the *lateral* (side-lying) position, the person lies on one side of the body (Figure 32-9D). Flexing the top hip and knee and placing this leg in front of the body creates a wide, triangular base of support that achieves greater stability. The greater the flexion of the top hip and knee, the greater the stability and balance. This flexion reduces lordosis and promotes good spinal alignment, making the lateral position optimal for resting and sleeping. The lateral position helps to relieve pressure on the sacrum and heels in people who sit much of the day or are confined to bed in Fowler's or dorsal recumbent positions. In the lateral position, most of the body's weight is borne by the lateral aspect of the lower scapula, the lateral aspect of the ilium, and the greater trochanter of the femur. People who have sensory or motor deficits on one side of the body usually find that lying on the uninvolved side is more comfortable.

Sims' Position

In *Sims'* (semiprone) position, the client assumes a posture halfway between the lateral and prone positions (see Figure 32-9E). The lower arm is positioned behind the client, and the upper arm is flexed at the shoulder and the elbow. Both legs are flexed in front of the client. The upper leg is more acutely flexed at both the hip and the knee than the lower one is.

Sims' position is occasionally used for unconscious clients because it facilitates drainage from the mouth and prevents aspiration of fluids. It is also used for paralyzed clients because it reduces pressure over the sacrum and greater trochanter of the hip. The Sims' position is often used for clients receiving enemas and occasionally for clients undergoing examinations or treatments of the perineal area. Many people, especially pregnant women, find Sims' position comfortable for sleeping. People with sensory or motor deficits on one side of the body usually find that lying on the uninvolved side is more comfortable.

Moving and Turning Clients in Bed

The level of assistance required depends on client mobility and health status. Nurses must be empathetic regarding the client's need for independence while assisting with movement (see Procedure 32-2).

When a nurse assists, correct body mechanics must be employed so the nurse is not injured. Correct client body alignment must be maintained to avoid excessive stress on the musculoskeletal system. Strategies for preventing strains and sprains in nurses are provided in Chapter 8 ⦾.

Transferring Clients

Many clients require assistance in transferring between bed and chair, wheelchair, toilet, or stretcher. The nurse must determine the client's capacity to participate and plan the maneuver before initiating a transfer. Methods of client transfer are given in Procedure 32-3 ■ on page 780.

Using a Hydraulic Lift

Hydraulic lifts, such as the Hoyer lift, are used primarily for clients who cannot assist or are too heavy for others to lift safely. The lift can be used in transferring the client between bed and wheelchair, bathtub, or stretcher. The *Hoyer lift* consists of a base on casters, a hydraulic mechanical pump, a mast boom, and a sling (Figure 32-11 ■). The sling may consist of a one-piece or two-piece canvas seat. The one-piece seat stretches from the client's head to the knees. The two-piece seat has one canvas strap to support the client's buttocks and thighs and a second strap extending up to the axillae to support the back. It is important to be familiar with the model used and the practices to accompany use. Before using the lift, the nurse ensures that it is in working order and that the hooks, chains, straps, and canvas seat are in good repair. Most agencies recommend that two nurses operate a lift. See Procedure 32-4 ■ on page 784 for instructions for using a Hoyer lift.

Providing ROM Exercises

When people are ill, they often need ROM exercises until they regain normal activity. *Active ROM exercise* is isotonic exercise in which the client moves each joint in the body

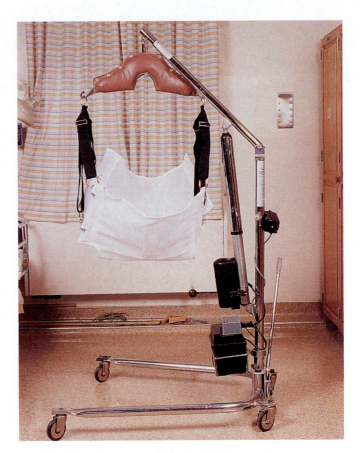

Figure 32-11. ■ A one-piece seat hydraulic lift. (Photographer: Jenny Thomas.)

through its complete range of movement, stretching all muscle groups as far as possible within each plane over the joint (see illustrations in Procedure 32-1 for muscle groups). They help to maintain cardiorespiratory function in an immobilized client and prevent deterioration of joint capsules, ankylosis, and contractures. See Box 32-2 for reminders about instructing clients to perform active ROM exercises.

The nurse may need to conduct passive ROM exercises until the client can accomplish these independently (see Procedure 32-1). During *passive ROM exercises,* the nurse (or an assistant) moves each of the client's joints through its complete range of movement, gently yet fully stretching all muscle groups over each joint. Passive ROM exercises are useful in maintaining joint flexibility. Passive exercises should be administered only when the client is unable to accomplish the movements independently.

Passive ROM exercises should be performed in a series, including each movement of the arms, legs, and neck that the client is unable to achieve. As with active ROM exercises, passive ROM should progress to the point of slight resistance, but never to the point of discomfort. Each exercise should consist of three repetitions, and the entire series is performed twice daily. One series should be performed during bath time.

During *active-assistive ROM exercises,* the client moves the immobile limb as far as possible, using the stronger arm or leg to move it. The nurse then continues the ROM to its maximal degree. Clients who begin with passive ROM exercises after disability generally progress to active-assistive ROM exercises and, finally, to active exercises.

Ambulating Clients

Ambulation (the act of walking) is a function most people take for granted. Prolonged bed rest (even 1 or 2 days) can make a person feel weak, unsteady, and shaky when first getting out of bed. Weakness is more pronounced in elderly and postoperative clients. Early ambulation greatly reduces the risks associated with immobility. Nurses should encourage clients to perform ADLs, maintain good body alignment, and carry out active ROM exercises to the maximum degree possible while on bed rest to prepare for ambulation.

Preambulatory Exercises

Clients on prolonged bed rest need exercises to strengthen the muscles used for walking before attempting to walk. One of the most important muscle groups is the quadriceps femoris, which extends the knee and flexes the thigh, enabling leg lifting, for example, to walk upstairs. To strengthen these muscles, the client consciously tenses them, drawing the kneecap upward and inward. The client pushes the popliteal space of the knee against the bed surface, relaxing the heels on the bed surface (Figure 32-12 ▪). On the count of 1, the muscles are tensed; they are held during the counts of 2, 3, 4; and they are relaxed at the count of 5. These exercises are called *quadriceps drills* or sets and should be performed within the client's tolerance, that is, without fatiguing the muscles. This simple exercise builds muscle strength when carried out several times an hour while the client is awake.

Assisting Clients to Ambulate

Clients who have been immobilized for even a few days may require assistance to ambulate. The level required depends on the client's condition, including age, health status, and length of inactivity. Assistance may mean walking along-

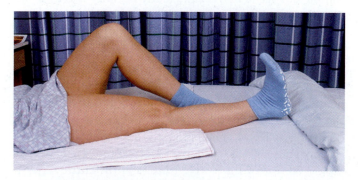

Figure 32-12. ▪ Tensing the quadriceps femoris muscles before ambulation.

BOX 32-4	CLIENT TEACHING

Controlling Postural Hypotension

- Sleep with the head of the bed elevated 8 to 12 inches (20.3–30.5 cm). This position makes the position change on rising less severe.
- Avoid sudden changes in position. Arise from bed in three stages:
  1. Sit up in bed for 1 minute.
  2. Sit on the side of the bed with legs dangling for 1 minute.
  3. Stand with care, holding onto the edge of the bed or another nonmovable object for 1 minute. Gradual changes in position stimulate *renin* (a kidney enzyme that has a role in regulating blood pressure), which prevents a dramatic drop in pressure.
- Never bend down all the way to the floor or stand up too quickly after stooping. *Baroreceptors* (sensory nerve endings in the walls of blood vessels) cannot accommodate rapid change.
- Postpone activities such as shaving and hair grooming for at least 1 hour after rising. Baroreceptor reflexes are slow to respond after a night of recumbency during sleep.
- Wear elastic stockings at night to inhibit venous pooling in the legs.
- Be aware that the symptoms of hypotension are most severe at the following times:
  - 30 to 60 minutes after a heavy meal
  - 1 to 2 hours after taking an antihypertension medication.
- Get out of a hot bath very slowly, because high temperatures can lead to venous pooling.
- Use a rocking chair to improve circulation in the lower extremities. Even mild leg conditioning can strengthen muscle tone and enhance circulation.
- Refrain from any strenuous activity that results in holding the breath and bearing down. This Valsalva maneuver slows the heart rate, leading to subsequent lowering of blood pressure.

---

side the client while providing physical support (see Procedure 32-5 ▪ on page 785) or providing instruction regarding the use of assistive devices such as a cane, walker, or crutches.

Clients may experience postural (*orthostatic*) hypotension and may exhibit the following symptoms: pallor, diaphoresis, nausea, tachycardia, and dizziness. If any of these are present, the client should be assisted to the supine position in bed and closely monitored. Box 32-4 ▪ provides client teaching for ways to manage postural hypotension.

EVALUATING

The goals established during the planning phase are evaluated according to specific desired outcomes, also established in that phase. If outcomes are not achieved the nurse, client, and support person (if appropriate) need to explore the reasons before modifying the care plan.

NURSING PROCESS CARE PLAN
Client in Traction

Kevin Andrews, a 17-year-old high school gymnast, fell from the parallel bars and fractured his left femur. Kevin has been on bed rest in skeletal traction since the injury. He is depressed and bored with the hospital routine of care. Because of painful muscle spasms, he often refuses to be turned or to move voluntarily. His appetite is poor, and he often refuses his hospital meals. He needs encouragement from the nursing staff to cough and deep breathe.

Assessment

- Height 175.3 cm (5′ 8″)
- Weight 70 kg (154 lbs) on admission
- 37°C (98.6°F)
- 80 bpm
- 16/minute
- BP 114/70 mm Hg
- Diagnostic data: chest x-ray negative, urinalysis negative, Hgb 13.3 g/dL, Hct 37%

Nursing Diagnosis. The following important nursing diagnosis (among others) is established for this client:

- *Risk for Disuse Syndrome* related to depression and reluctance to move secondary to painful muscle spasms.

Expected Outcomes. The expected outcomes specify that Mr. Andrews will:

- Perform ADLs within limitation of skeletal traction.
- Perform ROM exercises of upper limbs and unaffected lower limb tid.
- Use overhead trapeze every 3 h to strengthen muscles in upper limbs by day 3.
- Traction site remains free of drainage and odor.
- Homans' sign remains negative.

Planning and Implementation. The following nursing interventions are implemented for Kevin:

Traction/Immobilization Care

- Maintain proper position in bed to enhance traction.
- Ensure that the pull of ropes and weights remains along the axis of the fractured bone.

- Monitor pin insertion sites.
- Perform pin insertion site care.
- Monitor circulation, movement, and sensation of affected extremity.
- Monitor for complications of immobility.
- Administer appropriate skin care at friction points.
- Provide trapeze for movement in bed.
- Instruct Kevin on the importance of adequate nutrition for bone healing.

Exercise Therapy: Joint Mobility

- Determine Kevin's motivation level for maintaining or restoring joint movement.
- Explain to Kevin and his family the purpose and plan for joint exercises.
- Initiate pain control measures before beginning joint exercise.
- Assist Kevin to the optimal body position for each passive or active joint movement.
- Encourage active ROM exercises according to a regular schedule.
- Collaborate with a physical therapist in developing and executing an exercise program.

Evaluation. Goals partially met. Kevin performs active ROM exercises only once a day and refuses the other two sessions. He uses the overhead trapeze when repositioning frequently throughout the day but is reluctant to bathe and states "Just leave me alone for a while." His appetite has not improved and he eats approximately 40% to 50% of each meal. The skin surrounding the pin site remains odorless, dry, and intact. Homans' sign is negative; pulses are strong bilaterally.

Critical Thinking in the Nursing Process

1. What nursing intervention can be done for Kevin to relieve muscle spasms?
2. Kevin is refusing hospital meals. What can you do to improve Kevin's nutritional status needs to promote healing?
3. Describe diversion activities appropriate for a 17-year-old in traction.

Note: Discussion of Critical Thinking questions appears in Appendix I.

REST AND SLEEP

Rest and sleep are essential to health. Normal sleep is characterized by minimal physical activity, variable levels of consciousness, changes in the body's physiologic processes, and decreased responsiveness to external stimuli. Some environ-

mental stimuli, such as a smoke detector alarm, will awaken the sleeper, whereas other noises will not. Individuals respond to meaningful stimuli while sleeping and selectively disregard unmeaningful stimuli. Clients often complain that rest and sleep are difficult to achieve in the hospital environment. When deprived of sleep, clients become fatigued, depressed, or irritable. Nurses are responsible for providing an environment conducive to rest and sleep.

Physiology of Sleep

Sleep is a complex biologic rhythm. When a person's biologic clock coincides with sleep–wake patterns, the person is awake when the physiological and psychological rhythms are most active and is asleep when the physiological and psychological rhythms are most inactive. Infants are awake most often in the early morning and the late afternoon. After 4 months of age, infants enter a 24-hour cycle in which they sleep mostly during the night. By the end of the fifth or sixth month, infants' sleep–wake patterns are almost like those of adults.

Two types of sleep have been identified: non–rapid eye movement (NREM or non-REM) sleep and REM (rapid eye movement) sleep.

NREM SLEEP

Most sleep during a night is **NREM sleep**. It is a deep, restful sleep with some decreased physiological functions. NREM sleep is divided into four stages:

- Stage I is very light sleep. The person feels drowsy and relaxed. The sleeper can be readily awakened. This stage lasts only a few minutes.
- Stage II is light sleep during which body processes continue to slow down. The eyes are generally still, the heart and respiratory rates decrease slightly, and body temperature falls. Stage II lasts about 10 to 15 minutes.
- Stage III occurs when the heart and respiratory rates, as well as other body processes, slow further because of the domination of the parasympathetic nervous system. The sleeper becomes more difficult to arouse.
- Stage IV signals deep sleep, called delta sleep. The sleeper's heart and respiratory rates are 20% to 30% below waking rates. The sleeper is very relaxed, rarely moves, and is difficult to arouse. Stage IV is thought to restore the body physically. During this stage, the eyes usually roll, and some dreaming occurs.

REM SLEEP

REM sleep constitutes about 25% of the sleep of a young adult. It usually recurs about every 90 minutes and lasts 5 to 30 minutes. REM sleep is not as restful as NREM sleep. Most dreams take place during REM sleep. Box 32-5 ■ lists characteristics of sleep.

Functions of Sleep

Sleep exerts physiological effects on body systems and restores normal levels of activity and balance within the nervous system. The effects of sleep on the body are not fully understood.

BOX 32-5

Characteristics of Sleep

NREM Sleep

- Arterial blood pressure falls.
- Pulse rate decreases.
- Peripheral blood vessels dilate.
- Activity of the gastrointestinal tract occasionally increases.
- Skeletal muscles relax.
- Basal metabolic rate decreases 10% to 30%.

REM Sleep

- Active dreaming occurs, and dreams are remembered.
- The sleeper may be difficult to arouse or may wake spontaneously.
- Muscle tone is depressed.
- Heart rate and respiratory rate often are irregular.
- A few irregular muscle movements occur—in particular, rapid eye movements.
- The brain is very active.

Source: Adapted from A. C. Guyton and J. E. Hall, *Textbook of Medical Physiology,* 9th ed. Philadelphia: Saunders, 1996, pp. 762–763. Reprinted with permission.

However, it is known that the activity of the sympathetic nervous system is greater while the person is awake, as are impulses to the body's muscles, which increase muscle tone. During sleep, the activity of the parasympathetic nervous system increases, causing the physiological changes. Sleep is necessary for protein synthesis and cellular repair.

Research suggests that maintaining a regular sleep–wake rhythm (sleep hygiene) is more important than the actual number of hours slept. Some people, for example, can function well on as little as 5 hours' sleep each night. Reestablishing the sleep–wake cycle (e.g., after the disruption of surgery) is an important aspect of nursing.

Factors Affecting Sleep

Both the quality and the quantity of sleep are affected by a number of factors. Sleep quality refers to an individual's ability to stay asleep and to get appropriate amounts of REM and NREM sleep. Quantity of sleep is the total time the individual sleeps.

ILLNESS

Illness increases the need for sleep, but disease often disrupts normal sleep rhythms. Respiratory conditions affect sleep. Shortness of breath, nasal congestion, or sinus drainage and coughing disrupt sleep by causing frequent arousal.

People who have gastric or duodenal ulcers may find their sleep disturbed due to pain, the result of increased gastric secretions occurring during REM sleep. Endocrine disorders affect sleep. Hyperthyroidism lengthens presleep time, making it difficult to fall asleep. Hypothyroidism, conversely, decreases stage IV sleep. Elevated body temperatures can cause some reduction in stages III and IV NREM sleep and REM sleep.

The need to urinate during the night (*enuresis*) also disrupts sleep. People who awaken at night to urinate sometimes have difficulty getting back to sleep.

ENVIRONMENT

Environment can promote or hinder sleep. Changes in the level of sound, light, and room temperatures adversely affect sleep. Unfamiliar surroundings may contribute to anxiety, which disturbs sleep. Over time, however, most individuals adjust to these changes.

LIFESTYLE

Moderate exercise is conducive to sleep, but excessive exercise can delay sleep. The ability to relax before retiring is an important factor affecting the ability to fall asleep. Shift work affects the quality of rest and sleep. Night shift workers may experience effects of lack of synchronicity between the body's internal clock and waking/working hours. Moving shifts forward (day to evening; evening to night; night to day) can be helpful in preventing fatigue, illness, or work error.

EMOTIONAL STRESS

Anxiety and depression frequently disturb sleep. Anxiety increases the norepinephrine blood levels through stimulation of the sympathetic nervous system.

CULTURE

The hospital environment is strange to anyone who is newly admitted. However, cultural or ethnic customs may have an added impact on a client's ability to achieve rest and sleep (Box 32-6 ■).

ALCOHOL AND STIMULANTS

Excessive alcohol intake disrupts REM sleep, although it may hasten the onset of sleep. While making up for lost REM sleep after some of the effects of the alcohol have worn off, people often experience nightmares. Caffeine-containing beverages act as stimulants of the central nervous system, thus interfering with sleep.

SMOKING

Nicotine is a stimulant. Therefore, smokers generally suffer from poor sleep. Smokers have difficulty falling asleep and maintaining sleep. Avoiding tobacco after the evening meal improves sleep.

DIET

Weight change may affect sleep. Weight loss is associated with reduced total sleep time and early awakening. Weight gain is associated with fewer arousals, later awakening, and an increase in total sleep time.

The amino acid L-tryptophan is believed to enhance sleep. Milk and cheese are rich dietary sources of L-tryptophan, which may explain why warm milk helps some people fall asleep.

MOTIVATION

A strong desire to stay awake can counteract fatigue. An individual will find it easier to stay awake when engaged in an interesting activity, whereas boredom invites sleep.

MEDICATIONS

Medications affect the quality of sleep. Sedative-hypnotics (e.g., secobarbital) interfere with stages III and IV NREM sleep and suppress REM sleep. Beta blockers can cause insomnia and nightmares. Narcotics such as meperidine hydrochloride (Demerol) and morphine and tranquilizers suppress REM sleep and cause frequent awakenings and drowsiness. The following drugs may cause some of these sleep problems: disrupted REM sleep, delayed onset of sleep, decreased sleep time, nightmares, and increased daytime drowsiness:

- Amphetamines
- Antidepressants
- Beta blockers
- Bronchodilators
- Caffeine
- Decongestants
- Narcotics
- Steroids.

Common Sleep Disorders

INSOMNIA

Insomnia, the inability to obtain an adequate amount or quality of sleep, is the most common sleep disorder. People suffering from insomnia do not feel refreshed on arising.

Insomnia is most commonly caused by mental overstimulation due to anxiety, but may result from physical discomfort. Clients may become anxious because they think they might not be able to sleep. Drug and alcohol abusers generally suffer from insomnia.

BOX 32-6	CULTURAL PULSE POINTS

Effect of Culture on Rest and Sleep

Inability to rest or sleep in the hospital is one of the most frequent complaints from clients. Hospital noise, lights, and timing of procedures make it difficult to meet rest needs. Getting quality rest becomes more difficult when cultural issues are a factor. Some clients may be more comfortable resting or sleep on a mat on the floor, or sleeping with others in the same room or in the same bed. Others may be used to sleeping alone or in separate rooms. They may find it uncomfortable to share a room with one or more "strangers."

Women from Middle Eastern cultures may be uncomfortable leaving their rooms because of male clients who may be walking the hall in nightclothes. They may have difficulty sleeping, knowing that strange men are sleeping nearby.

Treatment for insomnia routinely includes a behavior modification plan in which the client learns new habits to foster sleep. The therapeutic value of sleep-inducing drugs is considered debatable because these drugs treat only the symptom and not the root cause of sleeplessness. Furthermore, prolonged usage creates drug dependency.

HYPERSOMNIA

Hypersomnia, or excessive daytime sleep (EDS), can result from many diseases. Central nervous system, kidney, liver, or metabolic disorders, such as diabetic acidosis and hypothyroidism, cause sleepiness. Hypersomnia can be linked to mental disorders; depressed persons may use sleep as an escape mechanism.

NARCOLEPSY

Narcolepsy is an underrecognized and poorly understood disorder believed to be genetic or autoimmune. Narcolepsy sufferers experience regular REM-onset sleep attacks lasting from a few seconds to several hours. Nighttime sleep may be fragmented by vivid dreams or nightmares. Central nervous system stimulants such as methylphenidate (Ritalin) or amphetamine may be prescribed to control excessive daytime sleepiness. Tricyclic antidepressants may be given to suppress REM sleep.

SLEEP APNEA

Sleep apnea is the periodic cessation of breathing during sleep. Apnea occurs most often in men over age 50 and postmenopausal women. Sufferers may experience up to 600 episodes per night during NREM sleep, each lasting from 10 seconds to 2 minutes. These multiple arousals cause fatigue and EDS.

An apneic episode begins with snoring. Breathing ceases, followed by gasping or snorting as breathing resumes. Breathlessness causes increased carbon dioxide levels in the blood, which trigger awakening.

Treatment is aimed at the cause of the apnea; for example, enlarged tonsils may be removed. The use of a nasal continuous positive airway pressure (CPAP) device at night is often effective.

Sleep apnea profoundly affects a person's work or school performance. In addition, prolonged sleep apnea can cause a sharp rise in blood pressure and may lead to cardiac arrest. Over time, apneic episodes can cause cardiac arrhythmias, pulmonary hypertension, and left-sided heart failure.

PARASOMNIAS

A **parasomnia** is behavior that may interfere with sleep. Examples of this are sleepwalking (*somnambulism*), sleep talking, bedwetting (*nocturnal enuresis*), nocturnal erection, and teeth grinding and clenching (*bruxism*).

SLEEP DEPRIVATION

Sleep deprivation is the reduction in the amount, quality, or consistency of sleep. This syndrome produces both physiological and behavioral symptoms whose severity depends on the degree and type of deprivation (i.e., REM or NREM sleep). Combined REM/NREM deprivation increases the severity of symptoms. Table 32-3 ▪ provides types, causes, and manifestations of sleep deprivation.

TABLE 32-3

Types, Causes, and Signs of Sleep Deprivation

TYPE	CAUSES	CLINICAL SIGNS
REM deprivation	Alcohol, barbiturates, shift work, jet lag, extended ICU hospitalization, morphine, meperidine hydrochloride (Demerol)	Excitability, restlessness, irritability, and increased sensitivity to pain Confusion and suspiciousness Emotional lability
NREM deprivation	All the above plus diazepam (Valium), flurazepam hydrochloride (Dalmane), hypothyroidism, depression, respiratory distress disorders, sleep apnea, and age (common in the elderly)	Withdrawal, apathy, hyporesponsiveness Feeling physically uncomfortable Lack of facial expression Speech deterioration Excessive sleepiness
Both REM and NREM deprivation	As above	Decreased reasoning ability (judgment) and ability to concentrate Inattentiveness Marked fatigue manifested by blurred vision, itchy eyes, nausea, headache Difficulty performing ADLs Lack of memory, mental confusion, visual or auditory hallucinations, and illusions

COLLABORATIVE CARE

Diagnostic Studies

Sleep may be measured objectively in a sleep laboratory by an electroencephalogram (EEG), electromyogram (EMG), and electro-oculogram (EOG) recorded simultaneously. This recording divides sleep into REM and NREM phases. Electrodes are placed on the scalp to record brain waves (EEG), at the outer canthus of each eye to record movement (EOG), and on the chin to record muscle contractions (EMG). Respiratory effort and airflow, ECG, leg movements, and oxygen saturation of arterial blood by pulse oximeter may also be monitored. Pulse oximetry and ECG recordings are of particular significance if sleep apnea is suspected. Video cameras may also be used to record the client's activity (movements, struggling, noisy respirations) during sleep.

NURSING CARE

ASSESSING

Sleep assessment includes a sleep history (sleep diary), physical examination, and review of diagnostic studies.

A brief general sleep history is obtained for all clients entering a healthcare facility. This enables the nurse to incorporate the client's needs and preferences in the plan of care.

Sleep Diary

A sleep diary may include all of the following information or selected aspects that pertain to the client's specific problem:

- Total number of sleep hours per day
- Activities performed 2 to 3 hours before bedtime (type, duration, and time)
- Bedtime rituals (e.g., ingestion of food, fluid, or medication, or ADLs such as prayer or bathing)
- Time of (1) going to bed, (2) trying to fall asleep, (3) falling asleep (approximate), (4) any instances of waking up and duration of these waking periods, and (5) waking up in the morning
- Any worries that the client believes may affect sleep
- Factors the client believes have a positive or negative effect on sleep.

Physical Examination

Examination includes observation of the client's physical appearance, behavior, and energy level. Evidence of a deviated nasal septum, enlarged neck, obesity, and snoring may indicate obstructive sleep apnea. Irritability, restlessness, inattentiveness, slowed speech, yawning, rubbing the eyes, confusion, incoordination, and physical weakness or lethargy also suggest sleep problems.

DIAGNOSING, PLANNING, AND IMPLEMENTING

Sleep Deprivation and *Disturbed Sleep Pattern* are NANDA nursing diagnoses that may be assigned to clients by the RN following assessment. See Appendix II ⬥ for a complete NANDA list. These diagnoses may include further descriptions such as "difficulty falling asleep."

Nursing interventions to enhance clients' sleep primarily involve nonpharmacologic measures. These include teaching sleep hygiene, supporting bedtime rituals, providing a restful environment, and providing comfort measures to promote relaxation and reduce anxiety.

Promoting client sleep during hospitalization is challenging to the nurse and requires organization, caring, and creativity to control the many external factors affecting sleep. Assistive techniques to promote rest are described in Box 32-7 ■.

Supporting Bedtime Rituals

Most people have developed presleep routines to help them relax. Altering or eliminating these routines can affect sleep. Common adult bedtime rituals include an evening stroll, listening to music, watching television, taking a bath, and praying. Children's rituals may include a bedtime story, hugging a favorite toy or blanket, and kissing everyone goodnight. Sleep is generally preceded by hygienic routines,

---

BOX 32-7	**NURSING CARE CHECKLIST**

Reducing Environmental Distractions in Hospitals

- ☑ Close window curtains if street lights shine through.
- ☑ Close curtains between clients in semiprivate and larger rooms.
- ☑ Reduce or eliminate overhead lighting; provide a night-light at the bedside or in the bathroom.
- ☑ Close the door of the client's room.
- ☑ Adhere to agency policy about times to turn off communal televisions or radios.
- ☑ Lower the ring tone of nearby telephones.
- ☑ Discontinue use of the paging system after a certain hour (e.g., 2100 hours), or reduce its volume.
- ☑ Keep required staff conversations at low levels; conduct nursing reports or other discussions in a separate area away from client rooms.
- ☑ Wear rubber-soled shoes.
- ☑ Ensure that all cart wheels are well oiled.
- ☑ Perform only essential nursing tasks during sleeping hours.

such as washing the face and hands (or bathing), brushing the teeth, and voiding.

In institutional settings, nurses can provide similar bedtime rituals. Talking about events such as a visit from friends or the weather can help clients relax.

Creating a Restful Environment

To create a restful environment, the nurse needs to ensure safety, reduce sleep interruptions and environmental distractions, and provide room temperature satisfactory to the client. Interventions to reduce environmental distractions, especially noise, are listed in Box 32-7.

Clients must also feel safe in order to rest comfortably. People who are not accustomed to narrow hospital beds may feel more secure with side rails.

Additional safety measures include:

- Placing beds in low positions
- Using night-lights
- Placing call bells within easy reach.

Promoting Comfort and Relaxation

Comfort measures are essential to help the client fall asleep and stay asleep, especially when disease interferes with sleep. A concerned, caring attitude, along with the following interventions, can significantly promote client comfort, relaxation, and sleep:

- Provide loose-fitting nightwear.
- Assist clients with hygienic routines and other bedtime rituals.
- Make sure the bed linen is smooth, clean, and dry.
- Assist or encourage the client to void before bedtime.
- Provide a back massage before sleep (see Procedure 32-6 ■ on page 787).
- Position dependent clients appropriately to aid muscle relaxation.
- Provide supportive devices to protect pressure areas.
- Schedule medications, especially diuretics, to prevent nocturnal awakenings.
- Manage pain by administering analgesics 30 minutes before sleep; change dressings and/or apply warm or cool compresses or splints to painful areas.
- Facilitate effective breathing by administering prescribed medications such as bronchodilators before bedtime and position clients appropriately (e.g., semi-Fowler's position).
- Encourage slow deep breathing followed by tonic muscle exercises (rhythmic contraction and relaxation) to promote relaxation.
- Encourage the client to share concerns; actively listen and address problems as they arise.

People, especially older adults, are unable to sleep well if they feel cold. Changes in circulation, metabolism, and

---

BOX 32-8	NURSING CARE CHECKLIST

Helping Older Clients Keep Warm in Bed

☑ Before the client goes to bed, warm the bed with hot water bottles or prewarmed bath blankets. Remove the hot water bottle before the client gets into bed to avoid the risk of a burn.

☑ Use 100% cotton flannel sheets, if possible, for warmth. Alternatively, apply thermal blankets between the sheet and bedspread.

☑ Encourage the client to wear own clothing, such as flannel nightgown or pajamas, loose-fitting jogging suit, thermal socks, leg warmers, long underwear, sleeping cap (if scalp hair is sparse), sweater, or a favorite quilt or blanket.

---

body tissue density reduce the older person's ability to generate and conserve heat. Interventions to keep elderly clients warm during sleep are listed in Box 32-8 ■.

Enhancing Sleep with Medications

Sleep medications (most often prescribed on a prn or as-needed basis) include sedative-hypnotics to induce sleep and tranquilizers (benzodiazepines) to decrease anxiety and tension. In institutional settings, the nurse shares responsibility with the client regarding when to administer them. Both nurses and clients must be aware of the actions, effects, and risks of medication prescribed. Medication should be administered only when indicated and once the client has demonstrated understanding of the drug's action and effects. Whenever possible, nonpharmacologic interventions (discussed earlier) are the preferred interventions.

EVALUATING

If the desired outcomes are not achieved, the nurse, client, and support people, if appropriate, should explore the reasons. In many facilities, a client care conference may be convened in order to discuss client progress, and analyze collected data. The desired outcome can be continued or revised at that time. If the goal is to be continued, a new timeline will be set.

CONTINUING CARE

Nurses can play a key role in teaching clients how to improve patterns of rest and sleep. This can speed recovery and add to quality of life. Box 32-9 ■ provides discharge teaching about promoting rest and sleep.

Note: The references and resources for this and all chapters have been compiled at the back of the book.

BOX 32-9   **CLIENT TEACHING**

Promoting Rest and Sleep

Sleep Pattern

- Establish a regular bedtime and wake-up time for all days of the week to prevent disruptions in your biologic rhythm. Eliminate lengthy naps, or if a daytime nap is necessary, take it at the same time each day and limit the time to 30 minutes, preferably once a day.
- Get adequate exercise during the day to reduce stress, but avoid excessive physical exertion 2 hours before bedtime.
- Avoid dealing with office work or family problems before bedtime.
- Establish a regular routine before sleep such as reading, listening to soft music, taking a warm bath, or doing some other quiet activity you enjoy.
- When you are unable to sleep, pursue some relaxing activity until you feel drowsy.
- If you have trouble falling asleep, get up and pursue nonstrenuous activity until you feel sleepy.
- Use the bed mainly for sleep, so that you associate it with sleep.

Environment

- Ensure appropriate lighting, temperature, and ventilation.
- Keep noise to a minimum; block out extraneous noise as necessary with soft music.

Diet

- Avoid heavy meals 3 hours before bedtime.
- Avoid alcohol and caffeine-containing foods and beverages (coffee, tea, chocolate) at least 4 hours before bedtime. These act as diuretics, creating the need to void during sleep time.
- Decrease fluid intake 2 to 4 hours before sleep if necessary to avoid the need to use the bathroom during sleeping hours.
- If a bedtime snack is necessary, consume only light carbohydrates or a milk drink. Heavy or spicy foods can cause gastrointestinal upsets that disturb sleep.

Medications

- Use sleeping medications only as a last resort. Take them judiciously (e.g., three times a week). Use over-the-counter medications sparingly because many contain antihistamines that cause daytime drowsiness.
- Take analgesics 30 minutes before bedtime to relieve aches and pains.
- Consult with your healthcare provider about adjusting other medications that may cause insomnia.

PROCEDURE 32-1 # Providing Passive Range-of-Motion Exercises

Purposes

- To maintain joint flexibility
- To provide exercise when the client is unable to accomplish movement actively

Equipment

- No special equipment is needed except a bed or exercise mat or table.

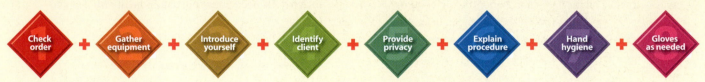

Check order + Gather equipment + Introduce yourself + Identify client + Provide privacy + Explain procedure + Hand hygiene + Gloves as needed

Interventions

1. Perform exercises in an organized format from head to toe. Repeat each movement three times, supporting the joint. *This allows the muscles to stretch and warm.*

2. Observe the client for nonverbal clues of pain. *This can reduce discomfort and prevent further injury.*

3. Neck
   - Remove pillow.
   - Flex and extend the neck (Figure 32-13 ■):
     a. Place palm of one hand under client's head and the other on the chin.
     b. Move head forward from an upright position until the chin rests on the chest.
     c. Move the head back to the resting supine position.
   - Lateral flexion of neck (Figure 32-14 ■):
     a. Place heels of the hands on each side of client's cheeks.
     b. Move head laterally toward the right and left shoulders.
   - Rotation (Figure 32-15 ■):
     a. Place heels of the hands on client's cheeks.
     b. Turn face as far as possible to the right and left.

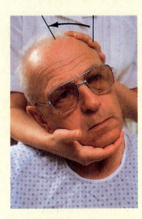

Figure 32-14. ■ Right/left lateral flexion.

4. Shoulder
   - Flexion/extension (Figure 32-16 ■):
     a. With client's arms at the side, grasp the arm beneath the elbow with one hand and beneath the wrist with the other hand.

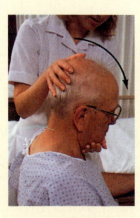
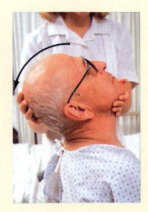

Figure 32-13. ■ Head flexion and extension.

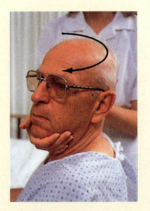
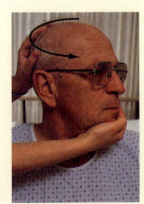

Figure 32-15. ■ Right/left rotation.

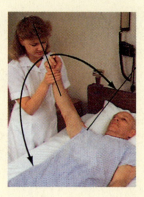

Figure 32-16. ■ Shoulder flexion and extension.

b. Raise the arm forward and upward to a position beside the head.
c. Move the arm from a vertical position beside the head forward and down to a resting position at the side of the body.
■ Abduction/adduction (Figure 32-17 ■):
a. Move arm laterally from the resting position at the side to a side position above the head, palm of the hand away from the head.
b. Move the arm laterally from beside the head downward laterally and across the front on the body as far as possible.
■ External/internal rotation:
a. With arm held out to the side at shoulder level and elbow at a right angle and fingers pointing downward, move the arm upward so that the fingers are pointing up and the back of the hand touches the bed or mat.
b. With arm held out to the side at the level of the shoulder and the elbow bent at a right angle, fingers pointing up, bring the arm forward and down so that the palm touches the mat.
■ Circumduction:
a. Move the arm forward and backward in a full circle.
5. Elbow
■ Flexion/extension (Figure 32-18 ■):
a. Bring lower arm forward and upward so that hand is at shoulder level.

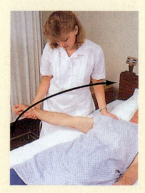

Figure 32-17. ■ Shoulder abduction and adduction.

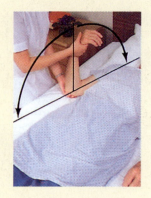

Figure 32-18. ■ Elbow flexion and extension.

b. Bring lower arm forward and downward, straightening the arm.
■ Rotation for supination/pronation (Figure 32-19 ■):
a. Grasp the client's hand with a handshaking motion and turn the palm upward. Make sure only the forearm and not the shoulder moves.
b. Turn the palm downward, moving only the forearm.
6. Wrist
■ Flexion/extension (Figure 32-20 ■):
a. Flex client's arm at the elbow until the forearm is at a right angle to the bed or mat. Support the wrist joint with one hand while manipulating the joint with your other hand.

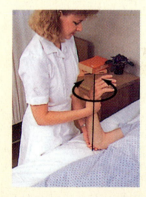

Figure 32-19. ■ Forearm pronation and supination.

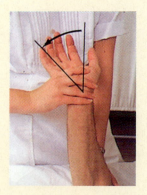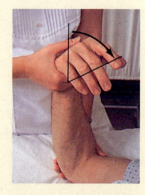

Figure 32-20. ■ Wrist flexion and extension.

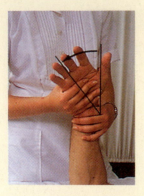
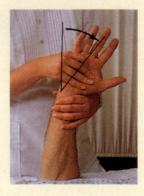

Figure 32-21. ■ Ulnar and radial deviation.

 b. Bring the fingers of the hand toward the inner aspect of the arm.
 c. Straighten the hand to the same plane as the arm.
 ■ Hyperflexion
 a. Bend fingers of the hand back as far as possible.
 ■ Radial flexion (abduction)/ulnar flexion (adduction) (Figure 32-21 ■):
 a. Bend wrist laterally toward the thumb side.
 b. Bend the wrist laterally toward the fifth finger.
7. Hand and fingers
 ■ Flexion/extension (Figure 32-22 ■):
 a. Make client's hand into a fist.
 b. Straighten the fingers.
 ■ Hyperextension:
 a. Gently bend fingers back.
 ■ Adduction/abduction (Figure 32-23 ■):
 a. Bring fingers together.
 b. Spread fingers of the hand apart.
8. Thumb
 ■ Flexion/extension:
 a. Move thumb across the palmar surface toward the fifth finger.
 b. Move the thumb away from the hand.
 ■ Abduction/adduction:
 a. Extend the thumb laterally.
 b. Move thumb back to the hand. *Note: Can be done when abducting and adducting fingers*.

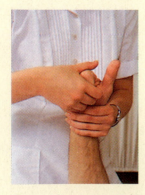
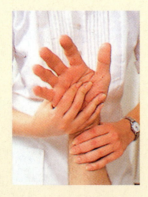

Figure 32-22. ■ Finger flexion and extension.

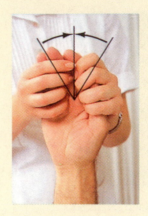
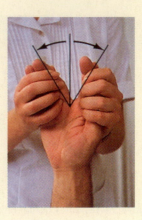

Figure 32-23. ■ Finger adduction and abduction.

 ■ Opposition (Figure 32-24 ■):
 a. Touch thumb to the top of each finger of the same hand.
9. Hip: To exercise hip and leg, place one hand under the client's knee and the other under the ankle.
 ■ Flexion/extension (Figure 32-25 ■):
 a. Lift the leg and bend the knee, moving the knee up toward the chest as far as possible.
 b. Bring leg down, straighten the knee, and lower the leg to the bed.

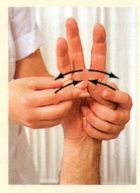

Figure 32-24. ■ Finger–thumb opposition.

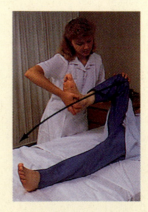

Figure 32-25. ■ Hip/knee flexion and extension.

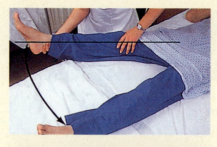

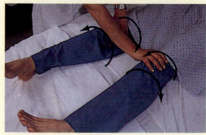

Figure 32-26. ■ Hip abduction and adduction.

- Abduction/adduction (Figure 32-26 ■):
  a. Move the leg to the side away from the client.
  b. Move leg back across and in front of the other leg.
- Slowly raise and lower leg (Figure 32-27 ■).
- Circumduction:
  a. Move the leg in a circle.
- Internal/external rotation:
  a. Roll the foot and leg inward.
  b. Roll foot and leg outward.
10. Knee
  - Flexion/extension (see Figure 32-25):
    a. Bend leg, bringing the heel toward back of thigh.
    Note: Can be done with hip flexion.
    b. Straighten the leg and return the foot to the bed.
11. Ankle
  - Extension/flexion (Figure 32-28 ■):
    a. Plantar flexion: Move the foot so that the toes are pointed downward.
    b. Dorsiflexion: Move foot so toes are pointed upward.

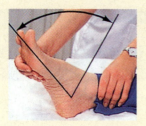

Figure 32-28. ■ Ankle dorsiflexion and plantar flexion.

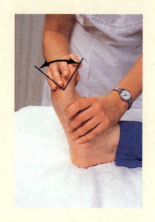
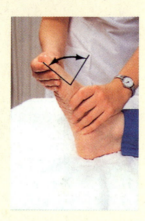

Figure 32-29. ■ Toe flexion and extension.

12. Foot
  - Eversion/inversion:
    a. Place one hand under the client's ankle and the other over the arch.
    b. Turn the whole foot outward.
    c. Turn the whole foot inward.
13. Toes
  - Flexion/extension (Figure 32-29 ■):
    a. Place one hand over arch.
    b. Place the fingers of the other hand over toes and curl downward.
    c. Place fingers under the toes and bend toes upward.
  - Abduction/adduction:
    a. Spread toes apart.
    b. Bring toes together.

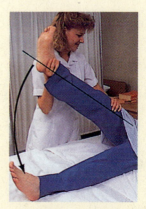

Figure 32-27. ■ Straight leg raising.

SAMPLE DOCUMENTATION

[date]   PROM to left lower extremity.

[time]   Knee flexion 110 degrees; no c/o
            discomfort. Full range on plantar
            flexion (50 degrees; 40 degrees
            yesterday).

_____ D. Smith, LPN

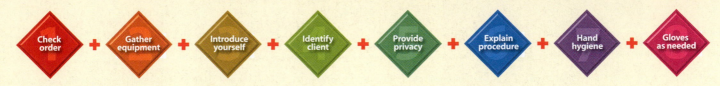

PROCEDURE 32-2 **Moving a Client in Bed**

Purpose

- To reposition clients who have slid down in bed from the Fowler's position or been pulled down by traction

Equipment

- None needed
- Second person may be needed to assist with some clients

Check order + Gather equipment + Introduce yourself + Identify client + Provide privacy + Explain procedure + Hand hygiene + Gloves as needed

Part A: Moving a Client in Bed

Interventions

1. Adjust the bed and the client's position.
   - Adjust the head of the bed to a flat position or as low as the client can tolerate. *Moving the client upward against gravity requires more force and can cause back strain.*
   - Raise the bed to the height of your center of gravity.
   - Lock the wheels on the bed and raise the rail on the side of the bed opposite you.
   - Remove all pillows, then place one against the head of the bed. *This pillow protects the client's head from inadvertent injury against the top of the bed during the upward move.*

2. Ask for the client's help in lessening your workload.
   - Ask the client to flex the hips and knees and position the feet so that they can be used effectively for pushing. *Flexing the hips and knees keeps the entire lower leg off the bed surface, preventing friction during movement, and ensures use of the large muscle groups in the client's legs when pushing, thus increasing the force of movement.*
   - Ask the client to:
   a. Grasp the head of the bed with both hands and pull during the move.
   or
   b. Raise the upper part of the body on the elbows and push with the hands and forearms during the move
   or
   c. Grasp the overhead trapeze with both hands and lift and pull during the move. *Client assistance provides additional power to overcome inertia and friction during the move. These actions also keep the client's arms partially off the bed surface, reducing friction during movement, and make use of the large muscle groups of the client's arms to increase the force during movement.*

3. Position yourself appropriately, and move the client.
   - Face the direction of the movement, and then assume a broad stance, with the foot nearest the bed behind the forward foot and weight on the forward foot. Incline your trunk forward from the hips. Flex hips, knees, and ankles.
   - Place your near arm under the client's thighs (Figure 32-30 ■). *This supports the heaviest part of the body (the buttocks).* Push down on the mattress with the far arm. *The far arm acts as a lever during the move.*
   - Tighten your gluteal, abdominal, leg, and arm muscles, and rock from the back leg to the front leg and back again. Then shift your weight to the front leg as the client pushes with the heels and pulls with the arms, so that the client moves toward the head of the bed. *Tightening your muscles helps to prevent strain. Moving the client as you shift your weight adds momentum.*

4. Ensure client comfort.
   - Elevate the head of the bed and provide appropriate support devices for the client's new position.

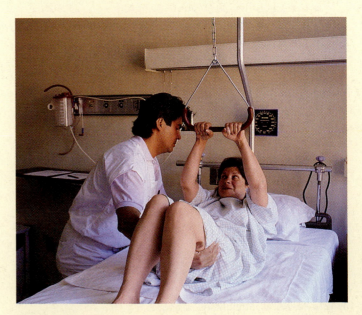

Figure 32-30. ■ Moving a client up in bed.

■ See the sections on positioning clients earlier in this chapter.

VARIATION: A CLIENT WHO HAS LIMITED STRENGTH OF THE UPPER EXTREMITIES

■ Assist the client to flex the hips and knees as in step 2 previously. Place the client's arms across the chest. *This keeps them off the bed surface and minimizes friction during movement.* Ask the client to flex the neck during the move and keep the head off the bed surface.

■ Position yourself as in step 3, and place one arm under the client's back and shoulders and the other arm under the client's thighs. *This placement of the arms distributes the client's weight and supports the heaviest part of the body (the buttocks).* Shift your weight as in step 3.

VARIATION: TWO NURSES USING A HAND–FOREARM INTERLOCK

Two people are required to move clients who are unable to assist because of their condition or weight. Using the technique described in step 3, with the second staff member on the opposite side of the bed, both of you interlock your forearms under the client's thighs and shoulders and lift the client up in bed.

VARIATION: TWO NURSES USING A TURN SHEET

Two nurses can use a turn sheet to move a client up in bed. *A turn sheet distributes the client's weight more evenly, decreases friction, and exerts a more even force on the client during the move. In addition, it prevents injury of the client's skin, because the friction created between two sheets when one is moved is less than that created by the client's body moving over the sheet.*

■ Place a drawsheet or a full sheet folded in half under the client, extending from the shoulders to the thighs. Each of you rolls up or fanfolds the turn sheet close to the client's body on either side.

■ Both of you then grasp the sheet close to the shoulders and buttocks of the client. *This draws the weight closer to the nurses' center of gravity and increases the nurses' balance and stability, permitting a smoother movement.* Then follow the method of moving clients with limited upper extremity strength, described earlier.

Part B: Turning a Client to a Lateral or Prone Position in Bed

Movement to a lateral (side-lying) position may be necessary when placing a bedpan beneath the client, when changing the client's bed linen, or when repositioning the client.

1. Position yourself and the client appropriately before performing the move.
   ■ Move the client closer to the side of the bed opposite the side the client will face when turned. *This ensures that the client will be positioned safely in the center of the bed after turning.* Use a pull sheet beneath the client's trunk and thighs to pull the client to the side of the bed. Roll up the sheet as close as possible to the client's body and pull the client to the side of the bed. Adjust the client's head and reposition the legs appropriately.
   ■ While standing on the side of the bed nearest the client, place the client's near arm across the chest. Abduct the client's far shoulder slightly from the side of the body. *Pulling the one arm forward facilitates the turning motion. Pulling the other arm away from the body prevents that arm from being caught beneath the client's body during the roll.*
   ■ Place the client's near ankle and foot across the far ankle and foot. *This facilitates the turning motion. Making these preparations on the side of the bed closest to the client helps prevent unnecessary reaching.*
   ■ Raise the side rail next to the client before going to the other side of the bed. *This ensures that the client, who is close to the edge of the mattress, will not fall.*
   ■ Position yourself on the side of the bed toward which the client will turn, directly in line with the client's waistline and as close to the bed as possible.
   ■ Incline your trunk forward from the hips. Flex your hips, knees, and ankles. Assume a broad stance with one foot forward and the weight placed on this forward foot.

2. Pull or roll the client to a lateral position.
   ■ Place one hand on the client's far hip and the other hand on the client's far shoulder (Figure 32-31 ■). *This position of the hands supports the client at the two heaviest parts of the body, providing greater control in movement during the roll.*

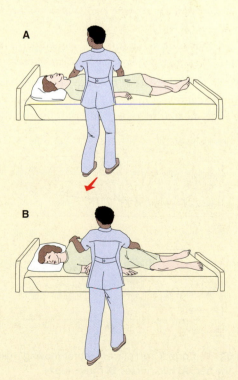

Figure 32-31. ■ A, B. Moving a client to a lateral position.

■ Tighten your gluteal, abdominal, leg, and arm muscles; rock backward, shifting your weight from the forward to the backward foot; and roll the client onto the side of the body to face you (see Figure 32-31B).

VARIATION: TURNING THE CLIENT TO A PRONE POSITION

To turn a client to the prone position, follow the preceding steps, with two exceptions:

■ Instead of abducting the far arm, keep the client's arm alongside the body for the client to roll over. *Keeping the*

arm alongside the body prevents it from being pinned under the client when the client is rolled.

■ Roll the client completely onto the abdomen. It is essential to move the client as close as possible to the edge of the bed before the turn so that the client will be lying on the center of the bed after rolling. Never pull a client across the bed while the client is in the prone position. Doing so can injure a woman's breasts or a man's genitals.

Part C: Logrolling a Client

Logrolling is a technique used to turn a client whose body must at all times be kept in straight alignment (like a log). *An example is the client with a spinal injury. Considerable care must be taken to prevent additional injury.* This technique requires two nurses or, if the client is large, three nurses. For the client who has a cervical injury, one nurse must maintain the client's head and neck alignment throughout the procedure.

1. Position yourselves and the client appropriately before the move.
   ■ Stand on the same side of the bed, and assume a broad stance with one foot ahead of the other.
   ■ Place the client's arms across the chest. *Doing so ensures that they will not be injured or become trapped under the body when the body is turned.*
   ■ Incline your trunk, and flex your hips, knees, and ankles.
   ■ Place your arms under the client as shown in Figure 32-32A ■ or B, depending on the client's size. *Each staff member then has a major weight area of the client centered between the arms.*
   ■ Tighten your gluteal, abdominal, leg, and arm muscles. *This provides support to your back muscles to prevent strain.*

2. Pull the client to the side of the bed.
   ■ One nurse counts, "One, two, three, go." Then at the same time, all staff members pull the client to the side of

the bed by shifting weight to the back foot. *Moving the client in unison maintains the client's body alignment.*
   ■ Elevate the side rail on this side of the bed. *This prevents the client from falling while lying so close to the edge of the bed.*

3. Move to the other side of the bed, and place supportive devices for the client when turned.
   ■ Place a pillow where it will support the client's head after the turn. *The pillow prevents lateral flexion of the neck and ensures alignment of the cervical spine.*
   ■ Place one or two pillows between the client's legs to support the upper leg when the client is turned. *This pillow prevents adduction of the upper leg and keeps the legs parallel and aligned.*

4. Roll and position the client in proper alignment.
   ■ All nurses flex the hips, knees, and ankles and assume a broad stance with one foot forward.
   ■ All nurses reach over the client and place hands as shown in Figure 32-33 ■. *Doing so centers a major weight area of the client between each nurse's arms.*
   ■ One nurse counts, "One, two, three, go." Then at the same time, all nurses roll the client to a lateral position.
   ■ Place pillows to maintain the client's lateral position. See the discussion of the lateral position.

VARIATION: USING A TURN OR LIFT SHEET

■ Use a turn sheet to facilitate logrolling. First, stand with another nurse on the same side of the bed. Assume a broad stance with one foot forward, and grasp half of the fanfolded or rolled edge of the turn sheet. On a signal, pull the client toward both of you (Figure 32-34 ■).

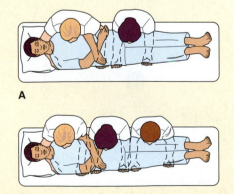

A

B

Figure 32-32. ■ Correct arm placement for moving a client to the side of the bed: **A.** two nurses; **B.** three nurses.

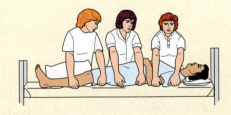

Figure 32-33. ■ Correct hand placement for logrolling a client.

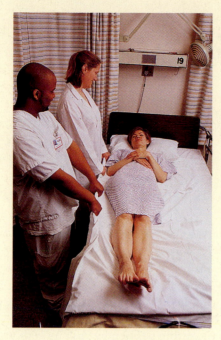

Figure 32-34. ■ Using the turn sheet, the nurses pull the sheet with the client on it to the edge of the bed. (Photographer: Jenny Thomas.)

■ Before turning the client, place pillow supports for the head and legs, as described in step 3 previously. *This helps maintain the client's alignment when turning.* Then go to the other side of the bed (farthest from the client),

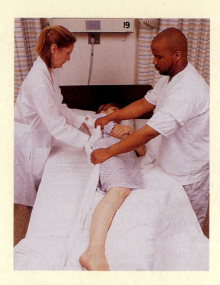

Figure 32-35. ■ The nurse on the right uses the far edge of the sheet to roll the client toward him; the nurse on the left remains behind the client and assists with turning. (Photographer: Jenny Thomas.)

and assume a stable stance. Reaching over the client, grasp the far edges of the turn sheet, and roll the client toward you (Figure 32-35 ■). The second nurse (behind the client) helps turn the client and provides pillow supports to ensure good alignment in the lateral position.

Part D: Moving a Client to a Sitting Position on the Edge of the Bed

The client assumes a sitting position on the edge of the bed before walking, moving to a chair or wheelchair, eating, or performing other activities.

1. Position yourself and the client appropriately before performing the move.
   ■ Assist the client to a lateral position facing you.
   ■ Raise the head of the bed slowly as high as it will go. *This decreases the distance that the client needs to move to sit up on the side of the bed.*
   ■ Position the client's feet and lower legs at the edge of the bed. *This enables the client's feet to move easily off the bed during the movement, and the client is aided by gravity into a sitting position.*
   ■ Stand beside the client's hips and face the far corner of the bottom of the bed (the angle in which movement will occur). Assume a broad stance, placing the foot nearest the client forward. Incline your trunk forward from the hips. Flex your hips, knees, and ankles (Figures 32-36A ■ and B).

2. Move the client to a sitting position.
   ■ Place one arm around the client's shoulders and the other arm beneath both of the client's thighs near the knees (see Figure 32-36A). *Supporting the client's shoulders prevents the client from falling backward during the movement. Supporting the client's thighs reduces friction of the thighs*

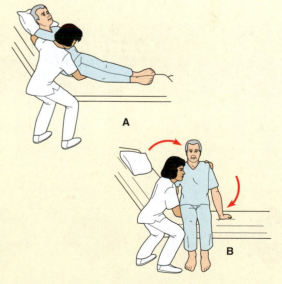

Figure 32-36. ■ **A, B.** Assisting a client to a sitting position on the edge of the bed.

against the bed surface during the move and increases the force of the movement.
   ■ Tighten your gluteal, abdominal, leg, and arm muscles. *This protects your own muscles from strain.*

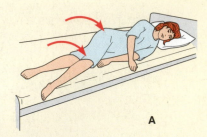
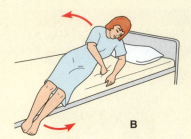
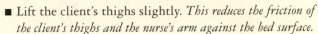

Figure 32-37. ■ **A, B.** Moving to a sitting position independently.

- Lift the client's thighs slightly. *This reduces the friction of the client's thighs and the nurse's arm against the bed surface.*
- Pivot on the balls of your feet in the desired direction facing the foot of the bed while pulling the client's feet and legs off the bed (see Figure 32-36B). *Pivoting prevents twisting of the nurse's spine. The weight of the client's legs swinging downward increases downward movement of the lower body and helps make the client's upper body vertical.*
- Keep supporting the client until the client is well balanced and comfortable. *This movement may cause some clients to faint.*
- Assess vital signs (e.g., pulse, respirations, and blood pressure) as indicated by the client's health status.

VARIATION: TEACHING A CLIENT HOW TO SIT ON THE SIDE OF THE BED INDEPENDENTLY

A client who has had recent abdominal surgery or who is weak may have too much abdominal pain or too little strength to sit straight up in bed. This person can be taught

to assume a "dangle" position without assistance. Instruct the client to

- Roll to the side and lift the far leg over the near leg (Figure 32-37A ■).
- Grasp the mattress edge with the lower arm and push the fist of the upper arm into the mattress (Figure 32-37B).
- Push up with the arms as the heels and legs slide over the mattress edge (Figure 32-37B).
- Maintain the sitting position by pushing both fists into the mattress behind and to the sides of the buttocks.

SAMPLE DOCUMENTATION

[date]   Client attempted dangling position,
[time]   felt faint, returned to supine.
           Reported to team leader.
                          _____ S. Courant, LVN

| PROCEDURE 32-3 | **Transferring a Client** |

Purpose

- To safely move a client from bed to chair, wheelchair, or stretcher

Equipment

- Transfer (walking) belt
- Stretcher (if transferring to stretcher)
- *Optional:* roller bar or long board (sliding board)

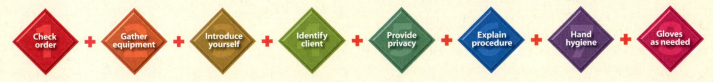

Check order + Gather equipment + Introduce yourself + Identify client + Provide privacy + Explain procedure + Hand hygiene + Gloves as needed

Part A: Transfer between a Bed and a Chair

Interventions

1. Position the equipment appropriately.
   - Lower the bed to its lowest position so that the client's feet will rest flat on the floor. Lock the wheels of the bed. *This helps to prevent risk of fall due to sudden movement.*
   - Place the wheelchair parallel to the bed as close to the bed as possible (Figure 32-38 ■). Lock the wheels of the wheelchair, and raise the footplate.

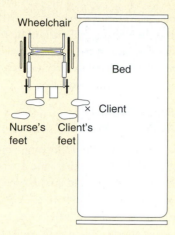

Figure 32-38. ■ The wheelchair is placed parallel to the bed as close to the bed as possible. Note that placement of the nurse's feet mirrors that of the client's feet.

2. Prepare and assess the client.
   - Assist the client to a sitting position on the side of the bed. See Procedure 32-2, Part D.
   - Assess the client for orthostatic hypotension before moving the client from the bed. *Changes in posture could result in fainting.*
   - Assist the client in putting on a bathrobe and nonskid slippers or shoes. *These provide comfort and safety when walking.*
   - Place a transfer belt snugly around the client's waist. Check to be certain that the belt is securely fastened.

3. Give explicit instructions to the client. Ask the client to
   - Move forward and sit on the edge of the bed. *This brings the client's center of gravity closer to the nurse's.*
   - Lean forward slightly from the hips. *This brings the client's center of gravity more directly over the base of support and positions the head and trunk in the direction of the movement.*
   - Place the foot of the stronger leg beneath the edge of the bed and put the other foot forward. *In this way, the client can use the stronger leg muscles to stand and power the movement. A broader base of support makes the client more stable during the transfer.*
   - Place the client's hands on the bed surface or on your shoulders so that the client can push while standing. *This provides additional force for the movement and reduces the potential for strain on the nurse's back. The client should not grasp the nurse's neck for support. Doing so can injure the nurse.*

4. Position yourself correctly.
   - Stand directly in front of the client. Incline the trunk forward from the hips. Flex the hips, knees, and ankles. Assume a broad stance, placing one foot forward and one back. Mirror the placement of the client's feet, if possible. *This helps prevent loss of balance during the transfer.*
   - Encircle the client's waist with your arms, and grasp the transfer belt at the client's back (Figure 32-39 ■) with thumbs pointing downward. *The belt provides a secure han-*

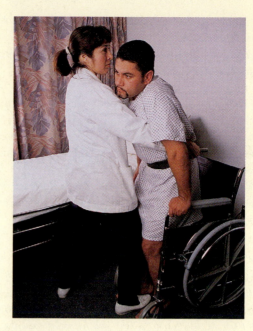

Figure 32-39. ■ Using a transfer (walking) belt. (Photographer: Elena Dorfman.)

dle for holding onto the client and controlling the movement. Downward placement of the thumbs prevents potential wrist injury as the nurse lifts. By supporting the client in this manner, you keep the client from tilting backward during the transfer.
   - Tighten your gluteal, abdominal, leg, and arm muscles.

5. Assist the client to stand, and then move together toward the wheelchair.
   - On the count of three:
     a. Ask the client to push with the back foot, rock to the forward foot, extend (straighten) the joints of the lower extremities, and push or pull up with the hands, while
     b. You push with the forward foot, rock to the back foot, extend the joints of the lower extremities, and pull the client (directly toward your center of gravity) into a standing position.
   - Support the client in an upright standing position for a few moments. *This allows the nurse and the client to extend the joints and provides the nurse with an opportunity to ensure that the client is all right before moving away from the bed.*
   - Together, pivot or take a few steps toward the wheelchair.

6. Assist the client to sit.
   - Ask the client to:
     a. Back up to the wheelchair and place the legs against the seat. *Having the client place the legs against the wheelchair seat minimizes the risk of the client's falling when sitting down.*
     b. Place the foot of the stronger leg slightly behind the other. *This supports body weight during the movement.*
     c. Keep the other foot forward. *This provides a broad base of support.*
     d. Place both hands on the wheelchair arms or on your shoulders. *This increases stability and lessens the strain on the nurse.*

- Stand directly in front of the client. Place one foot forward and one back.
- Tighten your grasp on the transfer belt, and tighten your gluteal, abdominal, leg, and arm muscles.
- On the count of three:
  a. Have the client shift the body weight by rocking to the back foot, lower the body onto the edge of the wheelchair seat by flexing the joints of the legs and arms, and place some body weight on the arms, while
  b. You shift your body weight by stepping back with the forward foot and pivoting toward the chair while lowering the client onto the wheelchair seat.
7. Ensure client safety.
   - Ask the client to push back into the wheelchair seat. *Sitting well back on the seat provides a broader base of support and greater stability and minimizes the risk of falling from the wheelchair. A wheelchair can topple forward when the client sits on the edge of the seat and leans far forward.*
   - Lower the footplates, and place the client's feet on them.
   - Apply a seat belt as required.

VARIATION: ANGLING THE WHEELCHAIR

For clients who have difficulty walking, place the wheelchair at a 45-degree angle to the bed. *This enables the client to pivot into the chair and lessens the amount of body rotation required.*

VARIATION: TRANSFERRING WITHOUT A BELT

- For clients who need minimal assistance, place the hands against the sides of the client's chest (not at the axillae) during the transfer (Figure 32-40 ■). For clients who require

more assistance, reach through the client's axillae and place the hands on the client's scapulae during the transfer. Avoid placing hands or pressure on the axillae, especially for clients who have upper extremity paralysis or paresis.
- Follow the steps described previously.

VARIATION: TRANSFERRING WITH A BELT AND TWO NURSES

- When the client is able to stand, position yourselves on both sides of the client, facing the same direction as the client. Flex your hips, knees, and ankles; grasp the client's transfer belt with the hand closest to the client; and with the other hand support the client's elbows.
- Coordinating your efforts, all three of you stand simultaneously, pivot, and move to the wheelchair. Reverse the process to lower the client onto the wheelchair seat.

VARIATION: TRANSFERRING A CLIENT WITH AN INJURED LOWER EXTREMITY

When the client has an injured lower extremity, movement should always occur toward the client's unaffected (strong) side. For example, if the client's right leg is injured and the client is sitting on the edge of the bed preparing to transfer to a wheelchair, position the wheelchair on the client's left side. In this way, the client can use the unaffected leg most effectively and safely.

VARIATION: USING A SLIDING BOARD

Have a client who cannot stand use a sliding board to move without nursing assistance. *This method not only promotes the client's sense of independence but preserves your energy* (Figure 32-41 ■).

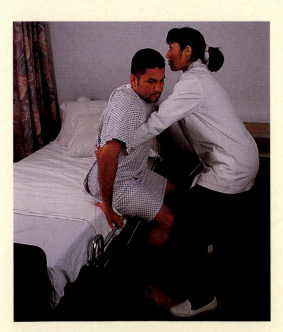

Figure 32-40. ■ Transferring without a belt. (Photographer: Elena Dorfman.)

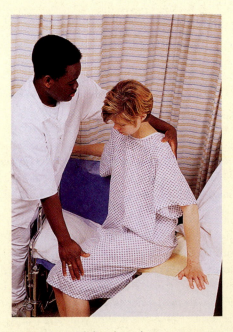

Figure 32-41. ■ Using a sliding board. (Photographer: Jenny Thomas.)

Part B: Transferring Client between a Bed and a Stretcher

The stretcher, or gurney, is used to transfer supine clients from one location to another. Whenever the client is capable of accomplishing the transfer from bed to stretcher independently, either by lifting onto it or by rolling onto it, the client should be encouraged to do so. If the client cannot move onto the stretcher independently, at least two nurses are needed to assist with the transfer. More are needed if the client is totally helpless or is heavy.

Interventions

1. Adjust the client's bed in preparation for the transfer.
   - Lower the head of the bed until it is flat or as low as the client can tolerate.
   - Raise the bed so that it is slightly higher than the surface of the stretcher. *It is easier for the client to move down an incline.*
   - Ensure that the wheels on the bed are locked.
   - Pull the drawsheet out from both sides of the bed.

2. Move the client to the edge of the bed, and position the stretcher.
   - Roll the drawsheet as close to the client's side as possible.
   - Pull the client to the edge of the bed, and cover the client with a sheet or bath blanket to maintain comfort.
   - Place the stretcher parallel to the bed, next to the client, and lock its wheels.
   - Fill the gap that exists between the bed and the stretcher loosely with the bath blankets (optional).

3. Transfer the client securely to the stretcher.
   - In unison with the other staff members, press your body tightly against the stretcher. *This prevents the stretcher from moving.*
   - Roll the pull sheet tightly against the client. *This achieves better control over client movement.*
   - Flex your hips, and pull the client on the pull sheet in unison directly toward you and onto the stretcher. *Pulling downward requires less force than pulling along a flat surface.*
   - Ask the client to flex the neck during the move, if possible, and place arms across the chest. *This prevents injury to these body parts.*

4. Ensure client comfort and safety.
   - Make the client comfortable, unlock the stretcher wheels, and move the stretcher away from the bed.
   - Immediately raise the stretcher side rails and/or fasten the safety straps across the client. *Because the stretcher is high and narrow, the client is in danger of falling unless these safety precautions are taken.*

VARIATION: USING A ROLLER BAR DURING THE TRANSFER

A roller bar is a metal frame covered with longitudinal rollers. Place the bar over the gap between the bed and the stretcher. Using a pull sheet, pull the client onto the roller bar, and roll the client easily onto the stretcher.

VARIATION: USING A LONG BOARD

The long board, which may be referred to as the Smooth Mover or Easyglide, is a lacquered or smooth polyethylene board measuring 45 to 55 cm (18 to 22 in.) by 182 cm (72 in.) with handholds along its edges. This device may be used by one nurse alone or up to four nurses together. Turn the client to a lateral position away from you, position the board close to the client's back, and roll the client onto the board. Pull the client and board across the bed to the stretcher. Safety belts may be placed over the chest, abdomen, and legs.

VARIATION: USING A THREE-PERSON CARRY (USE CAUTION)

Three people of about equal height stand side by side facing the client. Recommendations vary as to which staff member lifts a specific area of the client. Often, the strongest person supports the heaviest part of the client or the tallest person with the longest reach supports the head and shoulders. The stretcher or bed to which the client will be moved is placed at a right angle at the foot of the bed. The wheels of the bed and stretcher are locked. Each person flexes the knees and places the foot nearest to the stretcher slightly forward.

The arms of the lifters are put under the client at the head and shoulders, hips and thighs, and upper and lower legs. The lifters then, on the count of 3, roll the client onto their chests and step back in unison (Figure 32-42 ■). They then pivot around to the stretcher and lower the client by flexing their knees and hips until their elbows are on the surface of the stretcher. The client is then released on the stretcher surface and is aligned and covered, and the stretcher side rails are raised.

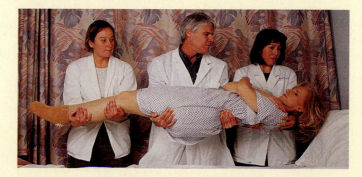

Figure 32-42. ■ The three-carrier lift. (Photographer: Elena Dorfman.)

PROCEDURE 32-4 | # Hoyer (Sling) Transfers Lift

Purpose

- To lift and transfer client from bed to chair and back

Equipment

- Hoyer lift base
- Canvas pieces: 1 large, 1 small
- Canvas straps

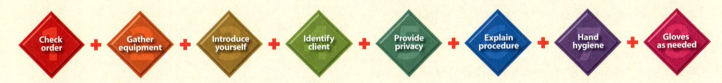

Check order + Gather equipment + Introduce yourself + Identify client + Provide privacy + Explain procedure + Hand hygiene + Gloves as needed

Intervention

1. Check orders and client care plan. Determine that lift can safely move the weight of the client.

2. Explain procedure to client. *Client may be frightened by use of a mechanical device.*

3. Bring lift to bedside. *Ensures safe elevation of client off bed.*

4. Lock wheels of bed. *Ensures that the bed will not move during transfer.*

5. Place client chair by the beside. Allow adequate space to maneuver the lift.

6. Raise bed to high position with mattress flat. Lower side rail on the side closest to you. *Maintains nurses' alignment during transfer.*

7. Keep bed side rail up on the opposite side. *Maintains client safety.*

8. Roll client on side away from you.

9. Place hammock or canvas strips under client to form sling. Place two canvas pieces so that lower edge fits under client's knees (wide piece), and upper edge fits under client's shoulder (narrow piece). *Two different types of seats are supplied. Hammocks are better for clients who are flaccid, weak, and need support; canvas can be used for clients with normal muscle tone. Hooks should face away from client's skin. Place sling under client's center of gravity and greatest portion of body weight.*

10. Raise bed rail. *Maintains safety.*

11. Go to opposite side and lower side rail. *Maintains safety.*

12. Roll client to opposite side and pull Hammock (strip) through. *Completes positioning of client on lift sling.*

13. Roll client supine onto canvas seat. *Sling should extend from shoulder to knees to support client's body weight equally.*

14. Remove client's glasses, if appropriate. *Swivel bar can break eyeglasses.*

15. Place lift's horseshoe bar under side of bed (on side with chair). *Positions lift efficiently and promotes smooth transfer.*

16. Lower horizontal bar to sling level by releasing hydraulic valve. Lock the valve. *Position hydraulic lift close to client. Locking valve prevents injury to client.*

17. Attach hooks to strap (chain) to holes in sling. Short chains or straps hook to top holes of sling; long chains hook to bottom of sling. *Secures hydraulic lift to sling.*

18. Elevate head of bed. *Puts the client in a sitting position.*

19. Fold client's arms over chest. *Prevents injury to paralyzed arms.*

20. Pump hydraulic handle using long, slow, even strokes until client is raised off of the bed.

21. Use steering handle to pull lift from bed and maneuver to chair. *Moves client from bed to chair.*

22. Roll base around chair. *Positions lift in front of chair to which client is to be transferred.*

23. Release valve slowly (turn to lift) and lower client into chair. *Safely guides client back of chair descends.*

24. Close valve as soon as client *is* on the chair or stretcher and straps can be released. *If valve is left open, boom may continue to lower and injure the client.*

25. Remove straps and lift. *Prevents damage to skin and underlining tissues from canvas or hooks.*

26. Check client's sitting alignment and correct if necessary. *Prevents injury from poor posture.*

27. Perform hand hygiene. *Reduces transmission of microorganisms.*

28. Evaluate client's tolerance and level of fatigue and comfort. *These clients may find transfer very fatiguing and will need post-transfer interventions to restore a level of comfort.*

29. Return client to bed using reverse method.

Reference: Sandra E. Smith, Donna J. Duell, Barbara C. Martin, *Clinical Nursing Skills,* Basic Advanced Skills, Sixth Edition, Pearson, Prentice Hall.

| PROCEDURE 32-5 | **Assisting a Client to Walk** |

Purpose
- To provide safety for the client who is weak

Equipment
- Walking belt (optional)

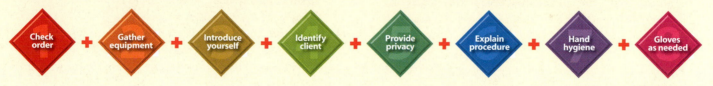

Interventions

1. Prepare the client for ambulation.
   - Apply elastic (antiemboli) stockings as required. See Procedure 24-6 ⊙⊙.
   - Assist the client to sit on the edge of the bed.
   - Assess the client carefully for signs and symptoms of orthostatic hypotension (dizziness, light-headedness, pallor, or a sudden increase in heart rate) prior to leaving the bedside.
   - Ensure that the client is appropriately dressed to walk and wears shoes or slippers with nonskid soles. *Proper attire and footwear prevent chilling and falling.*
   - Assist the client to stand by the side of the bed until the client feels secure.
   - Plan the length of the walk with the client, in light of the nursing or physician's orders. Be prepared to shorten the walk according to the person's activity tolerance.

One Nurse

2. Ensure client safety while assisting the client to ambulate.
   - Encourage the client to ambulate independently if the client is able, but walk beside the client.
   - Remain physically close to the client. *This gives you time to react in case assistance is needed at any point.*
   - Use a transfer or walking belt if the client is slightly weak and unstable. Make sure the belt is

pulled snugly around the client's waist and fastened securely. Grasp the belt at the client's back, and walk behind and slightly to one side of the client (Figure 32-43 ■).

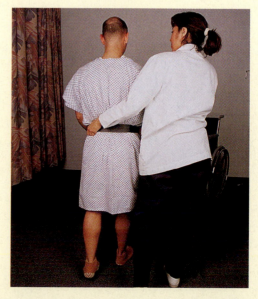

Figure 32-43. ■ Using a transfer (walking) belt to support the client. (Photographer: Elena Dorfman.)

- If it is the client's first time out of bed following surgery, injury, or an extended period of immobility, or if the client is quite weak or unstable, have an assistant follow you and the client with a wheelchair in case it is needed quickly.
- If the client is moderately weak and unstable, interlock your forearm with the client's closest forearm, and walk on the client's weaker side. Encourage the client to press the forearm against your hip or waist for stability if desired. In addition, have the client wear a transfer or walking belt so that you can quickly grab the belt and prevent a fall if the client feels faint.
- If the client is very weak and unstable, place your near arm around the client's waist, and with your other arm support the client's near arm at the elbow. Walk on the client's stronger side. Again, have the client wear a transfer or walking belt in case of an emergency.
- Encourage the client to assume a normal walking stance and gait as much as possible.

3. Protect the client who begins to fall while ambulating.
- If a client begins to experience the signs and symptoms of orthostatic hypotension or extreme weakness, quickly assist the client into a nearby wheelchair or other chair, and help the client to lower the head between the knees. *Lowering the head facilitates blood flow to the brain.*
- Stay with the client. *A client who faints while in this position could fall, head first, out of the chair.*
- When the weakness subsides, assist the client back to bed.
- If a chair is not close by, assist the client to a horizontal position on the floor before fainting occurs (Figure 32-44 ■). *A vertical position may increase feelings of faintness.*
  a. Assume a broad stance with one foot in front of the other. *A broad stance widens the nurse's base of support for stability. Placing one foot behind the other allows the nurse to rock backward and use the femoral muscles when support-*

ing the client's weight and lowering the center of gravity (see step b), thus preventing back strain.
  b. Bring the client backward so that your body supports the person. *Clients who do faint or start to fall and cannot regain their strength or balance usually drop straight downward or pitch slightly forward because of the momentum of ambulating; thus their head, hips, and knees are most vulnerable to injury. Bringing the client's weight backward against the nurse's body allows gradual movement to the floor without injury to the client.*
  c. Allow the client to slide down your leg, and lower the person gently to the floor, making sure the client's head does not hit any objects.

Two Nurses

4. Prepare the client.
- See step 1 above.

5. Ensure client safety.
- After the client stands, assume a position with one nurse at either side. Grasp the inferior aspect of the client's upper arm with your nearest hand and the client's lower arm or hand with your other hand (Figure 32-45 ■). *This provides a secure grip for each nurse.*
- *Optional:* Place a walking belt around the client's waist. Each nurse grasps the side handle with the near hand and the lower aspect of the client's upper arm with the other hand.
- Walk in unison with the client, using a smooth, even gait, at the same speed and with steps the same size as the client's. *This gives the client a greater feeling of security.*
- If the client starts to fall and cannot regain strength or balance, each nurse slips an arm under the client's axillae and grasps the client's hands, and together the nurses lower the person gently to the floor or to a nearby chair

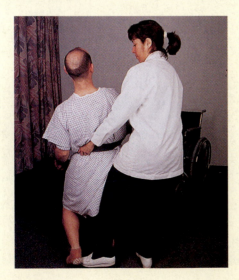

Figure 32-44 ■ Lowering a fainting client to the floor. (Photographer: Elena Dorfman.)

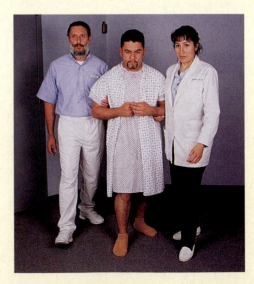

Figure 32-45. ■ Two nurses supporting an ambulatory client. (Photographer: Elena Dorfman.)

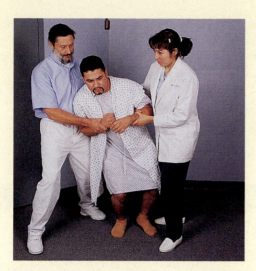

Figure 32-46. ■ Two nurses lowering a fainting client to the floor. (Photographer: Elena Dorfman.)

(Figure 32-46 ■). *Placing the nurses' arms under the client's axillae evenly balances the client's weight between the two nurses, preventing injury to both the nurses and the client.*

6. Document all relevant information.
   ■ Document the time of the walk, the distance walked or time taken, and all nursing assessments.

SAMPLE DOCUMENTATION

[date] [time]	Ambulated client from bed to nurse's station and returned. Client steady, no c/o dizziness. "Let's do more tomorrow!" _____ E. Ketterer, LPN

PROCEDURE 32-6 **Providing a Back Massage**

Purposes

■ To relieve muscle tension
■ To promote physical and mental relaxation
■ To relieve insomnia

Equipment

■ Lotion or oil

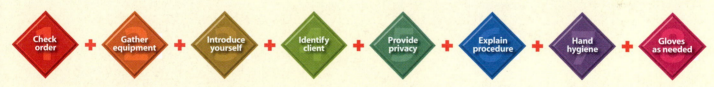

Check order + Gather equipment + Introduce yourself + Identify client + Provide privacy + Explain procedure + Hand hygiene + Gloves as needed

Interventions

1. Select an appropriate time free of interruptions and distractions.
   ■ Provide massage following the bath, before sleeping, and at other times as necessary to achieve relaxation and comfort for the client.
   ■ Assist the client to a prone or lateral position in bed. Remove the client's gown, or open the back of the gown.

2. Warm the massage lotion or oil before use. *This prevents the muscles from stiffening when it is used.*
   ■ Warm the lotion or oil by pouring and holding it in your hands or placing the container in warm water before applying it to the client's back. *Cold lotion may startle the client and increase discomfort.*

3. Massage the entire back. Two common types of massage strokes are **effleurage** (stroking the body; pronounced eh-

flu-RAJ) and **pétrissage** (kneading or making large quick pinches of the skin, subcutaneous tissue, and muscle; pronounced PET-ri-saj).
   ■ Place your hands on either side of the lower spine. Using your palms and fingers, slowly massage using a circular motion and moving upward to the neck, gradually decreasing pressure as you get close to the neck. Use the circular motion over the shoulder blades and then slowly move down the lateral surface of the back (Figure 32-47 ■). *Effleurage has a relaxing, sedative effect if slow movement and light pressure are used.*
   ■ Repeat this massage pattern for 3 to 4 minutes.
   ■ Maintain contact with the skin during the massage.
   ■ Use your thumbs to apply friction strokes (strong circular motions).

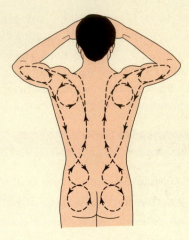

Figure 32-47. ■ A back rub pattern.

4. Optional: Pétrissage the back and shoulders of the client.
   ■ Pétrissage first up the vertebral column and then over the entire back. *Pétrissage is stimulating, especially if done quickly and with firm pressure.*
   ■ Observe the client carefully to ensure that pétrissage does not cause pain or discomfort. *If the client gri-*

maces or withdraws from the touch, ease the kneading pressure.
   ■ End the massage with long movements and tell the client you are finishing.
5. Optional: Effleurage and pétrissage the upper back and shoulders. *This area often experiences the most tension.*
6. Assist the client to a position of comfort.
7. Document the massage and your observations.

SAMPLE DOCUMENTATION

[date]	Client turned left laterally and
[time]	placed in Sims' position w/foam wedges. Back care including effleurage to lower lumbar and sacral area. "Very relaxing." Skin intact and pink.
	_____ J. Fontaine, LPN

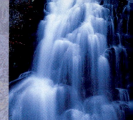

Chapter Review

 KEY TERMS by Topic

Use the audio glossary feature of either the CD-ROM or the Companion Website to hear the correct pronunciation of the following key terms.

Normal Movement
line of gravity, center of gravity, postural tonus, range of motion (ROM), equilibrium, labyrinth

Factors Affecting Body Alignment and Activity
vertigo

Effects of Immobility
osteoporosis, atrophy, ankylosed, thrombus, thrombophlebitis, emboli, infarction, vital capacity, atelectasis, urinary stasis, ambulation

Physiology of Sleep
NREM sleep, REM sleep

Common Sleep Disorders
insomnia, hypersomnia, narcolepsy, sleep apnea, parasomnia, effleurage, pétrissage

KEY Points

- The ability to move freely, easily, and purposefully in the environment is essential for people to meet their basic needs.

- Purposeful coordinated movement relies on the integrated functioning of the musculoskeletal system, the nervous system, and the vestibular apparatus of the inner ear.

- Body alignment and activity are influenced by growth and development, physical health, and prescribed limitations to movement. They are also influenced by mental health, personal values, and attitudes.

- Immobility adversely affects almost every body organ and system. It also can cause psychosocial problems.

- The nurse must (1) prevent the complications of immobility and reduce the severity of any problems resulting from immobility and (2) design exercise programs for clients to promote wellness.

- Positioning a client in good body alignment and changing the position regularly and systematically are essential aspects of nursing practice.

- Safety measures must always be employed when the nurse uses a wheelchair or stretcher to move and transfer clients.

- The nurse should prepare clients for ambulation by helping them become as independent as possible while in bed. Techniques that facilitate normal walking yet provide required physical support are most effective.

- Sleep is a naturally occurring altered state of consciousness in which a person's perceptions of and reactions to the environment are decreased.

- Many factors affect sleep, including illness, age, environment, lifestyle, emotional stress, culture, alcohol, smoking, diet, motivation, and medications.

- Nursing responsibilities to help clients sleep include (1) teaching sleep hygiene, (2) supporting bedtime rituals, (3) creating a restful environment, (4) promoting comfort and relaxation, and (5) enhancing sleep with prescribed medications.

- Nonpharmacologic measures to induce and maintain sleep are always the preferred interventions.

 EXPLORE Media Link

Additional interactive resources for this chapter can be found on the Companion Website at www.prenhall.com/ramont. Click on Chapter 32 and "Begin" to select the activities for this chapter.

For chapter-related NCLEX®-style questions and an audio glossary, access the accompanying CD-ROM in this book.

FOR FURTHER Study

Strategies for preventing strains and sprains in nurses are provided in Chapter 8.

See Chapter 11 for age-related considerations in regard to mobility.

See Chapter 22 for information on preventing and treating pressure ulcers.

See Chapter 23 for further discussion of the effects of immobility on the skin and risk for decubitus ulcer formation.

See Chapter 24 for information about oxygenation.

See Chapter 27 for bladder considerations.

See Chapter 28 for more about the effects of immobility on bowel elimination.

Critical Thinking Care Map

Caring for a Client with Sleep Problems
NCLEX-PN® Focus Area: Physiological Integrity: Basic Care and Comfort

Case Study: Gillian Marks, 51, states she has had a problem falling asleep since her mastectomy 2 months ago. She says fears of prognosis become prominent when she is not active and busy. She has tried reading or watching TV, but neither makes her sleepy or relaxed. She appears agitated and restless. She is receiving her last radiation treatment. A decision has not been made as to the need for chemotherapy.

Nursing Diagnosis: Disturbed Sleep Pattern; Insomnia

COLLECT DATA

Subjective	Objective
_____	_____
_____	_____
_____	_____
_____	_____
_____	_____
_____	_____
_____	_____

Would you report this data? Yes/No

If yes, to: _____

What would you report? _____

Nursing Care

_____
_____
_____
_____
_____
_____
_____
_____
_____
_____
_____
_____

How would you document this? _____

_____
_____

Data Collected
(use those that apply)

- Weight 126 lbs, 10-lb weight loss since surgery
- BP 128/86
- HR 84 and regular
- RR 16
- WBC 7,000
- H&H 12.8/36
- Skin pale; dark circles around eyes
- Surgical incision clean and healed well
- Radiation site irritated and red

Nursing Interventions
(use those that apply; list in priority order)

- Assess client's sleep patterns and usual bedtime rituals and incorporate these into the plan of care.
- Encourage client to express feelings to others.
- Monitor client's defense mechanisms and support healthy defenses.
- Assess for signs of new onset of depression, depressed mood state, statement of hopelessness, and poor appetite.
- Expect client to meet responsibilities; give positive reinforcement.
- Observe client's medication, diet, and caffeine intake. Look for hidden sources of caffeine.
- Identify causes for and observe client's expression of sorrow.
- Advise client to avoid use of alcohol or hypnotics to induce sleep.
- Assist to resolve ambivalent feelings about illness and management of therapeutic regimen.

Compare your documentation to the sample provided in Appendix I.

NCLEX-PN® Exam Preparation

1. The point at which all of the body's mass is centered and the base of support achieves balance is known as the:
   1. line of gravity.
   2. center of gravity.
   3. line of mobility.
   4. postural tonus.

2. Your client has been confined to bed following a musculoskeletal injury. The physician has ordered no weight bearing for an extended period of time. Which of the following conditions would be the biggest concern?
   1. contractures
   2. orthostatic hypotension
   3. osteoporosis
   4. disuse atrophy

3. Atelectasis, the collapse of a lobe or the entire lung in a bedridden client, is a result of:
   1. inflammation resulting from static secretions.
   2. reduced vital capacity.
   3. pulmonary emboli.
   4. decreased surfactant and mucous-blocked bronchioles.

4. Assistive mobility devices can present a safety hazard for an immobile client. Which of the following statements made by a client would demonstrate the need for additional teaching?
   1. "My crutches are adjusted to the proper length if the pads are touching my underarms."
   2. "It is important to remove throw rugs from around my bed until I am off these crutches."
   3. "I should wear a nonslip sturdy shoe on my unaffected foot."
   4. "The crutches need to have rubber tips to prevent slipping."

5. The position of choice for a client who has difficulty breathing or who is experiencing cardiac problems would be:
   1. dorsal recumbent.
   2. semi-Fowler's.
   3. orthopneic.
   4. Sims'.

6. During which stage of NREM (non–rapid eye movement) sleep are body processes dominated by the parasympathetic nervous system?
   1. stage I
   2. stage II
   3. stage III
   4. stage IV

7. Stage IV sleep is decreased by which of the following conditions?
   1. hyperthyroidism
   2. respiratory conditions
   3. hypothyroidism
   4. enuresis

8. Treatment for insomnia routinely includes:
   1. long-term use of sleep-inducing drugs.
   2. behavior modification.
   3. antidepressants.
   4. beta blockers.

9. Your client has a history of somnambulism; you understand that to be:
   1. sleepwalking.
   2. sleep talking.
   3. bedwetting.
   4. teeth grinding.

10. A home care client assigned to you has postural hypotension. The RN has recommended that she sit in a rocking chair when out of bed. A family member questions this. Which of the following rationales best explains the suggestion?
    1. Using a rocking chair can strengthen leg muscle tone and enhance circulation.
    2. The rocking motion increases the blood flow to the upper body.
    3. Because she needs help to stand when in the rocking chair, there will be less danger of her falling.
    4. Sitting in the rocking chair will take her mind off her health problems.

Answers and Rationales for Review Questions, as well as discussion of Care Plan and Critical Thinking Care Map questions, appear in Appendix I.

Chapter 33

Client Teaching

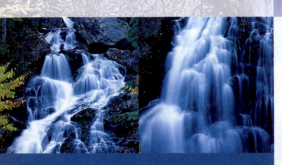

HISTORICAL Perspectives

Little emphasis was placed on formal client teaching until the late 1970s. At that time, organized programs such as cardiac rehabilitation and diabetic education were developed. Medicare reimbursement for home health care required that someone be taught to perform ongoing care. In the mid-1980s when DRGs became the standard for hospital reimbursement, and when HMOs came into being, the responsibility for providing care shifted to home health and self-care. Client teaching became imperative so that clients could remain out of the hospital. Accrediting bodies for hospitals began requiring documentation of client teaching and its effectiveness. In 1992, the Patient's Bill of Rights mandated client education as a client right.

BRIEF Outline

Learning
Teaching

LEARNING Outcomes

After completing this chapter, you will be able to:

1. Discuss the three main concepts of learning theory.
2. Describe the three domains of learning.
3. Identify factors that influence learning throughout life and factors that inhibit learning.
4. Contrast the nursing process and teaching process.
5. Identify the LPN's/LVN's role in client teaching.
6. Describe essential aspects of a teaching plan.
7. Identify effective teaching strategies.
8. Discuss the challenges of teaching clients of different cultures.
9. Identify methods to evaluate learning.
10. Demonstrate effective documentation of teaching–learning activities.

Client education is a major nursing responsibility—both legally and professionally. Legislation regarding nursing defines client teaching as an independent nursing function.

Learning

Client education is a dynamic, integrated, and multifaceted teaching–learning process in which the nurse and client work together to change client behaviors. Participants exchange information, emotions, perceptions, and attitudes.

Learning is a lifelong process of acquiring knowledge or skills that cannot be solely accounted for by human growth. This process is demonstrated by changes in behavior (Box 33-1 ■). Each client has unique learning needs regarding intellectual knowledge, skills, or behaviors.

An important aspect of learning is an individual's desire to learn and to act on the learning (Box 33-2 ■). In health care, **compliance** is the extent to which a person's behavior coincides with medical or health advice. Compliance is best demonstrated when the client embraces learning and then follows through with appropriate and expected behaviors. For example, a client who has been newly diagnosed with diabetes would show compliance by willingly studying the special diet and then planning meals accordingly. Areas for client education include health promotion, protection, and maintenance (Box 33-3 ■).

BOX 33-2

Attributes of Learning

Learning is:

- An experience that occurs inside the learner
- The discovery of the personal meaning and relevance of ideas
- A consequence of experience
- A collaborative and cooperative process
- An evolutionary process
- A process that is both intellectual and emotional.

BOX 33-3

Areas for Client Education

Promotion of Health

- Increasing a person's level of wellness
- Growth and development topics
- Fertility control
- Hygiene
- Nutrition
- Exercise
- Stress management
- Lifestyle modification
- Resources within the community

Prevention of Illness/Injury

- Health screening (e.g., blood glucose levels, blood pressure, blood cholesterol, Pap test, mammograms, vision, hearing, routine physical examinations)
- Reducing health risk factors (e.g., lowering cholesterol level)
- Specific protective health measures (e.g., immunizations, use of condoms, use of sunscreen, use of medication, umbilical cord care)
- First aid
- Safety (e.g., using seat belts, helmets, walkers)

Restoration of Health

- Information about tests, diagnosis, treatment, medications
- Self-care skills or skills needed to care for family member
- Resources within healthcare setting and community

Adapting to Altered Health and Function

- Adaptations in lifestyle
- Problem-solving skills
- Adaptation to changing health status
- Strategies to deal with current problems (e.g., home IV skills, medications, diet, activity limits, prostheses)
- Strategies to deal with future problems (e.g., fear of pain with terminal cancer, future surgeries, or treatments)
- Information about treatments and likely outcomes
- Referrals to other healthcare facilities or services
- Facilitation of strong self-image
- Grief and bereavement counseling

Nurses can use the following concepts about learners as a guide for teaching adult clients:

- As people mature, they move from dependence to independence (see Chapter 11 ∞).
- An adult's previous experiences can be used as a resource for learning.
- An adult's readiness to learn is often related to a developmental task or social role.
- People are more oriented to learning when the material is useful immediately, not sometime in the future.

LEARNING THEORIES

The three main theories of human learning are behaviorism, cognitivism, and humanism.

Behaviorism

Behaviorism is the belief that environment influences behavior, which is the essential factor determining human action. Edward Thorndike, who pioneered the twentieth-century behaviorist movement, asserted that learning should be based on the learner's behavior. B. F. Skinner introduced the importance of positive reinforcement to encourage a person to repeat a desired action. Alfred Bandura claimed that most learning comes from observation and instruction rather than personal trial and error; so, most people imitate or model observed behavior. Imitation and modeling of healthy behaviors are key goals of client teaching.

Cognitivism

Cognitivism defines learning largely as a complex thinking process. The learner constantly structures and processes information from many sources. Cognitivists emphasize the importance of individual perception and motivation, as well as the teacher–learner relationship and environment. Developmental readiness and individual readiness (called client *motivation*) are other key factors.

J. Piaget and B. Bloom are important cognitive theorists. Bloom (1956) identified three *domains* (or areas) of learning: cognitive, affective, and psychomotor. The **cognitive domain** includes knowing, comprehending, and applying. The **affective domain** includes feelings, emotions, interests, attitudes, and appreciations. The **psychomotor domain** includes motor skills (such as giving an injection). Nurses should address each domain in client teaching. For example, a three-point teaching session on colostomy care would include the following:

1. Demonstration of irrigation technique (*psychomotor* domain)
2. Discussion of safe fluid volume for irrigation (*cognitive* domain)
3. Discussion of the client's change in body image (*affective* domain).

Humanism

Humanism (humanistic learning theory) focuses on both cognitive and affective qualities of the learner. Leading humanists include Abraham Maslow and Carl Rogers. According to humanistic theory, each individual is a unique composite of biologic, psychological, social, cultural, and spiritual factors. Learning focuses on self-development, achieving full potential, and learning what the person needs (i.e., what is relevant). Autonomy and self-determination are most important. Learning is self-motivated, self-initiated, and self-evaluated. So, the learner is an active participant in every phase of the teaching process.

APPLYING LEARNING THEORIES

Each mode of teaching has benefits and drawbacks. Behaviorism is useful but may be hard to apply to complex learning situations. It also may limit the learner's role in the teaching process. Cognitivism recognizes complex and multiple learning domains. However, it may not address external factors that are beyond the nurse's control. Humanism addresses the client's first interest (him- or herself), but this may inhibit the teacher's role in the process. Table 33-1 ■ lists sample nursing applications for each mode of teaching.

FACTORS THAT FACILITATE LEARNING

Motivation

Motivation to learn is the desire to do so. It greatly influences how quickly and how much a person learns. Motivation is generally greatest when the client recognizes a need and believes he or she can meet it by learning. It is not enough for the need to be identified and verbalized by the nurse. The need must be experienced by the client. Often, the nurse's primary task in teaching is to help the client (or

TABLE 33-1	
Application of Learning Theory	
LEARNING THEORY	NURSING ACTIONS
Behaviorism	■ Encourage learner problem solving through trial and error. ■ Encourage repetitive practice and re-demonstration. ■ Praise the learner and provide positive feedback. ■ Provide role models of desired behavior.
Cognitivism	■ Assess the learner's developmental capacity and readiness to learn. ■ Adapt teaching strategies accordingly. ■ Recognize the role of personality in selecting teaching methods to target different learning styles. ■ Recognize the role of perception in learning by using multisensory teaching methods. ■ Provide an environment conducive to learning. ■ Encourage a positive teacher–learner relationship.
Humanism	■ Encourage self-directed and active learning by serving as a facilitator, resource, or mentor for the learner. ■ Encourage learners to establish and evaluate goals. ■ Expose the learner to relevant new information and ask appropriate questions to encourage fact seeking.

significant others) to recognize the need. For example, smokers with heart disease need to understand the effects of nicotine before they recognize the need to quit.

Readiness

Readiness to learn is the demonstration of behaviors or cues that reflect the learner's motivation to learn at a specific time. Readiness reflects not only desire or willingness but ability to learn at a given time. The nurse's role in teaching is to identify and develop client readiness. For example, a client may want to learn ostomy care, but postoperative pain or a change in body image may inhibit him. The nurse can provide pain medication and emotional support to enhance readiness.

Active Involvement

Active involvement in the learning process makes learning faster and more meaningful (Figure 33-1 ■). It also improves retention (holding, keeping; in the case of learning, retention means active remembering). *Active learning* promotes critical thinking and strengthens problem-solving ability. *Passive learning* (listening to lectures or watching television, for example) is much less effective. For example, clients who are actively learning about their therapeutic diets may be more able to apply the principles being taught to their cultural food preferences and their usual eating habits.

Relevance

Relevance is importance or applicability. The knowledge or skill to be learned must be personally relevant to the learner. The client can learn more easily if he can connect

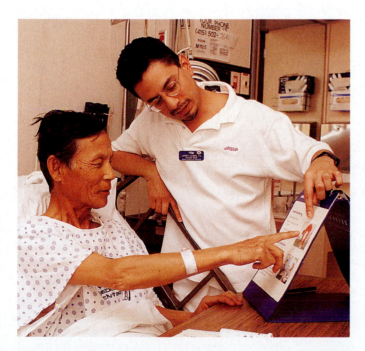

Figure 33-1. ■ Learning is facilitated when the client is interested and actively involved.

the new knowledge to what he already possesses. For example, a morbidly obese patient may be more motivated to lose weight if he remembers having more energy when he weighed less. The nurse should emphasize and validate the relevance of learning throughout the teaching process.

Feedback

Feedback is shared information that relates a person's performance to the desired goal. Feedback must accompany the practice of psychomotor skills; it must be meaningful to help the person learn those skills. Praise, redirection, constructive criticism, and advice are ways of providing *positive feedback. Negative feedback,* such as ridicule, anger, or sarcasm, inhibits learning. Such feedback is viewed as a type of punishment and may cause clients to avoid the teacher.

Nonjudgmental Support

People learn best when they believe they are accepted and will not be judged. Clients who expect to be judged (especially as "poor" students) will not learn as well as those who feel respected and accepted. Once learners have succeeded in accomplishing a task or understanding an idea, they gain self-confidence in their ability to learn. Self-confidence increases motivation and reduces anxiety and fear of failure.

Simple to Complex

Material that is logically organized and proceeds from the simple to the complex is easiest to learn. Such organization enables the learner to comprehend and assimilate knowledge to promote new understanding. Simple and complex are relative terms, however. What is simple for one client may be complex for another.

Repetition

Repetitive practice of key facts and skills aids retention of newly introduced concepts. When combined with positive feedback from the nurse, repetition improves skill performance and the client's ability to apply this knowledge to other settings.

Timing

People retain concepts best when the time between initial learning and active use is short. As time between learning and practicing increases, **retention** decreases. For example, if an asthmatic is prescribed an inhaler for prn use and effectively demonstrates "practice" use one time, this does not mean that he or she may remember how to use it 3 weeks later during an episode.

Environment

Environmental factors affect learning. The optimal learning environment promotes physical and psychological comfort (see Chapter 32 ⬤⬤). It is well lit (including glare-free lighting), well ventilated, neither too hot nor too cold, and with a minimum of noise and other distractions. Privacy is essential to some kinds of learning, such as when discussing confidential issues or demonstrating techniques such as perineal or ostomy care. Anxious or shy clients, however, may prefer to have a support person present. To ensure privacy, nurses should teach when visitors or other interruptions are unlikely.

FACTORS THAT INHIBIT LEARNING

Many internal and external factors can create barriers to the learning process (Table 33-2 ■).

Emotions

Emotions such as fear, anxiety, anger, and depression can impede learning. Clients experiencing intense emotions are preoccupied and unable to concentrate on incoming messages. Fear and anxiety may be minimized by providing factual information to counteract uncertainty or irrational thoughts. Severely depressed clients may require psychi-

atric and/or drug therapy to increase motivation and participation in the teaching process.

Physiological Events

Learning can be inhibited by physiological events such as a critical illness, pain, or sensory deficits.

clinical ALERT

The nurse must identify and reduce physiological barriers to learning *before* teaching. When a client cannot concentrate and apply energy to learning, the learning itself becomes impaired.

Cultural Barriers

Cultural barriers to learning include language and values. Foreign language is a common barrier. Western medicine may conflict with clients' native healing beliefs and cultural practices. For example, a client who comes from a culture that does not value slimness may have difficulty learning

TABLE 33-2
Barriers to Learning

BARRIER	EXPLANATION	NURSING IMPLICATIONS
Acute illness	Client requires all resources and energy to cope with illness.	Defer teaching until client is less ill.
Pain	Pain decreases ability to concentrate.	Deal with pain before teaching.
Prognosis	Client can be preoccupied with illness and unable to concentrate on new information.	Defer teaching to a better time.
Biorhythms	Mental and physical performances have a circadian (daily) rhythm.	Adapt time of teaching to suit client.
Emotion (e.g., anxiety, denial, depression, grief)	Emotions require energy and distract from learning.	Deal with emotions and possible misinformation first.
Language	Client may not be fluent in the nurse's language.	Obtain services of an interpreter or nurse with appropriate language skills.
Age—older adults	Vision, hearing, and motor control can be impaired.	Consider sensory and motor plan.
Age—children	Children have a shorter attention span.	Plan shorter and more active learning episodes.
Culture/religion	There may be cultural or religious restrictions on certain types of knowledge, for example, birth control information.	Assess the client's cultural/religious needs when planning learning activities.
Physical disability	Visual, hearing, sensory, or motor impairments may interfere with a client's ability to learn.	Plan teaching activities appropriate to learner's physical abilities. For example, provide audio learning tools for clients with visual impairments or who have trouble reading.
Mental disability	Impaired cognitive ability may affect the client's capacity for learning.	Assess client's capacity for learning, and plan teaching activities to complement the client's ability while planning more complex learning for the client's caregivers.

TABLE 33-3
Comparison of the Teaching Process and the Nursing Process

STEP	TEACHING PROCESS	NURSING PROCESS
1	Collect data; analyze client's learning strengths and deficits.	Collect data; analyze client's strengths and deficits.
2	Make educational diagnoses.	Make nursing diagnoses.
3	Prepare teaching plan.	Plan nursing goals/desired outcomes, and select interventions: ■ Write learning objectives. ■ Select content and time frame. ■ Select teaching strategies.
4	Implement teaching plan.	Implement nursing strategies.
5	Evaluate client learning based on achievement of learning.	Evaluate client outcomes based on achievement of goal criteria.

about a reducing diet. To be effective, the nurse should directly address such conflict. Support persons such as translators should be involved whenever there is a language barrier.

Psychomotor Ability

It is important that the LPN/LVN be aware of a client's psychomotor skills when collaborating with the RN to develop a teaching plan or in cooperation with other disciplines such as physical therapy. The following physical abilities are important for learning psychomotor skills:

1. *Muscle strength.* For example, an elderly client who cannot rise from a chair because of insufficient leg and muscle strength cannot be expected to learn to lift herself out of a bathtub.
2. *Motor coordination. Gross motor coordination* (coordination of large muscle groups) is necessary for walking. For example, a client who has advanced amyotrophic lateral sclerosis involving the lower limbs will probably be unable to use a walker. Likewise, fine motor coordination is needed when doing precise motions such as eating with a fork.
3. *Energy.* Learning psychomotor skills requires increased energy. The elderly and infirm often have limited energy resources, so practice sessions should be scheduled when the client's energy level is at its peak.
4. *Sensory acuity.* People depend on sight for most learning (e.g., walking with crutches, changing a dressing, drawing a medication into a syringe). Clients with visual impairments often need assistance to carry out such tasks.

Teaching

Teaching is a system of activities intended to produce specific learning. Individualized teaching emphasizes reducing health risks and taking specific action to increase the client's level of personal wellness.

The teaching process and the nursing process are much alike. Table 33-3 ■ compares the two processes.

TEACHING CLIENTS AND THEIR FAMILIES

Nurses teach clients and their families in varied environments such as the home, a hospital, assisted living, or a long-term care facility. Clients may be instructed in groups or in one-on-one sessions (Figure 33-2 ■). For example, a nurse may teach about diabetic foot care to several clients at once, or the nurse may teach privately about wound care while changing a client's dressing. Nurses are often responsible for teaching clients' spouses and other caregivers.

Despite time constraints caused by short hospital stays, nurses are expected to provide education that will ensure the client's safe transition from one level of care to another. Nurses must make appropriate plans for follow-up education in the client's home. Discharge plans must include documentation of all teaching before discharge, and the

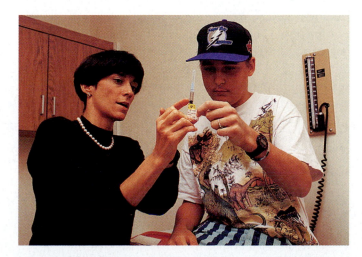

Figure 33-2. ■ Teaching activities may need to include hands-on client participation. (Photographer: Elena Dorfman.)

learning goals yet to be achieved. See Chapters 6 and 10, respectively, for more information about discharge and documentation.

TEACHING IN THE COMMUNITY

Nurses often participate in community health education programs. Teaching may be voluntary, such as for the Red Cross, or it may be compensated employment, such as for a government agency. Community teaching may be directed to large groups with a common interest in some aspect of health, such as nutrition, cardiopulmonary resuscitation (CPR), or bicycle and swimming safety. Community education programs can also be for small groups or individual learners, such as childbirth classes.

TEACHING HEALTH PERSONNEL

Nurses are responsible for supporting and maintaining the profession by teaching each other. In many facilities, nurses are required to present staff development sessions to colleagues. Experienced LPNs/LVNs may function as preceptors for new graduate LPNs/LVNs or for newly employed LPNs/LVNs. LPNs/LVNs reinforce teaching begun by the clinical nurse specialist and other members of the healthcare team. In some settings the LPN/LVN is responsible for all client teaching.

NURSING CARE

ASSESSING

Comprehensive assessment of learning needs incorporates data from the nursing history, physical assessment, and the client's support system. LPN/LVN observations are vital to the success of the overall assessment. Data collection should include information regarding all aspects of learning, including readiness, motivation, reading ability, and comprehension level. The nurse also comes to know the common learning needs that groups of people with similar health problems have. The LPN/LVN must be constantly aware of changes in the client's health status and report these observations as learning needs and health status change.

Several elements in the nursing history provide clues to learning needs:

- Age (and developmental status) dictates the choice of appropriate teaching strategies and health teaching content.
- Clients' perceptions of their current health problems and concerns may indicate knowledge deficits.
- A client's health beliefs and practices are always important to consider. Nurses must recognize that sometimes a client's health beliefs may interfere with healthful changes, and that it will not be possible to change that

individual's core beliefs. Clients who do make changes usually believe they are personally at risk; they believe that the risk is serious; and they believe that changes in lifestyle will help to prevent the undesired outcome.

- The client's cultural group may have beliefs and practices related to diet, health, illness, and lifestyle. It is important to know how a client's practices and values affect their learning needs and their willingness to learn. Although clients may understand the healthcare information being taught, they may avoid it in the home where folk medical practices prevail. It is important to know whether any advice or treatments given by the doctor conflict with their values or beliefs. If they seek the advice of traditional healers, or use herbs or folk treatments, it is important to verify whether their medical doctor knows about these. For additional information, see Chapter 2 ⬭, as well as the section on transcultural teaching later in this chapter.
- Economic factors can affect a client's learning. For example, elderly clients with diabetes may not have enough money to buy a large supply of sterile insulin syringes. The concern about cost may make it hard for them to focus on learning to administer the insulin.
- Learning styles vary. Some people are *visual learners* and learn best by watching or reading text. *Auditory learners* learn best by verbal explanations. Many learn best through touch and feel (*haptic learners*), such as by manipulating equipment to discover how it works. Some learn best in groups. For others, thinking about a skill and its logic promotes learning. The nurse should ask clients how they prefer to learn and have learned best in the past. The nurse can also discover a client's learning style by varying activities and techniques when teaching.
- In the client's support system, there may be others who can assist the client's learning. Family members or close friends may help reinforce health teaching to maintain lifestyle changes at home.

The physical examination provides useful clues to the client's learning needs, such as mental status, energy level, and nutritional status. The exam provides data about the client's physical capacity (such as vision, hearing, and muscle strength) to learn and perform self-care. This information is vital in developing the teaching plan.

Readiness to Learn

A client who is ready to learn may seek information by asking questions and requesting reading materials. The client who is not yet ready is unlikely to demonstrate these behaviors and may even engage in avoidance behavior. For example, the nurse may ask, "When would you like me to show you how to inject insulin?" and the client might respond, "Oh, my wife will take care of everything."

The nurse assesses for the following:

- *Physical readiness.* Is the client in pain, fatigued, or immobile? If so, the client may not be ready.
- *Emotional readiness.* Is the client motivated toward self-care? Clients who are anxious, depressed, or grieving over their health status are not ready.
- *Cognitive readiness.* What is the client's level of consciousness? Is disease (such as stroke) affecting the client's cognition? Are drugs affecting the client's judgment or concentration? If so, the client may not yet be ready to learn.

Nurses can promote learning readiness by providing physical and emotional support during the critical stage of recovery. As the client stabilizes physically and emotionally, the nurse can provide opportunities to learn.

Motivation

As discussed earlier, motivation is usually greatest when the client is ready, the learning need is recognized, and the information being offered is meaningful (relevant) to the client.

Nurses can increase a client's motivation by:

- Relating the learning to something the client values
- Creating a welcoming, nonthreatening learning environment in which the client is likely to succeed
- Encouraging autonomy and independence
- Demonstrating a positive attitude about the client's ability to learn
- Offering positive reinforcement and emotional support during the learning process.

Reading Level

The nurse should not assume that a client's reading level is equal to the level of formal education achieved. Nurses should ask clients about their reading proficiency. However, clients with literacy problems may be reluctant to discuss the issue. Reading materials for clients with low literacy should be at the eighth-grade level or lower.

To quickly determine the reading level of written materials, mark 10 sentences in a row at the beginning, middle, and end of the material. Then count every word within those 30 sentences with three or more syllables. If the same word appears more than once, count it each time it appears. Now total the number of words in all 30 sentences. For an eighth-grade reading level, you should have 21 to 30 multisyllable words.

DIAGNOSING, PLANNING, AND IMPLEMENTING

Three basic NANDA-approved nursing diagnoses directly relate to the learning process: *Deficient Knowledge, Health Seeking Behavior,* and *Noncompliance.* These diagnoses are used when a client's learning needs are the primary concern.

Whenever the diagnostic label *Deficient Knowledge* is used, either the client is seeking health information or the nurse has identified a learning need. An example of this would be *Deficient Knowledge: Low-Calorie Diet* related to inexperience with newly ordered therapy.

When the diagnostic label *Health Seeking Behavior* is used, the client is seeking health-related information. This diagnosis is especially appropriate for clients attending community health education programs. A sample NANDA label would be *Health Seeking Behavior: Exercise and Activity* related to desire to improve health behaviors and decrease risk of heart disease.

Whenever the diagnostic label *Noncompliance* is used, factors are present that prevent the person from following advice given by health professionals.

clinical ALERT

The diagnosis *Noncompliance* must be used with caution, because *failure to follow healthcare advice is not always the result of an unwilling attitude.*

Noncompliance, as a nursing diagnosis, is associated with the desire to comply, but the inability to do so because of intervening factors (Carpenito, 1997, p. 575). Intervening factors include communication barriers and financial limitations. A sample diagnosis is *Noncompliance: Hygienic Colostomy Care* related to insufficient funds to purchase necessary supplies.

A teaching plan is developed, using information collected during the nursing history and physical assessment, as well as observations from the LPN/LVN. Involving the client in this process is essential. Involved clients are more motivated and are more likely to achieve learning goals.

Determining Teaching Priorities

In the initial planning phase, the client and nurse collaborate to prioritize learning needs. For example, a client with heart disease may not be ready to learn about other lifestyle changes until she satisfies her need to learn how "to make food taste good without adding salt." Nurses can also use theoretical frameworks, such as Maslow's hierarchy of needs (see Figure 5-4 ⟲⟳), to establish priorities.

Setting Learning Objectives

Learning objectives are equivalent to desired outcomes for other nursing diagnoses. They are written in the same way. Like client outcomes, learning objectives would do the following:

1. State the client (learner) behavior or performance, not nurse behavior. For example, "Will identify personal risk factors for heart disease" (*client behavior*), not "Teach the client about cardiac risk factors" (*nurse behavior*).

2. Reflect an observable, measurable activity. The performance may be visible (e.g., walking) or invisible (e.g., adding a column of figures). The performance of an objective might be written: "Selects low-fat foods from a menu" (*observable*), not "understands low-fat diet" (*unobservable*). Verbs used for learning objectives would include *defines, describes, identifies, selects,* and so on. Outcomes would avoid words like *knows, understands, believes,* and *appreciates.* They are neither observable nor measurable.

3. Use modifiers as required to clarify what, where, when, or how the behavior will be performed. For example, "Irrigates colostomy independently as taught" tells how the client does the task.

4. Specify the time by which learning should have occurred. For example, "The client will state three things that affect blood sugar level by end of second class on diabetes."

Learning objectives can reflect the learner's command of simple to complex concepts. For example, the learning objective "The client will list cardiac risk factors" simply requires the learner to identify all cardiac risk factors. In contrast, the learning objective "The client will list *personal* cardiac risk factors" requires that the learner learn how general cardiac risk factors apply to his or her own behaviors.

Nursing Outcomes Classifications

Many different outcomes will be appropriate depending on what is being taught. However, some general nursing outcomes classifications could include:

1802	Knowledge: Diet
1803	Knowledge: Disease process
1805	Knowledge: Health behavior
1823	Knowledge: Health promotion
1824	Knowledge: Illness care
1808	Knowledge: Medication
1811	Knowledge: Prescribed activity
1814	Knowledge: Treatment procedure
1813	Knowledge: Treatment regimen

Choosing Content

The content of teaching is determined by learning objectives. For instance, "Identify appropriate sites for insulin injection" means the nurse must include content about the body sites suitable for insulin injections. Nurses can select among many sources of information including books, nursing journals, and other nurses and physicians. Whatever sources the nurse chooses, content should be:

■ Accurate
■ Current

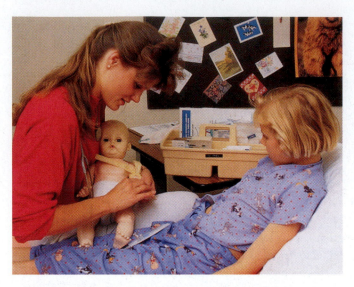

Figure 33-3. ■ Teaching materials and strategies should be suited to the client's age and learning abilities.

■ Based on learning goals (outcomes)
■ Adjusted for the learner's age, culture, and ability
■ Consistent with information the nurse is teaching
■ Selected with consideration of how much time and what resources are available for teaching.

Selecting Teaching Strategies

The method of teaching that the nurse chooses should be suited to the individual, to the material to be learned, and to the teacher (Figure 33-3 ■). For example, the person who cannot read needs to have material presented in other ways. The best strategy for teaching how to give an injection is not lecturing but demonstration. Teachers who lead group sessions should be poised, confident, and skilled at group facilitation. People who are visually oriented should be taught with visual aids. Table 33-4 ■ lists selected teaching strategies.

Ordering Learning Experiences

To conserve nursing resources, some health agencies have developed their own teaching guides. These guides feature standardized content and teaching methods that all staff nurses are expected to use when teaching. Standardized teaching plans are convenient. These guides ensure consistent content for the learner, and they reduce the confusion that might occur when more than one teacher is involved. Consistency of content is key whether the nurse develops an original teaching plan or uses a standardized format. For example, when teaching multistep procedures (such as ostomy care), the nurse should repeat the steps in the same sequence, without altering the order. If possible, the nurse should use the same brands and types of equipment the client will be

TABLE 33-4

Selected Teaching Strategies

STRATEGY	MAJOR TYPES OF LEARNING	CHARACTERISTICS
Explanation or description (e.g., lecture)	Cognitive	Teacher controls content and pace. Learner is passive; therefore retains less information than when actively participating. Feedback is determined by teacher. May be given to individual or group.
One-to-one discussion	Affective, cognitive	Encourages participation by learner. Permits reinforcement and repetition at learner's level. Permits introduction of sensitive subjects.
Answering questions	Cognitive	Teacher must understand question and what it means to learner. Learner may need to overcome cultural perception that asking questions is impolite and may embarrass the teacher. Can be used with individuals and groups. Teacher should confirm personal responses by asking the learner, "Does that answer your question?" Teacher controls most of content and pace.
Demonstration	Psychomotor	Often used with explanation. Can be used with individuals, small or large groups. Does not permit use of equipment by learners; learner is passive.
Discovery	Cognitive, affective	Teacher guides problem-solving situation. Learner is active participant; retention of information is high.
Group discussions	Affective, cognitive	Group members assist and learn from each other. Teacher needs to keep the discussion focused and prevent monopolization by one or two learners.
Practice	Psychomotor	Allows repetition and immediate feedback. Permits hands-on experience.
Printed and audiovisual materials	Cognitive	Forms include books, pamphlets, films, programmed instruction, and computer learning. Learners can proceed at their own speed. Nurse can act as resource person; need not be present during learning. Potentially ineffective if reading level of materials is too high. Teacher needs to select language that meets learner needs if English is a second language.
Role-playing	Affective, cognitive	Permits expression of attitudes, values, and emotions. Can assist in development of communication skills. Involves active participation by learner. Teacher must create supportive, safe environment for learners to minimize anxiety.
Modeling	Affective, psychomotor	Nurse sets example by attitude, psychomotor skill.
Computer-assisted learning programs	All types of learning	Learner is active. Learner controls pace. Learning programs provides immediate reinforcement and review. Use with individuals or groups.

using at home. Instructions for the nurse in client teaching were provided in Box 33-3.

The nurse needs to be flexible in implementing any teaching plan because the plan may need revising. The client may tire sooner than anticipated or be faced with too much information too quickly.

clinical ALERT

Report

The LPV/LVN should report any changes in the client's physical or psychosocial condition that might require alteration in the teaching plan.

The client's needs may change. External factors may intervene. For example, the nurse and the client may have planned for the client to self-irrigate his colostomy at 10 A.M., but when the time comes, he wants more information before actually doing it himself. In this case, the nurse would discuss the desired information, provide written information, and defer teaching until the next day. The LPN/LVN would collaborate with the team leader and document accordingly. (See Table 33-2 for barriers to learning.)

Implementation

Many nursing interventions classifications (NICs) can be used when implementing client teaching. Some general classifications that apply include:

5602	Teaching: Disease process
5606	Teaching: Individual
5603	Teaching: Group
5612	Teaching: Prescribed activity/exercise
5614	Teaching: Prescribed diet
5616	Teaching: Medication
5618	Teaching: Procedure/treatment
5620	Teaching: Psychomotor skill

Implementing Client Education

When structuring client teaching sessions, the nurse should keep the following eight principles in mind:

1. *The optimal time for each session depends largely on the learner.* Whenever possible, ask the client for help to choose the best time, for example, when she feels most rested or when no other activities are scheduled.
2. *The pace of teaching affects learning.* A very rapid pace may confuse or frustrate the learner. When the pace is too slow, the client may become bored and distracted. (Loss of interest may also indicate that the client is fatigued.)
3. *Position and location affect learning.* Most people associate their bed with rest and sleep, not with learning. A client who is shown a videotape while in bed is more

likely to become drowsy during instruction than a client who is sitting in a bedside chair.

4. *Teaching aids foster learning and attentiveness.* When selecting teaching aids, the nurse should choose identical products (such as ostomy pouches) to those the client will be using. When planning audiovisual presentations, the nurse should ensure that all equipment is functioning well before starting the session. Teaching aids should be appropriate to the client's developmental level (see Figure 33-3). For example, some anatomical models may contain tiny plastic parts that pose a choking hazard to young children. Box 33-4 ■ lists teaching tools that are specifically useful for children.

5. *Learning is more effective through self-directed activity.* The nurse can encourage independent learning by enabling the client to explore alternative sources of information. If the client chooses, the nurse may provide a list of related health topics to research.

6. *Repetition reinforces learning.* Summarizing content, rephrasing (using other words), and approaching the material from another point of view are ways of repeating and clarifying content. For instance, after discussing the kinds of foods that can be included in a diet, the nurse describes the foods again, but in the context of the three meals eaten during one day.

BOX 33-4   POPULATION FOCUS

Teaching Tools for Children

- **Visits.** Visiting the hospital and treatment rooms; seeing people dressed in uniforms, scrub suits, protective gear.
- **Dress-up.** Touching and dressing up in the clothing they will see and wear.
- **Coloring books.** Using coloring books to prepare for treatments, surgery, or hospitalization; shows what rooms, people, and equipment will look like.
- **Storybooks.** Storybooks describe how the child will feel, what will be done, and what the place will look like. Parents can read these stories to children several times before the experience. Younger children like this repetition.
- **Dolls.** Practicing procedures on dolls or teddy bears that they will later experience; gives a sense of mastery of the situation. For example, custom dolls are often available for inserting tubes and giving injections.
- **Puppet play.** Puppets can be used in role-play situations to provide information and show the child what the experience will be like; they help the child express emotions.
- **Health fairs.** Health fairs can educate children about their bodies and ways to stay healthy. Fairs can focus on high-risk problems children face, such as accident prevention, poison control, and other topics identified in the community as a concern.

7. *Organize the material; connect new information to what the client has already learned.* For example, "You understand how urine flows down a catheter from the bladder. Now I will show you how to push fluid up the catheter to rinse the bladder."

8. *Always use simple language.* If possible, eliminate medical jargon. Even common terms such as *urine* and *feces* may be unfamiliar to clients. Avoid common abbreviations such as RR (recovery room) or CAD (coronary artery disease).

Teaching Strategies

Nurses can choose from a number of special teaching strategies. Any strategy the nurse selects must be appropriate for the learner and the learning goals.

Client Contracting

A learning contract with a client specifies certain objectives and when they are to be met. Here is an example of a self-contract:

> I, Amy Martin, will jog for 20 minutes three times per week for a period of 2 weeks and will then buy myself six yellow roses.
>
> Amy Martin
> [date]

The contract, drawn up and signed by the client and the nurse, should specify learning objectives, responsibilities of the client and the nurse, and the methods of follow-up and evaluation. The learning contract allows for freedom, mutual respect, and mutual responsibility. Contracts may be revised when the client chooses to set new goals.

Group Teaching

Group instruction is economical, and it provides members with an opportunity to share and learn from others. A small group allows for discussion in which everyone can participate. A large group often requires a lecture technique or use of films, videos, slides, or role-playing by teachers. All members involved in group instruction should have a common need (e.g., prenatal health or preoperative instruction). It is also important to consider sociocultural factors when forming a group (see Chapter 2 ↺).

Computer-Assisted Instruction

Computer-assisted instruction is constantly advancing. Now, computers can be used to teach:

- Complex problem-solving skills
- Application of information
- Psychomotor skills.

"Virtual reality" programs and video clips can allow the client to "see" how the heart pumps blood or how nerves send messages to the brain. Learning is becoming increasingly visual.

Discovery/Problem Solving

In using the discovery/problem-solving technique, the nurse presents some initial information and then asks the learners a question or presents a situation related to the information. The learner applies the new information to the situation and decides what to do. Learners can work alone or in groups. This technique is well suited to family learning. The teacher guides the learners through the thinking process to reach the best solution or the best action to take in the situation. For example, the nurse-educator might present information on diabetes and glucose management. Then the nurse might ask the learners how they think their insulin and diet should be adjusted if their morning glucose reading was too low. In this way, clients learn what critical components they need to consider to reach the best solution to the problem.

Behavior Modification

Behaviorists believe that (1) human behaviors are learned and can be selectively strengthened, weakened, eliminated, or replaced and (2) a person's behavior is under conscious control. **Behavior modification** is a system of positive reinforcement in which desirable behavior is rewarded and undesirable behavior is ignored. For example, clients trying to quit smoking are not criticized when they smoke, but they are praised or rewarded when they go without a cigarette for a certain period of time. The effectiveness of a behavior modification plan may be increased by including a client contract. The contract outlines the behavior modification plan and lists specific rewards.

Transcultural Teaching

When the nurse and client come from different ethnic or cultural backgrounds, natural communication barriers may exist. These barriers include language, differing concepts of time, or cultural beliefs and practices that may influence compliance with client teaching and health care. It is important to keep these differences in mind when you are teaching clients about their health care. Treat the client's cultural healing beliefs with respect and try to identify whether they are in agreement or in conflict with what is being taught. Then focus on the ones in agreement to promote the integration of new learning with familiar health practices. Explain why certain folk healing practices are harmful, and how the recommended health practices will improve health. See Chapter 2 ↺ for more information on culturally proficient nursing. Guidelines for teaching clients from other ethnic or cultural groups are listed in Box 33-5 ∎.

EVALUATING

Evaluating Learning

Evaluation is both an ongoing and a final process in which the client, the LPN/LVN in collaboration with the RN, and

BOX 33-5   **POPULATION FOCUS**

Transcultural Teaching Guidelines

- **Enlist the aid of a translator when necessary.**
- **Obtain foreign language teaching materials.** The translator can assist by reading the materials to the nurse and can assist the nurse with adaptations of the material.
- **Use visual aids.** Many pictures, charts, and diagrams have universal meaning. Videos can allow the client to observe a skill or procedure, despite a language barrier. Audiovisual materials in which English is spoken slowly and clearly can benefit a client who may be learning English.
- **Use clear, simple language.** Avoid long sentences and big words. Use concrete rather than abstract terms. Avoid medical jargon.
- **Avoid slang or colloquialisms.** The client may think you mean these literally.
- **Present only one idea at a time.**
- **Phrase questions positively.** For example, "Do you understand how far you may bend your hip after surgery?" is a much better question than "You don't know how far you may bend your hip, do you?"
- **Validate verbal communication in writing.** This is especially important if understanding the client's speech is a problem. For example, during an assessment, write down numbers or phrases and have the client read them to verify accuracy.
- **Use humor very cautiously.** Meaning can change in the translation process.
- **Specifically invite the client to ask questions or request help.** In some cultures, expressing a need is not appropriate. Expressing confusion or asking to be shown something again may be considered rude. Some clients may feel that asking questions or stating a lack of understanding may cause the nurse to "lose face."
- **Confirm nonverbal cues.** A client who nods, uses eye contact, or smiles may not really understand what is being taught. In some cultures these signals are merely indicators of respect.
- **Identify cultural gender issues.** When explaining procedures or functioning related to personal areas of the body, it may be appropriate to have a nurse of the same sex do the teaching. Because of modesty concerns, and cultural taboos about male–female interaction, it is wise to have a female nurse teach a female client about personal care, birth control, sexually transmitted infections, and other potentially sensitive areas. If a translator is needed during explanation of procedures or teaching, the translator should also be female.
- **Include the family in planning and teaching.** This promotes trust and mutual respect. Identify the authoritative family member and incorporate that person into the planning and teaching to promote compliance and support of health teaching. In some cultures, the male head of household is the critical family member to include in health teaching; in other cultures, it is the eldest female member.
- **Consider the client's time orientation.** The client may be oriented to the past, present, future, or a combination of these. Cultures with a predominant orientation to the present include the Mexican American, Navajo Native American, Appalachian, Eskimo, and Filipino American cultures. Preventing future problems may be less significant for these clients, so teaching prevention may be difficult. For example, teaching a client why and when to take medications may be more difficult if the client is oriented to the present. In such instances, the nurse can emphasize preventing short-term problems. Schedules tend to be very flexible in present-oriented societies. Failure to keep clinic appointments or to arrive on time is common in clients who have a present-time orientation. The nurse can help by arranging transportation and by accommodating these clients when they do come rather than rescheduling an appointment that they probably will not keep. Teaching clients to take medications at bedtime or with a meal does not necessarily mean that these activities will occur at the same time each day. For this reason, the nurse should assess the client's daily routine before teaching the client to pair a treatment or medication with a daily event. When teaching a client when to take medication, the nurse should determine whether a clock or watch is available to the client and whether the client can tell time.

often the support people determine what has been learned. Learning is measured against the learning goals that were selected in the planning phase. For example, the objective "Selects foods that are low in carbohydrates" can be evaluated by asking the client to name such foods or to select low-carbohydrate foods from a list.

The best method for evaluating depends on the type of learning (cognitive, psychomotor, or affective). For cognitive learning, the client demonstrates the acquired knowledge. The client might:

- Select the solution to a problem using the new knowledge.
- Take written tests.
- Respond to oral questioning (e.g., restate information or give correct responses to questions).

- Self-report and self-monitor during follow-up phone calls, home visits, or computer-assisted instruction.

For psychomotor skills, evaluation is best done by observing how well the client carries out a procedure such as changing a dressing.

Affective learning is more difficult to evaluate. The nurse may listen to the client's responses to questions, note how the client speaks about relevant subjects, and observe the client's behavior that expresses feelings and values. For example, have parents learned to value health enough to have their children immunized?

Following evaluation, teaching may have to be modified or repeated. Follow-up teaching in the home or by phone may be needed.

Behavior change does not always take place immediately. Often, individuals accept change intellectually first and then change their behavior only periodically (for example, a person who knows that she must lose weight may diet and exercise off and on). If the new behavior is to replace the old behavior, it must emerge gradually; otherwise, the old behavior may prevail. The nurse can support behavior change by anticipating client vacillation and by providing encouragement.

Evaluating Teaching

It is important for nurses to evaluate their own teaching and the content of the teaching program, just as they evaluate the effectiveness of nursing interventions for other nursing diagnoses. Evaluation should include all aspects of teaching, including timing, teaching strategies, content quality, and so on. The nurse may find, for example, that the client was excited about understanding how to control her diabetes and was motivated to learn more.

Both the client and the nurse should evaluate the learning experience. The client should be asked for detailed feedback. Feedback questionnaires and videotapes of the learning sessions can be helpful.

The nurse should not feel ineffective as a teacher if the client forgets some of what is taught. Forgetting is normal and should be anticipated. Having the client write down information, repeating it during teaching, giving handouts on the information, and having the client be active in the learning process all promote retention (Box 33-6 ■).

Documenting

Documentation of the teaching process is essential. Charting provides a legal record that the teaching occurred, and it communicates the teaching to other health professionals. If teaching is not documented, legally it did not occur.

Responses to teaching should always be documented. What did the client or support person say or do to indicate that learning occurred? Has the client demonstrated mastery

---

BOX 33-6   NURSING CARE CHECKLIST

General Teaching and Client Teaching

General Teaching Guidelines

☑ **All teaching should be individualized.** If certain activities do not assist the learner, the nurse should make adaptations. For example, explanation alone may not be able to teach a client to handle a syringe. Actually handling the syringe may be more effective.

☑ **When the learner is involved in planning, the desire to learn is increased.**

☑ **Rapport between teacher and learner is essential.** The nurse should take time to establish rapport before teaching.

☑ **Teaching should build on the client's existing knowledge base.** For example, a person who already knows how to cook can use this knowledge when learning to prepare food for a special diet.

☑ **Communication must be clear, concise, and mutually understood.** For example, a client may understand the terms *damp* and *wet* to have very different meanings. So, when the nurse says, "Don't get the abdominal incision wet," the client may immediately understand that he may not shower or bathe, but may think that wiping the incision with a damp washcloth is allowed. The nurse should explain that no water or moisture should touch the incision.

☑ **Teaching that involves a number of the learner's senses often enhances learning.** For example, when teaching about changing a surgical dressing, the nurse can tell the client about the procedure (hearing), show how to change the dressing (sight), and show how to manipulate the equipment (touch).

☑ **Goal setting (determining learning objectives and outcomes) must be appropriate to the client's lifestyle and resources.** For example, it would be unreasonable to expect a woman to soak in a tub of hot water four times a day if she did not have a bathtub or hot running water.

Client Teaching Guidelines

☑ **Discover the client's knowledge or skill level.** Ask questions or have the client complete a written form, such as a pretest.

☑ **Identify fear, anxiety, or other barriers to learning. Address the source of anxieties before beginning to teach.** For example, a client's spouse may be reluctant to learn tracheostomy care due to fear of suffocating the client during suctioning.

☑ **Begin with relevant information in an area of client readiness.** For example, an adolescent may want to know how he may continue to play football before he can learn how to administer insulin to himself.

☑ **Teach the basics first.** Make sure the client demonstrates understanding of a procedure before you teach variations or give information on special circumstances or "troubleshooting." For example, when teaching a client to insert a retention catheter, explain the basic procedure in its entirety before discussing what to do if the catheter fails to drain properly.

☑ **Plan to review.** Schedule time to clarify content and to answer any questions the learner(s) may have.

of a skill or the acquisition of knowledge? Such documented responses provide evidence of learning. Many agencies have multiple-copy client teaching forms that include the medical and nursing diagnoses, the treatment plan, and the client education (see Figure 10-4 ⚭). After the teaching session is completed, the client and the nurse sign the form and a copy of the form is given to the client to reinforce content and provide a record of the teaching. A second copy of the completed and signed form is placed in the client's chart.

Key aspects of the teaching process to be documented in the client record include:

- Diagnosed learning needs
- Learning objectives
- Topics taught
- Client outcomes
- Need for additional teaching
- Resources provided.

The nurse's written teaching plan should include:

- Actual information and skills taught
- Teaching strategies used
- Time framework and content for each class
- Teaching outcomes and methods of evaluation.

NURSING PROCESS CARE PLAN
Client with Laceration

Kevin Brewer is a 24-year-old male college student admitted to the emergency department (ED) with a 7-cm (2.5-in.) laceration on the left lower anterior leg, which occurred during a hockey game. The laceration was cleaned, sutured, and bandaged. The client was given an appointment to return to the health clinic in 10 days for suture removal. Client states that he lives in a college dormitory and is able to care for the wound if given instructions. Client states he is able to read and understand English.

Assessment. Mr. Brewer complains of a pain level of 5 related to the laceration to his left leg. Thirty-five minutes after administration of prn pain medication, stated pain at a level of 1. Client is able to ambulate with a slow, steady gait. His roommate is on his way to the ED to drive the client home.

Nursing Diagnosis. The following important nursing diagnosis (among others) is established for this client:

- *Deficient Knowledge* related to wound care.

Expected Outcomes. The expected outcomes specify that Mr. Brewer will:

- Be able to describe signs and symptoms of wound infection.
- Respond to questions regarding wound care and perform return demonstration of wound cleansing and bandaging.
- Identify equipment needed for wound care.
- Describe appropriate action if complications arise.
- Identify date, time, and location of follow-up appointment for suture removal.

Planning and Implementation. The following nursing interventions are planned and implemented:

- Instruct client on what to look for regarding signs and symptoms of wound infection and appropriate action to take if complications arise.
- Demonstrate wound cleansing and bandaging, and allow time for a return demonstration by the client.
- Lay out equipment needed for wound care in front of client and encourage client to handle and become familiar with equipment.
- Provide written instructions for all implementations to client.
- Provide an appointment card for client with details for date, time, and location of suture removal appointment.

Evaluation. After teaching session, Mr. Brewer was able to fulfill all expected outcomes without difficulty.

Critical Thinking in the Nursing Process

1. Why is it necessary for Mr. Brewer to be able to identify the signs and symptoms of wound infection?
2. Why is it important for Mr. Brewer to be able to give a return demonstration of wound care?
3. Why should Mr. Brewer be allowed to handle the equipment needed for wound care?

Note: Discussion of Critical Thinking questions appears in Appendix I.

Note: The references and resources for this and all chapters have been compiled at the back of the book.

Chapter Review

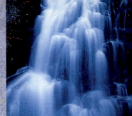

 KEY TERMS by Topic

Use the audio glossary feature of either the CD-ROM or the Companion Website to hear the correct pronunciation of the following key terms.

Learning
client education, learning, compliance, behaviorism, cognitivism, cognitive domain, affective domain, psychomotor domain, humanism, motivation, readiness, relevance, feedback, retention

Teaching
teaching, behavior modification

KEY Points

- Teaching clients and families about their health needs is a major role of the nurse.

- Learning is represented by a change in behavior.

- Three main theories of learning are behaviorism, cognitivism, and humanism.

- There are three learning domains: cognitive, affective, and psychomotor.

- Factors to facilitate learning include motivation, readiness, active involvement, relevance, feedback, nonjudgmental support, progression from simple to complex concepts, repetition, timing, and environment.

- Factors such as emotions, certain physiological events, cultural barriers, and psychomotor deficits may impede learning.

- Learning objectives guide the content of the teaching plan and are written in terms of client or learner behavior.

- Teaching strategies should be suited to the client, the material to be learned, and the teacher. They should be adjusted to the client's developmental level and health status.

- Teaching methods and materials must be adapted for clients who are illiterate, elderly, or from different cultural backgrounds.

- Documentation of client teaching is essential to communicate the teaching to other health professionals and to provide a record for legal and accreditation purposes.

 EXPLORE Media Link

Additional interactive resources for this chapter can be found on the Companion Website at www.prenhall.com/ramont. Click on Chapter 33 and "Begin" to select the activities for this chapter.

For chapter-related NCLEX®-style questions and an audio glossary, access the accompanying CD-ROM in this book.

FOR FURTHER Study

Further steps to improve culturally proficient nursing are discussed in Chapter 2.

For Maslow's hierarchy of needs, see Figure 5-4.

For more information on documentation of client teaching, see Chapter 6 and Figure 10-4.

For documentation methods and guidelines, see Chapter 6.

For more about client teaching at discharge, see Chapter 10.

For growth and developmental issues as they affect clients, see Chapter 11.

For environmental considerations, see Chapter 32.

Critical Thinking Care Map

Caring for a Client with Deficient Knowledge

NCLEX-PN® Focus Area: Physiological Integrity

Case Study: Mrs. Yorty, 59, is an African American bank vice president who is heavily relied on by her boss and coworkers. Three days ago she was admitted to the hospital with complaints of shortness of breath and mild chest pain. A diagnostic evaluation indicates that she has significant coronary artery disease but has not yet had a heart attack. Her physician indicated that Mrs. Yorty will need to make significant lifestyle changes to reduce her heart attack risk. Mrs. Yorty states that she rests a lot after work so she doesn't overwork her heart.

Nursing Diagnosis: Deficient Knowledge

COLLECT DATA

Subjective	Objective
_____	_____
_____	_____
_____	_____
_____	_____
_____	_____
_____	_____
_____	_____

Would you report this data? Yes/No

If yes, to: _____

What would you report? _____

Nursing Care

_____
_____
_____
_____
_____
_____
_____
_____
_____
_____
_____

How would you document this? _____
_____
_____

Compare your documentation to the sample provided in Appendix I.

Data Collected
(use those that apply)

- Weight: 180 lbs
- Height: 5′1″
- VS: T 98.5, P 80, BP 140/100
- Blood oxygen level 98%
- Lung sounds clear bilaterally
- Complains of shortness of breath on mild exertion
- Complains of occasional mild chest pain
- States she rests a lot after work so she doesn't overwork her heart
- States she has smoked one pack of cigarettes a day for 25 years

Nursing Interventions
(use those that apply; list in priority order)

- Explain to client that physical activity can reduce her risk of heart attack. However, her doctor will prescribe how much activity she may do based on the severity of her coronary artery disease.
- Instruct client that she will die of a heart attack if she doesn't stop smoking.
- Encourage client to make dietary changes. Stress importance of cutting back on fat, especially saturated fats, which may help reduce cholesterol.
- Explain to client that smoking is a major risk factor and that by quitting she can significantly cut her risk of a heart attack.
- Obtain a physician's order for the client to meet with the hospital dietitian.
- Encourage client to eat a well-balanced diet with at least five servings of fruits and vegetables a day.

NCLEX-PN® Exam Preparation

1   As you teach a client about a diabetic diet, you give praise and positive feedback each time the client makes an appropriate food choice. Which theory of learning are you applying?
1. behaviorism
2. cognitivism
3. humanism
4. health promotion

2   Information about tests, diagnosis, treatment, and medications would be covered in which area of client teaching?
1. promotion of health
2. prevention of illness/injury
3. restoration of health
4. adapting to altered health and function

3   Your client is scheduled for her first meeting with the physical therapist for mobility training following TKR. When you administer pain medication prior to the session, the client's family asks why. Your best response is:
1. "The next dose is due during the time physical therapy is scheduled. I don't want to interrupt them."
2. "The medication will take effect, so she will be able to rest following therapy."
3. "Your mother wants medication, so I need to give it to her."
4. "Pain decreases ability to concentrate, so the pain needs to be controlled before teaching begins."

4   You have just told your outpatient surgical client not to get the incision wet until after his follow-up visit. Which statement demonstrates a need for more instruction?
1. "I will not take a shower until I see the doctor."
2. "I will only wipe the area with a damp washcloth daily."
3. "I will be careful not to get the area wet while washing."
4. "The dressing should be kept clean and dry until I see the doctor."

5   You have been teaching your client self-administration of insulin. The first two times, she prepared the injection correctly. This morning she states, "I can't do it. How will I be able to take care of myself at home?" Which response is most appropriate?
1. You are right. I will arrange for a home health nurse to give you your insulin."
2. "You did it just fine yesterday. What's wrong with you today?"
3. "This may feel overwhelming. We'll keep working with you until you feel confident."
4. "Maybe we should have your daughter learn to do this in case you don't feel like it."

6   An elderly Vietnamese client does not maintain eye contact during discharge instructions. The nurse should interpret this behavior to mean that:
1. she does not understand the instructions.
2. she is not interested in what is being said.
3. she may feel eye contact is a sign of disrespect.
4. she prefers that the instructions be given by the physician.

7   You are assigned to teach a group of 4- and 5-year-olds about the Food Guide Pyramid. Using your understanding of appropriate client teaching, which method would you select for this group?
1. lecture and printed handouts
2. plastic foods to be placed appropriately on the pyramid
3. the "Hungry Caterpillar" story, plus a puppet and colorful pyramid and foods
4. cooking class using food from each group

8   An elderly man with dementia lives with family members who work full time. You are assigned to do a safety assessment of the client to ascertain if he can be alone during the daytime. Which statement demonstrates an understanding of your report by the family?
1. "We will tell him not to cook while we're out."
2. "There is a list of emergency numbers by the phone."
3. "We will be looking into a senior day care center where Dad can stay during our work hours."
4. "Dad has always been so independent; I can't bear to see him this way."

9   Feedback is necessary for successful learning to take place. Feedback can be positive or negative. Negative feedback:
1. is viewed as punishment and may cause clients to avoid the teacher.
2. is a way of getting the client's attention and works well in some instances.
3. can be used if presented in a joking manner.
4. is a form of behavioral modification.

10   You are teaching a client who has been newly diagnosed with diabetes how to do a fingerstick blood sugar and use a glucometer. When should you explain troubleshooting techniques for the glucometer?
1. As soon as you have explained how to use the glucometer, but before doing a fingerstick.
2. At the very beginning of instruction, in case there are problems with the glucometer during the lesson.
3. After the client performs one successful fingerstick blood sugar and glucometer reading.
4. After the client is comfortable performing the fingerstick blood sugar and glucometer reading.

Answers and Rationales for Review Questions, as well as discussion of Care Plan and Critical Thinking Care Map questions, appear in Appendix I.

Thinking Strategically About ...

You are a newly graduated LPN assigned to a medical-surgical unit. You have been assigned to three clients.

Mr. Ramos is a 58-year-old male who was admitted for a prostatectomy (TURP) this morning. He is predominantly Spanish speaking, though he knows a few words of English and understands a little if he is spoken to slowly. He has returned from surgery. Initially, he was sedated but begins to be more alert. He appears agitated and is yelling loudly at his roommate, who puts on his call light to summon the nurse. The roommate states, "Mr. Ramos is trying to climb out of bed and he is frightening me."

Mr. Drew is a 53-year-old male who was admitted directly from his physician's office with chest pain. His BP is 168/90 with tachycardia (heart rate 102). He is diaphoretic and is complaining of nausea.

Mr. Melezack is a 64-year-old male who had a colon resection 3 days ago. His NG tube has been clamped and he has been started on clear liquids. It was reported that he tolerated them well. The doctor has ordered that the tube can be removed if there is no nausea or vomiting.

TIME MANAGEMENT

You have received report. Using your knowledge of the three clients' diagnoses and present needs, prioritize your care for the shift.

CRITICAL THINKING

Mr. Drew's lab work has come back. You observe that his CPK values are within normal limits and that his chest pain is relieved with sublingual nitroglycerin spray. He will be discharged in the morning, and you are to begin his discharge planning. In your teaching plan, state what activities would decrease the chance of recurrent angina and the risk factors that need to be controlled to decrease effects of heart disease.

COMPASSIONATE CARING

Mr. Ramos is frightening his roommate and trying to climb out of bed. He has an IV line and a three-way catheter, which is draining dark red urine with clots. Outline the steps you would take to protect Mr. Ramos from himself and to relieve the concerns of the roommate.

COMMUNICATION AND TEAM BUIDLING

The client care assistant reports to you that Mr. Melezack is complaining of abdominal pain. He has vomited and asks to see you right away. After you go to his room to assess his present status, you will need to document and report your findings to the appropriate individuals. Write a medical record entry, using the focus charting method. State what information needs to be reported and to whom.

Promoting Health in Alternate Care Settings

UNIT V

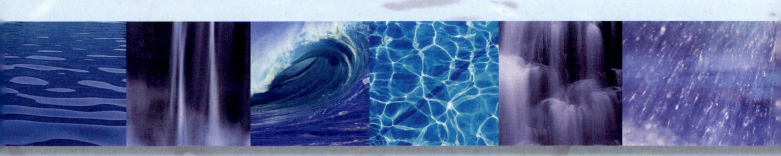

Chapter 34

Emergency and Urgent Care Nursing

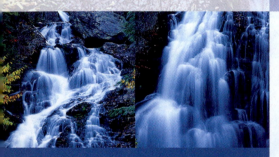

HISTORICAL Perspectives

The origins of emergency medical services (EMS) date back to the days of Napoleon, when the French army used horse-drawn "ambulances" to transport injured soldiers from the battlefield. One of the first civilian EMS services can be traced back to 1869, when Dr. Edward L. Dalton at Bellevue Hospital, then known as the Free Hospital of New York in New York City, started a basic transportation service for the sick and injured. The component of care on scene began in 1928, when Julien Stanley Wise started the Roanoke Life Saving and First Aid Crew in Roanoke, Virginia, which was the first land-based rescue squad in the nation. Over the years, EMS continued to evolve into much more than a "ride to the hospital."

BRIEF Outline

Emergency Care and Urgent Care
Initial Contact
Initial Protocols
Airway Management
Shock
Trauma in the Emergency Center
Burns
Poisoning

LEARNING Outcomes

After completing this chapter, you will be able to:
1. Identify the role of the LPN/LVN in emergency care/urgent care (EC/UC).
2. Discuss safety precautions used in the EC/UC setting.
3. Prioritize triage in the EC/UC setting.
4. Identify and describe airway management and CPR.
5. Recognize and describe types of shock and burn management.
6. Analyze important factors in care of clients with poisoning.
7. Discuss nursing care for different types of trauma in the EC/UC setting.

In today's rapidly changing healthcare system, the emergent and urgent care environments are increasingly demanding on nurses and staff. Rapid assessment skills, the ability to prioritize demands, and strong interpersonal communication skills (see Chapter 12 ⦿) are essential for ensuring the best client outcomes. This chapter discusses various areas of emergency and urgent care and the role of the LPN or LVN in them.

Emergency Care and Urgent Care

Emergency care (EC) and urgent care (UC) centers are a vital part of our healthcare system. **Emergency care** (also called ER for emergency room, or ED for emergency department) is a center where staffing is maintained around the clock to provide care for **high-acuity** (very urgent and possibly life-threatening) cases, such as trauma. It is also a place where a variety of clients receive primary care. This includes clients who have insurance for PPOs (see Chapter 7 ⦿), those receiving medical assistance, and those who are uninsured or underinsured (Box 34-1 ■). The **urgent care** center offers care for minor injuries and acute illnesses (e.g., strep throat) when clients cannot see their regular physician, such as when they are traveling. Major medical events are transferred from the UC facility to the EC. This chapter focuses primarily on the emergency care environment. Important differences in UC settings will be noted.

Practical and vocational nurses are a valuable part of the healthcare team in the emergent or urgent care setting (see Chapter 7 ⦿). They are primarily responsible for data collection, administering nursing interventions, and providing discharge planning (if applicable). Several states use certified LPNs/LVNs in more advanced roles. Once they

---

BOX 34-1   CULTURAL PULSE POINTS

Underserved Populations in the EC or UC Setting

Much of the health care for minority populations is delivered in emergency room or urgent care centers, especially in large urban areas, perhaps partially due to an increasing population of uninsured and underinsured clients. It is important that the nurse working in either of these areas consider the cultural needs of the client and his or her family. Lack of access to care is one reason for the increased use of the ER. Not having a regular healthcare provider makes follow-up and preventive health care almost impossible. The triage nurse in the EC or UC unit must be able to explain why a client with a nonurgent problem must wait, without making them feel that they do not deserve healthcare. It is also important for these clients to receive complete discharge instructions, including the need for follow-up. Community clinics may be a real alternative for people without a primary healthcare provider. The EC or UC nurse can be a source of referrals for future care. This information can be included in the teaching carried out at the end of the visit.

---

have received special certification, they can perform such tasks as intravenous (IV) cannulation, **phlebotomy** (drawing and dispensing blood), IV medication administration, and applying dressings. The LPN/LVN *always* works under the supervision of an RN or MD in the EC setting.

---

clinical ALERT

The LPN or LVN may not be able to accept verbal orders in the EC setting. This is determined by the state's nurse practice act, state board of nursing where the nurse is licensed, and facility policy. For their own and their clients' safety, nurses must identify and follow facility procedures and the guidelines of their state's nurse practice act.

SAFETY ISSUES

The EC setting presents many safety concerns for clients and staff. Clients may present with life-threatening conditions or highly contagious diseases. Client risk for infection may be heightened by diseases or open wounds. Risk for falls is increased with fainting, loss of blood, or fractures.

First and foremost, nurses must use Standard Precautions at all times in the EC setting (see Figure 9-2 ⦿). Standard Precautions include gloves, gown, masks, protective eyewear, face shields, and, of course, careful hand hygiene. The Centers for Disease Control and Prevention mandates clinical guidelines for safe practice. The careful and sensible use of Standard Precautions is especially important in the care of combative and confused clients. Such clients may be unable to identify areas of body/body fluids that can transmit disease or pathogens with initial contact. Without Standard Precautions, nurses or other staff could become infected.

The same protocols are employed within the UC settings for client care. Healthcare professionals are also at high risk for back injuries due to lifting or handling clients in an emergency situation. Safety must be the primary concern for the healthcare professional at all times.

Initial Contact

The EC setting can become overwhelmed with clients at a moment's notice. An efficient response to increased client numbers and high-acuity levels requires triage. **Triage** is the process used by healthcare providers to determine which person has the most emergent (pressing) problem. Usually, clients are prioritized by ABCD:

Airway
Breathing
Circulation
Deformity.

With triage, clients' conditions are prioritized from serious to stable.

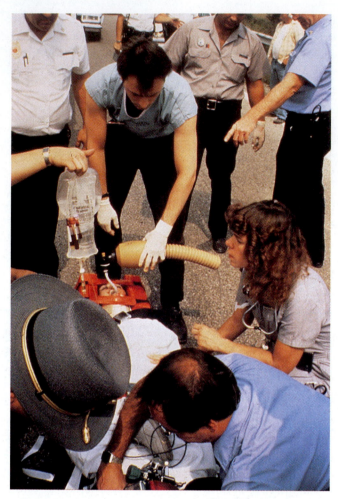

Figure 34-1. ■ Emergency medical technicians often provide the first treatment to victims outside the healthcare environment. (*Source:* Courtesy of University Air Core/University of Cincinnati Hospital.)

Note: In the event of a disaster internal or external to the EC (Figure 34-1 ■), the nurse would require additional assistance to manage appropriately the number of clients created by such a situation. (Part of staff training as an employee in this setting would be to know how to react in case of a major event.) The EC department would initiate a disaster plan or critical incident plan. This allows each individual within the EC and ancillary departments to prepare and assist a larger number of clients. It also allows various personnel from within and outside the facility (emergency medical staff, community law enforcement officials, etc.) to respond so that safe, effective care can be given to a large number of clients. Training and practice for disaster situations and knowing how to work with an incident command system are essential to effectively handling a disaster. It is also essential to understand the facility policy and emergency codes for such an event.

Urgent care also requires continuous monitoring of clients for acute changes. However, urgent care clients are generally treated on a first-come, first-served basis.

CONFIDENTIALITY

Prior to receiving treatment in the EC or UC setting, the client must sign consent for treatment and confidentiality forms. If the client is unable to sign, a legal responsible party may sign consent forms for the client. Consent for treatment includes forms for valuables (see Figure 10-2 ⬭), procedures, and the Health Insurance Portability and Accountability Act or HIPAA. (HIPAA regulations are described in detail in Chapter 3 ⬭.) All forms must be signed and documented in the client's chart. The staff is responsible for following protocols for standards of privacy and consent for treatment. The nurse must be mindful of who has a legal right to information obtained in the EC setting.

> ### clinical ALERT
>
> Privacy for the EC client is a challenging situation. It seems that many times the healthcare professional forgets that the EC client has rights to privacy. HIPAA regulations must be followed by all members of the healthcare team. Questions should be asked in a private area, away from others.

CONSENT FOR MINORS

In most cases, the nurse obtains the consent for minors from a parent or guardian. Exceptions to this rule are the following: a life-threatening situation, sexually transmitted infections, drug or alcohol abuse, or pregnancy. If no parent or guardian is present, then the decision to treat is really up to the provider. Follow your facility's policy for treating minors without a consenting adult present. Many times, if an adult's consent is needed but the adult can only be reached by phone, two nurses will listen to the adult give consent.

> ### clinical ALERT
>
> When a verbal telephone consent is obtained, BOTH nurses must document it in the chart.

BASIC DATA COLLECTION

On entering the EC, the client's basic data information will be obtained. Height and weight, vital signs, and, of course, the level of pain as the fifth vital sign must be obtained. (*Note:* Height is important because peak flow meter ranges are based on age and height. It is also helpful in determining growth and development norms.) Accuracy of data in an emergency situation is especially important. (See Figure 10-1 ⬭ for an adult admission assessment form.) Data collection is a systematic gathering of information about the client. The client is the primary source of information. Secondary sources of information include the client chart, family, and health team members. The nurse gathers subjective and objective data. Subjective data is the information the client or the caretaker tells the nurse during the nursing assessment. Subjective data can be called *symptoms.* Objective data is information collected by using the senses. Information may be observed, auscultated, percussed, or smelled. Objective data can be called *signs.* So subjective (S) data is what the patient says (S), and objective data (O) is what the nurse observes (O).

COLLECTING DATA

Data collection includes taking a health history by obtaining biographical data, the chief complaint, present illness, past history, current health information, and family history. Depending on the emergency a more focused collection of data may occur.

History

Medication history, allergies, over-the-counter (OTC) medications, vitamins, cultural treatments, and holistic medicines are vitally important information. Sometimes an OTC treatment can be the cause of the client's problem. However, clients often do not mention OTC products without prompting, because they do not think of them as medicine. Women using birth control may forget to mention that they are taking pills or injections. This information can be very important when reviewing test results or initiating a treatment. Most forms for emergency departments and urgent care centers have fill-in spaces for last menstrual period, medications, contraceptives, and so on.

Obtaining medication information during the data collection process is critical. This includes all medications routinely and occasionally taken by the person. Cardiac medications such as calcium channel blockers, digoxin, and diuretics are often heavily documented in cases of cardiac clients. Antibiotic use and pain medicines are also important to note, so that a complete evaluation by the primary physician can be performed.

A brief history of events, including the reason for admission, or chief complaint (C) is obtained and documented. Information should be obtained from the client, but may be obtained from family or friends if the client is unable to respond. Remember, the provider will treat the client according to the information obtained by the nurse. Information must be accurate and nonjudgmental. At this time a complete review of systems should be performed. This information is used to determine what to include in the head-to-toe physical exam. This is information that the client tells you as you ask about each of these areas. The physical assessment will be completed by the healthcare provider. Review of systems includes integumentary, head and neck, respiratory, cardiovascular, musculoskeletal, neurologic, genitourinary, reproductive, psychological, spiritual, social, and developmental.

The charge nurse will triage the clients and inform them of the EC procedures and protocols. Oftentimes ECs are overloaded with clients with various needs. Waiting times are often long due to the high volume of clients, limited client care areas, limited number of staff, and the *urgency* (acuity level) of client needs. The nurse should explain to the client that the waiting time to be seen may be from minutes to hours. The nurse must ask for patience and reassure clients that they will be seen. The nurse must also monitor previously admitted clients for acute changes and determine whether they need to be evaluated sooner by the physician.

PHYSICAL EXAMINATION AND ASSESSMENT

The physical examination and assessment will be performed by the healthcare provider, such as the physician, nurse practitioner, or physician's assistant. At this time a complete head-to-toe examination or a focused exam may be performed. The information obtained in the health history, including the review of systems aids the healthcare provider in the head-to-toe examination.

Initial Protocols

Depending on the nature of the problem causing admission to the EC, the nurse may initiate treatment while the client is in the waiting room, before evaluation by the physician. Examples include hot/cold packs to an injured area (see Chapter 23 ⚭). Bandages may be applied to minimal wounds (see Chapter 23 ⚭). The nurse utilizes the various treatment protocols and standing orders to initiate nursing care and also communicates with the attending physician.

> ### clinical ALERT
>
> Personnel should *always* follow Standard Precautions. Many times healthcare providers use poor judgment and do not protect themselves from body fluids from clients. There is no need to be heroic or a martyr. Use the necessary precautions and do not worry about what other professionals are doing. Remember, by following Standard Precautions you are protecting both yourself and your loved ones.

The nurse may administer medications to clients (usually to reduce fever) before the provider examines them. Fever is a sign of infection, and it is not necessary for clients to prove that they have a fever. Parents sometimes fail to medicate the child for fever so that providers can see that they are really ill. If this occurs, the nurse should educate the client that this is not necessary or helpful. Of course, it is important to find out what medicine and what dose was used and when, before administering medication. Medications for fever are usually administered according to weight and age in children (see Chapter 29 ⚭ and the nomogram of Figure 29-3 ⚭).

COLLABORATIVE CARE

The management of the client in the EC setting often requires communication and use of ancillary department staff.

The use of radiography, laboratory, and pharmacy consultation of healthcare professional/specialists results in a valuable network of services that assists in the care of the EC client.

Communication of ancillary services may be done with the use of informatics, computers (see Figure 6-6 ⬭), and traditional methods such as physician written orders and telephone chains. Continuous communication and updating of client services and information are necessary to ensure quality of care for the EC client. The healthcare team works collectively to assist in client recovery or rehabilitation.

Laboratory Tests

If a person presents with airway difficulty, a peak flow test may be ordered. A **peak flow test** evaluates maximum airflow during forced expiration and monitors bronchospasm in asthmatic clients. A nebulizer or metered-dose inhaler allows medication to be given via aerosol and inhaled for rapid treatment of airway difficulties. Peak flow measurements would be taken before and after use of the handheld nebulizer (Figure 34-2 ■). (See more about care of respiratory disorders in Chapter 24 ⬭.)

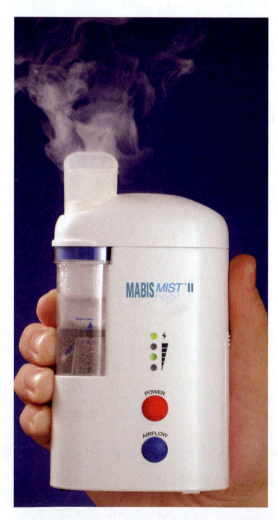

Figure 34-2. ■ A handheld nebulizer is used to assist the client. (*Source:* Courtesy of Mabis.)

If chest pain is present, an electrocardiography (ECG) monitor would be attached. **Stat** (immediate) labs for chest pain would include cardiac labs such as treponin levels, CPKs, LDH, and electrolytes.

Tests for trauma would include imaging techniques such as x-rays, positron-emission tomography (PET) scans, computerized tomography (CT) scans, and magnetic resonance imaging (MRI) if available in the EC.

Tests for infectious diseases would include a complete blood count with a differential count. Sedimentation rates are often helpful in pinpointing inflammation and infectious disease parameters.

Other tests would be ordered according to client symptoms.

Airway Management

The primary concern for any client in the EC setting is airway management. The nurse is responsible for assessing changes in the client's respiratory or breathing pattern at all times. Oxygen therapy and adjuncts are frequently utilized in maintaining airways. Apparatuses from oral and nasal airways, low-flow devices (nasal cannulas, Venturi masks, and simple face masks), and high-flow devices (nonrebreather, bag-valve-mask units, endotracheal tubes) are most often used. (See respiratory disorders and procedures for administering oxygen in Chapter 24 ⬭.) Saturation readings for O_2 are done frequently with clients requiring O_2, to monitor changes and to assess oxygen **titration** (determination of the correct volume for administration).

An initial survey of the ABCs (airway, breathing, circulation) is always conducted on a client in the EC. The airway must be maintained for *patency* (openness), airflow, and adequate ventilation. In cases of trauma, a client must have **cervical spine alignment** (*C spine*) performed. A cervical spine alignment is a manual maneuver performed by an individual to maintain spinal alignment. At times, this may include application of a cervical stabilizing collar device. A soft collar is not recommended because it is not effective in stabilizing a C spine. A chin-lift or modified jaw-thrust maneuver (discussed later in the CPR section) must be performed with clients who have experienced trauma. The mouth is inspected for bleeding, loose teeth, dentures, foreign objects, and emesis.

To keep the airway open, an apparatus may be placed into the nasopharyngeal or oral cavity. Endotracheal intubations (Figure 34-3 ■) may also be done. In severe cases a *cricothyroidectomy* (an incision into the trachea) may be performed by a physician or licensed professional in emergency care to make a direct opening into the trachea.

Breathing must be evaluated for rate, rhythm, and quality. Oxygen adjunct devices that deliver high-flow O_2 (nonrebreather, bag-valve-mask unit, endotracheal tube via

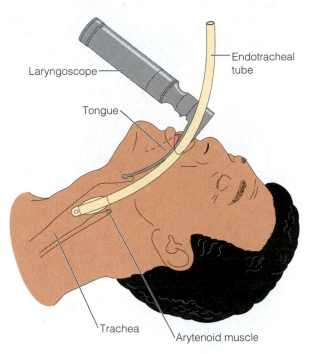

Laryngoscope

Tongue

Endotracheal tube

Trachea

Arytenoid muscle

Figure 34-3. ■ Endotracheal intubation maintains a patent airway for oxygen administration.

intubation) may be used. Low-flow devices such as nasal cannulas, Venturi masks, and face masks can also support ventilation in minor cases of compromise.

CARDIOPULMONARY RESUSCITATION

In clients with trauma and altered levels of consciousness (LOC), the carotid pulse is evaluated for quality, rate, and presence. **Cardiopulmonary resuscitation** (CPR, a combination of oral resuscitation and external cardiac massage) is always performed on clients in the EC who have an absent pulse. During times of inadequate tissue perfusion during cardiac arrest, CPR offers a small percentage of core circulation to the vital organs in order to sustain life during times of pulselessness. CPR can be administered to people of any age from newborn to geriatric (Figure 34-4 ■). CPR technique is varied with compressions, depth, and ratio in the adult, child, and infant. See general guidelines in Box 34-2 ■. Specific training is provided by the American Heart Association (AHA) and the Red Cross for certification in CPR. Continued education and training updates are an important part of providing quality, professional care.

BOX 34-2

First Steps to Prepare for Adult CPR

The following steps are based on instructions from the American Heart Association.

1. **Check for responsiveness.** Shake or tap the person gently. See if the person moves or makes a noise. Shout, "Are you OK?"
2. **Call 911 if there is no response.** Shout for help and send someone to call 911. If you are alone, call 911 even if you have to leave the person. Retrieve the automated external defibrillator (AED) and emergency equipment, if available.
3. **Carefully place the person on his or her back.** If there is a chance the person has a spinal injury, two people are needed to move the person without twisting the head and neck.
4. **Open the airway.** Lift up the chin with two fingers. At the same time, push down on the forehead with the other hand.
5. **Look, listen, and feel for breathing.** Place your ear close to the person's mouth and nose. Watch for chest rise and fall. Feel for breath on your cheek.
6. **If the person is not breathing:**
   - Cover the person's mouth tightly with your mouth.
   - Pinch the nose closed.
   - Keep the chin lifted and head tilted.
   - Give two slow, full breaths.
   - Use bag-mask unit with oxygen or barrier device whenever possible.
7. **If the chest does NOT rise, try the head-tilt/chin-lift maneuver again, and give two more breaths.** If the chest still doesn't rise, check to see if something is blocking the airway and try to remove it.
8. **Look for signs of circulation.** These signs include normal breathing, coughing, or movement. If these signs are absent, begin chest compressions.
   If there is circulation but no breathing:
      Provide rescue breathing (one breath every 4 to 5 seconds).

If no pulse or signs of circulation are present:
   If AED is available: power on, attach electrodes, and follow prompts.
   IF no AED, perform chest compressions.
9. **Perform chest compressions:**
   - Place the heel of one hand on the breastbone, right between the nipples.
   - Place the heel of your other hand on top of the first hand.
   - Position your body directly over your hands. Your shoulders should be in line with your hands. DO NOT lean back or forward. As you gaze down, you should be looking directly down on your hands.
   - Give 30 chest compressions. Each time, press down about 2 inches into the chest. These compressions should be FAST with no pausing. Count the 30 compressions quickly: "a, b, c, d, e, f, g, h, i, j, k, l, m, n, off."
10. **Give the person two slow, full breaths.** The chest should rise.
11. Continue cycles of 30 chest compressions followed by two slow, full breaths.
12. After about 2 minutes (five cycles of 30 compressions and two breaths), recheck for signs of circulation.
13. Repeat steps 11 and 12 until the person recovers or help arrives.

If the person starts breathing again, place him or her in the recovery position. Periodically recheck for breathing and signs of circulation until help arrives. **Remember, it is the nurse's responsibility to become certified and to maintain updated training in CPR.**

Source: Adapted from the *2005 American Heart Association Guidelines for Cardiopulmonary Resuscitation and Emergency Cardiovascular Care,* www.americanheart.org.

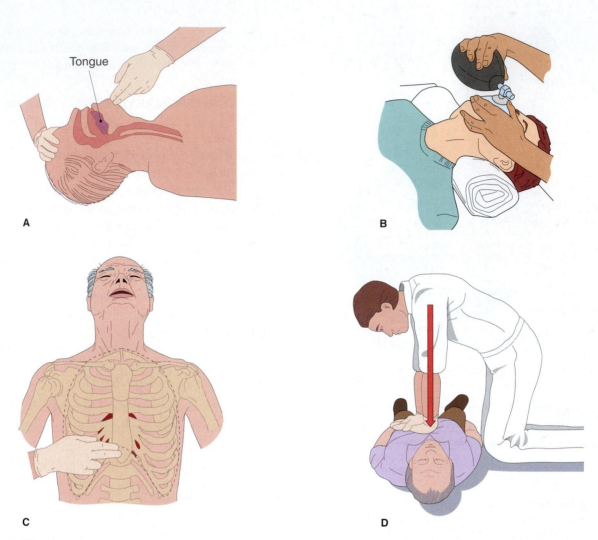

Figure 34-4. ■ CPR: **A.** Use the head-tilt/chin-lift method to open the airway. **B.** If client is not breathing, give two full breaths using a pocket mask, mouth shield, or bag-valve-mask unit. Observe the chest rise and fall during ventilation. **C.** Locate the compression site by following the edge of the rib cage to the notch where the ribs join the sternum. **D.** Position your hands and begin chest compressions with your arms vertical over the victim.

If the client has no pulse, CPR is administered immediately. Two-person CPR is generally performed in the EC, as staff participates in efforts to revive the client. Current AHA guidelines call for 30 chest compressions for every two rescue breaths. This applies to adults, children, and infants. Studies show that this creates more blood flow from the heart to the rest of the body until a defibrillator is available (American Heart Association, www.americanheart.org, November 28, 2005). The revised guidelines also recommend that emergency personnel cool the body temperature of cardiac arrest patients to 90 degrees for 12 to 24 hours; this results in improved survival and brain function for those who are comatose after initial resuscitation. Also, high-flow O_2 is always administered with a bag-valve-mask unit while compressions are performed.

Intravenous cannulation with a large-bore IV is initiated by a member certified with the EC to perform the function. IV lifelines provide access for medications to be administered hemodynamically, to improve the client's chances of survival. Should life-threatening dysrhythmia occur in cardiac arrest, a defibrillator may be used. A **defibrillator** is an instrument that provides various voltages of electricity (measured in joules) to trigger the electrical impulses of the heart (Figure 34-5 ■). If the client has a pulse initially, circulation is carefully monitored with frequent vital signs so that changes may be reported to the physician.

HEIMLICH MANEUVER

The Heimlich maneuver (see also Chapter 8 ⬭) is necessary for clients who have an airway obstruction due to ingestion of a foreign object. Food (such as a bolus of meat) is a common cause of choking. The tongue is the most common cause for obstruction in the unconscious client. Many

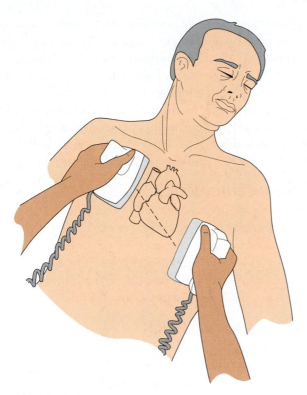

Figure 34-5. ■ Defibrillation.

times the relaxation of the muscle allows the tongue to fall back in the client's throat, obstructing airflow.

The universal sign for choking is typically demonstrated by the hand or hands at the throat, for an individual who is consciously choking (Figure 34-6 ■). Victims who are conscious and choking should not be touched if they can talk, cough, or speak in a high-pitched tone. If a client asks for assistance or becomes unconscious, abdominal thrusts are administered. Abdominal thrusts are given at the level of the midepigastric region, and below the xiphoid process (Figure 34-7 ■). If the client does not expel

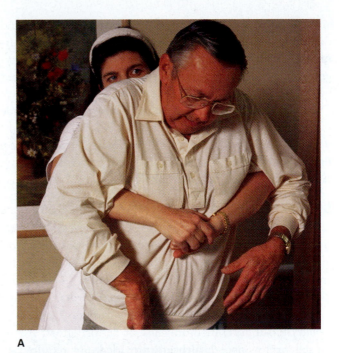

A

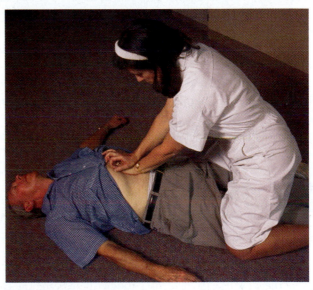

B

Figure 34-7. ■ Heimlich maneuver: **A.** thrust delivered on standing person with airway obstruction; **B.** position for Heimlich maneuver on unconscious client.

the object and becomes unresponsive, he or she should be assisted to the ground carefully. Examination of the mouth is done to see whether the airway has become patent from the position change. This examination is done again after a sequence of abdominal thrusts to determine whether the object has moved or the airway has become patent. Abdominal thrusts serve the purpose of an artificial cough. They produce force within the trachea to expel the object that is blocking the airway.

Within the EC setting, medical instruments such as Magill forceps may be used by the physician to remove objects in the

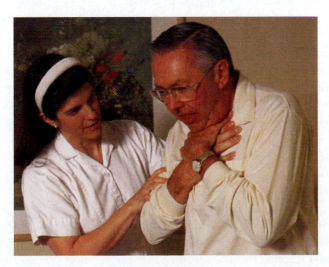

Figure 34-6. ■ Universal sign of choking.

airway if necessary. Suction should be readily available and the nurse should be prepared to assist with suctioning during the procedure. On successful removal of the object, oxygen therapy and airway management are always performed by the healthcare team until the client becomes stable.

Primary nursing diagnoses for these clients include *Ineffective Airway Clearance, Risk for Aspiration, Acute Confusion, Impaired Gas Exchange,* and *Ineffective Tissue Perfusion.* Practical and vocational nurses monitor airway, breathing, and circulation, and assist as noted earlier.

SKILL CERTIFICATIONS AND STAT TESTS

Given the severity and acuteness of clients in the EC setting, the nurse and other healthcare professionals are required by institutions to maintain standards of practice and certification in skill and competence. Certification must be maintained in ACLS (advanced cardiac life support), PALS (pediatric advanced life support), and BLS (basic life support) including use of defibrillators. All licensed professional healthcare providers are required to maintain proficiency in these areas while employed in the EC setting.

During a critical situation such as trauma or myocardial infarction, the ACLS, PALS, or BLS protocols are utilized. Twelve-lead ECGs are performed on clients to diagnose cardiac status and dysrhythmia so that appropriate treatments can be administered.

In cases of myocardial infarction (MI), cardiac labs (mentioned earlier under Collaborative Care) are often ordered in conjunction with diagnostics to verify a medical diagnosis. Most often labs are ordered *stat* (immediately) in the EC so that treatments can be given in a rapid sequence.

Shock

In the EC setting clients can have an array of wounds or injuries. One of the most urgent concerns is **shock** (life-threatening condition of inadequate tissue perfusion). Depending on the nature of the wound and the amount of blood or fluid volume loss, the nurse must identify changes in vital signs that indicate suspicion of shock. Vital signs include tachycardia, tachypnea, and hypotension. Figure 34-8 ■ shows the numerous effects of shock on body systems. Also monitor the possible effects of shock on the endocrine system, including decreased insulin production, increased blood sugar, and polyuria.

HYPOVOLEMIC SHOCK

Different types of shock can occur as a complication of trauma. Hypovolemic shock occurs when the body has sustained a severe amount of fluid deficit or loss. Reasons may include bleeding, burns, fluid and electrolyte imbalances related to excessive diarrhea or vomiting, or sepsis from trauma or injury. Signs and symptoms generally reveal pallor,

diaphoresis (sweating), hypotension, tachycardia, tachypnea, and decreased urine output (*oliguria*). There may also be changes in LOC. The symptoms may gradually become worse as fluid loss becomes greater, therefore creating obvious clinical manifestations. A pneumatic antishock garment (Figure 34-9 ■) or military antishock trousers (MAST) might be used to help maintain blood pressure. Hemorrhagic shock is a type of hypovolemic shock in which the patient has lost a significant amount of blood.

CARDIOGENIC SHOCK

Cardiogenic shock occurs when the heart sustains an injury or trauma resulting in pump failure. Acute MI, CHF, dysrhythmia, and blunt and penetrating chest trauma are known causes of cardiogenic shock. Signs and symptoms are similar to those for hypovolemic shock. In addition, clients may have pulmonary edema and distended (swollen) neck veins.

ANAPHYLACTIC SHOCK

Anaphylactic shock occurs in clients who experience hypersensitivity reactions to various antigens. Examples include medications, bee stings, blood products, natural rubber latex, and food ingestion. The signs and symptoms are similar to hypovolemic shock. In addition, however, the respiratory system becomes compromised. Dyspnea, laryngeal spasm and edema, and bronchospasm are often witnessed within minutes of onset. Clients will become extremely anxious and require immediate airway management to ensure safety.

> ### clinical ALERT
>
> Loss of life can ensue if the nurse does not have a client remain at the facility for 20 to 30 minutes after injections have been given to observe for anaphylactic shock. The client can wait in the waiting room if appropriate and report back to the nurse after the waiting period. Documentation of the person's condition at discharge and the time is crucial.

SEPTIC SHOCK

Septic shock is a condition that occurs from a systemic reaction and infection in the body. The body becomes overwhelmed with poisons (endotoxins) that cause the blood vessels to vasodilate. The body attempts to compensate for the fluid loss and *interstitial spacing* or **third spacing** (shunting of fluids into the extracellular space). Most often the causes are pathogens, such as gram-negative bacteria or viruses.

Septic shock is known for two phases of signs and symptoms. The first phase has normal BP, pulse, and urine output. Oftentimes the client becomes febrile with flushed skin tones and diaphoresis. The second phase reveals more obvious latent signs of shock: hypotension, bradycardia, oliguria, cold, clammy extremities, and a normal temperature (*afebrile*).

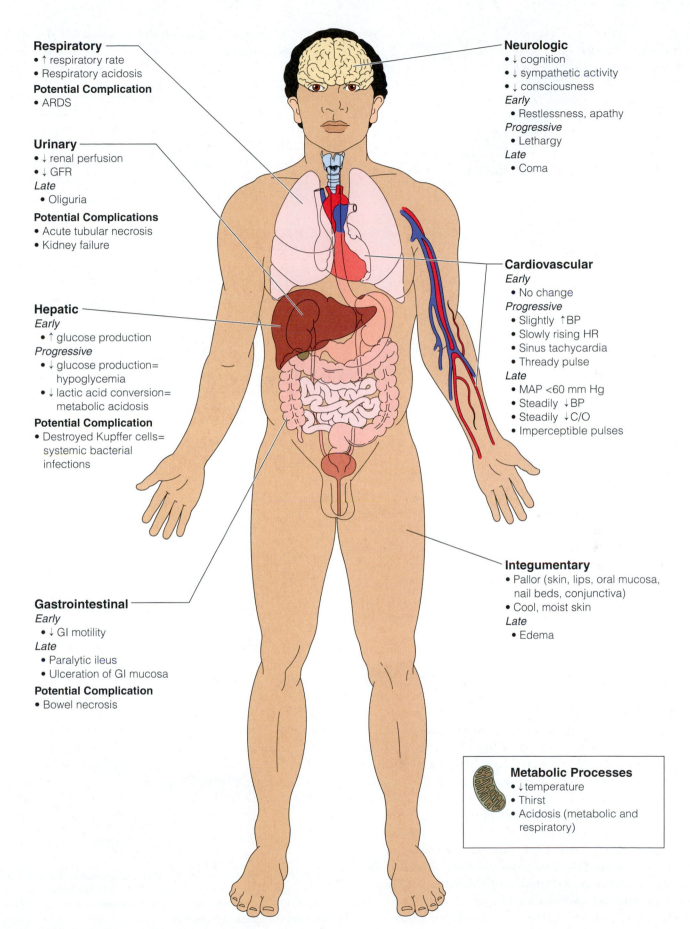

Respiratory
- ↑ respiratory rate
- Respiratory acidosis

Potential Complication
- ARDS

Urinary
- ↓ renal perfusion
- ↓ GFR

Late
- Oliguria

Potential Complications
- Acute tubular necrosis
- Kidney failure

Hepatic
Early
- ↑ glucose production

Progressive
- ↓ glucose production= hypoglycemia
- ↓ lactic acid conversion= metabolic acidosis

Potential Complication
- Destroyed Kupffer cells= systemic bacterial infections

Gastrointestinal
Early
- ↓ GI motility

Late
- Paralytic ileus
- Ulceration of GI mucosa

Potential Complication
- Bowel necrosis

Neurologic
- ↓ cognition
- ↓ sympathetic activity
- ↓ consciousness

Early
- Restlessness, apathy

Progressive
- Lethargy

Late
- Coma

Cardiovascular
Early
- No change

Progressive
- Slightly ↑BP
- Slowly rising HR
- Sinus tachycardia
- Thready pulse

Late
- MAP <60 mm Hg
- Steadily ↓BP
- Steadily ↓C/O
- Imperceptible pulses

Integumentary
- Pallor (skin, lips, oral mucosa, nail beds, conjunctiva)
- Cool, moist skin

Late
- Edema

Metabolic Processes
- ↓ temperature
- Thirst
- Acidosis (metabolic and respiratory)

Figure 34-8. ■ Multisystem effects of shock.

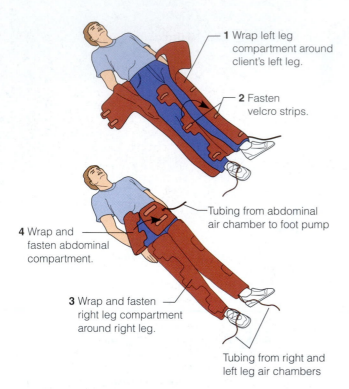

1 Wrap left leg compartment around client's left leg.

2 Fasten velcro strips.

Tubing from abdominal air chamber to foot pump

4 Wrap and fasten abdominal compartment.

3 Wrap and fasten right leg compartment around right leg.

Tubing from right and left leg air chambers

Figure 34-9. ■ Pneumatic antishock garment provides rapid, emergency treatment of shock.

NEUROGENIC SHOCK

Neurogenic shock occurs when there is trauma or malfunction to the nervous system. Most frequently known as spinal shock, neurogenic shock is related to gross injury to the spinal column. Motor vehicle crashes, household injuries, and falls are primary reasons for neurogenic shock. Some signs and symptoms are similar to those of hypo-volemic shock. However, in neurogenic shock, the skin is warm and dry and the heart rate falls (bradycardia). In addition, paralysis or limited extremity movement below the area of injury is seen.

NURSING CARE

PRIORITIES IN NURSING CARE

When caring for clients in shock, you must focus on recognizing the signs rapidly and implementing emergency measures quickly. Monitor vital signs in clients with suspected shock every 15 minutes or more often if the condition is changing rapidly. Position the client with shock in modified Trendelenburg position unless the client is in cardiogenic shock. This helps return blood to the heart. Be prepared to assist with immediate administration of IV fluids to increase blood volume and blood pressure. Be ready to obtain plasma expanders as ordered to keep blood volume increased. Administer oxygen as ordered to increase oxygen delivery to the brain, heart, and other vital

organs. Maintain an open airway, especially if the client loses consciousness.

ASSESSING

The treatment and management of shock includes rapid assessment and interventions for life-threatening situations in the EC. The LPN/LVN might assist the EC healthcare team in the initial stages until the client's condition has stabilized. Airway management, breathing, and circulation control ("the ABCs") are essential initial treatment.

clinical ALERT

Clients in nursing units may also go into shock. In fact, the LPN/LVN is often one of the first to recognize signs of shock, take immediate action to support the client's circulatory status, and call for help.

DIAGNOSING, PLANNING, AND IMPLEMENTING

Some common nursing diagnoses for clients with shock include the following:

- *Ineffective Airway Clearance*
- *Decreased Cardiac Output*
- *Impaired Gas Exchange*
- *Deficient Fluid Volume*
- *Ineffective Tissue Perfusion.*

The nurse must give close attention to clients with shock. Common interventions for all types of shock follow:

- Except for cardiogenic shock, place client in modified Trendelenburg position (supine with head of bed elevated 10 degrees and foot raised 20 degrees) (Figure 34-10 ■). *This position maintains blood flow to vital organs.*
- Monitor changes in level of consciousness. *These changes can signal further underlying changes that require medical attention. Report changes in LOC to the team leader or charge nurse.*

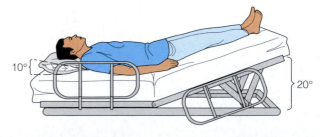

10° 20°

Figure 34-10. ■ Positioning of client for hypovolemic shock. The client in shock should be positioned with the lower extremities elevated about 20 degrees (knees straight), trunk horizontal, and the head elevated about 10 degrees.

- Administer oxygen and monitor breathing. Monitor cardiac circulatory status. *The ABCs are of primary importance in a client with shock.*
- Monitor IV fluids. *Increasing fluids helps replace blood volume and raise blood pressure. Clients with cardiac compromise may not be able to tolerate rapid fluid administration, so the nurse must monitor for signs of respiratory congestion. Vocational and practical nurses working in this environment can obtain a certification that qualifies them to administer IV fluids.*
- Report changes in vital signs. *In the severely compromised client, changes can occur rapidly. Prompt reporting can save a life.*
- Monitor I&O for deficits, especially urine decrease. *Reduction in the amount of urine may signal third spacing.*
- Treat symptoms appropriately and in a timely way as ordered by physician. Report all findings to the physician stat. *Communication among the emergency or urgent care staff is crucial to ensuring the best client outcomes.*

EVALUATING

The nurse checks vital signs, I&O, and LOC to determine whether the client's condition has become or remains stable. All changes must be reported promptly.

Trauma in the Emergency Center

Trauma is one of the most common reasons for visits within the EC setting. Two types of mechanisms of injury can be linked to life-threatening conditions and death if not treated promptly. The first is penetrating trauma (Figure 34-11 ■). This can be from a sharp object that penetrates the body rapidly. Penetrating trauma can range from minor (stepping on a nail) to life threatening (being stabbed with a knife). The second is blunt trauma or closed injury. This type of injury causes impact to an area (bone, tissue, organ) leading to internal bleeding or gross trauma at the point of origin. A blow from a baseball (see Figure 34-11A) or impact with a steering wheel in an automobile collision are two examples of blunt trauma.

HEAD TRAUMA

Trauma to the head can result in intracranial bleeding, intracranial pressure, and edema. Death may result if the client is not treated immediately. Assessment of the mechanism of injury is of utmost importance in determining how severe the injury is. Figure 34-12 ■ illustrates the double head injury that can occur in a car crash.

With head trauma, careful continuous monitoring of LOC is essential. The EC uses the Glasgow Coma Scale to evaluate level of consciousness (see Table 19-2 ⦿). The test scores range from 15 (alert and oriented) to 0. A score of less than 13 with head trauma is cause for concern and

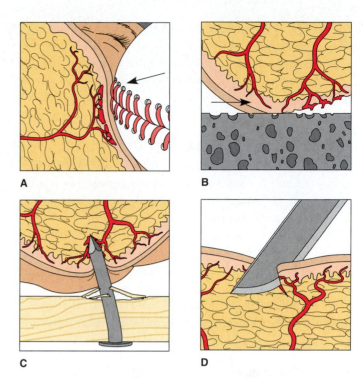

Figure 34-11. ■ Traumatic injuries to the skin: **A.** contusion; **B.** abrasion; **C.** puncture wound; **D.** laceration.

intervention. Lower scores may indicate increased intracranial pressure (IICP) and a potentially life-threatening situation for the client.

CHEST TRAUMA

Chest trauma occurs from injury to the thorax and mediastinal areas. Motor vehicle crashes, stab wounds, gunshot wounds, and sport injuries, for example, can cause chest trauma. Any type of injury to the chest area can result in a life-threatening situation. Complications of injuries to

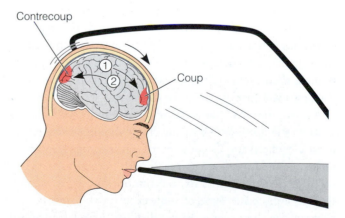

Figure 34-12. ■ A blow to the head, as from a car crash, can create more than one point of injury in the brain. This is called a *coup-contrecoup injury*. Following the initial injury (the coup), the brain rebounds within the skull and receives a second injury (contrecoup) in the opposite part of the brain.

the chest area can include pneumothorax, hemothorax, flail chest (see Chapter 20 ⬮⬮).

Interventions include high-flow O_2, IV administration/lifeline, frequent vitals, and O_2 saturations. The respiratory assessment is paramount in ensuring success in clients with chest trauma.

ABDOMINAL TRAUMA

Abdominal trauma can occur in the same manner as chest trauma. Careful consideration and assessment of vital organs must be done. The abdominal cavity encompasses many vascular organs that are not protected by bone structure, so injury can more easily occur in the abdomen than chest. Depending on the type and mechanism of injury (blunt or penetrating), rapid blood loss or volume can occur. The nurse must identify and monitor for signs and symptoms of shock that may indicate bleeding. Special attention is paid to the abdomen. Any signs of *ecchymosis* (bruising) and distention should be reported to the physician.

PRIORITIES IN NURSING CARE

When caring for trauma clients in the EC, focus your care on controlling external bleeding and monitoring for internal bleeding. Establish an airway and monitor breathing and circulation following the ABCs. Check vital signs every 15 to 30 minutes. Monitor for signs of shock and changes in LOC. Give emotional support to the client and family, because traumatic injuries are generally grave in nature and extremely upsetting to those who witness them. Give family members a private place to meet and support one another. Keep family informed of the condition of the client if changes occur.

EMERGENCIES OF EYES, EARS, OR NOSE

Any eye problem requires a visual acuity exam on a Snellen or other type of eye chart (Figure 34-13 ■). Most providers want documentation of the best corrected vision. If the client has contact lenses (and if the contacts are not part of the urgent problem), test the eyes before having the client remove them. Clients who wear glasses for distance vision (myopia) would wear them for the exam.

The top number to the left of the line of letters on an eye chart is the number of feet the client should stand from it. Most eye charts are 20-foot charts. The bottom number indicates how far (in feet) a person with normal vision could be from the chart and still read the line. There is usually a line or some other type of indication on the wall or floor near the eye chart that indicates distance. Check for this line so that you can avoid guessing at the distance. The client stands at the proper distance, covers the eye with an eye occluder or a solid object such as a piece of clean paper, and reads each line starting at the top.

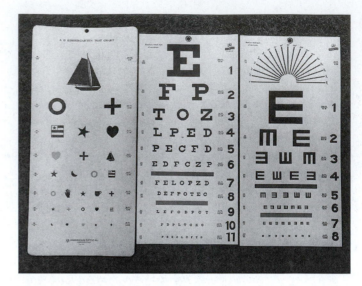

Figure 34-13. ■ Types of eye charts: preschool children's chart; Snellen's standard chart; Snellen E chart for clients who are not able to read.

clinical ALERT

Never have a client use the hand or fingers as an occluder. If an eye occluder is available, remember to clean it between uses to prevent transfer of eye infections or even foreign material from one client to another.

Check the right eye first, then the left eye, and finally both eyes. Stay in the same routine. *Note:* The Joint Commission on Accreditation of Healthcare Organizations (JCAHO) regulations state that documentation for eye tests must spell out "left eye, right eye, and both eyes." The abbreviations for eyes (OS, OD, and OU) are not to be used in charting in JCAHO-accredited institutions.

If a client presents with a chemical or foreign substance in the eye, an eye kit will need to be obtained. The eye kit includes a topical eye anesthetic (located in the refrigerator most often), a Wood's black light, fluorescing drops or strips, sterile needles, sterile applicators, a solution to flush the eye with such as Dacriose, a device to do a continuous irrigation when hooked to an IV line, ointments and drops, and eye patches.

Ear Lavage

Clients may need an ear lavage after the provider examines the client. Ear lavage is described in Chapter 29 ⬮⬮.

Foreign Object in the Nose

Children especially can put items in places where they will become trapped. The provider will need equipment necessary for viewing the particular site of the foreign object. Tweezers or small forceps may also be required.

Burns

Burns are a type of injury that is frequently seen in the EC setting. The three types of burns that can inflict injury are thermal, chemical, and electrical. Thermal burns are most common. They occur from everyday events, household scalds, fire, hot temperature contact with a substance or object, and even sun exposure. Chemical burns can occur within the household or outside environment. Chemical burns are either alkaline or acidic in pH, burning the mucous membranes on contact or exposure. Electrical burns can be caused by exposure to either high or low voltage or to a lightning strike while outdoors.

CLASSIFICATION OF BURNS

Burns are classified according to the thickness (Figure 34-14 ■). **Superficial burns** (also called first-degree burns) injure only the epidermis and may be caused by everyday events such as touching a hot element on the stove. Superficial burns may be pink and painful, but they generally heal within 3 to 6 days. **Partial-thickness burns** (also called second-degree burns) may be superficial or deep. If they are *superficial partial-thickness burns,* they involve the epidermal layer. They are generally painful to touch and are red in appearance.

Deep partial-thickness burns involve more injury to the skin. The areas involved include both the epidermis and dermis. The burn remains red in appearance. Blistered areas may lack some sensation but have a painful area of injury surrounding them.

Full-thickness burns (also called third-degree burns) are the most severe. The layers of the skin (dermis, epidermis, subcutaneous) are totally involved. The appearance is blackened, charred, and white to leathery. Full-thickness burns are painless, because the nerve endings have been destroyed. The surrounding tissues that may be partially burned may have some nerve sensation causing pain. However, the full-thickness burns do not generate discomfort.

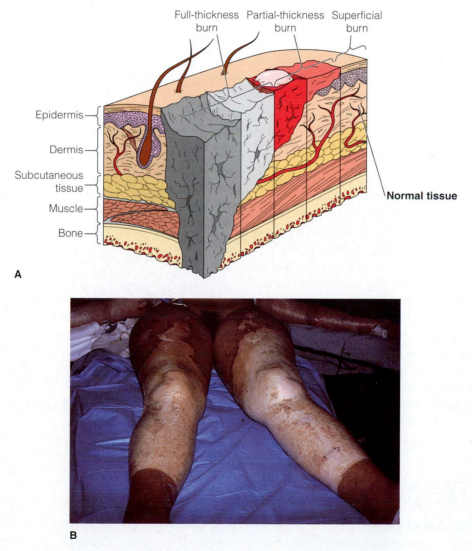

Figure 34-14. ■ A. Burn levels from superficial to full thickness. **B.** Client with a partial-thickness burn.

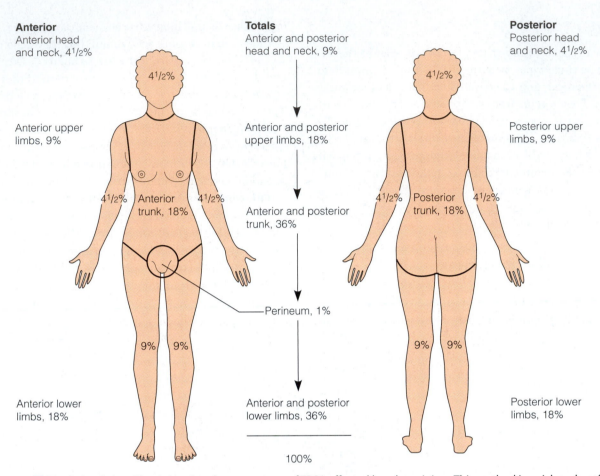

Anterior
Anterior head
and neck, 4¹/₂%

Anterior upper
limbs, 9%

4¹/₂%   Anterior
trunk, 18%   4¹/₂%

Anterior lower
limbs, 18%

Totals
Anterior and posterior
head and neck, 9%

Anterior and posterior
upper limbs, 18%

Anterior and posterior
trunk, 36%

Perineum, 1%

Anterior and posterior
lower limbs, 36%

100%

Posterior
Posterior head
and neck, 4¹/₂%

Posterior upper
limbs, 9%

4¹/₂%   Posterior
trunk, 18%   4¹/₂%

Posterior lower
limbs, 18%

4¹/₂%

9%   9%

4¹/₂%

9%   9%

Figure 34-15. ■ The "rule of nines" for estimating the percentage of TBSA affected by a burn injury. This method is quick and useful in emergency situations, but it is not accurate for short, obese, or very thin adults.

Skin affected by full-thickness burns may not recover from damage. Extensive skin grafting may be required.

The "rule of nines" is a measure of the total body surface area (TBSA) and is used to calculate an approximate percentage amount of burned area. The areas are divided into or are multiples of 9% (Figure 34-15 ■). Full-thickness burns and some partial-thickness burns are assessed and calculated to determine the TBSA involved.

Clients sustaining burns may be transported to a burn unit if the EC staff determines such a move would be beneficial for them. Burn centers specialize in the recovery and rehabilitation of severe burns. Treatment for clients with major burns includes aseptic technique for wound care and protective isolation. Burn centers provide the very specialized care needed to support wound healing, such as removing necrotic tissue (*debridement;* see also Chapter 23 ⊖⊙) and skin grafting.

NURSING CARE

PRIORITIES IN NURSING CARE

When caring for clients with burns, use meticulous aseptic technique to prevent infection. Monitor respiratory status and circulatory status closely, especially if the head and neck

are burned. Take vital signs every 15 to 30 minutes and watch for signs of shock. Administer pain medications as ordered and evaluate their effectiveness. The client with burns is generally in a great deal of pain and does not lose consciousness.

ASSESSING

In clients with burns, especially burns to the face and neck, it is crucial to focus on airway, breathing, and circulation. Increased edema and burns to the airway may be invisible, but they can be life threatening and critical to determine.

DIAGNOSING, PLANNING, AND IMPLEMENTING

Depending on the extent and location of the burn, the following nursing diagnoses might apply to a client with burns:

- *Impaired Skin Integrity*
- *Risk for Infection*
- *Ineffective Airway Clearance*
- *Ineffective Tissue Perfusion*
- *Acute Pain*

- *Deficient Fluid Volume*
- *Imbalanced Nutrition: Less than Body Requirements*
- *Disturbed Body Image*
- *Ineffective Coping*

Outcomes for clients with burns include, but are not limited to, the following:

- Respirations will remain within normal range and clear (**eupneic**).
- O_2 saturation will remain above 95%.
- Pain will be controlled by regularly administered medication.
- Client will maintain weight.
- Client will verbalize feelings about the injury and identify sources of support.

A client with a burn has lost the first line of defense against infection. Depending on the extent of the burn injury, a topical antimicrobial agent (silver nitrate, silver sulfadiazine, or mafenide acetate) and closed dressing may be applied (Figure 34-16 ■).

If the wound area is large, the client is also at risk for loss of fluid and loss of body heat (*Ineffective Thermoregulation*). Damage to tissues may interfere with circulation, leading to loss of fluid and decreased tissue perfusion. Increased demands for nourishment may cause imbalanced nutrition. In addition, the pain, trauma, and visible damage done to the body result in increased stress and psychosocial strain for the client. In the EC or UC setting, the primary concerns are airway, breathing, and circulation.

- In the EC or UC, the nurse's most important interventions support the client's ABCs. *Airway management and securing the airway when burns to the face and neck areas have been sustained are critical.*
- The nurse monitors O_2 administration and saturation whenever there are burns to the face and neck. *Edema and damage to the airway can be life threatening.*

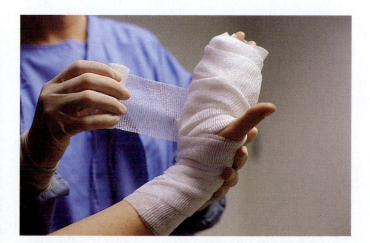

Figure 34-16. ■ Closed method of dressing a burn.

- Monitor IV therapy/lifeline. *A 16- to 18-gauge IV is routinely established in case of third spacing and shock.*
- Take vital signs frequently and monitor LOC for changes. These can be subtle. *The first sign is often missed. Changes may indicate impending shock.*
- Provide clients with sterile blankets or gowns if the percentage of estimated burns is severe and if heat loss occurs. *Full-thickness burn areas have lost the ability to retain or create heat related to the loss of skin; therefore, the nurse must keep the client's body temperature warm.*
- Maintain infection precautions. *The client's first line of defense has been injured or destroyed. Clients with burns are at risk for sepsis, infection, and death.*
- Provide or assist in treatment for minor burns including pain management, anti-infective medications (Silvadene, Flamazine), and wound care for the client (see Figure 34-16). Teaching is an important function in these cases. *The client, parent, or family member must continue treatment until the wound is healed. The nurse plays an important role in teaching the client what normal healing and trouble signs look like. The nurse also provides client education about ways to prevent future injuries.*

EVALUATING

The nurse evaluates the client's status frequently to be sure ABCs are stable. Changes in client condition are always reported stat to the physician.

NURSING PROCESS CARE PLAN
Client with a Burn

Mrs. Tompkins is a 51-year-old client admitted to the EC with burns to the face and neck. The nares (nostrils) are also singed. On review, the client complains of difficulty breathing and severe discomfort to the affected areas.

Assessment. VS: T 98.7, P 100, R 26, BP 110/60. The client is oriented to person, place, and time. Pain is rated an 8 on a scale of 1 to 10.

Nursing Diagnosis. The following important nursing diagnosis (among others) is established for this client:

- *Ineffective Airway Clearance* related to burns to the face, neck, and nares.

Expected Outcomes. The expected outcomes for the plan of care for Mrs. Tompkins are as follows:

- Respirations will remain within normal range.
- O_2 saturation will remain above 95%.
- Breath sounds will be clear and equal to auscultation.
- Pain will be managed at a mild level (i.e., less than a rating of 3).

Planning and Implementation. The following interventions are planned and implemented for Mrs. Tompkins:

- Administer O_2 as ordered; titrate as necessary via non-rebreather mask.
- Monitor respirations every 5 to 10 minutes for acute changes and report.
- Monitor O_2 saturations for changes in conjunction with respiratory rate, and report stat to physician.
- Administer analgesia for pain as ordered.
- Evaluate lung sounds every hour and prn for changes and report.
- Assist ventilation via bag-valve-mask unit if *bradypnea* (low respiration rate) occurs. Notify physician stat.

Evaluation. Client demonstrates ability to maintain safe effective respirations and rate. O_2 saturation level remains greater than 95%. Breath sounds are clear bilaterally. Pain management interventions effective; pain is controlled and reduced to a 2 at this time.

Critical Thinking in the Nursing Process

1. Identify factors that place Mrs. Tompkins at risk for airway ineffectiveness.
2. Discuss why pain management may be indicated with burns to the face and neck. Identify possible medications that may be administered for the client.
3. What are the potential risks Mrs. Tompkins may face during the rehabilitation process with burns to the upper torso? List three nursing diagnoses that may be applicable.

Note: Discussion of Critical Thinking questions appears in Appendix I.

Poisoning

Poisonings require rapid assessment and medical intervention within minutes. Poisoning can occur at any age. Poisons can be introduced into the body by inhalation, ingestion, and absorption and by venomous bites.

One of the primary concerns of assessment is to identify and report the method of exposure. A history of events must be taken and vital signs recorded.

Ingested poisons require rapid removal of the poison by two medications. Syrup of ipecac (for ingested poisons that will not erode the GI tract and that are not petroleum based) is administered by mouth. The standard recommended dose is 15 mL for children ages 1 to 5 and 30 mL for clients older than 6 years of age. Syrup of ipecac induces vomiting, and its administration is followed with large amounts of water. Ipecac is used less today than in the past. Now activated charcoal administration is more common. Activated charcoal is administered for medication overdoses and poisons that can cause esophageal damage if regurgitated. The dosage is normally 50 g by mouth or by nasogastric tube (if needed).

A secondary method for treatment of ingested poisons is gastric lavage. Lavage flushes the GI tract and may evacuate any remaining ingested poison.

Inhaled poisons require treatments with oxygen therapy and airway management.

INJECTED POISONS AND SNAKE BITES

Injected poisons or snake bites are serious situations that require rapid intervention. The source of the bite must be identified immediately if possible. These injuries can cause anaphylactic and respiratory impairment. If snakes bites are poisonous, treatment must focus on airway management and circulatory stabilization of the area of the body. Tourniquets are used to reduce blood flow or circulation to the involved area. However, tourniquets must not cut off circulation to a body part. The nurse should anticipate the need for antivenom and have it ready for use after initial airway stabilization and IV lifeline insertion by the healthcare team.

OTHER CONSIDERATIONS

Other procedures that the LPN/LVN may be required to know include fracture care; assisting with lacerations and stitching; splinting and casting; and measuring for crutches, canes, and walkers. Because a large number of x-rays are taken in the emergency setting, x-ray knowledge and safety are important. See Procedures 34-1 ■ and 34-2 ■.

Note: The references and resources for this and all chapters have been compiled at the back of the book.

PROCEDURE 34-1

PROCEDURE 34-1 Applying a Cast

Note: Cast application will be done by the healthcare provider unless you are specially trained to assist.

Purpose

■ To prepare the materials for casting and application

Equipment

■ Casting material; stockinette; padding, water, protective coverings (if needed)

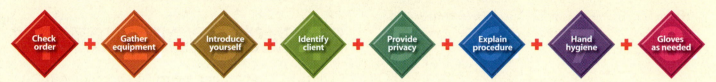

Check order ✛ Gather equipment ✛ Introduce yourself ✛ Identify client ✛ Provide privacy ✛ Explain procedure ✛ Hand hygiene ✛ Gloves as needed

Interventions

1. Determine the type of material the physician or technician will be using.

2. Gather supplies and cover area with protective covering if needed.

3. Position client supporting the extremity to be cast. *Position will be determined by type of cast and area.*

4. Explain the procedure to the client and that the cast may feel warm after application. *So the client will understand what to expect and cooperate.*

5. Assist the physician or technician during application by handing materials and holding the extremity.

6. When completed provide client and family with homecare instructions. *To ensure compliance with treatment plan.*

SAMPLE DOCUMENTATION

[date]
[time]
Short arm fiberglass cast applied to left arm, to treat colles fracture. Home care instruction given. Client to report increased pain, swelling or lack of circulation to physician.
_____ Ronald Smith, LPN

PROCEDURE 34-2 Measuring for Crutches, Canes, and Walkers

Purpose

■ To ensure proper fit for ambulation assistive devices.

Equipment

■ Measuring tape; hard sole street shoes

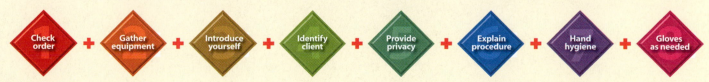

Check order ✛ Gather equipment ✛ Introduce yourself ✛ Identify client ✛ Provide privacy ✛ Explain procedure ✛ Hand hygiene ✛ Gloves as needed

Interventions

CRUTCHES

1. Explain the procedure to the client. *Explanation will help gain cooperation from the client.*

2. Have the client put on the shoes that will be worn when using the crutches. *So that crutches will be the proper length.*

3. Ask client to lay flat in bed with hands at side. *Will permit measuring without having client bear weight.*

4. Measure the distance from the client's axilla to a point 15–20 cm (6–8 in.) out from the heel. *This will determine the length of the crutch.*

5. Adjust the hand bar on the crutches so that the client's elbows are always slightly bent. *This is proper position for the elbows when crutch walking.*

6. Have client stand with crutches under the arm; *in order to check length.*

7. Measure the distance between the client's axilla and the crutch bar. *Crutches that do not fit the client correctly or crutches that are used incorrectly can damage the brachial plexus and cause paralysis of the arms.*

VARIATION FOR CANES

1. One cane *indicated for mild balance problems, fatigue with walking long distances, or increased weakness in one leg.*

2. Two canes *beneficial for further balance problems, or increased weakness in both legs.*

3. Place the device 15.2 cm (6 in.) away from the side of foot and with arm relaxed, adjust the device so it is even with the crease on the inside of the wrist, with a 25° elbow flexion. *To make sure cane fits correctly.*

VARIATION FOR WALKERS

Walkers help with more severe balance problems, progressive leg weakness in one or both legs, or fatigue.

1. Measure a walker in the same manner as a cane. *To provide correct size.*

2. Confer with client and therapist on the appropriate type of walker. *Different types of walkers are prescribed depending on the clients physical needs and environment.*

SAMPLE DOCUMENTATION

[date]
[time]   Crutches measured according to procedure; with client supine and standing. Hand bar adjusted. Crutch bar two finger widths from axilla.
                                    _____ S. Powell, LVN

Chapter Review

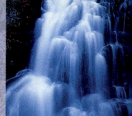

 ## KEY TERMS by Topic

Use the audio glossary feature of either the CD-ROM or the Companion Website to hear the correct pronunciation of the following key terms.

Emergency Care and Urgent Care
emergency care, high acuity, urgent care, phlebotomy

Initial Contact
triage

Initial Protocols
peak flow test, stat

Airway Management
titration, cervical spine alignment, cardiopulmonary resuscitation, defibrillator

Shock
shock, third spacing

Burns
superficial burns, partial-thickness burns, full-thickness burns, eupneic

KEY Points

- Triage is always performed in the EC setting. Triage is used to identify clients who should be treated as a priority. The UC setting generally treats clients on a first-come, first-served basis. The acuity of clients in the UC is less severe.

- The LPN/LVN assists the RN in the treatment and care of clients in the EC setting. The ability of the LPN to perform data collection and assigned nursing interventions is of critical importance. Practical and vocational nurses are a valuable part of the healthcare team within the EC setting.

- Inadequate tissue perfusion is an outcome of all types of shock. Changes in level of consciousness are generally the first sign of impending shock.

- The rule of nines is used in the EC setting to calculate percentage of burns and estimate outcomes.

- The identification of the substance responsible for a poisoning is the primary concern in determining positive treatment and outcomes for clients.

 ## EXPLORE MediaLink

Additional interactive resources for this chapter can be found on the Companion Website at www.prenhall.com/ramont. Click on Chapter 34 and "Begin" to select the activities for this chapter.

For chapter-related NCLEX®-style questions and an audio glossary, access the accompanying CD-ROM in this book.

FOR FURTHER Study

For in-depth details on HIPAA, see Chapter 3.

Documentation methods are discussed in Chapter 6.

Chapter 7 discusses the various types of healthcare systems.

For Standard Precautions, see Figure 9-2. For choking, asphyxiation, and Heimlich maneuver information, see also Chapter 8.

An adult admission form is shown in Figure 10-1, and a consent form for valuables is shown in Figure 10-2.

See Chapter 12 for a discussion of interpersonal communication skills that can ensure the best client outcomes.

The Glasgow Coma Scale is shown in Table 19-2.

For in-depth discussion of disorders of skin, see Chapter 23.

For more on hot/cold packs to an injured area, see Chapter 23.

Ear lavage is described in Chapter 29.

Medication administration is discussed in Chapter 29, and a nomogram is shown in Figure 29-3.

Critical Thinking Care Map

Caring for a Client with Hypovolemia
NCLEX-PN® Focus Area: Physiological Integrity

Case Study: Max Bayer is a 64-year-old male admitted to the EC with excessive nausea, vomiting, and diarrhea for 3 days. He is unable to tolerate PO fluids and is extremely weak with malaise. An IV of 1,000 mL of 0.9 normal saline is infusing via a 16-gauge catheter at 100 mL/h in his left arm.

Nursing Diagnosis: Deficient Fluid Volume

COLLECT DATA

Subjective	Objective
_____	_____
_____	_____
_____	_____
_____	_____
_____	_____
_____	_____

Would you report this data? Yes/No

If yes, to: _____

What would you report? _____

Nursing Care

_____
_____
_____
_____
_____
_____
_____
_____
_____
_____
_____

How would you document this? _____
_____
_____

Compare your documentation to the sample provided in Appendix I.

Data Collected
(use those that apply)

- VS: T 99.2, P 92, R 22, BP 90/58
- "I feel so weak, yet I'm hungry."
- "I'm so worried, my daughter hasn't called all day."
- Skin turgor greater than 3 seconds
- Complains of nausea
- Mucous membranes dry and cracked
- Increased thirst
- K^+ 3.5 mEq/L
- Complains pain at 8 (on a scale of 1 to 10) one-half hour before medication scheduled
- Decreased appetite

Nursing Interventions
(use those that apply; list in priority order)

- Monitor vital signs every 15 min.
- Encourage PO fluids.
- Instruct client on signs/symptoms of dehydration.
- Monitor IV site for infiltration.
- Notify physician regarding K^+ level.
- Administer antiemetics as ordered.
- Notify clergy.
- Assist PT with ambulation.
- Administer high-flow O_2.
- Order chest x-ray stat.
- Record I&O every shift.

NCLEX-PN® Exam Preparation

1 You are the nurse caring for a client in the EC after defibrillation from cardiac dysrhythmia. Which of the following observations is the highest priority for the nurse?

1. O_2 flow rate
2. airway management
3. changes in cardiac rhythm
4. level of consciousness

2 A nurse in the EC is preparing to discharge a client with congestive heart failure. The physician orders digoxin (Lanoxin) daily on discharge. In evaluating the client's level of understanding for the medication ordered, which of the following statements indicates reinforcement teaching is most necessary?

1. "I should call my doctor if my pulse goes above 100 or below 60."
2. "I should keep these pills separate and not mix them with my other medications."
3. "If I forget to take my pill, I'll just take two the next day."
4. "I know to call the doctor if I have any questions."

3 You are the nurse caring for a client with a partial-thickness burn to the face and neck areas. Which of the following is most important in caring for the client?

1. airway management
2. IV lifeline placement
3. sterile dressing application
4. maintenance of protective isolation

4 A 42-year-old female is admitted to the EC with a medication overdose. Vital signs are BP 118/70, P 84, R 20. Which of the following nursing interventions is required next?

1. insertion of a gastric lavage tube
2. identify the medication taken and report
3. administer syrup of ipecac as ordered
4. monitor vital signs for changes

5 You are the nurse caring for a combative, confused client in the EC. The client states he has been consuming alcohol and has a severe headache. The client is demanding pain medication for the headache. Which of the following statements is most appropriate when discussing the plan of care with the client?

1. "You are fourth on the triage list; it'll only be forty-five minutes longer."
2. "I will need to take your vital signs and report to the doctor first."
3. "What type of pain medicine do you normally take?"
4. "I know your headache is causing you discomfort. I will give you your pain medicine as soon as I talk to the doctor."

6 The nurse in the EC is collecting data on a client with heart failure and cardiogenic shock. Which of the following disorders by the client does not play a role in exacerbating the heart failure?

1. recent upper respiratory infection
2. nutritional anemia
3. peptic ulcer disease
4. atrial fibrillation

7 A nurse is caring for a client with full-thickness burns to the lower extremities. Which of the following positions is most appropriate for this type of burn injury?

1. dependent position
2. flat without elevation
3. elevation above the level of the heart
4. elevation of the knee gatched on the bed

8 A family member approaches a nurse to discuss the progress of her aunt who is being seen in the EC. Which of the following responses by the nurse is most appropriate?

1. "I would be glad to discuss this with you later in the shift."
2. "I apologize, but I am not at liberty to discuss your aunt's progress with you."
3. "If you would like to know more, please feel free to ask the physician."
4. "I know this must be difficult for you, but if your aunt agrees, I will share information."

9 A young mother brings her insulin-dependent diabetes mellitus 24-month-old child to the EC. The child is unresponsive. Vital signs are BP 70/40, P 130, R 60. Which of the following nursing interventions should the nurse perform next?

1. Administer high-flow O_2 via nonrebreather.
2. Initiate an IV lifeline.
3. Begin cardiopulmonary resuscitation.
4. Insert a Foley catheter for urine sample.

10 You are the nurse caring for an unresponsive client from a long-term facility. The client has an indwelling catheter; urine output is scant. Vitals reveal BP 100/58, P 62, R 24, and T 99.1°F. The client has recently been treated for a urinary tract infection by the primary physician and has not been feeling well for 5 days. Which of the following types of shock may be considered as evident?

1. hypovolemic
2. cardiogenic
3. septic
4. neurogenic

Answers and Rationales for Review Questions, as well as discussion of Care Plan and Critical Thinking Care Map questions, appear in Appendix I.

Chapter 35

Nursing Care in Ambulatory Settings

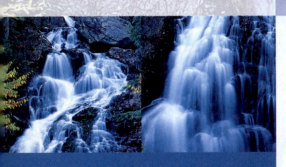

HISTORICAL Perspectives

During the 1940s and 1950s Helen Wells and Julia Tatum developed a series of books for young readers that chronicled the adventures of Cherry Ames. This series told Cherry's story from her days as a student through 25 different settings in which she delivered nursing care. Some of them were adventurous—Cherry Ames' Jungle Nurse—while others were ordinary—Cherry Ames' Rest Home Nurse. No matter what the setting, young future nurses had their horizons expanded as they learned of the many different opportunities nursing presented.

BRIEF Outline

Alternate Care Settings
Other Practice Areas

LEARNING Outcomes

After completing this chapter, you will be able to:

1. Describe the LPN/LVN scope of practice in the ambulatory setting.
2. Discuss reporting structure in an ambulatory setting.
3. Identify nursing responsibilities in planning ambulatory nursing care.
4. Identify HIPAA requirements that impact nursing care in an ambulatory setting.
5. Describe the client admission process in the physician's office or clinic.
6. Identify and describe several ambulatory client care settings.
7. Distinguish between the functions and responsibilities of the LPN/LVN and the medical assistant in the physician's office or clinic.
8. Describe client teaching opportunities in the ambulatory setting.
9. Identify assessment data that should be collected while preparing the client for the physician.
10. Identify additional skills needed to deliver nursing care in an ambulatory setting.

The opportunities for the LPN/LVN to deliver nursing care in alternate settings have increased during the past few years. In the not so distant past, LPN/LVN students could only look forward to jobs in skilled nursing facilities or in medical/surgical units of acute hospitals. Today, with the nursing shortage and higher client acuity, many other opportunities have become available. These practice settings require the ability to think critically and to function at times without direct supervision of a registered nurse. In this chapter you will learn about opportunities to use your nursing skills in alternate settings.

Alternate Care Settings

When **ambulatory care nursing** is considered, the primary location that comes to mind is the physician's office. In addition, you may wish to consider **clinics**, **urgent care offices** (see Chapter 34 🔗 for full coverage of emergency and urgent care nursing), **school health offices**, child and adult daycare, medical research offices, outpatient or **same-day surgery clinics**, cardiac rehab centers, physical and occupational therapy centers, dialysis centers, home care, and traveling and/or companion nursing (Figure 35-1 ■). A description of selected ambulatory settings is provided in Box 35-1 ■.

The scope of practice of LPNs and LVNs in these settings is delineated by the state board of nursing in the state where you are delivering care.

PHYSICIAN'S OFFICE

When the LPN/LVN is employed in a physician's office, he or she will be supervised by the physician or by a registered nurse. In smaller offices, there may not be a registered nurse. A medical assistant should not be given the authority to supervise the licensed nurse. Although the medical assistant may be designated as an office manager, in matters related to client care the LPN/LVN is responsible to the RN or directly to the physician. It is very important that the LPN/LVN understand the scope of practice and adhere to it at all times.

Some of the duties that the LPN/LVN may be called on to perform in the office are:

- Admitting new clients (Procedure 35-1 ■)
- Preparing clients for examination by the physician or nurse practitioner (Procedure 35-2 ■)
- Assisting with diagnostic and surgical office procedures (Procedures 35-3 ■ and 35-7 ■)
- Conducting electrocardiograms (Procedure 35-4 ■)
- Performing venipunctures and other lab tests (Procedures 35-5 ■ and 35-6 ■)
- Splinting (Procedure 35-8 ■).

(Step-by-step procedures appear at the end of this chapter.)

With the exception of the receptionist, the person who escorts the client from the waiting room to the exam room is responsible for the impression the entire experience has on

BOX 35-1

Selected Ambulatory Care Settings

Ambulatory care nursing: care provided to clients in a physician's office or clinic, in which the client obtains some medical service before returning home the same day.

Clinics: walk-in medical facilities where clients can obtain diagnostic testing or treatment before returning home the same day; also known as ambulatory care centers.

Urgent care office: walk-in medical facility where clients can obtain treatment for minor injuries and acute illnesses; they may be connected to or affiliated with a hospital.

School health office: room or area within a school where medications and first aid supplies are kept and distributed by qualified personnel.

Same-day surgery clinic: (also known as an outpatient surgical center): health facility in which the client arrives early in the day, has a surgical procedure, and returns home after he or she is fully recovered from anesthesia.

School-based health clinics: ambulatory care centers, located in a number of intercity school districts, which perform a higher level of care.

Summer day camp: a daytime program for children where LPNs/LVNs may obtain work; staff must be trained in first aid and CPR.

Mental health facility/clinic: medical facilities whose focus is on psychosocial issues and mental health status of its clients.

Adult day care facility: center that provides health and social services to the older adult who is still living at home.

Assisted living facility: facility that meets the needs of the ambulatory older adult; various degrees of personal care assistance may be provided.

Traveling nurse: companion nurse; a licensed nurse who accompanies a client who is traveling, usually for a limited length of time.

Correctional nurse: nurse who provides for the healthcare of inmates in correctional facilities such as juvenile offender homes, jails, prisons, and penitentiaries.

the new client. As a nurse you are responsible for maintaining not only your reputation, but also the reputation of the physician for whom you are working. New clients should always be greeted warmly, using their title and last name. During the admission period you may ask how the client wishes to be addressed. If the client prefers to be addressed less formally, she or he will let you know at that time.

It is common procedure to weigh clients prior to seating them in the exam room. Many clients are self-conscious about their weight. If the scale is in the hallway, be discrete if other staff or clients are in the area.

Although the physician's office may be very busy, when possible take a few minutes to introduce yourself, describe the office, and get to know the new client prior to beginning your assessment. Make the client comfortable and perform as much of the assessment as possible prior to having the client disrobe. This is an important consideration if there may be a delay before the physician sees the client.

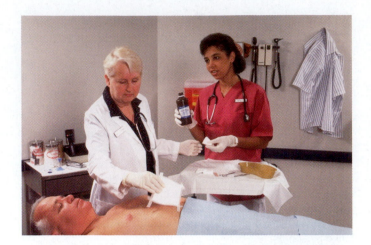

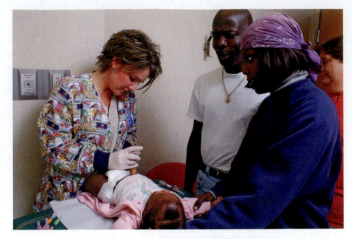

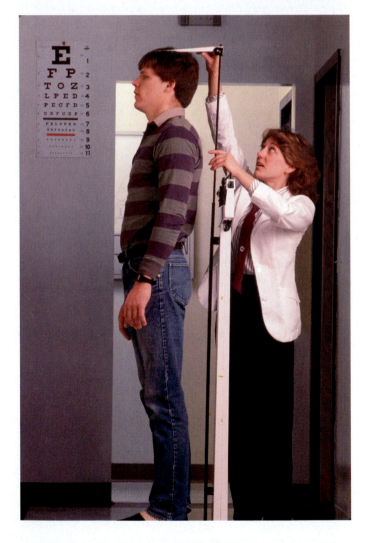

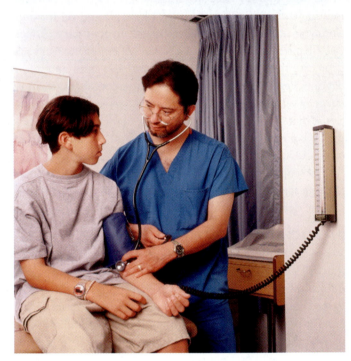

Figure 35-1. ■ Examples of alternate care settings in which LPNs/LVNs can practice.

Once the client has disrobed, be sure to inquire if he or she is warm enough. It the client is cool, provide a blanket.

After the physician has completed the consultation and examination, assist the client to dress if necessary. Be sure that the client has all prescriptions, referrals, and instructions prior to leaving the office.

Follow-Up

It is important that the client be notified of the results of any tests or lab work conducted during the visit. Inform the physician when results have been received. The physician decides who will contact the client with results. If office protocol demands it, the client will be contacted and instructed to make an appointment.

Confidentiality

The LPN/LVN employed in the physician's office must protect the client's privacy. This may be more difficult to ensure than in the hospital setting. Because the waiting room may be small and crowded, it is inappropriate to ask a client questions while standing at the reception window. If the receptionist or billing clerk is overheard discussing treatment or insurance issues where others can overhear the conversation, mention this to the office manager or physician.

HIPAA requirements apply to physicians' offices, just as they do to in-client settings. If you are responsible for calling test results to the client, take care not to leave private information on a home answering machine, on office voice mail, or with another person, not even a family member. If a message must be left, you could say something similar to this: "Mrs. Alvarez, this is Marie. Would you please call me at 555-1345 between 9 A.M. and 5 P.M. concerning your appointment." Be sure to inform the client during the office visit that you will be calling him or her with the results and how you will be leaving the message, so that your call is not confused with a telemarketing call.

OUTPATIENT SURGERY CENTERS

Outpatient or same-day surgery centers have become very popular in many areas of the country. The client arrives early in the morning and returns home after he or she is fully recovered from the anesthesia. Although registered nurses serve as the circulating nurse during surgery and in the postop recovery area, LPNs/LVNs are in demand for the admission area. In some states LPN/LVNs are also trained to assist in surgery as scrub techs.

In the admission area the LPN/LVN would be responsible for completing the admission paper work with the surgical client. (See the perioperative chapter, Chapter 31 ⚭, for an example of a pre-op checklist.) After the client is undressed and wearing the hospital gown, ask the client if he or she needs to use the restroom. The client will then be assisted onto the gurney so that the nurse can obtain vital signs and any other required assessment. Any collected data that is outside the normal parameters should be reported to the charge nurse, anesthesiologist, or surgeon immediately, because surgery may need to be postponed.

The LPN/LVN will also inquire about the last time clients ate or drank and if they have taken any medications this morning. Although the admission area can be fast paced due to the large number of early admissions, it is important that you take time to answer all the client's or family members' questions and inform them of all department procedures. Once the client is ready for surgery, document all of your findings and inform the clerk or transportation that the client is ready.

An LPN/LVN who is hired to work in the surgery suite or recovery area will be given additional training. Check with your state board of nursing to determine if the duties you will be performing are within your scope of practice.

SCHOOL HEALTH OFFICE OR CLINIC

In addition to physician's offices and surgery centers, LPNs/LVNs have been employed as health aides in school health offices or clinics. Many school districts are unable or unwilling to staff the health office at each school with a registered nurse. The district school nurse would serve as the supervisor for the LPN/LVN health aide. The school district will also retain a physician, who will serve as the medical director and will sign protocols for the school health office.

In this capacity the LPN/LVN administers basic first aid and conducts health screenings such as visual acuity tests (Procedure 35-9 ■), hearing tests (Procedure 35-10 ■), and scoliosis screening (Procedure 35-11 ■). (See procedures at the end of the chapter for step-by-step instructions.) He or she would also monitor health records such as immunizations. Having a licensed nurse on campus can offer the opportunity for health teaching for students as well as staff.

Working with minors in a school situation requires extra care in record keeping. A licensed nurse, no matter what the level of education, may not provide even over-the-counter medication to students without parental permission and physician's instructions. The LPN/LVN must follow office protocols that have been set up by the credentialed school nurse. This nurse will supervise the LVN/LPN who is employed as a health clerk or aide. The health aide should always contact the supervising nurse when an issue outside protocol presents itself.

A number of intercity school districts have **school-based health clinics** that perform a higher level of care. In many of these clinics a pediatric nurse practitioner is in charge of the clinic, and he or she follows the standards and protocols set forth by the medical director. When a high school has a health clinic, potential legal and ethical issues can arise. Students relate many of these issues to their involvement in sexual activity. The nurse must be aware of state laws and school district policies for providing information or treatment for sexually transmitted infections and referrals for pregnancy. The adolescent client may confide in the health clinic nurse. This presents ethical issues involving privacy and confidentiality, as well as the need for parent involvement in health issues of a minor.

School health clinic and health office staffs encounter many opportunities for preventive health education for both students and families. Involvement of the family in health education programs can provide a forum for students to communicate with parents on personal health issues they have previously been reluctant to discuss. Many parents do not know how to approach their teen about sexual activity and drug, alcohol, and tobacco use. The school nurse can provide training in this area for parents. The school health staff can be proactive in establishing communication about good health habits in the students and their families.

In addition to first aid services, school health office personnel perform several screenings. These are scheduled during years specified by state law and school regulations.

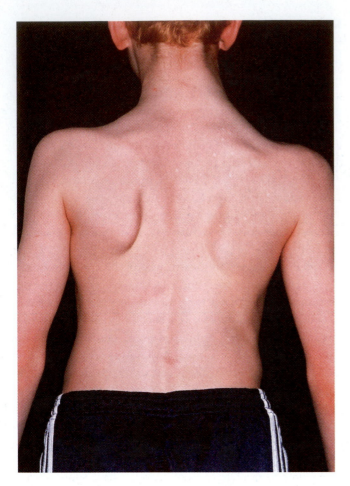

Figure 35-2. ■ Scoliosis.

Scoliosis is a lateral curvature of the spine (Figure 35-2 ■). Eighty-five percent of all cases have an unknown cause and are referred to as *idiopathic scoliosis.* This condition can be detected in children during the growth spurt period between the ages of 10 and 15 years. Girls are affected more often than boys.

About 2 in 100 people have a mild form of scoliosis. Scoliosis can be relatively easily detected by performing a 30-second scoliosis screen. If scoliosis is detected early, then treatment can be started before it becomes a physical or emotional disability. State requirements provide a method to ensure that all school-age children are screened for scoliosis, and to ensure that all children who fail the screening are referred for appropriate medical follow-up.

Screening Program

- *Qualifications of screeners:* Screeners shall be licensed physicians, individuals trained by a certified scoliosis screening instructor. School health personnel, volunteers, and other school employees will not perform scoliosis screening.
- *Guidelines for screening:* Girls in the 5th grade through the 10th grade should receive a scoliosis screening every year. Boys receive a scoliosis screening every other year from the 6th grade through the 10th grade.

- *Screening procedure:* The scoliosis screening procedure is used as the first stage of screening. If the scoliosis screening procedure indicates positive findings for possible scoliosis, the scoliometer will be used as the second stage of screening.
- *Recommendation for referral:* Refer a child with an abnormal screening and/or scoliometer (a device for measuring the amount of abnormal spinal curvature) reading of 7 degrees or more to a licensed physician. It is highly recommended that a child with a scoliometer reading of more than 8 degrees be referred to an orthopedist.
- *Referral system:* A certified scoliosis screening instructor or school health nurse shall contact the parents of a child who fails the screening by letter, telephone call, or in person to:
  1. Explain the findings
  2. Define and discuss scoliosis
  3. Discuss the need for referral to a licensed physician.
- The school provides a scoliosis screening report to the parent to take to the licensed physician. (Regulations of the Commissioner of Education Section 136.1–.3 March 2006)

clinical ALERT

Directions for Use of Scoliometer

An inclinometer (Scoliometer) measures distortions of the torso. The client is asked to bend over, with arms dangling and palms pressed together, until a curve can be observed in the thoracic area (the upper back). The Scoliometer is placed on the back and used to measure the apex (the highest point) of the curve. The client is then asked to continue bending until the curve in the lower back can be seen; the apex of this curve is then measured.

The measurements are repeated twice, with the client returning to a standing position between repetitions. The results of the Scoliometer can indicate problems, and some experts believe it is a useful device for widespread screening. Scoliometers, however, measure rib cage distortions in more than half of children who turn out to have very minor or no sideways curves. Scoliometers are not accurate enough to guide treatment, and, if results show a deformity, x-rays need to be performed.

Follow-Up

Students who were not screened because of absence should be scheduled within 90 days after the missed screening. Any reason for exclusion from the screening is documented. The school shall recontact the parents of students who failed the screening and were referred, but then missed that appointment. This contact is made by letter, telephone call, or in person at least one additional time to discuss the importance of follow-up. Refer to Procedure 35-11 ■ for the screening procedure.

The school nurse or health clerk is also responsible for keeping records of students' immunizations. An immunization record should be on file for each student in the school (Figure 35-3 ■). Students who do not have up-to-date

Vaccine Administration Record for Children and Teens

Client name: _____

Birthdate: _____

Chart number: _____

Vaccine	Type of Vaccine[1] (generic abbreviation)	Date given (mo/day/yr)	Source (F,S,P) [2]	Site[3]	Vaccine		Vaccine Information Statement		Signature/ initials of vaccinator
					Lot #	Mfr.	Date on VIS [4]	Date given [4]	
Hepatitis B[5] (e.g., HepB, Hib-HepB, DTaP-HepB-IPV) Give IM.									
Diphtheria, Tetanus, Pertussis[5] (e.g., DTaP, DTaP-Hib, DTaP-HepB-IPV, DT, Tdap, Td) Give IM.									
Haemophilus influenzae **type b**[5] (e.g., Hib, Hib-HepB, DTaP-Hib) Give IM.									
Polio[5] (e.g., IPV, DTaP-HepB-IPV) Give IPV SC or IM. Give DTaP-HepB-IPV IM.									
Pneumococcal (e.g., PCV, conjugate; PPV, polysaccharide) Give PCV IM. Give PPV SC or IM.									
Rotavirus (Rv) Give oral (po).									
Measles, Mumps, Rubella[5] (e.g., MMR, MMRV) Give SC.									
Varicella[5] (e.g., Var, MMRV) Give SC.									
Hepatitis A (HepA) Give IM.									
Meningococcal (e.g., MCV4; MPSV4) Give MCV4 IM and MPSV4 SC.									
Human papillomavirus (e.g., HPV) Give IM.									
Influenza[5] (e.g., TIV, inactivated; LAIV, live attenuated) Give TIV IM. Give LAIV IN.									
Other									

1. Record the generic abbreviation for the type of vaccine given (e.g., DTaP-Hib, PCV), **not** the trade name.
2. Record the source of the vaccine given as either F (Federally-supported), S (State-supported), or P (supported by Private insurance or other Private funds).
3. Record the site where vaccine was administered as either RA (Right Arm), LA (Left Arm), RT (Right Thigh), LT (Left Thigh), IN (Intranasal), or O (Oral).
4. Record the publication date of each VIS as well as the date it is given to the patient.
5. For combination vaccines, fill in a row for each separate antigen in the combination.

Technical content reviewed by the Centers for Disease Control and Prevention, Nov. 2006.

www.immunize.org/catg.d/p2022b.pdf • Item #P2022 (11/06)

Immunization Action Coalition • 1573 Selby Ave. • St. Paul, MN 55104 • (651) 647-9009 • www.immunize.org • www.vaccineinformation.org

Figure 35-3. ■ Sample immunization record for children and teens. (Courtesy of Immunization Action Coalition, St. Paul, MN.)

TABLE 35-1

Childhood Immunization Schedule

CHILD'S AGE	VACCINE AND DOSE	PROTECTS AGAINSTS
Birth to 2 months	Hepatitis B Dose 1 of 3	Hepatitis B virus (chronic inflammation of the liver, lifelong complications)
1 to 4 months	Hepatitis B Dose 2 of 3	Hepatitis B virus (chronic inflammation of the liver, lifelong complications)
2 months (part of well-baby visit)	DTaP Dose 1 of 5	Diphtheria, tetanus, whooping cough (pertussis)
	Hib Dose 1 of 4	Infections of the blood, brain, joints, or lungs (pneumonia)
	Polio (IPV) Dose 1 of 4	Polio
	Pneumococcal conjugate (PCV7) Dose 1 of 4	Infections of the blood, brain, joints, and inner ear
4 months (part of well-baby visit)	DTaP Dose 2 of 5	Diphtheria, tetanus, whooping cough (pertussis)
	Hib Dose 2 of 4	Infections of the blood, brain, joints, or lungs (pneumonia)
	Polio (IPV) Dose 2 of 4	Polio
	Pneumococcal conjugate (PCV7) Dose 2 of 4	Infections of the blood, brain, joints, and inner ear
6 months (part of well-baby visit)	DTaP Dose 3 of 5	Diphtheria, tetanus, whooping cough (pertussis)
	Hib Dose 3 of 4	Infections of the blood, brain, joints or lungs (pneumonia)
	Pneumococcal conjugate (PCV7) Dose 3 of 4	Infections of the blood, brain, joints, and inner ear
6 to 18 months	Hepatitis B Dose 3 of 3	Hepatitis B virus (chronic inflammation of the liver, lifelong complications)
	Polio (IPV) Dose 3 of 4	Polio
6 to 23 months	Influenza 1 dose every year	Flu and complications
12 to 15 months	Hib Dose 4 of 4	Infections of the blood, brain, joints, or lungs (pneumonia)
	Pneumococcal conjugate (PCV7) Dose 4 of 4	Infections of the blood, brain, joints, and inner ear
	MMR Dose 1 of 2	Measles, mumps, and rubella (German measles)
12 to 18 months	Varicella Dose 1 of 1	Chickenpox
15 to 18 months	DTaP Dose 4 of 5	Diphtheria, tetanus, whooping cough (pertussis)
2 to 5 years	Pneumococcal polysaccharide (PPV23) Dose 1 of 2 (*high risk only*)	Infections of the blood, brain, joints, and inner ear

TABLE 35-1		
Childhood Immunization Schedule (*continued*)		
CHILD'S AGE	**VACCINE AND DOSE**	**PROTECTS AGAINSTS**
5 years through 18 years	Pneumococcal polysaccharide (PPV23) Dose 2 of 2 (follows 3–5 years after dose 1 if needed)	Infections of the blood, brain, joints, and inner ear
2 to 18 years	Hepatitis A Dose 1 of 2	Hepatitis A (inflammation of the liver)
2½ years or older	Hepatitis A Dose 2 of 2 (follows 6 months after dose 1)	Hepatitis A (inflammation of the liver)
4 to 6 years	DTaP Dose 5 of 5	Diphtheria, tetanus, whooping cough (pertussis)
	Polio (IPV) Dose 4 of 4	Polio
	MMR Dose 2 of 2	Measles, mumps, and rubella (German measles)
11 to 12 years	Td booster 1 dose every 10 years	Tetanus and diphtheria

immunizations may be excluded from school. Some students cannot be immunized because of a compromised immune system (e.g., a child receiving chemotherapy). In the event of an identified case of measles, mumps, rubella, or chickenpox, these children would be excluded from school to protect them from exposure and possible health complications. Parents may sign a waiver for their child because of religious reasons or personal objection to immunizations. The school will honor the waiver, but the parents are informed in writing that their child may be excluded from school in the event that their lack of immunizations presents a health risk to students or staff. The American Academy of Pediatrics frequently reviews and updates the immunization schedules. Table 35-1 ■ illustrates such a schedule.

HOME CARE AND HOSPICE

Until a few years ago, home care and hospice agencies would not employee LPNs/LVNs until they had completed 2 or more years of acute hospital experience. The nursing shortage has resulted in some allowances being made in this area. A new graduate may be hired and be given on-the-job training under the direction of a case manager RN. An LPN/LVN with previous experience as a home health aide or a hospice caregiver may have more opportunities to be hired once licensed. Working in home care or home-based hospice care requires the nurse to have well-developed observational and critical thinking skills. Although your case manager is available by phone, home care re-

quires the nurse to assess the client and the situation independently. When a client is admitted to home care or hospice, a registered nurse will make an initial visit to do the admission. An RN case manager will make occasional visits, but regular visits may be assigned to an LPN/LVN or aide to carry out. The decision to assign a licensed nurse rather than a home health aide will be dependent on the level of care required.

The decision to work in hospice is one that needs to be considered carefully. The LPN/LVN working in this area needs to have well-developed communication skills and the ability to provide empathic care in crisis situations. Hospice agencies provide ongoing training and support for staff to assist them to provide quality care to clients who may not have long to live. Hospice care can be given in the client's home, but it can also continue if the client needs to be admitted into a skilled nursing facility. A nurse may see clients in both settings. A client who is eligible for hospice care has been given a terminal diagnosis with a prognosis of 6 months or less. The client's physician will certify the diagnosis and refer the client for admission. For additional information about hospice and end-of-life care, see Chapter 17 ⚭.

Other Practice Areas

Opportunities for LPNs/LVNs to use their skills are varied and interesting. With research and investigation, nurses can find a career opportunity that will interest and excite them. Some of these opportunities are described next.

The **correctional nurse** provides for the health care of inmates in correctional facilities such as juvenile offender homes, jails, prisons, and penitentiaries. An LPN/LVN would work under the supervising correctional nurse who is an RN.

Some of the health problems that will be addressed are trauma, influenza, and chronic health problems, including AIDS, substance abuse, mental illness, renal failure/dialysis, respiratory diseases, and terminal cancer. An LPN/LVN who has been trained to draw blood may be employed in an intake center. A nurse who has a desire to make a difference and establish long-term relationships can be rewarded with client gratitude. The age of the clients can range from young children to older adults.

The presence of guards, difficulty in establishing trust and confidential relationships, and bureaucratic red tape can be frustrating and would be considered the drawbacks of this type of job. An LPN/LVN who has medical-surgical, emergency, and trauma skills and who can function without direct supervision would be a good candidate for this job. Positions as correctional nurses are often appealing to male nurses.

Traveling nurse positions have become available to the LPN/LVN in recent years. Assignments vary in length; the normal assignment is 13 weeks. Traveler assignments can provide the nurse with an opportunity to assess a new location prior to making a commitment for a permanent move. Most traveler nurses do not have family ties or responsibilities, although it could provide an opportunity to be assigned to a location near a family member who is in the military or college. Traveler positions are obtained through employing agencies that provide benefits, relocation expense reimbursement, and a housing allowance. Travel assignments may sound really exciting, but the prospective traveler needs to consider if living and working in an unfamiliar area away from family and friends is desirable.

Adult day care or **assisted living facilities** are not required by law to have a licensed nurse on duty, but many employ LPNs/LVNs to have a qualified person to oversee the health and safety of their clients. A nurse who enjoys interacting with elders would be well suited to such a position.

Summer day camps can be a summer job opportunity for an LPN/LVN who works during the year in a school health office or clinic. Good first aid and CPR skills are a must. Many camps will allow a staff member's children to attend at a reduced rate, so this job could provide a summer income as well as summer activities for the nurse's children.

Some states have licensed psychiatric technicians who are employed **mental health facilities and clinics**. In other locations, other jobs in these facilities are open to LPNs/ LVNs.

Nurses with an interest in psychosocial health care could find working with these clients very rewarding. Mental health nursing courses in LPN/LVN programs are usually not comprehensive enough to prepare the LPN/LVN to work in a psychiatric facility without additional training. Some facilities may provide necessary training. Geropsych (an inpatient specialized unit, normally in a skilled nursing facility, that deals with the multiple aspects of normal and abnormal changes in cognition, personality, well-being, and mental health that occur with aging in the later years of life) units and facilities that care for children with developmental disabilities do have positions for the LPN/LVN. These are attractive positions, especially if they are state-supported institutions, because compensation and medical and retirement benefits are usually excellent.

The LPN/LVN who is considering advancing on the career ladder in the future may feel that acute hospital experience is essential. Opportunities are available although many hospitals are leaning toward all-RN staffs to meet state-imposed nursing ratios. Good experience can be obtained in sub-acute units and skilled nursing facilities that take Medicare clients. Hospital staff mixes change frequently due to supply and demand, so do not become discouraged if that "perfect" job seems to be eluding you as a new graduate. The LPN/LVN has a contribution to make to health care, and there are many opportunities available for the nurse who "looks outside the box" and is willing to stretch a bit and try something new.

NURSING PROCESS CARE PLAN
Same-Day Surgery Client (Postop Cataract Removal, Right Eye)

Dory Page is an 89-year-old female who lives with her husband in a retirement community. They have a homemaker aide four mornings per week to assist with showering, laundry, and light housekeeping. During the week they have senior meals delivered for lunch and dinner. One daughter lives locally, and she assists with shopping on weekends and takes them out for meals when they are up to it.

Mrs. Page also has a cataract on her left eye that will be removed surgically at a later date. Her daughter is present for discharge instructions and will provide transportation home.

Assessment. VS: T 97.8, P 84, R 28, BP 132/88. She is awake and stable. An eye patch/shield is in place over right eye. She has been up to the bathroom and has eaten half a sandwich and a cup of tea. Client has no c/o of pain. She is now ready for her instructions and discharge.

Nursing Diagnosis. The following important nursing diagnoses (among others) are established for this client:

- *Ineffective Coping* related to surgical experience
- *Risk for Injury* related to visual impairment
- *Deficient Knowledge* regarding home care related to unfamiliarity with information.

Expected Outcomes. The expected outcomes for the plan of care are as follows:

- Demonstrates knowledge of psychological responses to surgical procedures.
- Free from signs and symptoms of physical injury.
- Communicates purpose, dosage, route, and possible side effects of medication; provides return demonstration on proper medication administration; communicates proper storage of medication.
- Communicates concerns related to surgical procedure, next planned visit to healthcare provider, goals in realistic terms, sequence of postoperative events, and activities related to her care.
- Communicates sequences of wound healing related to surgical procedure; concerns about healing, dressing care, and wound management techniques; and goals of wound healing.

Planning and Implementation. The following nursing interventions are planned and implemented for Mrs. Page:

- Assess coping mechanisms based on psychological status.
- Identify individual's values and wishes concerning care.
- Note the following sensory impairments: Ask what the client can see with each eye. Implement protective measures to prevent injury. Orient the client to the environment and remove potential hazards.

- Evaluate environment for home care.
- Identify potential hazards such as throw rugs or extension cords and instruct family member to remove them.
- Provide instructions about prescribed medications.
- Identify expectations for home care; leave eye shield in place for 12 to 18 hours; put nothing into the eye unless instructed by surgeon; have companion stay with client; and contact physician if vision, pain, or nausea worsens or if vomiting occurs.
- Evaluate response to instructions.

Evaluation. Mrs. Page returns to the surgeon's office on the morning following surgery. She is free of any signs and symptoms of physical injury. She demonstrates proper procedures for instilling medication into eye and doing the dressing change. She demonstrates no psychological reaction to surgical procedure and is looking forward to having the other cataract removed, since her vision in her right eye has been poor since she was a child.

Critical Thinking in the Nursing Process

1. Discuss reasons for avoiding general anesthesia in a client of Mrs. Page's age.
2. Provide Mrs. Page and her daughter with discharge instructions for cataract removal.
3. Why was it recommended to first remove the cataract in the eye with the poorest vision?

Note: Discussion of Critical Thinking questions appears in Appendix I.

Note: The references and resources for this and all chapters have been compiled at the back of the book.

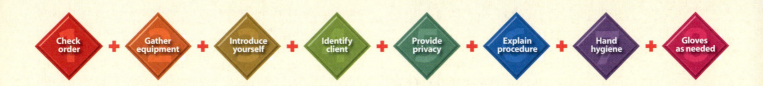

PROCEDURE 35-1	**Admitting a New Client**

Purpose

■ To complete a medical history form and gather necessary information for the physician

Equipment

■ Medical history form
■ Black and red pen
■ Vital sign equipment

Check order + Gather equipment + Introduce yourself + Identify client + Provide privacy + Explain procedure + Hand hygiene + Gloves as needed

Interventions

1. Gather supplies. *In order to not interrupt the procedure once it has begun.*

2. Review medical history form and client's chart. *Be familiar with the order of the questions and the type of information required and the information already given by the client, in order to facilitate communication.*

3. Escort the client to a private, comfortable area (Figure 35-4 ■). *A private place prevents distractions and ensures confidentiality for the client.*

4. Sit across from the client at eye level and make frequent eye contact. *Standing above the client may be perceived as threatening and hinder communication.*

5. Introduce yourself and explain the purpose of the interview. *This will establish a professional rapport with the client.*

6. Using language that the client can understand, ask appropriate questions and document the responses. *To obtain complete information for physician.*

7. Listen actively and look at the client when he or she is speaking. *Client can sense when the nurse is not listening, so be sure to show interest in what the client is saying.*

8. Regardless of the confidence the client shares, avoid displaying a judgmental attitude with words or actions. *Maintains professionalism and ensures the client's trust.*

9. Using open-ended questions, determine why the client is seeking medical care. *This will allow the client to explain his or her chief complaint (CC) in his or her own words.*

10. Determine the present illness (PI) using open-ended and closed-ended questions. *Use closed-ended questions to obtain specific data only after the client has responded to open-ended questions.*

11. Obtain client's vital signs (see Procedures 20-1 through 20-4 for complete steps.)

12. Document the CC, PI, and complete vital signs on the progress sheet in the client's chart. *Documentation should include date, time, CC, PI, TPR, BP, weight, and any other information obtained from the client and your signature and title. Use correct medical terminology and approved abbreviations.*

13. Thank the client for cooperating and explain that the physician will be in shortly to examine the client. *Courtesy encourages a positive attitude about the office. If you indicate a time frame in reference to the physician coming into the examination room, be honest.*

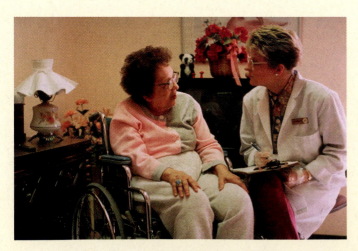

Figure 35-4. ■ Nurse conducting a client interview in a private place.

PROCEDURE 35-2

Preparing a Client for Examination by the Physician or Nurse Practitioner

Purpose

- To prepare the client for examination

Equipment

- Stethoscope
- Ophthalmoscope
- Otoscope
- Penlight
- Tuning fork
- Nasal speculum
- Tongue blade
- Percussion hammer
- Gloves
- Client gown and draping

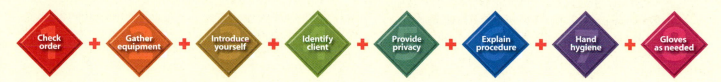

Check order + Gather equipment + Introduce yourself + Identify client + Provide privacy + Explain procedure + Hand hygiene + Gloves as needed

Interventions

1. Perform hand hygiene. *To aid in infection control.*

2. Prepare the examination room and assemble the equipment (Figure 35-5 ■). *A clean room free of contamination prevents transfer of microorganisms.*

3. Greet the client by name and escort him or her to the examination room. *Identifying the client by name prevents errors.*

4. Explain the procedure. *To reduce anxiety and help ensure compliance.*

5. Obtain and record the medical history and chief complaint. *To provide information for the examiner.*

6. Take and record vital signs, height, weight, and visual acuity. *The vital signs and other measurements give the examiner an overall picture of the client's health.*

7. If the physician requires it, instruct the client in the correct method of obtaining a urine specimen, then escort the client to the bathroom. *Even if the urine specimen is not a part of the physical examination, an empty bladder makes the abdominal examination more comfortable.*

8. Once the client has returned from the bathroom, instruct him or her in disrobing and how to put on the gown (open in the front or back). Leave the room while the client disrobes unless he or she needs assistance. *The gown must be open in the direction that provides accessibility for the examination. Older people and people with disabilities may need help disrobing and putting on the gown.*

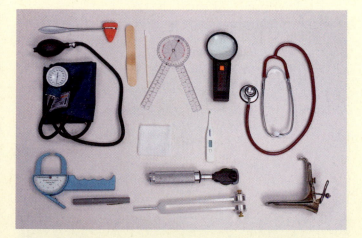

Figure 35-5. ■ Common equipment used in an adult physical examination.

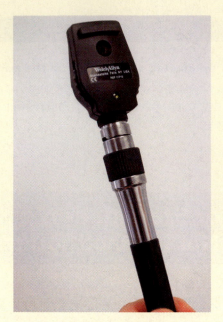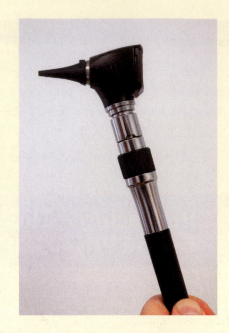

Figure 35-6. ■ Otoscope and ophthalmoscope.

9. Help the client sit on the end of the exam table and cover lap and legs with the drape. *The sitting position is often the first position used by the examiner.*

10. Place the medical record outside the examination room and notify the physician or RN practitioner that the client is ready. *Alerting the examiner helps prevent delays.*

11. Assist the examiner by handing him or her the instruments as needed and positioning the client appropriately. *Anticipating the examiner's needs promotes efficiency and saves time.*
    ■ Begin by handing the physician the instruments necessary for examining the following:
    a. Head and neck—stethoscope
    b. Eyes—ophthalmoscope (Figure 35-6 ■) penlight
    c. Ears—otoscope (see Figure 35-6), tuning fork, audioscope
    d. Nose—penlight, nasal speculum
    e. Sinuses—penlight
    f. Mouth—tongue blade, penlight
    Hand over the tongue blade holding it in the middle. When it is returned to you, grasp it in the middle again so that you do not touch the end that was in the client's mouth.
    g. Throat—gloves, tongue blade, laryngeal mirror, penlight
    Only the part of the body being examined should be exposed. Always preserve the clients' privacy and keep them covered as much as possible.
    ■ Help the client drop the gown to the waist for the examination of the chest and upper back. Hand the examiner the stethoscope.
    ■ Help the client to pull up the gown and remove the drape from the legs so the examiner can test reflexes. Hand the examiner the reflex hammer.

■ Help the client to lie supine, opening the gown at the top to expose chest again. Place the drape to cover the waist, abdomen, and legs. Hand the physician the stethoscope.
■ Cover the client's chest and lower the drape to expose the abdomen. Hand the physician the stethoscope.
■ Assist with the genital and rectal examinations. Hand the client a tissue following the examinations. *Tissue may be used to wipe off excessive lubricant.*

For Females
a. Assist the client to the lithotomy position and drape appropriately.
b. For examination of the genitalia and internal reproductive organs, provide a glove, lubricant, speculum (Figure 35-7 ■), microscope, slide or prep solution, and spatula or brush.
c. For the rectal exam, provide a glove, lubricant, and fecal occult blood test slide.

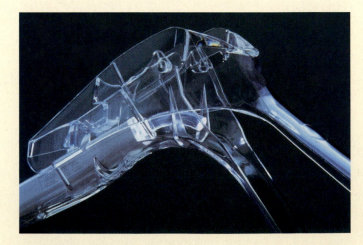

Figure 35-7. ■ Vaginal specula.

For Males

   a. Help the client to stand and have him bend over the examination table for a rectal and prostate examination.
   b. For a hernia examination, provide a glove.
   c. For a rectal examination, provide a glove, lubricant, and fecal occult blood test slide.
   d. For a prostate examination, provide a glove and lubricant.

   ■ With the client standing, the examiner can assess legs, gait, coordination, and balance.

12. Help the client sit on the edge of exam table. *The physician often discusses findings with the client at this time and may provide instructions.*

13. Perform any follow-up procedures and treatments.

14. Leave the room while the client dresses unless the client needs assistance. *Leaving the room provides privacy for the client.*

15. Return to the examination room when the client has dressed to answer any questions, reinforce instructions, and provide client education. *Compliance depends on full understanding of the treatment plan. Client education is the responsibility of all healthcare workers.*

16. Escort the client to the front desk. *You can clarify the appointment scheduling or billing issues.*

17. Properly clean or dispose of the equipment and supplies. Clean the room with a disinfectant and prepare for the next client. *All instruments, supplies, and equipment that came into direct contact with the client must be appropriately decontaminated or disposed.*

18. Perform hand hygiene and record any instructions from the physician. Also note any specimens and indicate the results of the tests or the laboratory where the specimens are being sent for testing. *Procedures and instructions are considered not to have been done if they are not recorded.*

SAMPLE DOCUMENTATION

[date] CC Annual physical examination
[time] completed per Dr. Chung. ECG done; results given to Dr. Chung. Blood drawn and sent to Merric lab for CBC, electrolytes, and liver panel. Instructed to return to the office in 3 weeks to discuss the results of the laboratory tests. Given written and verbal instructions regarding 1,800-calorie, low-sodium diet to follow as ordered by Dr. Chung; verbalized understanding.

_____ C. Ames, LVN

PROCEDURE 35-3 # Assisting with Office Surgical Procedures

Purpose

■ To prepare for and assist with procedure while maintaining sterile technique

Equipment

At-the-side equipment:

■ Sterile gloves
■ Local anesthetic
■ Antiseptic wipes
■ Adhesive tape
■ Specimen container
■ Completed laboratory request

Sterile field containing:

■ Basin for solutions
■ Gauze sponges and cotton
■ Antiseptic solution
■ Sterile drape
■ Dissecting scissors
■ Disposable scalpel
■ Blade of physician's choice
■ Mosquito forceps
■ Tissue forceps
■ Needle holder
■ Suture and needle of physician's choice

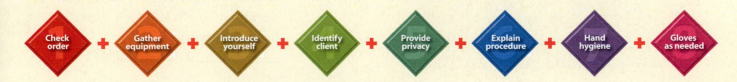

Check order + Gather equipment + Introduce yourself + Identify client + Provide privacy + Explain procedure + Hand hygiene + Gloves as needed

Part A: Excisional Surgery

Interventions

1. Perform hand hygiene. *To aid in infection control.*

2. Assemble equipment. *To ensure that everything will be available for the physician.*

3. Greet and identify client, explain procedure, and answer any questions. *This prevents errors in treatment, helps gain compliance, and eases anxiety.*

4. Set up a sterile field on a surgical stand with the at-the-side equipment close at hand. *Keeps sterile items separate and all items within easy reach.*

5. Position the client appropriately. *The required position depends on the location of the lesion.*

6. Put on sterile gloves or use sterile transfer forceps and cleanse the client's skin. *The antiseptic discourages the entrance of microorganisms into the wound. After cleansing skin, remove the gloves if used and perform hand hygiene.*

7. The physician will perform the procedure. You may be asked to assist by adding supplies as needed, watching closely for opportunities to assist the physician and comforting the client. *It is not necessary for you to wear sterile gloves during the procedure unless the physician requires you to handle sterile instruments or supplies.*

8. For lesions being referred to pathology for analysis, assist with collecting the specimen in the appropriate container. *Always follow Standard Precautions, wearing examination gloves when handling specimens. Have the container ready to receive the specimen.*

9. At the end of the procedure, perform hand hygiene and dress wound using sterile technique (according to Procedure 23-1). *The wound must be covered to protect the incision from contamination.*

10. Thank the client and give appropriate instructions for care of the operative site, changing the dressing, postoperative medications, and follow-up visits as ordered by the physician. *Courtesy encourages the client to have a positive attitude about the physician's office, and giving necessary instruction will ensure compliance from the client.*

11. Don gloves. Clean the examination room in preparation for the next client. Discard all used disposable items in appropriate biohazard containers. Return unused items to their proper place. Remove gloves and perform hand hygiene. *Standard Precautions must be followed.*

12. Record the procedure. *Procedures must to be documented to be considered done. Documentation of the procedure requires postoperative vital signs, care of the wound, instructions on postoperative care, and processing of any specimens.*

Part B: Incision and Drainage (I&D)

Additional Equipment

- Packing gauze
- Cultural tube
- Probe
  (Figure 35-8 ■)

Interventions

Follow the steps for excisional surgery. After the procedure the wound must be covered to avoid further contamination and to absorb drainage. The exudate is a hazardous body fluid requiring Standard Precautions.

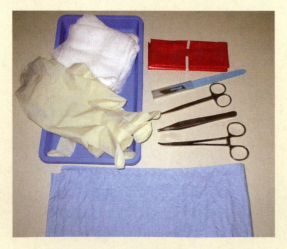

Figure 35-8.   ■ I&D surgical tray set up.

PROCEDURE 35-4

Performing a 12-Lead Electrocardiogram

Purpose

- To prepare client for and obtain a 12-lead ECG that is free of artifacts

Equipment

- ECG machine with cable and lead wires
- ECG paper
- Disposable electrodes that contain coupling gel
- Gown and drape
- Skin preparation materials including razor and antiseptic wipes

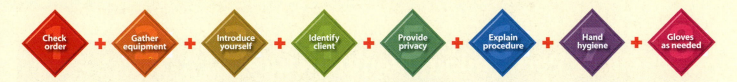

Check order + Gather equipment + Introduce yourself + Identify client + Provide privacy + Explain procedure + Hand hygiene + Gloves as needed

Interventions

1. Perform hand hygiene. *To aid in infection control.*

2. Assemble equipment.

3. Greet and identify the client. Explain the procedure. Ask for and answer any questions. *Identifying the client prevents errors. Explaining the procedure will relieve anxiety and ensure compliance.*

4. Turn the machine on and enter appropriate data, including the client's name and/or identification number, age, sex, height, weight, blood pressure, and medications. *Information will assist the physician in determining a proper diagnosis.*

5. Instruct the client to disrobe above the waist and provide a gown for privacy. Female client should also be instructed to remove any nylons or tights. *Clothing may interfere with proper placement of the leads. Clients wearing pants do not have to remove them if they can be pulled up to expose the lower legs.*

6. Position the client comfortably supine with pillows as needed for comfort. Drape the client for warmth and privacy. *If the client is uncomfortable, too cool, or improperly draped, movement is likely, which will result in artifacts on the ECG tracing.*

7. Prepare the skin as needed by wiping away skin oils or lotions with antiseptic wipes or shaving any hair that will interfere with good contact between the skin and the electrodes. *Skin preparation ensures properly attached leads and helps avoid improper readings and lost time repeating the test.*

8. Apply electrodes snugly against the fleshy, muscular part of the upper arms and lower legs according to the manufacture's directions. Apply the chest electrodes, V_1 through V_6. Electrodes that are not snug against the skin or are on bony prominences may cause improper reading

and artifacts. *In case of an amputation or otherwise inaccessible limb, place the electrode on the uppermost part of the existing extremity or on the anterior shoulder (upper extremity) and groin (lower extremity).*

9. Connect the lead wires securely according to the color-coded notations on the connectors (RA, LA, RL, LL, V_1–V_6). Untangle the wires before applying them to prevent electrical artifacts. Each lead must lie unencumbered along the contours of the client's body to decrease the likelihood of artifacts. Double check placement. *Improperly placed leads will result in time lost to an inaccurate reading and retesting.*

10. Determine the sensitivity, or gain, and the paper speed settings on the ECG machine before running the test. Set sensitivity or gain on 1 and paper speed on 25 mm/second. *A sensitivity setting of 1 and a paper speed of 25 mm/second are necessary to obtain an accurate ECG. These settings should not be changed without a direct order from the physician and the changes noted on the ECG tracing.*

11. Depress the automatic button on the machine to obtain the 12-lead tracing. The machine will automatically move from one lead to the next without your intervention. *If the physician wants only a rhythm strip tracing, use the manual mode of operation and select the lead manually.*

12. When the tracing is complete and printed, check the ECG for artifacts and a standardization. *With sensitivity set on 1, the standardization mark should be 2 small squares wide and 10 small squares high. The standardization mark documents accuracy of operation and provide reference points.*

13. If the tracing is adequate, turn off the machine and remove and discard the electrodes. Assist the client to a sitting position and help with dressing if needed. *Some clients become dizzy while lying supine.*

14. If a single-channel machine was used (each lead produced on a roll of paper, one lead at a time), carefully roll the ECG strips without using clips to secure the roll. The ECG must be mounted on 8½ × 11-inch paper or a form before going into the medical record according to the office policy and procedure. *Folding the ECG tracing or applying clips may make marks on the surface, obscuring the reading. Special forms may be purchased specifically for mounting a single-channel ECG strip and placing it in the medical record.*

15. Record the procedure in the client's medical record. *Procedures need to be documented in order to be considered done.*

16. Place the ECG tracing and the client's medical record on the physician's desk or give to the physician directly, as instructed.

SAMPLE DOCUMENTATION

[date]
[time]   Pre-op 12-lead ECG obtained and placed in chart. Given to Dr. Crane for evaluation. Discharged, no fol-low-up required at this time.
_____ S. Tensor, LPN

PROCEDURE 35-5   Performing a Venipuncture

Purpose

■ To obtain blood for diagnostic purposes and/or monitoring prescribed treatment

Equipment

■ Needle
■ Syringe and test tubes or evacuated tubes
■ Tourniquet
■ Sterile gauze pads
■ Bandages
■ Needle adapter
■ Sharps container
■ 70% alcohol pad or other antiseptic
■ Permanent marker or pen
■ Appropriate biohazard barriers (e.g., gloves, impervious gown, face shields)

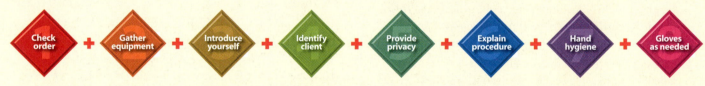

Check order + Gather equipment + Introduce yourself + Identify client + Provide privacy + Explain procedure + Hand hygiene + Gloves as needed

Interventions

1. Check the requisition slip to determine the tests ordered and specimen requirements. *To ensure proper specimen collection.*

2. Perform hand hygiene. *To aid in infection control.*

3. Assemble the equipment (Figures 35-9 ■ and 35-10 ■). Check expiration dates on the tubes. *To have all equipment close at hand. Expired tubes may not have a vacuum; additives may no longer be functional.*

4. Greet and identify the client. Explain the procedure. Ask for and answer any questions. *Identifying the client prevents errors. Explaining the procedure will relieve anxiety and ensure compliance.*

5. If a fasting specimen is required, ask the client the last time he or she ate. *For fasting specimens, client should not have eaten within 8 hours.*

6. Don nonsterile latex or vinyl gloves. *Standard Precautions must be followed. Determine if client has latex allergy; if so, use vinyl gloves and nonlatex tourniquet.*

7. Break the seal of the needle cover and thread the sleeved needle into the adapter, using the needle cover as a wrench (Figure 35-11 ■). Tap the tubes that contain additives to ensure that additive is dislodged from the stopper and wall of the tube. Insert the tube into the adapter until the needle slightly enters the stopper. Do not push the top of the tube stopper beyond the indentation mark. If the tube retracts slightly, leave it in the retracted position. If using a syringe, tighten the needle on the hub and breathe the syringe. *This ensures proper needle placement and tube positioning and prevents loss of vacuum in the evacuated tube or sticking of the plunger in the barrel of the syringe.*

8. Instruct the client to sit with a well-supported, straight arm and apply a tourniquet.
   ■ Apply the tourniquet around the client's arm 7.62–10.16 cm (3 to 4 in.) above the elbow (Figure 35-12 ■).

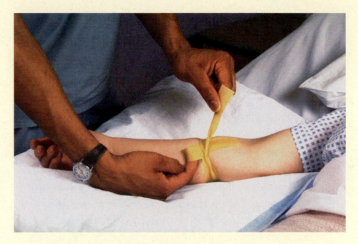

Figure 35-12. ■ Proper application of a tourniquet.

- Apply the tourniquet snugly, but not too tightly.
- Secure the tourniquet by using the half-bow knot.
- Make sure the tails of the tourniquet extend upward to avoid contaminating the venipuncture site.
- Ask the client to make a fist and hold it but not to pump the fist.

Veins in the antecubital fossa are most easily located when the arm is straight. The tourniquet makes the veins more prominent. Making a fist raises the vessels out of the underlying tissue and muscles.

9. Select a vein by palpating. Use your gloved index finger to trace the path of the vein and judge the depth. *The index finger is the most sensitive finger for palpating.*

10. Release the tourniquet after palpating the vein if it has been left on for more than 1 minute. *The tourniquet should not be left on for more than 1 minute at a time during the procedure.*

11. Cleanse the venipuncture site with an alcohol pad, starting in the center of the puncture site and working outward in a circular motion. Allow the site to dry or dry the site with sterile gauze. Do not touch the area after cleansing. *The circular motion helps avoid recontamination of the area. Puncturing a wet area stings and can cause hemolysis of the sample.*

12. If the blood drawn for culture will be used in diagnosing a septic condition, make sure the specimen is sterile. To do this, apply a 2% iodine solution in a wider circle. Never move the wipe back over the areas that have been cleansed; use a new wipe for each sweep across the area. *Ensuring sterility of the specimen will aid accurate diagnosis.*

13. Reapply the tourniquet if it was removed after palpation. Ask client to make a fist. *Tourniquet time greater than 1 minute may alter findings.*

14. Remove the needle cover. Hold the syringe or assembly in your dominant hand, thumb on top of the adapter and fingers under it. Grasp the client's arms with the other hand, using your thumb to draw the skin taut over the site. This anchors the vein about 2.54–3.08 cm (1 to 2 in.) below

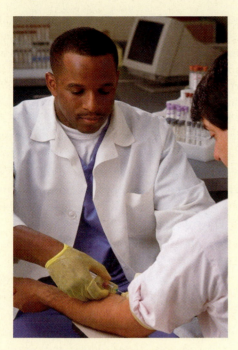

Figure 35-9. ■ Office blood drawing station.

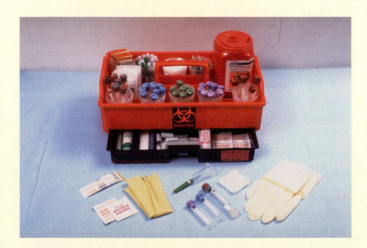

Figure 35-10. ■ Venipuncture equipment and supplies.

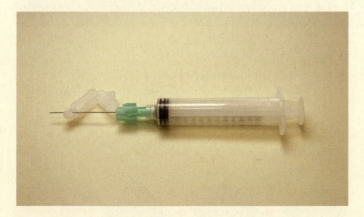

Figure 35-11. ■ Safety needle attached to syringe.

the puncture site and helps keep it in place during needle insertion. *Anchoring the vein allows for easier needle penetration.*

15. With the bevel up, line up the needle with the vein approximately one-quarter to half an inch (.14–1.27 cm) below the site where the vein is to be entered. At a 15- to 30-degree angle, rapidly and smoothly insert the needle through the skin. Remove your nondominant hand and slowly pull back the plunger of the syringe. Or place two fingers on the flanges of the adapter and with the thumb push the tube onto the needle inside the adapter. When the blood begins to flow into the tube or syringe, release the tourniquet and allow the client to release the fist. Allow the syringe or the tube to fill to capacity. When blood flow ceases, remove the tube from the adapter by gripping the tube with your nondominant hand and place your thumb against the flange during removal. Twist and gently pull out the tube. Steady the needle in the vein. Try not to pull up or press down on the needle while it is in the vein. Insert any other necessary tubes into the adapter and allow each to fill to capacity. *The sharpest point of the needle is inserted first. Proper tube filling ensures correct ratio of blood additive. Removal of tourniquet releases pressure on the vein and helps prevent blood from seeping into adjacent tissues and causing a hematoma.*

16. Remove the needle from the arm.
    - Place sterile gauze pad over the puncture site at the time of needle withdrawal. Do not apply pressure to the site until the needle is completely removed.
    - After the needle is removed, apply pressure or have the client apply direct pressure for 3 to 5 minutes. Do not bend the arm at the elbow.

    Removing the last tube from the adapter before removing the needle from the vein prevents any excess blood from dripping from the tip of the needle onto the client. Pressure decreases the amount of the blood escaping into the tissues. Bending the arm increases the chance of blood seeping into subcutaneous tissue.

17. Transfer the blood from a syringe into the tubes in the proper order of draw via the transfer device and allow the vacuum to fill the tubes. Do not hold the tube while using the transfer device; place it in a tube rack and carefully insert the device through the stopper. If the vacuum tube contains an anticoagulant, they must be mixed immediately by gently inverting the tube 8 to 10 times. Do not shake the tube. Label the tubes with the proper information. *Mixing anticoagulated tubes prevents clotting of the blood. Proper labeling of blood specimens avoids mixup of samples.*

18. Check the puncture site for bleeding. Apply a dressing (a clean 2 × 2 gauze pad folded in quarters) held in place by an adhesive bandage or 7.62 cm (3-in.) strip of tape.

19. Thank the client. Instruct the client to leave the bandage in place at least 15 minutes and not to carry a heavy object (such as a purse) or lift heavy objects with the arm for 1 hour. *Courtesy helps the client have a positive attitude about the procedure and the physician's office.*

20. Properly care for or dispose of all equipment and supplies. Clean the work area. Remove gloves and perform hand hygiene. *Standard Precautions must be followed throughout the procedure to prevent the spread of microorganisms.*

21. Test, transfer, or store the blood specimen according to the medical office policy.

22. Record the procedure. *In order for procedures to be considered done they must be documented.*

SAMPLE DOCUMENTATION

[date]   OP venipuncture for platelet count,
[time]   dx code ###. ## per Dr. Whiteman
           _____ J. Simpson, LVN

PROCEDURE 35-6

Obtaining a Capillary Blood Sample by Skin Puncture

Purpose

- To obtain blood for diagnostic purposes and/or monitoring of prescribed treatment

Equipment

- Sterile disposable lancet or automated skin puncture device
- 70% alcohol or other antiseptic
- Sterile gauze pad
- Micro-collection tubes or containers
- Heel-warming device (when obtaining sample from the heel of an infant)
- Appropriate biohazard barriers (gloves, gown, face shield, sharps container)

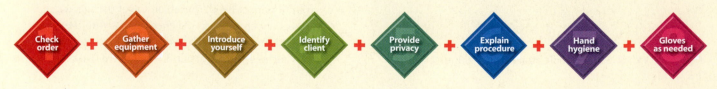
Check order + Gather equipment + Introduce yourself + Identify client + Provide privacy + Explain procedure + Hand hygiene + Gloves as needed

Interventions

1. Check the requisition slip to determine the test to be performed and specimen requirements. *This ensures proper specimen collection.*

2. Perform hand hygiene. *To aid in infection control.*

3. Assemble equipment. *Having equipment ready will speed collection so that the blood does not clot before the entire specimen has been collected.*

4. Greet and identify the client. Explain the procedure. Ask for and answer any questions. *Identifying the client prevents errors. Explaining the procedure helps ease anxiety and ensures compliance.*

5. Don gloves. *Standard Precautions must be observed.*

6. Select the puncture site (the lateral portion of the tip of the middle or ring finger of the nondominant hand; lateral curved surface of the heel or the great toe of an infant). The puncture should be made in the fleshy central portion of the second or third finger, slightly to the side of center, and perpendicular to the whorls of the fingerprint (Figure 35-13 ■). Perform heel puncture only on the plantar surface of the heel, medial to an imaginary line extending from the middle of the great toe to the heel, and lateral to an imaginary line drawn from between the fourth and fifth toes to the heel (Figure 35-14 ■). *Note:* When using heel of infant, apply a warm washcloth or heel warmer to the heel 10–15 minutes prior to procedure to stimulate blood flow. Use the appropriate puncture device for the site selected (Figure 35-15 ■). *The ring and middle finger are less calloused then the forefinger. The lateral tip is the least sensitive part of the finger. A puncture made across the fingerprints will produce a round, large drop of blood. In an infant skin puncture, the area and the depth designed reduce the risk of puncturing the bone.*

7. Make sure the site selected is warm and not cyanotic or edematous. Gently massage the finger from the base to the

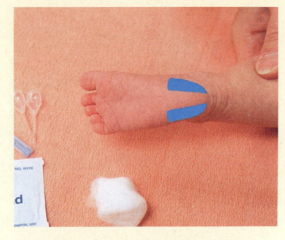

Figure 35-14. ■ Acceptable areas for heel puncture on newborns.

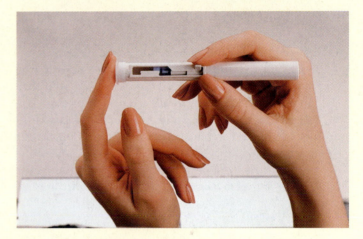

Figure 35-15. ■ Finger puncture lancets. Client obtained self sample.

tip. *Massaging the area increases the blood flow. Good circulation at the chosen site yields a better blood sample for analysis.*

8. Grasp the finger firmly between your nondominant index finger and thumb, or grasp the infant's heel firmly with your index finger wrapped around the foot and your thumb wrapped around the ankle. Cleanse the selected area with 70% isopropyl alcohol and wipe dry with a sterile gauze pad or allow to air dry. *Maintaining your hold at the site prevents the client from contaminating the cleansed puncture area and allows you to have control of the puncture site. The area must be dry to eliminate alcohol residue, which can cause the client discomfort and interfere with test results.*

9. Hold the client's finger or heel firmly and make a swift, firm puncture. Perform the puncture perpendicular to the whorls of the fingerprint or footprint. Dispose of the used puncture device in a sharps container (Figure 35-16 ■).
   - Wipe away the first drop of blood with sterile dry gauze (Figure 35-17 ■). *The first discarded drop may be contaminated with tissue fluid or alcohol residue.*
   - Apply pressure toward the site but do not milk the site. *Milking the site will dilute the specimen with tissue fluid.*

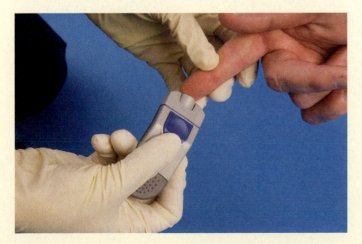

Figure 35-13. ■ Recommended site and direction of finger puncture.

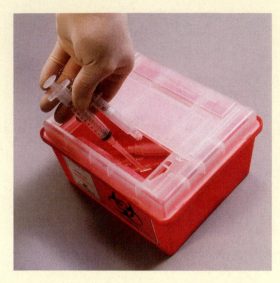

Figure 35-16. ■ Proper disposal of used venipuncture supplies.

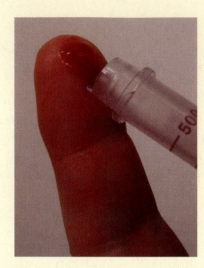

Figure 35-18. ■ Touch only the tip of the collection tube to the drop of blood.

10. Collect the specimen in the chosen container or slide. Touch only the tip of the collection device to the drop of blood (Figure 35-18 ■). Blood flow is encouraged if the puncture site is held downward and gentler pressure is applied near the site. Cap micro-collection tubes with the cap provided and mix additives by gently tilting or inverting the tube 8 to 10 times. *Scraping the collection device on the skin activates platelets and may cause hemolysis. Touching the tube to the site may cause contamination. Mixing the specimens prevents clotting.*

11. When collection is complete, apply clean gauze to the site with pressure (Figure 35-19 ■). Hold pressure or have the client hold pressure until bleeding stops. Label the containers with the proper information. Do not apply a dressing to a skin puncture of an infant under 2 years of age. Never release a client until the bleeding has stopped. *Proper labeling prevents mixup of specimens. Younger children may develop skin irritation from the adhesive bandage. Also young children may put the bandage in their mouths and choke.*

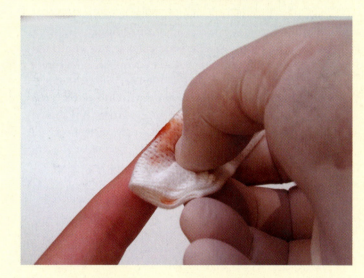

Figure 35-19. ■ Apply pressure with clean gauze.

12. Thank the client. Instruct the client to leave the bandage in place for at least 15 minutes. *Courtesy helps the client have a positive attitude about the procedure and the facility.*

13. Properly care for or dispose of equipment and supplies. Clean work area. Remove gloves and perform hand hygiene. *Standard Precautions must be followed throughout the procedure.*

14. Test, transfer, or store specimen according to the facility policy.

15. Document the procedure.

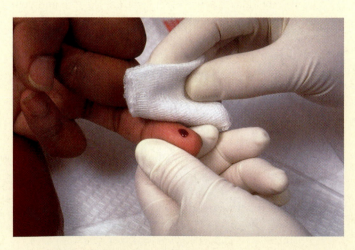

Figure 35-17. ■ Wipe away first drop of blood.

SAMPLE DOCUMENTATION

[date]   OP fingerstick for prothrombin
[time]   time per Dr. Rubin.
                     _____ C. Wasson, LPN

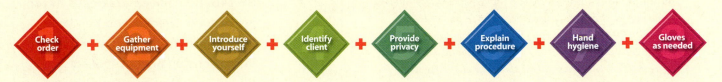

PROCEDURE 35-7   # Assisting with a Sigmoidoscopy

Purpose

- To prepare the client and assist with an endoscopic colon procedure

Equipment

- Flexible or rigid sigmoidoscope
- Water-soluble lubricant
- Gown and drape

- Cotton swabs
- Suction if not part of the scope
- Biopsy forceps
- Specimen container and preservative
- Completed lab requisition form
- Personal wipes or tissue
- Equipment for assessing vital signs
- Examination gloves

Check order + Gather equipment + Introduce yourself + Identify client + Provide privacy + Explain procedure + Hand hygiene + Gloves as needed

Interventions

1. Perform hand hygiene. *To aid in infection control.*

2. Assemble equipment and supplies. Write the name of the client on the specimen container label and complete the requisition slip. *The name of the client must be clearly marked on the container and the requisition for accurate identification.*

3. Check the light source if a flexible sigmoidoscope (Figure 35-20 ■) is being used. Turn off the power after checking for working order to avoid a buildup of heat in the instrument. *If heat is permitted to build up in the scope, the client may be burned.*

4. Greet and identify the client and explain the procedure. Inform the client that a sensation of pressure or need to

defecate may be felt during the procedure and that pressure is from the instrument and will ease. The client may also feel gas pressure when air is insufflated during the sigmoidoscopy. *Note:* The client may have been ordered to take a mild sedative before the procedure. *Identifying the client prevents errors in treatment. Explaining the procedure helps to ease anxiety and ensure compliance.*

5. Instruct the client to empty the urinary bladder. *Pressure from the instrument may injure a full bladder. Urine in the bladder increases discomfort.*

6. Assess the vital signs and record in the medical record. *Colon examination procedures may cause cardiac arrhythmias and change in blood pressure in some clients. Baseline vital signs will allow you to detect variations from the client's normal vital signs.*

7. Have the client undress completely from the waist down and put on a gown. Drape appropriately.

8. Assist the client on to the examination table. If a fiber optic device is being used, Sims' position is the most comfortable for the client (Figure 35-21 ■). If a rigid instrument is used, the client will be placed in the knee–chest position when the physician is ready to begin. *These positions facilitate the procedure by moving the abdominal organs up into the abdominal cavity rather than the pelvis.*

9. Assist the physician as needed with lubricant, instruments, power, swabs, and specimen container.

10. During the procedure, monitor the client's response and offer reassurance. Instruct the client to breathe slowly through pursed lips to aid in relaxation if necessary.

11. When the physician is finished, assist the client to a comfortable position and allow a rest period. Offer

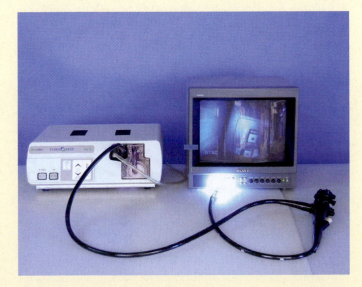

Figure 35-20. ■ A flexible sigmoidoscope.

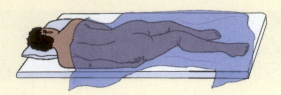

Figure 35-21. ■ Sims' positions

personal cleaning wipes or tissues. Take the vital signs before allowing the client to stand and assist the client from the table and with dressing as needed. Give the client any instructions regarding care after the procedure and follow-up as ordered by the physician. *A drop in blood pressure on standing is common after lying in any of these positions for an extended period. If clients complain of dizziness or light-headedness after sitting up, have them lie down again. If any biopsy samples were taken, the client may have slight rectal bleeding.*

12. Clean the room and route the specimen to the laboratory with the requisition. Disinfect or dispose of the supplies

and equipment as appropriate and wash your hands. *Follow Standard Precautions throughout the procedure.*

13. Document the procedure.

SAMPLE DOCUMENTATION

[date] VS: T 98.4, P 100, R 22, BP 144/84.
[time] Sigmoidoscopy performed by Dr. Narang and specimen obtained. Procedure tolerated well. Specimen to Quest Laboratories, VS after procedure: P 112, R 24, BP 146/86. Denies dizziness after procedure. Discharged per Dr. Narang with verbal and written instructions on procedural care. Client verbalizes understanding.
_____ S. Lewan, LPN

PROCEDURE 35-8 # Applying a Splint

Purpose

■ To immobilize an injured extremity to prevent further injury until swelling decreases and a cast can be applied

Equipment

■ Ready-made or customized splint appropriate for the area of injury
■ Velcro® straps or elastic bandage
■ Clips or tape

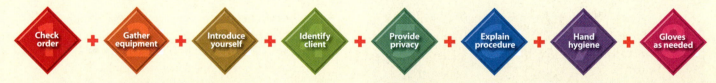

Interventions

1. Assemble equipment. *Organizing supplies and equipment before beginning will help procedure to proceed smoothly.*

2. Perform hand hygiene. *Hand hygiene assists in infection prevention.*

3. Greet and identify the client. Explain the procedure. Ask for and answer any questions. *Identifying the client prevents errors. Explanations relieve anxiety and help to gain cooperation of the client.*

4. Assist the client to the examination table. Place in a comfortable position supporting injured extremity. *In order for the splint to be applied properly, the client must be seated or lying down. Supporting the extremity can lessen the pain.*

5. Pad the inside of the splint and check for proper fit on the extremity. *Ready-made splints (Figure 35-22 ■) are already padded; on a custom splint the padding will need to be added to support the extremity properly.*

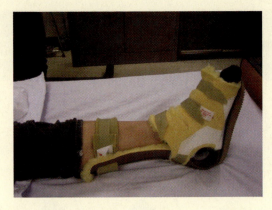
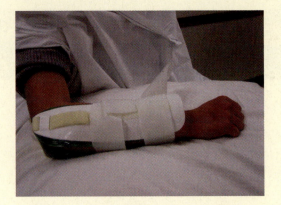

Figure 35-22. ■ Ready-made leg and arm splints.

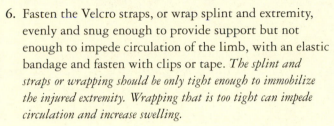

6. Fasten the Velcro straps, or wrap splint and extremity, evenly and snug enough to provide support but not enough to impede circulation of the limb, with an elastic bandage and fasten with clips or tape. *The splint and straps or wrapping should be only tight enough to immobilize the injured extremity. Wrapping that is too tight can impede circulation and increase swelling.*

7. Instruct the client to keep the extremity elevated and apply ice. *Elevating the extremity above the level of the heart and applying ice aid in decreasing swelling.*

8. Apply a sling for an arm splint (Figure 35-23 ■). *The sling will help the client support the injured arm and keep it elevated.*

9. If a leg splint has been applied, provide client with crutches and instructions for use. An elderly client may need a wheelchair rather than crutches. *The client should not bear weight on the splinted leg. Crutches can be used if the client is agile enough to use them and keep weight off the injured extremity. Otherwise the client should use a wheelchair until the limb is casted and weight bearing is allowed.*

10. Provide verbal and written instructions for follow-up care. *Instructions need to be given that include when the follow-up visit for casting is scheduled and how to care for injury until that time. Written instructions serve as a reminder when the client is at home.*

11. Document procedure.

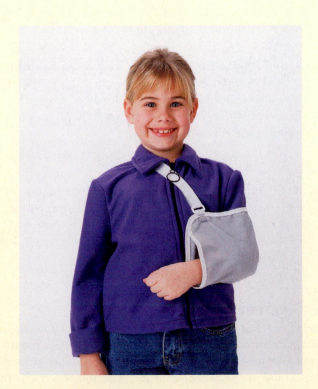

Figure 35-23. ■ Arm sling.

SAMPLE DOCUMENTATION

[date] Splint applied to right lower leg;
[time] and wrapped with elastic bandage, per Dr. Morrison, following x-ray that revealed tibia/fibula fracture. To return to orthopedic clinic on [date] for application of a cast. Verbal and written instructions given and client verbalized understanding. Crutches measured and fitted by PT and instructions for use given. Rx for Motrin 600 mg every 4 h prn pain.

_____ B. Rodgers, LVN

Purpose

- To assess and document the distance visual acuity of a student in both eyes, with or without corrective lenses, according to required health assessment timelines

Equipment

- Snellen eye chart
- Paper cup or eye paddle

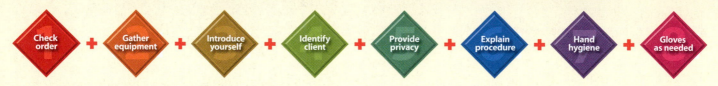

Interventions

1. Perform hand hygiene. *To aid in infection control.*

2. Prepare the examination area. Make sure the area is well lighted, a distance marker is placed exactly 20 feet from the Snellen chart (Figure 35-24 ■), and the chart is at eye level. *All distance visual testing is done at 20 feet for consistency of results.*

3. Greet and identify the student and explain the procedure. *A student who understands the procedure is likely to be compliant and produce accurate results.*

4. Position the student at the 20-foot mark. *The student may stand or sit as long as the chart is at eye level and 20 feet away.*

5. Observe whether the student is wearing glasses. If not, ask if he or she is wearing contact lenses and mark the results of the test accordingly. *The visual acuity examination is usually performed with students who need corrective lenses wearing them. If that is the case, the record must indicate that the lenses were worn for the test.*

6. Have the student cover the left eye with the paper cup or eye paddle. Instruct the student to keep both eyes open during the test. *The test starts with the left eye covered for consistency. The hand should not be used to cover the eye, because pressure against the eye or peeking through the fingers affects the results. Closing one eye will cause squinting of the other, which changes the vision and skews the findings.*

7. Stand beside the chart and point to each row as the client reads aloud the indicated lines, starting with the 20/200 line. The line numbers are shown on the right side of the chart next to each line. *It is generally best to start about the second or third row to judge the student's response. If these lines are read easily, move down to smaller figures. If the student has difficulty reading the larger lines, inform the parents so student can be taken for follow-up exam.*

8. Record the smallest line that the student can read with either 1 or no errors, according to policy. If line 5 is read with one error with the right eye, it will be recorded as Rt. eye 20/40-1. If no errors are read at 20/40 line, it is recorded as Rt. eye 20/40.

9. Repeat the procedure with the right eye covered and record as in step 8 using left eye.

10. If the student squints or leans forward while testing either eye, record this observation on the health record. *As the health clerk it is important that testing be documented, including the notification to the parent, in order to comply with student health screening requirements.*

11. Perform hand hygiene and document results.

ALTERNATE PROCEDURE

If student is not yet reading or is unable to identify letters, an E chart or picture chart should be used. In step 7 ask the student to use his or her hand to indicate in which directions the legs of the E are pointing on the indicated line or to name the pictures on the indicated line.

Figure 35-24. ■ Snellen charts used to assess distance vision.

PROCEDURE 35-10   # Conducting Audiometric Testing

Purpose

- To accurately assess and document a hearing test using audiometry and comply with mandated health screening

Equipment

- Audiometer
- Otoscope or audioscope

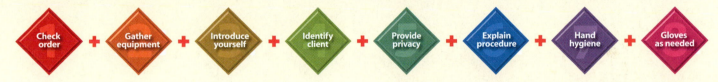

Check order + Gather equipment + Introduce yourself + Identify client + Provide privacy + Explain procedure + Hand hygiene + Gloves as needed

Interventions

1. Perform hand hygiene. *To aid in infection control.*

2. Greet and identify the student. Explain the procedure. Take the student to a quiet room for testing. *Students who understand the procedure are likely to be compliant, producing accurate results. A quiet room allows for accurate results without distraction. Determine the signal (raising the hand or saying yes) to indicate that the tones are heard.*

3. Using an otoscope or audioscope with a light source, visually inspect the ear canal and tympanic membrane before testing. *Looking in the ear canal verifies that there are no obstructions, such as cerumen, to interfere with the test. If you see an obstruction, refer the student to have the ear irrigated.*

4. Choose the correct size tip for the end of the audiometer (Figure 35-25 ■). Attach a speculum to fit the student's external auditory meatus, making sure the ear canal is occluded with the speculum in place. *The design of the tip or speculum obviates bulky earphones; the tip should block any environmental noise during the test.*

5. With the speculum in the ear canal, retract the pinna, down and back for a child. (For older students, pull pinna up and back). *Pulling the pinna down and back for a child straightens the ear canal.*

6. Turn the instrument on and select the screening level. There is a pretest tone for practice if necessary. Press the start button and observe the tone indicators and the client's response. *The signal (raising the hand, saying yes) was determined before starting to test. The audiometer will proceed down each tone with a light indicator.*

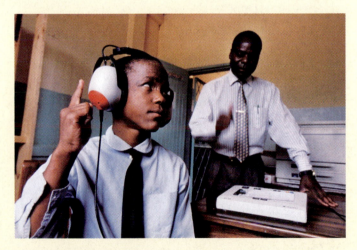

Figure 35-25. ■ Audiometer.

7. Screen the other ear.

8. If the student fails to respond at any frequency, rescreening is required. If a particular tone does not illicit a response, a second opportunity should be given.

9. If the student fails rescreening, notify the parents so they can take the child to their family physician. *A student who fails to hear one or more tones may need to be referred to an audiologist.*

10. Record the results in the student health record. *Hearing test are mandated by state law a various grade levels; these need to be recorded in the student's health record.*

PROCEDURE 35-11 Screening for Scoliosis

Purpose

■ To meet school health guidelines for scoliosis screening and identify students who need medical evaluation for spinal curvature

Equipment

■ Scoliometer

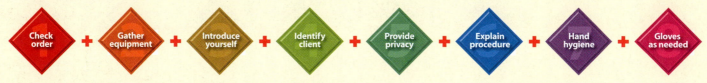

Check order + Gather equipment + Introduce yourself + Identify client + Provide privacy + Explain procedure + Hand hygiene + Gloves as needed

Interventions

1. Explain the procedure to the group or each student individually. *A general explanation can be given class by class as long as the student is given the opportunity to ask questions privately.*

2. Have child remove outer garments. Deformity, if any will be easier to identify through a t-shirt.

3. Instruct student to bend over with arms dangling while standing with feet together and knees straight. *The curve of structural scoliosis is more apparent when bending over.*

4. Observe an imbalanced rib cage, with one side being higher than the other. *The lateral curve of scoliosis will cause ribs to be nonsymmetrical.*

5. Observe for other deformities if present. *The hip opposite the deviation will be higher with scoliosis, resulting in what appears to be unequal leg lengths.*

6. Confirm diagnosis using additional physical test. The student is requested to walk on the toes, then the heels, and then is asked to jump up and down on one foot. *Such activities indicate leg strength and balance.*

7. Additional screening can be performed with the inclinometer (scoliometer). An inclinometer, also known as a scoliometer, measures distortions of the torso. The procedure is as follows:
   ■ The student bends over, arms dangling and palms pressed together, until a curve can be observed in the *upper* back (thoracic area).
   ■ The scoliometer is placed on the back and measures the apex (the highest point) of the upper back curve.

■ The student continues bending until the curve can be seen in the *lower* back (lumbar area). The apex of this curve is also measured.

Some experts believe the scoliometer would make a useful device for widespread screening. Scoliometers, however, indicate rib cage distortions in more than half of children who turn out to have very minor or no sideways curves. They are therefore not accurate enough to guide treatment.

8. Document findings and notify parent if medical follow-up is needed. *Provide parents with result of screening to take to family physician.*

Chapter Review

 KEY TERMS by Topic

Use the audio glossary feature of either the CD-ROM or the Companion Website to hear the correct pronunciation of the following key terms.

Alternate Care Settings
ambulatory care nursing, clinics, urgent care office, school health office, same-day surgery clinic, traveling nurse, school-based health clinic

Other Practice Areas
correctional nurse, adult day care, assisted living facility, summer day camp, mental health facility and clinic

KEY Points

- A variety of opportunities are available for LPNs/LVNs to use their skills.

- Although a medical assistant may be designated as the office manager in a physician's office, the LPN/LVN never defers to an unlicensed person for treatment questions.

- Privacy and confidentiality are more difficult to ensure in a medical office, but nevertheless all HIPAA regulations must be followed closely.

- School health offices and school-based clinics are providing care for minors, so laws and district policies must be followed.

- School health personnel are a great source for health education for students and families.

- Home care and hospice opportunities are opening up for the LPN/LVN.

- Same-day surgery clinics employ the LPN/LVN to admit clients and prepare them for surgery.

- LPNs/LVNs assist the physician or the nurse practitioner with many procedures in the physician's office.

 EXPLORE Media Link

Additional interactive resources for this chapter can be found on the Companion Website at www.prenhall.com/ramont. Click on Chapter 35 and "Begin" to select the activities for this chapter.

For chapter-related NCLEX®-style questions and an audio glossary, access the accompanying CD-ROM in this book.

FOR FURTHER Study

See Chapter 17 for information about hospice and end-of-life care.

See the procedures in Chapter 20 for assessing vital signs.

See Chapter 31 for an example of a pre-op checklist.

See Chapter 34 for information about emergency and urgent care nursing.

Critical Thinking Care Map

Caring for a Client with Scoliosis Who Attends School with a Milwaukee Brace

NCLEX-PN® Focus Area: Psychological Integrity

Case Study: J. J. Smith is a 16-year-old male who will be returning to his junior year in high school with a Milwaukee brace for treatment of scoliosis. "JJ" is to wear the brace 23 of 24 hours per day. Last year he was the forward on the water polo team and was a competitive swimmer. JJ is reluctant to return to school because the "brace is very visible and I know the guys will make fun of me." He also states that he is "bummed that he won't be on the water polo team, and I am not sure I will be ready to compete for the swim team in the spring." After conferring with his parents, physician, and coach, they are contemplating allowing him to practice with the team as long as he wears the brace the remainder of each day.

Nursing Diagnosis: Disturbed Body Image r/t Milwaukee Brace

COLLECT DATA

Subjective	Objective
_____	_____
_____	_____
_____	_____
_____	_____
_____	_____
_____	_____
_____	_____

Would you report this data? Yes/No

If yes, to: _____

What would you report? _____

Nursing Care

_____
_____
_____
_____
_____
_____
_____
_____
_____
_____

How would you document this? _____
_____
_____

Compare your documentation to the sample provided in Appendix I.

Data Collected
(use those that apply)

- Weight: 178 lbs
- Height: 5'11"
- 35° lateral spinal curve
- Will not make eye contact
- Wearing Milwaukee brace over t-shirt; reluctant to remove jacket
- C/o pain and requesting to call mother and go home
- VS: T 98.4, P 72, R 24, BP 110/74
- Did not eat lunch, complains that brace is putting pressure on abdomen so he cannot eat

Nursing Interventions
(use those that apply; list in priority order)

- Assist JJ to develop new interests that he can be involved in while still in a brace.
- Establish a contract with JJ that he will wear brace at all times except during practice and workout in the pool and shower time.
- Regularly monitor height and weight.
- Evaluate brace for pressure areas.
- Consider JJ's developmental level and how wearing the brace at school can affect it.
- Arrange meeting with counselor, coach, parents, and physician to discuss available options.
- Obtain order for pain medication during school as needed.
- Allow JJ to come to health office or see the counselor if he has the need to talk.

NCLEX-PN® Exam Preparation

TEST-TAKING TIP   Remember the order of priority of AIRWAY, BREATHING, and CIRCULATION!

1 Practice areas for the LPN/LVN are many and varied. To determine if the job duties are within the scope of practice for the LPN/LVN, he or she should check:

1. the facility's policy and procedure manual.
2. the job description for the position.
3. the Nurse Practice Act for the state.
4. the state board of nursing.

2 You are an LPN/LVN working in a physician's office. In matters related to client care, who is considered to be the LPN/LVN's supervisor?

1. the office manager
2. the back office medical assistant
3. the medical assistant with the most seniority
4. the RN

3 Scoliosis screening is mandated by law. The initial screening for male students is in what grade?

1. 5th
2. 6th
3. 10th
4. 11th

4 You are employed by a home health agency that offers hospice services. One of your clients is inquiring about hospice services. You explain the requirements for admission into hospice to the client and his daughter. Which of the following statements would alert you that more teaching is needed?

1. "Our physician is not supporting our decision to seek hospice care but we want to sign up anyway."
2. "Hospice can provide multidisciplinary care to improve the quality of Dad's life for the time he has left."
3. "I know that Dad may have less than six months to live but I want him to be as comfortable as possible."
4. "I am so glad that hospice care can be given in our home or in the nursing home if there comes a time that Dad needs more care than I can give him."

5 The LVN/LPN can perform all of the following duties in a same-day surgery center except:

1. admission nurse.
2. scrub tech.
3. circulating nurse.
4. recovery room nurse.

6 You are employed by a physician as his office LPN/LVN. A client is scheduled for a surgical office procedure. During the procedure all of the following may be your duties except:

1. setting up the sterile field and instruments.
2. positioning the client.
3. administering the local anesthetic.
4. completing laboratory requisitions.

7 A 4-year-old child is scheduled for a school physical. One of the required tests is a visual acuity test for distance vision. The mother tells you that they child does not know the alphabet. What would be your appropriate action?

1. State on the physical form that the acuity could not be tested.
2. Assess the child to see what letters she knows and use a line that contains only those letters.
3. Ask the mother if the child has any vision problems and list her response on the form.
4. Use the Snellen E chart and explain the procedure to the child.

8 You have assisted the physician with a sigmoidoscopy. Following the procedure you should:

1. assist the client into a comfortable position and allow a rest period.
2. leave the room so the client can have privacy for dressing.
3. tell the client to meet you at the desk for discharge instructions.
4. help the client to stand and then leave the room.

9 A client was treated in the walk-in clinic where you work for a fracture of his radius. The nurse practitioner instructs you to immobilize the arm, since there is too much swelling to permit cast application today. Which of the following is the best intervention?

1. Tightly wrap the arm from the wrist to below the elbow.
2. Splint the arm from below the wrist to above the elbow, apply a sling to keep the arm elevated, and apply ice.
3. Apply ice and apply a sling.
4. Apply a splint until the swelling is resolved.

10 You are working in a school health office. You are checking immunization records for incoming kindergarten students. In order for students to meet the recommended immunization requirements they should have had how many doses of DTaP, polio, and MMR?

1. DTaP, 5; polio, 3; MMR, 2
2. DTaP, 4; polio, 4; MMR, 2
3. DTaP, 5; polio, 4; MMR, 2
4. DTaP, 5; polio, 4; MMR, 1

Answers and Rationales for Review Questions, as well as discussion of Care Plan and Critical Thinking Care Map questions, appear in Appendix I.

Thinking Strategically About ...

You have just started a job as a health clerk in a health clinic at Wilson Middle School. You and one other LPN–health clerk and a nurse practitioner staff the clinic. The RNP covers this school as well as the local high school. It is Monday morning, and the schedule for today includes scoliosis screening on all the girls in the sixth grade; a parent orientation for the incoming student for the fall; health checks for the students going to outdoor education camp and an Individual Education Plan (IEP) meeting for Billy Suarez, a 7th grader with Down syndrome who attends the special education class.

The RNP is at the high school assisting with athletic physicals. She may not be back in time for the IEP meeting. The parents do not speak English, and you do not speak Spanish. The other LPN called in sick, and she was supposed to interpret for the meeting. You are responsible for running the clinic and completing all the tasks on the schedule until the RNP returns.

COMMUNICATION AND TEAM BUILDING

Using your knowledge of communication and team building, what solutions could you discuss with the RNP by phone? List several possibilities.

CRITICAL THINKING

All scheduled activities for, as well as care of, students with acute health problems need to be addressed. Prioritize all activities and develop a plan for dealing with each.

CONFLICT RESOLUTION

You notify the school psychologist that you are the only nurse on campus this morning. The interpreter will not be available for the Suarez IEP meeting, and the RNP may be late. The psychologist becomes very upset and blames you saying, "We will have to cancel the meeting. This is a problem since the parents took time off work for the meeting." What solutions could you suggest to correct the problem and the conflict with the psychologist?

CULTURAL COMPETENCY

The school population is very diverse: 40% of the students are Hispanic, 10% Korean, 15% Caucasian, 10% African American, 10% Middle Easterners, the remaining 15% other. It is very important that your orientation to the health services be sensitive to the different cultures present. Describe how you would accomplish this.

Becoming a Licensed Nurse

UNIT VI

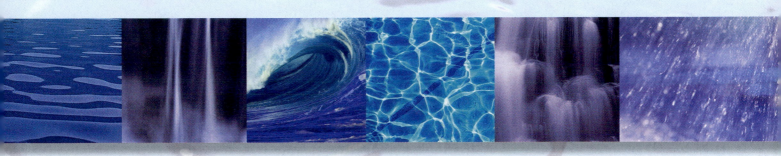

Chapter 36

Leadership and Professional Development

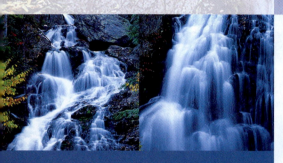

BRIEF Outline

Licensure
Leadership Styles
Team Leading
Reporting Techniques
Paperwork
Conflict Resolution
Nursing Care Delivery Trends
Surveyors and Accreditation
Community Service

HISTORICAL Perspectives

Take a look at nurses' duties in 1887: In addition to caring for your fifty patients, each nurse will follow these regulations:

1. *Daily sweep and mop the floor of your ward, dust the patient's furniture and window sills.*
2. *Maintain an even temperature in your ward, by bringing in a scuttle of coal for the day's business.*
3. *Light is important to observe the patient's condition. Therefore, each day fill kerosene lamps, clean chimneys, and trim wicks. Wash windows once a week.*
4. *The nurse's notes are important in aiding the physician's work. Make your pens carefully; you may whittle nibs to your individual taste.*

LEARNING Outcomes

After completing this chapter, you will be able to:

1. Discuss factors that govern the licensure process.
2. Describe the purpose of nurse practice acts.
3. Identify important attributes of effective leaders.
4. Understand the various reporting techniques and types of paperwork involved in the nursing process.
5. Define conflict and discuss conflict resolution strategies.
6. Describe the advantages of each method of nursing care delivery.
7. Demonstrate an understanding of the 14 national patient safety goals.

Licensure

A graduate of a practical/vocational nursing program cannot use the title of licensed practical/vocational nurse until the licensing exam has been taken, passed, and the **license** issued. **Licensure** is a process by which a government agency gives permission for an individual to engage in an occupation or profession. It certifies that the individual has attained the minimum requirements necessary to protect the public safety and welfare. These requirements for a nursing license are outlined in the nurse practice act for each state.

The requirements for obtaining a license vary from state to state. In general, the applicant must (1) have completed a minimum of 2 years of high school or its equivalent (many states now require a high school diploma), (2) have completed an approved course in practical/vocational nursing, and (3) be a citizen of the United States or have a current visa. If these requirements have been met, the applicant will be eligible to take the examination. Following the exam the state board of nursing will review the application and issue the license.

All the work you have done up to this point has been in preparation for taking the licensing exam. The exam is designed to measure your knowledge in a number of areas. Passage of the exam certifies that you have enough knowledge to practice safely as an entry-level licensed practical/vocational nurse.

At one time each state had its own licensing exam; today there is a national exam developed by the National Council of State Boards of Nursing. The exam is the NCLEX-PN® (National Council Licensure Examination for Practical Nurses). The examination is a computer adapted test (CAT) that is administered by testing agencies throughout the community. The agency provides the state board of nursing with the names of the individuals who have passed the examination. The board is responsible for issuing the license. Licenses may not be issued to persons convicted of certain crimes, a person who is mentally ill, or a person who is addicted to alcohol or other drugs. In Texas and California the license is for vocational nursing; in all other states, such nurses are known as licensed practical nurses.

Licenses are issued for a specific period of time, which is determined by the board that issued the license. It is the responsibility of the licensee to keep his or her license current and to meeting any continuing education requirements. It is a violation of the nurse practice act to function as an LPN/LVN without a current license.

SUSPENSION OR REVOCATION

The state board of nursing has a responsibility to protect the public. The board has the authority, under the state nurse practice act, to suspend or revoke a nursing license if the licensee is found guilty of an offense. Box 36-1 ■ lists examples of cause for license suspension or revocation.

BOX 36-1

Causes of License Suspension or Revocation

- Conviction of
  - Felony
  - Moral turpitude or gross immorality
- Guilty of
  - Fraud or deceit in obtaining a license
  - Willful neglect of a patient
- Mental incompetence
- Chemical dependence or abuse including alcohol
- Suspended or revoked license in another jurisdiction
- Unfit by reason of neglect

When action is taken against a licensee, the nurse must be notified of the charges and given a hearing before the board. The individual, either in person or through an attorney, has the right to enter a defense.

The board, in addition to suspension and revocation, can, for just cause, place a licensee on probation, refuse to issue or renew a license, or issue a letter of reprimand.

Actions taken against a licensed nurse are a matter of public record. In many states the information can be obtained by any community member by telephone or from the board's website.

STANDARDS OF CARE

Standards of care are used to determine what a nurse should or should not do. All healthcare professionals must adhere to certain standards. A physician's standards of care are different from those of a registered nurse and an LPN's/LVN's standards differ from those of the RN. Each nurse must be aware of the standards of care to which they will be held accountable because they can be sued to determine if appropriate action was taken. Standards of care come from various sources: state licensing laws, nurse practice acts, nursing organizations, journal articles, or policies and procedures for individual facilities.

NURSE PRACTICE ACTS

Nurse practice acts, in general, provide a definition for *nurse,* establish a board of nursing, outline the requirements for licensure, and provide the circumstances for suspension and revocation of the license. These acts are specific for each state or territory and facilitate recognition of possible conflict between the scope of practice and the tasks being performed by the LPN/LVN.

Although the acts differ from state to state, some standardized terminology is used. The understandings of these terms maybe helpful as you assume the role of a licensed nurse within your state. Table 36-1 ■ lists some common terms and their explanation.

TABLE 36-1	
Common Terms used in Nurse Practice Acts	
TERMS	**EXPLANATION**
Basic nursing care	Nursing care which is predictable and with which modifications are unnecessary, based on the knowledge and skills obtained during an educational program, and those which can be safely performed by an LPN/LVN.
Basic patient situation	Situations in which the client's condition is predictable and the clinical condition requires only basic nursing care. Medical and nursing orders are continuously changing and do not contain complex modifications. The situation is determined by the RN.
Complex nursing situation	Client's clinical condition is not predictable and requires frequent changes in medical or nursing orders or complex modifications. Nursing care expectations are beyond that learned by the LPN/LVN during the educational program.
Delegated medical act	Doctor's orders given to the RN or LPN/LVN.
Delegated nursing act	Nursing orders given to an RN or LPN/LVN by an RN.
Direct supervision	Supervisor is continuously present to coordinate, inspect, or direct nursing care.
General supervision	Supervisor regularly coordinates, inspects, or directs nursing care. The supervisor is available within the building or by telephone.

The National Association for Practical Nurse Education and Service issued the statement shown in Box 36-2 ■, listing the responsibilities of practice of the LPN/LVN, in its 1998 Code of Ethics for the Licensed Practical/Vocational Nurse. Statements from professional organizations are not state law; they merely serve as guidelines for practice.

BOX 36-2	

Code of Ethics for the Licensed Practical/Vocational Nurse

The Licensed Practical and Licensed Vocational Nurses shall ...

- Consider as a basic obligation the conservation of life and the prevention of disease
- Promote and protect the physical, mental, emotional, and spiritual health of the patient and his/her family
- Fulfill all duties faithfully and efficiently
- Function within established legal guidelines
- Accept personal responsibility for his/her acts, and seek to merit the respect and confidence of all members of the health team
- Hold in confidence all matters coming to his/her knowledge, in the practice of his/her profession, and in no way at no time violate this confidence
- Give conscientious service and charge just remuneration
- Learn and respect the religious and cultural beliefs of his/her patient and of all people
- Meet the obligation to the patient by keeping abreast of current trends in health care through reading and continuing education
- As a citizen of the United States of America, uphold the laws of the land and seek to promote legislation that will meet the health needs of its people.

Source: Reprinted by permission of the National Association for Practical Nurse Education and Service.

Leadership Styles

The transition from graduate to licensed nurse happens quickly. You will need to begin to think differently about yourself. **Leadership** is a process used to move a group toward setting and achievement of goals. This definition is compatible with nursing leadership. The process can be used by anyone; therefore anyone can, in theory, be a leader. As you begin your career you will have the opportunity to observe nursing leaders; as you watch and learn you will begin to develop your own leadership style. There are several leadership styles and each one has good and not so good characteristics. There are situations where one style may be more effective than another. Leaders will change their style in order to maximize their leadership effectiveness.

TYPES OF LEADERS

The Autocrat

The **autocratic** leader makes unilateral decisions while dominating the team members. This approach can result in passive resistance from team members. It requires constant control from the leader in order to have the singular objective met. The authoritarian approach is generally not successful in getting the best performance from a team. There are, however, some instances when the autocratic style is appropriate. When there is a need for immediate action, this style may be the most effective. Most people are familiar with the autocratic style and have little trouble adopting it. In some situations subordinates may actually prefer being directed by an autocrat.

The Laissez-Faire Leader

The **laissez-faire** leader exercises little control over the group. Team members are left alone to tackle their work, sort out their roles, and solve problems. This approach leaves the team floundering with little motivation or direction.

There are situations in which the laissez-faire approach is effective. It can be appropriate with highly motivated and skilled team members, who have produced excellent work in the past. Once the leader has established the team as competent, confident, and motivated it may be appropriate to back off and allow the team to function. By handing over ownership of the project, the leader empowers the team and they can take ownership and will most likely achieve the goals.

The Democrat

The **democratic** leader makes decisions after consulting with team members. Although, the team participates in the decision-making process, the leader still maintains control. The team is allowed to decide how the task will be accomplished and who will be responsible for each task.

The democratic leader can be viewed in two ways. The good democratic leader delegates wisely and encourages participation, but the leader never loses sight that the ultimate responsibility belongs to him or her. The leader values group discussion and input. The leader draws from the team members' strengths and knowledge in order to obtain the best performance from the team. However, the democratic leader can also be seen as being unsure of himself and his relationship with his subordinates. It appears that everything is a matter of group decision. This type of leader is seen as not leading at all.

Team Leading

The first leadership role you might experience as an LPN/LVN may be that of a team leader. In this role you will be responsible for guiding and directing the care for a group of clients. You will also be responsible for supervising the members of the team, which includes nursing assistants.

The duties of the team leader include:

- Making assignments
- Taking report
- Making rounds and assessing clients
- Giving report to team members on assigned clients
- Assisting in administration of medications and treatments
- Facilitating team conferences
- Collaborating with an RN supervisor or clinical nurse specialist.

DELEGATION

The sign of a good leader is to know how and when to delegate. The leader will understand the scope of all team members so that delegation of tasks will be appropriate.

The first step in the **delegation** (the distribution of tasks in a way that prioritizes activities and available resources)

process is to prioritize activities, with available resources. The purpose of delegation is efficiency. No one person can do it all, therefore some work must be passed on. It is important to remember that even though a task has been delegated, the ultimate responsibility for the task belongs to the nurse-leader.

Some leaders have difficulty delegating. This presents several problems. The leader who does not delegate becomes overworked, tired, and ineffective. When delegation is not utilized, some team members become lazy or bored. Team members who are never given responsibility through delegation may feel that the leader is unappreciative of their contribution and thinks they are incapable; this leads to a breakdown of the team.

Group leaders who have a leader who makes use of delegation benefit in the following ways:

- Their sense of responsibility increases.
- Their job satisfaction in heightened.
- Their knowledge is increased.

Ultimately, delegation will promote happiness within the group; morale will improve as will productivity. In other words the team will likely be functioning at its peak.

The reason why leaders may delegate poorly or not at all may be that they simply do not know how. Delegation skills can be learned and perfected. Delegation works best when assignments are specific. Team members may be afraid to accept the assignment from fear of failure. They need to be given the opportunity to ask questions and seek clarification prior to being expected to take on the task. They also need to know they can trust the leader to support them in their efforts. The leader should be ready to reward the group for successful completion of delegated activities. Group members whose contributions are appreciated will be motivated to accept further responsibility. A simple word of thanks can go a long way.

Reporting Techniques

In nursing giving report is very much related to delegation. Reporting to other nurses at the change of shifts is both delegation of responsibility and an accounting as to what has been done.

Shift report is the most effective way to pass information from one shift to another. The report can take on many forms. It may be oral face to face with the staff arriving for the next shift. It may be done in a room or as a part of walking rounds. The report may be taped by the nurse going off duty to be listened to by the on-coming nurse or the report may be written. There are advantages and disadvantages of each. No matter which form the facility uses, some important issues need to be established. Each form of report will be discussed giving both the advantages and disadvantages.

Taped report has been adopted by many facilities in an effort to save time and provide floor coverage during report. The nurses going off duty can tape report on their clients one

BOX 36-3

Clinical Alert: Taped Report

1. Give your name/shift/date
2. Room number
3. Client's full name
4. Age of client
5. Diagnosis/admission date/surgical date
6. Primary or admitting physician's name
7. Proceed with information. Remember that the nurse coming on may not know the client as well as you do. Be complete. Don't drag. Give pertinent information. Most nurses follow the Kardex and then add changes. For example,
   - C/o of gas pains. What did you do?
   - BP was elevated. What was it? What did you do?
   - No code
   - Specimens needed
   - Accucheck AC/HS. What were the blood sugars and was insulin coverage given?
   - Drainage from NGT/JP/Hemovac. How much?
   - Teaching. Did client demonstrate/understand?
   - Dressing change
   - *Pet peeves:* Don't belittle the client on tape. If you don't like a client, keep it to yourself. Personal comments about clients make the nurse look unprofessional.
8. Remember not to mumble or yawn too much. You can always stop the tape if you forget something. Put the tape on pause, gather information, and restart the tape.
9. If you have had a particularly hard shift and haven't finished something like a dressing which was not a priority, make sure you let the next shift know; don't let them find it. You need to be honest. Try not to let it become a habit to leave things undone.
10. *Insight:* Clients sometimes like to play nurse against nurse, shift against shift. Don't play into it. Remember nursing is continuity of care and it is a team effort even if it happens on someone else's shift. It is the client who suffers or gains.
11. End on a good note—"Have a good day!"

BOX 36-4

Helpful Hints for Listening to a Taped Report

- It can be difficult to hear at first. You have to tune out the other noise and concentrate. It may be necessary to let the staff know you can't hear, especially if they are socializing. They usually know their clients and have a trained ear.
- Listen for pertinent data and changes
  - Age/diagnosis
  - Temperature elevation, BP changes
  - Altered mental status
  - Dressing changes
  - Unusual problems
  - Pain/whether medication is controlling it
- If you can get diet/VS/I&O, great, but you can also get that information from the Kardex.

at a time, leaving the other staff to provide coverage for all the clients. Nurses coming on shift can listen to the tape while the previous shift continues to cover the patients. Some disadvantages of taped report are that sometimes they are difficult to hear or understand and questions must be tabled to the end when they must be addressed with the nurse who may be anxious to go off duty. Box 36-3 ■ provides an outline for making a taped report and Box 36-4 ■ gives helpful hints for listening to a taped report.

An **oral report** is very much like a taped report in that it can be delivered in a report room or while making client rounds. Advantages are that questions can be addressed immediately and, if on rounds, clients can be checked at the same time. Disadvantages are that the report cannot start until all staff have arrived. If clients are in semiprivate rooms, confidentiality may be breeched when report is given on rounds.

Written report is frequently used in long-term care facilities. Each nurse's station will have a report or communication book. Because residents have a lower acuity there is less to report. The nurses are well acquainted with the residents, because they been under their care for a long time. Written report should be concise. State the resident's name, the problem, what has been done, and what if anything needs to be done by the on-coming shift. Before the entry, list time and date. If more details are needed, the on-coming nurse can be referred to the chart.

HANDOFF PROCEDURE

In addition to the end of shift report, it is important for nurses to provide information on their assigned clients at other times in order to enhance client safety. Such times include, but are not limited to when a nurse takes a break or lunch, when a nurse leaves the unit to attend a meeting or in-service, when a nurse leaves the floor with one client who is being transferred or discharged or when a client leaves the unit for diagnostic test or procedures.

It is imperative that the procedure be efficient and not create additional paperwork for the nursing staff. One system of standardized communication technique that seems to be showing promising results and acceptance by JCAHO is SBAR (situation, background, assessment and recommendation). This technique was originally developed by the U.S. Navy as a way to improve communication of critical information. Kaiser Permanente of Colorado by use of a multidisciplinary team adapted the technique for use by healthcare organizations.

The technique follows an established pattern of communication, so that deviation will be readily apparent. This will help to prevent errors and omissions.

SBAR components can be described as two objective components: situation and background. The situation includes information such as the client name, room number and what is presently going on with the client.

Example: Mrs. Warren in room 224 returned from recovery 1 hour ago, following an R TKR. (*Situation*)

Background includes admitting diagnosis and progress related to the diagnosis.

Example: She was admitted with DJD and scheduled knee replacement, which was completed today. (*Background*)

The assessment and recommendation components are that allow delivery of subjective information, including opinion and specific recommendation.

Example: She has a PCA and her pain level is 2 on a scale of 10. She is drifting in and out of sleep. (*Assessment*)

Example: She will need another set of vital signs in 15 minutes and reassess her pain. (*Recommendations*)

Many facilities have created a form that can be used. In addition the information should be provided orally giving the accepting nurse an opportunity to repeat the information to establish understanding.

Client safety has become an ongoing concern within health care organizations. Using procedures such as these will improve teamwork, communication and client care.

Students should make use of these techniques using them whenever care of a client is relinquished to another student or a licensed nurse.

Paperwork

You may have heard seasoned nurses complain about the increasing amount of paperwork. Over the years changes have been made to control the amount of writing a nurse must do. Narrative notes have been replaced with flow sheets and other forms of abbreviated charting. Increased regulations, licensing requirements, and government restrictions have created additional need for documentation. See Chapter 6 🔗 for more information about documentation.

PHYSICIAN'S ORDERS

Physician's orders are a part of the client medical record. As a nurse you need to have an order for all areas of client care. The client cannot even be admitted to the hospital without an order from a physician. Physician's orders take different forms:

- Handwritten by the physician during hospital rounds
- Verbal orders
- Preprinted or standing orders to cover admissions for certain conditions or surgeries (e.g., postpartum care following an uncomplicated delivery or total knee replacement surgery)
- Telephone orders.

Transcription of Orders

Some facilities employee a clerical person to transcribe physician's orders. This individual may have the title of ward or unit secretary or ward clerk. Unit secretaries might not be employed for the evening and night shifts or in long-term care facilities, so the LPN/LVN may be expected to carry out this task.

Handwritten orders may be difficult to read. With practice you will learn the commonalities of a physician's handwriting and will be able to read what has been written. It is important to seek a second opinion if you are having trouble deciphering an order—never guess. When in doubt seek clarification from the physician. Never carry out an unclear order until it has been clarified. Medication orders can present a particular problem. When the spelling of a medication is in question, refer to a current drug reference or a list of commonly prescribed medications. With the number of new drugs being developed and the use of both generic and trade names, it is impossible to know all drugs by sight. Use available resources to protect your clients from error.

Verbal and telephone orders are taken by a licensed nurse and recorded on the physician order sheet. Policies regarding verbal and phone orders differ from facility to facility. It is important for the LPN/LVN to know the state board policy on verbal and phone orders. These policies vary from state to state. Federal Hospital Certification Regulation 42 CFR 482.223 (c)(2)(i) states that when telephone or oral orders must be used they must be "Accepted only by personnel that are authorized to do so by the medical staff policies and procedures, consistent with Federal and State laws."

Orders given via the telephone or verbally have an increased opportunity for error. Clarify the order by repeating it back to the physician. This will give the nurse and the physician the opportunity to hear the order and make corrections if necessary. Verbal or telephone orders should be written down immediately. Verbal and phone orders must be signed by the physician. The facility will have a policy as to when the orders must be signed; policies differ with the type of facility.

INCIDENT REPORTS

An **incident report** or occurrence report is completed when client care was not consistent with standards for expected care. Issues involve omitted medications or treatments or medication administration that violated one of the "Five rights." Any unusual occurrence, one that did or may have caused harm, needs to be documented on an incident report. Injuries to client, employee, or visitor also require a report. The incident report does not become a part of the client medical record. They are usually filed with the risk management department.

When completing an incident report, be sure to include all pertinent details. List time, date, and an objective observation of the incident. Guilt should not be admitted. Other staff members who witnessed the incident or were involved should also be listed. The completed report should be turned over to the supervisor or individual designated by the facility to investigate. The purpose of the incident report is to help the facility prevent future problems through correction and education.

When the incident is reported in the medical chart, the completion of an incident report is usually not documented. Figure 36-1 ■ is an example of an incident report.

CONFIDENTIAL REPORT OF UNUSUAL OCCURRENCE
NOT a part of the Medical Record - Please forward to RISK MANAGEMENT

I. (COMPLETE IF ADDRESSOGRAPH UNAVAILABLE)

PATIENT/VISITOR _____ PHYSICIAN _____

MEDICAL RECORD # _____ DATE OF BIRTH _____

ADDRESSOGRAPH

II. DATE OF OCCURRENCE _____ TIME OF OCCURRENCE _____ LOCATION (ROOM OR FLOOR) _____

NAME OF M.D. NOTIFIED _____ PATIENT AWARE OF OCCURRENCE: YES___ NO___ FAMILY AWARE OF OCCURRENCE: YES___ NO___

REPORT COMPLETED BY _____ OTHERS FAMILIAR WITH OCCURRENCE _____

III. ADMITTING DIAGNOSIS _____

PATIENT CONDITION PRIOR TO OCCURRENCE: ALERT _____ ASLEEP _____ ANESTHETIZED _____ DISORIENTED _____ OTHER _____

IF SEDATIVE/NARCOTICS/DIURETICS GIVEN IN LAST 12 HOURS (WHERE APPLICABLE) PLEASE COMPLETE: (MED, DOSE, TIME)

IV. EVENT

FALLS
- 100 Unobserved Fall
- 101 Assisted to Floor
- 102 Fell from Bed
- 103 Fell from Table/Equipment
- 104 Fell in Bathroom
- 105 Walking/Standing/Slip & Fall
- 106 Sitting Commode/Wheelchair
- 107 Restrained Prior to Fall
- 108 Restrained After Fall
- 109 Bed Rails Up (1 2 3 4)
- 110 Bed Rails Down (1 2 3 4)
- 112 Visitor Fall
- 113 Outpatient Fall
- 119 Other_____

BURNS
- 120 Electrical/Chemical Burn
- 121 Spill
- 122 Fire
- 129 Other_____

ALTERCATION/COMPLAINTS
- 130 Pt/Family/Employee/Visitor
- 131 Complaint-Waiting Time
- 132 Complaint-Billing Services
- 133 Complaint-Food Services
- 134 Complaint-Housekeeping/Ancillary
- 135 Complaint-Nursing
- 136 Complaint-Medical Staff
- 137 Complaint-Security
- 139 Other_____

MISCELLANEOUS
- 140 Suicide/Attempt
- 141 Left AMA/Elopement
- 142 Equipment-Struck/Failure
- 143 Property Loss/Damage
- 144 Unexpected Death
- 145 Non-Compliant Smoking
- 148 Development of Pressure Ulcer
- 149 Other_____

MEDICATIONS   Drug_____
- 150 Order (Computer Entry)
- 151 Wrong Time
- 152 Wrong Dosage
- 153 Wrong Route
- 154 Wrong Drug
- 155 Wrong Patient
- 156 Omission
- 157 Adverse Drug Reaction
- 158 Prescribing Error
- 159 Other_____

INTRAVENOUS Sol._____
- 160 Infiltration
- 161 Wrong Rate
- 162 Wrong Solution
- 163 Wrong Time
- 164 Order (Computer Entry)
- 165 Infected Site/Phlebitis
- 169 Other_____

BLOOD TRANSFUSION
- 170 Allergic/Adverse Reaction
- 171 Delay in Administration
- 172 Incorrect Flow Rate
- 173 Infiltration
- 174 Omitted/Patient Refusal
- 175 Wrong Amount
- 176 Wrong/Omitted Filter
- 177 Wrong Component
- 178 Biological Product Deviation
- 179 Other_____

PATHOLOGY
- 180 Reference Laboratory Error
- 181 Lost/Mishandled Specimen
- 182 Specimen Collection Error
- 183 Cytology/Biopsy Discrepancy
- 184 Biopsy/Resection Discrepancy
- 185 Autopsy Suggests Serious Clinical Discrepancy
- 186 Frozen Section/Pathological Discrepancy
- 187 Error Performing Test/Error Reporting Results
- 188 Delayed Draw
- 189 Hematoma Following Draw
- 190 Other_____

OR/PACU/OPS/WOR
- 200 Removal Foreign Body
- 210 Incorrect Count-Sponge/Needle/Instr
- 202 X-rays Taken/Deferred
- 203 Arrest
- 204 Wrong Pt/Side/Site/Procedure
- 205 OPS Pt Admitted Post-Op
- 206 Unplanned Organ Repair/Removal
- 207 Lac/Tear/Puncture-Organ/Body Part
- 208 Canceled Surg-Prep/Equipment Problem
- 209 Unplanned Return to OR
- 210 Surgery Delayed
- 211 Consent Incorrect/Incomplete/Not Done
- 212 Reddened Area
- 213 Unsterile Situation
- 214 Specimen Problem
- 215 Eye Irritation/Injury
- 216 Post Arterial Hematoma
- 217 Improper Discharge
- 219 Other_____

ANESTHESIA
- 220 Unexpected Arrest
- 221 Canceled Surgery After Induction
- 222 Injury/Death Post Induction
- 223 Tooth/Face/Lip/Mandible Damage
- 224 CNS Injury/Brain Damage
- 225 Unplanned Transfer to Special Care Unit
- 226 Aspiration
- 229 Other_____

EMERGENCY DEPARTMENT
- 230 Arrives DOA After Discharge/Seen in ED within Past 7 Days
- 231 Seen for Complication Post Treatment/Procedure from Prev. Hospitalization
- 232 Left AMA
- 239 Other_____

OB/GYN/INFANT CARE
- 240 Delivery Occurred Outside L&D Area
- 241 Mother Transferred to ICU
- 241 Unplanned Return to Surgery
- 243 Stirrup Related Injury
- 244 Delivery Unattended by any Physician
- 245 Blood Loss > 1500 cc
- 246 Cord Blood Gas pH <7.0
- 247 Cardiac/Respiratory Arrest
- 248 Infant Seizures in Delivery Room
- 249 Apgar Score 5 or Less at 5 Minutes
- 250 Unusual Condition - Child
- 251 Infant Injury-skull fx/paralysis/palsy
- 252 Transfer From NB Nursery to ISC/NICU
- 253 Instrumented Delivery-Injury
- 259 Other_____

ADULT/PEDIATRIC CARE
- 260 Unexpected Tx – Higher Care Level
- 261 Significant Neurosensory/Functional Deficit/Intractable Pain not Present upon Admit
- 262 Acute MI/CVA within 48 hours of Surgery/Procedure
- 263 Death within 48 hours of Surgery/Procedure
- 264 Nosocomial Infection Prolonging Stay or Complicating Pt's Condition > 5 days
- 265 Patient Found Unresponsive
- 266 Self Extubation
- 267 Arrest – Code Team Activation
- 268 Soft Tissue Injury
- 269 Other_____

TESTS/TREATMENTS
- 270 Wrong Patient
- 271 Wrong Test/Treatment
- 272 Treatment Delayed
- 273 MD Ordered-Not Done
- 274 Complication Resulting in Injury
- 275 Computer Entry
- 276 Infection Control issue
- 279 Other_____

RADIOLOGY/RAD ONC/IMAGING
- 280 Complication Requiring Surgical Correction
- 281 New Onset Nerve Deficit
- 282 Reaction to Contrast Agent
- 283 Overexposure to Radiation
- 284 Cardiac/Respiratory Arrest
- 285 Treatment Delayed Worsening Condition
- 286 Unplanned Repeat Diagnostic Procedure
- 287 Monitored Inadequately
- 288 X-ray Inaccurately Read
- 289 Equipment Failure
- 290 Lack of Prep-Cancel Procedure
- 291 Wrong Pt/Side/Site/Prodedure
- 299 Other_____

V. OUTCOME

SEVERITY OF OUTCOME
- 350 No Injury/Unaffected
- *351 Minor Injury
- *352 Major Injury/Consequential

*_SPECIFY INJURY BELOW –

GENERAL
- 300 Delay in Therapy
- 301 Embolism
- 302 Reaction/Toxic Effect
- 303 Death
- 304 Prolonged Hospital Stay
- 305 Neurological Sensory
- 306 Decubitus
- 307 Arrest/CPR
- 309 Other_____

OBSTETRICAL
- 310 Unusually Low Apgar
- 311 Fetal Injury
- 312 Fetal Death
- 313 Maternal Injury
- 314 Maternal Death
- 319 Other_____

SKELETAL
- 320 Fracture
- 321 Dislocation
- 322 Teeth
- 323 Sprain
- 329 Other_____

TISSUE
- 330 Hematoma/Contusion
- 331 Necrosis
- 332 Laceration
- 333 Fistula
- 334 Dehiscence
- 335 Abrasion/Blister
- 336 Swelling
- 337 Reddened Area/Ecchymosis
- 338 Skin Tear
- 339 Other_____

VI. BRIEF COMMENTS IF NECESSARY _____

1004952 (9/01)

Figure 36-1. ■ Example of an incident report.

Conflict Resolution

Conflict can be defined as a disagreement or antagonism between groups, individuals, or ideas. The presence of conflict is not necessarily a negative situation. Well-managed conflicts can stimulate competition, can bring new ideas to the table, and can identify legitimate differences and problems within an organization. As children we were taught to manage conflicts passively; we were sent to the corner or "time-out" when we couldn't get along. In nursing conflicts cannot be ignored, but instead must be dealt with and managed no matter how difficult that might be.

Several common approaches are used for conflict resolution. The ability to manage conflicts is a critical skill, which a nurse must develop. Use of these skills can help the nurse to be more productive. It is important to select a strategy that is appropriate to the situation. Frequently, nurses select strategies that are more comfortable rather than effective. Table 36-2 ■ lists various approaches to conflict resolution and situations in which they are used.

STAGES OF CONFLICT

On-the-job conflicts produce reactions within the person, much like any other psychosocial problem. There are six stages of conflict:

1. *Disbelief* is an initial emotional reaction. This frequently happens when values that are held in high regard are disagreed with or discounted.
2. *Disconnectedness.* This stage follows the shock of the first stage. The individual feels confused and taken aback.
3. *Obsession.* The individual becomes obsessed with the situation, and soon it is all the person can think about. Many times, this results in inability to sleep; wakeful nights are spent thinking about what to do.
4. *Frenzied activity* follows. Many people find this a way of reducing the bitterness, pain, and frustration they feel. The conflicted person may acquire boundless energy, working endlessly to seek information that will help him or her understand the problem. Colleagues are consulted one after another, trying to redefine the situation. The individual aggressively takes on new tasks or may be involved in numerous activities simultaneously.

TABLE 36-2

Conflict Resolution Strategies

STRATEGIES	DESCRIPTION	SITUATION
Competition	Winner takes all; results in a win–lose situation.	During an emergency when there is no time for discussion. **Situation:** During a code blue situation; someone must direct the code team without discussion.
Accommodation	One person or a group is willing to yield to the other.	When preserving relationships; or encouraging others to express themselves and learn by actions. **Situation:** Used by two team leaders when deciding who will get the extra float nurse.
Avoidance	Lose–lose; one side denies that the problem exists or withdraws so that there is no active resolution.	When others may resolve the conflict more effectively; both sides see issue as minor or the negative impact is too costly to meet issue head on. **Situation:** After a heated discussion with a physician, a nurse asks another to make rounds until the nurse has had time to calm down. Nurses use avoidance as primary strategy for resolution of conflicts.
Compromise	Negotiation, trade-offs; each person gets something and gives up something; win–lose/win–lose for both sides.	When there is a need to reach an agreement between equally empowered sides. Conflicts resolved by finding common ground. **Situation:** A nurse volunteers to stay over to cover a shift if another colleague agrees to come in early.
Collaboration	Both parties meet problem on an even playing field. Each has equal concern for the issues, allows everyone to win by identifying areas of agreement and differences. Alternatives are evaluated and solutions are selected. There is full support and commitments from both sides.	Can be used to solve previously irreconcilable and long-standing problems. **Situation:** A manager assigns two feuding nurses to work together to solve chronic unit problems.

5. *Balance or burnout.* As the frenzied search for clues subsides, the individual either begins to reestablish balance or succumbs to symptoms of burnout—withdrawal, depression, and apathy. In intense conflicts, the individual may turn the negative feelings inward. When this occurs, purposeful alienation follows: The individual places emotional and perhaps even physical space between self and colleagues. This is a self-preservation move.

6. *Caution* is adopted as the individual controls verbalization and self-preservation. This move provides a rest or refuge for all involved parties. Once the conflict is resolved positively, the individual may gain personal insight into how to handle future conflicts.

Nurses will have to be prepared to deal with conflicts in all areas of nursing practice. Knowing how and when to use appropriate strategies will promote successful conflict resolution.

Nursing Care Delivery Trends

Throughout the years the delivery of nursing services has continued to change. It is important that nursing professionals understand these trends and be proactive as far as making personal changes to meet the needs of their careers.

The oldest delivery method of nursing services is the **case method,** in which a nurse is responsible for care provided for clients during one shift. Intensive care units frequently operate under the case method. Private duty nurses and home care can also be described as nursing by the case method.

In the **functional nursing** system, each team member is assigned specific tasks or functions. Although functional nursing is efficient, it can create fragmented delivery of client care. Establishing a therapeutic relationship between nurse and client is somewhat more difficult because of the large number of care professionals interacting with the client.

In **primary nursing** a professional nurse has total responsibility for a group of clients. It is a more recent development in delivery methods. Primary nursing in the purest sense gives responsibility to the nurse 24 hours a day 7 days a week, from admission through discharge. The purpose of this method is to provide continuity and coordination of care. If the RN is not physically in attendance, the care may be delegated to an associate who may be another RN or and LPN/LVN. Many hospitals ascribe to primary nursing, but in a way that resembles the case method. While the nurse is working, the responsibility to the assigned client is his or hers.

Team nursing has been used since the early 1950s. It was replaced with primary nursing in the 1970s. The purpose of this concept was to reduce fragmentation, which was present in the functional method. Team nursing is again becoming increasingly popular given the nursing shortage and small nurse-to-client ratios. An RN usually directs the nursing team in the acute hospital. The remainder of the team is made up of LPNs/LVNs and unlicensed

---

> **BOX 36-5**
>
> ### Roles and Responsibilities of the LPN/LVN
>
> - Recognizes the LPN's/LVN's role in the healthcare delivery system and articulates that role with those of other healthcare team members.
> - Maintains accountability for one's own nursing practice within the ethical and legal framework.
> - Serves as a client advocate.
> - Accepts role in maintaining developing standards of practice in providing health care.
> - Seeks further growth through educational opportunities.

---

personnel (e.g., nursing assistants, client care technicians). A nursing unit may have two or more nursing teams caring for 10 or more clients. Team members work together to use their diverse skills and education to best care for the assigned clients. Care planning is done in team meetings in which all members have input.

MEN IN NURSING

Throughout history men have made significant contributions to the nursing profession. Current trends show increased numbers of men entering the profession. At one time men sought positions in specialty areas such as psychiatry, emergency and trauma nursing, correctional institutions and rehabilitation, and the medical-surgical area. They sought administration positions. More recently there has been increased interest by men in hospice, pediatric, and neonatology nursing and in teaching in schools of nursing. The increased number of men entering the profession has brought a different perspective and an increase in salary and benefits.

Regardless of whether the nurse is a male or a female, whether he or she works in an acute hospital, ambulatory care, a specialty area, or long-term care, it is important to be aware of current trends. Being well informed will help you to be a more effective nurse and a valuable member of the healthcare community, as you carry out the roles and responsibilities of an LPN/LVN. Box 36-5 ■ explains these roles and responsibilities.

Surveyors and Accreditation

Two words that seem to send a wave of fear through a healthcare facility are *surveys* and *accreditation.* Meeting standards such as those put forth by the Joint Commission on Accreditation of Healthcare Organizations (JCAHO) have become increasingly important. Healthcare consumers are becoming more involved in their healthcare choices, so a facility that achieves accreditation will be one that is sought after by prospective clients. Whether you are the bedside nurse in an acute hospital or have more responsibility in a subacute area, when the surveyors visit you will be a vital part of the team.

TRACER METHODOLOGY

Tracer methodology is an evaluation method used by JCAHO surveyors. They select a resident or client and use that individual's record as a road map to move through the organization to assess and evaluate the organization's compliance with selected standards and the organization's systems of providing care and services. If the surveyor identifies problems, the facility has 45 days from the end of the survey to submit evidence of standards compliance and identify measures of success.

NATIONAL PATIENT SAFETY GOALS

In May 2005, the JCAHO's Board of Commissioners approved 2006 national patient safety goals. Fourteen goals have been identified that have accreditation program applicability. Table 36-3 ■ summarizes these safety goals.

TABLE 36-3

JCAHO's 2006 National Patient Safety Goals

GOAL	SUBGOAL	FACILITY-TYPE AFFECTED
Goal 1 Improve the accuracy of patient identification.	**1A** Use at least two patient identifiers (neither can be room number). **1B** Prior to invasive procedure verify correct patient, procedure, site, and availability of appropriate documents.	**[1A]** Ambulatory, assisted living, behavioral health care, critical access hospitals, disease-specific care, home care, hospital, lab, long-term care **[1B]** Assisted living, disease-specific care, home care, lab, long-term care
Goal 2 Improve the effectiveness of communication among caregivers.	**2A** "Read back" complete verbal or telephone orders or reporting of critical test results. **2B** Standardize a list of abbreviations, acronyms, and symbols that will not be used throughout an organization. **2C** Improve the timeliness of reporting and receipt of critical test results and values. **2D** Critical labs reported to responsible care provider within time frame set by lab and have a mechanism for notifying an alternate responsible caregiver if primary is unavailable. **2E** Implement a standardized approach to "hand off" communication, including an opportunity to ask and respond to questions.	**[2A]** Ambulatory, assisted living, behavioral health care, critical access hospitals, disease-specific care, home care, hospital, lab, long-term care, office-based surgery **[2B]** Ambulatory, assisted living, behavioral health care, critical access hospitals, disease-specific care, home care, hospital, lab, long-term care, office-based surgery **[2C]** Ambulatory, behavioral health care, critical access hospitals, disease-specific care, home care, hospital, lab, office-based surgery **[2D]** Lab
Goal 3 Improve the safety of using medications.	**3B** Standardize and limit the number of drug concentrations available in the organization **3C** Identify and annually review list of look-alike/sound-alike drugs and take action to prevent errors. **3D** Label all medications, medication containers, or other solutions on and off the sterile field in perioperative and other procedural settings.	**[3B]** Ambulatory, behavioral health care, critical access hospitals, disease-specific care, home care, hospital, long-term care, office-based surgery **[3C]** Ambulatory, behavioral health care, critical access hospitals, disease-specific care, home care, hospital, long-term care, office-based surgery **[3D]** Ambulatory, critical access hospitals, hospital, office-based surgery
Goal 4 Eliminate wrong-site, wrong-patient, wrong-procedure surgery.	**4A** Create and use a preoperative verification process to confirm appropriate documents are available. **4B** Implement a process for marking surgical site, which involves the patient.	**[4A]** Disease-specific care **[4B]** Disease-specific care
Goal 5 Infusion pump safety (Goal 5 retired in 2005)	None	None
Goal 6 Improve the effectiveness of clinical alarm systems.	**6A** Implement regular preventive maintenance and testing of alarm system. **6B** Ensure alarms are activated and audible.	**[6A]** Disease-specific care **[6B]** Disease-specific care
Goal 7 Reduce the risk of healthcare-associated infections.	**7A** Comply with current CDC hand hygiene guidelines.	**[7A]** Ambulatory, assisted living, behavioral health care, critical access hospitals, disease-

(continued)

TABLE 36-3

JCAHO's 2006 National Patient Safety Goals (*continued*)

GOAL	SUBGOAL	FACILITY-TYPE AFFECTED
	7B Manage as sentinel event all identified cases of unanticipated death or major permanent loss of function associated with healthcare-associated infections.	specific care, home care, hospital, lab, long-term care, office-based surgery **[7B]** Ambulatory, assisted living, behavioral health care, critical access hospitals, disease-specific care, home care, hospital, lab, long-term care, office-based surgery
Goal 8 Accurately and completely reconcile medications across the continuum of care.	**8A** Implement a process for obtaining and documenting a complete list of patient's current medications on admission to healthcare facility. **8B** A complete list of patient's medications is communicated to the next provider of service when a patient is referred or transferred to another setting service, practioner or level or care within or outside the organization.	**[8A]** Ambulatory, assisted living, behavioral health care, critical access hospitals, disease-specific care, home care, hospital, long-term care, office-based surgery **[8B]** Ambulatory, assisted living, behavioral health care, critical access hospitals, disease-specific care, home care, hospital, long-term care, office-based surgery
Goal 9 Reduce risk of patient harm resulting from falls.	**9B** Implement a fall reduction program and evaluate effectiveness.	**[9B]** Assisted living, critical access hospital, disease-specific care, home care, long-term care
Goal 10 Reduce the risk of influenza and pneumococcal disease in institutionalized older adults.	**10A** Develop and implement protocol for administration and documentation of flu vaccine. **10B** Develop and implement protocol for administration and documentation of pneumococcus vaccine. **10C** Develop and implement protocol to identify new cases of influenza and manage outbreaks.	**[10A]** Assisted living, disease-specific care, long-term care **[10B]** Assisted living, disease-specific care, long-term care **[10C]** Assisted living, disease-specific care, long-term care
Goal 11 Reduce risks from surgical fires.	**11A** Educate staff on how to control heat source and manage fires and establish guidelines to minimize oxygen concentration under drapes.	**[11A]** Ambulatory, office-based surgery
Goal 12 Implement applicable national safety goals and associated requirements by components and practitioner sites.	**12A** Inform and encourage components and practitioner sites to implement the national safety goals.	**[12A]** Networks
Goal 13 Encourage the active involvement of patients and their families in patient's care as a patient safety strategy.	**13A** Define and communicate the means for patients to report concerns about safety and encourage them to do so.	**[13A]** Assisted living, disease-specific care, home care, lab
Goal 14 Prevent healthcare-associated pressure (decubitus) ulcers.	**14A** Assess and reassess each patient's risk for developing a pressure ulcer and take action to address any identified risks.	**[14A]** Long-term care

Community Service

Your community has provided you with many opportunities. If you received your training in a public institution, your community has supported you in reaching your goal to become a nurse. It is now time for you to do the same for other citizens. Community service is one very important way to fulfill this challenge. You can volunteer to use your skills at schools, community activities, senior centers, or churches. You can provide community healthcare education or you can become involved with activities such as Race for the Cure, Relay for Life, or a Memory Walk. These events give you the opportunity to raise money for the sponsoring agencies, educate your sponsors, and provide you with an opportunity to exercise.

Note: The references and resources for this and all chapters have been compiled at the back of the book.

Chapter Review

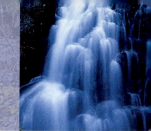

 KEY TERMS by Topic

Use the audio glossary feature of either the CD-ROM or the Companion Website to hear the correct pronunciation of the following key terms.

Licensure
license, licensure, standards, nurse practice acts

Leadership Styles
leadership, autocratic, laissez-faire, democratic,

Team Leading
delegation

Reporting Techniques
shift report, taped report, oral report, written report

Paperwork
incident report

Conflict Resolution
conflict

Nursing Care Delivery Trends
case method, functional nursing, primary nursing, team nursing

KEY Points

- Graduates of an LPN/LVN program cannot use the title licensed practical/vocational nurse until the licensing exam has been passed.

- The licensing exam is a national test developed by the National Council of State Boards of Nursing.

- Each state board of nursing has a responsibility to protect the public.

- Nurse practice acts are specific for each jurisdiction and recognize possible conflicts between the scope of practice and task being performed by the LPN/LVN.

- Leadership styles need to be adapted to the situation.

- The leadership role most often assumed by the LPN/LVN is the role of team leader.

- The ability to delegate is a sign of a good leader.

- Shift report is a form of delegation. Not only does it pass responsibility from one nurse to another, but reports what has been done.

- Even if clerical staff are responsible for transcribing physicians' orders, the license nurse is ultimately responsible for the transcription being correct.

- The incident does not become a part of the medical record.

- Conflicts should not be encouraged or discouraged.

- Well-managed conflicts can stimulate competition and identify legitimate differences and problems within the organization.

- Methods of delivery of nursing services continue to change. Keeping up with current trends is very important for the working nurse.

 EXPLORE Media Link

Additional interactive resources for this chapter can be found on the Companion Website at www.prenhall.com/ramont. Click on Chapter 36 and "Begin" to select the activities for this chapter.

For chapter-related NCLEX®-style questions and an audio glossary, access the accompanying CD-ROM in this book.

FOR FURTHER Study

See Chapter 6 for more information about documentation.

NCLEX-PN® Exam Preparation

1 The most frequent conflict resolution strategy used by staff nurses is:

1. collaboration.
2. accommodation.
3. avoidance.
4. competition.

2 A new LPN is assigned to your unit. She appears to have a great need to be liked. Which of the following conflict resolution strategies is this individual likely to use?

1. collaboration
2. accommodation
3. avoidance
4. competition

3 Your hospital has begun to hire unlicensed assistive personnel (UAPs) to alleviate some of the workload of the licensed nurses. You will be delegating some activities to the UAPs. The most frequent reason delegated activities are not completed as expected is:

1. the need to avoid conflict.
2. inappropriate supervision.
3. poor UAP attitudes.
4. inadequate communication.

4 Which of the following job titles require a license to practice?

1. care partner
2. nursing assistant
3. LPN or LVN
4. orderly

5 You have been studying accountability in nursing as it relates to delegation of tasks. One of your classmates asks you to define the term. Of the following definitions, which most accurately describes accountability?

1. the provision of guidance, direction, evaluation, and follow-up by a licensed nurse
2. being responsible and answerable for actions of self and others in the context of delegation
3. delegating nursing activities to be performed by an individual consistent with his or her licensed scope of practice
4. transferring to a competent individual the authority to perform a selected nursing task in a selected situation

6 You are working as a certified nursing assistant on weekends while enrolled in your vocational nursing program. Your supervisor knows that you are a student and asks you to pass medications, which she had prepared. Of the following, which is the best response to her request?

1. "I can't do that because I am not licensed yet. I would think you would know better than to ask me."
2. "I have been trained to pass medications in my program. I can pass them, but you will have to sign the M.A.R."
3. "I have my own work to do, I don't have time."
4. "I'm sorry; medications are not within the scope of practice for a nursing assistant. Perhaps I could assist you by giving your clients their baths or making their beds."

7 You have been discussing leadership styles in class. Your instructor describes a manager who leaves the unit staff alone to tackle their work, sort out their roles, and solve problems, leaving the team floundering with little motivation or direction. You know that this is a description of which style of management?

1. autocratic
2. laissez-faire
3. authoritative
4. democratic

8 The nursing system in which establishing a therapeutic relationship between nurse and client is somewhat more difficult because of the large number of team care professionals interacting with the client is known as:

1. team nursing.
2. primary nursing.
3. functional nursing.
4. case method.

9 Under the nurse practice act, who has the responsibility to suspend or revoke a nursing license?

1. the National Council for Licensure Examination for Practical Nurses (NCLEX-PN®)
2. the attorney general of the state in which the license was issued
3. the state board of nursing in the state in which the license was issued
4. the superior court judge if the nurse is convicted of a felony

10 You are assigned to a nursing team that consists of an RN, two unlicensed assistive personnel (UAPs), and yourself (the LPN). You observe that both assistants have left the floor for their lunch break at the same time. What is your most appropriate action to remedy the situation?

1. Have them paged on the overhead pager to return to the floor, and tell them never to do that again.
2. When they return, inquire as to why they both left at the same time, and discuss with them the floor policy and the safety issues, which may have occurred.
3. When they return, tell them that you will have to report them to the RN.
4. Report their behavior to the RN, mentioning how irresponsible they are being.

Answers and Rationales for Review Questions, as well as discussion of Care Plan and Critical Thinking Care Map questions, appear in Appendix I.

Chapter 37

Preparing to Take the Licensure Exam

BRIEF Outline

Development of the NCLEX-PN®
Understanding the NCLEX-PN® Plan
Preparing and Reviewing for the Exam
Evaluating Your Readiness to Take the Examination
Applying to Take the NCLEX-PN®
Coping with Test Anxiety
Taking the Examination
Waiting for Your Results

LEARNING Outcomes

After completing this chapter, you will be able to:

1. Describe the purpose of the examination.
2. Explain how the National Council of State Boards of Nursing develops the test plan and the test.
3. Identify how to get a copy of the current NCLEX-PN® test plan.
4. Explain the concept of a multistate compact.
5. Describe the four categories of client needs and their subcategories.
6. Describe selected aspects of the test itself.
7. Develop an individualized plan for reviewing for the NCLEX-PN®.
8. Assess personal readiness for the examination.
9. Explain how to apply to take the examination.
10. Describe how to overcome test anxiety.
11. Describe what to do the day before, day of, and during the examination to increase the chances of success on the examination.

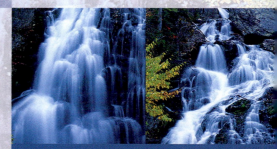

HISTORICAL Perspectives

The history of LPN/LVN testing and licensure is relatively short. In the 1950s regulatory laws governing nurses began to address LPNs/LVNs as well as registered nurses. Licensure examinations in the 1950s were developed and administered by the individual state boards of nursing and were paper-and-pencil tests, usually offered in one or more selected locations in the state, once or twice a year with many students testing in the same room. Test question security was a major concern.

From the minute you enter nursing school until you graduate, you must be aware that, in order to practice as a licensed practical/vocational nurse:

1. You need to acquire a certain body of nursing knowledge and nursing skills.
2. You must pass the National Council Licensure Examination for Practical/Vocational Nurses (NCLEX-PN®).

The purpose of this examination is to protect the public by ensuring that all licensed entry-level nurses have the competencies they need to practice safely and effectively.

Development of the NCLEX-PN®

The National Council of State Boards of Nursing, Inc. (NCSBN), is a not-for-profit organization comprised of the boards of nursing in the 50 states, the District of Columbia, and five United States territories: American Samoa, Guam, Northern Mariana Islands, Puerto Rico, and the Virgin Islands.

NCSBN develops a test plan on which the NCLEX-PN® is based. In developing the test plan, the NCSBN considers the legal scope of practical/vocational nursing practice, as governed by each state's laws and regulations, including the various nurse practice acts. The NCSBN also conducts a vocational nursing job analysis study every 3 years. This analysis is used to develop the framework for the current NCLEX-PN®. Test questions on the NCLEX-PN® focus on the job tasks identified as those normally carried out by entry-level LPNs/LVNs in their first year of nursing employment. The test plan provides a summary of the content and the scope of the exam.

The NCSBN currently (2005) contracts with Pearson Professional Testing for the development and administration of the NCLEX-PN®. NCSBN retains oversight and provides volunteer test item writers. These item writers are professional faculty members in schools of nursing who have been approved and recommended to NCSBN by their respective state boards of nursing and screened for test-writing ability. Item writers receive additional training in item writing and write test questions based on the test plan. Expert item reviewers review all items written by item writers. Accepted items then go to panel judges for additional review and edit. New items are pilot tested on the NCLEX-PN® and these items do not count for or against the test taker.

AVAILABILITY OF THE NCLEX-PN®

The NCLEX-PN® is available in the District of Columbia, every state in the United States, in the various territories of the United States, and three foreign countries: Seoul, South Korea; London, England; and Hong Kong, Special Administrative District of China.

Because the boards of nursing from the United States and its territories, as well as these other countries, use the NCLEX-PN® to assist them in making licensure decisions, you may be able to get licensure by endorsement from a state board of nursing in a state or territory and possibly a country other than the one in which you took the examination, should you decide to work somewhere other than the state or country where you took your exam.

Multistate Compact

In addition to endorsement, the concept of a **multistate compact** became reality when, in 2000, Utah became the first state to enact multistate licensure legislation. Arkansas, Maryland, North and South Carolina, Texas, Iowa, Nebraska, South Dakota, Wisconsin, Mississippi, Maine, Delaware, and Idaho quickly joined Utah. If the state where you pass your NCLEX-PN® is part of this multistate compact, you can practice in another state that is part of the compact, as long as you follow the nurse practice act and the rules and regulations pertaining to the act. See also Chapter 3 ⬭.

Understanding the NCLEX-PN® Plan

COGNITIVE LEVELS OF QUESTIONS

The NCLEX-PN® questions are developed at the cognitive levels of knowledge, comprehension, application, and analysis. Table 37-1 ■ describes the cognitive levels of testing and provides some examples. Your nursing instructors will give you tests and examinations at these cognitive levels throughout your nursing courses. These will help prepare you for the examination and be more comfortable with each level of question.

TEST PLAN FRAMEWORK

"Client needs" was chosen as the framework of the test plan. Client needs is a universal concept that is applicable to a variety of clients in a wide spectrum of healthcare settings.

Client Needs

The NCLEX-PN® is organized around four categories of client needs across the life span in a variety of settings:

1. Safe, effective care environment
2. Health promotion and maintenance
3. Psychosocial integrity
4. Physiological integrity.

Box 37-1 ■ lists the categories and subcategories of the test. The percentage of questions given for each category for the 2005–2006 test are also shown in Box 37-1. Percentages of questions from each of the 10 subcategories are set by the NCSBN. These percentages can be obtained by visiting the NCSBN website or by writing to the NCSBN for a test plan. Percentages can change from one test plan revision to the next.

TABLE 37-1	
Cognitive Levels of Testing (Bloom's Taxonomy)	
COGNITIVE LEVEL	**DESCRIPTION AND EXAMPLE**
Knowledge	Questions at a knowledge level test a person's memory of a fact or recall of a given piece of information. *Example:* Which of the following numbers of questions is the maximum number of questions a test taker can receive when taking the NCLEX-PN®? *Answer:* 205. This tests simple memory of this fact.
Comprehension	Comprehension questions test a person's understanding of concepts or principles. It is an understanding of what something means or how something is related to something else. It can involve reorganizing or restating learned information to demonstrate understanding. *Example:* After completing the teaching of insulin injection to a diabetic client, the nurse will have the most confidence in the client's understanding of the teaching if the client does which of the following things? *Answer:* Demonstrates self-injection principle; most people learn better by doing rather than seeing or hearing.
Application	Application questions test a person's ability to use information such as concepts, theories, principles, and formulas in new situations, or to come up with a solution to a problem. *Example:* The LPN is admitting a new client to the pediatric clinic. The mother asks if the 15 month old child is due for any immunization today. The most appropriate answer would be _____. *Answer:* Since Varicella was not given at your 12 month visit it should be given today. The nurse applies knowledge of the immunization schedule to answer the mother's questions.
Analysis	Analysis questions provide information that needs to be separated, sorted, and examined by looking at the various parts and a conclusion drawn to clarify meaning or show how something is structured. *Example:* The physician orders: Vistaril 20 mg IM every 4–6 hours prn nausea for a child, who weighs 44 lbs. The medication resource indicates that the usual IM dosage is 0.5 mg to 1 mg/kg/dose every 4 to 6 hours as needed. Is this a safe dosage for this child's weight? *Answer:* Yes, this child's safe range is 10 to 20 mg/dose.

A number of concepts and processes that students learn well before graduation are integrated throughout the categories of client needs. They include (1) clinical problem solving process (i.e., the nursing process; see Chapter 4 ⚭), (2) caring, (3) communication and documentation, and (4) teaching/learning.

NCLEX-PN® QUESTIONS BY CLIENT NEEDS.   The questions in Box 37-2 ■ will give you some idea of the format of the NCLEX-PN® questions. Provided in the discussion of the answer is the category of client needs as well as the subcategory (see Box 37-1). Students do not need to know how to identify the categories and subcategories listed in Box 37-1 to

BOX 37-1	

Framework of the NCLEX-PN Exam

Client Needs Categories and Percentage of Questions

1. Safe, effective care environment:
   a. Coordinated care (11–17%)
   b. Safety and infection control (8–14%)
2. Health promotion and maintenance (7–13%)
3. Psychosocial integrity (8–14%)
4. Physiological integrity:
   a. Basic care and comfort (11–17%)
   b. Pharmacologic therapies (9–15%)
   c. Reduction of risk potential (10–16%)
   d. Physiological adaptation (12–18%)

Additional Concepts and Processes

- Nursing process
- Caring
- Communication
- Documentation
- Cultural awareness
- Self-care
- Teaching/learning

Test Plan Contact Information

Information on the current test plan can be found on the NCSBN website or you can write to National Council of State Boards of Nursing, 676 St. Clair Street, Suite 550, Chicago, Illinois 60611-2921.

BOX 37-2

Sample NCLEX-PN® Type Questions by Client Needs Category

1. Your assigned client asks you for something for pain. The physician has ordered meperidine (Demerol) 125 mg and promethazine hydrochloride (Phenergan) 25 mg every 4 hours prn. In addition to checking for allergies and when the last dose of the medication was given, it would be most important to do which of the following?
   1. Check the client's respiration rate before giving the injection.
   2. Put the side rails up after the injection.
   3. Teach client not to wait until pain is bad to ask for medication.
   4. Identify the location and intensity of the pain.
   Answer: 1. Since Demerol is likely to depress respirations, the nurse must check the respiratory rate to ensure that it is 12 breaths per minute or above before giving the pain medication. *This question is at the client need category of physiological integrity and subcategory of reduction of risk potential.*

2. When working with a client who has been admitted with a diagnosis of alcohol dependency, the nurse asks the client to describe the problems that caused him to be admitted. The client says that he does not have any problems and it is his spouse who has the problems. The nurse realizes that the client is using which of the following defense mechanisms?
   1. denial
   2. suppression
   3. rationalization
   4. identification
   Answer: 1. The client is using denial. Persons with alcohol or other drug abuse or dependency most often use the defense mechanism of denial. They frequently deny that they have a problem to avoid getting treatment. *This question is at the level of evaluation in nursing process. It is in the client needs category of psychosocial integrity and the subcategory of coping and adaptation.*

3. The nurse is doing some teaching on recognizing the early warning signs of diabetes. Which of the following warning signs will the nurse include as an early warning sign of diabetes?
   1. pain on urination
   2. lack of appetite
   3. increased thirst
   4. scant voidings
   Answer: 3. The early warning signs of diabetes include increased urination, increased hunger, and increased thirst. *This question is in the health promotion and maintenance category of client needs and the subcategory of prevention and early detection of disease.*

---

test well. You will not be asked to identify them. This information is provided for those students who want an example of the various categories and subcategories of client needs on the test plan. It would be helpful to look at the categories and the lists of related content that is included under each category of client needs, for example, under the category "safe, effective care environment," you will find the content includes advance directives, advocacy, informed consent, and much more. Under psychosocial integrity there is abuse or neglect, coping mechanisms, grief and loss, and much more. Looking at information on content under the four categories of client needs might help you in planning your studies and help you realize the wide scope of content on the NCLEX-PN®. You can find this information on the NCLEX Examination Candidate Bulletin at the NCSBN website.

Computer Adaptive Testing (CAT)

Prior to April 1994, the examination for licensure as a licensed practical/vocational nurse was a paper-and-pencil test administered by each state board of nursing. Large numbers of candidates for licensure took the exam in a room monitored by proctors. Examinations were usually given only twice a year. Test security was a major concern, with large numbers of people taking the same examination at the same time and with versions of the test being administered again from time to time.

In April 1994, candidates for licensure began to take the licensure examination on the computer. The computer uses a method called **computer adaptive testing (CAT)** to provide each student a unique examination, selecting the test questions as the student takes the examination. In April 2001, those taking the exam could use a computer mouse for the first time, and a drop-down calculator became available.

The test questions for the NCLEX-PN® exams are stored in an extremely large test bank. Questions are categorized according to their fit into various categories of the test plan structure. In addition, questions are categorized according to the level of difficulty. Each candidate is given a unique examination to test her or his knowledge and abilities while meeting the test plan requirements.

When you take this exam and answer a question correctly, the computer will scan the test bank and give you a more difficult question. On the other hand, if you select an incorrect answer, the computer will scan the test bank and give you an easier question.

In addition to the "real" questions that will determine if you are a safe practitioner or not, you will be given an additional 25 questions that will not count for or against you. These 25 additional questions are often referred to as "try-out" questions. These questions are being field tested or "pilot tested." In other words, they are being tested or tried out on real exam takers to see if they are appropriate questions for future NCLEX® examinations.

The maximum testing period is 5 hours. These 5 hours include a tutorial, sample questions, and breaks as well as answering the examination questions. If you are still testing at the end of 5 hours, you will receive no more questions. The maximum number of questions you can receive is 205. If you are testing and finish the 205th question, you will get no more questions. That is the end of your testing. The minimum number of questions you can receive is 85 carefully chosen questions. The NCSBN believes that this is the minimum number of questions that can determine whether you are a safe practitioner or not.

You will test until (1) the computer program determines that you have clearly met the test plan requirements or (2) you have failed or (3) you have run out of time. You can pass or fail with either the minimum number or the maximum number or any number between 85 and 205.

To understand how you can pass or fail with the same number of questions, it is helpful to realize that if you answer a question correctly, you will be given a harder question. If you answer a question incorrectly, you will be given an easier question. The computer ends your examination when it calculates with a 95% degree of confidence that you have tested in a way that indicates you are a safe/competent practitioner or you are not.

Alternate Format Questions

The majority of items on the NCLEX-PN® are four-option, multiple-choice questions. Initially the exam offered only this type of question, but beginning in April 2003, alternate item formats were introduced into the examination. Alternate items are based on the current test plan and do not have an effect on the length of the test. Initially, less than 2% of the items in the question pool were of the alternate type. A candidate taking the minimum length examination might receive one item in the alternate format. This alternate format type of question gives the candidate the opportunity to demonstrate entry-level nursing competence in ways that are different from the standard multiple-choice items. Some of the alternate format question types ask the candidates to perform calculations without the benefit of selecting the answer from four answer options. Another form is a fill-in-the-blank question, which requires the candidate to type in an answer to the question. Some of the new items present four or more response options, and they may require the candidate to select more than one correct option. The final question type can be used to evaluate the candidate's skill. This type is referred to as a "Hot Spot." This item includes an anatomic drawing and requests the candidate to identify the appropriate spot for obtaining assessment information.

Specific example questions can be viewed at the NCSBN website or in the NCLEX® Examination Candidate Bulletin.

Preparing and Reviewing for the Exam

PREPARING FOR THE EXAM

Have you ever been in a class where some of the students asked the instructor to cover only what would be on the exam, suggesting that if it is not on the exam, it is not important? This is not the way to prepare yourself for the licensure exam or to prepare yourself to provide good nursing care. Preparation begins the day you start your first nursing class and includes but is not limited to the following:

- Reading assignments for class
- Completing practice quizzes at the end of assigned chapters
- Using the computerized test banks that come with the texts to practice taking tests of key concepts
- Participating in class
- Learning **mnemonics** (techniques for developing memory).

Mnemonics can help you remember key concepts that you need to recall for the NCLEX-PN®, as well as important information for giving safe care to your clients. An example of a mnemonic for blood pressure readings is using the words "sit down." "Sit" stands for systolic as the first/top number; "down" stands for diastolic or the bottom/last number in a blood pressure reading. When you say "sit down," you think, "**s**it" is for **s**ystolic (the first number and the one on top); **d**own is for **d**iastolic (the bottom and last number in the blood pressure reading). Mnemonics are useful for any key things that you must remember quickly and retain forever, not just for a quiz, midterm, or final exam.

Box 37-3 ■ provides tips for preparing for the NCLEX-PN® if English is not your first language.

BOX 37-3   **CULTURAL PULSE POINTS**

English as a Non-Native Language

Preparing for the licensure examination should begin early in nursing school. Many instructors incorporate NCLEX®-style questions into their tests. Studying for quizzes and final exams will also help you to prepare for the NCLEX®. If English is not your native language, you may encounter words, phrases, or expressions that are confusing. Create a section in your notebook to record these things that you do not understand from lecture reading or conversation. Leave space so that you can later record an explanation. It is not appropriate to interrupt the instructor for each one of these; but the instructor will be happy to explain them after class, especially if you have tried to sort them out for yourself.

The following is one example of confusing wording: The nurse *wound* a gauge bandage around the client's arm to hold the dressing over the *wound*.

REVIEWING FOR THE EXAM

Review for the NCLEX-PN® examination needs to begin early. Plan to devote some time each day or a certain number of hours per week to such activities as working in an NCLEX-PN® review book or studying with a study group. Closer to the time of the examination, you can consider taking a professional review course for the NCLEX-PN® and taking a mock NCLEX® examination. Some schools of nursing require students to take a mock NCLEX® examination.

NCLEX-PN Review Books

A variety of NCLEX-PN® review books have been published by major nursing publishing companies. These books do not contain the questions from the NCLEX-PN® itself. (The questions in that test bank are confidential.) However, these review books do contain similar questions and cover the key concepts as well as the areas and categories that are tested in the licensing exam. While the review books may vary in their presentation, most are divided into units of specialized content, each with a review of key concepts, a practice exam on the content, and a section of answers with rationales for the correct answer.

To maximize your readiness to take the exam, you need to begin using a review book long before you take the licensing exam (Figure 37-1 ■). You could start at least 6 months before the exam and try to review a set number of pages each day or each week so you will have sufficient time to firm up the key concepts in your mind. You would benefit from reviewing more than one NCLEX-PN® book. You and a fellow student might each buy different review books and trade books at some point.

Study Groups

In addition to using NCLEX-PN® review books, many students find they benefit from a study group. The study group can be used not only for course tests, but also to review and discuss the rationales for answers to questions in the review books. Setting aside time to work with a study group each week will benefit most students.

Some students claim that a study group only confuses them. Why is this? Occasionally, one or two students in a group monopolize the group's time or say things that are incorrect or not needed by the others in the group. Several alternative solutions to this problem come to mind. One solution is for other members of the group to insist on members taking turns in the group or speaking up when the topic has been sufficiently covered. Another solution is to join a different group, and a third solution is to study with just one strong student. If group study simply does not work for you, try setting aside time to study in the library or a quiet place alone.

Professional Review Courses

Professional review courses are usually 1 to 2 days in length, requiring advanced registration and payment of a course fee. Your instructor, director of your program, or your state board of nursing will usually be able to advise you of dates and costs of these review courses.

Mock NCLEX® Examination

Some programs of practical/vocational nursing require, or offer a chance for, students to take a mock NCLEX-PN® examination just prior to graduation. Although these examinations are not free, they do provide a student with a percentile score for each category of client needs found on the examination. The student receives information on questions he or she got wrong and a list of the correct answers, along with an explanation and the rationales for the correct answers and for the distracters for each question. If you can take a mock NCLEX-PN® exam, the information you receive on completion will help you to identify the areas where you need to focus your study time.

Evaluating Your Readiness to Take the Examination

You have finished your formal nursing program and received your diploma. Are you ready to take the NCLEX-PN®, or do you suppose putting off taking the exam would improve your chances of passing? Usually, people completing practical nursing programs are anxious to take the NCLEX-PN® soon after completing the program for several reasons. Taking the exam soon means you are taking it while you are accustomed to testing and while much of what you have learned is fresh in your mind. From a practical and economic standpoint, you may also want to get your license so you can make more money. You probably want to

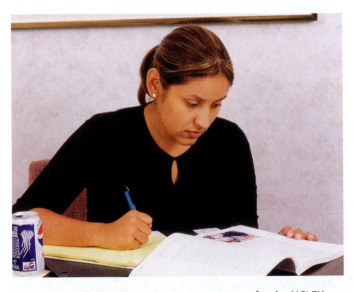

Figure 37-1. ■ Taking regular times to prepare for the NCLEX-PN® will help you study better and remember more.

get to work as a licensed practical/vocational nurse and sign your name with LPN (LVN if in Texas or California). If you did well on the mock NCLEX-PN® and/or if you have done well in answering most or all of the questions from all the various sections of your NCLEX-PN® review book or books, you will probably decide that you are ready to take the examination. You have many indicators that you have a great chance of passing the examination.

If you have indicators that you may not do well on the NCLEX-PN® exam, you should consider taking a review class. There are two types of classes. The first format reviews course work; the other is designed to prepare you to take the test. It provides test-taking tips and assistance in dealing with different types of questions. Time is also devoted to working through some of the psychological aspects of testing, such as test anxiety.

Delaying the exam does not necessarily improve your chances of passing the examination. In fact, there is some evidence that the probability of failure increases the longer a graduate waits.

It is important to remember that the NCLEX-PN® exam is testing your ability to be a safe entry-level practitioner. Don't let your fears prevent you from being successful.

Applying to Take the NCLEX-PN®

The National Council of State Boards of Nursing website has information on scheduling your NCLEX-PN® examination. You can also get this information by writing to NCSBN for a copy of the test plan. In general, you will do the following:

1. Fill out an application for a license to the board of nursing of your state or the state in which you wish to take the examination. The director of your nursing program or the faculty will probably provide you with an application for your state and will instruct you on the fees and size and type of pictures that must be submitted with the application and any other requirements that must be met.

2. Meet all the board of nursing's eligibility requirements in order to get permission to take the NCLEX-PN® exam. Prospective student nurses need to know the eligibility requirements prior to enrolling in nursing school and need to review these early in their nursing education. After processing your application as satisfactory, the board of nursing of your state will advise the testing service selected by NCSBN to administer the examination of your eligibility to test.

3. Receive from the testing service an Authorization to Test and a booklet, which will tell you about the test centers and how to schedule your examination.

4. Register with, and schedule an appointment with, the testing service that has been selected by NCSBN to administer the examination, and pay the required fee for taking the examination. Beginning October 1, 2002, candidates scheduled with Pearson Professional Testing to take the licensing examination.

Coping with Test Anxiety

Test anxiety seems to occur among students, as if on a continuum from low to high: from a normal mild level of uneasiness, which can be controlled easily and used as energy to do well on the exam, to a level of uneasiness and fear that immobilizes the test taker. Some students have a great deal of test anxiety before and/or during every quiz, midterm, and final exam and find themselves having difficulty focusing on the quiz or exam. Grades may suffer because of test anxiety. Other students seem to enjoy exams, concentrate fully, and look at them as a challenge.

WAYS TO OVERCOME TEST ANXIETY

If you are one of the students who are very nervous before or during tests, you need to start now to reduce your nervousness and anxiety around test taking. (See also Chapter 16 ⚭.) You would probably benefit from working with a counselor on these issues. If your test anxiety is not overwhelming, some simple strategies may reduce it. Sit down in a quiet place and write down 10 things you think would help you to reduce your test anxiety. You are the expert on you and may be able to come up with exactly what you need. Perhaps you will have on your list some of the following suggestions:

1. Learn some relaxation techniques, such as closing your eyes and tensing then relaxing each part of your body beginning at the head and neck and working downward. Think thoughts like "I am relaxing deeper and deeper" while breathing slowly and feeling your muscles relaxing. You are capable of relaxing yourself rather than saying things to yourself that create tension and uneasiness. Check with your library to see if they have a relaxation tape and some books on relaxation that you can check out.

2. Try picturing yourself taking the exam, being in control, and doing well with the answers to the questions.

3. Imagine your mind as a blackboard and erase any negative thoughts that lead to believing you might not do well. Write on your imaginary board, "I will do well on the test/exam."

4. Refuse to think about anything that you can't see, smell, feel, or touch. You can't see, feel, smell, or touch a worry about not doing well.

5. Desensitize yourself about your fear of failing a test. Take some short tests until you are doing well and seeing your success. Build up to bigger tests. You could enlist the help of an instructor.

6. Count from 10 to 1 when you begin to feel nervous.

Taking the Examination

Preparation on the day before and the day of the examination can help you arrive at the test prepared and relaxed. Try following these suggestions:

1. Do not cram the night before the examination. Relax your body and your mind. This could mean a pleasant movie or light reading. Some people relax by doing relaxation exercises or yoga or relaxing in warm water.

2. It is usually best to avoid using stimulants or depressants the evening before the examination. This includes caffeine drinks, alcohol, and other forms of stimulants and depressants.

3. Select some comfortable clothing for the next day. Perhaps something "layered" so you can take something off or put something on in case it is too warm or too cool for your comfort in the testing room.

4. Lay out anything you will have to take to the examination with you. This includes your instructions, required forms of identification, and your vehicle keys. You don't want to be searching for your vehicle keys when it is time to leave for the examination. You may want to take a power snack and a bottle of water to the examination with you to consume on your 10-minute break during the examination.

5. Get sufficient sleep the night before taking the test. Go to bed at the usual time and arise at the usual time. If crises are apt to occur at your home, make plans to sleep in a more restful environment. Getting into an argument with your roommate, significant other, or spouse the night before the exam will almost always not help you do well on the exam.

The day of the examination:

1. Eat moderately and finish your meal at least 1 to 2 hours before the exam. Avoid sugared foods, and include some protein in your meal. This will mean that you will have a more stable blood sugar than you would from just eating sugared foods. Do not rush your meal or overeat before the examination. If you overeat, blood will leave your brain to aid in digestion. This is blood you need to keep your brain working.

2. Be certain you have the required identification with you as you leave home to go to the examination.

3. Wear a watch. When taking the NCLEX-PN® computer examination, you can take as long as you wish to review a question (also referred to as an item) and select an answer. Consider two things in deciding how long to take in reviewing a question and trying to determine the answer: (a) Once you have recorded your answer, the question will disappear and you cannot get it back. You will have to answer the question on the screen before you can get another question. Even if you need to guess, you must answer each question. (b) You will have 5 hours for the exam, so while you don't have to rush, you cannot afford to take a half hour or more per question. Taking an extremely long time to answer a question will not increase your chances of getting the right answer and will probably increase your anxiety.

4. Push negative thoughts out of your mind. Replace negative thoughts with positive ones.

5. You will receive instructions and practice questions before the actual exam begins. You will not need prior computer experience to take the examination because you will only be using the cursor, the space bar, and the enter key and there are no other functional keys. The use of the computer has been made very simple.

6. Don't waste time looking for a pattern to the answers or making your educated guesses based on a pattern. All answers are random.

7. There will be very few if any questions that ask you to determine the answer that is "not correct" or the action that is "inappropriate." However, you need to read your questions very carefully to determine exactly what the question is asking. Answer what is being asked. The choices may include a correct statement that does not answer the question. Reading the question carefully will help you avoid selecting the statement that is correct but is not the right answer.

8. When answering questions, discipline yourself to answer based on the idea that the vast majority of the time your selected answer is true or best. Some test takers miss questions because they are searching for the one instance they know of, or have heard of, in which this answer might not be true or best.

9. If you find yourself not liking the question or wishing it were reworded, put your feelings aside and just do your best to answer the question as it is.

10. Concentrate fully on the exam. If you find yourself being distracted, tell yourself to focus and concentrate deeper.

Waiting for Your Results

Stay calm while waiting for your results. Your state board of nursing will mail your results in about a month. Only your board of nursing can release your exam results to you. Some states provide a 900-telephone number that the candidate can call for a fee. If your state participates, you will be given the information on when and how to obtain results by phone.

During the waiting period you may find that you are recalling and worrying about some questions you feel certain that you missed on the examination. While looking up the answers so you will have this knowledge, you want to try to avoid worrying because some of the questions you missed are likely to be the pilot questions that do not count against you and almost everyone will miss some of the "real" questions.

The best news that you can receive is that you have passed the examination. In this event, you are now a licensed practical nurse (or, if you are testing in Texas or California, you are a licensed vocational nurse). Congratulations! You now have all the benefits and responsibilities of being an LVN/LPN. Your lifelong learning continues.

The only other news you could receive is that you have failed the examination. Failing the exam means two things: One is that you need to identify any factors that you could change to increase your chances of passing. The other is that you need to develop a plan to prepare yourself better to take the examination.

A **diagnostic profile** is provided to candidates who fail the examination. The diagnostic profile is mailed to these candidates by their respective boards of nursing, along with the results of the examination. The profile aids the candidate in determining their areas of relative strength and weakness based on the test plan and in designing their study accordingly, prior to retaking the exam.

Stop any worrying that you are doing and begin to prepare. Do not say anything negative to or about yourself. This only wastes energy you need in preparing to take and pass the examination. You might make and hang some posters saying "SUCCESS" or "I WILL BE SUCCESSFUL" in your study area. If that isn't possible, then put sticky notes with that message in your study book.

There is a minimum number of days set by the NCSBN that you must wait before retaking the NCLEX-PN®. Your state board of nursing can set a longer period of time, but not a shorter period. This time period is of course designed to allow you time to prepare yourself for success.

If you failed the examination, you will benefit from doing some or all of the following:

- Talking with the director of your nursing program
- Working on a plan to be prepared when you retake the examination
- Getting a tutor
- Taking a review course
- Obtaining another NCLEX® review book
- Spending more time reviewing
- Getting professional help for test anxiety.

Note: The references and resources for this and all chapters have been compiled at the back of the book.

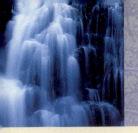

Chapter Review

 KEY TERMS by Topic

Use the audio glossary feature of either the CD-ROM or the Companion Website to hear the correct pronunciation of the following key terms.

Development of the NCLEX-PN®
multistate compact

Understanding the NCLEX-PN® plan
computer adaptive testing (CAT)

Preparing and Reviewing for the Exam
mnemonics

Coping with Test Anxiety
test anxiety

Waiting for Your Results
diagnostic profile

KEY Points

- Preparation for the NCLEX-PN® examination needs to begin when a student first enters the school of nursing.

- Students must pass the NCLEX-PN® test in order to practice. The plan takes into consideration the legal scope of practical/vocational nursing of each state and a practical/vocational nursing job analysis.

- The purpose of the NCLEX-PN® examination is to protect the public by ensuring that all who pass and receive a license to practice have the entry-level competencies needed to practice safely and effectively.

- Test questions on the NCLEX-PN® are at the cognitive levels of knowledge, comprehension, application, and analysis.

- The test plan is organized around four categories of client needs across the life span in a variety of settings. The categories of human needs are safe, effective care environment, health promotion and maintenance, psychosocial integrity, and physiological integrity.

- The maximum testing period is 5 hours with the maximum number of questions being 205 and the minimum 85. A student can pass or fail with the minimum or maximum number of questions or any number in between.

- Mnemonics are a way to help a person recall key concepts.

- It is a good idea to get an NCLEX® review book and begin using this book at least 6 months before taking the NCLEX-PN® examination. Study groups and review groups also help most students do better on the NCLEX-PN®.

- Readiness for the NCLEX-PN® can be judged by looking at one's performance on tests and examinations in the nursing program, performance on mock NCLEX® examinations, and results of practice tests in an NCLEX-PN® review book.

- Learning techniques for reducing test anxiety can greatly improve your NCLEX-PN® results.

- Prepare before the examination by avoiding stimulants or depressants the night before the test, determining the route to the examination, laying out everything needed for the examination ahead of time, relaxing, and getting enough sleep.

- Pace yourself during the exam so you can finish within 5 hours. Don't waste time looking for patterns to answers. Select the best answer, and concentrate fully on the examination.

 EXPLORE MediaLink

Additional interactive resources for this chapter can be found on the Companion Website at www.prenhall.com/ramont. Click on Chapter 37 and "Begin" to select the activities for this chapter.

For chapter-related NCLEX®-style questions and an audio glossary, access the accompanying CD-ROM in this book.

FOR FURTHER Study

For further study about legal and ethical issues, see Chapter 3.

For in-depth discussion about the nursing process, see Chapter 4.

For more information about stress and coping, see Chapter 16.

NCLEX-PN® Exam Preparation

1 When is the best time for a student who is enrolled in a practical nursing program to begin preparing for the NCLEX-PN®?

1. on the first day of the nursing program
2. after the completion of the first nursing course
3. six months before completion of the program
4. as soon as the nursing program is completed

2 You have been asked to answer this question: When is the best time for a student who is enrolled in a practical nursing program to begin preparing for the NCLEX-PN®? This question is an example of testing at which of the following levels of comprehension?

1. knowledge
2. comprehension
3. application
4. analysis

3 The NCLEX-PN® examination is revised periodically with the time period for review based on:

1. an annual analysis of how secure the test questions in the test bank are.
2. completion of a new job analysis of the tasks of licensed vocational nurses.
3. a vote of the member states of the National Council of State Boards of Nursing.
4. when substantial changes in the nurse practice acts of the states have occurred.

4 To prepare for the NCLEX-PN®, a nursing student needs what degree of computer expertise?

1. extensive
2. above average
3. average
4. none

5 A student finds that he is worrying before, during, and after tests in his nursing courses because the tests are so difficult. Which of the following actions would be best on this student's part?

1. Use the grievance procedure and complain about the test difficulty.
2. Seek help in designing effective methods of studying and relaxing.
3. Talk with peers about how much you are worried and how you worry.
4. Wait and see if it gets easier in another course with another teacher.

6 The night before the examination, it is usually best to go to bed at which of the following times?

1. about 8 to 10 hours before time to awaken
2. no later than midnight
3. the usual time you normally go to bed
4. whenever you feel tired

7 In taking the tests in nursing courses and answering questions in the NCLEX-PN® review books, you find that even though you memorize a lot of things, the questions don't seem to test these facts. The best explanation for this is:

1. you are not studying the facts needed for these questions.
2. you are having difficulty memorizing enough.
3. the teacher is not very good at writing tests on what was taught.
4. the level of the testing is at comprehension, analysis, or synthesis.

8 You must not forget to take which of the following things to the NCLEX-PN® testing location with you?

1. watch
2. calculator
3. identification
4. scratch paper

9 The maximum testing period during which you can answer questions on the NCLEX-PN® is which of the following?

1. 1 hour
2. 3 hours
3. 4 hours
4. 5 hours

10 The minimum number of questions you could be given on the NCLEX-PN® is _____.

Answers and Rationales for Review Questions, as well as discussion of Care Plan and Critical Thinking Care Map questions, appear in Appendix I.

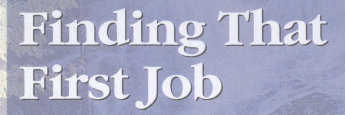

Chapter 38

Finding That First Job

BRIEF Outline

Portfolio
Interviews
Job Search
The Hiring Process

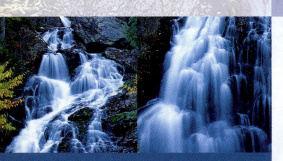

HISTORICAL Perspectives

Here are some nurses' duties in 1887:

1. *Each nurse on day duty will report every day at 7:00 A.M. and leave at 8:00 P.M., except on the Sabbath, on which day you will be off from 12 noon to 2:00 P.M.*

2. *Each nurse should lay aside from each payday a goodly sum of her earnings for her benefits during her declining years so that she will not become a burden. For example, if you earn $30 a month, you set aside $15.*

3. *Any nurse who smokes, uses liquor in any form, gets her hair done at a beauty shop, or frequents dance halls will give the Director of Nurses good reason to suspect her worth, intentions, and integrity.*

LEARNING Outcomes

After completing this chapter, you will be able to:

1. Describe the components of a portfolio.
2. Develop a cover letter for an entry-level job.
3. Prepare a résumé.
4. Define professional behavior.
5. Describe a career ladder for the nursing profession.

There are many differences between student and graduate nurses. Once you are out of school, reality hits. Like most new graduates you probably feel unprepared, overwhelmed, and scared. The good news is that no employer, whether a hospital or other agency, expects you to know everything. You will continue to learn as you begin your first job. You may even come to think of that first position as being another phase of your education.

You may be realizing a lifelong dream to be a nurse, embarking on a new career, or returning to the workforce. No matter what it was that brought you to this place, you are now a new member of a profession who has much to contribute to it. This chapter provides you with a survival plan as you transition from student to licensed practical/vocational nurse. To make the transition from student to licensed nurse, you will need to make preparations. It is not unlike planning a trip to Europe. You need to decide where you want to go, be sure you have all your documents, prepare the appropriate wardrobe, and have your timeline and contact persons well in mind.

You may have a facility in mind, where you would like to work. It may be one you were assigned to as a student, where you have worked as an unlicensed healthcare worker or one that was recruiting at a job fair. Learn as much as you can about the facility and its parent company before making application.

Portfolio

Your next step is to review your **portfolio**. A portfolio is defined as an itemized visual account of your skills and best practices that are related to the position you are seeking. It is a working portfolio so that when you leave your schooling you are prepared to walk into an interview with all the information needed to emphasize your strengths, education, and experience and to present yourself as a professional LPN/LVN. You will compile your portfolio so that it demonstrates your capabilities and competencies. Compiling your portfolio does not happen overnight. Ideally, you should begin developing it about halfway into your nursing program.

A leather-type, three-ring binder is an appropriate way to display your personal portfolio. A complete portfolio includes:

- Title page
- Table of contents
- Cover letter/introduction letter
- Application
- Résumé
- Work samples (two):
  - Nursing care plans
  - Narrative charting samples
  - Lesson plan

- Writing samples (one):
  - Case studies
  - Module research projects
  - Observation studies
- Student reflection
- Community service
- Clinical evaluations
- Awards/achievements
- Recommendation letters
- Sample thank-you letter
- Sample resignation letter.

The portfolio is an idea place to store copies of your license, CPR card, or other certifications (e.g., intravenous or blood withdrawal). You also may wish to include a list of references with their contact information and a sample completed application. These will be helpful when asked to fill out an application on site.

THE COVER LETTER

The **cover letter** you write will contain essential information that gives you the opportunity to sell yourself. This letter is what potential employers read about you and it helps them determine whether they want to find out more about your qualifications. It should be brief and to the point, but highlight your best professional and educational attributes. This concise one-page letter must reflect correct grammar, spelling, and appropriate format.

Do your homework, find out who you are addressing, make a point to correctly spell the person's name, and establish their title or position. The cover letter is a first impression—think about what you do with mail that is addressed to "occupant." It usually gets tossed in the round file and that is not what you want done with your cover letter and résumé.

The introductory paragraph should immediately explain the letter's purpose. Begin by introducing yourself. Explain your intent to apply for the position of licensed practical/vocational nurse. Give the details of your response to an ad, job listing, website, or other source that disclosed this job offering. A new graduate should include the school attended and date of graduation.

The body or second paragraph is where your highlighted qualifications are contained. This is where your enthusiasm for this particular job is addressed. State how you have been prepared by your education. Describe briefly the skills and strengths that you will contribute to the position. Write about what sets you apart from the other applicants. Include a statement about the organization and why you want to be part of a "recognized staff and organization." This is the time to write about your experience and competencies. If you have limited clinical experience, mention your diverse clinical rotations. Include major accomplishments and awards. Remember this is your first position in this capacity

BOX 38-1

Sample Cover Letter

Mary J. Fuller, LPN
4123 W. Green Street
Martinsville, Iowa 92222
(999) 555-1212
e-mail mjf24@aol.com

[date]

Roseanne Blake, RN
Director of Nurses
St. Catherine's Hospital
1002 Main Street
Marysville, Iowa 92223

Dear Ms. Blake:

It is with great interest that I apply for the licensed practical nurse position advertised in the *Marysville Times* on Sunday. I am a recently licensed practical nurse, having completed the nursing program at the Waterloo Vocational and Technical School.

I have more than 7 years of experience as a certified nursing assistant in the acute care setting. My background as a nursing assistant and the clinical experience obtained during my practical nursing program have built a firm foundation for my first nursing position.

I graduated first in my class and received the faculty award for clinical excellence. I received a silver medal in practical nursing skills at the Health Occupation Students of America National Leadership Conference in June. I will consider any clinical area, depending on your needs. I am enthusiastic and dependable and I am committed to quality client care.

I have enclosed my résumé for your consideration. If you need additional information, please feel free to contact me at my home number listed above. Thank you for your time and consideration. I will call your office next week to discuss further the possibilities of employment.

Sincerely,

Mary J. Fuller, LPN

Mary J. Fuller, LPN

Enclosure

---

and avoid using words like *best, expert,* and *excellent* to describe yourself. Avoid flowery words or phrases that are not reflective of a professional nurse. Write out any industry-specific abbreviations you may be using.

The closing paragraph restates your interest and conveys your anticipation in obtaining an interview. Indicate when and how you will follow up your letter. Refer to your enclosed résumé.

Include your name, address, and telephone number. Printed letterhead is acceptable. Use the same quality bond paper for both your cover letter and résumé. Cream, beige, or light gray paper is suggested. Review your letter for errors and have some else read it. If it is computer generated, use the spelling and grammar checks. Box 38-1 ■ shows a sample cover letter

APPLICATION

Filling out an application may seem like an easy task; however, the more attention you pay to details, the better you represent yourself to your potential employer. Practice completing an application; never leave lines blank. If something is not applicable to you, write "N/A" in the space provided. Type the application if you can; if you are completing it in the office, be neat, legible, avoid abbreviations, and use ink. Have all the information required at your fingertips—being prepared is to your advantage. If you plan to apply to a facility you have worked at as a student, ask for an application and practice completing it. Some employers have their applications online.

RÉSUMÉ

The **résumé** is a concise systematic summary of your professional experience and educational background. This is a marketing tool to give your potential employer a snapshot glimpse into your nursing background and experience. A one-page document is preferred, with two pages being the maximum. Remember, if you are too wordy or if the employer has to search to find required information, your résumé may end up being ignored. This document needs to be well planned, informative, and organized. Take the time necessary to be precise, neat, and accurate.

There are three types of résumé formats: chronological, functional, and a combination of the two. The chronological format highlights your employment in reverse chronological order and is the most traditional. The functional format emphasizes skills. The combination uses both. Chronological style is discussed in the following paragraphs.

To prepare your résumé, you first need to assemble data that illustrates your professional qualifications. It is important for a new graduate to evaluate accomplishments that would give a potential employer insight into your work ethic and commitment. Include areas in community service or service as a class officer. Listing Health Occupations Students of America competitive event awards, scholarships, or honors would be appropriate. Employment experience includes dates, positions, and employing agency. Educational history includes years of education attendance, graduation, school name, location, certification, and diploma information. Usually it is presented in a reverse chronological order. The first entry is the most current and you work backward from there. Note that references are available upon request. You should have a copy of your references, their addresses, and phone numbers typed/computer generated on a single sheet of paper that you keep handy in your portfolio in case of a request. Three to four references are adequate. Be sure to contact them to obtain permission to use their names and phone numbers. Two should be professionals connected to the type of job you are seeking. The others can be personal references.

Most résumés are computer generated today, but at the very least, it must be typed on quality paper and should be on the same light-colored paper (off white, beige, light gray) that you used for your cover letter. Many computer résumé programs are available; you may want to start there. However, you want it individualized to you. Many students have learned to used graphics from computer files, but remember to keep your résumé professional—no hearts or stethoscopes to detract from the purpose and content. Have an experienced professional nurse review your résumé for spelling, grammatical errors, and appearance. Use action words to describe your qualifications. (Box 38-2 ■ lists action words.) This is not a document to be taken lightly and will take more than one draft to complete. Use a consistent format and follow it throughout the document.

Résumé Components

A sample résumé is shown in Figure 38-1 ■. The heading includes your name, complete address, phone number, and an e-mail address. Remember when you have sent a résumé, you may receive a call, so make sure your message machine is working properly and there is a professional message left for callers. Additionally, if your e-mail address is not professional, you may want to have a separate address for work-related business.

A job objective is next, although not everyone agrees that you need an objective on your résumé today. In your

BOX 38-2	
Action Words	
Accomplished	Observed
Achieved	Organized
Analyzed	Planned
Built	Presented
Chaired	Prevented
Collaborated	Provided
Communicated	Reduced
Created	Reorganized
Delegated	Served
Designed	Simplified
Developed	Standardized
Devoted	Studied
Dispensed	Taught
Ensured	Transformed
Evaluated	Unified
Expanded	Validated
Focused	Worked
Formulated	Wrote
Implemented	

objective you are stating your professional career goal. You can be general in your goal or more specific. This will help the Human Resource Department determine whether you may be qualified for the position they need to fill. Your job objective should be one sentence.

A summary is used to assist a new nurse to stress strong points but be sure to include why you are qualified to meet your objective. You can bullet it for easier reading.

EDUCATION. In this section you will want to start with your most recent education. Include the name of the school, and then enter city and state. List your certification, license, degree or focus of education, and graduation date. Follow through with other educational background.

EXPERIENCE. Again, start with your most recent or current work experience. Include full-time and part-time employment; clearly state the position succinctly and dates employed. Describe the duties and responsibilities assigned. Your work history is important to employers and they look for gaps in time. Use the same format as you did with your education.

ACHIEVEMENT. This section highlights your value to the employer. As a student, your accomplishments are important; use them to your advantage. Perfect attendance, faculty awards for clinical excellence, academic excellence awards, and Health Occupations Students of America competitive awards would demonstrate value. Include community service; it displays personal commitment and involvement. Intravenous therapy and blood withdrawal and telemetry classes are additional skills that may increase your marketability.

Luz Marina Balderas
555 Main Street
Any Town, CA 99999
(555)555-1234
lmbalderas@internet.com

OBJECTIVES:

To obtain a challenging position in the Nursing QI/QM field where I can utilize my clinical knowledge and quality management experience in an environment that will promote career and educational opportunities.

SKILLS:

Project
Management:
- Time management and project deadline compliance
- Critical thinking and conflict resolution
- Data collection and statistical data analysis
- Delegation and team work management

Business:
- Accurately type and enter data, 120 words per minute.
- Computer proficiency in Word, Excel, Access, PowerPoint, E-Z Cap, SPSS, MedCore
- Strong customer relations background
- Public speaking and project presentation experience
- Employee training and compliance assurance
- Policy and procedure development and implementation

EXPERIENCE:

Position:	Market Research Analyst
Company:	MedPartners, Inc.
Location:	Long Beach, California
Employment:	September 1999 through July 2005

Position:	IPA Quality Improvement Coordinator
Company:	MedPartners, Inc.
Location:	Long Beach, California
Employment:	June 1993 through September 1999

Position:	QI Nursing Representative
Company:	MedPartners, Inc.
Location:	Long Beach, California
Employment:	May 1991 through June 1993

Position:	Specialty Clinic – Back Office Medical Assistant
Company:	MedPartners, Inc.
Location:	Long Beach, California
Employment:	July 1988 through May 1991

Figure 38-1. ■ Sample résumé.

Luz Marina Balderas
555 Main Street
Any Town, CA 99999
(555)555-1234
lmbalderas@internet.com

Page 2

EDUCATION:

North Orange County ROP:	Licensed Vocational Nursing Program	Aug. 2003 - July 2005
Cypress Community College:	Limited X-Ray Technician Program	Sept. 1987 - Sept. 1989
Cerritos Community College:	Medical Assisting Program	Sept. 1985 - Sept. 1987
Downey Adult Ed. Program:	Nurses' Assistant Program	July 1985 - Dec. 1986
University of Calif., Irvine:	Bachelor's in Science - Psychology	Sept. 1981 - June 1985

AWARDS & ACHIEVEMENTS:

Kaiser Permanente Health Care Issues State Scholarship: 1st Place, March 2005
HOSA State Leadership Conference: Gold Medallist - Pathophysiology, March 2005
HOSA State Leadership Conference: Bronze Medallist - Bio Medical Debate, March 2005
Kaiser Permanente Health Care Issues National Scholarship: 1st Place, June 2005
HOSA National Leadership Conference: Gold Medallist - Pathophysiology, June 2005
HOSA National Leadership Conference: 1st Place - Health Education Pilot Event, June 2005
Class Valedictorian: NOCROP – LVN Program, Graduating Nursing Class A, July 2005

PRESENTATIONS:

"Cushing's Syndrome"	NOCROP – LVN Program, Pharmacology Module, October 2004
"Traumatic Head Injuries"	NOCROP – LVN Program, Neurology Module, May 2005

CERTIFICATIONS & LICENSES:

Basic Cardiac Life Support Certification
Phlebotomy Certified
Medical Assistant Certification
Limited X-Ray License: Expired
Nursing Assistant Certification: Expired

REFERENCES:

Available upon request

Figure 38-1. ■ Sample résumé. (*continued*)

You may be allowed to e-mail résumés to prospective employers, which is a quick and efficient way to cover a lot of ground electronically. Human Resources can keep you on file for positions that become available. Keep your e-mail short and concise; let your prospective employer know if you are willing to relocate. Identify the position for which you are applying. Don't forget to attach your résumé to your e-mail.

Interviews

Being asked to do an interview means that the employer is interested in what they have read in your cover letter and résumé. This is where you sell yourself to the employer. A face-to-face meeting gives a first impression. Whether it results in employment or not it is an experience that will provide you with insight into your ability to speak logically and think critically. Did you get your message across? Did your nervousness get the best of you or did practice pay off? One-on-one interviews are less nerve wracking, but nowadays you may be faced with two or three interviewers firing questions at you during one interview.

TIPS TO A SUCCESSFUL INTERVIEW

Professional dress means different things to different people. What does it mean to you? For a male, it is a conservative suit, dress shirt, and tie. Men should be clean-shaven or beards must be trimmed and neat. For the female it means a medium-length skirt with a blouse and jacket. (If you are tugging at your skirt when you sit, it is too short. If you have to ask, "Is this appropriate?" find something else to wear.) A pantsuit, however, is permissible. Avoid plunging necklines and skirts with thigh-high slits. Clothes should be neatly pressed. Closed toed shoes with hose/nylons are proper dress. Wearing your uniform is regarded sufficient; however, remember you are trying to make an impression. A clean, controlled hairstyle is paramount. One set of stud earrings and neutral moderate makeup and nails are essential. Hygiene is understood.

Arrive at the interview at least 15 minutes early. Identify yourself at the front desk or with the secretary and state who you are to meet with.

You are in charge of your attitude. Be positive, polite, and confident. Your enthusiasm for the position comes across to the panel and even if you are not the most qualified and experienced, that refreshing attitude can have an effect on your rating. Convince the interviewer(s) about your commitment and motivation. Be aware of your verbal and nonverbal communication. Avoid the phrases "You guys," "Like, you know," and be aware of how many "umms" you might say. If your hands tend to shake, put them in your lap. Also avoid touching and playing with your hair.

The previous interview may extend into your assigned time. If that happens, be patient. Review what you know

about the facility and staff. Show sincere interest and articulate why you have chosen this facility for application, if and when the opportunity arises. For example, it might be the compassionate care that you observed firsthand as a student. It may possibly be the renowned staff and cutting-edge cancer research or may be the physician–nurse respect and interdisciplinary approach used to care for clients. If you don't have firsthand information about the facility, you might want to research it via its website or speak with staff members.

When you enter the interview offices, use a firm handshake with each panel member. Smile to break the ice, and once again state your name clearly. Address the panel members by Miss, Mrs., Mr., respectively. Remain standing until you are asked to take a seat. Avoid fidgeting, sit upright and a little forward in the chair, and be attentive. Do not chew gum during an interview; it leaves a negative impact. Eye contact conveys confidence and credibility in your answers. Answer questions succinctly but completely; use examples if appropriate. Roughly 6 to 10 questions will be asked. Be interesting and avoid rambling. The usual time period for an interview is 15 to 20 minutes. Discuss your qualifications and experiences related to the position. As a new graduate you can use your clinical rotation and any associated work experiences. Offer your portfolio for their review; point out highlights that you feel would be of particular interest.

When the interview is finished, the interviewer will ask you about any questions you may have. Have at least two questions ready to pose. Suitable questions to be considered might be:

- What is the normal staffing to client ratio?
- What type of continuing education or classes are offered, and is there is a fee?
- Does this organization offer tuition reimbursement for higher education?
- How long is the new graduate orientation and what is the process?
- What are full-time benefits?
- Are there job advancement or level changes?
- When and how will you be notified about their decision concerning the position?
- What is the involvement of the nursing staff in community service?

Points of view differ on asking questions about salary. One view is that it isn't discussed until the job is offered. However, if you have a salary requirement and entry level is unacceptable, it is better to clarify this early in the process.

Express your appreciation for the interviewers' time and for the opportunity to interview for this position. Shake hands with the panel and exit promptly. Write a short thank-you note following the interview; it reminds the interviewer of your interest. To be effective, the note should

BOX 38-3

Examples of Interview Questions

- Initially the interviewer will ask you to describe your education and experience as it relates to the position.
- What is one quality you like about yourself?
- How would you handle an irritated family member?
- What can you bring or contribute to this company or facility?
- What interested you in applying for this facility?
- Where do you see yourself in 5 years?
- How would you handle a combative client?
- How do you view yourself as a worker?
- What skill, personal or professional, do you feel you need improvement on to make you a better employee?
- How do you rate yourself in the area of problem solving on a scale of 1 to 5, with 5 being the highest? Describe the process used and give an example. Remember to use the nursing process!
- What are your strengths/weaknesses and elaborate on each?
- What do you like most about your job?
- What are some things you have learned from clients?
- What would you do if you believed a doctor was causing harm to a client?
- If you were asked to do something out of your scope of practice, what would be your course of action?
- If you could change one thing in nursing, what would it be and why?
- As a new graduate, why would I hire you over someone with 2 years of experience?
- What is the biggest issue facing nursing today?
- How do you feel about floating to an area unfamiliar to you?

be received within a week of the interview. To be prepared for an interview, you must practice and rehearse a variety of questions. Mock interviews will help you gain poise and allow you to think about what you need to modify before you are in the midst of an actual interview. Box 38-3 ■ lists examples of interview questions. Refer to Box 38-4 ■ for a rubric on interview skills. Reviewing this rubric will assist you to self-evaluate your abilities in this area.

Illegal Questions

Some questions cannot be legally asked by interviewers. The Federal Civil Rights Act and state laws protect citizens against these questions, and you are not required to answer them. However, should such a question be asked, be prepared to tactfully decline to answer or veer the discussion to another topic. Avoid putting the panel on the defensive. If you point out an illegal question, the interview—and your chance at a position—may be terminated early.

Examples of illegal questions include:

- Are you married?
- What are you child care arrangements?
- What is your religion?
- How old are you? What is your birth date?

- Where were you born?
- Race-related questions.

There are ways to reply to such questions that will not alienate the interviewer. Reply to unlawful questions in a controlled manner. Do not offer more personal information than is necessary. Maintain a positive attitude; keep your voice conversational and upbeat. If an interviewer consistently asks personal questions, think twice about taking that job.

Suggested responses to this type of questioning include:

- I'm not sure how that question pertains to this position.
- Child care arrangements are not an issue. Please do not be concerned.
- If you mean am I over 18, yes I am.

Now that you have completed the interview process, you will need to patiently wait for the panel to make their decision and check your references. If during the interview they told you when they would be making their decision, it is permissible to call the human resource or nursing office after that time to check on the status of the position. Making this call can be difficult, but it will let you know if you are still being considered or if you should pressure other options.

Job Search

There are many ways to look for potential practical/vocation nurse positions. Many companies advertise on the Internet, and you can check the newspaper ads, job boards, nursing magazines, and where you currently work. Some job fairs are just for nursing positions. Make a list of questions before applying to an organization. Decide what priorities you want in a position. These are a few examples:

- What information does the advertisement give you on the organization?
- What experience is required?
- Is there a hiring-on benefit?
- Do nurses work 8- or 12-hour shifts?
- Starting pay?
- Is there advancement for an LPN/LVN?
- Is there a plan for school reimbursement?
- Does the organization provide continuing education classes and is there a fee for employees?
- What benefits are available?
- Who is the contact person?

On the Internet, you can find the average salaries for LPN/LVNs. This will help you determine where the organization stands in comparison to the average for the county, state, and nation in which you are applying.

Work Samples

Work samples are items used in the workplace. Individualized nursing care plans you have developed are an excellent way to

---

BOX 38-4

Interview Rubric

Interview Skills

A successful interview …

- Exhibits professional dress and demeanor.
- Arrives early for the interview, with all necessary documents.
- Speaks clearly and confidently about skills and qualifications.
- Uses effective verbal and nonverbal communication skills.

Advanced
- Student arrives early for the interview, with all necessary documents, and exhibits professionalism in both appearance and demeanor.
- The student can list important documents that may be requested at the interview, including the following: résumé; letters of reference; work samples; and photocopies of diplomas, awards, certificates, driver's license, Social Security card, and any military papers.
- Student demonstrates appropriate verbal and nonverbal communication before, during, and after the interview, shaking hands and making eye contact with all interviewers. He/she demonstrates a high degree of knowledge of the company and/or position and demonstrates interest by asking a minimum of two appropriate questions.
- All interview questions are answered in an organized, professional manner, using supporting details and/or examples.
- Language is appropriate to the available position, and student's demeanor and voice tone are pleasant.
- The student demonstrates interview follow-up by writing a thank-you letter to the interviewer and/or calling the company to inquire about the company's hiring decision in a sophisticated, professional manner.
- Understands the importance of following up the interview.

Proficient
- Student arrives early for the interview, with all necessary documents, and exhibits professionalism in both appearance and demeanor.
- The student can explain the purpose of a job interview. Questions are answered clearly and confidently, using language appropriate to the available position.
- Supporting details and/or examples may be missing.
- Oral delivery is clear but needs improvement in one to two of the following areas: tone of voice, pace, energy, and/or nonverbal communication.
- The student demonstrates interview follow-up, including writing a thank-you letter to the interviewer and/or calling the company to inquire about the company's hiring decision.
- Demonstrates some interest in asking a question about the position or company.

Basic
The student does not demonstrate a basic understanding of the job interview, as indicated by any of the following behaviors:
- He/she does not arrive early and/or is missing necessary documents.
- Dress and demeanor are not professional.
- Questions are not answered completely; supporting details and/or examples are weak or absent.
- Oral delivery demonstrates deficiencies in three or more of the following areas: tone of voice, pace, energy, and/or nonverbal communication. Asks no questions of the interviewer.
- There is no interview follow-up.

Source: Courtesy of Lynne Porter, RN, North Orange County, RUP, Anaheim, CA.

---

display your critical thinking skills. Charting is a most important presentation of your writing skills related to the workplace. It demonstrates your flexibility in charting using different methods and strategies of documentation. Lesson plans for client teaching under the direction of the RN will establish further evidence of problem-solving and intervention skills. Compile this information as you progress through your program to underscore your strengths in the nursing field.

Writing Samples

Effective writing that is organized, clear, and uses correct grammar and spelling is a meaningful workplace skill. Use a sample of your work that is researched and includes a bib-

liography. This item stresses your ability to write in a logical order using correct format and shows your attention to details. Journaling or a student reflection piece would serve as an additional writing sample.

Community Service

This is documentation of your giving back to the community. Society looks to the nursing professions for leadership and guidance. Health professionals' involvement in community service demonstrates commitment and dedication to organizations that contribute to the well-being of the community. An employer would consider this a positive attribute.

Clinical Evaluation

Provide a copy of your best evaluation signed by your clinical instructor. This instructor may also be on your recommendation list.

Sample Thank-You Letter

A brief thank-you letter for the interviewers can remind them of you and your abilities. Be positive about the interview process and thank them for their time and consideration; use correct grammar and spelling. Having a sample letter in your portfolio will make this a simple task when needed.

Letter of Resignation

It is customary to write a letter of resignation for your position when you are leaving. Two weeks of notice is appropriate. Be positive about your work environment and position; thank your employers for the experience and professional growth you have gained. The first person you notify about your resignation should be your manager; it is not wise to have him or her hear it through the grapevine. The appropriate reasons for leaving are new challenges, increase in pay, relocation, family matters, or career advancements.

The Hiring Process

When you receive on offer of employment, you will be very excited. Contain yourself long enough to get all the details as well as time and dates of your orientation. If you have received more than one job offer and need time to make a decision, thank the caller for the offer and state that you will get back to them at a specific time with your answer.

ORIENTATION

Orientation is the program or time period provided for newly hired individuals to prepare themselves to take on the responsibilities of the position for which they were employed.

Most facilities have new hires complete paperwork during the first day of orientation, although you may be required to complete a physical, drug test, or fingerprinting prior to that date. It is a good idea to ask about proper dress for the first orientation day—business attire or a nursing uniform? Be sure you know where to park and the exact time and place to report. Plan to spend the full day. You may be finished early, but that is not something you can count on. Most facilities provide several weeks of orientation. Some may offer a longer new graduate program. The first week is normally on the day shift, with additional time provided on the shift to which you are assigned. It is a good idea to arrive for orientation with a notebook. You will be given a lot of information and it is wise to write it down so you can refer to it later.

You have now made that transition from student to licensed nurse. Congratulations—all of your hard work and dedication have paid off! You are now a member of a worthy profession.

BOX 38-5

Professional Characteristics and Behaviors

A practicing nurse (LPN/LVN) should possess professional qualities of warmth and empathy. These characteristics include but are not limited to:

- Ability to develop relationships that exhibit a caring philosophy.
- An ethic of caring reflected by appropriate emotional responses, communication, punctuality, hygiene, and attire that seeks to preserve the wholeness of dignity of self and others.
- Adherence to confidentiality of clients and others.
- Behavior that reflects responsibility and accountability for safety of clients, self, and others.
- Demonstration of knowledge regarding scope of practice of the LPN/LVN.
- Demonstration of interpersonal skills needed to function as an effective team member.
- Demonstration of problem-solving skills applying the concepts of the nursing process within the scope of the LPN/LVN.
- Development of an awareness of available resources for continued personal and professional growth.

PROFESSION/PROFESSIONALISM

A **profession** is defined as an occupation to which one devotes oneself and in which one has specialized expertise (Becker & Fendler, 1994). Licensed practical/vocational nursing is an integral part of the profession. As an LPN/LVN working in a hospital or other healthcare agency, you will be expected to demonstrate certain characteristics and behaviors that demonstrate **professionalism**. Box 38-5 ■ lists examples of professional characteristics and behaviors. By emulating these behaviors you will be well on you way to being a successful licensed nurse. See Box 38-6 ■ for "Tips to Thrive"—not just survive—the first year as an LPN/LVN.

PROBATIONARY PERIOD AND PERFORMANCE EVALUATION

Each healthcare facility has a **probationary period** for newly hired employees. During this time your immediate supervisor will be evaluating your performance. At the end of this time you will be given a **performance evaluation** and most likely a small increase in salary. Your attendance and promptness will be an important consideration, as will your ability to work as a team member, complete your assignments in a timely manner, and perfect your skills. After the initial evaluation, most facilities evaluate employees on an annual basis. Annual evaluations may include skills testing and renewal of CPR or other certifications. It is important that the staff nurse keep track of these requirements, because expired certifications may prevent you from working.

BOX 38-6

Thriving During the First Year on the Job

- **Be patient.** It takes time to gain experience. Some say it takes up to 2 years to be able to handle most situations.
- **Be positive.** Everyday write down something good you did or learned; review your list often. Focus on the positive; it will become your reality.
- **Be a seeker.** Don't wait for someone to tell you to do a procedure. Seek out opportunities to do new things. If you don't know how, request the opportunity to observe a more experienced colleague. Show your willingness to learn.
- **Be a helper.** It is never too soon to lend a hand to a coworker. Be sure to be available to students—you were there once.
- **Be a buddy.** Buddy up with a coworker after whom you would like to model yourself. Remember someone doesn't have to have the same position in order for you to learn from him or her.
- **Be a team player.** Introduce yourself to coworkers on all shifts, to physicians, and to other hospital personnel. Have lunch with someone you don't know. Become a part of the team.
- **Be a lifelong learner.** Use references and policy and procedure manuals. Ask questions and do your homework at the end of each day by looking up things that are new to you.
- **Be a joiner.** Become a member of a professional organization; develop close ties with colleagues on a state and national level. Organizations provide cutting-edge information.
- **Be a tracker.** Track your progress. Don't lose track of the progress you have already made. Review this often; see how far you have come.
- **Be a stress buster.** Stress should be managed not just tolerated. Make time for yourself to socialize, for leisure activities, for hobbies—take care of yourself so you can give care to others.
- **Be focused.** Keep moving forward. You can do it!

CONTINUING EDUCATION

All state boards of nursing have continuing education requirements for licensed nurses. The number of hours varies with the individual board. It is your responsibility to know the requirements for your state. Requirements can be met with on-site classes, professional conferences, home study courses, or courses on the Internet. It is important that classes be completed prior to the renewal date of your license. Once completed keep the certificates on file. Your portfolio is an excellent storage location for a copy, since state nursing boards conduct random audits of license holders. Continuing education courses are designed to help keep you current in the field, but such courses can also introduce you to new skills or even a new specialty. The possibilities are only limited by your time and interest.

CAREER LADDER

A **career ladder** can be described as progression from one level in a profession to another through educational pursuits and professional experience (Figure 38-2 ■).

Career ladder programs offer a variety of options. An individual who already has a practical or vocational nursing license can enter an associate nursing degree (AND) program by taking a transition course. Some training programs have direct articulation with schools of registered nursing, so that LPN/LVNs can receive advanced placement when they wish to pursue additional education. Another option is to enroll in a 2-year AND program and exit after the first year after completing the practical nurse option. These options may better meet some individuals' needs for employment and continuing education.

Many LPN/LVNs have a desire to progress beyond the AND level of registered nursing. The availability for lifelong learning and advanced practice opportunities are many. New graduates may be ready to dive right into additional schooling, others need to seek full-time employment to support themselves or family, and others may need a well-deserved break from school. With nursing the option is always there, either now or in the future. Your career goal may be fulfilled as an LPN/LVN or you may wish to continue up the ladder. Whatever your professional goal, it is important never to stop learning and to strive to be a competent and compassionate nurse.

PROFESSIONAL ORGANIZATIONS

The first professional nursing organization was established in 1893. Nurses found that if they united to achieve common goals and missions they would be more likely to have an impact on their chosen profession. The National League for Nursing (NLN) was established under the name of the American Society of Superintendents of Training Schools for Nurses in the United States and Canada. In 1912 the name was changed to NLN. Its purpose was to standardize and improve nursing education. There are two levels of membership in the NLN, individual and agency. Schools of nursing and other agencies that provide nursing care are eligible for agency membership. In 1943, lay members were permitted to join the organization, which had previously been open only to nurses. The NLN is the accrediting organization for nursing programs. A graduate of an NLN-accredited program will be recognized nationally and credits will be recognized by other NLN-approved programs when the nurse chooses to continue his or her education.

The American Nurses Association is the professional organizations for the RN. Membership is limited to registered nurses. The National Federation of Licensed Practical Nurses and the National Association for Practical Nurse Education and Service are the professional organizations for the LPN/LVN. Membership in a professional organization provides the licensed nurse with many services; they are your representative on a national level, providing continuing education opportunities and opportunities for networking.

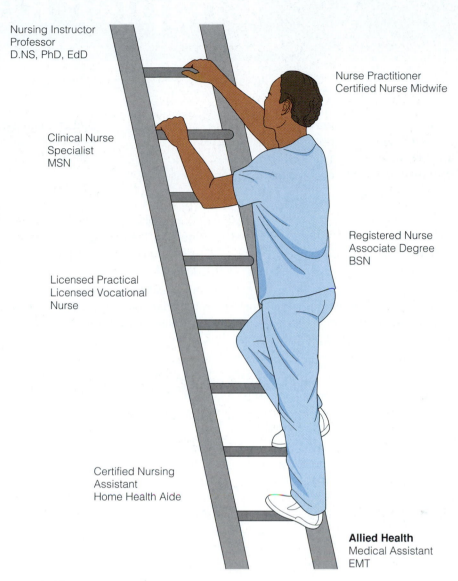

Nursing Instructor
Professor
D.NS, PhD, EdD

Nurse Practitioner
Certified Nurse Midwife

Clinical Nurse
Specialist
MSN

Registered Nurse
Associate Degree
BSN

Licensed Practical
Licensed Vocational
Nurse

Certified Nursing
Assistant
Home Health Aide

Allied Health
Medical Assistant
EMT

Figure 38-2. ■ Nursing career ladder.

There are specialty organizations for nurses working in pediatrics, geriatrics, or obstetrics to name a few. Participation in a local or national organization is a worthwhile activity for a graduate nurse.

NETWORKING AND COLLABORATION

Nursing is not a career that one can pursue in a vacuum. **Networking** is described as the deliberate attempt to make connections among people for a variety of interests, including employment opportunities. Networking may be causal or formal (Kurzen, 2004).

Collaborative nursing practice or interdependent nursing practice is working jointly with other healthcare professionals, including physicians, in the performance of nursing roles within the scope of practice. Learning to network and collaborate with other nurses and healthcare providers is extremely important. You can begin to learn these skills by participating in staff or unit minutes. In the beginning you may feel you have little to contribute, but as you listen to your colleagues and progress in your nursing practice you will see ways to improve client care and unit operations. Once you are comfortable in a small group, volunteer for a hospital or system-wide committee. As a member of a professional organization, your networking and collaborative opportunities will increase as your circle of professional associates increases.

Note: The references and resources for this and all chapters have been compiled at the back of the book.

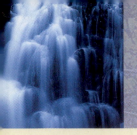

Chapter Review

 KEY TERMS by Topic

Use the audio glossary feature of either the CD-ROM or the Companion Website to hear the correct pronunciation of the following key terms.

Portfolio
portfolio, cover letter, résumé
The Hiring Process
orientation, profession, professionalism,
probationary period, performance evaluation, career ladder, networking, collaborative

KEY Points

- You will continue to learn as you begin your first job. You may even come to think of that first position as being another phase of your education.

- Learn as much as you can about the facility and its parent company before making application.

- A portfolio is an itemized visual account of your skills and best practices that are related to the position you are seeking.

- Most résumés are computer generated today, but at the very least, it must be typed on quality paper and is normally the same light-colored paper that you used for your cover letter.

- A face-to-face meeting gives a first impression. Whether it results in employment or not, it is an experience that will provide you with insight into your ability to speak logically and think critically.

- Continuing education is required by all state boards of nursing. The licensed nurse needs to be aware of the specific requirements of the state in which he or she is licensed.

- Professional organizations represent the members' interests nationally as well as providing educational and networking opportunities.

 EXPLORE Media Link

Additional interactive resources for this chapter can be found on the Companion Website at www.prenhall.com/ramont. Click on Chapter 38 and "Begin" to select the activities for this chapter.

For chapter-related NCLEX®-style questions and an audio glossary, access the accompanying CD-ROM in this book.

1 A cover letter should contain three paragraphs. The first paragraph is where you would:
1. highlight your particular qualifications.
2. identify yourself and the job that is being sought.
3. convey your anticipation in obtaining an interview.
4. express your enthusiasm for this particular job.

2 You have a significant time gap in your work history, following a layoff from a previous job. Which of the following is the best way to address the time gap on an employment application?
1. Skip that time period; prospective employers are not interested in times when you were not employed.
2. Leave the area blank on the application where it asks why you left that job.
3. Identify the time period and highlight educational or volunteer activities during that time.
4. Write an explanation about why you were laid off, so they know it was not your fault.

3 If subjected to a question concerning the applicant's religion, which of the following would be the best response?
1. "Civil rights law prohibits you from asking me personal questions."
2. "I would really rather not answer that question."
3. "I will need time off on religious holidays to fulfill my personal obligations. I hope that won't be a problem."
4. "My religious beliefs will not interfere with my ability to carry out the responsibilities of this position."

4 One of your fellow students has applied to several healthcare facilities but has not received even one call back. You notice that her cover letter and résumé are generic and are addressed "To Whom It May Concern. Which of the following is the most likely reason for the lack of response?
1. The facilities do not like to hire new graduates.
2. Her cover letter and résumé did not demonstrate an effort on her part to find out pertinent information about the facility and staff.
3. The facility knew she was applying to others and did not want to waste their time if she really wasn't interested.
4. Because the letter was not addressed to a person it did not reach the person doing the hiring.

5 A profession can be described in many ways. The definition that best describes nursing as a profession is:
1. an occupation to which one devotes oneself and in which one has specialized expertise.
2. a job that requires post-baccalaureate education.
3. a lifelong career that provides upward mobility.
4. an occupation that has a continuing education requirement.

6 You are scheduled for an interview at a hospital where you were employed as a nursing assistant during your nursing program. The interview is scheduled at 9 A.M. after you have worked the night shift. Which is the most appropriate view about attire for the interview?
1. "I will wear my uniform. That way I will not be rushed and can relax before the meeting."
2. "Since the director of nursing and human resource director already know me, it won't matter how I am dressed."
3. "I will go home, shower and dress in business attire, in order to show respect for the interview team, and the position for which I am applying."
4. "I will tell my supervisor I need to leave early, because this interview is really important."

7 Which of the following would be considered to be casual networking?
1. attending a presentation with classmates on a new facility who is recruiting LPNs
2. attending a job fair at a local college
3. while having coffee with a friend, the advantages of her new job come up in conversation
4. discussing job opportunities on a hospital Internet website

8 There are several types of résumé formats. Which of the following formats emphasizes skills?
1. chronological
2. functional
3. combination
4. e-résumé

9 It is important to include writing samples in your portfolio because they demonstrate:
1. your ability to write in a logical order using correct format and show your attention to details.
2. that academic skills were a part of your nursing program.
3. your ability to chart effectively.
4. your level of computer skills.

10 The first professional nursing organization, American Society of Superintendents of Training Schools for Nurses in the United States and Canada, was established in 1893. Its name was later changed to:
1. the American Nurses Association
2. the National Association for Practical Nursing
3. the North American Nursing Diagnosis Association
4. the National League for Nursing.

Answers and Rationales for Review Questions, as well as discussion of Care Plan and Critical Thinking Care Map questions, appear in Appendix I.

Thinking Strategically About ...

You are a recent graduate from a vocational nursing program. You successfully passed your licensure exam and have been hired as night shift charge nurse for a skilled nursing facility. Your orientation went well, and now this is your first night alone on the unit.

A client from the assisted living unit was sent to the ED of the local hospital for IVs to treat dehydration resulting from several days of nausea and vomiting. The IV line has been placed. He will be discharged from the ED and will be coming to your unit. You are not yet IV certified but are planning to take the class after receiving your first paycheck.

You attempt to reach the director of nursing (DON) by phone and find that she is out of town. You call the assistant DON and inform her that no nurse in the building is IV certified. You request that the client be kept at the hospital until morning. You explain your lack of certification to the ADON. She hesitates, then asks what care will be needed during the night. There is no medication to be given IV, but fluids will need to be added to the IV at about 5 A.M. You have watched the procedure many times and realize that although you are not legally qualified, it is a relatively easy procedure.

COMMUNICATION AND TEAM BUILDING

Using your knowledge of communication and team building, what solutions could you suggest to the ADON? List several possibilities.

CRITICAL THINKING

The ADON says, "Well, you've watched these things being done a dozen times. It's not that big a deal. Can't you just do it?" When you hesitate, she lashes out and states, "I knew there would be a problem hiring you new grads. If you can't solve your problems, maybe we need to rethink your charge nurse position." What responses would be appropriate in this situation?

CONFLICT RESOLUTION

After this conflict, you are concerned about your relationship with the ADON. You want to try to resolve the tension over the IV issue. How might you approach the ADON to change the situation? If you are concerned that the ADON might try to get you fired, what steps should you take to protect your position?

Appendix I

Answers and Rationales for Care Plans, Care Maps, and NCLEX-PN® Questions

CHAPTER 1

NCLEX-PN® ANSWERS 1. (3) Application. Questions of knowledge simply test facts. Comprehension questions require you to understand the meaning of a work (such as *cathartic*) and to use the knowledge to arrive at an answer. Application involves knowledge and comprehension, plus use of that information in a fresh situation. Analysis questions are more complex than application questions. 2. (3) The NCLEX-PN® is a computer adaptive test that is mostly multiple-choice questions. The questions are used to determine whether a person can function safely and effectively as an entry-level LPN/LVN. 3. (3) When a student is unsure of how to proceed, he or she must ask for help in order to ensure client safety. When students know how to proceed but feel hesitant or nervous, they should recognize the feeling but go ahead. 4. (3) The terms *client, patient, customer,* and *consumer* are all used in healthcare discussions. The term *client* is often preferred because it implies the person's involvement in decisions about care; the client is not just passively accepting help and decisions from others. 5. (2) Florence Nightingale contributed to many aspects of nursing and public health. However, it is because of her attempts to define what nursing is and is not that she is sometimes called the first nurse scientist-theorist. 6. (1) 1950s. 7. (3) Provided federal funding for practical nurse education. 8. (3) Operating under the umbrella of an overseeing organization distinguishes a profession from an occupation. 9. (3) Lillian Kuster started the National Federation of Licensed Practical Nurses. Lillian Wald founded the Henry Street Settlement and Visiting Nurses Service. 10. (2) Each state has its own nurse practice act, which provides the scope of nursing for its jurisdiction. Nurses are responsible for knowing the limits of practice whenever they work.

CHAPTER 2

NCLEX-PN® ANSWERS 1. (1) Stereotyping is an oversimplification of conceptions, opinions, or beliefs about some aspect of a group of people. Ethnocentrism means interpreting the beliefs and behavior of others in terms of one's own cultural values and traditions. It assumes that one's own culture is superior. Acculturation is the modification of the culture of a group as a result of contact with another group. Cultural awareness is the increasing of one's consciousness of cultural diversity. 2. (3) Madeline Leininger developed the Sunrise model as part of her cultural diversity and universality theory. Although the others are nursing theorists, their theories do not focus on culture.

3. (2) Cultural competency includes five concepts including ability to adapt practice skills to fit the cultural context of the client. Although it helps to be able to communicate in the client's native language, culturally competent care can be delivered without this ability. Complementary alternative medicine is becoming more readily accepted in mainstream Western medicine, but its use is not required for culturally competent nursing care. Ignoring a client's culture decreases one's ability to provide competent care. Cultural differences exist. Their consideration is an important part of treating the client holistically. 4. (3) Many cultural beliefs are closing tied to religious practices and belief. For example, an individual of some culture may follow strict religious practices such as fasting especially during religious holy days. Adherence to these practices could compromise their recovery. 5. (3) In health care, ethnocentrism can include the view that the only valid healthcare beliefs and practices are those held by healthcare professionals. 6. (1) Classifying clients' responses to care and treatment by ethnicity is considered to be stereotyping. 7. (2) In some families the man is considered to be the provider and the decision maker. The woman may need to consult her husband prior to making decisions about medical treatment for her child. 8. (3) Always consider the client's culture before assuming that people do not understand or are being resistant. Modesty is a real issue with hospitalized clients of many cultures. 9. (4) Many religious groups have specific dietary laws that they must follow. These needs can be met while hospitalized by consulting with the dietitian. 10. (2) The nurse should avoid using family members to interpret to limit biased responses. Interpreters who are the same sex as the client are preferred to provide translation.

CHAPTER 3

NCLEX-PN® ANSWERS 1. (1, 4) Your first responsibility is to be sure all legal requirements have been met; a client who changes his or her mind after signing consent may not have made an informed decision. Healthcare professionals should always consider the principle of beneficence. Although it would be better for family and client to agree, it is not essential for the nurse to consider the family's opinion about treatment. Even if the client has signed the consent, he or she can revoke that consent. 2. (2) Restraint without an order, or failing to follow facility policies on restraints, constitutes false imprisonment. Negligence and ethical considerations may enter into the discussion, but they are not the best answer in this situation. Defamation has to do with false communication, not restraints. 3. (3) Negligence is practice that is below the accepted standard expected by an ordinary, reasonable, prudent practitioner. A prudent nurse will always recheck a physician's order if the client has questions about medication or treatment. 4. (2) Slander is defamation by the spoken word. Libel is defamation in the form of a printed or written word or picture. Invasion of privacy and breach of confidence have to do with confidentiality. When a nurse discredits another staff member, he or she is guilty of defamation. 5. (2) Failure to observe and take appropriate action is malpractice related to failure to report a client's complaint or concern. 6. (3) The National League for Nursing is a private agency responsible for the accreditation of basic nursing programs. The individual state boards of nursing are responsible for the other tasks. 7. (3) Completion of an incident report is the duty of the nurse who discovers the incident. This may be the nurse involved in the incident, but does not have to be. The supervisor and the risk management department will review the report. 8. (2) The ADA prohibits discrimination on the basis of disability in employment, public service, and public accommodations. This act is enforced by the federal government. 9. (2) The concept of autonomy involves people's right to make their own decisions. 10. (2) Computerized medical records present specific security concerns. The best thing staff members can do to preserve confidentiality is protect their personal security codes and follow the facility's policies for use.

CHAPTER 4

NCLEX-PN® ANSWERS 1. (2) The art of thinking about thinking represents critical thinking. Choice 1: Although the word *critical* can mean fault finding, in this context critical means discerning. Choices 3 and 4 are characteristics of natural rather than critical thinking. 2. (1) During the assessment/data collection phase the nurse must consider personal assumptions or biases that may affect judgment. 3. (1) A nurse who is using critical thinking skills will evaluate the client's cognitive ability or limitations prior to beginning health-related teaching. 4. (3) The process of seeking alternatives involves identifying all possibilities for meeting the criteria. 5. (1) With inductive reasoning, certain bits of information suggest a particular interpretation when viewed together. 6. (2) Choice 2 infers that aspirin is the cause of Reye's syndrome, so any child receiving it would have a risk of developing Reye's syndrome. Choice 1 is a statement of fact; 3 is a judgment; and 4 is an opinion. 7. (3) Environment (according to Nightingale) is related to internal and external factors such as light and excessive noise. Choice 1 represents health; 2 represents person/client; and 4 represents nursing. 8. (2) Newman's theory focuses on reaction to stress in the environment; Roy focuses on the adaptation to the changes in the environment; Orem's theory focuses on self-care; and Leininger focuses on cultural care. 9. (1) Environmental theory, Nightingale; adaptation model, Roy; systems model, Newman; and cultural care diversity, Leininger. 10. (4) Leininger's theory is based on universal human caring, although ways of caring vary across cultures.

CHAPTER 5

NCLEX-PN® ANSWERS 1. (3) Assessment involves data collection related to the client's current health status, while evaluation is concerned with accomplishment of the goals. 2. (3) The second phase of nursing process is diagnosing. During this phase collected data are analyzed and problems are identified. 3. (2) Goals must have a subject (*client*), verb (*walk*), condition or modifier (*the length of the hall*), criteria for desired outcome (*with assistance of two staff members, 2 times per day*), and time line (*in 2 days*). The other choices are missing one or more required components. 4. (1) Rationales are the reason why a particular intervention was tried. They identify the scientific basis for the intervention. 5. (4) The care plan is the culmination of the planning phase. Choosing interventions occurs before the care plan, and evaluation of effectiveness of interventions is part of the evaluation phase. Delegating interventions is part of implementation. 6. (3) Explain why an intervention of vital sign and pulse oximeter readings should be included. Choice 1 is an intervention; choices 2 and 4 are statements of evidence for evaluation. 7. (2) Although the care plan is written in the planning stage, it is put into action in the implementation stage. 8. (3) Once the care plan has been implemented, the licensed nurse will decide what tasks can be carried out by other nursing personnel and also how much supervision they will need to complete them. 9. (1) Evaluations must include a conclusion (goal met, not met, or partially met) and data that provide evidence for the stated conclusion. 10. (3) Although the other choices contribute to the nursing process, choice 3 provides a clear definition of the nursing process as an organized framework for professional nursing practice.

CARE PLAN HINTS

1. Assess respiratory effort; ausculate lung sounds; position to facilitate breathing (e.g., high-Fowler's position); complete check of vital signs, temperature, and heart rate; determine intensity of pain; call the physcian with your findings.

2. To identify the organism that has caused the infection, results are used to choose the appropriate antibiotic to fight the microorganism. Culture should be obtained prior to beginning therapy so that accurate results can be obtained.

3. Remain calm and appear confident; encourage slow deep breathing; demonstrate cough, deep breathing, and use of incentive spirometer; administer anlagesic as needed; encourage client to express concerns; explain condition and all procedures prior to beginning.

4. Avoid exposure to people with cold/flu; drink plenty of fluids (at least 8 glasses/day) to help thin secretions and facilitate expectoration; good hand hygiene techiques and

proper disposal of secretions; teach importance of good oral care to clear mouth of pathogens to help prevent pneumonia; consider being immunized with the pneumoccal vaccine and/or receiving year influenza vaccine, since she may be more susceptiable to respiratory infection in the future; get plenty of rest, eat a well-balanced diet, and exercise.

CRITICAL THINKING CARE MAP

Subjective Data He doesn't know her. Says they won't give him any food. "It was a bad idea to plan this trip. I should stay and take Charles home with me."

Objective Data Alzheimer's disease $\times 3$ years. Articef. Coreg 6.125 mg. every day (hold if SBP $<$ 110). Ativan 1 mg prn every 6 h for anxiety. Regular insulin per sliding scale ac and at bedtime. NPH Humulin 30 units every am. Diet: mechanical soft diet. VS: 98.2/68/16, BP 104/60. Wife crying during visit.

Report Yes, BP 106/60; Coreg held. Report to physician if blood pressure continues to be outside the parameters.

Nursing Interventions Assist significant person with expanding repertoire of coping skills. Help family members recognize the need for help and teach them how to ask for it. Encourage family members to verbalize feelings. Validate the family's feelings regarding the impact of client's illness on family lifestyle.

Documentation **D**—Wife crying. Client upset does not think Mrs. Weldon is his wife. Telling wife he is not being fed. Wife talking of canceling trip and taking client back to their apartment. **A**—Encouraged wife to verbalize feelings and talk about concerns about her trip. Reviewed client's food intake with wife. Provide wife with information on Alzheimer Support Group. **R**—Wife able to talk about need for some personal relaxation, although expresses guilt for not being able to care for husband. Wife expressed interest in support group attendance when she returns from trip. A. Harper, LPN

UNIT I WRAP-UP

COMMUNITY Long-term care is "home" for many of the residents. A nurse who seems abusive may be creating an environment that affects all the people who live there. He or she may make them all more anxious about how they might be treated. In this sense, a staff member who is abusive is equivalent to a "neighborhood bully."

CRITICAL THINKING

- Whistle-blowers are people who expose negligence, abuse, or dangers (such as professional misconduct or incompetence) in the organization in which they work. They become whistle-blowers because normal quality control is neglected by those in charge.
- This situation has both ethical and legal implications. Carlos was motivated by his concern for the client and the nursing code of ethics. Depending on the jurisdiction in

which Carlos works, there may be legal ramifications if he does not report his observations. It may be necessary to report the abuse outside of the organization. In many jurisdictions, legislation requires that child abuse or abuse of vulnerable adults be reported.

- It would probably be difficult for Carlos to prove that he was being ostracized by the staff. If other staff members would testify to the racial slurs, he may have some recourse, although legal action would not improve his work situation.

COMMUNICATION Role-playing these scenes negatively and discussing the feelings that they raise can be useful. However, it is even more important to role-play positive alternatives to these scenarios, because these are what nurses will need. Making a long list of possible alternatives is also a valuable class activity.

CONFLICT RESOLUTION Carlos could have done several things differently. He could have gathered facts about the situation and ascertained the risks, then spoken privately to other staff members and to the resident to determine whether abuse had occurred. He could have sought relevant information directly from the nurse whose behavior or practice raised concerns. ("Is this client giving you problems?") The nurse may not have realized that her behavior was viewed by others as abusive. He could have modeled good nursing behavior in relation to the client. As charge nurse, he could have called a team conference to discuss aspects of this client's care. He could have requested in-service training for all nurses to help in dealing with client behavior issues.

CHAPTER 6

NCLEX-PN® ANSWERS 1. (3) This answer is most accurate and reflects the need to inform the doctor of the client's emotional status. 2. (4) There is no reason to discuss a client's condition with someone not directly involved with care. Choice 3 would respect client confidentiality as you are explaining to a visitor what the contact isolation means, not what is wrong with the client. 3. (2) You would initial the original medication administration record, not the copy. The other statements are reasonable requests to ensure confidentiality of information. 4. (1) This is the correct procedure for most agencies. While the chart does belong to the facility, the client generally has a right to a copy after making a request. There may be a copy fee. 5. (3) It is not necessary to cross out an entry or entries so that your notes are in chronological order. A late entry made with the event's time and labeled as a late entry is appropriate. 6. (3) Requesting assistance from your charge nurse is appropriate because he or she may be more familiar with the physician's handwriting. If you and your charge nurse are unable to read the orders, you would then call the doctor for clarification. 7. (4) Every facility defines the duties of its LPNs/LVNs in a job description, which may or may not be similar to job descriptions at other facilities. 8. (1) You should always use the time that the event happened when making your entry. **9. (2)** Faxing information to a physician's office is appropriate (if permitted by your agency), but should be followed up with a call to the office to ensure that they received the fax. You should also get the name of the person you spoke with and include an entry in the nurse's notes that you called to verify receipt of the fax. **10. (2)** Walking rounds are common in many facilities but care must be taken to ensure that your comments are appropriate and that your voices are not overheard by people in the hall. Caution must also be taken when speaking in front of the client, because medical terminology may be misunderstood or misinterpreted by the client.

CARE PLAN HINTS

1. Maintain aseptic/neutropenic environment. Maintain freedom from infection.
2. Wearing a mask reduces Amy's risk of contracting a disease since her immune system is compromised.
3. Notify the physician. These are signs and symptoms of infection.
4. The steroids suppress the immune system and permit the chemotherapeutics to work more effectively.

CRITICAL THINKING CARE MAP

Subjective Data States "I don't know how to cook for one person"; decreased social activity; crying; talks as if spouse alive.

Objective Data Weight loss since admission. Not wearing makeup. Hair not combed. Decreased interest in surroundings.

Report Yes, to attending physician and care coordinator

Nursing Interventions Obtain referrals to grief counselor and appropriate grief support group. Arrange dietitian consult for meal planning on discharge. Suggest to family that the client's priest should visit regularly. Schedule time during the shift to spend one-on-one time with client. Encourage client to talk about spouse.

Documentation

Date	Time	Nurse's Notes
[date]	[time]	Client ate 25% of supper, declined supplement. States not hungry. —S. Randall, LVN
[date]	[time]	Family here to visit. Reports changes in client eating habits with weight loss over last 2 years. Also reports client cries frequently over death of husband dead 2 yrs. Family also reports that client's current lack of interest in church or grooming was not present prior to death of spouse. —S. Randall, LVN
[date]	[time]	Dr. Jones here to see client. Notified of weight loss and family reports (see note above). New orders noted for grief counselor referral and dietitian consult. —S. Randall, LVN
[date]	[time]	Dietary notified of consult order. Client and family notified of orders and of presence of two grief counselors in their area. Son states will choose one and call back in A.M. with choice. —S. Randall, LVN

CHAPTER 7

NCLEX-PN® ANSWERS **1. (2)** Included in this bill are the right of clients to considerate and respectful care; privacy for the clients, confidentiality of records and communications regarding their care; and the right to make decisions about their care, including right to refuse treatment. **2. (1)** OBRA instituted requirements for nurse's aide training. Specifically, they include a minimum of 75 hours of training and competence evaluation of aides. **3. (3)** All of these may be an issue with a homeless client. However, the living environment and the exposure to disease, poor nutrition, and the elements would be the major concern. **4. (4)** Team nursing is a collaborative effort of direct client care, with healthcare workers from two or more levels. Care is allocated according to the scope of practice of the individual team members. **5. (4)** The 1965 Medicare amendments (Title 18) to the Social Security Act provided for national and state health insurance for older adults. Medicaid and Medi-cal are health insurance for individuals needing federal and/or state assistance. Medicare is a federal program; Medi-cal is one of numerous state programs. **6. (3)** In 1983 the U.S. Congress passed legislation putting the prospective payment system into effect. Reimbursement is made according to a classification system called diagnostic-related groups. **7. (4)** Paramedical is defined as having some training to do with medicine. A spiritual support person attends to the client's spiritual needs, but is not required to have healthcare training. Occupational therapists, physiotherapists, and laboratory technicians are interdisciplinary team members specially trained to meet specific health needs. **8. (1)** Although managed care may mean that the number of hospital days may be reduced and allocation of services may be more efficient, the purpose of managed care is to provide the client with the most effective treatment. Managed care can be used with any nursing model. **9. (2)** Health maintenance organizations provide capitated care. In other words, a monthly fee is paid for each member, whether or not they received treatment during that time period. **10. (1)** Primary care includes preventive care, health education, environmental protection, and early detection and treatment. Secondary care includes acute care and diagnosis and treatment. Tertiary care includes rehabilitation and care of the terminally ill.

CHAPTER 8

NCLEX-PN® ANSWERS **1. (3)** Children are curious and have not developed the judgment needed to understand danger. Bad behavior and parent neglect can cause injury, but unfounded accusation should not be made. New walkers frequently fall, but a child-safe environment can protect from injury. 2. (2) A mitt restraint will prevent the client from pulling at IV lines, but will not restrict overt movements. A vest restraint and bed alarms are used to keep the client in bed, but will not prevent the client from disturbing IV lines. Arm restraints would keep the client from pulling out IV lines, but they would unnecessarily restrict movement. 3. (2) The MSDS provides all necessary information to the nurse to safely work with chemicals in the workplace. The name of the chemical, years of experience using the chemical, and previous exposure are not as important as having access to the MSDS. 4. (3) The walker will need to be used at all times until he is fully recovered. The other choices show good understanding of his discharge needs. 5. (2) Body mechanics is a safe and efficient way to move the body. Physical therapy is treatment of large muscle groups; occupational therapy deals with small muscle groups. Nursing interventions are nursing actions to help clients meet goals. 6. (2) OSHA, the Occupational Safety and Health Administration, is the government agency responsible for safe work environments. CDC is the Centers for Disease Control and Prevention. The Department of Labor is concerned with all work-related issues, not specifically safety. JCAHO is not a government agency; it is responsible for accreditation of healthcare organizations. 7. (3) The CDC recommends that isolation linens be removed promptly from the room by bagging them. Linens are not disposable, so they should not be placed in a refuse container. 8. (2) Items such as paper and cloth could easily ignite if they come in contact with heating appliances. Appropriate use of electric heaters does not present an increased fire hazard. Bars over windows cannot prevent intruders from entering a home, but in the event of a fire, can prevent windows from being used as an exit. Fire extinguishers are normally stored in the kitchen for quick access in case of fire. 9. (4) During transfer, holding the client close to your center of gravity and standing with a wide base of support is the safest position for client and nurse. Keeping the client at arm's length and having feet close together are not appropriate use of body mechanics by the nurse. Unless client is independently ambulatory, the nurse should support and assist the client during transfer using proper body mechanics. 10. (1, 3, 4) In the event of a fire in a client's room, remove the client to a safe place, close the door to contain the fire, and activate the alarm. It is not necessary to contact the client's physician.

CARE PLAN HINTS

1. Restraints should only be used as a last resort. Studies have not shown that restraining a client prevents falls or injury. Restraints reduce the client's movement and independence, which infringes on their rights. The restraints can cause injury (e.g., pressure ulcers, skin tears, or death from strangulation). Restraints can interfere with treatment. Restraints can increase health problems such as poor circulation. They can be embarrassing to both the client and family members.

2. He has been physically and socially active and independent; he has a strong family support system (his son will visit daily); he has access to community resources; his rooms are on one level and his home is small; he has pets to decrease his loneliness; he has no other chronic illnesses that would interfere with his healing process.

3. Several factors could affect Mr. Moore's safety. These include, but are not limited to, age greater than 65; history of falls; recent hip surgery to repair fracture, which might impair his mobility; and the possibility that he is weaker now than before surgery. He may resume normal activities before he is strong enough. Mr. Moore may not be able to meet his nutritional needs because he will be preparing all meals but one each day. He is a greater risk for injury while preparing his own food. He may not understand the precautions necessary to protect his own safety.

CRITICAL THINKING CARE MAP

Subjective Data Client's wife expressed concerns about his upcoming discharge. Lives alone in a two-story house. Does yard work. Socializes with the neighbors. Daughter and three grandchildren live 75 miles away. Mrs. Whitman and the daughter feel the couple should move to a retirement apartment. Mr. Whitman expressed, "Selling the house would be a sign that I am just giving up."

Objective Data Rigidity due to the Parkinson's. Difficulty in swallowing. Large bruise on his left leg and right forearm. VS: T 98.2, P 76, R 20, BP 140/88. H&H 13.2 40.4, PT 13.5 sec, PTT 90 sec.

Report Bruising on left leg and right arm. Would report to M.D.—client is on anticoagulation therapy.

Nursing Interventions Take temperature, pulse, and blood pressure every 4 h. Observe nutritional status. Work with dietitian to increase nutritional status. Monitor risk for bleeding. Teach client and family signs of bleeding, precautions to take to prevent bleeding.

Documentation Areas of bruising on left thigh and right forearm. Client resting in bed. H&H 13.2 40.4, PT 13.5 sec, PTT 90 sec. 9 A.M. heparin held, physician notified. K. Smartt, LPN

CHAPTER 9

NCLEX-PN® ANSWERS 1. (4) The wound and the dressing are contaminating the environment, and because it is wet it may be transmitting other organisms to the wound itself. The physician would not ordinarily order medications for a temperature below 101°F. Elevation of the leg and placing the client in isolation may be done later. 2. (2) The tuberculosis organism is transmitted through the air in droplets. Tier 2 or Transmission-based Precautions are specific for this condition. Tier 1 or Standard Precautions and the use of clean gowns do not address airborne organisms. The nurse would use the mask to prevent inhalation of the tuberculosis organism. 3. (3) Metal and glass items are autoclaved. Plastic and rubber items are gas sterilized to prevent melting. The items must be put into separate, properly labeled bags. The bags must be impervious to drainage and are usually colored (red). None of the items can be disposed of in an ordinary fashion because they would contaminate the environment. 4. (1) The items are contaminated so they must be cleaned. However, throwing toys and clothes away is costly and unnecessary. Exposing them to air will not kill any of the organisms. Washing the items in hot water will clean them before they are used again and destroy most bacteria. 5. (1) Covering the client will not prevent the spread of airborne organisms, nor will the wearing of gloves. The client, not the transporter, should wear the mask to prevent the spread of organisms when they cough or sneeze. Informing the radiology department that the client is still infectious will allow them to take appropriate precautions. 6. (4) Using sterile forceps is appropriate, but not reaching across the field, since organisms could fall on it and contaminate it. Only sterile gloves are worn while handling the contents of the tray so as to not contaminate them. All sterile trays and materials should be covered with sterile towels immediately if they are not in use. 7. (3) The gloves are contaminated and must be removed first in sequence before the ties of the mask or gown are touched. Otherwise, the person's head, neck, and back can become contaminated. Only the ties of the mask are handled, and they are undone next. Finally, the ties of the gown are loosened and the gown is removed. 8. (2) A compromised host is someone who is already at high risk for getting infections because of one or more reasons. The client is elderly and has a history of emphysema, two other predisposing problems. A susceptible host is just at risk for developing an infection. 9. (2) Choices 1 and 3 are part of the assessment phase of the nursing process, and choice 4 is part of the implementation phase. Only choice 2 describes a goal in the planning stage. 10. (3) Itching is not considered part of the inflammatory process but a possible result. The hallmark signs of inflammation are swelling or edema, and redness as well as heat due to increased circulation in the area. Bruising generally does not occur with inflammation, and the wound does not need to be weeping to be inflamed.

CARE PLAN HINTS

1. Because Mrs. Chase is elderly and has a history of emphysema, she is at risk for respiratory infection. In addition she smokes, which decreases ciliary function and makes infection more likely. By caring for her grandchild who was ill with a strep infection, she was exposed to bacteria that her immune system was unable to fight off.
2. Microorganisms from Mrs. Chase's respiratory tract are transmitted to the tissues through mucus and saliva. Because the tissues have touched the bed linens, the linens are now also contaminated. The nurse who removes the tissues must wear gloves while doing so to avoid further transmission of microorganisms.
3. Mrs. Chase has an elevated temperature, is coughing up yellow/green-tinged mucus, and has an elevated white count. Her abnormal chest x-ray indicates pneumonia.

CRITICAL THINKING CARE MAP

Subjective Data Complains of burning pain in area of wound. Says his foot is cold. Says he hasn't washed right leg in several days. States he left wound open because "air is good for it,"

Objective Data Yellow/green secretions. Foul odor from wound and secretions. Poor pedal pulses. Feet appear slightly cyanotic.

Report Yes, to RN, charge nurse, and physician. Report poor pedal pulses and edema.

Nursing Interventions Administer analgesics as ordered by physician. Elevate feet. Cleanse wound and apply wound dressings as ordered. Keep feet warm. Teach patient about airborne contamination. Consult with dietician regarding diet.

Documentation [date] [time] On admission ulcerated area noted on lower, inner aspect of right leg. No apparent dressing. Moderate amount of thick yellow/green drainage observed. Foul odor noted. Area 15 cm long, 6 cm wide, 1.5 cm deep. Pedal pulses present but weak, foot slightly cyanotic with +2 edema. Wound edges red, surrounding skin hot. States wound has "stinging pain." Charge nurse notified. Wound cleansed with sterile normal saline, wet-to-dry dressing applied. Foot elevated and supported, covered with blanket for warmth. 500 mg acetaminophen given PO. Medicated for pain per physician's order. Started on high-protein diet. Teaching about wound contamination done. M. Penn, LVN

CHAPTER 10

NCLEX-PN® ANSWERS 1. (4) The nurse refers to the client properly by her last name, does not relay health information, and does not refer to the client as a diagnosis. Choice 1 is incorrect because the nurse refers to the client as a diagnosis; this can result in a loss of self-identity. In choice B, the nurse refers to the client by his first name, which some people find offensive. Choice 3 is incorrect because the client is referred to by room number and not by last name. 2. (4) During the initial interview, language skills and understanding should be assessed and arrangements made for an interpreter. Choice 1 is wrong because Indian was an incorrect name for native people that was adopted early in our country's history. Choice 2 is incorrect because in some cultures, the informal use of a client's first name is offensive. Choice 3 is incorrect; it is important to speak clearly and use simple words without slang, but nurses need not speak above their normal tone. 3. (1) Individualized client care during admission, transfer, and discharge reduces anxiety; it also promotes safety and improved health status. Choice 2 is incorrect because discharge planning does not require a physician's order and should begin on admission. Choices 3 and 4 are incorrect; the client's coping skills and knowledge deficit should be incorporated into the individualized plan for care. 4. (4) Lack of oxygen is life threatening, so breathing is always a priority consideration. The nurse should anticipate that the client's oxygen need will increase with activity and anxiety. Oxygen delivery can be maintained during transfer by securing a portable oxygen tank. Choices 1 and 3 are good, but they are not the priority interventions. In terms of choice 2, the LPN/LVN may answer questions related to the transfer and would call the RN if the client or significant other has unanswered questions. 5. (3) The JCAHO requires that a registered nurse perform the admission assessment. Choices 1 and 4 are incorrect because formulation of nursing diagnoses and development of the treatment plan are RN responsibilities. Choice 2 is also incorrect. The LPN/LVN may collect data related to the confused client but should report findings to the charge nurse, not apply a restrictive device. 6. (2) The first choice should be to send any valuables home with a significant other. If this is not possible, the valuables may be able to be stored in the hospital safe. Choice 1 is incorrect; only the personal items that a client needs (such as glasses, dentures, and hearing aids) should stay by the client's bedside. They should be recorded on the inventory list. Choices 3 and 4 are not the best solution. 7. (3) All clients need discharge planning to begin at admission. The nurse can anticipate a client with a language barrier will need additional planning and coordination. The LPN/LVN will need to collaborate with the RN to clarify teaching and discharge goals for this clients. Choices 1, 2, and 4 are incorrect because the LPN/LVN would be able to clarify goals and discharge planning needs independently for these clients. 8. (1) Client safety should be the nurse's first concern. The nurse should check the identification band before performing any procedure or giving any medication. Choice 2 is incorrect because the LPN/LVN does not need to consult with the RN before replacing an unreadable identification band. With choice 3 or 4, a medical error might occur. 9. (1) Children may experience separation anxiety if the parent is not allowed to stay through the admission process. Choice 2 is incorrect because the nurse is a stranger; trying to hold the child may increase the child's anxiety. Choice 3 is correct, but it is not the best answer because the priority goal is to reduce the client's anxiety related to the admission process. Choice 4 is incorrect because the nurse–client relationship is harmed when the nurse does not tell the truth. 10. (3) The nursing actions during transfer should be directed toward managing the transfer process in an efficient and calm manner. When the nurse shares information, anxiety is decreased and compliance increased. Choice 1 is incorrect because placing the client on their side may not be possible. Choice 2 is incorrect because

the nurse should introduce the client using the first and last name. Choice 4 is incorrect because the client may not understand the information presented and become more anxious.

CARE PLAN HINTS

1. The reason for Mr. Reynolds' admission (potential myocardial infarction) led Janet to address nursing care issues related to his physical status. Specifically, she observed his color and level of pain, monitored his vital signs, and completed the required systems assessment. She also observed and listened to his reaction to his medical situation. Mr. Reynolds gave evidence of having emotional as well as physical nursing care issues. Janet routinely informs the nursing team leader that a new client's admission has been completed, and reports particular problems requiring the team leader's attention. Regarding Mr. Reynolds, Janet reported that he was experiencing a high degree of anxiety. There were several considerations in making her report. Janet understood that fear and anxiety could exacerbate his symptoms. The physician may have ordered anxiety-reducing medication that would be administered by the nursing team leader (an RN). Janet did not have meds certification. She would also discuss with the nursing team leader the nature of Mr. Reynolds' concerns because the anxiety they produced represented a nursing care issue that would be noted in the nursing care plan and require a team response.

2. There were several verbal and nonverbal indications that Mr. Reynolds was experiencing fear and anxiety. Certainly what Mr. Reynolds said and how he said it would indicate that he thought he was having a heart attack, that he might die, and that he might never see his wife again. His sentences were short and clear. His behavior could also be interpreted as anxious. Mr. Reynolds seemed to be taking his carotid pulse. His face was grimaced. Janet observed Mr. Reynolds' nonverbal behavior and listened to what he said in order to anticipate and recognize clues related to anxiety and fear. Janet empathically understood that anyone in Mr. Reynolds' situation would most likely experience some degree of fear and anxiety.

3. Arranging a room might seem insignificant, but Janet realized that chaos tends to increase anxiety. She understood that establishing order does not in itself reduce fear and anxiety. However, giving Mr. Reynolds choices and listening to his preferences could enable him to feel that he has more control over his situation. It could help him settle in physically and emotionally and prepare him to face his health issues.

CRITICAL THINKING CARE MAP

Subjective Data "My cats need me, and I can make do." Chart indicates noncompliance with discharge plan to assisted living facility.

Objective Data Unsafe environment at home (outdoor entry and metal stairs). Daughter says client very independent.

Report Yes, inform charge nurse of client's non-compliance with discharge plan.

Nursing Interventions Assess level of understanding regarding discharge and transfer. Explain purpose of transfer to assisted living. Allow time to answer questions about the assisted living facility. Demonstrate firmness in seeking cooperation. Maintain a calm, quiet manner. Encourage statement of concerns. Inquire about family members who live in the area.

Documentation [date] [time] Discharge interview for transfer to rehab attempted. Daughter did not arrive as scheduled. Client resistant to discussion of rehab, even as temporary. Stated "I'm not going there! I'm going home," turned chair to window. Told client would talk after dinner. Reported to charge nurse. R. Perry, LPN

UNIT II WRAP-UP

CRITICAL THINKING Remember ABC priority when seeing clients in an emergency situation. Mr. Suarez's breathing is compromised; this will be the priority nursing concern. Based on information gained from the intake inquiry, he may have a communicable disease. Mr. and Mrs. Suarez should be escorted to a private holding area in the emergency department, where Mr. Suarez can rest and his vital signs can be taken. Until Mr. Suarez is removed to an isolated area, he will need to wear a mask. Anyone attending to Mr. Suarez would utilize strict respiratory and contact isolation precautions.

COLLABORATIVE CARE The triage nurse would be called immediately. A radiology technician and lab technician would be required. The IV team or assigned RN should be notified to start a peripheral line. An infectious control consult would be called. The infectious control manager of the hospital should be alerted. It might also be necessary to contact the county Public Health Department.

CULTURAL COMPETENCY A translator should be summoned stat to speak to Mr. Suarez and to obtain further information from Mrs. Suarez. The nurse should be sensitive to the fact that Mr. Suarez gave all information, in spite of difficulty breathing. His role may be threatened if caregivers refer questions and decisions to his wife.

COMPASSIONATE CARING Nursing care for clients with significant respiratory complications focuses on maintaining airway clearance, ease of breathing, and adequate rest. The head of Mr. Suarez's bed should be elevated and he should be offered oxygen delivered by nasal cannula, according to unit standing orders. Mr. Suarez should be monitored for coughing and ability to clear sputum. Offer Mr. Suarez cool liquids to drink, to promote hydration until the IV has been started.

CHAPTER 11

NCLEX-PN® ANSWERS 1. (2) The best response is to explain how development occurs cephalocaudally, and that it is very individualized. False reassurance such as in choice 1 or generalized statements as in choices 3 and 4 do not serve to relieve the mother's concerns. 2. (3) Your client's developmental needs are not being met and thus despair is being expressed. Choice 1 coincides with the toddler year, 2 occurs during middle adult years, and 3 is related to the young adult period. 3. (2) A child between the ages of 6 and 11 is in Erikson's stage of industry vs. inferiority. Children at this age want to be productive and need to feel that they can do a task well. 4. (3) An infant's weight at 5 months will be approximately double the birth weight. Choice 4 would be the approximate weight at 1 year. 5. (3) Although growth has slowed somewhat by the preschool period, the extremities tend to grow a bit faster than the trunk. 6. (3) Right behavior is obeying the law and following the rules. At this stage, the circumstances are not taken into account. 7. (4) The individual becomes less dogmatic at this stage and is aware of truth from a variety of viewpoints. 8. (4) This is one of the six developmental tasks described by Havighurst during the age period of later maturity. 9. (4) During maturity, an individual whose developmental needs have been met will be able to accept the uniqueness of one's own life and death. If needs are not met, the individual will experience a sense of loss and despair. 10. (1, 3, 4) Intimacy vs. isolation relates to the young adult period. Generativity vs. stagnation applies to the middle adult, and integrity vs. despair relates to older adults. Identify vs. role confusion is the adolescent.

CARE PLAN HINTS

1. Mrs. Peterson's burns could be an attempt to get attention from her family. Her behaviors have been alienating her children, but because they love her and are concerned, they will respond to the injuries. Self-inflicted injuries can also be a way of releasing tension or anxiety. Depression can result in a lack of concentration, so her injuries may be a result of not concentrating on a task when she is in the kitchen. It is also possible that the injuries are a result of some physiological problem. She should have a complete medical workup, including hormone levels.

2. Now that Mrs. Peterson's children are grown and she has less responsibility, she will need to become involved in activities that will give her a feeling of self-worth. Social or civic responsibilities can be a source of self-worth. Leisure activities will help her to establish new friendships and help to relieve tension. Mrs. Peterson and her husband need to relate to each other as individuals. Now that their parenting roles and responsibilities have changed, their relationship may have changed also.

3. Avoiding contact with Mrs. Peterson will only increase her critical attitude toward her family. She and her children should begin making changes in their relationship. Inter-

acting with each other as adults is difficult but very necessary if they are to have a harmonious relationship. Mrs. Peterson needs to bring herself to look at her children as adults with families of their own. It is very important that parents, especially mothers, work at these adult interactions prior to the arrival of grandchildren.

CRITICAL THINKING CARE MAP

Subjective Data Lives with parents. Half-sister, child of father's previous marriage, visits alternate weekends. Both parents work outside the home. Is cared for by maternal grandmother during the week. Diet: appetite fair. Grandmother has trouble getting him to sit down for meals, usually resorts to finger food. Takes a bottle at night. Mother states opened medicine bottles from home medicine cabinet. Able to open patio door near backyard Jacuzzi. Mother states she is worn out from chasing Todd.

Objective Data Two year-old male child. VS: T 98.8 (tympanic), P 80, R 18. Weight 29 lbs. Height 34 inches. Climbing on furniture, opening cupboard, pull paper from exam table. Mother chasing child around room.

Report Yes, report mother's concerns about home safety and her own physical state and stress level to the physician.

Nursing Interventions Teach caregiver the need for close supervision of young children. Provide poison control number to mother. Instruct parent to keep syrup of ipecac in home first aid kit. Assist parents in devising a plan to childproof home. Inform parents of available CPR and first-aid training in the community.

Documentation Two-year-old active, well-developed child to see physician for follow-up for antibiotic therapy (amoxicillin 500 mg tid × 10 days) course completed 2 days ago. Mother expressed concerns for child safety related to ability to open medicine bottles from cabinet and patio door leading to Jacuzzi area. Mother questioned if degree of activity is normal for a 2-year-old. Marge Smith, LPN

CHAPTER 12

NCLEX-PN® ANSWERS 1. (2) Personal space is the distance people prefer in interaction with others; sitting on the bed invades that space. 2. (3) Closed-ended questions frequently can be answered with a yes or no or a single word (e.g., "How old are you?" "Seventy-three.") 3. (1) The opening sets the tone for the whole interview. The closing states appreciation for what has been accomplished. During the body of the interview is when the client can communicate what she or he thinks, feels, knows, or perceives, and the orientation gives the nurse the opportunity to state the purpose of the interview. 4. (2) Interpreting nonverbal behavior is done by a systematic assessment of physical appearance, posture, gait, facial expression, and

gestures. Interpreting nonverbal behaviors does not contradict the client's verbal communication, although it may identify some incongruencies. The client, not the nurse, is communicating nonverbally. The nurse's observations are designed to interpret the client's action, not make judgments. 5. (1) Telling the client that you are available and how much time you have will help to establish a therapeutic relationship. 6. (2) Changing the subject, ignoring your mistake, and ending the session quickly will set up barriers to a therapeutic relationship. 7. (2) Active listening demonstrates an interest in what the client is saying with eye contact, posture, and gestures. Interrupting, making notes, and looking at your watch or away do not demonstrate an interest on the part of the nurse. 8. (3) A leading question is one where the questioner inadvertently gives the answer with the question. 9. (4) The body is the time when the client can communicate what she or he thinks, feels, knows, or perceives in response to the nurse's questions. 10. (2) Expressing enjoyment for the time together and appreciation for what was accomplished is an excellent way to allow the client to know the interview is coming to an end. Abruptly cutting off conversation or changing position will not allow the client to express additional needs or wants. Telling the client you have other people you must see may make him or her feel unimportant and place a barrier for future communication.

CARE PLAN HINTS

1. Sat with client; asked questions; expressed compassion.
2. Lucy did not validate Mrs. Levowitz's feelings when she said, "The news can't be that bad"; she used false reassurance when she said, "Everything will be OK for you. It will turn out just fine." She did not think before she spoke; did not sit quietly and listen attentively.
3. Pulling up a chair conveyed that she was not in a hurry, although her words and nonverbal communication were not congruent.

CRITICAL THINKING CARE MAP

Subjective Data Feels she is fat; lost 15 pounds in 2 months. LMP 3 months ago. Regularly exercises more than 2 hours per day. Mother's relationship with client appears very controlling. Mother seems to be in denial about eating disorder; "eats lunch at school." Mother thinks client may be pregnant. Takes laxative for constipation.

Objective Data Height 5′9″. Weight 98 lbs. VS: T 96.8, P 100, R 18, BP 90/66.

Report Yes. Significant weight loss; amenorrhea × 2 months. Mother does not seem to recognize eating disorder. Client's life seems to be planned and controlled by mother. Report to physician for possible referral to counselor.

Nursing Interventions Establish open and trusting relationship within the family. Facilitate modeling and role-playing for family regarding healthy ways to communicate and interact. Provide sufficient knowledge to support family decisions regarding therapeutic regimens. Review with family members the congruence and incongruence of family behaviors and health-related goal. Review symptoms of specific disorder and work with family toward developing a greater awareness of symptoms. Collaborate with other consultants regarding strategies for working with families.

Documentation 18-year-old female with anorexia nervosa; appointment for college physical. Mother reluctant to allow daughter to be seen without her being present. Mother questioned if client could be pregnant, amenorrhea × 2 months. Client and mother unaware of seriousness and symptoms of disorder. 15-lb. weight loss; c/o constipation; taking laxative. Suggested that client see physician alone while mother and nurse discuss proper diet for active teenager. R. Dunheim, LVN

CHAPTER 13

NCLEX-PN® ANSWERS   **1.** (2) The stimulus acts on nerve receptors. Choice 1 is the receptor, choice 3 is the impulse, and choice 4 is perception. **2.** (3) The client who is not oriented to time, place, and person is disoriented. The client with reduced awareness who is easily bewildered is confused. A semicomatose individual can be aroused by extreme or repeated stimuli. **3.** (4) Conversing in a foreign language may cause sensory deprivation for the clients, this should be explained to the staff, since they may not be aware of it. **4.** (3) Placing an activity list in type large enough for the resident to easily read and a clock will allow the individual to be independent. Referring him to the activity board may cause confusion and it is not readily available for him to check. Sending someone for him will not promote independence. Overhead paging can cause sensory overload for the residents as well as others. It should be avoided in residential care facilities. **5.** (2) Hearing many times is still intact even when a client is unconscious, talking to the client and explaining what you are doing can help relieve anxiety. **6.** (1) Always give your arm to a client who is visually impaired, allowing her to choose the dominant or nondominant arm. Walking about 1 foot ahead will allow you to evaluate hazards and promote safe ambulation. **7.** (2) Sudden loss of a loved one is one of the primary causes of confusion in the elderly who are cared for in their own homes. **8.** (1) Safety and preventing sensory deprivation are the priorities. The other things will have little bearing if a safe, stimulating environment is not maintained. **9.** (1) All adults over age 40 years should have a visual exam every 3 to 5 years; however, if there is a family history of glaucoma they should be examined more frequently. Waiting until symptoms occur may result in irreversible deficits. **10.** (3) Reorient the client and offer to stay with her until she falls asleep and offer to make contact with husband in the morning. Threatening the client with restraints or medication is never an acceptable solution. The nurse should never tell a client that a family member has been contacted and that everything is fine, unless it has actually been done.

CARE PLAN HINTS

1. She is being bombarded by the noise of her monitors and ventilator, which may be distorted and meaningless due to the sedation she is receiving. Her pain and inability to communicate also contribute to her sensory overload because they contribute to her feelings of being overwhelmed and out of control.

2. Interventions include, but are not limited to, reducing lights; decreasing noise to the degree possible (close curtains or doors); orienting the client to person, place, and time; speaking in a soft, unhurried manner; and limiting visitors.

3. A client at home may experience either sensory deprivation or overload depending on the environment. If it is a busy, active environment with several family members, the client may experience overload. If the client lives alone, has few supportive family members, or is seldom contacted, she is more likely to experience social isolation and become withdrawn or uncommunicative or lose interest in her usual activities. Interventions for home care or ICU clients are similar and adapted to the specific needs of the client, regardless of setting.

CRITICAL THINKING CARE MAP

Subjective Data She states "I'm afraid of all of these strange creatures in this orphanage." Cared for herself independently for 15 years in her own home. Her children were concerned about her physical safety, lack of socialization.

Objective Data Height: 63″. Weight 122 lbs. VS: T 98.6, P 72, R 18, BP 128/74. Underwent surgery for removal of cataracts. Rinne test: negative. Experienced more difficulty with hearing. Chest x-ray, CBC, and urinalysis all negative. Somewhat confused and disoriented to person, place, and time. Appears restless, withdrawn, and her syntax is sometimes inappropriate.

Report Yes, report altered mental status to physician.

Nursing Interventions Obtain Mrs. Hagstrom's attention through touch. Facilitate use of hearing aids, as appropriate. Provide a consistent physical environment and a daily routine. Provide low-stimulation environment for Mrs. Hagstrom because disorientation may be increased by overstimulation. Provide caregiver who is familiar to Mrs. Hagstrom. Provide for adequate rest, sleep, and daytime naps.

Documentation [date] [time] 80-year-old female admitted 3 days ago to extended care facility, disoriented to person, place and time. States "I am afraid of all these strange creatures in this orphanage." Bilateral cataract removal status post × 2 weeks. C/o of increased difficulty with hearing. Reoriented to person, time, and place. Is able to identify primary nurse by name and expresses a desire to go home for Thanksgiving in 3 weeks. Asked that batteries be checked in her hearing aid. M. Smythe, LPN

CHAPTER 14

NCLEX-PN® ANSWERS 1. (2) Self-concept has four dimensions: self-knowledge: the knowledge that one has about oneself, including insights into one's abilities, nature, and limitations; self-expectation: what one expects of oneself; may be a realistic or unrealistic expectation; social self: how a person is perceived by others and society; and social evaluation: the appraisal of oneself in relationship to others, events, or situations. 2. (3) Psychosocial development theory was developed by Erikson. Sigmund Freud's theory was psychosexual development, Kohlberg was concerned with the theory of moral development, and Aaron Beck was concerned with cognitive theory. 3. (4) Self-concept is established when the inborn tendencies of the individual connect with reality and are brought into compliance with the demands of society. 4. (2) Although any of these diagnoses could be used for this medical diagnosis, *Disturbed Body Image* is evident when the individual does not recognize serious weight loss when viewing own body. 5. (4) Making eye contact and a gentle touch can convey caring and let the client know you are available to him or her. Lack of eye contact and a reluctance to touch a client may give the client the feeling of being unworthy. 6. (2) "I can't" statements reinforce negative self-concept. Worry or concerns about health or status changes are normal and demonstrate the client's efforts to cope with the change. 7. (3) Validating the client's feelings and offering to be there for the client is the best way to show empathy. The other choices discount feelings and offer false reassurance. 8. (1) Self-esteem can be assessed in terms of the goals a client can set for him- or herself. 9. (2) Therapeutic relationships should be client centered and aimed at assisting the client to evaluate his or her own behavior and initiate change. 10. (1, 3, 5) Choices 1, 3, and 5 are considered to be body image stressors. The others are related to self-concept, but not specifically body image.

CARE PLAN HINTS

1. Brian needs to feel that what is said will be kept confidential, and that the nurse will respond nonjudgmentally. Provide a private area for Brian to talk. Listening attentively, without interrupting. Be careful not to offer approval or disapproval. This subject may be uncomfortable for you; it is all right to let him know that you are somewhat uncomfortable, but express your desire to learn more about his feelings. If you are unable to get past your own feelings, help him to make contact with someone who is better suited to establish this relationship. Validate his feelings; state implied feelings and thought. This will let him know you are paying attention and that you care and are willing to help.

2. Brian is an adult, but apparently his family and their response to his feelings are very important to him. Explain to the father that you cannot discuss Brian's treatment plan with him, but that Brian wishes his family to be involved in decisions that he needs to make. Suggest that he take the opportunity to speak with the counselor by attending the session with Brian, but also let him know that he can make arrangements with the counselor to be seen privately if the need arises. Reassure him that the session is an opportunity to talk about concerns that both he and Brian may have in a nonthreatening atmosphere. Thank him for his concern and encourage him to be supportive of his son.

3. Decisions such as the ones Brian is considering are life altering. He needs to be provided with correct reliable information. Encourage him to seek additional opinions and to discuss his feelings with the counselor and other trusted professionals. The nurse needs to be supportive of whatever decision the client makes and let him know that no matter the outcome, he is still a very important, worthy individual and that you want the best for him. Be sure to provide him with crisis intervention resources, since decisions such as this can cause severe anxiety and even thoughts of suicide. Make sure he knows that life is always the best option.

CRITICAL THINKING CARE MAP

Subjective Data Mother very supportive. Father is grief stricken and having difficulty dealing with Craig's condition because Craig was captain of his college basketball team; shared aspirations of becoming a professional basketball player. Usually an outgoing individual.

Objective Data 20-year-old male student. Automobile accident 3 days ago. Mother at bedside. Traumatic amputation of his left lower leg. Condition is stable. Rehabilitation program to begin immediately. To be fitted for a leg prosthesis. Somber and untalkative. Does not look at his leg when dressings are being changed. Refuses to discuss rehabilitation.

Nursing Interventions Accept client's own pace in working through grief and crisis situation. Assess client's support system. Assess for unhealthy coping mechanisms such as substance abuse. Have client list strengths. Actively listen to, demonstrate respect for, and accept the client. Provide information about support groups.

Report Yes, report following to the primary physician or a mental health professional: Usually an outgoing individual, Craig is somber and unntalkative. He does not look at his leg when dressings are being changed and he refuses to discuss his rehabilitation program.

Documentation Sample Documentation Focus: Body image. D—Somber, untalkative, unwilling to look at surgical site or discuss rehab. program. A—Dressing changed approached in unthreatening manner. Procedure explained. Encouraged to ask questions. **R**—Was able to look at residual limb after redressed. Asked if swelling and pain is normal. S. Garcia, LVN

CHAPTER 15

NCLEX-PN® ANSWERS   1. (4) Alcohol is a relaxant and central nervous system depressant. Chronic alcoholism is associated with impotence. While alcohol may lower inhibitions and impair judgment, it is not a sexual stimulant. 2. (1) The position that offers the most pleasure and is acceptable to both partners is the correct one. 3. (2) During early adolescence primary and secondary sex characteristics develop for boys. This involves an increase in the size of the testes and scrotum and the darkening of the skin over the scrotum. 4. (3) All states have child abuse laws that require professionals, including nurses, to report suspected child abuse. 5. (3) In 1996 the U.S. Congress passed legislation making practicing any form of female genital mutilation, including closure of the vagina (infibulation), on girls under age 18 a federal criminal offense. 6. (1) Females are more at risk of cervical cancer if they have human papillomavirus or multiple sexual partners. 7. (2) Coitus interruptus should be taught as far less effective than the other methods listed. 8. (4) Gender determination can be made by the 11th to 14th week of gestation. 9. (3) Most cases of orgasmic dysfunction have psychological causes. 10. (2) The nurse will teach the client who has had heart surgery or been hospitalized for alterations in heart function to avoid sexual intercourse after large meals and/or consumption of alcoholic beverages.

CARE PLAN HINTS

1. Mr. Stevens was engaged in sexual intercourse when he experienced a myocardial infarction. This is likely to make him concerned about sexual activity. He may be making inappropriate sexual suggestions as a way of denying to himself that his sexual activity must change because of his condition. However, he also directly expresses his concern that his sexual relationship with his wife won't be the same. Mr. Stevens' remarks may be a way of asking for help.

2. It would have been helpful to know Mr. Stevens' activities prior to his MI (e.g., hours and activity at work) and prior to other episodes of chest pain. Family history of heart disease is also important.

3. Mrs. Stevens should be involved in all discussions about Mr. Stevens' health and condition. This is important both because of the way the condition affects his sexual activity and because the experience may be overwhelming for him. Having a second person there to listen will be useful. Contact with others who have recovered from MIs and with a counselor will also be beneficial.

CRITICAL THINKING CARE MAP

Subjective Data States she will never be the same. States husband deserves more.

Objective Data Looks down when speaking. Holds robe tightly around chest. Ate 10% of breakfast and lunch. Stayed in bed with face covered all morning. Refused to ambulate in the hall. Looked through mail brought to room by volunteer.

Report Yes, report client expressing grief reaction to the nurse in charge of the unit and physician.

Nursing Interventions Encourage client to express feelings about the way she feels about sexuality related to loss of the breast. Discuss the usual feelings of clients who are postoperative mastectomy and ways to cope. Discuss with client importance of Reach for Recovery follow-up. Instruct in the importance of communication with husband to work through feelings toward acceptance. Discuss available support groups in the community and obtain necessary contacts for follow-up (American Cancer Society). Encourage client to discuss sexuality issues with the primary healthcare provider.

Documentation [date] [time] States "I'll never be the same" and "My husband deserves more." Discussed with client why she stated "I'll never be the same." Client expressed concern over her appearance and working in the office. Questioned about Reach for Recovery Program contact and client states she does not need their assistance. Reported to charge nurse and physician. Discussed the purpose of Reach for Recovery and assistance provided. Agreed to call and schedule follow-up. Janie Miller, LVN

CHAPTER 16

NCLEX-PN® ANSWERS   1. (4) A mentally healthy individual is able to cope with life while working and forming relationships. The other responses are symptoms of an individual who is experiencing a mental illness or emotional imbalance. 2. (4) Denial is an unconscious refusal to accept situations as they are. 3. (1) The client has temporarily separated the painful situation from consciousness. 4. (1) Mild anxiety heightens the person's response; a higher level of anxiety decreases the person's ability to respond and cope. 5. (4) A client experiencing physical symptoms related to anxiety needs to have support from the nurse. Ignoring the anxiety or discounting it will not validate the importance of the client's feelings. The episode should be documented, but it is not necessary to immediately notify the physician. 6. (2) The nurse in order to prevent burnout must first recognize his or her stress. The other interventions will need to follow. 7. (3) Regardless of the cause, circumstances, or psychological interpretation of a demanding situation, the response is a pattern of physiological responses known as the general adaptation syndrome. 8. (1) Adolescents have rapid physical and sexual development; this coupled with identity and role confusion issues are major stressors during the adolescent period. 9. (3) The fight-or-flight response is a physiological response to the release of adrenaline, when an individual feels in personal danger. 10. (1) Compensation is a defense mechanism that allows an individual to make up for inadequacies in one area of life by substituting attributes or behaviors from another area.

CARE PLAN HINTS

1. Ms. Levitt's stressors may include the fact that she has sole responsibility for three children; lack of financial assistance from her husband; the demands being placed on her by her job, school, and community activities; the lack of emotional support systems; possible financial problems; weight gain; and not having adequate time for rest and leisure.
2. Mrs. Levitt seems to have predominantly physiological manifestations to stress—physical problems with no apparent cause.
3. None of the data support that Mrs. Levitt is angry; however, she may not be expressing anger. Any of her stressors could provoke anger on her behalf, and suppression of that anger could result in physical signs and symptoms.
4. Some of the changes that would serve as cues to positive adaptation include decreased or absence of symptoms produced by stress, lifestyle changes such as decreased activities, change in diet, balancing leisure with work, or taking time for herself.

CRITICAL THINKING CARE MAP

Subjective Data He says, "I'm scared about this. My dad died of a heart attack when he was forty-eight years old." Severe chest pain.

Objective Data Lungs clear. Pale; skin cool and diaphoretic. Nail bed pink. ECG—normal sinus rhythm. Alert and oriented to time, place, and person. VS: T 99.6, P 88, R 28, BP 140/82. Peripheral pulse strong and equal. Capillary refill less than 3 seconds. Appears restless. Questions everything that is going on. Hyperventilating.

Report Yes, to the physician.

Nursing Interventions Assess client's level of anxiety and physical reaction to anxiety. Validate observations by asking client, "Are you feeling anxious now? Allow and reinforce client's personal reaction to or expression of pain, discomfort or threat to well-being. Explain all activities, procedures and issues that involve the client; use nonmedical terms and calm, slow speech. Do this is advance of procedures when possible, and validate client's understanding. Explore coping skills previously used by the client to relieve anxiety; reinforce these skills and explore other outlets. Provide back rub to decrease anxiety.

Documentation Client presented at the ER c/o chest pain, Nitro sublingual given ×1, hyperventilating, other VS within normal limits. ECG—normal sinus rhythm. Stated, "My father died of a heart attack, and having chest pain really scares me." Demonstrated relaxation techniques. Explained the importance of stress control. E Keene, LPN

CHAPTER 17

NCLEX-PN® ANSWERS 1. (2) In mutual pretense, the family and health personnel know the prognosis but no one talks about it. With closed awareness, the client and the family are unaware of the impending death. In open awareness, the client and the people around know about the impending death and feel comfortable discussing it, even though it is difficult. 2. (1) When the client is in the denial stage there is a refusal to believe that the loss is happening. The client may be artificially cheerful to prolong denial. 3. (3) A notarized document that outlines the client's wishes should be followed. In some states the wishes of a domestic partner cannot overrule the wishes of the family. The ER physician's assessment determines the status of the client; once this has been determined, the notarized durable power of attorney will be the basis for the decisions. 4. (3) Expressing feelings to an understanding listener helps to facilitate the grieving process. Communication helps people deal openly with their emotions and feelings, which is healthier than suppressing them. Being sent home or changing assignment would not help promote grieving. Asking the CNA to perform postmortem care in the emotional state would show disregard for the trauma the individual may be experiencing. 5. (1) Dying clients tend to become isolated and deserted by the staff. The primary objective in this case should be to provide a physical presence to listen and support the client as death draws near. All other choices involve leaving the client alone to die. 6. (4) When the parents wish to see their stillborn baby, the baby can be cleaned and wrapped in a baby blanket. The mother and father of the baby should be allowed to see, touch, and hold their baby. Although some parents may not wish to view the baby, doing so allows them to close the cycle of birth and death and accept the fact that their baby is dead. 7. (3) Hospice is care usually in the home or specialized facility dedicated to the care of clients with terminal illnesses. It is designed to provide quality of life when quantity is not possible. It is not done as a cost-saving measure or because of special equipment. Although hospice nurses have special training, they do not have more or less skill than hospital nurses. 8. (2) A client on life support must have an absence of electric currents from the brain (measured by an electroencephalogram) for at least 24 hours. Clients continue to have respirations as long as the respirator is functioning. A court order is not necessary unless the client has left no instructions or there is a disagreement between family members. 9. (4) Dysfunctional grieving is characterized by physical and psychological reactions and thoughts of suicide. 10. (3) Children from 9 to 12 years old express an interest in the afterlife; 5-year-olds look at death as reversible or temporary; 5- to 9-year-olds believe that unrelated events can be responsible for the death; 12- to 18-year-olds view it in religious or philosophic terms.

CARE PLAN HINTS

1. Mrs. Smith should be encouraged to participate in her own care and make personal health decisions as long as she

is able to, in order to give her power over her life, care, and dying process.

2. Decreased appetite occurs for many reasons. First, she has tumor growth in her abdomen, giving a feeling of fullness. Second, toxins from liver involvement (which gives rise to his jaundice) and tumor growth may cause nausea and decreased appetite. Third, during the dying process, body systems are failing, activity decreasing, and nutritional needs are greatly diminished.

3. The long-acting morphine is designed to decrease pain over a long period of time, eliminating the need for frequent doses of pain medication. Because there are sometimes episodes of acute pain, known as breakthrough pain, short-acting morphine is often made available. Ideally, breakthrough pain medication should only be required two to three times a day.

CRITICAL THINKING CARE MAP

Subjective Data Easily fatigued. Reports poor appetite. States pain 9 on scale of 1 to 10.

Objective Data Short of breath. Skin color dusky. Drowsy. BP 90/40.

Report Yes; report shortness of breath, blood pressure, and pain level to charge nurse.

Nursing Interventions Auscultate breath sounds with RN. Administer pain medications as ordered around the clock. Administer oxygen as needed. Position client for comfort. Use therapeutic touch and encourage family communication. Observe family response to grieving and offer appropriate support. Set up for a bed bath. Moisten client's lips as needed. Encourage client to eat.

Documentation [date] [time] Breath sounds irregular on auscultation, nostrils flared, skin color dusky, oxygen administered per M.D. order. Positioned for comfort. Pain medication administered for breakthrough pain as ordered. Family members at the bedside encouraged to communicate with client once he has experienced some relief from pain. Roger Hadrick, LVN

UNIT III WRAP-UP

CULTURAL COMPETENCY

- In many cultures, it is common for the family to keep the diagnosis from a client with a serious diagnosis, such as cancer. It is thought that knowing the diagnosis may create a sense of hopelessness and hasten the death.
- Often, the dying client knows the truth but is reluctant to discuss it with the family. A sensitive nurse can be open to providing a therapeutic environment for the client so he or she can discuss concerns when the family is not around. The nurse can also make time to listen to family members' concerns out of earshot of the client.

CRITICAL THINKING With the current federal laws under the Health Insurance Portability and Accountability Act (HIPAA), information cannot be given to anyone other than the client without prior permission. The scenario described here would occur only if the client had signed a document saying that a designated family member would be the primary decision maker, or if the physician or other caregivers ignored HIPAA. Ethically, it is difficult not to give a dying person the opportunity to bring closure to his or her life. Most people value the chance to say goodbye and resolve unfinished business. Healthcare institutions and workers must develop a means for handling such situations in a legal and ethical manner.

COMPASSIONATE CARING If you suspect that the client is aware of the diagnosis, you can encourage him or her to make a journal or to record messages for the family on tape. You can listen while clients talk about their life, and encourage them to express to family any wishes they want carried out when death comes. If sufficient time is available, the nurse may be able to support the client so that he or she will be able to raise the subject with family and say goodbyes in person.

COMMUNITY CARE STRATEGIES Remember, the "experts" in caregiving learn every day from their clients. You don't need to have all the answers when you begin to practice. Good listening skills and a caring attitude will help you learn ways to give excellent nursing care.

CHAPTER 18

NCLEX-PN® ANSWERS 1. (2) Smooth endoplasmic reticulum serves as the site of lipid and cholesterol synthesis. 2. (2) Homeostasis is a state of balance within the body. 3. (4) The cavity of the front of the body is the ventral cavity, which consists of the thoracic and abdominopelvic subdivisions. 4. (1) The respiratory system, which consists of the lungs and associated passages, is responsible for the transport of oxygen into and carbon dioxide out of the body. 5. (4) Mitosis, a form of cell division, occurs in this order: prophase, metaphase, anaphase, and telophase. 6. (2) The sagittal plane cuts the body in two from front to back, separating it into right and left portions. 7. (1) A ligament consists of fibrous connective tissue in which the fibers are all arranged in the same direction and connects bones to other bones. 8. (3) When cells are arranged in two or more layers, the term used to describe them is *stratified.* 9. (2) Endocrine glands do not have ducts and their secretions, known as hormones, are transported away from the gland by blood flowing through the gland. 10. (3) Ribosomes, which are the site of protein synthesis, are often found on the surface of the endoplasmic reticulum.

CHAPTER 19

NCLEX-PN® ANSWERS 1. (2) Clients with eating disorders frequently have dental caries and skin excoriation on hands, which result from contact with gastrointestinal acid from forced vomiting. **2.** (2) All assessments are designed to focus on the client's complaints. Nursing diagnoses are developed in response to problems identified in the assessment phase. Physician and nursing orders are carried out during the implementation stage of the nursing process. **3.** (3) McBurney's pain is in the LRQ, and where area is depressed and released the client will experience pain with appendicitis. **4.** (2) Tonsils will be visibly inflamed when client has tonsillitis. Inflammation is seen when the tongue is depressed and the area visualized using a direct light source. **5.** (3) Assessment of perfusion, capillary refill, vital signs, and pulses are performed when a cast application has been completed. DVTs are assessed with Homans' sign. Hip fracture in traction and TKR with CPM is assessed with circulation, movement, and sensation. **6.** (2) A reading of 100/60 is considered to be normal and should be charted. **7.** (2) Gurgles are continuous, low-pitched, coarse, gurgling, harsh, loud sounds with a moaning or snoring quality. Best heard on expiration but can be heard on both inspiration and expiration. May be altered by coughing. *Crackles (rales)* are fine, short, interrupted crackling sounds; alveolar rales are high pitched. Sound can be simulated by rolling a lock of hair near the ear. Best heard on inspiration but can be heard on both inspiration and expiration. May not be cleared by coughing. *Friction rub* is superficial grating or creaking sounds heard during inspiration and expiration. Not relieved by coughing. *Wheezes* are continuous, high-pitched, squeaky musical sounds. Best heard on expiration. Not usually altered by coughing. **8.** (1) It appears that the client may have scabies. The nurse should complete the assessment wearing gloves because scabies can be spread by direct skin-to-skin contact. **9.** (4) The phenomenon of skin retaining a pinch's shape and returning slowly to normal shape is described as *tenting;* this is seen in dehydration. Normal skin turgor is soft and elastic and normal skin returns to shape quickly. Loose skin has lost it elasticity from aging or significant weight loss. Tight skin results from edema. **10.** (2) Moods, affect, judgment, abilities, and lifestyle are part of a psychosocial assessment. A history and physical records previous and present health issues, a focused assessment concentrates on body systems, and a family health history records pertinent family health problems that have a bearing on the client.

CARE PLAN HINTS

1. Ms. Franklin's blood pressure was low and her pulse elevated due to blood loss. As her blood pressure dropped, her pulse increased to compensate and force more blood to the vital organs.
2. Because Ms. Franklin's blood pressure was low, the blood was reaching her head slowly, resulting in dizziness.
3. *Risk for Interrupted Family Processes* is an appropriate diagnosis because it is possible that breastfeeding would be interrupted due to Ms. Franklin's intolerance to activity and the possibility that she would need to be off the postpartum floor for a procedure to control the bleeding.

CRITICAL THINKING CARE MAP

Subjective Data Family not present, uninvolved in care of client. Client unmotivated to get better. Complains of dizziness on standing.

Objective Data Blood pressure 128/80—110/72—90/50, lying/sitting/standing. Pitcher of water is on the left side of the bed and is full. Saline lock in place and patent. Complains of loss of appetite over the past week. Crackles noted in lower lobes of lungs, bilaterally. Nonproductive cough. Pulse 89. Temp 99.0°F. Respiratory rate at rest 18 and shallow; 26 and shallow on exertion. Skin is pale and client is diaphoretic.

Report Yes, report the change in blood pressure, complaint of dizziness, and crackles noted in lower lobes of lungs, bilaterally, to team leader

Nursing Interventions Place water pitcher on client's right side, within reach. Instruct client to sit up in bed for a few minutes before standing. Put a bed alarm in place according to agency policy. Check physician's orders for IV fluid administration and discuss with RN. Encourage client to increase clear fluid intake. Instruct client to call for assistance before ambulating. Use a walking belt when ambulating client. When mobilizing client monitor for orthostatic hypotension accompanied by dizziness and/or fainting. Encourage client to change positions slowly. Slow pace of care, allowing client extra time to carry out activities.

Documentation [date] [time] Complains of dizziness on standing, blood pressure 128/80—110/72—90/50, lying/sitting/standing, skin dry and flaky, oral mucosa dry. Crackles noted in lower lobes of lungs, bilaterally. Blood oxygen level 98%, nonproductive cough noted. Encouraged increased fluid intake. Bed alarm placed on bed. Instructed client to call for assistance before ambulating. K. Hirota, LVN

CHAPTER 20

NCLEX-PN® ANSWERS **1.** (3) A temperature of 101.8 (A) is considered to be one degree lower than an oral temp. A temperature of 102.8 would warrant immediate reporting. A blood pressure above 140 should be compared to the patient's last reading. A pulse of 100 or above should be reassessed after the patient has rested. **2.** (2) Blood pressure should not be taken on the arm on the side of a mastectomy. It also should not be taken on an arm that has sustained and injury. It is best to obtain a larger cuff and take the pressure on the thigh. **3.** (1) A cuff with a bladder that is too narrow will provide an erroneously high blood pressure reading. **4.** (2) Phase 5 of the Korotkoff's sounds is considered to be the adult diastolic pressure, which is followed by a period of silence. **5.** (4) When converting Celsius temperature to Fahrenheit, 38.6 converts to 101.48; 101.5 is the closest. **6.** (4) Pulse for children under 3 years of age is more frequently assessed apically. **7.** (1) Normal systolic blood pressure for a child is 80 + 2 × the child's age. 8. (1) Orthostatic hypotension will be evident when blood pressure drops as the patient's position changes. 9. (3) Prior to administration of digoxin, the apical pulse must be assessed. The medication is held if the apical pulse is less than 60 or more than 100. 10. (3) Morphine sulfate depresses respirations, so they need to be assessed for 30 seconds following administration.

CARE PLAN HINTS

1. It is important to perform activities of daily living as independently as possible. Perform activities at a comfortable pace, and take a rest break as soon as you get tired. Plan to walk twice daily at a comfortable pace, increasing the distance weekly until you are able to walk 1 to 2 miles without shortness of breath. You should be able to do 2 miles in 40 minutes, within 6 weeks. After distance is reached, decrease time to 30 minutes, with no dyspnea.

2. Caution Mrs. Munson to discuss the herbal medicine with her physician. "Mrs. Munson, even though the herbs you are taking are natural, they can cause interaction with food and other medication. Notify your physician if any side effects occur. You should have your blood pressure monitored 1 time each week. Report any abnormal readings to your physician. (An abnormal BP would be 30 mm Hg above or below your baseline.) Continue to adhere to your diet and report any headaches or visual disturbance to the physician immediately."

3. These are warning signs of stroke. If the client experiences one or more of the following, she should go to an emergency room to be evaluated: (a) sudden numbness or weakness of the face, arm, or leg, especially on one side of the body; (b) sudden confusion or trouble speaking or understanding; (c) sudden trouble seeing in one or both eyes; (d) sudden trouble walking, dizziness, or loss of balance or coordination; or (e) sudden severe headache with no known cause.

CRITICAL THINKING CARE MAP

Subjective Data Chest pain, radiating to back and down arm 9/10. Pain 5/10 following medication. "I probably won't live to an old age. I have bad genes for heart attack and stroke." Mother stroke at 60. Father died at age 56 of a heart attack. "I normally eat fast food for lunch. My wife does make healthy dinners." Lives with wife; one son nearby. Employed as history teacher at local college. Head injury 1 week ago in motor vehicle crash (MVC).

Objective Data African American male. VS: T 99.8, P 100, R 24, BP 158/90. Height 5'10", weight 295 lbs. Sinus tachycardia with occasional PVC.

Report Yes, report head injury 1 week ago MVC to physician.

Nursing Interventions Assess client's feelings, values, and reasons for not following prescribed plan of care. Discuss client's

beliefs about health and his ability to maintain health. Identify barriers and benefits to being healthy. Encourage client to eat a diet with fresh foods, low saturated fat, and no added salt. Compare client's height and weight to standards for age and height. Assess for the influences of cultural beliefs, norms, and values on the client's beliefs about health.

Documentation

Focus		
Health-Seeking Behavior	1120	D Family hx of CVA and MI. Pt. being treated for hypertension, Verapamil 180 mg bid. VS 99.8/ 100/24 158/90. Pt. describes diet as fast food regularly for lunch, healthy dinners.
		A Provided information on cardiac diet to enhance treatment of hypertension. Discussed food likes and dislikes.
		R Pt able to explain benefits of appropriate diet and choose daily menu that meets the prescribed criteria. K. Turner, LVN

D = Data; A = Action; R = Results.

CHAPTER 21

NCLEX-PN® ANSWERS 1. (3) The client is the best source of information about the pain being experienced. Choices 1 and 2 place the responsibility for control on the healthcare professional; participation in the plan by the client will result in a more satisfying experience; choice 4 discounts the client's input and understanding. 2. (2) Using a numerical pain rating scale is the most effective way of assessing the severity of the pain. Choice 1 is a closed-ended question, which rarely provides good data for the assessment. Choices 3 and 4 are vague and subjective. 3. (4) Acute pain lasts only through the expected recovery period, whether its onset is sudden or slow and regardless of the intensity. Chronic pain lasts beyond the typical healing time period. Chronic pain that persists despite therapeutic interventions is classified as intractable. Referred pain is pain felt in a part of the body that is considerably removed from the tissues causing the pain. 4. (1) Constipation is a side effect and occurs frequently with opioids. Rashes and anaphylaxis are symptoms of an allergic reaction. Respiratory depression can occur with opioids and can be a life-threatening reaction. 5. (3) Many clients have had good response to anticonvulsants when dealing with nerve pain. NSAIDs work well for muscle pain and inflammation. Nonopioids are effective for mild pain; opioids are more appropriate for severe pain (7–10 on a rating scale). 6. (2) Time of onset, duration, and recurrence or intervals without pain are referring to the pain pattern. Intensity and severity are rated with a pain scale; duration refers to how long the pain episode lasts. 7. (3) Duragesic, an opioid analgesic, comes in the form of a patch that is placed on the skin (transdermal). Patient-controlled analgesia is IV pain control that is accessed by a push button available to the client. It has a lockout mechanism to prevent overdose. Intravenous analgesia is usually given IV push by the RN. Intraspinal analgesia is delivered via catheter into the subarachnoid or epidural space. 8. (4) Level 4 of sedation is characterized by minimal or no response to stimuli. Level 1 is easily arousable; level 2 is awake and alert; and level 3 is frequently drowsy, arousable, and drifts off to sleep during conversation. 9. (2) Tissue ischemia is a chemical type of pain stimuli. Tumors and trauma to body tissues (e.g., surgery) and blockage of a body duct are mechanical stimuli. 10. (3, 7, 2, 9, 1, 4, 6, 9, 5, and 8) When the client request medication perform a pain assessment and then check the physician's order and establish the time of the last injection in order to establish what can be given and when. Wash hands and prepare the medication, don gloves and administer the medication to the client, wash hands again and document on the MAR or Chart. Reassess the client in 30 minutes.

CARE PLAN HINTS

1. Subjective data (rating pain as 5) and objective data (vital signs, position, holding abdomen, lying in rigid position) are present to support that Mrs. Lundahl is experiencing pain; however, no conclusions can be drawn about the intensity, location, quality, or pattern of her pain.

2. It would be incorrect to assume that Mrs. Lundahl needs no interventions for her pain. People rate their pain differently based on their past pain experiences, their pain tolerance, and their ethnic/cultural values. Mrs. Lundahl should be asked if she needs pain intervention.

3. Mrs. Lundahl is most likely experiencing acute pain from her surgery. Depending on the amount of manipulation of bowel, blood vessels, and so on within her abdomen. She may also be experiencing visceral pain.

4. Numerous interventions, in addition to pain medication, may be helpful, such as changing her position, a back massage, use of a cutaneous stimulator, and distraction (e.g., soft music).

5. The most reliable method of determining that Mrs. Lundahl's pain has been relieved is for her to tell you that her pain has been relieved. Objective data may include decreased blood pressure and respirations when compared to preintervention values; Mrs. Lundahl resting quietly or sleeping; pink color, absence of perspiration; and relaxed facial expression.

CRITICAL THINKING CARE MAP

Subjective Data C/o of pain (7 on a scale of 1–10). "I am cold and tired, I wish I could sleep." C/o being thirsty. C/o nausea but no vomiting.

Objective Data Height: 188 cm (6'3"). Weight: 90.0 kg (200 lbs). Temperature: 37°C (98.6°F). Lying in dorsal recumbent position with legs drawn up. Pulse: 90 bpm. Respirations: 24/minute.

Blood pressure: 158/82 mm Hg. Skin pale and moist, pupils dilated. NPO, intravenous infusion of D_5 1/2 NS at 125 mL/h left arm, nasogastric tube to low intermittent suction. Restless. Midline abdominal incision, sutures dry and intact. Chest x-ray and urinalysis negative. WBC 12,000.

Report No.

Nursing Interventions Instruct client to request prn pain medication before the pain is severe. Medicate before an activity to increase participation. Determine analgesic selections (narcotic, non-narcotic, or NSAID) based on type and severity of pain. Institute safety precautions as appropriate if receiving narcotic analgesics. Evaluate the effectiveness of the pain control measures used through ongoing assessment. Create a quiet, nondisruptive environment with dim lights and comfortable temperature when possible.

Documentation [date] [time] Client restless; lying in bed with legs drawn up. C/O pain 7/10 in abdomen. Abdomen distended, NG to low intermittent suction. c/o thirst and nausea. NG irrigated with 30 cc NSS. Reconnected to low suction, 300 CC of brown fluid drained. Demerol 75 mg IM given. G. Nugent, LVN

[date] [time] Abdomen soft, reports pain decreased to 2/10. no c/o of nausea. NG draining. Resting comfortably. Asked "Please turn off the TV and pull the curtain. I think I can take a nap now." G. Nugent, LVN

CHAPTER 22

NCLEX-PN® ANSWERS 1. (3) Early A.M. care includes washing the face and hands and giving oral care or assisting the client in doing these hygiene tasks. It also includes offering the urinal or bedpan if the client is on bed rest. 2. (1) It is best to follow the client's preferences as long as they are compatible with client's health and equipment. This action on the part of the nurse provides the client with a sense of participation and control and helps the client's self-esteem. Also, having a familiar routine is comforting to the client. 3. (1) Loose bed linen and wrinkles can cause irritation and possible skin breakdown. Massaging with alcohol will dry the skin further. It is not recommended that feet be rubbed briskly. Top sheets should be tucked in loosely or with toe pleat in order to keep feet in proper alignment and to prevent pressure in feet. 4. (3) The nursing staff and others caring for elderly clients need to offer water throughout the day as well hydrated skin is less prone to injury and breakdown. 5. (2) Position the unconscious client in a side-lying position, with the head of the bed lowered. In this position, the saliva automatically runs out by gravity rather than being aspirated into the lungs. This position is the one of choice for the unconscious client receiving mouth care. If the client's head cannot be lowered, turn it to one side. The fluid will readily run out of the mouth or pool in the side of the mouth, where it can be suctioned. 6. (4) Sebum is an oily substance secreted by the skin that not only lubricates the skin, but also prevents heat loss, kills bacteria, produces and absorbs vitamin D, and has other beneficial qualities. 7. (3) When the client is not going to be using the hearing aid for several days, the batteries need to be removed. 8. (2) Students with tinea pedis can spread it by going barefoot in the shower room and students can get it by going barefoot in the shower room where others with the fungus have walked barefoot. 9. (2) The nurse needs to use a different cotton ball for each wipe. The nurse needs to use normal saline not tap water and wipe from inner to outer canthus. The eye shield is used if the corneal reflex is absent and the doctor gives an order for it. 10. (2) It is important to hold dirty linens away from your uniform, and it is important not to shake the linens as that could spread harmful microorganisms.

CARE PLAN HINTS

1. Mr. Bucholz stated that no one "ever told me I shouldn't cut my nails." Although he may have been told this when he was first diagnosed with diabetes he may have been overwhelmed with all the information that comes with a new diagnosis. Giving a client an easy to follow pamphlet regarding important subjects such as foot care may help reinforce the instructions given.
2. Getting into the habit of having a podiatrist cut his nails may help deter Mr. Bucholz from attempting to cut them at home.
3. If peripheral circulation is not improved and extremities are not protected from injury, the client will be at risk for amputation. Amputation is a frequent and serious consequence of inadequate peripheral circulation in the client with diabetes mellitus.

CRITICAL THINKING CARE MAP

Subjective Data States, "I can't remember when I last saw a dentist."

Objective Data VS: T 99.2, P 78, R 20, BP 134/82. Pulse ox 98% on room air. Teeth stained from heavy smoking. One large cavity evident in second lower left molar. Tartar buildup along gum margins. Pronounced halitosis. Gums are reddened in some areas and bleed when flossed.

Report Yes, evidence of gum disease to admitting physician.

Nursing Interventions Inspect oral cavity at least once daily and note any discoloration, lesions, edema, bleeding, exudate or dryness. Use foam sticks to moisten the oral mucous membrane, clean out debris and swab while client is NPO. Use tap water or normal saline to provide oral care; do not use commercial mouthwash containing alcohol or hydrogen peroxide. Keep lips well lubricated using petroleum jelly or a similar product. Determine client's usual method of oral care and address any concerns related to oral care. Identify reasons client has not seen a dentist.

Documentation [date] [time] Focus: Oral mucosa. D—Teeth stained. Gums are reddened in some areas and bleed when flossed. One large cavity evident in second lower left molar. Tartar buildup along gum margins. Pronounced halitosis. A— Oral care provided with foam stick. Rinsed, cautioned not to swallow due to NPO status. Flossed. Petroleum jelly applied to lips. R—no evidence of bleeding from flossing. Mucosa dry; no exudates. Maureen Stiefle, LPN

CHAPTER 23

NCLEX-PN® ANSWERS 1. (2) The first intervention would be to change position as a preventive measure. Every 2 hours is the standard recommendation for repositioning an immobile client. An airflow mattress and protective pads are preventive measures but not the nurse's immediate response. 2. (4) When the dry dressing is removed, it eliminates necrotic debris, which has been softened by the dressing solution. Cooling is an effect of a wet dressing. The purpose of this type of dressing is to debride. Antipruritic medication stops itching. A nevus is a mole. 3. (1) The open wound becomes a portal for microorganisms to enter the body. An open wound is susceptible to infection and can become contaminated at the time of injury or as healing progresses. Vitamin D synthesis, lubrication, and excretion are functions of the integumentary system. 4. (4) Stage IV includes full-thickness skin loss with necrosis and/or damage to muscle, bone, or other supporting structures. Sinus tracts can also be associated with the stage IV ulcer and are not always easily identified. 5. (1) Maceration is a softening of the skin, which can lead to further skin breakdown. Frequent dressing changes occur with wet dressings. Debridement is the desired outcome of a wet-to-dry dressing. Ischemia is decreased blood flow to the area. 6. (1) The second phase of healing includes granulation tissue. Capillaries grow across the wound bringing oxygen and nutrients. The tissue is a translucent red color and bleeds easily. Phagocytosis is a process to ingest and digest bacteria and cellular debris. Necrosis is blackened dead tissue. Exudate is drainage of fluid and cells from a wound. 7. (4) Shearing force is caused by skin that is not moving in relationship to a downward-sliding body movement in bed. Evisceration describes the protrusion of the internal viscera through an incision. Hematoma is a localized collection of blood underneath the skin that appears as a reddish-blue swelling. Reactive hyperemia occurs once pressure has been relieved, the area is flooded with extra blood to compensate for the blood flow that was impeded. 8. (3) Hand washing is healthcare personnel's primary defense against nosocomial infections. Incisions open to air promote healing. Surgical and clean techniques are utilized in dressing changes. Incisions are cleaned from clean to contaminated areas. 9. (1) Diabetes is a systemic disease and affects organs and blood vessels of the body. Peripheral vascular disease decreases the blood flow and contributes to the formation of ulcers. 10. (2) Alcohol has a drying effect on the skin and evaporates rapidly. Maceration softens the skin. Suppuration is pus formation.

CARE PLAN HINTS

1. It is important to reinforce diabetes teaching to encourage regimen compliance. Diabetes is a systemic disease and is difficult to control under normal conditions. When the body is compromised with an open wound, the blood sugars rise, causing vascular changes and slowing healing. Diabetes hastens atherosclerotic changes in (hardening and closing of) blood vessels and decreases blood flow. When monitoring blood sugars, it is important to have Mrs. Lee keep a record of her glucose levels. She becomes an active participant in her care and records her blood sugar progress. Remind her of the healing process and the role that blood flow plays in healing.

2. Stage III involves a full-thickness skin loss involving damage or necrosis of subcutaneous tissue that may extend down to, but not through, underlying fascia. The ulcer presents as a deep crater with or without undermining of adjacent tissue. The stage IV ulcer is also full-thickness skin loss with extensive destruction, tissue necrosis, or damage to muscle, bone, or supporting structures. Undermining and sinus tracts are associated with this stage. Treatment for necrosis can involve enzymatic medications to break down the dead tissue for easier removal. Necrosis needs to be removed because it contains bacteria and must be eliminated to allow healing to take place. Use of a wet-to-dry dressing with a cleansing solution allows for mechanical debridement. Wound packing strategies vary. With a stage III ulcer, the whole wound is visible. In a stage IV ulcer, the wound may have sinus tracts, which, if allowed to heal over, can develop pockets of infection and prolong the healing process. Grafting can be another method of treatment.

3. Nutritional needs increase with a pressure ulcer. Protein, vitamin C, and multivitamins assist in healing by enhancing tissue repair and normal growth. The wound stage is correlated with the severity of nutritional deficits. Ensure that teeth are in good condition and dentures fit correctly.

CRITICAL THINKING CARE MAP

Subjective Data Difficulty ambulating. Client states, "I'm not hungry most of the time." General malaise. Decreased sensation to his entire right side.

Objective Data Height: 6 ft. Weight: 135 lbs. Incontinent of urine. Deeply reddened coccyx, right hip, and peritoneal area. Right-sided weakness.

Report Yes, report the reddened coccyx, rt. hip, and peritoneal area to both the charge nurse and physician.

Nursing Interventions Turn client every 2 hours. Steadily increase ambulation. Monitor reddened area. Offer urinal frequently.

Documentation [date] [time] Client has reddened coccyx (2 × 2), rt. hip (2 × 3), and peritoneal area, no open areas noted, physician notified. Client turned every 2 h and ambulated 6 feet to the restroom. Urinal offered at frequent intervals, incontinent × 1 this shift. Will continue to monitor reddened areas and offer urinal. D. Stormer, LVN

CHAPTER 24

NCLEX-PN® ANSWERS 1. (4) High-Fowler's position (~90 degrees) allows gravity to aid in lowering the diaphragm, allowing greater chest expansion. Choice 1: Trendelenburg is a head-down, feet-up position. Abdominal contents would be pushed up on the diaphragm resulting in *less* chest expansion. Choice 2: In low-Fowler's position, the head of the bed is only elevated ~30 degrees. The gravitational pull is significantly less than in the high-Fowler's position. Choice 3: Sims' position is a side-lying position and, as a result, restricts the movement of the chest on the dependent side. 2. (1) Kussmaul's is the pattern described in this question. Choice 2: Tachypnea refers solely to respiratory rate; specifically a faster than normal rate. Choice 3: dyspnea refers to difficulty breathing. Choice 4: Eupnea is normal breathing: regular, quiet, effortless. 3. (4) All three of these assessments are essential elements of a respiratory assessment. Restlessness can be an early sign of hypoxia (lack of oxygen to the brain). Choice 1: None of these data are a priority, with the possible exception of pain. Pupil size is more a neurologic concern; sneezing is not a priority complaint. Choice 2: BP and sweating would be more significant for a patient with a cardiac diagnosis. Choice 3: Capillary refill is more directly related to perfusion. Trembling is irrelevant. The amount of sputum is important, but not the *most* important. 4. (2) An open airway with adequate gas exchange takes the highest priority (airway and breathing always take priority; then circulation). Choice 1: Reducing anxiety is a desired goal but should not receive the highest priority. Choice 3: Talking about feelings is an important goal, but is superseded by the need for a patent airway. Choice 4: Maintaining fluid balance is important, but not the most essential element to sustain life. 5. (4) Orthopnea is a respiratory condition in which the client complains of difficulty breathing in any position except sitting or standing. It is seen in heart failure, pulmonary edema, and severe emphysema. The client may be in respiratory distress, be acidotic, and have periods of apnea as well, but the question asked for a definition of orthopnea. Choice 1: This is not the definition of orthopnea; it more closely defines dyspnea. Choice 2: Not a definition of orthopnea. Choice 3: Not a definition of orthopnea. 6. (3) A tracheostomy tube is inserted into the trachea to create an artificial airway. Choice 1: A tracheostomy tube cannot be used for nutrition; it is inserted in the airway, not the esophagus. Choice 2: A tube to remove flatus would be inserted in the rectum. Choice 4: A tracheostomy tube decreases dead space. 7. (1) The ABC's (*a*irway, *b*reathing, *c*irculation) are always the first priority. Rapid, irregular respirations of 32/min require immediate intervention. Choice 2: Skin that is warm, flushed, and dry does not take priority over increased respirations. Choice 3: This is a slight temperature elevation and is not a priority. Choice 4: A dry, nonproductive cough is not a priority. 8. (4) *Dyspnea* means difficult breathing or difficulty breathing (taken from the Latin *dys* for "difficult" and *pnea* for "breath"). Choice 1: Shallow respirations do not necessarily mean that the patient's gas exchange is compromised. Choice 2: Rapid breathing is called tachypnea and could be a physiological compensatory mechanism. Choice 3: This is a definition of orthopnea. 9. (2) Oxygen is a highly combustible gas that can easily ignite on contact with a spark. Posting "No Smoking" signs promotes client safety. Choice 1: All rooms should be well ventilated, regardless of oxygen use. Choice 3: One liter difference in flow rate does not increase combustibility of oxygen. Choice 4: Skin lotions do not interfere with oxygen administration, nor do they pose a danger. 10. (2) Hypoxia is a diminished oxygen supply to the cells of the body resulting in the symptoms listed. The respiratory control center is located in the brain, therefore judgment can also be impaired. Choice 1: Hypertension is a *late* sign of hypoxia. Choice 3: Cyanosis is a *late* sign of hypoxia. Choice 4: Crowing respirations are characteristic of an obstructed airway.

CARE PLAN HINTS

1. Mr. Markert is at risk for respiratory complications related to his chest trauma. The pulse can detect changes in oxygen status such as hyperemia, before clinical manifestations develop. If complications are noted early in their development, actions can be taken to stop progression of the problem.

2. Important nursing care involves frequent monitoring of Mr. Markert's respiratory and cardiac status and his oxygen saturations; monitoring the patency of his drainage system; maintaining the integrity of his water-seal drainage; never raising the drainage system above his chest; implementing emergency measures should an air leak develop; and providing Mr. Markert with information and reassurance.

3. Mr. Markert would benefit from sitting or lying in a position that enhances respiration, engaging in deep breathing exercises, ambulating or exercising, and maintaining adequate fluid intake.

CRITICAL THINKING CARE MAP

Subjective Data Fatigue. Bad cold for several weeks that just wouldn't go away. Dieting for several months and skipping meals. Works full time and is attending college. Smoked one pack of cigarettes per day since 18 years of age.

Objective Data Height: 66″. Weight: 120 lbs. VS: T 103, P 82, R 24, BP 118/70. Skin pale; cheeks flushed; chills; nasal flaring; use of accessory muscles; inspiratory crackles with diminished breath sounds right base; thick, yellow sputum. Chest x-ray: right lobar infiltration. WBC 14,000. pH 7.48. HCO_3: 20 mEq/L. $PaCO_2$: 80 mm Hg.

Report Yes, diminished breath sounds, fever, productive cough to the physician.

Nursing Interventions Encourage her to take a deep breath, hold for 2 seconds, and cough two or three times in succession.

Encourage use of incentive spirometry, as appropriate. Monitor rate, rhythm, depth, and effort of respirations. Auscultate breath sounds, noting area of decreased or absent ventilations and presence of adventitious sounds. Monitor respiratory secretions. Monitor increased restlessness, anxiety, and air hunger.

Documentation [date] [time] Focus: Cough. **D**—Yellow thick sputum, expectorated following C/DB and respiratory treatment. C/o of discomfort right chest. Pale; lips cyanotic; diaphoretic. **A**—Breath sounds assessed; assisted to high-Fowler's position; cough preparation administered per physician's order. **R**—Color improved, lips pink, sitting up in bed. Stated "My chest doesn't hurt as much now." W. Poole, LPN

CHAPTER 25

NCLEX-PN® ANSWERS 1. (1) The protein in a diet provides amino acids, the structural material for building body tissues. Although protein intake is related to fat intake, this answer does not satisfy the question being asked. Calories are primarily gained from consumption of carbohydrates, not proteins. Calcium may be present in protein, but supplements are often given to those at risk for decreased bone density. 2. (3) When clients believe that they can make a difference in the outcome of their health, they are more likely to succeed at making dietary changes. Relying on others, looking for approval, or lacking belief that dietary changes can influence health outcome all suggest less likelihood of success. 3. (less than 4) The pH of gastric fluid is normally 6 or lower. 4. (2) Cream sauces tend to be high in fat, which would increase LDL cholesterol. It is not necessary to shop in specialty stores. The substitutes in choice 4 contain salt and may promote hypertension. 5. (3) A person who is 20% over IBW is obese and remains at risk even though he or she may be physically active. 6. (2) No feeding is to be started until placement is clearly and positively identified. There is no prioritized need to weigh the client before restarting tube feeding. Do not give the client trials of eating food without evidence of safety in swallowing, including swallow studies and physician orders; feeding food without first checking for ability to swallow could lead to aspiration. 7. (1) Insulation is a function of fats. Protein provides building blocks for body repair. Although carbohydrates may supply fiber, their primary function is to provide energy for the body. 8. (2) The milkshake, apricot nectar, and creamed soups are not transparent. 9. (3) Choice 1: The smaller blue part is for air exchange. Giving medications through it may cause inadequate functioning of the tube. Choice 2 would be unsafe and unacceptable nursing practice; do not give the client medications orally unless a physician's order precisely directs you to do this. Choice 4: Medications must continue to be given even in the presence of a NG tube. 10. (1,3,4)

CARE PLAN HINTS

1. The nurse would attempt to encourage the client to consume a greater part of the diet provided. If the nurse can

establish a trusting relationship, it may be possible to identify some foods that would be preferred, and to discuss the client's self-perception of being overweight. Although other means would be attempted first, it may be necessary to provide parenteral nutrition to the client to maintain or restore electrolyte balance.

2. Anorexia is a psychological disorder. A trained psychologist might be able to help the client understand what caused the feelings of being overweight to occur, and what other feelings might be standing in the way of a healthier self-image.

3. *Disturbed Body Image* is appropriate because the client feels huge, ugly, and overweight when she is in fact in danger of starving to dearth. At this point, she is not capable of seeing her real image clearly.

CRITICAL THINKING CARE MAP

Subjective Data Complaint of being thirsty. Client states "My chest hurts when I breathe."

Objective Data Height: 150 cm (4'11"). Weight: 39.55 kg (87 lbs). Temperature: 39°C (102.6°F). Pulse: 86 bpm. Respirations: 30/min, labored. Blood pressure: 130/82 mm Hg. Skin pale and moist. NPO, nasogastric tube 150 mL/h Glucerna. Blood glucose 236 7 A.M. Foley catheter in place draining dark amber urine. Chest x-ray and urinalysis done—results pending. WBC 28,000.

Report Yes, temperature, labored breathing to physician.

Nursing Interventions Check tube placement and residual each shift and prn. Hold tube feeding for residual <150 mL. VS every 4 h. Tylenol gr. × for temp < 101.6. Cooling measures for temp < 102. Blood glucose monitoring a.c. and h.s. Insulin per sliding scale. Flush tube with 100 mL water following medication administration. Encourage coughing and deep breathing. Elevate head of bed 30°.

Documentation [date] [time] Temp 102.6. NG tube in place, residual 90 mL Tylenol gr × liquid via NG tube flushed with 100 mL water. Glucerna 150 mL/h via pump. K. Scranton, LPN

CHAPTER 26

NCLEX-PN® ANSWERS 1. (**respiratory alkalosis**) When a client breathes rapidly, CO_2 (an acid) is blown off, causing a decrease in $PaCO_2$ and elevated pH. This occurs when pain, anxiety, or fever causes hyperventilation. 2. (1) Insensible losses occur through the skin in the form of perspiration and diffusion and from the lungs in exhaled air. 3. (2) To calculate the answer, you add the urine output and the amount of emesis to gain an accurate result. 4. (2) The most common type of a hypotonic solution is 0.45% sodium chloride (1/2 NS), a solution that has an osmolarity that is lower than blood serum. 5. (3) Redness and swelling could be a sign of phlebitis. Depending on the grade, the treatment will be different so the LVN should confer with the RN to determine intervention and if the physician needs to be notified. 6. (2) Fluid intake includes oral intake that is liquid at room temperature; pureed foods do not meet this criteria. 7. (4) Isotonic fluids have the same concentration as blood serum and other body fluids. They expand the intravascular compartments of the body without causing a shift in fluids. 8. (1) When fatty acids change to ketone bodies, diabetes mellitus metabolic acidosis may occur. 9. (2) Potassium helps maintain ECF and ICF water balance and acid–base balance and is vital for skeletal, cardiac, and smooth muscle activity. A deficiency can affect cardiac function. 10. (1) Sodium is the most abundant cation, and its function is to control and regulate water balance.

CARE PLAN HINTS

1. Sodium levels may appear normal due to increased water retention, which dilutes the blood.

2. Uremia is the usual cause of disorientation and confusion in clients with renal failure, although it is important to rule out any other possible causes. It also is important to establish if confusion or disorientation was present prior to the allergic reaction to the contrast dye for the IVP.

3. It would be important to establish what the client has been told about dialysis by the physician. Explain that dialysis is ordered when medical management of renal failure is insufficient. Dialysis is a process for eliminating toxins and retained fluid from the body, when the kidneys are unable to do this. Dialysis must be done on a regular basis, from daily to three times per week depending on the buildup of toxins. Dialysis will need to be continued as long as the kidneys are unable to eliminate waste products. When medical treatment is not effective, the destruction of nephrons continues. Dialysis usually is a lifelong process unless the client is a candidate for renal transplant.

CRITICAL THINKING CARE MAP

Subjective Data Mood: irritable, anxious. States she is very thirsty.

Objective Data Weight: 145 lbs; BP 98/62; P 110, regular; R 16; oxygen saturation: 93% on room air. Nausea and vomiting present. Mucous membranes dry. Skin turgor poor. Urine dark amber, 50 mL in last voiding.

Nursing Interventions Monitor and report abnormal lab results. Monitor and document intake and output. Encourage fluid intake. Teach client to stand slowly. Monitor color, amount, and frequency of fluid loss. Assess for vertigo and hypotension. Take daily weights. Give and monitor effectiveness of antinausea medication as ordered. Give and monitor effectiveness of antidiarrheal medications as ordered. Monitor orthostatic blood pressure every 4 h. Administer IV therapy as ordered. Provide frequent oral care.

Report Yes, nausea and vomiting, diminished urine output, poor skin turgor to physician and/or charge nurse.

Documentation Client states thirsty; mucous membranes dry. Instructed on intake/output. Safety precautions instructed; rise slowly. Provided oral care for comfort. IV fluids initiated per orders. Orthostatic BP, pulse as ordered. I. Sharpsaddle, LPN

CHAPTER 27

NCLEX-PN® ANSWERS 1. (2) Women are prone to UTIs because of their short urethra and the proximity of the urinary meatus to the vagina and anus. 2. (4) Diuresis is the production and excretion of large amounts of urine. Oliguria is low urine output; anuria refers to a lack of urine production, without effective urinary output. Polydipsia is excessive thirst. 3. (3) The kidneys produce urine at a rate of approximately 60 mL per hour or about 1500 mL per day. 4. (1) Urine culture is ordered to identify microorganisms causing UTI. 5. (2) At the start of the collection period, have the client void and discard this first urine. 6. (3) Clamp the catheter for 30 minutes; this allows fresh urine to collect in the catheter. 7. (2) The specific gravity of water is 1.000; the specific gravity of urine is between 1.010 and 1.025 and is a measure of its concentration. 8. (3) Increasing fluid for a client with kidney disease may be contraindicated related to the functional ability of the kidneys. Renal calculi and UTI would require increasing fluid intake. 9. (4) Increase the acidity of urine by the consumption of vitamin C or by drinking cranberry juices. This inhibits bacterial formation. Increase fluids, showering rather than bathing, and the use of cotton underclothes are preventive measures. 10. (4) The suprapubic catheter is inserted through the abdominal wall above the symphysis pubis and into the urinary bladder.

CARE PLAN HINTS

1. Wash hands prior to any procedure—this is the single most effective practice to inhibit contamination. Use disposable gloves and cleanse the area where the needle will be inserted with a disinfectant. This will remove microorganisms on the surface of the catheter. Be careful not to puncture the tube, compromising the closed system. When transferring the urine to the specimen container, do not allow the needle to touch the side of the container; this would contaminate the sterile container

2. Measures to prevent the development of a UTI are to increase fluid intake and wipe the perineal area from front to back following urination or defecation. Catheter care will prevent organisms from traveling up the catheter into the bladder. Encourage fluids that increase the acidity of urine through intake of vitamin C and cranberry juices, which inhibit bacterial growth. Early removal of the catheter per physician's order will decrease the risk for infection.

3. St. cath (straight catheter) for residual is performed to determine if the client is able to fully empty the bladder. This may be ordered following removal of an indwelling catheter to determine client ability to void prior to discharge.

CRITICAL THINKING CARE MAP

Subjective Data Diabetes out of control. Weakened. Tired. Thirst. Diabetic care compliance.

Objective Data Incontinent. Foul-smelling urine. Cloudy urine. Mucous threads in urine. Diminished pedal pulses. Glucose 440. Temp. 99. Catheter to gravity drainage.

Report Yes. Notify the physician about the glucose result of 440 and client complaining of thirst. Urine is foul smelling with mucous threads and cloudy. Temperature is low grade at 99. Pedal pulses are diminished.

Nursing Interventions Monitor lab tests. Observe urine for output. Assess urine for abnormal constituents. Maintain catheter asepsis. Take vital signs every 4 hours.

Documentation [date] [time] Client's urine is cloudy, foul smelling with mucous threads. 18-in. urinary catheter placed, per order. Output spontaneous 300 mL. Patient tolerated procedure well. Temp. 99. Glucose 440; physician notified. Medicated patient with 10 units of regular insulin. Lab results pending. D. Haus, LVN

CHAPTER 28

NCLEX-PN® ANSWERS 1. (4) Surgery that involves direct handling of the intestines can cause the intestinal movement to cease temporarily. It usually lasts 24 to 48 hours. Constipation is defined as fewer than three bowel movements per week. The stool becomes dry and hardened. Volvulus is a twisting of the bowel. Ulcerative colitis is a disease of the colon, causing inflammation of the bowel wall resulting in severe diarrhea. 2. (3) Rectal stimulation is contraindicated for those with cardiac disease because it may result in cardiac arrhythmias. 3. (4) Wavelike motion that propels intestinal contents forward occurs with both circular and longitudinal muscle contraction, known as peristalsis. 4. (3) An oil retention enema lubricates and softens the stool prior to manual removal. 5. (1) Digestive enzymes break down large molecules to simple chemicals; therefore, if these enzymes come in contact with the skin, it would cause breakdown and irritation. 6. (2) The guaiac test is used to determine blood in the stool, as is testing for occult (hidden) blood. 7. (2) Fluid and electrolytes (potassium) are not being reabsorbed, they are being eliminated from the body. 8. (2) Codeine decreases gastrointestinal motility. Colace is a stool softener, while Catapres and clonidine are antihypertensives. 9. (3) Ambulation increases peristalsis and therefore can facilitate gas movement. Use of a straw may increase gulping air, adding to the problem. Lomotil is an antidiarrheal medication. 10. (3) When the skin is irritated the site should be treated and assessed every 24 to 48 hours. Five days would be the length of time that the appliance remains intact.

CARE PLAN HINTS

1. The expulsion of feces from the anus and rectum is known as defecation. The frequency is individual and can vary from daily to every third day or more. Peristalsis moves feces into the sigmoid colon and rectum, the sensory nerves in the rectum are stimulated, and the individual becomes aware of the need to defecate. Expulsion of feces is assisted by contraction of the abdominal muscles and the diaphragm. This causes intra-abdominal pressure, which moves the feces through the anal canal.

2. Diet is important in providing bulk, which stimulates peristalsis to move the feces along the canal. Activity and exercise increase peristalsis. Fluid intake is a factor that affects the consistency of the stool; 2,000 to 3,000 mL/day promote normal soft stool. Individuals who eat at the same times every day usually have a regularly timed physiological response to the food intake and regular pattern of peristaltic activity in the colon.

3. Continuous use of laxatives and/or enemas will cause a dependency. Client will eventually not be able to have a spontaneous bowel movement.

CRITICAL THINKING CARE MAP

Subjective Data Client not looking at stoma. Pain. Anxious. Fearful.

Objective Data Ileostomy rt. abdomen. Stoma brick red. Effluent watery, dark brown, flecks of blood. Peristomal area reddened. Weight: 110 lbs. Hemoglobin 10. WBC 12,000. Temperature 99.4. Skin turgor slow.

Report Yes. Make the physician aware of low-grade temp, WBC 12,000, hemoglobin 10, flecks of blood, reddened peristomal area, slow skin turgor, clients' denial regarding ostomy. Also inform the enterostomal nurse regarding the peristomal area.

Nursing Interventions Monitor intake and output. Assess skin turgor. Take daily weights. Take VS every 4 hours. Increase fluid intake. Assess stoma. Inspect peristomal skin. Include family in teaching. Refer to ostomy association. Monitor lab values. Assess coping mechanisms.

Documentation [date] [time] Client is having difficulty accepting ileostomy, evidenced by covering head when staff empties bag, encouraged verbalization. Enterostomal nurse changed appliance at 1330. Included family members when reinforcing ostomy care. Client assisting minimally with ostomy. Temp. 99.4, skin turgor slow; encouraged fluids. Monitoring daily wts. Stoma brick red color, peristomal area reddened, no breakdown. Effluent drk. brown with flecks of blood. Fecal output at 500 mL. Physician notified. D. Haus, LVN

CHAPTER 29

NCLEX-PN® ANSWERS 1. (3) When a portion of a unit dose of a controlled substance is not used it must be disposed of in the presence of another licensed person. Both must acknowledge the wasting in writing. Never dispose of a controlled substance in the sharps container; it could be retrieved and used illicitly. Allowing a client to remain without medication could be considered neglect. 2. (1) The nurse is responsible for his or her actions. Although the error could have been discovered by any of the other parties, the responsibility belongs to the nurse. 3. (3) The reason a drug is prescribed is the therapeutic effects. The other choices are adverse effects of the drug. 4. (2) The idiosyncratic effect is an unexpected individualized reaction. Drug tolerance occurs when more drug is required to cause the same effect. Drug interaction is the effect that occurs when two or more drugs interact with each other. An iatrogenic disease is a disease caused unintentionally by medical therapy. 5. (2) A "stat" order is one that is to be given immediately and only once. An order that is to be given as needed is a prn order. An order that has no d/c date is known as a standing order. The times at which a drug is given may be by facility policy, but the order must be written by the physician (e.g., "4 times a day" could be 9, 13, 17, and 21, or 6, 11, 18, and 24). 6. (2) Grain = 1 mg. On hand you have 1 mg/mL so you would give 0.2 mL to equal 1/300. All the others would be too much: 1 mL would equal 5 times the ordered dose, and 2 mg would be 10 times the dose. 1/3 mL would be approximately 0.33 mL, which would be about 1½ times the ordered dose. 7. (4) Using a medicine cup is the most accurate way for the mother to measure the medication. A household teaspoon can over measure by almost a half more. Mixing medication with essential food can alter the taste and the child may be reluctant to eat the food in the future. The medication is ordered every 6 hours, which means it needs to be given around the clock. Giving it with meals and at bedtime would not be the appropriate times. 8. (2) A tuberculin syringe can be used for medication when less than 1 mL is to be given Sub-Q. 4,000 units would equal 0.8 mL. The attached needle is of the appropriate length and gauge for a Sub-Q injection. Insulin syringes are used only for insulin; insulin units and heparin units are not equal. Two- and 3-mL syringes are difficult to exactly measure less than 1 mL, and the needle gauge or length is not appropriate for a Sub-Q injection. 9. (1) The primary reason for wearing gloves is to prevent the spread of microorganisms from the skin. Some topical medications can cause an effect in the nurse; for example, nitro patches can cause headaches if the nurse comes in contact with the medication. The typical medication will not be passed on to another client if the nurse follows Standard Precautions and washes hands between clients. Unless there are open wounds (e.g., severe burns), topical application of medication is not usually done as a sterile procedure. 10. (2) The gluteal muscles are developed by walking, so they should not be used for injections until the child has been walking for at least 1 year. All muscles absorb medication at the same rate. Bruising results from technique and type of medication rather than location. A child must be held securely to prevent injury no matter what site you use.

CARE PLAN HINTS

1. Side effects are not related to an allergic reaction and do not produce the same symptoms as allergies do. Allergic reactions have a distinct pattern of reaction (e.g., skin rash, pruritus, rhinitis, tearing, nausea, vomiting, wheezing, dyspnea, or diarrhea).

2. The appropriate injection site depends on factors such as client's body weight, the healthiness of the muscle tissue, access to the site, the frequency with which the site has been used for previous injections, the condition of the skin over the site, and the client's preference. The ventrogluteal site is generally preferred because the area contains no large nerves or blood vessels and has less fat than the buttocks area.

3. Some drugs are better absorbed when given on an empty stomach; others cause gastrointestinal irritation and should be given with meals or after meals.

CRITICAL THINKING CARE MAP

Subjective Data "It will be hard to follow the diet at home, I don't eat on a regular schedule on my school nights and my roommates are big snackers." States, "I have been so tired, but it is probably because I am working and going to school." C/o excessive thirst and frequent urination. Client hesitant to perform monitoring and injections herself.

Objective Data Weight: 156 lbs. Fasting blood sugar 164 mg/mL. Urine shows presence of ketones. VS: T 99, P 132, R 28, BP 100/54. Started on insulin injection and BGM. 1,800-calorie ADA diet.

Report Yes, to the diabetes educator and the physician.

Nursing Interventions Provide information about the therapeutic regimen in various formats (video, brochures, written instructions). Deliberate with the client on changes that are possible to meet therapeutic goals. Demonstrate and allow client to perform monitoring and self-injection under supervision.

Documentation [date] [time] Has completed diabetic education program. BGM performed by client. Able to complete all steps accurately. Prepared insulin injection per sliding scale and routine NPH order under supervision. Client still hesitant to inject self. Discussed reluctance. Expressed concern with associated pain. Stated "I am just a chicken." Injection given by nurse in abdomen. Client admitted to very little discomfort, and stated she will try to do it herself next time. V. Dawson, LPN

CHAPTER 30

NCLEX-PN® ANSWERS **1.** (1) An 18-gauge cannula should be selected, so that no hemolysis of the blood will occur. In addition a large vein that will accommodate this cannula is advisable.

2. (4) The use of 0.9% sodium chloride (NS) with transfusion therapy is established in policies and procedures. Isotonic solutions have the same osmolarity as that of normal body fluids. **3.** (2) An intermittent infusion device is used for many purposes. It is used for vascular access for the client receiving medications, and to enable the staff to draw blood. It can also be used for emergency medication administration, and reduces the client's cost while increasing mobility and comfort. **4.** (2) Moist rales, increased respiratory rate, dyspnea, and 3+ edema are highly suspicious for *Excess Fluid Volume.* **5.** (1) The peripheral vein that is most appropriate for blood administration and medications that are irritating is the cephalic vein. The size of this vein accommodates a large-gauge needle. **6.** (2) The lungs effectively regulate the blood levels of CO_2, while the kidneys reabsorb or excrete acids and bases into the urine. **7.** (3) The symptoms exhibited by the client—irritability, fatigued muscles, nausea, and anorexia, including a K level of 3.1—are indicative of hypokalemia. **8.** (3) A minidrip administration set that delivers 60 gtt/minute is used for pediatric or critically ill clients to monitor the fluid infused. **9.** (4) Bicarbonate excess, or metabolic alkalosis, is exhibited by symptoms of dizziness, decreased respirations, tingling of fingers and toes, cardiac dysrhythmias, and hyperventilation. **10.** (2) Septicemia is a central line complication exhibited by fever, profuse sweating, low blood pressure, and nausea.

CARE PLAN HINTS

1. Isotonic solutions have the same osmolarity as that of normal body fluids. They have no effect on the volume of fluid within the cell. Isotonic solutions are used to expand the ECF compartments. Hypotonic solutions contain less sodium than the intracellular space. Hypotonic solutions move water into the cell, causing the cell to swell and possibly burst. Body fluids shift out of the blood vessels into the interstitial tissue and cells. Hypotonic solutions hydrate cells and can deplete the circulatory system. The isotonic solutions used in dehydration are D_5W, or 0.9% normal saline.

2. Common signs and symptoms include weight gain, edema, puffy eyelids, hypertension, I&O variances, shortness of breath, crackles, and distended neck veins. Nursing Implications include these: monitor IV flow rates, monitor I&O, place clients in high-Fowler's position, monitor VS, and administer oxygen as ordered. Use microdrip administration set for accurate infusion.

3. $$\frac{100 \text{ mL } (15)}{60 \text{ min}} = \text{drops per minute}$$

$$\frac{100 \ (1)}{4} = \frac{100}{4} = 25 \text{ gtt/minute}$$

CRITICAL THINKING CARE MAP

Subjective Data Lethargic. C/o pain.

Objective Data Surgery right hip replacement. Pulse 110, BP 90/55. Hemoglobin 6 g/dL. Hematocrit 22%. Hemovac 150 mL, serosanguineous drainage.

Report Yes, H/H to physician.

Nursing Interventions Reinforce surgical dressing. Monitor I&O. Drain Hemovac and record drainage.

Monitor H/H. Transfuse client with 1 unit PRBCs if H/H is <7 g/dL or 22%. Monitor VS every 4 hours.

Documentation [date] [time] **D**—Client pulse 110, BP 90/55, drainage from Hemovac at 150 mL of serosanguineous drainage. H/H 6 g/dL/ 22%; client complains of lethargy. **A**— Dressing to rt hip reinforced, monitor Hemovac for drainage. Notified physician regarding H/H including dressing drainage. Will proceed with transfusion 1 unit of PRBCs. Client prepared for pending transfusion with information for use and procedure. **R**—Client understands transfusion need and procedures. M. Taban, LVN

CHAPTER 31

NCLEX-PN® ANSWERS **1.** (3) Good preoperative teaching by the nurse can decrease the client's postoperative pain and give the client coping mechanisms to deal with postoperative discomfort. **2.** (4) Clients who are scheduled for a radical mastectomy usually are scheduled for lymph node dissection in the affected side, which may lead to swelling of the affected extremity. **3.** (3) Hypotension and depressed respirations indicate potential postoperative complications or an allergic reaction to pain medication and must be treated as a medical emergency. **4.** (3) Clients who have had spinal anesthesia must lie flat for 8 to 12 hours or as ordered by the anesthesia care provider. **5.** (2) This procedure is called splinting and is effective in decreasing postoperative pain when moving or coughing. **6.** (4) This is the accepted pain rating scale used and understood by healthcare professionals. **7.** (3) Providing a rationale for the client about why you are asking him or her to do something is the best way to communicate. **8.** (3) The client has to be aware of the surgical procedure and cannot sign the surgical consent unless he or she fully understands what procedure is scheduled and the risks involved for the procedure and anesthesia. **9.** (3) Positioning the tubing lower than the stomach will prevent reflux of gastric contents into the NG tubing. **10.** (3) Evisceration occurs when the surgical incision opens and the bowel is visible or protrudes from the incisional site.

CARE PLAN HINTS

1. Factors that may increase Mr. Teng's risk include these: Mr. Teng is 77 years old, placing him at a greater risk than younger adults; his respiratory status is compromised and he runs a greater risk for developing postoperative atelectasis or lung infection; he may be taking medications that will slow healing such as corticosteroids.
2. A major disadvantage of general anesthesia is that it depresses the respiratory and the circulatory systems, so regional anesthesia was probably chosen so as not to further compromise his respiratory status.

3. Specific precautions may include promoting adequate hydration to replace fluids lost during surgery or fluid limitations prior to surgery; early movement and ambulation to foster maximum lung expansion, and prevent lung infection; deep breathing exercises to remove mucus and prevent stasis of lung secretions; pain control so that he can ambulate and cough more effectively; and leg exercises to prevent thrombophlebitis.

CRITICAL THINKING CARE MAP

Subjective Data Complains of pain. "I wish I had died in the accident; life will never be the same."

Objective Data Vital signs stable. Refuses to respond to nurse's questions about pain level. Will not look at limb during dressing change. Dressing dry and intact. Wound healing without signs of infection

Report Yes, to social worker.

Nursing Interventions Contact physician for social worker or psychologist referral. Acknowledge denial, anger, or depression as normal. Encourage client to make own decisions, participate in plan of care, and accept both inadequacies and strengths. Allow client gradual exposure to body change. Help client to accept help from others. Teach family appropriate care of surgical site.

Documentation Client turned toward wall during dressing change. Refused to look at limb. Stated "I wish I had died in the accident; life will never be the same." Complaining of pain, unable to describe the level. H. Mobley, LVN

CHAPTER 32

NCLEX-PN® ANSWERS **1.** (2) The center of gravity is where the body's mass and base of support are centered and balance is achieved. The line of gravity is an imaginary vertical line through the center of gravity. Postural tonus is muscle contraction needed to maintain an upright position. **2.** (3) Osteoporosis is a demineralization process of the bones, which occurs without the stress of weight-bearing activity. Contractures are permanent shortenings of the muscles that cause permanent fixation of joints. Orthostatic hypotension is a drop in blood pressure following a rapid change in position. Disuse atrophy is loss of normal strength and function and size of unused muscles. **3.** (4) Bed rest decreases the production of surfactant, which enables the alveoli to remain open. This, along with mucous-plugged bronchioles, can cause a lung to collapse. **4.** (1) Crutches must be adjusted so that weight is on the forearm, not the axilla, since pressure on the underarm can damage the brachial plexus. Understanding the need for nonslip shoes and rubber tips on the crutches and removal of hazards in the home demonstrates successful learning. **5.** (3) The orthopneic position is modified Fowler's, which aids in air exchange in respiratory and heart clients. **6.** (3) Stage III occurs when heart and respiratory rates and other body processes slow and are dominated by the parasympathetic nervous system. The sleeper becomes more difficult to arouse. Stages I and II are light sleep; stage IV is deep sleep. 7. (3) Hypothyroidism decreases stage IV sleep. Hyperthyroidism lengthens presleep time, making it difficult to fall asleep. 8. (2) Treatment of insomnia routinely includes behavior modification in which the client learns new habits to foster sleep. Long-term sleep-inducing medication is not recommended because it does not treat the cause and can result in dependency. Antidepressants and beta blockers can cause nightmares and daytime drowsiness. 9. (1) *Somnambulism* is a term meaning sleepwalking; bedwetting is enuresis, and teeth grinding is bruxism. 10. (1) Even mild conditioning can strengthen the legs and increase circulation, which will help relieve postural hypotension.

CARE PLAN HINTS

1. Check traction for proper alignment and ensure that weights are hanging free. Traction will maintain the position of the fracture and help relieve muscle spasms. Encourage Kevin to do active ROM exercises to unaffected extremities. Encourage position changes with the aid of a trapeze.

2. Once Kevin's bowel sounds have returned, he should be permitted a regular diet. Request the physician to write an order that food can be brought in from home. Have dietitian talk with Kevin about food likes and dislikes; provide nutritious snacks, fresh fruit, dairy products, and protein. Discuss the need for calcium and protein to promote healing. Allow Kevin to make informed choices.

3. Distractions might include handheld video games, DVD movies, music, Internet access (if possible) to help him keep up with school work, and interactions with family and peers. Roommate selection is very important if long-term hospitalization is necessary. It is important for Kevin to have contact with his peers at his developmental level.

CRITICAL THINKING CARE MAP

Subjective Data States she has a problem falling asleep since her mastectomy 2 months ago. Says fears of prognosis becomes prominent when she is not active and busy. Has tried reading or watching TV but neither make her sleepy or relaxed.

Objective Data Weight 126 lbs. 10-pound weight loss since surgery. R 16; skin pale; dark circles around eyes. Radiation site irritated and red. Appears agitated and restless.

Report Yes, sleeplessness, weight loss, and agitation to physician.

Nursing Interventions Assess client's sleep patterns and usual bedtime rituals and incorporate these into the plan of care. Assess for signs of new onset of depression, depressed mood state, statement of hopelessness, poor appetite. Observe client's diet and medication and caffeine intake. Look for hidden sources of caffeine. Advise client to avoid use of alcohol or hypnotics to induce sleep.

Documentation [date] [time] Focus: Insomnia. **D**—Anxious and agitated, states she has not been sleeping well since surgery; admitted to dwelling on prognosis. **A**—Discussed bedtime rituals and caffeine intake. Suggested keeping a sleep diary until next visit. **R**—Agreed to keep diary and replace bedtime tea with decaffeinated or herbal tea. M. Tunny, LPN

CHAPTER 33

NCLEX-PN® ANSWERS 1. (1) In behaviorism, correct choices are rewarded and behaviors that are incorrect and need to be avoided are ignored. 2. (3) Restoration involves information about what is being done as well as self-care skills and resources. 3. (4) Pain is a barrier to learning because it decreases concentration. Pain needs to be dealt with prior to initiating teaching. 4. (2) It is important to use words that the client understands, e.g., that bathing and shower, as well as washing the incision with soap and water, could interfere with the healing process. 5. (3) The nurse needs to validate the client's feeling and help restore her or his self-confidence by assisting her or him to practice skills. 6. (3) Many cultural groups, especially from east Asia, are reluctant to maintain eye contact with professionals, feeling that it is a lack of respect. It does not mean that they are confused or that they are not interested. The client probably would not make eye contact with the physician either if he or she were giving the instructions. 7. (3) Young school-age children relate to and learn better from imaginary figures. They tend to give life to inanimate objects (*animism*). Stories, puppets, and colorful items are the best reinforcement of learning in this age group. Lecture and handouts are better used with individuals who can read and who have a longer attention span. Food that can be manipulated and placed on the pyramid can be used with school-age children as a return demonstration. Cooking class works well for older school-age children as they enter the stage of industry. 8. (3) Understanding that it is not safe to leave the client alone for extended periods each day is important to home safety. When a client suffers from dementia, he may forget that he should not use the stove, or forget to turn it off after use. Posting a number is a good idea, but in an emergency the client with dementia will not be able to process quickly who should be called. Although it is hard for the family to see their loved one like this, this statement does not address the safety issues. 9. (1) Negative feedback will cause the client to avoid the nurse. It is never appropriate and should not be used in a teaching situation. 10. (4) Troubleshooting should be delayed until client is comfortable with the procedure so that client does not become overwhelmed and unable to process all of the information.

CARE PLAN HINTS

1. Early detection of the signs and symptoms of infection may decrease the need for very aggressive treatment of the infection. If the infection is not discovered until it is se-

vere, the client may need to be readmitted to the hospital and aggressive action taken.

2. In order for the nurse to be sure the client is able to clean and dress his wound correctly, he or she must see the client perform these actions.

3. If a client is familiar with the equipment needed for wound care, he will be less likely to have difficulty performing his wound care once he is at home.

CRITICAL THINKING CARE MAP

Subjective Data Complains of shortness of breath on mild exertion. Complains of occasional mild chest pain. States she rests a lot after work so she doesn't overwork her heart. States she has smoked one pack of cigarettes a day for 25 years.

Objective Data Weight: 180 lbs. Height: 5′1″. VS: T 98.5, P 80, BP 140/100. Blood oxygen level 98%. Lung sounds clear bilaterally.

Report Yes, report blood pressure, any present complaint of chest pain to RN.

Nursing Interventions Encourage client to make dietary changes. Stress importance of cutting back on fat, especially saturated fats, which may help reduce cholesterol. Encourage client to eat a well-balanced diet with at least five servings of fruits and vegetables a day. Obtain a physician's order for the client to meet with the hospital dietitian. Explain to client that physical activity can reduce her risk of heart attack. However, her doctor will prescribe how much activity she may do based on the severity of her coronary artery disease. Explain to client that smoking is a major risk factor and that by quitting she can significantly cut her risk of a heart attack.

Documentation Complains of shortness of breath on exertion and occasional, mild chest pains. Blood pressure 140/100, pulse 80, temperature 98.5, blood oxygen level 98%. Lungs clear bilaterally. Weight 180 lbs, height 5′1″. M. Taban, LVN

UNIT IV WRAP-UP

TIME MANAGEMENT After report, the nurse should first visit each client's room to introduce himself or herself and make a quick assessment of each client. The LPN can assess vital signs and surgical sites at this time (or delegate vital signs to UAP). It is important to check the MAR, Kardex, or chart for any new orders. Since Mr. Drew and Mr. Melezack are quiet at the moment, it will be a priority to deal with Mr. Ramos's agitation. Check to see if he can be medicated for anxiety. Make sure his catheter irrigation is running, and determine if the irrigation needs to be increased to flush out clots, which may be causing him discomfort. Bring in someone to sit with Mr. Ramos until he is calm again, and administer medication. Then inform his doctor of the agitation; discuss the need for physical restraints if he cannot be controlled by other means.

At this point, if you are informed of Mr. Melezack's nausea and vomiting and pain, this will become your priority. While documenting, review lab work. When you find that Mr. Drew has not had an MI, you will need to schedule time to begin his discharge teaching. This is of lower priority, and may be accomplished at the end of visiting hours while you are providing HS care.

CRITICAL THINKING Teach Mr. Drew some of the things that can be done to decrease recurrent angina: avoid overexertion; decrease anxiety and stress (causes blood vessels to constrict); avoid overeating (increases workload of the heart); avoid cold weather (constricts blood vessels to conserve heat); avoid hot, humid conditions (increase workload of the heart); avoid walking uphill and/or against the wind (increases workload of the heart). Also teach ways to control risk factors: stop smoking; decrease intake of fat content foods/cholesterol; decrease weight; increase exercise (gradually if not used to exercise); decrease hypertension by above activities; decrease stressors (some stress is normal), especially if they precipitate chest discomfort; take medication as prescribed by physician.

COMPASSIONATE CARING Although the first concern is for the physiological status of Mr. Ramos, the nurse must also be concerned with the stress the roommate is experiencing because of his behavior. While you are assessing your client, the nurse assigned to the roommate should (if possible) remove him from the area. He could be taken to the solarium in a wheelchair, if necessary, while arrangements are made to move him to a different room. It will be necessary to obtain an interpreter in order to assess Mr. Ramos's pain and anxiety level properly. It will be important to take the client's vitals signs and observe the catheter bags for the condition of the drainage. It will be necessary to have a Spanish-speaking sitter stay with the client until he can be calmed down, since climbing out of bed could result in a fall and injury, and he could dislodge his IV or catheter if he climbs out of bed. Client safety is a priority—it will be necessary to medicate or temporarily restrain the client to prevent injury.

COMMUNICATION AND TEAM BUILDING [date] [time] Focus: NG tube. **D**—NGT clamped since 12 noon, clear liquid lunch; 50% consumed and tolerated. C/o stabbing abdominal pain 8/10. Vomited 500 mL dark brown emesis. **A**—NGT unclamped; irrigated with 100 mL of NSS, connected to low intermittent wall suction. Medicated for pain Meperidine 75 mg with Vistaril 25 mg IM. Dr. Sample notified, order to continue suction. **R**—Client resting comfortably; pain 2/10. No c/o of nausea. NGT drain moderate amt. of dark brown emesis. L. Fellows, LPN

Report client's condition to the charge nurse or RN team leader. Since NG tube cannot be removed, MD should be notified. Discuss client's needs with the care assistant and give instructions to provide mouth care, ice chips, partial bath, and gown and bed change as necessary.

CHAPTER 34

NCLEX-PN® ANSWERS **1.** (2) Airway management with clients in the EC and especially cardiac disturbances is the primary intervention requiring the attention of the healthcare staff first. **2.** (3) The client's comprehensive understanding of the correct medication administration is vital for safety. **3.** (1) Clients with burns to the face and neck areas are at risk for airway compromise related to edema and third spacing. Airway management and maintenance are always chief concerns with burns to the upper torso. **4.** (2) Data collection of the specific agent is required as soon as possible. The sooner the agent is identified, the more rapidly effective treatment may be administered for a safe and effective outcome. **5.** (2) Reassuring the client and obtaining pertinent objective data may be necessary elements that must be considered first in order for accurate medical care to be administered by the physician. **6.** (2) The diagnosis of nutritional anemia has no direct effect on cardiogenic shock or heart failure. The other medical diagnoses listed can have a direct effect on the client's cardiac status. **7.** (3) Keeping the client's extremity above the level of the heart improves circulation. By reducing the opportunity for dependent edema to the extremity, blood flow can be improved to the area, and lessen third spacing/dependent edema. **8.** (2) According to HIPAA, client confidentiality must be maintained at all times. **9.** (1) The ABCs of resuscitation must be initiated with clients with compromised vital organs. Airway management for the unresponsive client with high-flow O_2 is the first line of treatment in the EC. **10.** (3) An indwelling Foley catheter can be a primary source of infection in a client, especially in long-term care settings. The vital signs indicate septic shock because vascular compromise and infection are indicated.

CARE PLAN HINTS

1. Client may suffer from edema to throat and neck related to third spacing. There is a major risk of infection, which could interfere with breathing. Pain would reduce ability to breathe effectively. Reduction in mobility related to area of injury or trauma may result in pooling of secretions and difficulty breathing.
2. Pain management can improve mobility and enhance ability to breathe by reducing the pain threshold and increasing comfort. Common medications for such a client would be Demerol or morphine.
3. Risks include infection, pain, and altered body image. Nursing diagnoses include, but are not limited to, *Risk for Infection, Disturbed Body Image, Self-Esteem, Self-Care Deficit,* and *Deficient Knowledge.*

CRITICAL THINKING CARE MAP

Subjective Data "I feel so weak, yet I'm hungry." Complains of nausea; increased thirst; decreased appetite.

Objective Data VS: P 92, R 22, BP 90/58. Skin turgor greater than 3 sec. Mucous membranes dry and cracked. K^+ 3.5 mEq/L.

Report Yes, to the RN and the physician directly.

Nursing Interventions Monitor vital signs every 15 min. Instruct client on signs and symptoms of dehydration. Monitor IV site for infiltration. Administer antiemetics as ordered. Assist PT with ambulation. Administer high-flow O_2. Record I&O every shift.

Documentation [date] [time] Admitted for nausea and vomiting for 3 days. Denies any pain; states "I feels weak…." Alert and oriented to person, place, time. Skin turgor less than 3 sec. IV of 1000 mL of 0.9 NSS infusing via 16-gauge catheter in R arm. Site intact, no S/Sx of infiltration. J. Tompkins, LPN

CHAPTER 35

NCLEX-PN® ANSWERS **1.** (3) The Nurse Practice Act provides information as to scope of practice for the LPN/LVN. A facility's policies and procedures do not delineate scope of practice for licensed nurses. Choice 2: The job description describes the expected duties, but it is the responsibility of the licensed nurse to be sure the duties he or she performs are within their scope of practice. Although the state board of nursing establishes the scope of practice, it cannot be expected to answer individual questions concerning scope of practice. Instead, the nurse will be referred to the Scope of Practice Document. **2.** (4) The LPN/LVN working in the physician's office reports to an RN or the physician for clinical issues. Choices 1, 2, and 3 refer to unlicensed medical assistants, and it is not appropriate for an unlicensed person to supervise a licensed nurse. **3.** (2) Scoliosis screening is mandated by law and calls for the initial screening for males to be given in the 6th grade and every other year until the 10th grade since this period of time coincides with their rapid growth period. Choice 1: The 5th grade is when girls are initially assessed, since their growth spurt begins earlier than boys. Choice 3: The 10th grade is when the every other year screening is completed for male students and yearly screening for girls. Choice 4: School screenings for scoliosis are completed before the 11th grade. **4.** (1) When a client is admitted to hospice, a physician's order is necessary with a second physician's certification. The family stating that they want to sign the patient up without these items demonstrates the need for additional teaching. The other statement demonstrates an understanding of hospice and no additional teaching is needed. **5.** (3) The circulating nurse is considered to be the charge nurse of the operating room; this job is within the scope of the registered nurse. The LPN/LVN can (choice 1) admit the patient and (choice 4) provide observation of the patient and provide needed care during the immediate post-op period. Choice 2: With specialized training the LPN/LVN can carry out the duties of a scrub tech. **6.** (3) Anesthesia will be administered by the physician. The LPN/LVN office nurse can (choice 1) set up the surgical tray, (choice 2) position the client, and (choice 4) complete the lab slips; these all are within the scope of the LPN's/LVN's duties. 7. (4) With proper instructions the child should be able to identify the position of the E and accomplish the screening test. Choice 1: Because there are other methods for testing the visual acuity, they should be exhausted before stating on the physical form that the test could not be completed. Choice 2: Unless the child has the ability to read letters on all lines the results of the test would not be accurate. Choice 3: The mother's assessment of the child's vision is not a replacement for a visual acuity screening. 8. (1) The client may be light-headed and dizzy after the procedure so he or she should be allowed to rest prior to getting up. Choice 2: Don't leave the client alone to dress until you are sure that he or she is stable. Choice 3: Discharge instructions should be given in the room or another private place to ensure confidentiality once the client is stable and ready to go home. Choice 4: Client should not be allowed to stand until vital signs and client's condition have been assessed. 9. (2) Splinting the arm from below to above the joints that surround the location of the injury will immobilize the fracture. Applying the sling to elevate the arm above the level of the heart and application of ice will help to decrease the swelling. Choice 1: Tightly wrapping the arm from the wrist to below the elbow with an elastic bandage can constrict the blood flow and increase swelling above the wrap. Choice 3: Ice and a sling can help reduce swelling, but will not immobilize the fracture. Choice 4: The splint will immobilize the fracture but will not decrease swelling. 10. (3) Between ages 4 and 6, the child should have the 5th of five DTaP; the 4th of four polio, and the 2nd of two MMR immunizations. Choice 1 does not provide adequate protection from polio; choice 2 does not provide adequate protection from diphtheria, tetanus and pertussis; and choice 4 does not provide adequate protection from measles, mumps and rubella.

CARE PLAN HINTS

1. General anesthesia cannot be used if a client is young, has a hearing impairment or a mental impairment (e.g., dementia, severe anxiety), has a language barrier, or is sensitive to local anesthesia. General anesthesia has the potential for postop nausea and vomiting, which can increase intraocular pressure. Older adults often have concurrent disease processes that would preclude general anesthesia.

2. She should have a responsible adult remain with her for 24 to 48 hours after surgery; continue presurgery diet and fluids; keep eye shield in place for 12 to 18 hours to protect eyes; continue presurgery activities with caution due to the change in depth perception caused by having a shield covering the eye; limit the number of trips up and down the stairs for a few days. If the patient has not had a bowel movement by the third day postop, she should take a laxative to prevent straining. Do not put eyedrops in the eye unless instructed to do so by the surgeon. She should return to the physician's office the next day for an appointment and she should call the physician

if over-the-counter medication does not relieve pain, if she experiences nausea or vomiting, or if there is a sudden worsening of her vision.

3. Removing a cataract from the eye with the poorest vision will aid the physician by giving him or her information as to the difficulty of removing the cataract, and the patient will better understand the reaction and recovery from surgery. Removing the cataract from the eye with the best vision first might compromise vision in the event of complications.

CRITICAL THINKING CARE MAP

Subjective Data C/o pain and requesting to call mother and go home. Did not eat lunch; complains that brace is putting pressure on abdomen so he can't eat.

Objective Data Weight: 178 lbs. Height: 5′11″. VS: T 98.4, P 72, R 24, BP 110/74. Lateral spinal curve of 35°. Will not make eye contact. Wearing Milwaukee brace over t-shirt; reluctant to remove jacket.

Report Yes, place a call to his physician to inform him of JJ's issues.

Nursing Interventions Evaluate brace for pressure areas. Consider JJ's developmental level and how wearing the brace at school can affect it. Allow JJ to come to health office or see the counselor if he has the need to talk. Arrange meeting with Counselor, coach, parents and physician to discus available options. Establish contract with JJ that he will wear brace at all times except during practice and workout in the pool and shower time. Regularly monitor height and weight. Assist JJ to develop new interests that he can be involved in while still in brace.

Documentation [date] [time] 16-year-old student presented at the health office on first day back at school following an application of Milwaukee brace for the treatment of a 35° lateral spinal curve. Showing signs of disturbed body image. Expresses concerns that his friends may not accept him with the brace and that he will not be able to participate in sports this year. C/o pain and discomfort when he tried to eat lunch. As he was given opportunity to talk c/o lessened. Receptive to a conference with coach, parents, and physician to investigate possibility of practicing with team. M. Howard LVN, School Health Clerk

UNIT V WRAP-UP

COMMUNICATION AND TEAM BUILDING I would contact the RNP immediately to notify her of the situation and report that I am in the clinic alone. Discuss the schedule with her and see if anything can be rescheduled. Suggest that you notify the principal to see if it would be possible to secure a substitute LPN health clerk, or, if not, a sub or a parent volunteer to answer the phone and check students in. Determine the approximate time the RNP will come to your campus. Follow through with any suggestions that she gives you.

CRITICAL THINKING   Any activities that involve parents need to go ahead as scheduled. Parents have had to make arrangements to attend and if a meeting or orientation were canceled it would create a negative view of the school. It is difficult enough to get parents to participate in school activities, so it is imperative that this remain as scheduled. Student acute health problems need to be handled; first aid and contagious conditions could put students at additional risk. Determine with the teacher who is coordinating the outdoor science trip when the students will be leaving. It is determined that the buses are scheduled to leave at 10 A.M. tomorrow. Reschedule the health check at 8:30 A.M. tomorrow morning, and secure some extra help to take temperatures and record the students' health status. Reschedule the scoliosis screening for Wednesday. Since most of the seventh graders will be off campus at Outdoor Ed, the workload should be less. Also secure volunteers to assist with escorting students from the classroom to the screening area and to assist with paperwork.

CONFLICT RESOLUTION   The psychologist is very upset; make an attempt to defuse the situation by coming up with a solution to the problem that has been created by the crisis that developed in the health clinic today. Inform the psychologist that you have spoken to the RNP and she will return to campus to participate in the IEP although she may be a few minutes late. Let her know that you will be available for health questions if any arise prior to the RNP's arrival. Also inform him that another interpreter will attend the meeting,

CULTURAL COMPETENCY   The preadolescent period is very difficult for many families, and many families from other cultures find the media, social, and peer influences on their children to be disturbing. Also there are many differences between cultures as to what is acceptable in terms of discussing health-related issues in public, and in some cultures this age group is considered to still be children. The orientation program should consider all of these issues. The important thing is to explain that all health services and presentations at the school will require parental permission and that parents are invited to participate with their child.

CHAPTER 36

NCLEX-PN® ANSWERS   1. (3) Although it is not the best way to resolve conflicts, avoidance is the most frequently used; many staff nurses feel if it is ignored it will resolve itself. Both sides see the issue as minor or consider the negative impact to be too costly to meet the issue head on. 2. (2) Accommodation is used when one person or a group is willing to yield to the other and when preserving relationships is the most important task. A staff member who wants others to like him or her would use this strategy, either consciously or unconsciously. 3. (4) Lack of communication, especially incomplete instructions, is the most frequent reason why delegated tasks are not completed as expected. An UAP cannot be expected to perform unless he or

she has been adequately prepared to complete the task. Avoidance of conflict, lack of supervision, and poor attitudes can have an effect but they are not the primary reason. 4. (3) Care partners, nursing assistants, and orderlies are unlicensed assistive personnel. The LPN/LVN is the only job title listed that requires a license. 5. (2) Accountability is related to responsibility and being responsible for one's own action and the actions of those you have delegated to. The other choices have to do with supervision and delegation. 6. (4) Politely decline to carry out tasks that are outside of the job for which you were hired. Offering to assist with tasks that you can do will relieve the nurse so that she can complete work that you cannot do for her. Choices 1 and 3 are rude responses and should not be made from a subordinate to a supervisor. Choice 2 should never be considered. Skills learned as a student can only be done under the supervision of an instructor and when in the capacity of a student. Performing these duties while working as an UAP could jeopardize your future license and the facility. 7. (2) A management style that is unstructured and leaves the decisions up to the group is known as laissez-faire. The autocratic leader makes unilateral decisions while dominating the team members. The democratic leader makes decisions after consulting with team members. Authoritative is another term for autocratic. 8. (3) Although functional nursing is efficient, it can create fragmented delivery of client care. In primary nursing, a professional nurse has total responsibility for a group of patients. The case method is when a nurse is responsible for providing care to clients during one shift. The purpose of team nursing was to reduce fragmentation which was present in the functional method. 9 (3) The state boards of nursing have a duty to protect the public. When a licensed nurse violates the provisions of the license, the state board has jurisdiction over that license. NCLEX® is responsible for the licensing exam. If a crime has been committed, the attorney general and the courts will become involved but the decision regarding the license is up to the state board. 10. (2) Dealing with the supervision of UAPs can be difficult; it is always best to discuss the issue and determine why the incident happened. Counsel with regard to facility policies and the importance of adequate staffing for the safety of the clients. Although the RN may need to be informed, reporting them should not be handled as a threat. It is also not a good idea to report them without first talking to them, because this may adversely affect your working relationship with them, as will overhead paging.

CHAPTER 37

NCLEX-PN® ANSWERS   1. (1) Reviewing and studying as you move through the program will help you retain the knowledge and information you are learning. It also will prevent "cramming" just before you take the examination. 2. (1) You are being asked to recall a fact or statement presented to you. 3. (2) Although ongoing review and analysis do occur, the revision is based on completion of a new job analysis of the tasks of licensed vocational nurses. Changes in the nurse practice acts of the states may occur at any time and are not linked to test revision. 4. (4) The test is set up so that any student can follow the computer instructions and take the test. 5. (2) Taking a proactive approach is most helpful. There are useful techniques that can improve both your study methods and your ability to relax. 6. (3) A sudden change in sleep time can disturb your biorhythms and cause you to feel more tired and less alert. 7. (4) Questions of comprehension, analysis, or synthesis require you to do more than memorize facts. They require you to put information together and think more in depth. 8. (3) Identification is essential in order to sit for the exam. The computer program for the test contains a pull-down calculator. Most likely, there will be a clock in the exam room. 9. (4) Depending on your answers, you may complete the test in much less time than 5 hours. However, if 5 hours pass and you have not completed enough questions to pass, the exam will end. 10. (85) You will receive 25 pilot questions, along with a minimum of 60 test questions. Sixty questions were determined to be the minimum a person had to answer correctly in order to prove competence and awareness of safety.

CHAPTER 38

NCLEX-PN® ANSWERS   1. (2) Use the first paragraph to identify yourself and the job you are interested in; this will facilitate your letter reaching the correct person. The other choices are found in paragraphs 2 and 3. 2. (3) Employers will be concerned with time gaps on applications. By highlighting your activities during the gap, it will demonstrate your interest in improving your skills or contributing to the community. It is never appropriate to leave blanks on an application or ignore large time gaps on an application. Writing an explanation is not necessary and appears like an excuse. 3. (4) Although you are not required to answer personal questions, an answer that could alleviate concerns of the interviewer without revealing personal information is the best solution. Quoting the law or stating that you won't answer the question or use it to make stipulations on the job may put the interviewer on the defense and prevent you from being considered. 4. (2), although any of these reasons are possible. Nonspecific résumés and letters not addressed to a name and title show lack of research into the position for which the applicant is applying. 5. (1) A profession is characterized by devotion and expertise. Most nurses consider themselves to be part of the profession even after retirement, and although continuing education is necessary is it not the definer of the profession. 6. (3) The best response is to shower and dress professionally. Wearing your uniform is acceptable unless it is soiled, which is a possibility after working all night. Even though the interviewers know you,

you want them to look at you as a professional nurse; dressing appropriately will help them see you in that way. 7. (3) Having coffee with a friend can provide valuable job search information, in a causal setting. The other choices are planned activities and are considered to be formal networking. 8. (2) The functional résumé focuses on the skills an individual possesses, while a chronological résumé presents education and skills in reverse chronological order. An e-résumé highlights keywords and employers file résumés by these keywords. 9. (1) The main reason for including a writing sample is to highlight your ability to write in a logical order using correct format and to show your attention to details. 10. (4) The NLN was the name given in 1912 to the American Society of Superintendents of Training Schools for Nurses in the United States and Canada.

UNIT VI WRAP-UP

COMMUNICATION AND TEAM BUILDING   You can tell her you looked at the schedule and an IV-certified nurse will be coming in at 6 A.M. You could call him, asking him to come in 1 hour early, and offer to relieve him an hour early the next day. You could ask the ADON to come in to do the IV. You could repeat your suggestion to have the client stay at the hospital another day. You could ask her to approve having a registry nurse or a home health nurse come in to do the IV.

CRITICAL THINKING   No matter what the result, do not jeopardize your hard-earned license. The ADON is not demonstrating good managerial or leadership skills by asking you to do a procedure that is outside your scope of practice. Let her know that you are unwilling to break the law and that if a solution is not reached prior to the time the solution must be added, you will be forced to call the administrator. If no one has arrived to add the IV fluids at the prescribed time, call the administrator and leave the matter in his or her hands.

CONFLICT RESOLUTION   You could tell the ADON that you intend to take the IV certification class as soon as you get paid. (Most facilities do not provide training but may front the cost for newly graduated employees.) Tell her that you want to be fully prepared for your job.

For your own records, document the interaction as exactly as possible and keep it in your home file, along with any further related exchanges. Do your job well and document carefully. Chances are, the situation will be forgotten. If, however, the ADON wants you fired, you need to have your own documentation of consequences, including changed assignments, imbalanced scheduling, denials of requests for time off, constant criticisms without balancing encouragement, and so on.

Appendix II

2007–2008 NANDA-Approved Nursing Diagnoses

Activity Intolerance
Activity Intolerance, Risk for
Adaptive Capacity: Intracranial, Decreased
Airway Clearance, Ineffective
Allergy Response, Latex
Allergy Response, Risk for Latex
Anxiety
Anxiety, Death
Aspiration, Risk for
Attachment, Parent/Infant/Child, Risk for Impaired
Blood Glucose, Risk for Unstable
Body Image, Disturbed
Body Temperature: Imbalanced, Risk for
Bowel Incontinence
Breastfeeding, Effective
Breastfeeding, Ineffective
Breastfeeding, Interrupted
Breathing Pattern, Ineffective
Cardiac Output, Decreased
Caregiver Role Strain
Caregiver Role Strain, Risk for
Comfort, Readiness for Enhanced
Communication, Readiness for Enhanced
Communication: Verbal, Impaired
Confusion, Acute
Confusion, Chronic
Confusion, Risk for Acute
Constipation
Constipation, Perceived
Constipation, Risk for
Contamination
Contamination, Risk for
Coping: Community, Ineffective
Coping: Community, Readiness for Enhanced
Coping, Defensive
Coping: Family, Compromised
Coping: Family, Disabled
Coping: Family, Readiness for Enhanced
Coping (Individual), Readiness for Enhanced
Coping, Ineffective
Decision Making, Readiness for Enhanced
Decisional Conflict (Specify)
Denial, Ineffective
Dentition, Impaired
Development: Delayed, Risk for
Diarrhea

Disuse Syndrome, Risk for
Diversional Activity, Deficient
Dysreflexia, Autonomic
Dysreflexia, Autonomic, Risk for
Energy Field Disturbance
Environmental Interpretation Syndrome, Impaired
Failure to Thrive, Adult
Falls, Risk for
Family Processes, Dysfunctional: Alcoholism
Family Processes, Interrupted
Family Processes, Readiness for Enhanced
Fatigue
Fear
Fluid Balance, Readiness for Enhanced
Fluid Volume, Deficient
Fluid Volume, Deficient, Risk for
Fluid Volume, Excess
Fluid Volume, Imbalanced, Risk for
Gas Exchange, Impaired
Grieving
Grieving, Complicated
Grieving, Risk for Complicated
Growth, Disproportionate, Risk for
Growth and Development, Delayed
Health Behavior, Risk-Prone
Health Seeking Behaviors (Specify)
Home Maintenance, Impaired
Hope, Readiness for Enhanced
Hopelessness
Human Dignity, Risk for Compromised
Hyperthermia
Hypothermia
Identity: Personal, Disturbed
Immunization Status, Readiness for Enhanced
Infant Behavior, Disorganized
Infant Behavior: Disorganized, Risk for
Infant Behavior: Organized, Readiness for Enhanced
Infant Feeding Pattern, Ineffective
Infection, Risk for
Injury, Risk for
Insomnia
Knowledge, Deficient (Specify)
Knowledge (Specify), Readiness for Enhanced
Lifestyle, Sedentary
Liver Function, Risk for Impaired
Loneliness, Risk for

Memory, Impaired
Mobility: Bed, Impaired
Mobility: Physical, Impaired
Mobility: Wheelchair, Impaired
Moral Distress
Nausea
Neglect, Unilateral
Neurovascular Dysfunction: Peripheral, Risk for
Noncompliance (Specify)
Nutrition, Imbalanced: Less than Body Requirements
Nutrition, Imbalanced: More than Body Requirements
Nutrition, Imbalanced: More than Body Requirements,
    Risk for
Nutrition, Readiness for Enhanced
Oral Mucous Membrane, Impaired
Pain, Acute
Pain, Chronic
Parenting, Impaired
Parenting, Readiness for Enhanced
Parenting, Risk for Impaired
Perioperative Positioning Injury, Risk for
Poisoning, Risk for
Post-Trauma Syndrome
Post-Trauma Syndrome, Risk for
Power, Readiness for Enhanced
Powerlessness
Powerlessness, Risk for
Protection, Ineffective
Rape-Trauma Syndrome
Rape-Trauma Syndrome: Compound Reaction
Rape-Trauma Syndrome: Silent Reaction
Religiosity, Impaired
Religiosity, Readiness for Enhanced
Religiosity, Risk for Impaired
Relocation Stress Syndrome
Relocation Stress Syndrome, Risk for
Role Conflict, Parental
Role Performance, Ineffective
Self-Care, Readiness for Enhanced
Self-Care Deficit: Bathing/Hygiene
Self-Care Deficit: Dressing/Grooming
Self-Care Deficit: Feeding
Self-Care Deficit: Toileting
Self-Concept, Readiness for Enhanced
Self-Esteem, Chronic Low
Self-Esteem, Risk for Situational Low
Self-Esteem, Situational Low
Self-Mutilation
Self-Mutilation, Risk for
Sensory Perception, Disturbed (Specify: Visual, Auditory,
    Kinesthetic, Gustatory, Tactile, Olfactory)

Sexual Dysfunction
Sexuality Pattern, Ineffective
Skin Integrity, Impaired
Skin Integrity, Risk for Impaired
Sleep Deprivation
Sleep, Readiness for Enhanced
Social Interaction, Impaired
Social Isolation
Sorrow, Chronic
Spiritual Distress
Spiritual Distress, Risk for
Spiritual Well-Being, Readiness for
    Enhanced
Stress Overload
Sudden Infant Death Syndrome, Risk for
Suffocation, Risk for
Suicide, Risk for
Surgical Recovery, Delayed
Swallowing, Impaired
Therapeutic Regimen Management: Community,
    Ineffective
Therapeutic Regimen Management, Effective
Therapeutic Regimen Management: Family,
    Ineffective
Therapeutic Regimen Management, Ineffective
Therapeutic Regimen Management, Readiness
    for Enhanced
Thermoregulation, Ineffective
Thought Processes, Disturbed
Tissue Integrity, Impaired
Tissue Perfusion, Ineffective (Specify: Renal, Cerebral,
    Cardiopulmonary, Gastrointestinal, Peripheral)
Transfer Ability, Impaired
Trauma, Risk for
Urinary Elimination, Impaired
Urinary Elimination, Readiness for
    Enhanced
Urinary Incontinence, Functional
Urinary Incontinence, Overflow
Urinary Incontinence, Reflex
Urinary Incontinence, Risk for Urge
Urinary Incontinence, Stress
Urinary Incontinence, Total
Urinary Incontinence, Urge
Urinary Retention
Ventilation, Impaired Spontaneous
Ventilatory Weaning Response, Dysfunctional
Violence: Other-Directed, Risk for
Violence: Self-Directed, Risk for
Walking, Impaired
Wandering

Appendix III

Sample Critical Pathway for Client Following Total Mastectomy

ASSESSMENT DATA

NURSING ASSESSMENT FOR HELEN MORTON Mrs. Helen Morton, 36 years old, was admitted for a right mastectomy. She had a positive biopsy for breast cancer two weeks prior to admission. On admission to ambulatory surgery, Mrs. Morton asked the nurse, "Will I ever look normal again?" She also told the nurse, "I don't want any visitors after surgery; I don't want anyone to see how I look." The day following surgery, Mrs. Morton states, "I don't want to look at it," when the physician starts the dressing change.

Physical Examination
  Height: 167.6 cm (5'6")
  Weight: 65 kg (143 lbs)
  Temperature: 37°C (98.6°F)
  Pulse rate: 76 bpm
  Respirations: 20/minute
  Blood pressure: 120/80 mm Hg

Skin warm, dry, pink, and pale
Mastectomy incision clean, dry, and well approximated

Diagnostic Data
  RBC: 4.2 million/μL
  Hgb: 10.2 g/dL
  Hct: 39%
  Urine: negative
  Expected length of stay: 3 to 4 days
  Daily outcomes
  Tests and treatments
  Knowledge deficit
  Diet
  Activity
  Medications
  Body image
  Psychosocial
  Transfer/discharge plans

Expected Length of Stay: 3 to 4 Days

	DATE _____ FIRST 24 HOURS POSTOPERATIVE	DATE _____ 48 HOURS POSTOPERATIVE	DATE _____ 3–4 DAYS POSTOPERATIVE
Daily outcomes	Client will ■ Be afebrile. ■ Have clean, dry dressing. ■ Recover from anesthesia as evidenced by vital signs return to baseline; being awake, alert, and oriented. ■ Verbalize understanding and demonstrate cooperation with turning, coughing, deep breathing, and splinting. ■ Tolerate ordered diet without nausea and vomiting. ■ Verbalize control of incisional pain. ■ Verbalize ability to cope.	Client will ■ Be afebrile. ■ Have clean, dry wound with edges well approximated, healing by first intention. ■ Demonstrate cooperation with turning, coughing, deep breathing, and splinting. ■ Tolerate ordered diet without nausea and vomiting. ■ Ambulate 4 times per day in hallway. ■ Verbalize control of incisional pain. ■ Verbalize beginning ability to cope with changes in body image. ■ Verbalize ability to cope. ■ Verbalize beginning understanding of home care instructions.	Client will ■ Be afebrile. ■ Have clean, dry wound with edges well approximated, healing by first intention. ■ Manages pain with oral medications and/or nonpharmacologic measures. ■ Be independent in self-care. ■ Be fully ambulatory. ■ Have resumed preadmission urine and bowel elimination pattern. ■ Verbalize home care instructions. ■ Tolerate usual diet. ■ Verbalize ability to cope with changes in body image and ongoing stressors. ■ Demonstrate progressive upper extremity exercises that include external rotation and abduction of the affected shoulder when the stitches are removed 7 to 10 days after surgery.

Expected Length of Stay: 3 to 4 Days (*continued*)

	DATE _____ **FIRST 24 HOURS POSTOPERATIVE**	DATE _____ **48 HOURS POSTOPERATIVE**	DATE _____ **3–4 DAYS POSTOPERATIVE**
Tests and treatments	Vital signs and O$_2$ saturation, neurovascular assessment, dressing and wound drainage assessment q15min × 4; q30min × 4; q1h × 4 and then q4h if stable. NO BLOOD PRESSURES OR VENIPUNCTURE ON AFFECTED ARM. Assess respiratory status q4h and prn. Incentive spirometer q2h. Intake and output q shift. Assess voiding—if unable to void, try suggestive voiding techniques or catheterize q8h or prn.	Vital signs and dressing and wound drainage assessment q4h. NO BLOOD PRESSURES OR VENIPUNCTURE ON AFFECTED ARM. Assess respiratory status q4h. Incentive spirometer q2h until fully ambulatory. Intake and output q shift. Assess voiding pattern q shift. Dressing change by surgeon.	Vital signs and dressing and wound drainage assessment q4h–8h. NO BLOOD PRESSURES OR VENIPUNCTURE ON AFFECTED ARM. Assess respiratory status q4h–8h. Assess wound and apply dry sterile dressing q day and prn.
Knowledge deficit	Orient to room and surroundings. Provide simple, brief instructions. Review preoperative preparation, including hospital and specific postoperative care: turning, coughing, deep breathing, incentive spirometer, mobilization, intravenous infusions, pain management.	Review plan of care and importance of early mobilization. Begin discharge teaching regarding wound care/dressing change, diet, and activity. Review written discharge instructions with client and support person.	Complete discharge teaching to include wound care, diet, follow-up care, signs and symptoms to report, activity, and medication: frequency, dose, route, and side effects. Provide client with written discharge instructions including upper arm and shoulder exercises for affected arm.
Diet	Clear to full liquids as tolerated.	Full liquids to usual diet to tolerance.	Usual diet to tolerance.
Activity	Provide safety precautions. Ambulate 4 times in room. Encourage finger, wrist, and elbow movement and use of affected arm for ADLs and personal hygiene.	Fully ambulatory in room. Walk in hall 4 to 6 times per day. Encourage finger, wrist, and elbow movement and use of affected arm for ADLs and personal hygiene. Instruct client in progressive upper arm exercises.	Fully ambulatory. Encourage finger, wrist, and elbow movement and use of affected arm for ADLs and personal hygiene. Reinforce instructions regarding progressive exercises.
Medications	IM or IV/PCA analgesics. IV antibiotics. IV fluids.	PO, IM, or IV/PCA analgesics. IV antibiotics. Intermittent IV device.	PO analgesics. Discontinue IV device.
Body image	Establish a trusting relationship with client. Encourage client and significant others to verbalize their feelings about the mastectomy. Listen to client and significant others and show interest and concern rather than giving advice. Allow the client to respond to loss of body part and changed body image with denial, shock, anger, depression, and other grieving behaviors. Support the client's strengths and assist her to look at herself in totality.	Maintain trusting relationship with client. Encourage client and significant others to verbalize their feelings about the mastectomy. Listen to client and significant others and show interest and concern rather than giving advice. Allow the client to respond to loss of body part and changed body image with denial, shock, anger, depression, and other grieving behaviors. Support the client's strengths and assist her to look at herself in totality.	Provide opportunities to verbalize ongoing concerns regarding changes in body image and self-concept. Encourage and provide opportunities for self-care of wound and dressing. Provide opportunity for client to meet with volunteer from Reach to Recovery. Assist client to obtain temporary breast prosthesis. Answer questions and provide information on breast reconstruction. (*continued*)

Expected Length of Stay: 3 to 4 Days (*continued*)

	DATE _____ **FIRST 24 HOURS POSTOPERATIVE**	DATE _____ **48 HOURS POSTOPERATIVE**	DATE _____ **3–4 DAYS POSTOPERATIVE**
Psychosocial	Assess coping status. Use active listening. Provide a nonthreatening environment. Determine support people and resources available to the client. Assess responses of support people. Allow for client's input regarding sequence of care. Be supportive of client's effective coping behaviors.	Assess coping status. Use active listening. Provide a nonthreatening environment. Assist client to identify and develop support system and resources. Assess responses of support people. Allow for client's input regarding sequence of care. Be supportive of client's effective coping behaviors.	Assess coping status. Use active listening. Provide a nonthreatening environment. Determine support people and resources available to the client. Assess responses of support people. Allow for client's input regarding sequence of care. Be supportive of client's effective coping behaviors.
Transfer/ discharge plans	Determine discharge needs with client and support people. Begin home care instructions.	Review progress toward discharge goals. Finalize discharge plans. Refer to Reach to Recovery.	Complete discharge instructions.

Appendix IV

Weapons of Mass Destruction Awareness Training

Source: WMD Awareness Level Training
Student Manual AWR-160
U.S. Department of Homeland Security

INTRODUCTION

OBJECTIVE   Designed to prepare individuals who, in the course of their everyday duties, "are likely to witness or discover a hazardous substance release . . ." (OSHA 1910.120.(q)(6)(i)).

DEFINITIONS

CBRNE: **C**—chemical agent, **B**—biological hazard, **R**—radiological hazard, **N**—nuclear hazard, **E**—explosives

Terrorism: A criminal act intended to intimidate or coerce the civilian population or influence a government. Activities include, but are not limited to, acts dangerous to human life or having the potential for destruction of critical infrastructure or any key resource.

Weapons of mass destruction (WMD): Any weapon that is designed or intended to cause death or serious bodily injury through the release, dissemination, or impact of toxic or poisonous chemicals or their precursors. Any weapon involving a disease organism or that is designed to release radiation or radioactivity at a level dangerous to human life.

AWARENESS

FACTORS OF THREAT

Means of attack: Limited to the terrorist's imagination. According to federal authorities, the most likely scenario is an improvised explosive device.

Surprise: The element of surprise in a terrorist attack allows more reward to the terrorist.

Target of the attack: Targets may vary; however, the goal is mass casualties.

POTENTIAL TARGETS

- Schools
- High-rise residences
- Hospitals
- Transportation systems
- Emergency services

INITIAL ACTIONS

RAIN   RAIN is an acronym used by individuals to quickly gather and process information and to synthesize the information in order to facilitate life safety actions in a WMD incident.

- **Recognize** the hazard/threat (What do I see, hear, or smell?)
  - Multiple victims with the same signs and symptoms may indicate a potential WMD release (convulsions, dyspnea, or vomiting.)
  - Listen for hissing sounds that may indicate pressure releases. Listen to what people are saying.
  - The sense of smell may detect odors, but may be dangerous if you are too close to the source.
  - Do not touch or taste anything that has not been identified.
- **Avoid** the hazard/contamination/injury (What do I stay away from?)
  - **"Time, distance, and shielding"**: Avoid exposure time, put distance between you and the threat, and put protective equipment/barriers between you and the threat.
- **Isolate** the hazard area (Whom do I protect?)
  - Evacuate the area *or*
  - Shelter in place if evacuation is not possible. This is done by seeking a safe place in the building.
  - Close all windows, doors, and shut off ventilation systems.
  - Sheltering in place is often used by hospitals and facilities with nonambulatory patients.
- **Notify** the appropriate support (Whom do I call?)
  - Follow your employer's policies and procedures.

RECOGNITION OF WMD AGENTS

Biological agents as WMD: Biological attacks may mimic naturally occurring diseases. The first clues to a biological attack may be large numbers of patients with the same illness within a few days; occurrence of an unusual disease for a region; the appearance of an illness "out of season" or one that was thought to have been eradicated (smallpox.)

Chemical agents as WMD: Chemical incidents are characterized by the rapid onset of medical symptoms (minutes to hours) and easily observed signatures (colored residue, dead foliage, pungent odor, and dead insect and animal life.)

Explosive devices as WMD: According to the FBI, approximately 70% of all terrorist incidents involve the use of explosives and incendiary agents. These devices are designed to cause injury and/or death through burn or inhalation injuries and through penetrating injury from shrapnel. When involved in an incident with explosives, remember one thing: *If you can see the explosive device, then it can see you!* Many people have been severely or fatally injured as a result of their curiosity.

Radiological materials and nuclear weapons: Signs and symptoms will vary based on the type of material that a person is exposed to, the amount of time the patient was exposed, and whether there was any protection in place during the exposure. The patient may be either exposed or actually contaminated. This will also dictate the level of symptoms. Get a history of the exposure.

References and Resources

CHAPTER 1

Baer, E. D., D'Antonio, P., Rinker, S., & Lynaugh, J. E. (Eds.) (2000). *Enduring issues in American nursing*. Philadelphia: Springhouse Corporation.

Barber, M. F. (1992). In R. Smolan (Ed.), *The power to heal: Ancient arts & modern medicine*. Upper Saddle River, NJ: Prentice Hall.

Creighton, J. (1998, December 28). Nurse on cap hunt. *The Toronto Sun*, p. A-28.

Dolan, J. A., Fitzpatrick, M. L., & Herrmann, E. K. (1983). *Nursing in society: A historical perspective* (15th ed.). Philadelphia: W. B. Saunders.

Edmonds, S. E., & Leonard, E. D. (1999). *Memoirs of a soldier, nurse and spy: A woman's adventures in the Union Army*. DeKalb, IL: Northern Illinois University Press.

Ellis, J. R., & Hartley, C. L. (2001). *Nursing in today's world: Challenges, issues & trends* (7th ed.). Philadelphia: Lippincott Williams & Wilkins.

Hamilton, P. M. (1999). *Realities of contemporary nursing* (2nd ed.). Menlo Park, CA: Addison-Wesley.

Kelly, L. Y., & Joel, L. A. (1999). *Dimensions of professional nursing* (8th ed.). New York: McGraw-Hill.

Kowalski, K., Burton, L., & Rehwaldt, M. (1997, September/October). Revisioning, re-educating, regenerating, and recommitting nursing for the twenty-first century. *Nursing Outlook, 45*, 220–223.

Lang-Otsuka, P. A. (Ed.). (2002). *Pathophysiology made incredibly easy*. Philadelphia: Springhouse–Lippincott William & Wilkins.

National Federation of Licensed Practical Nursing. (2003). *Nursing practice standards for the licensed practical/vocational nurse*. Garner, NC: Author.

Nelson, S. (2002). The fork in the road: Nursing history vs. the history of nursing. In *Nursing history review* (Vol. 10). Lanoka, NJ: American Association for the History of Nursing, Inc.

Nightingale, F. (1860). *Notes on nursing: What it is, and what it is not* (commemorative ed.). Philadelphia: Lippincott.

Norman, E. (2000). *We band of angels*. New York: Pocket Books.

Porter, L. (n.d.). *Notes on how to read a textbook* (unpublished). Anaheim, CA: North Orange County Regional Occupational Program.

Ramsom, C. B. (2003). *Clara Barton history maker bios*. Berkeley, CA: Lerner Publication Company.

Sandelowski, M. (2000). *Devices & desires: Gender, technology and American nursing*. Chapel Hill: University of North Carolina Press.

Schorr, T. M., with Kennedy, M. S. (1999). *100 years of American nursing*. Philadelphia: Lippincott.

Schuyler, C. B. (1992). Florence Nightingale. In F. Nightingale, *Notes on nursing: What it is, and what it is not* (commemorative ed., pp. 3–17). Philadelphia: Lippincott.

Sorel, N. C. (2000). *The women who wrote the war*. New York: Harper Perennial.

Wake, R. (1998). *The Nightingale Training School 1860–1996*. London: Haggerstown Press.

Wood, W. (Ed.). (1999, December 13). Century in review. *Nurseweek, 12*(25), 1.

Zerwekh, J., & Claborn, J. C. (2002). *Nursing today: Transition and trends* (3rd ed.). Philadelphia: W. B. Saunders.

CHAPTER 2

Adler, R. B., Rosenfeld, L. B., Towne, N., & Proctor, R. F., III. (1998). *Interplay: The process of interpersonal communication*. Fort Worth, TX: Harcourt Brace College Publishers.

American Association of Colleges of Nursing. (1999). *Nursing educational agenda for the 21st century*. Washington, DC: Author.

American Nurses Association. (2000). *New position statement: Adolescent Health Task Force*. Washington, DC: Author.

Anderson, M. M., & Boyle, J. S. (1999). *Transcultural concepts in nursing care* (3rd ed.). Philadelphia: Lippincott.

Bakker, l. (1995). Communicating across cultures. *Nursing 95, 25*(1), 79–80.

Banks, C., & Banks, J. (1995). Equity pedagogy: An essential component of multicultural education. *Theory into Practice, 34*(3).

Bengiamin, M. I., Downey, V. W., & Heuer, L. J. (1999). Transcultural healthcare: A phenomenological study of an educational experience. *Journal of Cultural Diversity, 6*(2), 60–68.

Bowers, P. (2000). *Cultural perspectives in childbearing* (Nursing spectrum self-study module). Retrieved July 27, 2003, from http://nsweb.nursingspectrum.com/ce

Boyd, M. D., Gleit, C. J., Graham, B. A., & Whitman, N. I. (1997). *Health teaching in nursing practice: A professional model* (3rd ed.). Upper Saddle River, NJ: Prentice Hall.

Butler, J. P. (1994). Of kindred minds: The ties that bind. In M. A. Orlandi (Ed.), *Cultural competence for evaluators: A guide for alcohol and other drug abuse prevention practitioners working with ethnic/racial communities: Theory and practice*. Washington DC: U.S. Department of Health and Human Services.

Clark, L., Zuk, J., & Baramee, J. (2000). A literacy approach to teaching cultural competence . . . reading of the book *The Spirit Catches You and You Fall Down. Journal of Transcultural Nursing*, 11, 199–203.

Cross, T., et al. (1989). *Towards a culturally competent system of care*. Washington, DC: Georgetown University Child Development Center for Child Health and Mental Health Policy.

Davidhizar, R., & Giger, J. (1997, November/December). Pain and the culturally diverse patient. *Today's Surgical Nurse*, pp. 36–39.

Denboba, D. (1993). *MCHB/DSCSHCN guidance for competitive applications*. Maternal and Child Health Improvement Projects for Children with Special Health Care Needs.

Finucane, M. (2000). Presented at Second National Conference on Quality Health Care for Culturally Diverse Populations: Strategy and Action for Communities, Providers and a Changing Health System, Los Angeles, CA, October 11–14, 2000.

Flaskerud, J. H. (2002). *Culturally competent neuropsychiatric NP program*. Los Angeles: UCLA School of Nursing. Retrieved July 27, 2003, from http://bhpr.hrsa.gov/nursing/fy02grants/abstracts

Galanti, G. A. (1997). *Caring for patients from different cultures: Case studies from American hospitals*. Philadelphia: University of Pennsylvania Press.

Giger, J. N., & Davidhizar, R. E. (2000). *Transcultural nursing: Assessment and intervention* (3rd ed.). St. Louis, MO: Mosby.

Leininger, M. (1997). Understanding cultural pain for improved health care. *Journal of Transcultural Nursing, 9*(1), 32–35.

Leininger, M., McFarland, M., & McFarlane, M. (2002). *Transcultural nursing* (3rd ed.). New York: McGraw-Hill Professional.

Mbiti, J. B. African religions and philosophies. Garden City, NY: Anchor Books, as cited in W. Nobles, African philosophy: Foundations for Black psychology, in R. H. Jones (Ed.). (1972). *Black psychology*. New York: Harper & Row.

National Association of Neonatal Nurses. (1999). Position Paper on Cultural Competence #3037 Glenview, IL: Author. Retrieved July 27, 2003, from www.nann.org/files/public/3037.doc

O'Brien, J. (2000). Presented at Second National Conference on Quality Health Care for Culturally Diverse Populations: Strategy and Action for Communities, Providers and a Changing Health System, Los Angeles, CA, October 11–14, 2000.

Pachter, L. M. (1996). Cultural issues in pediatric care (pp. 16–17). In W. E. Nelson, R. E. Behrman, R. M. Kinegman, & A. M. Arvin (Eds.), *Nelson's textbook of pediatrics* (15th ed.). Philadelphia: W. B. Saunders.

Purnell, L. D., & Paulanka, B. J. (1998). *Transcultural health care: A culturally competent approach.* Philadelphia: F. A. Davis.

Roberts, R., et al. (1990). *Developing culturally competent programs for families of children with special needs.* Washington, DC: Georgetown University Child Development Center.

Robinson, J. H. (2000). Increasing students' cultural sensitivity: A steep toward greater diversity in nursing. *Nurse Educator, 25*(3), 131–135.

Ryan, M., Carlton, K. H., & Ali, N. (2000). Transcultural nursing concepts and experiences in nursing curricula. *Journal of Transcultural Nursing, 11*(4), 300–307.

Steelfel, L. (2003, June 1). No cookie cutter approach to postpartum culture care. *Nursing Spectrum* [Online]. Retrieved July 26, 2003, from http://community.nursingspectrum.com/MagazineArticle

Taylor, D., Polan, E., & Weitzman, J. P (2003). *Journey across the life span: Human growth and development and health promotion* (2nd ed.). Philadelphia: F. A. Davis.

U.S. Department of Health and Human Services. (2000). *Health People 2010.* Washington, DC: Author.

HRSA, Office of Minority Health, Cultural Competence Workgroup; 1998.

CHAPTER 3

American Nurses Association (1998). *Standards of clinical nursing practice* (2nd ed.). Washington, DC: Author.

Anderson, M. A. (2001). *Nursing leadership, management, and professional practice for the LPN/LVN* (2nd ed.). Philadelphia: F. A. Davis.

Burke, L., & Weill, B. (2000). *Information technology for health care professionals.* Upper Saddle River, NJ: Prentice Hall.

Brent, N. J. (1997). *Nurses and the law.* Philadelphia: W. B. Saunders.

Centers for Disease Control and Prevention. (2001). *Guidelines for HIV counseling, testing and referral.* Atlanta, GA: Author.

Equal Employment Opportunity Commission. (1980). Sex discrimination guidelines. In *EEOC Rules and Regulation.* Chicago: Commerce Clearing House.

Nightingale, F. (1992). *Notes on nursing.* Philadelphia: J. B. Lippincott (original work published 1859).

Norman, J. C. (2000). HIV/AIDS: Epidemic update. *CME Resources, 67*(7), 12–36.

Smith, K. V. (1996). Ethical decision-making by staff nurses. *Nursing Ethics: An International Journal for Health Care Professionals, 3*(1), 17–25.

Taylor, P., & Ferszt, G. (1998, August). The nurse as patient advocate. *Nursing 98, 28*(8), 70–71.

Wood, L. C., & DelPapa, L. A. (1996). Nurses' attitudes, ethical reasons, and knowledge of the law concerning advance directives. *Image: Journal of Nursing Scholarship, 28*(4), 371.

CHAPTER 4

Andrews, M. M., & Boyle, J. S. (1999). *Transcultural concepts in nursing care* (3rd ed.). Philadelphia: Lippincott.

Fawcett, J. (1995). *Analysis and evaluation of conceptual models of nursing* (3rd ed.). Philadelphia: F. A. Davis.

Johnson, D. E. (1980). The behavioral system model in nursing. In J. P. Riehl & C. Roy (Eds.), *Conceptual models for nursing practice* (2nd ed.). New York: Appleton-Century-Croft.

Kurzen, C. (2001). *Contemporary practical/vocational nursing* (4th ed.). Philadelphia: J. B. Lippincott.

Neuman, B. (1989). In conclusion—transition. In B. Neuman (Ed.), *The Neuman systems model* (2nd ed.). Norwalk, CT: Appleton & Lange.

Orem, D. E. (1991). *Nursing: Concepts of practice* (4th ed.). St. Louis, MO: Mosby-Year Book.

Paul, R. W., & Elder, L. (2001). *Critical thinking.* Upper Saddle River, NJ: Pearson Education.

CHAPTER 5

Ackley, B. J., & Ladwig, G. B. (2005). *Mosby's guide to nursing diagnosis.* St. Louis, MO: Mosby.

Ackley, B. J., & Ladwig, G. B. (2006). *Nursing diagnosis handbook: A guide to planning care* (7th ed.). St. Louis, MO: Mosby.

Alfaro-LeFevre, R. (2005). *Applying the nursing process: A tool for critical thinking.* Philadelphia: Lippincott.

American Nurses Association. (1998). *Standards of clinical nursing practice* (2nd ed). Kansas City, MO: Author.

Anderson, M. A. (2005). *Nursing leadership, management, and professional practice for the LPN/LVN: In nursing school and beyond.* Philadelphia: F. A. Davis.

Boucher, M. A. (1998, February). Delegation alert. *American Journal of Nursing, 98*(2), 26–32.

Carpenito, L. J. (2005a). *Handbook of nursing diagnosis* (11th ed.). Philadelphia: Lippincott Williams & Wilkins.

Carpenito, L. J. (2005b). *Nursing diagnosis: Application to clinical practice* (11th ed.). Philadelphia: Lippincott Williams & Wilkins.

Johnson, M., et al. (2005). *Nursing diagnosis, outcomes, & interventions: NANDA, NOC, & NIC Linkages, nursing interventions classification 4e, Nursing Outcomes Classification 3e* (2nd ed.). St. Louis, MO: Mosby.

Joint Commission on Accreditation of Healthcare Organizations. (2002). *Accreditation manual for hospitals.* Chicago: Author.

McCloskey, J. C., & Bulechek, G. M. (Eds.). (2003). *Nursing interventions classification (NIC).* (4th ed.). St. Louis, MO: Mosby-Year Book.

North American Nursing Diagnosis Association. (2005). *Nursing diagnoses: Definitions & classification, 2005–2006.* Philadelphia: Author.

Wilkinson, J. M. (2001). *Nursing process: A critical thinking approach* (p. 4). Menlo Park, CA: Addison Wesley.

Wilkinson, J. M. (2004). *Nursing diagnosis handbook with NIC interventions and NOC outcomes* (7th ed.). Upper Saddle River, NJ: Prentice Hall.

CHAPTER 6

American Nurses Association. (1985). *Code for nurses.* Kansas City, MO: Author.

Austin, S. (2006). "Ladies & Gentlemen of the jury, I present . . . the nursing documentation." *Nursing, 36*(1), 56–62.

Coty, E., Davis, J., & Angell, L. (2002). *Documentation: The language of nursing.* Upper Saddle River, NJ: Prentice Hall.

Iyer, P. W., & Camp, N. H. (2005). *Nursing documentation: A nursing process approach* (4th ed.). Flemington, NJ: Med League Support Services, Inc.

Joint Commission on Accreditation of Healthcare Organizations. (2000). *2000 accreditation manual for hospitals.* Chicago: Author.

Joint Commission on Accreditation of Healthcare Organizations. (2002). *Management of information update 3/14/02.* Chicago: Author.

Malestic, S. L. (2003). A Quick Guide to Verbal Reports. *RN, 66*(2), 47–49.

Marrelli, T. M. (2000). *Nursing documentation handbook.* St. Louis, MO: Elsevier.

Springhouse Corporation. (1995). *Mastering documentation.* Springhouse, PA: Author.

Springhouse Corporation. (2002a). *Charting made incredibly easy!* Springhouse, PA: Author.

Springhouse Corporation. (2002b). *Skillmasters: Better documentation.* Springhouse, PA: Author.

Springhouse Corporation. (2006). *Chart smart: The A–Z guide to better nursing documentation.* Springhouse, PA: Author.

White, L. (2002). *Documentation and the nursing process, a review.* Clifton Park, NY: Thomson Delmar Learning.

Yocum, R. F., (2002). Documenting for quality patient care: Chart a course for productivity, quality, and efficiency. *Nursing, 32*(8), 58–63.

CHAPTER 7

Abrams, W., Beers, M., & Berkow, R. (Eds.). (2004). *The Merck manual of health and aging* (3rd ed.). Whitehouse Station, NJ: Merck.

American Hospital Association. (1992). *A patient's bill of rights.* Chicago: Author.

American Hospital Association. (2006). *Protecting and improving care for patients and communities: Coordinating care for the chronically ill.* Retrieved from www.aha.org/content/2006

Avery-Wall, V. (2006). Are you religious sensitive? *AHA News Now.* Retrieved August 21, 2006, from www.ahanews.com

Stoker, J. (2000, February). The Omnibus Consolidation Appropriation Act of 2000. *Home HealthCare Nurse, 18*(2), 84.

Thomas, K. K. (1999). American Academy of Nursing's Women's Health Expert Panel recommendations for women's health and women's health care. *Nursing Outlook, 47*(1), 43.

U.S. Department of Health and Human Services. (2000). *Healthy people 2010: Understanding and improving health* (2nd ed.). Washington, DC: U.S. Government Printing Office.

U.S. Department of Health and Human Services. (2002). *Confronting the new health care crisis: Improving health care quality and lowering costs by fixing our medical liability system.* Washington, DC: U.S. Government Printing Office.

U.S. Department of Justice and Federal Trade Commission. (2004). *Improving health care: A dose of competition.* Washington, DC: U.S. Government Printing Office.

U.S. Department of Labor, Bureau of Labor Statistics (1999 and various years). *Employee benefit survey.* Washington, DC: U.S. Government Printing Office.

Whelchel, C. (2004). Patient first when budging. *Nursing Management, 35*(2), 16.

CHAPTER 8

American Heart Association. (2005). Highlights of the 2005 American Heart Association guidelines for cardiopulmonary resuscitation and emergency cardiovascular care, *Currents in Emergency Cardiovascular Care, 16*(4), 9–16. Retrieved February 18, 2006, from www.americanheart.org/downloadable/heart/1132621842912 Winter2005.pdf

Arias, K. M. (Ed.). (2000). *Quick reference to outbreak investigation and control in health care facilities.* New York: Aspen.

Bonder, B., & Wagner, M. B. (2001). *Functional performance in older adults.* Philadelphia: F. A. Davis.

Brenner, Z. R. (1998). Toward restraint-free care. *American Journal of Nursing, 98*(12), 16F–16I.

Centers for Disease Control and Prevention. (1987, August 21). *Recommendations for prevention of HIV transmission in health-care settings.* Retrieved March 17, 2005, from http://wonder.cdc.gov/wonder/prevguide/p0000318/p0000318.asp

Charney, W. (Ed.). (1999). *Handbook of modern hospital safety.* Boca Raton, FL: Lewis Publishing.

Doenges, M. E., & Moorhouse, M. F. (2003). *Application of nursing process and nursing diagnoses: An interactive text for diagnostic reasoning* (4th ed.). Philadelphia: F. A. Davis.

Edelman, C. L., & Mandle, C. L. (2002). *Health promotion throughout the lifespan* (5th ed.). St. Louis, MO: Mosby.

Hutton, J. T., Elias, W., Shroyer, J. A., & Curry, Z. (2000). *Preventing falls: A defensive approach.* Amherst, NY: Prometheus Books.

Kobs, A. (1998). Questions and answers from the JCAHO. Restraints revisited. *Nursing Management, 29*(1), 17–18.

Occupational Safety and Health Administration. (1992, July 1). *Intro to 29 CFR Part 1910, Occupational Exposure to Bloodborne Pathogens.* Retrieved March 17, 2006, from www.osha-slc.gov/pls/oshaweb/owadisp.show_document?p_table=PREAMBLES&p_text_version=FALSE

Springhouse Corporation. (1998). *Healthcare professionals guide: Safety and infection control.* Springhouse, PA: Author.

Tai, E. (2000). *OSHA compliance management: A guide for long-term health care facilities.* Boca Raton, FL: Lewis Publishing.

Tideiksaar, R. (2002). *Falls in older persons.* Baltimore, MD: Health Professions Press.

Wagner, K. D., Rounds, C. D., Spurgin, R., & Biello, L. (1998). *Environmental management in healthcare facilities.* Philadelphia: W. B. Saunders.

Wilkinson, J. M. (2005). *Nursing diagnosis handbook* (8th ed.). Upper Saddle River, NJ: Prentice Hall.

CHAPTER 9

Carpenito, L. J. (2005). *Handbook of nursing diagnosis* (11th ed.). Philadelphia: Lippincott.

Carrico, R. (Ed.). (2005). *APIC text of infection control and epidemiology: Principles of microbial pathogenicity and host response* (2nd ed.). Washington, DC: Association for Professionals in Infection Control and Epidemiology.

Centers for Disease Control and Prevention. (1996). Guidelines for isolation precautions in hospitals, Part 1: Evolution of isolation practices. *American Journal of Infection Control, 24*(1), 24–31.

Centers for Disease Control and Prevention. (1998). *Guidelines for infection control in health care personnel.* Atlanta, GA: Author.

Centers for Disease Control and Prevention. (2001, June 29). Updated U.S. Public Health Service guidelines for the management of occupational exposures to HBV, HCV, and HIV and recommendations for postexposure prophylaxis. *MMWR.*

Centers for Disease Control and Prevention. (2002, October 25). Guidelines for hand hygiene in health care settings: Recommendations of the Healthcare Infection Control Practices Committee. *MMWR, 51*(RR16), 1–44.

Centers for Disease Control and Prevention. (2005, September 30). *Controlling tuberculosis in the United States.* Atlanta, GA: Author.

Centers for Disease Control and Prevention. (2005, December 30). *Guidelines for preventing the transmission of Mycobacterium tuberculosis in health-care settings.* Atlanta, GA: Author.

Harkness, G. A., & Dincher, J. K. (1999). *Medical-surgical nursing: Total patient care* (10th ed.). St. Louis, MO: Mosby.

LeMone, P., & Burke, K. M. (2000). *Medical-surgical nursing: Critical thinking in patient care* (2nd ed.). Upper Saddle River, NJ: Prentice Hall.

Needlestick Prevention Act, U.S. Congress, March 2000.

Nettina, S. M. (Ed.). (2000). *The Lippincott manual of nursing practice* (7th ed.). Philadelphia: Lippincott Williams & Wilkins.

North American Nursing Diagnosis Association. (2005). *Nursing diagnoses: Definitions & classification, 2005–2006.* Philadelphia: Author.

OSHA Enforcement Procedure for Bloodborne Pathogens Regulation, CPL 2–2. 69, November 27, 2001.

Smith, S. F., Duell, D. J., & Martin, B. C. (2000). *Clinical nursing skills: Basic to advanced* (5th ed.). Upper Saddle River, NJ: Prentice Hall.

Springhouse Corporation. (1998). *Healthcare professional guides: Safety and infection control.* Springhouse, PA: Author.

Timby, B. K., Scherer, J. C., & Smith, N. E. (1999). *Introductory medical-surgical nursing* (7th ed.). Philadelphia: Lippincott.

CHAPTER 10

Grubbs, P., & Blasband, B. (2000). *The long-term care nursing assistant* (2nd ed.). Upper Saddle River, NJ: Prentice Hall.

Kellter, P. G., & Sucher, K. P. (1990). Diet counseling in a multicultural society. *Diabetes Education, 39,* 127–134.

Kongstvedt, P. R. (2001). *The managed health care handbook* (4th ed.). Sudbury, MA: Jones and Bartlett Publishers.

Pulliam, J. (2002). *The nursing assistant: Acute, subacute and long-term care* (3rd ed.). Upper Saddle River, NJ: Prentice Hall.

Wyler-Lawm, P. (2002). Legal nurse consulting—Hospital regulations, *Nursing Economics, 18*(6), 312.

CHAPTER 11

Barkauskas, V., Bauman, L. C., Stoltenberg-Allen, K., & Darling-Fisher, C. (1998). *Health and physical assessment* (2nd ed.). St. Louis, MO: Mosby.

Cicchetti, D. (2000). *The promotion of wellness in children and adolescents: Issues in children's and families' lives.* Stamford, CT: Appleton & Lange.

Edelman, C., & Mandle, C. L. (2006). *Health promotion throughout the life span* (6th ed.). St. Louis, MO: Mosby.

Eliopoulos, C. (2001). *Gerontological nursing* (5th ed.). Philadelphia: Lippincott.

Erikson, E. H. (1963). *Childhood and society* (2nd ed.). New York: Norton.

Erikson, E. H. (1982). *The life cycle completed: A review.* New York: Norton.

Erickson, E. H., & Joan M. (1997). *The life cycle completed.* New York: W. W. Norton and Company.

Fontaine, K. L. (2003). *Mental health nursing* (5th ed.). Upper Saddle River, NJ: Prentice Hall.

Piaget, J. (1966). *Origins of intelligence in children.* New York: Norton.

U.S. Bureau of the Census. (2000). Washington, DC: U.S. Government Printing Office.

Wold, G. (1999). *Basic geriatric nursing* (2nd ed.) St. Louis, MO: Mosby-Year Book.

Zator-Estes, M. E. (2001). *Health assessment & physical examination* (2nd ed.). Clifton Park, NY: Delmar Publishing.

CHAPTER 12

Ackley, B. J., & Ladwig, G. B. (2005). *Mosby's guide to nursing diagnosis* (6th ed.). St. Louis, MO: Mosby.

Anderson, M. A. (2001). *Nursing leadership, management and professional practice for the LPN/LVN* (2nd. ed.). Philadelphia: F. A. Davis.

Anderson, M. A. (2005). *Nursing leadership, management and professional practice for LPN/LVN: In nursing school and beyond.* Philadelphia: F. A. Davis.

Anderson, M. A., & Helm, L. B. (2000). Talking about patients: Communication and continuity of care. *Journal of Cardiovascular Nursing, 14*(3), 15.

Arnold, E., & Boggs, K. U. (2003). *Interpersonal relationships: Professional communication skills for nurses* (4th ed.). Philadelphia: W. B. Saunders.

Bateson, G. (2002). *Mind and nature—A necessary unity (advanced systems theory, complexity and the human sciences).* New York: Hampton Press.

Buresh, B., & Gordon, S. (2006). *From silence to voice: What nurses know and must communicate to the public (the culture and politics of health care work).* Ottawa, Ontario: Canadian Nurses Association.

Carpenito, L. J. (2005). *Nursing diagnosis: Application to clinical practice* (11th ed.). Philadelphia: Lippincott.

Deering, C. G. (1999). To speak or not to speak? Self-disclosure with patients. *American Journal of Nursing, 99*(1), 34–39.

Eby, L., & Brown, N. J. (2005). *Mental health nursing care.* Upper Saddle River, NJ: Prentice Hall.

Egan, G. (2002). *The skilled helper: A problem-management and opportunity development approach to helping* (7th ed.). Pacific Grove, CA: Brooks/Cole.

Fontaine, K. L. (2003). *Mental health nursing* (5th ed.). Upper Saddle River, NJ: Prentice Hall.

Hersey, P., Blanchard, K. H., & Johnson, D. E. (2001). Effective communication, Chap. 13 in *Management of organizational behavior: Leading human resources* (8th ed.) Upper Saddle River, NJ: Prentice Hall.

Hodes, R. J. (2004). *Working with your older patient—A clinician's handbook.* Washington, DC: National Institutes of Health, National Institute on Aging.

Purnell, L. D., & Paulanka, B. J. (2004). *Transcultural health care—A culturally competent approach* (2nd ed.). Philadelphia: F. A. Davis.

Reynolds, J. (2004). Letters: Tips for talking to patients. *Nursing 2004, 34*(12), 10.

Sheldon, L. K. (2004). *Communication for nurses: Talking with patients.* Boston: Jones and Bartlett.

Stewart, C. J., & Cash, W. B. (2006). *Interviewing: Principles and practice* (11th ed.). New York: McGraw-Hill.

Tannen, D. (2001). *You just don't understand: Women and men in conversation* (1st Quill ed.). New York: Balantine.

Ufema, J. (2004). Insights on death and dying: Three keys to communication. *Nursing 2004, 34*(10), 12.

CHAPTER 13

Bernstein, D. K., & Tiegerman-Farber, E. (2001). *Language and communication disorders in children* (5th ed.). Boston: Allyn & Bacon.

Bohannon, R. W. (2003). Evaluation and treatment of sensory and perceptual impairments following stroke. *Topics in Geriatric Rehabilitation,19*(2), 87–97.

Bylsma, F. W., & Doninger, F. (2004). Neuropsychological assessment in individuals with severe visual impairment. *Topics in Geriatric Rehabilitation, 20*(3), 196–203.

Centers for Disease Control and Prevention, National Center for Birth Defects and Developmental Disabilities. (2001). *Early Hearing Detection and Intervention Program: What is EHDI?* Retrieved October 15, 2001, from www.cdc.gov/ncbddd/ehdi/ehdi.htm

Clinical do's and don'ts: Talking with a hearing-impaired patient. (2002). *Nursing 2002, 32*(8), 20.

Ebersole, P., & Hess, P. (2001). *Geriatric nursing & healthy aging.* St. Louis, MO: Mosby.

Hasselkus, A., Tenenholtz, E., & Brown, J. (2002). Speech-language pathologists add value to home care. *Home Healthcare Nurse, 20*(6), 393–398.

Jarvis, C. (2000). *Pocket companion for physical examination and health assessment.* Philadelphia: W. B. Saunders.

Lucas, L. J., & Matthews-Flint, L. J. (2003). Hospital nursing—Heed the word about hearing impairment. *Nursing 2003, 33*(10), 32nh1–32hn4.

North American Nursing Diagnosis Association. (2005). *Nursing diagnoses: Definitions & classification, 2005–2006.* Philadelphia: Author.

Pankow, L., Luchins, D., Studebaker, J., & Chettleburg, D. (2004). Evaluation of a vision rehabilitation program for older adults with visual impairment. *Topics in Geriatric Rehabilitation, 20*(3), 223–232.

Papalia, D. E., Olds, S. W., & Feldman, R. D. (2001). *Human development* (8th ed.). Columbus, OH: McGraw-Hill.

CHAPTER 14

Arnold, E., & Boggs, K. U. (2003). *Interpersonal relationships—Professional communication skills for nurses* (4th ed.). Philadelphia: W. B. Saunders.

Carpenito-Moyet, L. J. (2005). *Handbook of nursing diagnosis* (11th ed.). Philadelphia: Lippincott.

Eby, L., & Brown, N. J. (2005). MENTAL HEALTH NURSING CARE. Upper Saddle River, NJ: Prentice Hall.

Edelman, C. L., & Mandle, C. L. (2002). *Health promotion throughout the life span* (5th ed.). St. Louis, MO: Mosby.

Erikson, E. H. (1963). *Childhood and society* (2nd ed.). New York: Norton.

Erikson, E. H., & Erikson, J. M. (1997). *The life cycle completed*. New York: Norton.

Kear, M. (2002, November). Concept analysis of self-efficacy. *Graduate Research in Nursing On-line Journal*. Retrieved March 29, 2005, from www.graduateresearch.com

Neeb, K. (2006). Fundamentals of mental health nursing (3rd ed.). Philadelphia: F. A. Davis.

North American Nursing Diagnosis Association. (2005). *Nursing diagnoses: Definitions & classification, 2005–2006*. Philadelphia: Author.

CHAPTER 15

American Cancer Society. (2001). *Cancer facts and figures—2001*. Atlanta, GA: Author.

Anderson, K. N. (Ed.). *Mosby's medical, nursing, and allied health dictionary (2002).* (6th ed., p. 808). St. Louis, MO: Mosby.

Ball, J., & Bindler, R. (2005). *Pediatric nursing: Caring for children* (2nd ed.). Upper Saddle River, NJ: Prentice Hall.

Brady, M. (1998). Female genital mutilation. *Nursing 98, 28*(9), 50–51.

Carpenito, L. J. (2005). *Handbook of nursing diagnosis* (11th ed.). Philadelphia: Lippincott Williams & Wilkins.

Centers for Disease Control and Prevention. (2002, April 12). *CDC effort to eliminate racial & ethnic disparity in health care*. Atlanta, GA: Author.

Clark, M. J. (2003). *Community health nursing: Caring for the population* (4th ed.). Upper Saddle River, NJ: Pearson Education.

Clayton, B. D., & Stock, Y. (2001). *Basic pharmacology for nurses* (12th ed.). St. Louis, MO: Mosby.

Hofland, S. L., & Powers, L. (1996). Sexual dysfunction in the menopausal woman: Hormonal causes and management issues. *Geriatric Nursing, 17*(4), 161–165.

Masters, W. H., & Johnson, V. E. (1966). *Human sexual response*. Boston: Little, Brown.

Masters, W. H., Johnson, V. E., & Kolodny, R. C. (1995). *Human sexuality* (5th ed.). New York: HarperCollins College.

Nettina, S. (2001). *The Lippincott manual of nursing practice* (7th ed., p. 1115). Philadelphia: Lippincott Williams & Wilkins.

Novak, J. C., & Broom, B. L. (1999). *Ingalls and Salerno's maternal and child health nursing*. St. Louis, MO: Mosby.

Porth, C. M. (2003). *Pathophysiology: Concepts in altered health states*. Philadelphia: Lippincott Williams & Wilkins.

Sherwin, L. N., Scalawen, M. A., & Weingarten, C. T. (1999). *Maternity nursing*. Norwalk, CT: Appleton & Lange.

Towle, M. & Adams, E. (2008). Maternal-child nursing care. Upper Saddle River, NJ: Prentice Hall.

CHAPTER 16

Carpenito, L. J. (2005). *Nursing diagnosis: Application to clinical practice* (11th ed.). Philadelphia: Lippincott.

Fontaine, K. L., & Fletcher, J. S. (2003). *Mental health nursing* (5th ed.). Upper Saddle River, NJ: Prentice Hall.

Freud, S. (1946). The ego and the mechanisms of defense. New York: International Universities Press.

Holmes, T. H., & Rahe, R. H. (1967). The Social Readjustment Scale. *Journal of Psychosomatic Research II,* pp. 213–218.

Jacobs, G. D. (2001). The physiology of mind–body interactions: The stress response and the relaxation response. *Journal of Alternative and Complementary Medicine, 7*(supplement), 89–93.

Kurzen, C. R. (2001). *Contemporary practical/vocational nursing* (4th. ed.). Philadelphia: Lippincott.

Lazarus, R. S. (1965). *Psychological stress and coping process*. New York: McGraw-Hill.

Lazarus, R. S. (1993). Psychological stress to the emotions: A history of changing outlook. *Annual Review of Psychology, 44,* 1–21.

LeMone, P., & Burke, K. M. (2004). *Medical-surgical nursing: Critical thinking in client care* (3rd ed.). Upper Saddle River, NJ: Prentice Hall.

Monat, A., & Lazarus, R. S. (1991). *Stress and coping: An anthology* (3rd ed.). New York: Columbia University Press.

Neeb, K. (2005). *Fundamentals of mental health nursing* (3rd. ed.). Philadelphia: F. A. Davis.

Selye, H. (1976). *The stress of life* (revised ed.). New York: McGraw-Hill.

Sherman, D. W. (2004). Nurses' stress 7 burnout: How to care for yourself when caring for patients, families experiencing life-threatening illness. *American Journal of Nursing, 104*(5), 48–56.

Thomas, C. L. (Ed.). (2006). *Taber's cyclopedic medical dictionary* (20th ed.). Philadelphia: F. A. Davis.

Townsend, M. C. (2005). *Essentials of psychiatric mental health nursing* (3rd ed.). Philadelphia: F. A. Davis.

Wicks, R. J. (2006). *Overcoming secondary stress in medical and nursing practice: A guide to resilience and personal well being*. Oxford, UK: Oxford University Press.

CHAPTER 17

Anweiler, N. (2000). Another dying patient. *Nursing, 30*(11), 32.

Benton, R. E. (1978). *Death and dying: Principles and practices in patient care*. New York: Van Nostrand.

Carpenito, L. J. (2005). *Handbook of nursing diagnosis* (11th ed.). Philadelphia: Lippincott.

Engel, G. L. (1964). Grief and grieving. *American Journal of Nursing, 64,* 93–98.

Furman, J. (2002). What you should know about chronic grief. *Nursing 02, 32,* 56.

Hospice and Palliative Nurses Association. (1999). *Hospice and palliative nursing practice review* (3rd ed.). Dubuque, Iowa: Kendall/Hunt.

Kübler-Ross, E. (1969). *On death and dying*. New York: Macmillan.

Kübler-Ross, E. (1974). *Questions and answers on death and dying*. New York: Macmillan.

Kübler-Ross, E. (1975). *Death: The final stage of growth*. Englewood Cliffs, NJ: Prentice Hall.

Kübler-Ross, E. (1978). *To live until we say good-bye*. Englewood Cliffs, NJ: Prentice Hall.

North American Nursing Diagnosis Association. (2005). *Nursing diagnoses: Definitions & classification, 2005–2006*. Philadelphia: Author.

Ross, H. (2001). Islamic tradition at the end of life. *Medsurg Nursing, 10*(2), 83.

Ufema, J. (2002, various). Monthly column: Insights on death and dying. *Nursing 02*.

Wrede-Seaman, L. (1999). *Symptom management algorithms: A handbook for palliative care* (2nd ed.). Washington, DC: Intellicard, Inc.

CHAPTER 18

Cohen, B. J., et al. (2000). *Memmler's the human body in health and disease* (9th ed.). Philadelphia: Lippincott Williams & Wilkins.

Marieb, E. N. (2001). *Human anatomy & physiology* (5th ed.). Upper Saddle River, NJ: Pearson Education.

Scanlon, V. C., & Sanders, T. (2003). *Essentials of anatomy and physiology* (4th ed.). Philadelphia: Davis.

Seeley, R. R., et al. (2006). *Anatomy & physiology* (7th ed.). New York: McGraw-Hill Higher Education.

Spence, A. P., et al. (1992). *Human anatomy & physiology* (4th ed.). Eagan, MN: West Publishing Company.

Tortora, G. J., Derrickson, B. (2006). *Principles of anatomy and physiology* (11th ed.). Hoboken, NJ: John Wiley & Sons.

Van De Graff, K. M., Fox, S. I. (1999). *Concepts of human anatomy & physiology* (5th ed.). New York: WCB/McGraw-Hill.

CHAPTER 19

Barkauskas, V., Bauman, L. C., Stoltenberg-Allen, K., & Darling-Fisher, C. (1998). *Health and physical assessment* (2nd ed.). St. Louis, MO: Mosby.

Berman, A., Snyder, S., Kozier, B., & Erb, G. (2003). *Kozier and Erb's techniques in clinical nursing* (5th ed.). Upper Saddle River, NJ: Prentice Hall.

Bickley, L. S. (2005). *Bates' guide to physical examination and history taking* (9th ed.). Philadelphia: Lippincott.

Fuerst, E. V., & Wolff, L. (1964). *Fundamentals of nursing* (3rd ed., p. 135). Philadelphia: J. B. Lippincott.

Leifer, G. (1999). *Thompson's introduction to maternity and pediatric nursing* (3rd ed.). Philadelphia: W. B. Saunders.

Lewis, S. M., Heitkemper, M. M., & Dirkson, S. R. (2004). *Medical-surgical nursing assessment and management of clinical problems* (6th ed.). St. Louis, MO: Mosby.

Memmler, R. L., Cohen, B. J., & Wood, D. L. (2000). *Structure and function of the human body* (7th ed.). Philadelphia: Lippincott-Raven.

O'Hanlon-Nichols, T. (1998, April). Basic assessment series: Gastrointestinal system. *American Journal of Nursing, 98*(4), 48–53.

O'Hanlon-Nichols, T. (1998, June). Basic assessment series. A review of the adult musculoskeletal system: A guide to a key aspect of client care. *American Journal of Nursing, 98*(6), 48–52.

Owen, A. (1998, April). Respiratory assessment revisited: Refresh your technique for spotting pulmonary problems. *Nursing 98, 28*(4), 48–49.

CHAPTER 20

Ackley, B. J., & Ladwig, G. B. (2006). *Nursing diagnosis handbook* (7th ed.). St. Louis, MO: Mosby.

American Heart Association. (1993). *Recommendations for human blood pressure determination by sphygmomanometers* (6th ed., Product No. 88:2460–2467). Dallas, TX: Author.

American Heart Association. (1997, January). Consult stat. Guidelines for monitoring BP at home. *RN, 60,* 57.

Bickley, L., & Szilagyi, P. C. (2002). *Bates' guide to physical examination and history taking* (7th ed.). Philadelphia: Lippincott, Williams and Wilkins.

Erickson, R. S., Meyer, L. T., & Woo, T. M. (1996, Spring). Accuracy of chemical dot thermometers in critically ill adults and young children. *Image, 14,* 23–28.

Guyton, A. C., & Hall, J. (2000). *Textbook of medical physiology* (10th ed.). Philadelphia: W. B. Saunders.

Jones, D., Engelke, M. K., Brown, S. T., et al. (1996). A comparison of two noninvasive methods of blood pressure measurement in the triage area. *Journal of Emergency Nursing, 22*(2), 111–115.

Ladewig, P. W., London, M. L., Moberly, S. M., & Olds, S. B. (2002). *Maternal-newborn nursing care: The nurse, the family, and the community* (5th ed.). Upper Saddle River, NJ: Prentice Hall.

Marieb, E. N. (2001). *Human anatomy and physiology* (5th ed.). Menlo Park, CA: Benjamin/Cummings.

Roper, M. (1996, August). Back to basics: assessing orthostatic vital signs. *American Journal of Nursing, 96,* 43–46.

Thomas, D. O. (1996, April). Assessing children—it's different. *RN, 59,* 38–45, 53.

CHAPTER 21

Ackley, B. J., & Ladwig, G. B. (2006). *Nursing diagnosis handbook* (7th ed.). St. Louis, MO: Mosby.

American Academy of Pain Medicine. (2002). The use of opioids for the treatment of chronic pain (Joint consensus statement from the American Academy of Pain Medicine and the American Pain Society). Retrieved from www.productpub/statements.painmed.org

Blanchard, R. (2002). Why study pain? A qualitative analysis of medical and nursing faculty and students' knowledge of and attitudes to cancer pain management. *Journal of Palliative Medicine, 5*(1), 57.

Briggs, E. (2002). The nursing management of pain in older people. *Nursing Older People, 14*(7), 23–29.

Bucknall, T., Manias, E., & Botti, M. (2001). Acute pain management: Implications of scientific evidence for nursing practice in the postoperative context. *International Journal of Nursing Practice, 7*(4), 266.

Carr, D. B., et al. (1992). *Acute pain management: Operative or medical procedures and trauma (Clinical practice guidelines).* Rockville, MD: Agency for Health Care Policy and Research, Public Health Services, U.S. Department of Health and Human Services.

Edwards, H. E., et al. (2001). Determinants of nurses' intention to administer opioids for pain relief. *Nursing & Health Sciences, 3*(3), 149.

Guyton, A., & Hall, J. E. (2000). *Textbook of medical physiology* (10th ed.). Philadelphia: W. B. Saunders.

Houldin, A. D. (2002). *Patients with cancer: Understanding the psychological pain.* Philadelphia: Lippincott Williams and Wilkins.

Kanner, R. (2001). *Pain management secrets.* Philadelphia: Lippincott Williams and Wilkins.

McCaffery, M. (1979). *Nursing management of the patient with pain* (2nd ed.). Philadelphia: Lippincott.

McCaffery, M. (2002). *Pain management revised—The nurse's active role in opioid administration* [CD-ROM]. Philadelphia: Lippincott Williams & Wilkins.

McCaffery, M., & Beebe, A. (1989). *Pain: Clinical manual for nursing practice.* St. Louis, MO: Mosby.

McCaffery, M., & Pasero, C. L. (1998). Pain control. Talking with patients and families about addiction. *American Journal of Nursing, 98*(3), 18–21.

Melzack, R., & Wall, P. (1965). Pain mechanism: A new theory. *Science, 150,* 171–179.

North American Nursing Diagnosis Association. (2005). *Nursing diagnoses: Definitions & classification, 2005–2006.* Philadelphia: Author.

Pasero, C. L. (1997). Using the Faces scale to assess pain. *American Journal of Nursing, 97*(7), 19–20.

Pinnell, N. (1996). *Nursing pharmacology.* Philadelphia: W. B. Saunders.

Schechter, N. L., Berde, C. B., & Yaster, M. (2002). *Pain in infants, children and adolescents.* Philadelphia: Lippincott Williams & Wilkins.

Slaughter, A., Pasero, C., & Manworren, R. (2002). Unacceptable pain levels: A process to prompt pain relief. *American Journal of Nursing, 102*(5), 75.

Unacceptable pain levels. (2002, May). *American Journal of Nursing, 102*(5), 75–77.

Vega-Stromberg, T., Holmes, S., Gorski, L., & Johnson, B. P. (2002). Road to excellence in pain management: Research, outcomes and direction (ROAD). *Journal of Nursing Care Quality, 17*(1), 15.

Wong, D. L. (2001). *Whaley and Wong's essentials of pediatric nursing* (6th ed.). St. Louis, MO: Mosby.

CHAPTER 22

Berman, A., Snyder, S., Kozier, B., & Erb, G. (2002). *Kozier and Erb's techniques in clinical nursing.* Upper Saddle River, NJ: Prentice Hall.

Beuscher, T. L. (1998). Community outreach: Foot care for the elderly: A winning proposition. *Home Healthcare Nurse, 16*(1), 37–44.

Calianno, C. (2002). Patient hygiene part 2—Skin care: Keeping the outside healthy. *Nursing2002, 32*(6). Page supplement.

Carpenito, L. J. (2002). *Handbook of nursing diagnosis* (9th ed.). Philadelphia: Lippincott.

Claphan, L. (1997, September). Preventing foot problems in patients with diabetes. *Professional Nurse, 12*(12), 851–853.

Dugan, M. B. (2003). *Living with hearing loss.* Washington, DC: Gallaudet University Press.

Effects of hydrogen peroxide rinses on the normal oral mucosa (1993). *Nursing Research, 6,* 332–337.

Eshleman, J., & Davidhizar, R. (2002). When your patient complains of hair loss. *Home Health Care Nurse, 20*(12), 778–782.

Kydd, A. (2002). Focusing nursing care on the older person. *Nursing Times, 98*(33), 13.

Lassieur, A. (2000). *Head lice (my health).* New York: Frank Watts, Inc.

Little, J. W. (Ed.). (2002). *Dental management of medically compromised patients.* St. Louis, MO: Mosby.

Marieb, E. N. (2001). *Human anatomy and physiology* (5th ed.). Menlo Park, CA: Pearson/Benjamin Cummings.

Mauizio, S. J., & Rogers, J. L. (1997). Prevention update: Oral hygiene to the home care patient. *Caring, 16*(3), 54–55.

North American Nursing Diagnosis Association. (2005). *Nursing diagnoses: Definitions & classification, 2005–2006.* Philadelphia: Author.

Reed, S. (2002). Implementing best practices in pressure ulcer prevention. *Nursing Times, 97*(24), 69.

Wilkinson, J. M. (2004). *Nursing diagnosis handbook with NIC interventions and NOC outcomes* (7th ed.). Upper Saddle River, NJ: Prentice Hall.

Wilkinson, J. (2001). Patient hygiene. Part I, oral care: The inside story. *Nursing, 31*(5), 1.

CHAPTER 23

Capobianco, M. L., & McDonald, D. D. (1996, November/December). Factors affecting the predictive validity of the Braden Scale. *Advances in Wound Care: The Journal for Prevention and Healing, 9,* 32–36.

Carpenito, L. J. (2005). *Handbook of nursing diagnosis* (11th ed.). Philadelphia: Lippincott.

Duimel-Peeters, I. (2005). Wound wise: Preventing pressure ulcers with massage. *American Journal of Nursing, 105*(8), 31–32.

Hahn, J. F., Olsen, C. L., Tomaselli, N., & Goldberg, M. (2000, revised 2002). *Wounds: Nursing care and product selection—Part I* [Electronic version]. *Nursing Spectrum.*

Hess, C. T. (2002). *Clinical guide to wound care* (4th ed.). Philadelphia: Lippincott Williams & Wilkins.

International Committee on Wound Management. (1996). ICWM World Council consensus statement on cost effective wound care. Evaluating your supply use to prepare for managed care. *Ostomy/Wound Management, 42*(2), 72, 74–76.

Maklebust J., & Sieggreen, M. (2000). *Pressure ulcers: Guidelines for prevention and nursing management* (2nd ed.). Springhouse, PA: Springhouse Corporation.

McConnell, E. A. (1997). Clinical do's and don'ts: Using dry heat to promote healing. *Nursing, 27*(5), 22.

Mendez-Eastmann, S. (2005, May). Using negative-pressure wound therapy for positive results. *Nursing 2005,* pp. 48–50.

North American Nursing Diagnosis Association. (2005). *Nursing diagnoses: Definitions & classification, 2005–2006.* Philadelphia: Author.

Pieper, B., Sugrue, M., Weiland, M., Sprague, K., & Heiman, C. (1998). Risk factors, prevention methods, and wound care for patients with pressure ulcers. *Clinical Nurse Specialist, 12*(1), 7–14.

Sieggreen, M. Y. (2005, October). Stepping up care for diabetic foot ulcers. *Nursing 2005,* 36–39.

Sisk, B. (2002). *Pressure sore update* [Electronic version]. *Nurse Scribe.*

Sterling, C. (1996). Methods of wound assessment documentation: A study. *Nursing Standard, 11*(10), 38–41.

Stotts, N. A. (1990). Seeing red, yellow, and black: The three-color concept of wound care. *Nursing 90, 20,* 59–61.

U.S. Department of Health and Human Services, PPPPUA. (1992). *Clinical practice guideline #3: Pressure ulcers in adults: Prediction and prevention* (AGCPR Publication No. 92-0047, p. 8). Rockville, MD: Public Health Service.

Van Rijswijk, L. (1996). The fundamentals of wound assessment. *Ostomy/Wound Management, 42*(7), 40–42, 44, 46, 48–50.

WEBSITES

KCI. (2006a). *How V.A.C.® therapy works.* Retrieved January 11, 2006, from www.kci1.com/82.asp

KCI. (2006b). *V.A.C.® Therapy System.* Retrieved January 11, 2006, from http://www.kci1.com/35.asp

National Decubitus Foundation. www.decubitus.org. Describes wound care.

National Pressure Ulcer Advisory Panel (NPUAP). www.npuap.org/default.htm. Current research, newsletter, conferences, and information about pressure ulcers.

Wound Care Information Network. www.medialedu.com/default.htm. Site maintained by two MDs: A. Freedline and T. Fishman; information based on national guidelines.

CHAPTER 24

Brown, P. (2000). DVT: What every nurse should know. *RN, 63*(4), 58–62.

Burke, K. M., LeMone, P., & Mohn-Brown, E. L. (2003). *Medical-surgical nursing care.* Upper Saddle River, NJ: Prentice Hall.

Carroll, P. (2001). How to intervene before asthma turns deadly. *RN, 64*(5), 52–58.

Davies, P. (2002). Guarding your patient against ARDS. *Nursing 2002, 32*(3), 36–41.

Fort, C. W. (2002). Get pumped to prevent DVT. *Nursing 2002, 32*(9), 50–52.

Lazzara, D. (2002). Eliminate the air of mystery from chest tubes. *Nursing 2002, 32*(6), 36–43.

McConnell, E. A., (2002). Applying antiembolism stockings. *Nursing 2002, 32*(4), 17.

Perkins, L. A., & Shortall, S. P. (2000). Ventilation without intubation. *RN, 63*(1), 34–38.

Pope, B. B. (2002). Asthma: Patient education series. *Nursing 2002, 32*(5), 44.

Siomko, A. J. (2000). Demystifying cardiac markers. *American Journal of Nursing, 100*(1), 36–40.

U.S. Department of Health and Human Services. (2000). *Healthy people 2010: Understanding and improving health* (2nd ed.). Washington, DC: U.S. Government Printing Office.

West, J. B. (2001). *Pulmonary physiology and pathophysiology: An integrated, case-based approach.* Philadelphia: Lippincott Williams & Wilkins.

CHAPTER 25

Como, D. (Ed.). (2002). *Mosby's medical, nursing, and allied health dictionary.* St. Louis, MO: Mosby.

Lane, K. (Ed.). (1999). *The Merck manual.* West Point, PA: Merck.

Nettina, S. M. (Ed.). (2001). *The Lippincott manual of nursing practice.* Philadelphia: Lippincott-Raven.

Pagana, K. D., & Pagana, T. J. (2003). *Mosby's diagnostic and laboratory test reference.* St. Louis, MO: Mosby.

Whitney, E. N., Cataldo, C. B., & Rolfes, S. R. (2002). *Understanding normal and clinical nutrition.* Belmont, CA: Wadsworth/Thomson Learning.

Wilkinson, J. M. (2000). *Nursing diagnosis handbook.* Upper Saddle River, NJ: Prentice Hall Health.

CHAPTER 26

Como, D. (Ed.). (2002). *Mosby's medical, nursing, and allied health dictionary.* St. Louis, MO: Mosby.

Lane, K. (Ed.). (1999). *The Merck manual.* West Point, PA: Merck.

McPhee, A. T. (1997). *Fluids and electrolytes made incredibly easy.* Springhouse, PA: Springhouse Corporation.

Nettina, S. M. (Ed.). (2001). *The Lippincott manual of nursing practice.* Philadelphia: Lippincott-Raven.

Pagana, K. D., & Pagana, T. J. (2003). *Mosby's diagnostic and laboratory test reference.* St. Louis, MO: Mosby.

Phillips, L. (2001). *Manual of I.V. therapeutics.* Philadelphia: F. A. Davis.

Wilkinson, J. M. (2000). *Nursing diagnosis handbook.* Upper Saddle River, NJ: Prentice Hall Health.

CHAPTER 27

Ackley, B. J., & Ladwig, G. B. (2006). *Nursing diagnosis handbook: A guide to planning care* (7th ed.). St. Louis, MO: Mosby.

Carpenito, L. J. (2003). *Nursing care plan and documentation* (4th ed.). Philadelphia: Lippincott.

Demarest, L. (2006, February). A common diversion. *Nursing Spectrum* [Online]. Retrieved April 6, 2007, from http://community.nursingspectrum.com/MagazineArticles/article.cfm?AID=19722

Kinsley, M. (2005, October). Gotta go: Overactive bladder. *Nursing Spectrum* [Online]. Retrieved April 6, 2007, from http://community.nursingspectrum.com/MagazineArticles/article.cfm?AID=17979

McUsic, T. (2005, October). Texas nurses help tackle incontinence uncertainties. *Nursing Spectrum* [Online]. Retrieved June 2006 from http://community.nursingspectrum.com

Nettina, S. M. (2001). *Lippincott manual of nursing practice* (7th ed.). Philadelphia: Lippincott Williams and Wilkins.

Newman, D. K. (2002). *Managing and treating urinary incontinence* (1st ed.). Baltimore, MD: Health Professions Press.

Polick, T. Slaying the myths concerning women and urinary incontinence. *Nursing Spectrum* [Online].

Springhouse Corporation. (2004). *Fluids and electrolytes made incredibly easy* (3rd ed.). Springhouse, PA: Author.

Williams, L., & Hopper, P. (2003). Understanding medical surgical nursing (2nd ed.). Philadelphia: F. A. Davis.

WEBSITES

National Association for Continence, www.nafc.org
Simon Foundation for Continence, http://www.simonfoundation.org

CHAPTER 28

Blackwood, H. S. (2005, February). Help your patient downsize with bariatric surgery. *Nursing 2005, 35*(9), (Supplement Medical-Surgical Insider), 4–5.

Bryant, D., & Fleischer, I. (2000, November). Changing an ostomy appliance. *Nursing* [Online], *30*(11), 51.

Carpenito, L. J. (2005). *Handbook of nursing diagnosis* (11th ed.). Philadelphia: Lippincott.

Day, A., & Bean, K. B. (2006). LPN's mission: Where do LPNs go from here? *Gastroenterology Nursing, 29*(2), 157.

Gauthier, P., & Bean, K. B. (2006). Fundamentals of GI. *Gastroenterology Nursing, 29*(2), 160.

Guyton, A. C., & Hall, J. E. (2005). *Textbook of medical physiology* (11th ed.). Philadelphia: Elsevier/Saunders.

Nettina, S. M. (2001). *Lippincott manual of nursing practice* (7th ed.). Philadelphia: Lippincott Williams and Wilkins.

North American Nursing Diagnosis Association. (2005). *NANDA nursing diagnoses: Definitions and classification 2005–2006.* Philadelphia: Author.

Rushing, C. (2005). Clinical dos and don'ts: Inserting a nasogastric tube. *Nursing 2005, 35*(5), 22.

SGNA position statement: Role delineation of LPN/LVN in gastroenterology. (2006). *Gastroenterology Nursing, 29*(1), 60–61.

Vickery, G. (1997). Basics of constipation. *Gastroenterology Nursing, 20*(4), 125–128.

WEBSITES

National Association for Continence, www.nafc.org
National Institute of Diabetes & Digestive & Kidney Diseases, www.niddk.nih.gov/health/digest/nddic.htm. See listings for constipation, diarrhea, ileostomy, colostomy, and ileoanal reservoir surgery and digestive disease statistics.
Simon Foundation for Continence, http://simonfoundation.org

CHAPTER 29

Ackley, B. J., & Ladwig, G. B. (2006). *Nursing diagnosis handbook: A guide to planning care* (7th ed.). St. Louis, MO: Mosby.

Beyea, S., & Nicoll, L. (1996). Back to basics: Administering IM injections the right way. *American Journal of Nursing, 96*(1), 34–35.

Cohen, M. R. (2002). *Medication errors.* Huntingdon Valley, PA: American Pharmaceutical Association.

Deglin, J. H., & Vallerand, A. H. (2003). *Davis's drug guide for nurses* (8th ed.). Philadelphia: F. A. Davis.

edruginfo.com. (2002). *Clinical pearls.* Philadelphia: Lippincott Williams & Wilkins.

Glazer, G. (2002, February 28). Legislative column: Medication administration interventions that must be performed by a registered nurse. *Journal of Issues in Nursing* [Online]. Retrieved from www.nursingworld.org/ojin/tpclg/leg_12.htm

Highleyman, L. (2002, September). *Preventing HCV transmission in personal care settings.* San Francisco: Hepatitis Support Project.

Marieb. E. N. (1997). *Human anatomy* (2nd ed.). Menlo Park, CA: Benjamin/Cummings.

McCloskey, J. C., & Bulechek, G. M. (2000). *Nursing interventions classification (NIC).* (3rd ed.). St. Louis, MO: Mosby-Year Book.

Miller, D. (2000). *Nurse's clinical guide: Medication administration.* Philadelphia: Springhouse–Lippincott Williams & Wilkins.

Moses, S. (2000). Cation-exchange resin. In *Family practice notebook* [Online]. Retrieved January 29, 2003, from www.fpnotebook.com/REN101.htm

National Institute for Occupational Safety and Health (1999, November). *Alert—Preventing needlestick injuries in health care settings* (Publication No. 2000–108). Cincinnati, OH: Author.

National League for Nursing (2001). *Basic proficiency in medication administration* (4th Version). New York: Author.

Sifton, D. W. (Ed.). (2001). *Physician's desk reference* (56th ed.). Montvale, NJ: Medical Economics.

Smith, S. F., Duell, D. J., & Martin, B. C. (2000). *Clinical nursing skills: Basic to advanced skills.* Upper Saddle River, NJ: Prentice Hall.

Wilson, B. A., Shannon, M. T., & Stang, C. L. (2003). *Nurse's drug guide.* Upper Saddle River, NJ: Prentice Hall.

Wolfe, S. (Ed.). (2001). Safer needle devices, part 1. *RN, 62*(10), 59.

Woodrow, R. (2002). *Essentials of pharmacology for health occupations* (4th ed.). Clifton Park, NY: Delmar.

Worthington, K. A. (2002). Hazardous drugs: Handling medications can pose danger to nurses. *American Journal of Nursing, 102*(5), 120.

CHAPTER 30

Berman, A., Snyder, S., Kozier, B., & Erb, G. (2002). *Techniques in clinical nursing* (5th ed.). Upper Saddle River, NJ: Prentice Hall.

Boyer, M. J. (2006). *Math for nurses* (6th ed.). Philadelphia: Lippincott Williams & Wilkins.

Josephson, D. (2004). *Intravenous infusion therapy for nurses: Principles and practice* (2nd ed.). Clifton Park, NY: Thomson Delmar Learning.

Phillips, L. (2005). *Manual of I.V. therapeutics* (4th ed.). Philadelphia: F. A. Davis.

Smith, S. F., Duell, D. J., & Martin, B. C. (2000). *Clinical nursing skills: Basic to advanced skills.* Upper Saddle River, NJ: Prentice Hall.

Smith, S. F., Duell, D. J., & Martin, B. C., (2002). *Photo guide of nursing skills,* Upper Saddle River, NJ: Prentice Hall.

Springhouse Corporation. (2004). *Fluids and electrolytes made incredibly easy* (3rd ed.). Springhouse, PA: Author.

Wikipedia. (2006). Jehovah's Witnesses and blood transfusions. Retrieved June 2006 from http://en.wikipedia.org/wiki/Jehovah's_Witnesses_and_blood

Wikipedia (2006). Bloodless surgery. Retrieved June 2006 from http://en.wikipedia.org/wikiBloodless_surgery

Williams, L., & Hopper, P. (2003). *Understanding medical surgical nursing* (2nd ed.). Philadelphia: F. A. Davis.

CHAPTER 31

Ackley, B. J., & Ladwig, G. B. (2006). *Nursing diagnosis handbook* (7th ed.). St. Louis, MO: Mosby.

Benko, T., Cooke, E. A., McNally, M. A., & Mollan, R. (2000). Graduated compression stockings—knee length or thigh length. *Clinical Orthopaedics and Related Research, 383,* 197–203.

Brown, B. (2001). Promoting patient safety through preoperative patient verification. *AORN Journal, 74*(11), 690.

Busen, N. H. (2001). Perioperative preparation of the adolescent surgical patient. *AORN Journal,739*(2), 464.

Carroll, P. (1993). Deep venous thrombosis: Implications for orthopaedic nursing. *Orthopaedic Nursing, 12*(3), 33–43.

Church, V. (2000). Staying on guard for DVT & PE. *Nursing 2000, 30*(2).

Dealey, C. (2000). *The care of wounds: A guide for nurses* (2nd. ed.). Boston: Blackwell Science.

Garbee, G. (2001). Creating a positive surgical experience for patients. *AORN Journal 74*(9), 333.

Meeker, M. H., & Rothrock, J. C. (1999). *Alexander's care of the patient in surgery* (11th ed.). St. Louis, MO: Mosby.

Munden, J. (2002). *Pathophysiology made incredibly easy* (2nd ed.). Springhouse, PA: Lippincott Williams & Wilkins.

North American Nursing Diagnosis Association. (2005). *NANDA nursing diagnoses: Definitions and classification 2005–2006.* Philadelphia: Author.

Smith, S. F., Duell, D. J., & Martin, B. C. (2000). *Clinical nursing skills: Basic to advanced* (5th ed.). Upper Saddle River, NJ: Prentice Hall.

Tappen, C. (2001). Perioperative assessment and discharge planning for older adults undergoing ambulatory surgery. *AORN Journal 73*(2), 464.

Walton, J. (2001). Helping high-risk surgical patients beat the odds. *Nursing 2001, 31*(3), 54.

Winslow, E. H., & Crenshaw, J. T. (2002). Preoperative fasting: Old habits die hard. *American Journal of Nursing, 102*(5), 36–44.

CHAPTER 32

Ackley, B. J., & Ladwig, G. B. (2006). *Nursing diagnosis handbook: A guide to planning care* (7th ed.). St. Louis, MO: Mosby.

Carpenito, L. J. (2005). *Handbook of nursing diagnosis* (11th ed.). Philadelphia: Lippincott.

Clinical rounds: Bedrest may not be best after all. (2005). *Nursing 2005, 35*(8), 33.

Duimel-Peeterrs, L. (2005). Wound wise: Preventing pressure ulcers with massage? Some say it works others disagree; ay, there's the rub. *American Journal of Nursing, 76*(8), 31–33.

Graves, G. (1998, March). The 9 habits of highly successful sleepers. *Good Housekeeping,* pp. 82, 84, 88.

Guyton, A. C., & Hall, J. E. (2005). *Textbook of medical physiology* (11th ed.). Philadelphia: W. B. Saunders.

Haigh, C., & Peacok, L. (1998). Dilemmas in moving and handling patients. *Community Nurse, 4*(1), 26–28.

Krahn, L., Black, J., & Silber, M. (2001). Subspecialty clinics: Sleep disorders: Narcolepsy—New understanding of irresistible sleep. *Mayo Clinic Proceedings, 76,* 185–194.

Photo guide: Performing passive range of motion. (2006). *Nursing 2006, 36*(3), 50–51.

Richardson, S. (2003). Effects of relaxation and imagery on sleep of critically ill adults. *Dimensions of Critical Care Nursing, 22*(4), 182–190.

Thomason, M., Huggins, M., Beier, S., & Watkins, T. (2002). *The autoimmune hypothesis in narcolepsy.* Retrieved July 16, 2002, from www.tonto.stanford.edu/^john/205/watkins.pdf

Trupp, R. J. (2004). The heart of sleep: Sleep-disordered breathing and heart failure. *Journal of Cardiovascular Nursing, 19*(6), 567–574.

CHAPTER 33

Bandura, A. (1971). Analysis of modeling processes. In A. Bandura (Ed.), *Psychological modeling.* Chicago: Aldine.

Bloom, B. S., et al. (1956). *Bloom's taxonomy of educational objectives, Handbook I: Cognitive domain.* Boston: Allyn & Bacon.

Byrnes, J. P. (2001). *Cognitive development and learning in instructional context.* Boston: Allyn & Bacon.

Carpenito, L. J. (2005). *Handbook of nursing diagnosis* (11th ed.). Philadelphia: Lippincott.

Doak, C. C., Doak, L. G., & Root, J. H. (1996). *Teaching patients with low literacy skills* (2nd ed.). Philadelphia: Lippincott.

McCloskey, J. C., & Bulechek, G. M. (Eds.). (2003). *Nursing interventions classification (NIC).* (4th ed.). St. Louis, MO: Mosby-Year Book.

Messner, R. I. (1997). Patient teaching tips from the horse's mouth. *RN, 60*(8), 29–31.

Moorehead, S., Johnson, M., & Maas, M. (2003). *Nursing outcomes classifications* (3rd ed.). St. Louis, MO: Mosby.

Rankin, S. H., & Stallings, K. D. (1996). *Patient education: Issues, principles, practices* (3rd ed.). Philadelphia: Lippincott.

Redman, B. K. (1993). *The process of patient education* (7th ed.). St. Louis, MO: Mosby.

Robinson, A., & Miller, M. (1996). Making information accessible: Developing plain English discharge instructions. *Journal of Advanced Nursing, 24*(3), 528–535.

Rutledge, D. N., & Donaldson, N. E. (1998, June). Improving readability of print materials in patient care and health services. *Journal of Clinical Innovations, 1*(3), 1–27.

Stephens, S. T. (1992). Patient educational materials: Are they readable? *Oncology Nursing Forum, 19*(1), 84.

CHAPTER 34

Lemone, P., & Burke, K. (2004). *Medical-surgical nursing* (3rd ed.). Upper Saddle River, NJ: Prentice Hall.

Lewis, S. M., Heitkemper, M. M., & Dirksen, S. R. (2003). *Medical surgical nursing.* St. Louis, MO: Mosby.

Paradiso, C. (1995). *Fluid and electrolytes.* Philadelphia: Lippincott.

Williams, L. S., & Hopper, P. D. (1999). *Understanding medical-surgical nursing* (2nd ed.). Philadelphia: F. A. Davis.

CHAPTER 35

Ackley, B. J., & Ladwig, G. B. (2006). *Nursing diagnosis handbook* (7th ed.). St. Louis, MO: Mosby.

North American Nursing Diagnosis Association. (2005). *NANDA nursing diagnoses: Definitions and classification 2005–2006.* Philadelphia: Author.

Regulations of the Commissioner of Education. (2006, March). Section 136.1–.3 March 2006.

WEBSITE

Childhood Immunization Support Program, www.cispimmunize.org

CHAPTER 36

Anderson, M. A. (2005). *Nursing leadership, management, and professional practice for LPN/LVNs* (3rd ed.). Philadelphia: F. A. Davis.

Hansten, R. I., & Washburn, M. J. (2004). *Clinical delegation skills—A handbook for professional practice* (3rd ed.). Gaitherburg, MD: Aspen Publishing.

Hill, S. S., Howlett, H. S., & Howlett, H. A. (2001). *Success in practical/vocational nursing from student to leader* (4th ed.). Philadelphia: W. B. Saunders.

Hohenhaus, S., Powell, S., & Hohenhaus, J. T. (August). Enhancing patient safety during hand-offs: "Standardized communication and teamwork using 'SBAR' method." *American Journal of Nursing, 106*(8), 72A–72C.

Kurzen, C. R. (2001). *Contemporary practical/vocational nursing* (4th ed.). Philadelphia: Lippincott.

Walczak, M. B., & Absolon, P. L. (2001). Essentials for effective communication in oncology nursing: Assertiveness, conflict management, delegation and motivation. *Journal of Nursing Staff Development, 17*(3), 159–162.

CHAPTER 37

Gronlund, N. (2000). How to write and use instructional objectives. Upper Saddle River, NJ: Prentice Hall.

Hill, S. S., Howlett, H. S., & Howlett, H. A. (2001). *Success in practical/vocational nursing from student to leader* (4th ed.). Philadelphia: W. B. Saunders.

Is Puerto Rico's Nurse Licensing Exam Equivalent to the NCLEX-RN®? (2005). Retrieved February 20, 2005, from www.minoritynurse. com/vitalsigns/july04-6.html

National Council of State Boards of Nursing, Inc. (2002). *NCLEX-PN® examination effective date: April 2002.* Chicago: Author.

Smith, S. (1997). *Review questions for the NCLEX-PN CAT* (3rd ed.). Upper Saddle River, NJ: Prentice Hall.

Wilson, B., Shannon, S., & Strang, C. (2002). *Prentice Hall's nurse's drug guide 2002.* Upper Saddle River, NJ: Prentice Hall.

WEBSITES

For information on international testing in three countries, go to http://biz.yahoo.com/iw/040601/067961.html (accessed February 20, 2005).

For information on the NCLEX-PN® April 2005 test plan, go to www.ncsbn.org/pdfs/PN_test_plan_05_Web.pdf (accessed February 20, 2005).

For an NCLEX candidate bulletin, go to www.ncsbn.org/pdfs/Web_Bulletin_05.pdf (accessed February 20, 2005).

CHAPTER 38

Anderson, M. (2000). *To be a nurse—Personal/vocational relationships for the LPN/LVN.* Philadelphia: F. A. Davis.

Anderson, M. A. (2005). *Nursing leadership, management, and professional practice for LPN/LVNs* (3rd ed.). Philadelphia: F. A. Davis.

Becker, B. G., & Fendler, D. T. (1994). *Vocational and personal adjustment in practical nursing* (7th ed.). St. Louis, MO: Mosby.

Claywell, L., & Corbin, B. (2003). *LPN to RN transition.* St. Louis, MO: Mosby.

Dunne, G. D. (2002). *The nursing job search handbook.* Philadelphia: University of Pennsylvania Press.

Hill, S. S., Howlett, H. S., & Howlett, H. A. (2001). *Success in practical/vocational nursing from student to leader* (4th ed.). Philadelphia: W. B. Saunders.

Kurzen, C. R. (2001). *Contemporary practical/vocational nursing* (4th ed.). Philadelphia: Lippincott.

Makely, S. (2004). *Professionalism in health care: Primer for success* (2nd ed.). Upper Saddle River, NJ: Brady/Prentice Hall.

Porter, L. (n.d.). *Notes on how to read a textbook* (unpublished). Anaheim, CA: North Orange County Regional Occupational Program.

Taylor, J., & Hardy, D. (2004). *Monster careers: How to land the job of your life.* New York: Penguin Press.

Glossary

A

Ablation: removal by surgery (e.g., of a diseased body part) **(31)**

Absorption: process by which the drug passes into the blood stream **(29)**

Acceptance: coming to terms with loss; may have decreased interest in physical surroundings and support people **(17)**

Accommodation: alternating change in pupil size (pupils constrict when looking at near objects, dilate when looking at distant ones) **(19)**

Acculturation: the modification of a group's or individual's culture as a result of contact with another group **(2)**

Acid–base balance: regulation of hydrogen ion concentration of body fluids **(30)**

Active range of motion: full normal movement of the extremities and joints by the client through a systematic series of motions **(19)**

Active transport: the movement of electrolytes from an area of low concentration to an area of high concentration **(30)**

Acute pain: pain that lasts only through the expected recovery period **(21)**

Adenosine triphosphate (ATP): energy compound of cells **(18)**

Admission: process a client undergoes when entering a hospital for treatment **(10)**

Adult day care: center that provides health and social services to the older adult who is still living at home **(35)**

Adventitious breath sounds: abnormal breath sounds **(19)**

Adverse effects: severe side effects or drug reactions **(29)**

Advocate: one who expresses and defends the cause of another **(3)**

Afebrile: without fever **(20)**

Affective domain: aspects of learning that include feelings, emotions, interests, attitudes, and appreciations **(33)**

Afternoon care: care of client that often includes providing a bedpan or urinal, washing the hands and face, and assisting with oral care **(22)**

Against medical advice: situation in which a client leaves the hospital or healthcare facility without the written permission of a physician **(10)**

Algor mortis: gradual decrease of the body's temperature after death **(17)**

Alopecia: hair loss **(22)**

Ambulation: act of walking **(32)**

Ambulatory care nursing: care provided to clients in a physician's office or clinic, in which the client obtains some medical service before returning home the same day **(35)**

Amino acids: end products of protein digestion **(25)**

Ampule: clear glass container with a distinctive shape usually designed to hold a single dose of a drug **(29)**

Anabolism: process of building tissue **(25)**

Analgesics: pain relievers **(21)**

Analyze: process of interpreting a variety of data and recognizing the commonalities, differences, and interrelationships among ideas **(1)**

Anatomic position: normal standing position; body is upright, facing front, arms at the sides with the palms facing forward, and feet parallel **(18)**

Anatomy: study of body structure **(18)**

Anemia: condition of too few red blood cells that contain too little or abnormal hemoglobin **(24)**

Anesthesia: alteration in the level of sensation and consciousness; classified as *general* (comprehensive) or *regional* (specific) **(31)**

Anger: emotional state that includes feelings of animosity or strong displeasure **(16)**

Angina pectoris: chest pain, usually caused by lack of oxygen to the coronary vessels **(24)**

Ankylosed: permanently immobile **(32)**

Anticipatory grieving: state in which an individual or group experiences reactions in response to an expected significant loss **(17)**

Antiemboli stockings: firm elastic hose that compress the veins of the legs and facilitate the return of venous blood to the heart **(31)**

Antigens: markers that identify the type of cell and help the immune system determine whether the cell is foreign to the organism **(9)**

Antiseptics: agents that inhibit the growth of some microorganisms **(9)**

Anuria: lack of urine production, with no effective urinary output **(27)**

Anxiety: state of mental uneasiness, apprehension, dread; feeling of helplessness related to an unidentified threat to self or significant relationships **(16)**

Apical: at the apex of the heart **(20)**

Apnea: periods of no breathing **(24)**

Apothecaries' system: system of measurements that predates the metric system **(29)**

Appliance: pouch or bag **(28)**

Application: utilizing knowledge and understanding in a particular case **(1)**

Approximates: brings together the two sides of skin **(31)**

Asepsis: absence of disease-causing microorganisms **(9)**

Aseptic technique: method used to prevent the transmission of microorganisms from one place or person to another **(9)**

As-needed (prn) care: care provided as required by the client **(22)**

Assault: an attempt or threat to touch another person unjustifiably **(3)**

Assessment: systematic collection, organization, *validation* (proving or supporting), and documentation of *data* (information) **(5)**

Assisted living facility: facility that meets the needs of the ambulatory older adult; various degrees of personal care assistance may be provided **(35)**

Atelectasis: collapse of the alveoli, of a lobe, or of an entire lung **(31)**

Atherosclerosis: narrowing and obstruction of circulatory vessels; most common cause of ischemia **(24)**

Atherosclerotic plaque: fat deposits within blood vessels **(24)**

Atrophy: unused muscles atrophy (decrease in size), losing most of their normal strength and function **(32)**

Attitudes: mental positions or feelings toward a person, object, or idea **(3)**

Auditory: hearing **(13)**

Auscultation: process of listening to sounds produced within the body **(19)**

Autocratic: making unilateral decisions while dominating team members **(36)**

Autologous: when client provides his or her own blood for donation **(30)**

Autonomy: the right to make one's own decisions **(3)**

Autopsy: postmortem examination; examination of the body after death **(17)**

B

Bacteria: most common microorganisms that cause disease in humans **(9)**

Bactericidal agent: agent that destroys bacteria **(9)**

Bacteriostatic agent: agent that prevents growth and reproduction of only some bacteria **(9)**

Bagging: means of enclosing dirty, contaminated, or hazardous materials in plastic bags for safe removal and disposal **(8)**

Bargaining: when client promises a change in behavior to avoid loss **(17)**

Basal metabolic rate (BMR): rate at which the body metabolizes (burns) food to maintain energy **(20)**

Battery: the willful and unjustifiable touching of a person or personal items; it may or may not cause harm **(3)**

Bed cradle: (Anderson frame) a device designed to keep the top bedclothes off the feet, legs, and even abdomen of a client **(22)**

Bedpan: receptacle for urine or feces **(28)**

Behavior modification: system of positive reinforcement in which desirable behavior is regarded and undesirable behavior is ignored **(33)**

Behaviorism: belief that environment influences behavior, which is the essential factor determining human action **(33)**

Beliefs: interpretations or conclusions that people accept as being true; they do not necessarily involve values **(3)**

Bereavement: subjective response experienced by the surviving loved ones after the death of a person with whom they have shared a significant relationship **(17)**

Bevel: the slanted part of the tip of a needle **(29)**

Biocultural ecology: involves the assessment of skin color and biologic variations **(2)**

Bioethics: ethics as applied to life **(3)**

Blood pressure: measure of the pressure exerted by the blood as it flows through the arteries **(20)**

Body image: how a person perceives the size, appearance, and functioning of the body and its parts **(14)**

Body mechanics: term used to describe safe, efficient use of the body to move objects and carry out activities of daily living **(8)**

Body temperature: reflects the balance between the heat produced and the heat lost from the body **(20)**

Bradypnea: abnormally slow respiratory rate **(24)**

Buccal: pertaining to the cheek; in medication administration, it means next to the mucous membranes of the cheek **(29)**

Buffers: chemicals that help maintain acid–base balance by neutralizing excess acids or bases **(26)**

C

Calculi: stones **(27)**

Calories: units of heat energy **(25)**

Cannula: shaft part of a needle, which is attached to the hub **(29)**

Capillary refill: return of blood to tissue (such as the nail bed) after being pressed; return of normal color to tissue **(19)**

Cardiac output: amount of blood pumped by the heart in 1 minute **(20)**

Cardiopulmonary resuscitation (CPR): combination of oral resuscitation (mouth-to-mouth breathing) and external cardiac massage (chest compression); procedure is intended to provide oxygen to the lungs and reestablish cardiac function and blood circulation **(24)**

Care plan: written guide that organizes information about the client's care **(5)**

Career ladder: progression from one level in a profession to another through educational pursuits and professional experience **(38)**

Caries: cavities **(22)**

Carrier: person or animal that has a pathogenic microorganism living inside the body **(9)**

Case management: range of models for integrating healthcare services for individuals or groups **(7)**

Case method: system in which one nurse is responsible for the comprehensive care of a group of clients during an 8- or 12-hour shift **(7)**

Catabolism: process of breaking down tissue **(25)**

Cathartics: medication that stimulates bowel activity and assists fecal elimination **(28)**

Catheterization: introduction of a catheter through the urethra into the urinary bladder **(27)**

Cell: basic unit of all life **(18)**

Cell membrane: "skin" of a cell; plasma membrane **(18)**

Center of gravity: point at which all of the body's mass is centered; the base of support of the foundation on which the body achieves balance **(32)**

Cerumen: earwax **(22)**

Cervical spine alignment: a manual maneuver performed by an individual to maintain spinal alignment; also called *C spine* **(34)**

Change-of-shift report: a report given to all nurses on the incoming shift **(6)**

Channels: openings that permit the passage of certain materials into or out of a cell **(18)**

Charting: recording; documenting; process of making an entry on a client's record **(6)**

Chronic illness: caused by a disease that produces signs and symptoms within a variable period of time, develops slowly and runs a long course, allows only partial recovery, and imposes an enormous financial burden on a family **(17)**

Chronic obstructive pulmonary disease (COPD): persistent obstruction of bronchial airflow **(24)**

Chronic pain: pain that lasts beyond the typical healing period **(21)**

Chyme: waste products that leave the stomach through the small intestine and then pass through the ileocecal valve **(28)**

Cilia: hairlike projections on the surface of some cells **(18)**

Circumcision: removal of the foreskin of the penis **(15)**

Cleaning baths: baths given chiefly for hygiene purposes **(22)**

Client: (in this text) recipient of nursing care; includes individuals, families, and communities **(1)**

Client education: integrated and multifaceted teaching–learning process in which the nurse and client work together to change unhealthy client behaviors **(33)**

Client-focused care: delivery model that brings all services and care providers to the clients **(7)**

Clinical pathway: method for tracking the client's progress, planning care, and providing client teaching and discharge planning **(7)**

Clinical record: chart; client record; formal, legal document that provides evidence of a client's care **(6)**

Clinics: walk-in medical facilities where clients can obtain diagnostic testing or treatment before returning home the same day; also known as *ambulatory care centers* **(35)**

Closed-ended questions: questions that generally require only "yes" or "no" or short factual answers **(12)**

Closed wound drainage system: a drain connected directly from the wound or from an incision near the wound to a suction device; it promotes healing by allowing excess serosanguineous fluid and purulent material to drain **(31)**

Code of ethics: formal statement of a group's ideals and values **(3)**

Cognitive: related to awareness; perceiving; thinking **(11)**

Cognitive development: a result of interaction between an individual and the environment **(11)**

Cognitive domain: area of learning that includes knowing, comprehending, and applying **(33)**

Cognitivism: definition of learning as largely a complex thinking process; emphasizes individual perception and motivation, as well as the teacher–learner relationship and environment **(33)**

Coitus: copulation; heterosexual genital intercourse **(15)**

Collaborative: working jointly with other healthcare professionals in the performance of nursing roles within the scope of practice **(38)**

Collaborative interventions: nursing activities that reflect the overlapping responsibilities among healthcare personnel **(5)**

Colostomy: an opening into the *colon* (large bowel) **(28)**

Communicable disease: disease spread or transmitted by direct or indirect contact **(9)**

Communication: exchange of information or thoughts between two or more people through language, the arts, or body actions **(12)**

Compliance: extent to which a person's behavior coincides with medical or health advice **(33)**

Comprehension: knowledge and understanding of information **(1)**

Computerized adaptive testing (CAT): method of testing in which the computer selects a unique set of test questions for each test taker from a large test bank of questions. It provides a set percentage of questions from predetermined categories **(37)**

Confer: to consult another person for advice, information, ideas, or instructions **(6)**

Conflict: competitive or antagonistic state; mental state resulting from opposing needs, wishes, or demands **(36)**

Connective tissue: supporting fabric of the body **(18)**

Conscious sedation: a minimal form of anesthesia in which a client is conscious and has an increased pain threshold during surgery **(31)**

Consensual response: constriction of one eye when a bright light is shown into the opposite pupil, removed, and shown a second time **(19)**

Constipation: fewer than three bowel movements per week **(28)**

Consumer: individual, group of people, or community that uses a service or commodity **(1)**

Contact lenses: thin, curved disks of hard or soft plastic that fit on the cornea of the eye directly over the pupil; used to improve vision **(22)**

Continuous feedings: feedings generally administered over a 24-hour period using an infusion pump that guarantees a constant flow **(25)**

Coping: dealing with problems and situations successfully **(16)**

Coping behavior: behavior by people in times of crisis or stress, in an attempt to deal with their feelings **(10)**

Coping mechanism: inborn or learned way of responding to a changing environment, specific problem, or situation **(13)**

Correctional nurse: nurse who provides for the health care of inmates in correctional facilities such as juvenile offender homes, jails, prisons, and penitentiaries **(35)**

Cover letter: concise, one-page letter that highlights professional and educational attributes for a potential employer **(38)**

Crime: act committed in violation of public (criminal) law and punishable by a fine or imprisonment **(3)**

Crisis: stage in fever marked by excessive sweating and hot, flushed skin due to sudden vasodilation; acute, time-limited state of emotional imbalance resulting from sources of stress **(16)**

Critical thinking: process of examining one's own thinking and assumptions to arrive at a broader viewpoint **(4)**

Cultural awareness: knowing about the similarities and differences among cultures **(2)**

Cultural competence: the knowledge, skill, and ability to provide safe and effective health care regardless of population or setting **(2)**

Cultural empathy: ability to experience "as" the client experiences rather than "how" they experience themselves; ability to show caring without being involved in the same emotions as the client **(2)**

Cultural sensitivity: having an understanding on one's own culture while understanding and respecting the cultures of others **(2)**

Cumulative effect: buildup of a drug in the blood because of impaired metabolism or excretion **(29)**

Cutaneous pain: pain that originates in the skin or subcutaneous tissue **(21)**

Cyanosis: bluish tinge of skin that usually indicates poor oxygenation **(19)**

Cytoplasm: main substance filling the inside of the cell; a colloidal (jelly-like) suspension **(18)**

D

Dandruff: diffuse scaling of the scalp **(22)**

DAR: diagnosis (**D**), action (**A**), and response (**R**); means of organizing progress notes into data **(6)**

Database: baseline data; information about a client gathered from many sources; a reference point to assess changes in a client's condition **(5)**

Date rape: situation in which one person manipulates a social interaction in order to have nonconsensual intercourse with another **(15)**

Debride: removal of necrotic material **(23)**

Deductive reasoning: reasoning from the general to the specific **(4)**

Defamation: communication that is false, or made with careless disregard for the truth, and that results in injury to the reputation of a person **(3)**

Defecation: bowel movement; expulsion of feces from the anus and rectum **(28)**

Defense mechanisms: psychologic adaptive mechanisms that develop as the personality attempts to defend itself, establish compromises among conflicting impulses, and allay inner tensions **(16)**

Defibrillator: an instrument that provides various voltages of electricity (measured in joules) to trigger the electrical impulses of the heart **(34)**

Dehisced: opened on the suture line **(31)**

Dehiscence: partial or total rupturing of a sutured wound **(23)**

Dehumanization: process in which unique human qualities are ignored (as in hospitalized clients having to surrender their belongings, privacy, and independence) **(10)**

Delegation: distribution of tasks in a way that prioritizes activities and available resources **(36)**

Democratic: making decisions that reflect input from team members **(36)**

Denial: when a client refuses to believe that the loss is happening and is not ready to deal with practical problems **(17)**

Dentures: a "plate" of artificial teeth for one jaw **(22)**

Depression: common reaction to overwhelming or negative events **(17)**

Designated blood: blood that is donated by friends and relatives of the client **(30)**

Development: an increase in the complexity of function and skill progression and in adaptation to the environment **(11)**

Diagnosing: second phase of nursing process; uses critical thinking skills to interpret assessment data and identify client strengths and problems **(5)**

Diagnostic: used to confirm or establish a diagnosis **(31)**

Diagnostic profile: information provided to students who fail the NCLEX-PN®, giving them data on performance in the various categories of the test **(37)**

Diagnostic-related groups (DRGs): classification of clinical conditions used for reimbursement by Medicare to healthcare provider or facility **(7)**

Diarrhea: passage of liquid feces and increased frequency of defecation **(28)**

Diastole: period in which the ventricles of the heart relax **(19)**

Diastolic pressure: pressure when the ventricles are at rest; the lower pressure that is present at all times within the arteries **(20)**

Diffusion: the movement of gases or other particles from an area of greater pressure or concentration to an area of lower pressure or concentration **(24)**

Direct response: constriction or tightening of a pupil when a bright light is shown into it **(19)**

Discharge: official procedure by which a client leaves a healthcare facility and returns home or to another setting **(10)**

Discrimination: differential treatment of individuals or groups based on categories such as race, ethnicity, gender, social class, or exceptionality **(2)**

Disease: process with distinctive signs and symptoms of infection **(9)**

Disinfectants: agents that destroy pathogens other than spores **(19)**

Diuresis: production and excretion of large amounts of urine **(27)**

Diuretics: chemicals that increase urine formation by preventing the reabsorption of water and electrolytes from the tubules of the kidney into the bloodstream **(27)**

Documenting: process of making an entry on a client record **(6)**

Do-not-resuscitate (DNR) order: order given for clients who are in a stage of terminal, irreversible illness or expected death **(17)**

Drug allergy: immunologic reaction to a drug **(29)**

Drug interaction: problem that occurs when the administration of one drug alters the effect of another drug **(29)**

Drug tolerance: occurs when a person requires increases in dosage to maintain the therapeutic effect **(29)**

Drug toxicity: deleterious effects of a drug on an organism or tissue resulting from overdosage or from ingestion of a drug intended for external use **(29)**

Durable power of attorney for health care: written statement appointing someone else to manage healthcare treatment decisions when the client is unable to do so **(17)**

Dysfunctional grieving: grieving characterized by extended time of denial, depression, severe physiologic symptoms, or suicidal thoughts **(17)**

Dysmenorrhea: painful menstruation **(15)**

Dyspareunia: pain during sexual activity and intercourse **(15)**

Dyspnea: difficult or labored breathing **(24)**

Dysrhythmias: abnormalities of the heart rate and rhythm **(24)**

Dysuria: painful or difficult urination **(27)**

E

Early morning care: care provided to clients as they awaken in the morning **(22)**

Edema: presence of excess interstitial fluid in tissue; causes a puffy appearance **(19)**

Effleurage: technique used in massage to promote relaxation and rest; light massage **(32)**

Effluent: fecal material **(28)**

Elective surgery: surgery performed when a condition is not immediately life threatening or to improve the client's life **(31)**

Electrocardiography: graphic recording of the heart's electrical activity **(24)**

Electrolytes: charged ions that can conduct electricity; present in all body fluids and fluid compartments **(26)**

Emboli: clots moved from their place of origin, causing circulatory obstruction elsewhere; may lodge in vessels supplying vital organs **(32)**

Embolus: thrombus that has broken loose **(24)**

Emergency care: care given for an urgent or life-threatening illness or accident; also called *ER* (for emergency room) **(34)**

Emergency surgery: surgery performed immediately to preserve function or the life of the client **(31)**

Endocrine glands: glands that do not have ducts; secretions (hormones) are transported away from the gland by blood flowing through the gland **(18)**

Endogenous opioids: naturally occurring opioids (enkephalins, dynorphins, and beta endorphins) that bind to opiate receptor sites in the central and peripheral nervous system, decreasing or blocking any pain impulse **(21)**

Endoplasmic reticulum: network of membrane-bound tubules that extend from the cell membrane to the nuclear membrane **(18)**

Enema: solution introduced into the rectum and large intestine to distend the intestines and sometimes to irritate the intestinal mucosa to promote peristalsis and remove feces and flatus **(28)**

Enteral nutrition (EN): nutrients provided when the client is unable to ingest or absorb foods; also called *total enteral nutrition* (TEN) **(25)**

Enuresis: urinary incontinence usually occurring at night in children, commonly known as bedwetting **(27)**

Environments: internal and external surroundings that affect the client **(4)**

Enzymes: proteins that speed up chemical reactions that occur at the cell membrane **(18)**

Epiglottis: inlet to the larynx that closes during swallowing, routing food to the esophagus **(24)**

Epithelium: tissue that forms a covering or lining **(18)**

Equilibrium: sense of balance **(32)**

Erectile dysfunction: see *Impotence* **(15)**

Eructation: belching or burping **(28)**

Erythema: redness associated with a variety of rashes **(19)**

Erythrocytes: red blood cells **(24)**

Eschar: scar tissue **(23)**

Ethics: method of inquiry that helps people to understand the morality of human behavior; the practices or beliefs of a certain group; the expected standards of moral behavior of a particular group **(3)**

Ethnocentrism: the view that the beliefs and values of one's own culture are superior to those of other cultures **(2)**

Etiology: identification of factors contributing to, or probable causes of, a health problem **(5)**

Eupnea: normal respiration; it is quiet, rhythmic, and effortless **(24)**

Eupneic: having characteristics of normal respiration **(34)**

Evaluation: review of interventions to determine their effectiveness **(5)**

Evisceration: protrusion of internal viscera and tissue through an incision **(23)**

Exacerbation: flare-ups of a chronic disease **(17)**

Examination: physical assessment; a systematic method of collecting physical data about a client **(5)**

Exocrine glands: glands that secrete substances through ducts that reach the epithelial surface inside the body or on the skin **(18)**

Exogenous opioid: analgesics (e.g., morphine) that bind to receptor sites to provide pain relief **(21)**

Expected outcomes: goal; a description, in terms of observable client responses, of what the nurse hopes the client will achieve by implementing the nursing orders **(5)**

Expiration: exhalation; air moving out of the lungs as part of ventilation **(24)**

External disasters: events outside the hospital that produce a large number of victims (e.g., fires, plane or train accidents, earthquakes, or violent civil disturbances) **(18)**

External respiration: refers to the interchange of oxygen and carbon dioxide between the alveoli of the lungs and the pulmonary blood **(20)**

Extracellular fluid (ECF): fluid found outside the cells; accounts for about one-third of total body fluid **(26)**

Exudate: material that has escaped from blood vessels during the inflammatory process and is deposited in tissue or on tissue surfaces **(23)**

F

False imprisonment: unlawful restraint or detention of another person against his or her wishes **(3)**

Fecal diversion: an alternate route for feces elimination **(28)**

Feces: excreted waste products; also called *stool* **(28)**

Feedback: shared information that relates a person's performance to the desired goal **(33)**

Fight-or-flight response: a generalized body response to an emergency situation **(16)**

Filtration: the transfer of water and dissolved substances from a region of high pressure to a region of low pressure **(30)**

Fistula: abnormal passage between a hollow organ and the skin or between two hollow organs **(23)**

Flagellum: long whiplike extension from a cell that is used to move the cell itself **(18)**

Flatulence: presence of excessive *flatus* (gas) in the intestines **(28)**

Flatus: air and by-products of the digestion of carbohydrates within the bowel; gas **(28)**

Flow sheets: abbreviated progress notes that enable nurses to record nursing data quickly and concisely and provide an easy-to-read record of the client's condition over time **(6)**

Fluid: divided into intracellular and extracellular compartments **(26)**

Fontanelles: gaps in the bone structure of an infant's skull that close gradually **(11)**

Friction: force acting parallel to the skin surface **(23)**

Frontal plane: runs from one side of the body to the other, separating the body into front and back portions **(18)**

Fulcrum: fixed point about which a lever moves **(8)**

Full-thickness burns: third-degree burns that involve all the layers of skin and may extend into subcutaneous fat, connective tissue, muscle, and bone **(34)**

Functional method: delivery model that focuses on the jobs to be completed, using personnel with less preparation than the professional nurse to perform less complex care requirements **(7)**

Functional nursing: system in which each team member is assigned specific tasks or functions **(36)**

Fungi: microorganisms classified as either yeasts or molds **(9)**

G

Gametes: sperm or egg cells **(18)**

Gastrostomy: surgical creation of an artificial opening into the stomach **(25)**

Gate control theory: theory stating that peripheral nerve fibers carrying pain to the spinal cord can have their message modified at the spinal cord level (the "gate") before transmission to the brain **(21)**

General adaptation syndrome (GAS): three stages of changes in the body in the presence of stress: alarm reaction, resistance, and exhaustion **(16)**

Generic: family name of a drug **(29)**

Gestures: body movements **(12)**

Gingiva: the gums **(22)**

Glands: tissue that produces some form of secretion **(18)**

Glycogen: stored form of glucose **(25)**

Goals: see *Expected outcomes* **(5)**

Golgi apparatus: site where materials are synthesized and sorted for secretion from the cell **(18)**

Granulation tissue: translucent red tissue that grows in a wound **(23)**

Grief: total response to the emotional experience related to loss **(17)**

Grieving: process of reacting to loss; natural human response involving psychosocial and physiological reactions to an actual or perceived loss **(11)**

Group: two or more people who have shared needs and goals, who take each other into account in their actions, and who thus are held together and set apart from others because of their interactions **(12)**

Growth: physical change and increase in size, including height, weight, bone size, and dentition **(11)**

Guaiac test: a test for occult blood **(28)**

Gustatory: dealing with the sense of taste **(13)**

H

Half-life: time interval required for the body's elimination processes to reduce the concentration of the drug in the body by one-half **(29)**

Halitosis: bad breath **(22)**

Health: degree of wellness or well-being that the client experiences **(4)**

Health maintenance organization (HMO): group healthcare agency that provides basic and supplemental health maintenance and treatment services to voluntary enrollees; fee is set without regard to the amount or kind of services provided **(7)**

Healthcare system: totality of services offered by all health disciplines **(7)**

Hearing aid: battery-powered, sound-amplifying device used by people with hearing impairments **(22)**

Helpful communication: communication that encourages a sharing of information, thoughts, or feelings between two or more people **(12)**

Hematocrit: measurement of the percentage of erythrocytes in the blood **(24)**

Hematuria: evidence of blood in the urine **(27)**

Hemoglobin: oxygen-carrying red pigment in the red blood cells **(24)**

Hemoptysis: blood in the sputum **(24)**

Hemorrhage: persistent bleeding **(23)**

Hemostasis: the arrest of bleeding **(23)**

Hemothorax: blood in the pleural space **(24)**

Hermaphroditism: presence of both testicular and ovarian tissue in an infant at birth **(15)**

High acuity: very urgent and possibly life threatening **(34)**

Hirsutism: growth of excessive body hair **(22)**

Holistic: approach that takes into account the client as a physical, mental, emotional, and spiritual being **(4)**

Homeostasis: state of balance, when all the components of a system are working properly; normal ranges of fluids and electrolytes and of acids and bases **(18)**

Homologous: a blood donation by someone other than the person receiving the blood **(30)**

Hormones: secretions of (ductless) endocrine glands **(18)**

Hour of sleep care (HS): care provided to clients before they retire for the night **(22)**

Household system: measures commonly used in the home, including drops, teaspoons, tablespoons, cups, and glasses **(29)**

Hub: part of the needle that fits onto the syringe **(29)**

Humanism: humanistic learning theory; focuses on both cognitive and affective qualities of the learner **(33)**

Hygiene: science of health and its maintenance **(22)**

Hypercapnia: accumulation of excessive carbon dioxide in the blood; also called *hypercarbia* **(24)**

Hypercarbia: see *Hypercapnia* **(24)**

Hypersomnia: excessive daytime sleep **(32)**

Hyperthermia: body temperature above the usual range; fever **(20)**

Hypertonic: having a greater concentration of solutes than plasma **(26)**

Hyperventilation: increased rate and depth of respirations **(24)**

Hypervolemia: excess blood volume such as might result from fluid retention or kidney failure **(24)**

Hypothermia: core body temperature below the lower limit of normal **(20)**

Hypotonic: having a lesser concentration of solutes **(26)**

Hypovolemia: inadequate blood volume such as might result from hemorrhage or severe dehydration **(24)**

Hypoxia: condition of insufficient oxygen anywhere in the body **(24)**

I

Iatrogenic disease: disease caused unintentionally by medical therapy **(29)**

Iatrogenic infection: infection directly caused by any diagnostic or therapeutic source **(9)**

Idiosyncratic effect: unexpected unique bodily response that causes unpredictable abnormal symptoms in clients **(29)**

Ileostomy: an opening into the *ileum* (small bowel) **(28)**

Illness: highly individualized response to disease **(1)**

Immunity: resistance of the body to infection **(9)**

Impaction: mass or collection of hardened, putty-like feces in the folds of the rectum **(28)**

Impaired nurse: a nurse whose practice has been negatively affected by chemical abuse, specifically the abuse of alcohol and drugs **(3)**

Implementation: fourth step of nursing process, in which selected nursing interventions (actions) are performed **(5)**

Impotence: erectile dysfunction; the inability to achieve or maintain an erection sufficient for sexual satisfaction for oneself or one's partner **(5)**

Impulse: travels along nerve pathways to the spinal cord or directly to the brain **(13)**

Incident: any unexpected event **(6)**

Incident report: occurrence report; form completed when client care was not consistent with standards for expected care **(36)**

Incontinence: inability to control excretion **(27)**

Independent practice association (IPA): similar to an HMO or PPO except that an IPA's clients pay a fixed prospective payment to the IPA, and the IPA pays the provider **(7)**

Inductive reasoning: forming generalizations from a set of facts or observations **(4)**

Infarction: death of tissue **(32)**

Infection: invasion and growth of microorganisms in a body tissue **(9)**

Infertility: inability to conceive a child **(15)**

Infibulation: excision of the clitoris, the labia minora, and the labia majora, or closure of the vagina **(15)**

Inflammatory response: local nonspecific defense reaction of tissues when they are exposed to infection or injury **(9)**

Insomnia: inability to obtain an adequate amount or quality of sleep; is the most common sleep disorder **(32)**

Inspection: visual examination; assessing by using the sense of sight **(19)**

Inspiration: inhalation; air flowing into the lungs as part of ventilation **(24)**

Intake and output (I&O): measurement and recording of all fluid taken in and excreted during a 24-hour period **(26)**

Integrated delivery system: incorporates acute care services, home health care, extended and skilled care facilities, and outpatient services to provide care throughout the life span **(7)**

Integumentary system: skin and its associated structures (hair, nails, oil and sweat glands, blood vessels, nerves, and sensory organs) **(18)**

Intercourse: the sexual union of two persons **(15)**

Intercultural communication: process that occurs when members of two or more cultures exchange messages in a manner that is influenced by their different cultural perceptions **(2)**

Intermittent feeding: administration of 300–500 mL of enteral formula several times per day **(25)**

Internal disasters: events within the hospital that interrupt services and produce victims (e.g., utility interruption or chemical spill) **(8)**

Internal respiration: interchange of oxygen and carbon dioxide between the circulating blood and the cells of the body tissues **(20)**

Interstitial fluid: fluid between cells; transports wastes from cells via lymph system, as well as directly into blood plasma through capillaries **(26)**

Interventions: actions performed by a nurse. 1. *Independent interventions:* activities nurses are licensed to initiate on the basis of their knowledge and skills. 2. *Dependent interventions:* activities carried out under the physician's orders or supervision, or according to specified routines **(5)**

Interview: planned communication; conversation with a purpose **(5)**

Intracellular fluid (ICF): fluid within the cells of the body; about two-thirds of the total body fluid in adults **(26)**

Intractable pain: chronic pain that persists despite therapeutic interventions **(21)**

Intradermal (ID): injection into the dermis or skin **(29)**

Intramuscular (IM): injection into the muscle **(29)**

Intravenous (IV): injection into the vein **(29)**

Invasion of privacy: direct wrong of a personal nature that injures the feelings of the person and does not take into account the effect of revealed information on the standing of the person in the community **(3)**

Irrigation: flushing or washing out with a specified solution; lavage **(27)**

Ischemia: lack of blood supply to tissues and organs due to obstructed circulation **(23)**

Isotonic: having the same concentration of solutes as blood plasma **(26)**

J

Jejunostomy: surgical creation of a permanent opening through the abdominal wall into the jejunum **(25)**

K

Kardex: a widely used, concise method of organizing and recording data about a client **(6)**

Keloid: hypertrophic (progressively enlarging) scar **(23)**

Kinesthetic: awareness of the position and movement of body parts **(13)**

Knowledge: recall of information **(1)**

Kussmaul's breathing: hyperventilation that accompanies metabolic acidosis; rapid, deep breaths that attempt to rid the body of excess body acids by blowing off the carbon dioxide **(24)**

L

Labyrinth: inner ear; consists of the cochlea, vestibule, and semicircular canals **(32)**

Laissez-faire: exercising little control or guidance over a group **(36)**

Lanugo: fine hair on the body of the fetus; downy or woolly hair **(22)**

Law: "rules made by humans that regulate social conduct in a formally prescribed and legally binding manner" (Bernzweig, 1996, p. 3) **(3)**

Laxative: medication that stimulates bowel activity and assists fecal elimination; less potent than a cathartic **(28)**

Leadership: process used to move a group toward setting and achieving goals **(36)**

Learning: lifelong process of acquiring knowledge or skills that cannot be solely accounted for by human growth; it is demonstrated by changes in behavior **(33)**

Lesion: alteration in normal skin appearance **(19)**

Level of consciousness (LOC): state of alertness; LOC can range from alert and oriented to coma **(19)**

Liability: being legally responsible for one's acts and omissions **(3)**

Libel: defamation by means of print, writing, or pictures **(3)**

License: issued after passing the licensing exam **(36)**

Licensure: process by which a government agency gives permission for an individual to engage in an occupation or profession **(36)**

Line of gravity: imaginary vertical line drawn through the body's center of gravity **(32)**

Lipids: organic substances that are greasy and insoluble in water but soluble in alcohol or ether **(25)**

Living will: a type of advanced medical directive that provides specific instructions about what medical treatment the client chooses to omit or refuse (e.g., CPR, intubation, ventilatory support) in the event that the client is unable to make those decisions **(17)**

Livor mortis: discoloration of tissues after blood circulation has ceased **(17)**

Local infection: illness caused by microorganisms that are only in a specific part of the body **(9)**

Loss: an actual or potential situation in which someone or something that is valued is changed, no longer available, or gone **(17)**

M

Maceration: softening of tissue by prolonged wetting **(23)**

Malpractice: negligence that occurs while a person is performing as a professional **(3)**

Managed care: healthcare system that provide cost-effective, quality care for groups of clients **(7)**

Manifestations: combination of subjective and objective data **(5)**

Matrix: network of nonliving, intracellular material **(18)**

Meatus: opening of the urethra on the external body **(27)**

Medicaid: federal public assistance program paid out of general taxes to people who require financial assistance **(7)**

Medical asepsis: all practices used to confine a specific microorganism to a specific area **(9)**

Medicare: amendment to the Social Security Act that provided a national and state health insurance program for older adults **(7)**

Medication: substance administered for the diagnosis, cure, treatment, relief, or prevention of disease; a drug **(29)**

Meiosis: type of cell division responsible for the formation of sex cells **(18)**

Menstruation: monthly uterine bleeding **(15)**

Mental health facility/clinic: medical facilities whose focus is on psychosocial issues and the mental health status of its clients **(35)**

Metabolic acidosis: condition that occurs when bicarbonate is lost or acid is increased within the plasma **(26)**

Metabolic alkalosis: condition that occurs when the plasma loses hydrogen ions (acid) and gains bicarbonate **(26)**

Metric system: decimal system based on units of ten **(29)**

Micturition: process of emptying the urinary bladder **(27)**

Midsagittal plane: plane running from front to back, separating the body into equal left and right portions **(18)**

Midstream voided: term for a clean-catch urine specimen collected after voiding a small amount of urine to clear the urethra **(27)**

Mitochondria: large organelles where adenosine triphosphate (ATP) is produced **(18)**

Mitosis: division of a single parent cell into two genetically identical daughter cells **(18)**

Mnemonics: techniques for developing memory **(37)**

Moral: having to do with judgments of right or wrong **(11)**

Moral development: includes six stages of learning "right" and "wrong" **(11)**

Morning care: care provided after clients have breakfast **(22)**

Motivation: desire **(33)**

Motor development: the development of abilities to move and to control the body **(11)**

Mourning: behavioral process through which grief is eventually resolved or altered **(17)**

Multistate compact: an agreement among several state boards of nursing that a nurse licensed in one of these states can work in any other state that has signed the agreement without having to obtain a separate license **(37)**

Myocardial infarction (MI): heart attack **(24)**

N

Narcolepsy: poorly understood disorder, possibly genetic or autoimmune; sufferers experience regular REM onset sleep attacks lasting from a few seconds to several hours **(32)**

NCLEX-PN®: National Council Licensure Examination for Practical/Vocational Nurses; a test given to ensure that graduates of practical/vocational nursing schools meet the minimum standards to practice safely as LPNs/LVNs **(1)**

Negligence: misconduct or practice that is below the standard expected of an ordinary, reasonable, and prudent practitioner, which places another person at risk for harm **(3)**

Networking: deliberately making connections among people with common interests and for employment opportunities **(38)**

Neuropathic pain: pain felt as the result of a disturbance of the nerve pathways either from past or continuing tissue damage **(21)**

Nitrogen balance: measure of intake and loss of nitrogen **(25)**

Nociceptors: receptors that transmit pain sensation **(21)**

Nomogram: body surface area determined by using a child's height and weight; considered to be the most accurate method of calculating a medication dose for a child **(29)**

Nonspecific defenses: defenses that protect the body against all microorganisms **(9)**

Nonverbal communication: uses other forms of communication such as gestures, facial expressions, and touch **(12)**

Nosocomial infections: infections that occur as a result of healthcare delivery in a healthcare setting **(9)**

NPO: nothing by mouth **(29)**

NREM sleep: non–rapid eye movement sleep; a deep, restful sleep with some decreased physiological functioning **(32)**

Nucleus: most prominent organelle; control center that contains a cell's genetic material (DNA) **(18)**

Nurse practice acts: acts that legally define and describe the scope of nursing practice and that protect the public; legal acts that regulate the practice of nursing in the United States and Canada **(1)**

Nursing care conference: meeting of a group of nurses to discuss possible solutions to client problems **(6)**

Nursing diagnosis: clinical judgment about individual, family, or community responses to actual and potential health problems or life processes **(5)**

Nursing process: systematic, logical method of providing individualized nursing care; includes assessment, diagnosis, planning, implementation, and evaluation **(5)**

Nursing rounds: procedures in which a group of nurses visit selected clients at each client's bedside **(6)**

Nutrients: organic, inorganic, and energy-producing substances found in food **(25)**

Nutrition: result of the interaction between nutrients and the human body **(25)**

O

Obesity: body weight that exceeds ideal by more than 20% **(25)**

Objective data: signs that are detectable by an observer or can be tested against an accepted standard **(4)**

Observation: process of gathering data by using the senses **(5)**

Occult blood: hidden blood, as in stool **(28)**

Olfactory: having to do with the sense of smell **(13)**

Oliguria: low urine output **(27)**

Omnibus Budget Reconciliation Act (OBRA): legislation to bring a measure of quality improvement to the nursing home and extended care facility industry **(7)**

Open-ended questions: questions that invite a client to explore his or her thoughts or feelings **(12)**

Ophthalmics: preparations for the eye (29)

Oral report: taped report delivered in a report room or while nurses are making client rounds (36)

Orchiectomy: removal of the testicles (15)

Organ system: organs that function together for the same general purpose (18)

Orgasmic dysfunction: the inability of a woman to achieve orgasm (15)

Orientation: introduction of clients to the people and facility into which they have been admitted; awareness of place and time and family members; program or time period provided for newly hired individuals to prepare them for their position (10)

Orthostatic hypotension: sudden decrease in central blood pressure with position changes (20)

Osmolarity: the total number of osmotically active particles; refers to the concentration of a solute in a volume of solution (30)

Osmosis: passage of water from an area of lower particle concentration toward an area of higher concentration of particles (30)

Osmotic pressure: develops as solute particles collide against each other (30)

Osteoporosis: demineralization process, continues during immobility; bones become spongy and deformed, and they fracture easily (32)

Ostomy: an opening in the abdominal wall for the elimination of feces or urine (28)

Otics: ear preparations (29)

P

Pain: sensation that is highly subjective and individual; one of the body's defense mechanisms indicating that there is a problem (21)

Pain reaction: responses that include those of the autonomic nervous system and behavioral responses (21)

Pain threshold: amount of pain stimulation a person requires in order to feel pain (21)

Pain tolerance: maximum amount and duration of pain that an individual is willing to endure (21)

Palliative care: for relief or reduction of symptoms of a disease; does not produce a cure (17)

Pallor: pale appearance caused by lack of circulating blood or hemoglobin, which results in reduced amounts of oxygen being carried to body tissues (19)

Palpation: examination of the body using the sense of touch (19)

Paralytic ileus: temporary cessation of intestinal movement (28)

Parasites: microorganisms that live on other living organisms (9)

Parasomnia: behavior that may interfere with sleep, such as sleepwalking (32)

Parenteral: injectable medications (29)

Parenteral nutrition: nutrients provided, usually intravenously, when the client is unable to ingest or absorb foods (25)

Partial-thickness burns: second-degree burn that involves the entire dermis and may also involve the hair follicles (34)

Passive diffusion: the movement of molecules randomly in all directions from a region of high concentration to one of low concentration (30)

Passive range of motion: movement of the client's extremities and joints by a caregiver (19)

Pathogens: microorganisms that cause disease (9)

Patient: person who is waiting for or undergoing medical treatment and care (1)

Peak flow test: test that evaluates maximum airflow during forced expiration and monitors bronchospasm in asthmatic clients (34)

Pediculosis: infestation with lice (22)

Percussion: act of striking a part with short, sharp blows (1) to help gather data about internal organs; (2) to assist in massage; (3) to help a client to clear the respiratory tract (19)

Performance: relates what a person does in a particular role to the behaviors expected of that role (14)

Performance evaluation: a review (usually annual) of on-the-job activity (including attendance and promptness, skills, work as a team member, and ability to complete assignments in a timely manner) (38)

Perfusion: blood supply to an area (19)

Perioperative period: time surrounding a surgery, consisting of the *preoperative phase* (prior to surgery), *intraoperative phase* (during surgery), and *postoperative phase* (following surgery) (31)

Peripheral pulse: pulse located in the periphery of the body (foot, hand, or neck) (20)

Peripheral vascular system: all of the blood vessels that carry oxygenated blood to body tissues and organs and that return deoxygenated blood to the heart and lungs (19)

Peristalsis: wavelike motion that propels intestinal contents forward (28)

Peristomal: skin around stoma opening (28)

PERRLA: pupils equally round and reactive to light and accommodation (19)

Personal identity: conscious sense of individuality and uniqueness that continually evolves throughout life (14)

Personal space: the distance people prefer in interactions with others (12)

Petrissage: technique used in massage to stimulate muscles; deep massage (32)

Phagocytosis: engulfing of microorganisms and cellular debris by white blood cells known as phagocytes (23)

Phantom pain: a painful sensation perceived in a body part that is missing (21)

Phlebotomy: a procedure for drawing and dispensing blood (34)

Physical assessment: one of three types of examination of the body: (1) complete assessment, (2) focused assessment by body systems, or (3) focused assessment of a body part (19)

Physiological: having to do with physical processes in the human body (11)

Physiology: study of how the body functions (18)

Plane: imaginary flat surface that divides a structure into two portions (18)

Planning: third step of nursing process; consists of decision making, prioritizing, and problem solving to achieve desired client outcomes (5)

Pleural effusion: fluid in the pleural space (24)

Pneumothorax: air in the pleural space (24)

Polyuria: production of abnormally large amounts of urine by the kidneys (27)

Portfolio: itemized visual account of skills and best practices related to the position one is seeking (38)

Postural tonus: sustained muscle contraction required to maintain the upright position (32)

Preemptive analgesia: administration of analgesics prior to an invasive or operative procedure; also includes around-the-clock (ATC) analgesia (21)

Preferred provider arrangement (PPA): similar to a PPO but can be contracted with individual healthcare providers, rather than an organization of healthcare providers (7)

Preferred provider organization (PPO): group of physicians and perhaps a healthcare agency (often hospitals) that provide an insurance company or employer with health services at a discounted rate (7)

Prejudice: a strongly held positive or negative opinion about some topic or group of people; it may be based on experience, fear, or misinformation (2)

Prescription: written direction for the preparation and administration of a drug (29)

Pressure ulcers: decubitus ulcers, pressure sores, or bedsores; lesions caused by unrelieved pressure that results in damage to underlying tissue (23)

Primary nursing: system in which one nurse is responsible for total care of a number of clients 24 hours a day, 7 days a week (7)

Primary prevention: practices and education that prevent healthy individuals from becoming ill or developing a disorder (17)

prn order: "as-needed order"; permits the nurse to give a medication when the client requires it (29)

Probationary period: time during which an immediate supervisor evaluates a new employee's performance (38)

Problem-oriented medical record (POMR): arrangement of data according to individual problems the client has rather than by the source of the information; also called *problem-oriented record* (POR) (6)

Procedures: technical, *psychomotor* (hands-on) skills that involve nursing actions such as manipulating equipment, giving injections, or repositioning clients (5)

Profession: occupation to which one devotes oneself and in which one has specialized expertise (1)

Professionalism: a courteous, conscientious, and generally business-like manner in the workplace (38)

Prospective payment system: legislation that limits the amount paid to hospitals that are reimbursed by Medicare (7)

Prosthesis: artificial limb or part (31)

Protein-calorie malnutrition: significant problem of clients with cancer and chronic disease; characterized by weight loss, and visible muscle and fat wasting (25)

Psychomotor domain: area of learning that includes motor skills (such as giving an injection) (33)

Psychosocial: having to do with relationships with oneself and others (11)

Puberty: period in which sexual organs mature and secondary sexual characteristics develop (11)

Pulmonary function tests: testing done to measure lung volume and capacity (24)

Pulse: heartbeat (19)

Pulse deficit: differences between the apical and radial pulse rates (20)

Pyrexia: hyperthermia, fever, body temperature above the usual range (20)

R

Radiating pain: pain perceived at the source of the pain that extends to nearby tissues (21)

Rales: crackle sounds (19)

Range of motion (ROM): maximum movement possible for that joint (32)

Rape: sexual intercourse in which one person is an unwilling or unconsenting party (15)

Rationale: scientific principle given as the reason for selecting a particular nursing intervention (5)

Reactive hyperemia: reaction in which skin takes on a bright red flush when pressure is relieved (23)

Readiness: motivation to learn at a specific time (33)

Receptor: point of attachment for materials on the surface of the cell membrane; nerve cells that receive a stimulus and convert it to a nerve impulse (13)

Reconstructive (surgery): performed to restore function or appearance that has been lost or reduced (31)

Record: a written or computer-based collection of data (6)

Referred pain: pain felt in a part of the body that is considerably removed from the tissues causing the pain (21)

Reflexes: unconscious, involuntary responses that are neither learned nor consciously carried out; nervous system responses to stimuli (11)

Rehabilitation: process of learning to live one's maximum potential with a chronic impairment, disability, or substance dependency (17)

Relevance: importance or applicability (33)

REM sleep: rapid eye movement sleep; part of sleep in which dreams occur (32)

Remission: time period in a chronic illness when the disease is present, but there are no symptoms (17)

Report: a means of conveying information about changes in a client's condition promptly (6)

Reservoir: place where a microorganism naturally lives (9)

Resident flora: microorganisms that are normal in a particular body area (9)

Residual urine: urine remaining in the bladder following voiding (27)

Respiration: the act of breathing (20)

Respiratory acidosis: a state of excessive carbon dioxide in the body; hypercapnia (26)

Respiratory alkalosis: a state of excessive loss of carbon dioxide in the body (26)

Response: an effect from an illness or stimulus (16)

Résumé: concise systematic summary of professional experience and educational background (38)

Retention: holding, keeping; in the case of learning, active remembering (33)

Rigor mortis: stiffening of the body that occurs about 2 to 4 hours after death (17)

Role: set of expectations about how the person occupying one position behaves toward a person occupying another position (14)

S

Sagittal plane: separates into left and right **(18)**

Same-day surgery clinic: health facility in which the client arrives early in the day, has a surgical procedure, and returns home after he or she is fully recovered from anesthesia; also known as an *outpatient surgical center* **(35)**

Sanguineous: hemorrhagic; consisting of large amounts of red blood cells **(23)**

Scabies: contagious skin infestation by the itch mite **(22)**

School-based health clinic: ambulatory care centers, located in a number of intercity school districts, that perform a higher level of care than the regular school health office **(35)**

School health office: room or area within a school where medications and first aid supplies are kept and distributed by qualified personnel **(35)**

Scope of practice: document developed by the board of nursing that governs practice within each state **(3)**

Sebum: oily skin secretion that softens and lubricates the hair and skin **(22)**

Secondary prevention: early diagnosis and treatment to prevent negative outcomes **(17)**

Secondary sex characteristics: traits associated with gender but not directly necessary for reproduction **(18)**

Segregation: physical separation of housing and services based on race **(2)**

Self-concept: a complex idea that includes all aspects of how one perceives oneself **(14)**

Self-esteem: one's judgment of one's own worth **(14)**

Sensory deficit: impaired reception, perception, or both, of one or more of the senses **(13)**

Sensory deprivation: decrease in or lack of meaningful stimuli **(13)**

Sensory overload: excessive stimulation; generally occurs when a person is unable to process or manage the amount or intensity of sensory stimuli **(13)**

Sensory perception: the conscious organization and translation of data or stimuli into meaningful information **(13)**

Sepsis: presence of infection **(9)**

Septicemia: condition that exists when bacteria enter the bloodstream and spread through all of the body's systems **(9)**

Sequential compression device (SCD): device such as elastic stockings that promotes venous return from the legs **(31)**

Serosanguineous: blood tinged **(23)**

Serous: exudates consisting chiefly of serum derived from blood **(23)**

Sex: term most commonly used to denote biologic male or female status; also, sexual intercourse **(15)**

Sexual abuse: any involvement of a child in an act designed to provide sexual gratification to an adult **(15)**

Sexual dysfunction: undesired, altered sexual function **(15)**

Sexual harassment: "unwelcome sexual advances, requests for sexual favors, and other verbal or physical conduct of a sexual nature" (EEOC) **(3)**

Sexual orientation: preference of a person for one sex or the other **(15)**

Sexuality: dimension of personality, broader than one's capacity for erotic response alone **(15)**

Sexually transmitted infections (STIs): infections spread by sexual activity **(15)**

Shearing force: combination of friction and pressure **(23)**

Shift report: report to other nurses at the change of shifts to delegate responsibility and describe what has been done **(36)**

Shock: a life-threatening condition of inadequate tissue perfusion **(34)**

Shortness of breath (SOB): feeling of being unable to get enough air **(24)**

Side effects: unintended drug action **(29)**

Sigmoidoscopy: diagnostic procedures for visualizing the sigmoid colon **(28)**

Single order: "one-time order"; medication is given once at a specified time **(29)**

Sitz bath: therapeutic bath for soaking a client's pelvic area **(23)**

Slander: defamation by the spoken word; making false statements that can cause damage to a person's reputation **(3)**

Sleep apnea: periodic cessation of breathing during sleep **(32)**

Somatic pain: diffuse pain that arises from ligaments, tendons, bones, blood vessels, and nerves **(21)**

Source-oriented record: a record in which information about a particular problem is documented under different sources **(6)**

Specific defenses: immune defenses; antibody-mediated and cell-mediated defenses against identified foreign proteins such as bacteria, fungi, viruses, and other infectious agents **(9)**

Specific gravity: a measure of concentration, or the amount of solutes present in the solution (e.g., urine) **(27)**

Spiritual: having to do with relationship with God or a higher power **(11)**

Spiritual development: includes six stages of establishing spiritual beliefs **(11)**

Sputum: mucous secretion from the lungs, bronchi, and trachea **(24)**

Standard Precautions: precautions used with all clients to prevent spread of microorganisms; applied to all body fluids, blood, secretions, excretions (except sweat), mucous membranes, and nonintact skin **(9)**

Standards: used to determine what a nurse should or should not do **(36)**

Standing order: may or may not have a termination date; medication can be given indefinitely **(29)**

Stat: immediate or immediately **(34)**

Stat order: medication to be given immediately and only once **(29)**

Statute of limitations: limit to the amount of time that can pass between recognition of harm and the bringing of a suit **(3)**

Stereognosis: ability to recognize objects by touching or manipulating them **(13)**

Stereotypes: assumption that all members of a culture or ethnic group are alike **(2)**

Sterile field: microorganism-free area **(9)**

Stimuli: agent or act that stimulates a nerve receptor **(13)**

Stress: universal phenomenon described as tension between two opposing forces **(16)**

Stressors: sources of stress that are classified as either internal or external **(16)**

Stridor: harsh, high-pitched sound **(24)**

Subcutaneous (SC or SQ): below the skin **(29)**

Subjective data: symptoms, facts, perceptions, or sensations apparent only to the person affected **(4)**

Sublingual: administration of a medication under the tongue **(29)**

Suctioning: aspirating secretions through a catheter connected to a suction machine or wall suction outlet **(24)**

Suffocation: asphyxiation; lack of oxygen due to interrupted breathing **(8)**

Summer day camp: a daytime program for children where LPNs/LVNs may obtain work; staff must be trained in first aid and CPR **(35)**

Superficial burns: first-degree burns that involve only the epidermal layer of the skin **(34)**

Supplemental Security Income (SSI): special benefits for people with disabilities or who are blind and not eligible for Social Security; payments are not restricted to healthcare costs **(7)**

Suppuration: process of pus formation **(23)**

Surgery: a unique experience of a planned physical alteration **(31)**

Surgical asepsis: sterile technique; practice that keeps an object or an area completely free of microorganisms and spores **(9)**

Susceptible host: individual who has difficulty combating microorganisms and is at risk for developing an infection **(9)**

Sutures: threads used to sew body tissues together **(31)**

Syringes: equipment used to administer parenteral medications **(29)**

Systemic infection: illness caused by microorganisms that spread to and damage other body areas **(9)**

Systole: period in which the ventricles of the heart contract **(19)**

Systolic pressure: pressure of the blood as a result of contraction of the ventricles; the pressure of the height of the blood wave **(20)**

T

Tachypnea: rapid breathing rate **(24)**

Taped report: report spoken into a tape recorder by nurses going off duty **(36)**

Tarry: red or black stool **(28)**

Teaching: system of activities intended to produce specific learning **(33)**

Team nursing: delivery of individualized nursing care to clients by a nursing team led by a professional nurse; members use diverse skills and education to deliver client care **(7)**

Tertiary prevention: care activities aimed at preventing further disability **(17)**

Test anxiety: range of feelings from uneasiness about an upcoming test or uneasiness during a test, to extreme and excessive worry about failing **(37)**

Theories: ways of looking at a discipline—such as nursing—in clear, explicit terms that can be communicated to others **(4)**

Therapeutic baths: baths given for physical effects, such as to soothe irritated skin or to treat an area **(22)**

Therapeutic communication: client-centered, goal-directed, and time-limited communication **(12)**

Therapeutic effect: desired effect; reason the drug is prescribed **(29)**

Third spacing: shunting of fluids into the extracellular space **(34)**

Thrombophlebitis: one or more clots loosely attached to an inflamed vessel wall **(32)**

Thrombus: blood clot **(24)**

Tissue: cells with similar structures and functions **(18)**

Tissue perfusion: passage of oxygen-carrying blood through the vessels to tissues **(31)**

Titration: determination of the correct volume for administration **(34)**

Tort: civil wrong committed against a person or a person's property **(3)**

Tracheostomy: surgical incision in the trachea just below the larynx through which a tracheostomy tube is inserted **(24)**

Transactional: focuses on individual differences in response to stress, rather than to events or reactions **(16)**

Transfer: move to another unit or to a different facility as a result of a client or physician request **(10)**

Transmission: manner in which a microorganism gets to the host. (1) *Direct:* infected person has direct contact with another person through touch, droplets, kissing, or sexual intercourse. (2) *Indirect:* requires a vector or vehicle to carry the microorganism to the host. (3) *Airborne:* droplet nuclei (remains of droplets coming from an infected person) are spread to another person **(9)**

Transmission-based Precautions: used in addition to Standard Precautions for any client with known or suspected infections that are spread by airborne or droplet transmission, or by physical contact **(9)**

Transplant: surgical replacement of a malfunctioning structure **(31)**

Traveling nurse: companion nurse; a licensed nurse who accompanies a client who is traveling, usually for a limited length of time **(35)**

Triage: means of assessing a large number of emergency victims quickly. Victims are prioritized according to their care needs, from most severe to least **(8)**

Triglycerides: fatty acids **(25)**

Turgor: elasticity (fullness) of the skin **(19)**

Twisting: rotation of the thoracolumbar spine **(18)**

U

Undernutrition: nutrient intake insufficient to meet daily energy requirements **(25)**

Unhelpful communication: communication that hinders or blocks the transfer of information and feelings **(12)**

Urgent care: care provided for minor injuries and acute illnesses **(34)**

Urgent care office: walk-in medical facility where clients can obtain treatment for minor injuries and acute illnesses; the office may be connected to or affiliated with a hospital **(35)**

Urinary diversion: surgical rerouting of urine from the kidneys to a site other than the bladder **(27)**

Urinary retention: accumulation of urine in the bladder and inability of the bladder to empty itself **(27)**

Urinary stasis: stagnation of urine flow **(32)**

V

Vagus nerve: located in the rectal wall **(28)**

Validation: form of feedback that provides confirmation that both parties have the same basic understanding of the message and the feedback **(12)**

Valsalva maneuver: straining associated with constipation; often accompanied by holding the breath **(28)**

Values: freely chosen, enduring beliefs or attitudes about the worth of a person, object, idea, or action **(3)**

Vector: object or animal by which organisms are transmitted (an insect, or a used drinking glass, for instance) **(9)**

Ventilation: (breathing) movement of air between the atmosphere and the alveoli of the lungs **(24)**

Vertigo: strong sensation of spinning around in space, which impairs balance **(32)**

Vial: small glass bottle with a sealed rubber cap; contains medication **(29)**

Virulence: microorganism's ability to produce disease **(9)**

Viruses: microorganisms made primarily of a substance called nucleic acid; they must enter living cells in order to reproduce **(9)**

Visceral: having to do with any large interior organ **(13)**

Visceral pain: pain that results from stimulation of pain receptors in the abdominal cavity, cranium, and thorax **(21)**

Viscosity: physical property that results from friction of molecules in a fluid **(20)**

Vital capacity: maximum volume of air that can be exhaled after maximum inhalation **(32)**

Vital signs: measurements of temperature, pulse, respirations, and blood pressure; assessment of pain is sometimes called the fifth vital sign **(19)**

Vitamin: organic compound that cannot be manufactured by the body and is needed in small quantities to *catalyze* (or trigger) metabolic processes **(25)**

Voiding: urination; the process of emptying the urinary bladder **(27)**

W

Wellness: state of well-being **(1)**

Wheezes: continuous, high-pitched musical squeak or whistling sound occurring on expiration and sometimes on inspiration when air moves through a narrowed or partially obstructed airway **(19)**

Written report: report, frequently used in long-term care facilities, that is written in a communication or report book **(36)**

Index

(*Note:* Figures and tables, denoted by *f* and *t,* are generally cited only when they appear outside the text discussion.)

SINGLE PC LICENSE AGREEMENT AND LIMITED WARRANTY

READ THIS LICENSE CAREFULLY BEFORE OPENING THIS PACKAGE. BY OPENING THIS PACKAGE, YOU ARE AGREEING TO THE TERMS AND CONDITIONS OF THIS LICENSE. IF YOU DO NOT AGREE, DO NOT OPEN THE PACKAGE. PROMPTLY RETURN THE UNOPENED PACKAGE AND ALL ACCOMPANYING ITEMS TO THE PLACE YOU OBTAINED THEM. *THESE TERMS APPLY TO ALL LICENSED SOFTWARE ON THE DISK EXCEPT THAT THE TERMS FOR USE OF ANY SHAREWARE OR FREEWARE ON THE DISKETTES ARE AS SET FORTH IN THE ELECTRONIC LICENSE LOCATED ON THE DISK:*

1. GRANT OF LICENSE and OWNERSHIP: The enclosed computer programs and data ("Software") are licensed, not sold, to you by Pearson Education, Inc. ("We" or the "Company") and in consideration of your purchase or adoption of the accompanying Company textbooks and/or other materials, and your agreement to these terms. We reserve any rights not granted to you. You own only the disk(s) but we and/or our licensors own the Software itself. This license allows you to use and display your copy of the Software on a single computer (i.e., with a single CPU) at a single location for academic use only, so long as you comply with the terms of this Agreement. You may make one copy for back up, or transfer your copy to another CPU, provided that the Software is usable on only one computer

2. RESTRICTIONS: You may not transfer or distribute the Software or documentation to anyone else. Except for backup, you may not copy the documentation or the Software. You may not network the Software or otherwise use it on more than one computer or computer terminal at the same time. You may not reverse engineer, disassemble, decompile, modify, adapt, translate, or create derivative works based on the Software or the Documentation. You may be held legally responsible for any copying or copyright infringement which is caused by your failure to abide by the terms of these restrictions.

3. TERMINATION: This license is effective until terminated. This license will terminate automatically without notice from the Company if you fail to comply with any provisions or limitations of this license. Upon termination, you shall destroy the Documentation and all copies of the Software. All provisions of this Agreement as to limitation and disclaimer of warranties, limitation of liability, remedies or damages, and our ownership rights shall survive termination.

4. LIMITED WARRANTY AND DISCLAIMER OF WARRANTY: Company warrants that for a period of 60 days from the date you purchase this SOFTWARE (or purchase or adopt the accompanying textbook), the Software, when properly installed and used in accordance with the Documentation, will operate in substantial conformity with the description of the Software set forth in the Documentation, and that for a period of 30 days the disk(s) on which the Software is delivered shall be free from defects in materials and workmanship under normal use. The Company does not warrant that the Software will meet your requirements or that the operation of the Software will be uninterrupted or error-free. Your only remedy and the Company's only obligation under these limited warranties is, at the Company's option, return of the disk for a refund of any amounts paid for it by you or replacement of the disk. THIS LIMITED WARRANTY IS THE ONLY WARRANTY PROVIDED BY THE COMPANY AND ITS LICENSORS, AND THE COMPANY AND ITS LICENSORS DISCLAIM ALL OTHER WARRANTIES, EXPRESS OR IMPLIED, INCLUDING WITHOUT LIMITATION, THE IMPLIED WARRANTIES OF MERCHANTABILITY AND FITNESS FOR A PARTICULAR PURPOSE. THE COMPANY DOES NOT WARRANT, GUARANTEE OR MAKE ANY REPRESENTATION REGARDING THE ACCURACY, RELIABILITY, CURRENTNESS, USE, OR RESULTS OF USE, OF THE SOFTWARE.

5. LIMITATION OF REMEDIES AND DAMAGES: IN NO EVENT, SHALL THE COMPANY OR ITS EMPLOYEES, AGENTS, LICENSORS, OR CONTRACTORS BE LIABLE FOR ANY INCIDENTAL, INDIRECT, SPECIAL, OR CONSEQUENTIAL DAMAGES ARISING OUT OF OR IN CONNECTION WITH THIS LICENSE OR THE SOFTWARE, INCLUDING FOR LOSS OF USE, LOSS OF DATA, LOSS OF INCOME OR PROFIT, OR OTHER LOSSES, SUSTAINED AS A RESULT OF INJURY TO ANY PERSON, OR LOSS OF OR DAMAGE TO PROPERTY, OR CLAIMS OF THIRD PARTIES, EVEN IF THE COMPANY OR AN AUTHORIZED REPRESENTATIVE OF THE COMPANY HAS BEEN ADVISED OF THE POSSIBILITY OF SUCH DAMAGES. IN NO EVENT SHALL THE LIABILITY OF THE COMPANY FOR DAMAGES WITH RESPECT TO THE SOFTWARE EXCEED THE AMOUNTS ACTUALLY PAID BY YOU, IF ANY, FOR THE SOFTWARE OR THE ACCOMPANYING TEXTBOOK. BECAUSE SOME JURISDICTIONS DO NOT ALLOW THE LIMITATION OF LIABILITY IN CERTAIN CIRCUMSTANCES, THE ABOVE LIMITATIONS MAY NOT ALWAYS APPLY TO YOU.

6. GENERAL: THIS AGREEMENT SHALL BE CONSTRUED IN ACCORDANCE WITH THE LAWS OF THE UNITED STATES OF AMERICA AND THE STATE OF NEW YORK, APPLICABLE TO CONTRACTS MADE IN NEW YORK, AND SHALL BENEFIT THE COMPANY, ITS AFFILIATES AND ASSIGNEES. HIS AGREEMENT IS THE COMPLETE AND EXCLUSIVE STATEMENT OF THE AGREEMENT BETWEEN YOU AND THE COMPANY AND SUPERSEDES ALL PROPOSALS OR PRIOR AGREEMENTS, ORAL, OR WRITTEN, AND ANY OTHER COMMUNICATIONS BETWEEN YOU AND THE COMPANY OR ANY REPRESENTATIVE OF THE COMPANY RELATING TO THE SUBJECT MATTER OF THIS AGREEMENT. If you are a U.S. Government user, this Software is licensed with "restricted rights" as set forth in subparagraphs (a)-(d) of the Commercial Computer-Restricted Rights clause at FAR 52.227-19 or in subparagraphs (c)(1)(ii) of the Rights in Technical Data and Computer Software clause at DFARS 252.227-7013, and similar clauses, as applicable.

Should you have any questions concerning this agreement or if you wish to contact the Company for any reason, please contact in writing: Prentice-Hall, New Media Department, One Lake Street, Upper Saddle River, NJ 07458.

Guide to Special Features

Guide to Special Features

NURSING PROCESS CARE PLANS

POPULATION FOCUS BOXES